David Clark

David Clark

TEXTBOOK OF PEDIATRIC NUTRITION

Second Edition

TEXTBOOK OF PEDIATRIC NUTRITION

Second Edition

EDITORS

Robert M. Suskind, M.D.
Professor and Chairman,
Department of Pediatrics
Louisiana State University School of Medicine
New Orleans, Louisiana

Leslie Lewinter-Suskind, M.S.S.
Director, International Program
Departments of Psychiatry and Pediatrics
Louisiana State University School of Medicine
New Orleans, Louisiana

RAVEN PRESS ● NEW YORK

Raven Press, Ltd., 1185 Avenue of the Americas, New York, New York 10036

© 1993 by Raven Press, Ltd. All rights reserved. This book is protected by copyright. No part of it may be reproduced, stored in a retrieval system, or transmitted, in any form or by any means, electronic, mechanical, photocopying, recording, or otherwise, without prior written permission of the publisher.

Made in the United States of America

Library of Congress Cataloging-in-Publication Data

Textbook of pediatric nutrition/editors, Robert M. Suskind and
  Leslie Lewinter-Suskind.—2nd ed.
    p. cm.
  Includes bibliographical references and index.
  ISBN 0-88167-896-1
  1. Nutrition disorders in children. 2. Children—Diseases—
Nutritional aspects. 3. Diet therapy for children. 4. Infants—
Nutrition. 5. Nutrition disorders in infants. I. Suskind, Robert
M., 1937-   . II. Lewinter-Suskind, Leslie.
  [DNLM: 1. Child Nutrition. 2. Child Nutrition Disorders. 3. Diet
Therapy—in infancy & childhood. 4. Infant Nutrition Disorders.
WS 115 T3552]
RJ399.N8T49 1992
618.92'39—dc20
DNLM/DLC
for Library of Congress   91-45634

The material contained in this volume was submitted as previously unpublished material, except in the instances in which some of the illustrative material was derived.

Great care has been taken to maintain the accuracy of the information contained in the volume. However, neither Raven Press nor the editors can be held responsible for errors or for any consequences arising from the use of the information contained herein.

Materials appearing in this book prepared by individuals as part of their official duties as U.S. Government employees are not covered by the above-mentioned copyright.

9 8 7 6 5 4 3 2 1

To Dana, Sydnie, David, and Michael—the strength and love of our lives, and with love and appreciation, to our parents Ida and Philip Suskind and Dorothy and Martin Lewinter for everything they have done to make us able to do what we do.

Contents

Contributing Authors xi
Preface xvii
Acknowledgments xix

I. Infant Nutrition

1. Nutritional Factors in Pregnancy Affecting Fetal Growth and Subsequent Infant Development 1
Ronald A. Chez

2. Nutritional Requirements of the Term Newborn 9
Fernando R. Moya

3. Nutritional Requirements of the Premature and Small for Gestational Age Infant 23
David A. Clark

4. Human Milk and Infant Formula 33
Cutberto Garza, Nancy F. Butte, and Armond S. Goldman

5. Mother-Infant Interaction: Relationship to Early Infant Nutrition and Feeding 43
Helen Britton

II. Nutritional Deficiency States

6. Disorders of the Fat-Soluble Vitamins A, D, E, and K 49
Robert E. Olson

7. Disorders of the Water-Soluble Vitamin B-Complex and Vitamin C 73
Harry L. Greene

8. Nutritional Anemias in Childhood: Iron, Folate, and Vitamin B_{12} 91
Peter R. Dallman

9. The Effects of Iron Deficiency, Food Additives, and Other Nutrients on Behavior 107
David A. Levitsky and Barbara J. Strupp

10. Trace Element Deficiencies in Childhood 115
Michael Hambidge

11. The Malnourished Child 127
Leslie Lewinter-Suskind, Dana Suskind, Krishna K. Murthy, and Robert M. Suskind

12. Malnutrition and the Immune Response 141
Ricardo U. Sorensen, Lily E. Leiva, and Solo Kuvibidila

13. Endocrine Changes in Malnutrition 161
    Alfred Tenore and Alfonso Vargas

14. Malnutrition and Mental Development 173
    Janina R. Galler and Robert N. Ross

15. Nutritional Implications of Vegetarianism for Children 181
    Johanna T. Dwyer

III. Nutritional Support of the Hospitalized Child

16. Clinical and Laboratory Assessment of the Malnourished Child 191
    Reinaldo Figueroa-Colon

17. Nutritional Support of Children in the Intensive Care Unit 207
    Murray M. Pollack

18. Energy and Protein Metabolism in the Pediatric Burn Patient 217
    Hugo F. Carvajal

19. Parenteral Support of the Hospitalized Child 225
    William C. Heird

20. Enteral Support of the Hospitalized Child 239
    George J. Fuchs III

21. Nutrient-Drug Interactions in Children 247
    Mark J. S. Miller

IV. Clinical Nutrition

22. Nutrition and the Adolescent 257
    Johanna T. Dwyer

23. Nutritional Considerations in the Treatment of Anorexia Nervosa and Bulimia 265
    Michael J. Pertschuk

24. Nutritional Considerations in the Development and Treatment of Psychosocial-Deprivation Dwarfism 275
    Alfonso Vargas and Alfred Tenore

25A. Childhood Obesity 279
    William H. Dietz

25B. Treatment of Childhood Obesity 285
    Reinaldo Figueroa-Colon, T. Kristian von Almen, and Robert M. Suskind

26. Dyslipidemia in Childhood 295
    Raynorda F. Brown, Cynthia Cole Franklin, Binh Dac Ho, and Frank A. Franklin, Jr.

27. Nutritional Considerations in the Therapy of the Child with Diabetes Mellitus 309
    Allan L. Drash and Dorothy J. Becker

28. Nutritional Considerations in the Treatment of Acute and Chronic Diarrhea   325
    Shimon Reif and Emanuel Lebenthal

29. Nutritional Treatment of Growth Failure and Disease Activity in Children with Inflammatory Bowel Disease 341
    Ernest Seidman

30.	Nutritional Considerations in the Prognosis and Treatment of Liver Disease in Children	353
	John B. Watkins	
31.	Nutritional Considerations in the Prognosis and Treatment of Children with Pancreatic Disease	363
	J. Armando Madrazo-de la Garza and Emanuel Lebenthal	
32.	Nutritional Management of Children with Cystic Fibrosis	375
	Robert L. Hopkins	
33.	Nutritional Considerations in the Prognosis and Treatment of Children with Congenital Heart Disease	383
	Amnon Rosenthal	
34.	Nutritional Considerations in the Prognosis and Treatment of Children with Renal Disease	393
	Warren E. Grupe	
35.	Nutritional Considerations in the Diagnosis and Treatment of Children with Juvenile Arthritis	407
	Daniel J. Lovell	
36.	Nutrition and Childhood Malignancies	417
	Lolie C. Yu	
37.	Nutritional Support of Children with Sickle-Cell Disease and Thalassemia	425
	Solo Kuvibidila and Rajesekharan P. Warrier	
38.	Nutritional Management of Immunodepressed Children	437
	Ricardo U. Sorensen, Solo Kuvibidila, and Robert M. Suskind	
39.	Pediatric AIDS and Nutrition	447
	Anthony R. Mawson, Rajesekharan P. Warrier, Solo Kuvibidila, and Robert M. Suskind	
40.	Food Allergy in Children	457
	Ricardo U. Sorensen, Mary Catherine Porch, and Lan C. Tu	
41.	Nutritional Treatment of Children with Inborn Errors of Metabolism	471
	Joyce M. Bradburn and Emmanuel Shapira	
42.	Nutritional Support of the Developmentally Disabled Child	485
	Ann C. H. Tilton and Marilyn D. Miller	
43.	Nutritional Support for Optimizing Children's Dental-Oral Health	493
	Kenneth C. Troutman	
44.	Characterizing Children's Eating Behavior	505
	Rosanne Perlman Farris and Theresa A. Nicklas	
45.	Nutritional Surveillance and Supplemental Food Programs in the United States	517
	David M. Paige	

Appendix A
    Pediatric Nutrition Guidelines ... 531
    Rosanne Perlman Farris

Appendix B
    Exchange Lists for Meal Planning from the American Diabetes Association, Inc. and the American Dietetic Association ... 549

Subject Index ... 557

Contributing Authors

Dorothy J. Becker, M.B., B.Ch.
Department of Pediatrics
University of Pittsburgh Children's Hospital
3705 Fifth Avenue
Pittsburgh, Pennsylvania 15213

Joyce M. Bradburn
Human Genetics Program
Hayward Genetics Center
Tulane University School of Medicine
1430 Tulane Avenue
New Orleans, Louisiana 70112

Helen Britton, M.D.
Department of Pediatrics
University of Utah School of Medicine
50 North Medical Drive
Salt Lake City, Utah 84132

Raynorda F. Brown, M.D.
Department of Pediatrics
Louisiana State University School of
  Medicine
1542 Tulane Avenue
New Orleans, Louisiana 70112

Nancy F. Butte, Ph.D.
United States Department of Agriculture/
  Agricultural Research Service
Children's Nutrition Research Center
1100 Bates Street
Houston, Texas 77030

Hugo F. Carvajal, M.D.
Division of Pediatric Critical Care Unit
Humana Women's and Children's Hospital
8109 Fredericksburg
San Antonio, Texas 78229

Ronald A. Chez, M.D.
Department of Obstetrics and Gynecology
University of South Florida College of
  Medicine, Suite 500
Four Columbia Drive
Tampa, Florida 33606

David A. Clark, M.D.
Department of Pediatrics
Louisiana State University School of
  Medicine
1542 Tulane Avenue
New Orleans, Louisiana 70112

Peter R. Dallman, M.D.
Department of Pediatrics
University of California at San Francisco
505 Parnassus Avenue, Box 0106
San Francisco, California 94143

William H. Dietz, M.D., Ph.D.
Department of Pediatrics
Tufts University School of Medicine
750 Washington Street
Boston, Massachusetts 02111

Allan L. Drash, M.D.
Division of Endocrinology, Metabolism, and
  Diabetes Mellitus
University of Pittsburgh Children's Hospital
3705 Fifth Avenue
Pittsburgh, Pennsylvania 15213

Johanna T. Dwyer, D.Sc., R.D.
Frances Stern Nutrition Center
750 Washington Street
Boston, Massachusetts 02111

Rosanne Perlman Farris, M.S. Hyg., LDN
Department of Pediatrics
Louisiana State University School of
   Medicine
1542 Tulane Avenue
New Orleans, Louisiana 70112

Reinaldo Figueroa-Colon, M.D.
Departments of Pediatrics and Nutrition
   Sciences
Division of Pediatric Gastroenterology and
   Nutrition
University of Alabama at Birmingham
Children's Hospital of Alabama
1600 Seventh Avenue South
Birmingham, Alabama 35233

Cynthia Cole Franklin, BSN-CPNP, MPH
c/o Departments of Pediatrics and
   Nutritional Services
Division of Pediatric Gastroenterology and
   Nutrition
University of Alabama at Birmingham
   School of Medicine
Children's Hospital of Alabama
1600 Seventh Avenue South
Birmingham, Alabama 35233

Frank A. Franklin, Jr., M.D., Ph.D.
Departments of Pediatrics and Nutritional
   Services
Division of Pediatric Gastroenterology and
   Nutrition
University of Alabama at Birmingham
   School of Medicine
Children's Hospital of Alabama
1600 Seventh Avenue South
Birmingham, Alabama 35233

George J. Fuchs III, M.D.
Department of Pediatrics
Louisiana State University School of
   Medicine
1542 Tulane Avenue
New Orleans, Louisiana 70112

Janina R. Galler, M.D.
Center for Behavioral Development and
   Mental Retardation
Boston University School of Medicine
80 East Concord Street
Boston, Massachusetts 02118

Cutberto Garza, M.D., Ph.D.
Division of Nutritional Sciences
Cornell University
127 Savage Hall
Ithaca, New York 14853

Armond S. Goldman, M.D.
Department of Pediatrics
University of Texas Medical Branch
Galveston, Texas 77555

Harry L. Greene, M.D.
Bristol Meyers Squibb Company
Mead Johnson Nutritional Group
2400 West Lloyd Expressway
Evansville, Indiana 47721 (R 20)

Warren E. Grupe, M.D.
Division of Medical and Health Sciences
   Education
Project HOPE Health Sciences Education
   Center
Millwood, Virginia 22646

Michael Hambidge, M.D.
Department of Pediatrics
University of Colorado Health Sciences
   Center
4200 East Ninth Avenue
Denver, Colorado 80262

William C. Heird, M.D.
Department of Pediatrics
Baylor College of Medicine
Children's Nutrition Research Center
United States Department of Agriculture/
   Agricultural Research Society
1100 Bates Street
Houston, Texas 77030

Binh Dac Ho, BSEN
Department of Biomedical Engineering
Tulane University School of Medicine
1430 Tulane Avenue
New Orleans, Louisiana 70118

Robert L. Hopkins, M.D.
Department of Pediatrics
Section of Critical Care
Tulane University School of Medicine
1430 Tulane Avenue
New Orleans, Louisiana 70112

Solo Kuvibidila, Ph.D.
Department of Pediatrics
Louisiana State University School of
  Medicine
1542 Tulane Avenue
New Orleans, Louisiana 70112

Emanuel Lebenthal, M.D.
Department of Pediatrics
International Institute for Infant Nutrition
  and Gastrointestinal Disease
Hahnemann University Hospital
Broad and Vine Streets
Philadelphia, Pennsylvania 19102

Lily E. Leiva, Ph.D.
Department of Pediatrics
Louisiana State University School of
  Medicine
1542 Tulane Avenue
New Orleans, Louisiana 70112

David A. Levitsky, Ph.D.
Division of Nutritional Sciences and
  Department of Psychology
Cornell University
112 Savage Hall
Ithaca, New York 14853

Leslie Lewinter-Suskind, M.S.S.
Departments of Psychiatry and Pediatrics
Louisiana State University School of
  Medicine
1542 Tulane Avenue
New Orleans, Louisiana 70112

Daniel J. Lovell, M.D., MPH
Department of Pediatrics
University of Cincinnati
Children's Hospital Medical Center
Elland and Bethesda Avenues
Cincinnati, Ohio 45229-2899

J. Armando Madrazo-de la Garza, M.D.
Departments of Gastroenterology and
  Ophthalmology
Hospital de Pediatria
Mexico City, Mexico 06725

Anthony R. Mawson, M.A., P.H.
Department of Ophthalmology
Louisiana State University School of
  Medicine
1542 Tulane Avenue
New Orleans, Louisiana 70112

Marilyn D. Miller, R.N., MSN
Department of Nursing
Children's Hospital
200 Henry Clay Avenue
New Orleans, Louisiana 70118

Mark J. S. Miller, Ph.D.
Department of Pediatrics
Louisiana State University School of
  Medicine
1542 Tulane Avenue
New Orleans, Louisiana 70112

Fernando R. Moya, M.D.
Department of Pediatrics, Obstetrics and
  Gynecology
University of Texas Southwestern Medical
  Center
5323 Harry Hines Boulevard
Dallas, Texas 75235

Krishna K. Murthy, DVM, Ph.D.
Department of Virology and Immunology
Southwest Foundation for Biomedical
  Research
7620 Northwest Loop 410
San Antonio, Texas 78227

Theresa A. Nicklas, Dr. P.H., LDN
Department of Medicine
Louisiana State University School of
  Medicine
1542 Tulane Avenue
New Orleans, Louisiana 70112

Robert E. Olson, M.D., Ph.D.
Departments of Medicine and Pharmacology
Health Sciences Center
State University of New York at Stony Brook
Stony Brook, New York 11794-8651

David M. Paige, M.D., M.P.H.
Department of Maternal and Child Health
The Johns Hopkins University School of
  Public Health
615 North Wolfe Street
Baltimore, Maryland 21205

Michael J. Pertschuk, M.D.
Department of Psychiatry
University of Pennsylvania
  Graduate Hospital
1740 South Street
Philadelphia, Pennsylvania 19146

Murray M. Pollack, M.D.
Departments of Anesthesiology and
 Pediatrics
Critical Care Medicine
George Washington University and
 Children's Neonatal Medical Center
111 Michigan Avenue, N.W.
Washington, D.C. 20010

Mary Catherine Porch, R.N., M.P.H.
Department of Pediatrics
Louisiana State University School of
 Medicine
1542 Tulane Avenue
New Orleans, Louisiana 70112

Shimon Reif, M.D.
Department of Pediatrics
Tel Aviv University
Tel Aviv, Israel

Amnon Rosenthal, M.D.
Department of Pediatrics
University of Michigan School of Medicine
C.S. Mott Children's Hospital
1500 East Medical Center Drive
Ann Arbor, Michigan 48109

Robert N. Ross, Ph.D.
Center for Behavioral Development and
 Mental Retardation
Boston University School of Medicine
80 East Concord Street
Boston, Massachusetts 02118

Ernest Seidman, M.D.
Department of Pediatrics and Nutrition
Pediatric Gastroenterology Division
Hôpital Saint Justine
University of Montreal
3175 Côte Sainte Catherine Road
Montreal, Québec H3T 1C5, Canada

Emmanuel Shapira, M.D., Ph.D.
Human Genetics Program
Hayward Genetics Program
Tulane University School of Medicine
1430 Tulane Avenue
New Orleans, Louisiana 70112

Ricardo U. Sorensen, M.D.
Department of Pediatrics
Louisiana State University School of
 Medicine
1542 Tulane Avenue
New Orleans, Louisiana 70112

Barbara J. Strupp, Ph.D.
Division of Nutritional Sciences and
 Department of Psychology
Cornell University
112 Savage Hall
Ithaca, New York 14853

Dana Suskind, M.D.
Department of Otolaryngology
University of Pennsylvania School of
 Medicine
3800 Spruce Street
Philadelphia, Pennsylvania 19104

Robert M. Suskind, M.D.
Department of Pediatrics
Louisiana State University School of
 Medicine
1542 Tulane Avenue
New Orleans, Louisiana 70112

Alfred Tenore, M.D.
Department of Pediatrics
University of Udine
Udine, Italy 33100

Ann C. H. Tilton, M.D.
Department of Pediatric Neurology
Tulane University School of Medicine
1430 Tulane Avenue
New Orleans, Louisiana 70112

Kenneth C. Troutman, D.D.S., M.P.H.
Department of Pediatric Dentistry
Columbia University
Columbia-Presbyterian Medical Center
630 West 168th Street
New York, New York 10032

Lan C. Tu, M.D.
Department of Pediatrics
Louisiana State University School of
 Medicine
1542 Tulane Avenue
New Orleans, Louisiana 70112

Alfonso Vargas, M.D.
Department of Pediatrics
Louisiana State University School of
 Medicine
1542 Tulane Avenue
New Orleans, Louisiana 70112

T. Kristian von Almen, Ph.D.
Department of Pediatrics
Children's Hospital of New Orleans
200 Henry Clay Avenue
New Orleans, Louisiana 70118

Rajesekharan P. Warrier, M.D.
Department of Pediatrics
Louisiana State University School of
 Medicine
1542 Tulane Avenue
New Orleans, Louisiana 70112

John B. Watkins, M.D.
Department of Pediatrics
Washington University School of Medicine
St. Louis Children's Hospital
400 South Kingshighway Boulevard
St. Louis, Missouri 63110

Lolie C. Yu, M.D.
Department of Pediatrics
Louisiana State University School of
 Medicine
1542 Tulane Avenue
New Orleans, Louisiana 70112

Preface

The Textbook of Pediatric Nutrition is a carefully designed tool for medical professionals, including pediatricians, family physicians, surgeons, nutritionists, and dieticians. It is a compendium of the latest knowledge in pediatric nutrition geared to provide optimum nutritional care of normal children, prenatally through adolescence, as well as of children with a variety of disease states.

For the healthy child, it is often the quality of nutrition that determines the meeting of potential. The first two years are the ones of greatest growth, physically as well as developmentally. In extreme deprivation, these parameters can be severely influenced, affecting not only the child but adult potential as well. Although most children in industrialized countries do not experience the episodes of severe malnutrition common in third world countries, mild forms of deficiencies may also affect, more subtly, both growth and development. More common, however, in countries where day-long grazing has replaced mealtimes, and eating is more to assuage boredom than hunger, obesity and its long-term negative ramifications predominate.

For the child with primary disease states, including cancer, diabetes, and sickle-cell anemia, nutrition often makes the difference in prognosis and outcome. Awareness of this fact is an important factor in acknowledging nutrition's essential role in the management of children with these disease states. Ignoring this fact often results in a state of severe malnutrition, not unlike that found in third world countries, which impacts significantly on ultimate morbidity as well as mortality.

Research in nutrition has produced a body of knowledge both broadened and refined since the first edition of this book was published. The first edition highlighted not only primary nutritional deficiencies in children, but also the important role that nutrition plays as a secondary factor in the majority of disease states which effect children. This volume is comprised of the most recent findings in the world of pediatric nutrition, compiled by many of the world's leading experts. It is divided into 4 sections, *Infant Nutrition, Nutritional Deficiency States, Nutritional Support of the Hospitalized Child,* and *Clinical Nutrition,* totalling 45 chapters. Appendices with formulas for enteral and parenteral feeding are also included.

We hope this book successfully meets the needs of those medical professionals who understand the importance of optimal nutrition to the normal, healthy child, as well as to those children with secondary nutritional deficiencies. We also hope *The Textbook of Pediatric Nutrition* further establishes nutrition as an essential subspecialty in the practice of pediatrics and an essential adjunct to other pediatric subspecialties.

Robert M. Suskind
Leslie Lewinter-Suskind

Acknowledgments

We should like to thank Mr. Louis Castaing, Ms. Judy C. Lua, and Ms. Virginia Howard for their superb efforts during the preparation for this textbook as well as Lisa Berger, Robyn Flusser, and Susan Berkowitz, and all of the staff at Raven Press for their support and understanding during the editing of this text. We are also appreciative of the excellent work, investigating and writing, which was done by each author. It has produced a volume that is not only the final word in pediatric nutrition, but eminently readable, as well. To everyone, thank you.

CHAPTER 1

Nutritional Factors in Pregnancy Affecting Fetal Growth and Subsequent Infant Development

Ronald A. Chez

The fundamental requirement of a species is the ability to reproduce. The female body is designed to reproduce; toward that end the physiological and biochemical aspects of a woman's life are appropriately modified to accommodate and support a pregnancy when it occurs.

The role of the health care team is to foster the health and well-being of the mother, fetus, infant, and family (1). Although this is done, in large part, during the perinatal period, optimally, care should extend from preconception through pregnancy, labor, delivery, and the postpartum period.

The components of perinatal care include early and continuous risk assessment to evaluate the need for special care, promotion of health via patient education, and medical and psychosocial interventions that support maternal and fetal tolerance to the pregnancy (1,2).

A dominant focus of each of these components of perinatal care is maternal nutrition. The normal-weight woman who enters pregnancy well nourished and then maintains good nutritional health throughout pregnancy and lactation has markedly improved her potential of experiencing a favorable outcome. Obtaining this goal is the shared responsibility of the patient and her health care team.

Clinical guidelines to follow derive from both scientific research and observational studies. Adaptation to pregnancy in the human has been studied primarily at the macroscopic and descriptive level. Changes at the cellular level are less well understood. This chapter provides an overview of what is, and what is not, known about the role of nutrition in determining pregnancy outcome.

R. A. Chez: Department of Obstetrics and Gynecology, University of South Florida College of Medicine, Tampa, Florida 33606.

ENERGY REQUIREMENTS OF PREGNANCY

Maternal and Fetal Components

At term, the normal pregnant woman will have accumulated tissues and fluids sufficient for the development of a fetus of appropriate weight for the gestational age. She will also have made the necessary biologic adjustments required to sustain her through labor, delivery, and lactation.

The end results of these changes include a 3,500 g fetus, a 650 g placenta, 800 ml of amniotic fluid, a 970 g uterus, breasts that now weigh 400 g, and an increase in circulating blood volume of 1,200 ml. Retention of approximately 1,700 ml extravascular volume also occurs; this may appear as dependent edema. The presence of generalized edema can add as much as 6,600 ml more fluid (3–5).

The normal weight pregnant woman also stores fat. This is presumed to be for maternal caloric needs in the third trimester and lactation. Estimates of accumulated body fat, derived from measurements of lean tissue density and skinfold thickness, range from 1,300 to 5,400 g (6,7). The total weight gain of the woman who does not have generalized edema is approximately 13 kg (5).

Maternal physiological adaptation to pregnancy begins in the first trimester during fetal organogenesis (8). These changes are preparatory for the subsequent role of sustaining the growth and development of the fetus while preserving maternal well-being in this and any future pregnancies.

The extent of the specific changes in maternal body composition of fat, lean tissue mass, and other non–fat tissue components is difficult to discern (9). The clinician measures only the end results of any composition change as incremental weight gain and total weight gain.

It has been difficult to find a dependable clinical tool to measure body composition. The technologies available for measuring the distribution of fat are dependent on the accuracy of the determination of lean body mass. This in turn can be a function of lean tissue hydration with body water.

Changes in fat and lean tissue distribution occur early in the first trimester. Skinfold thicknesses can be considered only estimates of change in fat content because the technique is difficult to reproduce; results vary according to the site chosen and are influenced by water retention (10). In addition, a determination of how much body fat is accumulated during pregnancy will be inaccurate if a prepregnancy measurement has not been obtained. Further confounding variables are maternal utilization of fat as a caloric source and retention of body water, both of which are features of normal third trimester metabolism.

Caloric Needs

Energy is necessary to supply the caloric requirements of the pregnant woman's daily activity, her own weight gain, and fetal growth. Endogenous maternal fat stores and increased consumption of calorie-rich nutrients are required to provide this energy.

The main portions of the energy expenditure requirement include basal and resting metabolic rate of the mother, thermogenesis, and physical activity. Although there is wide variation in the range of reported basal and resting metabolic rates, these rates do increase on average. The increment appears to be between 20,000 and 30,000 kilocalories (Cal) during the course of the pregnancy (11). There does not appear to be a change in thermogenesis.

Physical activity was thought to decrease because of an increase in sedentary behaviors of pregnant women. This has not been found, however, either in developed or developing countries. The increase in body mass during pregnancy requires more energy to meet the requirements for the activities of daily living as most women continue to work in the home, factory, or field (11).

The increment in total energy expenditure and therefore the requirement for dietary supplementation was thought to be 85,000 Cal per pregnancy or 300 Cal per day (5). It appears more likely that the overall cost is in the range of 55,000 Cal, or an increased need of about 200 Cal per day (11).

DETERMINANTS OF NEWBORN WEIGHT

Normal Birth Weight

Maternal weight gain during pregnancy reflects the weight of the products of conception, the accumulation of maternal tissue and retained water, and the length of the pregnancy. There are maternal characteristics that statistically influence the weight gain including food access and intake, and fundamental changes in physiology or some other mechanism (12).

Birth weight at term is directly and linearly related to maternal weight gain. It is similarly related to prepregnant weight. These relationships are both independent and additive. The risk of a low birth weight newborn at term decreases as prepregnant body mass index increases. It also decreases as total weight gain, net weight gain, and net weight gain per week after 20 weeks gestation increases. The highest incidence of normal birth weight infants occurs in women of normal prepregnant weight who gain between 25 and 35 lb during pregnancy (13–16).

In the United States, lesser weight gain during pregnancy occurs in unmarried women, black women, multiparas, women older than 30 years of age, those with an increased body mass index, those less than 67 inches tall, cigarette smokers, and women with less than a 12-year education. However, in each of these categories, birth weights between 3,000 and 4,000 g at 39 to 41 weeks gestation do occur, making it difficult to indict any one behavior or demographic feature (12).

Low Birth Weight

Low birth weight is a dominant factor in newborn and infant morbidity and mortality (16,17). It also has a direct, adverse impact on subsequent childhood somatic growth, neuropsychological development, infant mortality, and infant morbidity. Low birth weight is a result of premature birth and of intrauterine growth retardation.

The single and most prominent direct determinant of premature birth is cigarette smoking (18). Cigarette smoking also increases the risk of spontaneous abortion, third trimester placental bleeding, and premature rupture of the membranes. Other direct determinants include low prepregnancy weight and a history of prior premature birth and spontaneous abortions. Maternal age and socioeconomic status are indirect established determinants (19).

The direct determinants of intrauterine growth retardation include maternal height less than 62 inches, low prepregnant weight, low maternal weight gain, cigarette smoking, alcohol consumption, and general maternal morbidity. Indirect determinants include race, parity, maternal age, and socioeconomic status (19).

Adolescence per se does not have an adverse impact on pregnancy or birth weight outcome if the young woman is of normal weight and gains appropriately. Thus, adolescents and mature women share the same determinants for birth weight (20).

The risk of preterm birth increases with poor weight gain. This is particularly true when the decreased weight gain occurs after the 20th week of gestation. It is not clear if the etiology is a direct function of maternal dietary intake, incomplete changes in maternal body composition or physiology, increased energy expenditure, and/or psychosocial stress (21). Even when specific causes have not been ascertained, decreased weight gain during pregnancy does alert the provider to the need for intervention. Some interventional strategies may be introduced by the health professional, whereas others, more societal in scope, may be more difficult to initiate.

The appropriate solution for achieving satisfactory weight gain in an underfed pregnant woman would seem to be increasing the daily caloric intake. However, a relationship between an increase in energy intake and maternal weight gain and/or birth weight has not been consistently found. This may be a function of maternal nutritional vulnerability. Undernourished women who receive supplements can demonstrate an increase in birth weight, whereas women with less of a deficit between energy intake and requirements do not (9). Explanations for the inconclusive data predominantly relate to flaws in scientific method (22). Regardless, food as the therapy for malnutrition and undernutrition makes clinical sense.

Interestingly, mothers with a high body mass index have an increase in low birth weight with weight gains in excess of 20 lb. This may result from the increased incidence of illnesses in women with moderate and marked obesity. In women with normal or low body mass index, the risk of low birth weight begins to increase after a total weight gain of 45 pounds (12).

Women, Infants, and Children (WIC), a program of the United States Department of Agriculture, provides nutritional supplementation and counseling for pregnant and breast-feeding women and children up to age 5. Eligibility is based on nutritional status and financial need. Women who use the program are less likely to deliver low birth weight infants (23).

The WIC program is essentially supplementation with dairy products and cereals. This type of supplementation should be differentiated from supplementation with a high protein-to-calorie ratio diet, which may result in a negative effect on fetal growth and an increase in premature delivery (24).

High Birth Weight

Macrosomia is arbitrarily defined as a birth weight greater than 4,000 g. The rate of high birth weights has been increasing for the past decade. Most of the increase reflects a shift to the right of the entire curve of birth weights over time. Most high birth weights, therefore, may be considered secondary to normal biologic variation. Associations that result in a relatively higher proportion of macrosomic newborns include multiparity, history of a previous macrosomic baby, large maternal stature, and postdatism. Direct determinants include prepregnant obesity, excess weight gain in pregnancy, and poorly controlled gestational and preexisting diabetes mellitus.

Macrosomia results in an increased incidence of dysfunctional labor, fetopelvic disproportion, shoulder dystocia, instrument delivery, birth trauma, and cesarean section delivery. Consequently, macrosomic infants have an increased perinatal mortality and morbidity with adverse sequelae into childhood. Obese infants of diabetic mothers tend to remain obese into adolescence and also have a higher risk of developing diabetes mellitus.

Between 15% and 40% of reproductive-age women are obese. Fecundity is not impaired by obesity; the incidence of twins actually increases. The primary antepartum complications associated with maternal obesity are hypertension and gestational diabetes. Intrapartum complications in the obese woman are those associated with delivery of a macrosomic infant (25).

Macrosomia secondary to maternal glucose intolerance has been recognized for several decades (26). The shift in the birth weight curve to the right in infants of diabetic women directly relates to the mean circulating maternal plasma glucose level during pregnancy. Maintenance of fasting and postprandial levels in the normal nonglucose intolerant range, by a regime consisting of daily, split doses of insulin, a proportioned diet, and exercise, will result in an infant of normal birth weight.

Twins

Twin gestation occurs in approximately 1.2% of births in the United States. Twin pregnancy is at increased risk of intrauterine growth retardation, premature delivery, discordance, congenital anomalies, gestational diabetes, pregnancy-induced hypertension, and perinatal acute and chronic asphyxia. Because of these associations, there is an increased incidence of perinatal mortality.

The lowest perinatal mortality of twins occurs in the 3,000 to 3,500 g range; this is associated with a total weight gain of 44 lb in the pregnant underweight woman and 41 lb in the normal-weight woman. The birth weights of twins increase linearly with the prenatal weight gain of women who were either underweight or normal weight prior to conception. Also, and independently, the proportion of low birth weight twin infants decreases as prepregnant weight increases. The lowest incidence of low birth weight occurs in women who were obese and very obese in their prepregnant state (27).

As a result of the increasing use of diagnostic ultrasound, multiple gestations are more frequently being identified in the first half of pregnancy. This should result in guidelines specifying greater incremental and total weight gain for multiple gestations over those for singleton pregnancies.

BIRTH DEFECTS

Minerals

Fetal exposure to high maternal blood lead levels coupled with an increase in postnatal blood levels can result in a decline in linear growth rates in the second year of life as well as slowed cognitive development (28,29). Food contaminated with methyl mercury ingested during pregnancy has resulted in infants with cerebral palsy, mental retardation, and systemic organ damage (30).

Iodine deficiency in pregnancy is not found in the United States. It is associated with cretinism, stillbirth, congenital anomalies, and hearing loss.

There is a lack of consistency in the studies that link zinc deficiency with adverse pregnancy outcome. It is, therefore, difficult to associate zinc intake and maternal serum levels of zinc with congenital anomalies. However, the possibility of nutrient-zinc interactions and associated changes in cell and circulating zinc levels cannot be readily dismissed (31).

Vitamins

There are potential risks from large overdoses of some vitamins during pregnancy. Excess vitamin D has been associated with infantile hypercalcemia syndrome. Vitamin A overdosage has been related to anomalies of bone, the urinary tract, and central nervous system. However, there is little evidence that vitamin C overdose during pregnancy will induce a relative deficiency in the newborn by increasing the metabolic clearance of the vitamin (9).

Nutritional deficiencies during the first half of organogenesis, particularly of folic acid, have been linked to the occurrence of neural tube defects. A number of studies have affirmed that the use of multivitamins containing folic acid during the first 6 weeks of pregnancy will prevent by more than half the recurrence of neural tube defects in the woman at risk (32).

Diabetes Mellitus

There is an increased incidence of congenital anomalies in the offspring of diabetic women. This occurrence has been directly related to the degree of control of blood sugar levels at the time of conception and during organogenesis (33). Maintaining euglycemia in the periconception period and then during the first trimester results in rates of congenital anomalies similar to those found in the normal population. Other potential adverse outcomes that are increased in a poorly controlled diabetic pregnancy include stillbirth, neonatal death, neonatal morbidity, birth injury, intellectual delay and impairment, and childhood obesity. As manifestations of a metabolic derangement, all are preventable by supervised control of blood glucose levels (34).

Ketonuria has been associated statistically with lower mental, motor, and intelligence quotient scores in the children of both normal and diabetic pregnancies analyzed in the Perinatal Collaborative Study (35). However, additional analyses of these data, controlling for nonnutritional factors, have not confirmed these associations (36). Further, ketonuria occurs sporadically in most normal pregnant women (37).

CLINICAL IMPLICATIONS FOR PRENATAL CARE

Preconception Care

Prepregnant weight is an important clue to nutritional health. Body mass indices are independent of adult stature and permit reference points for the determination of under-, normal, and overweight categories. The Quetelet index for body mass is determined by dividing weight in kilograms by height in meters squared. The body mass index cutoffs are <17.9 for extreme underweight, <19.8 for underweight, >26.0 for overweight, and >29.1 for extreme overweight. Weight or weight-for-height cannot determine proportion or distribution of fat content and lean body mass; physical examination is more helpful.

Weight and nutrition do not necessarily relate. Historical factors and physical examination provide more specific information about nutritional status. Particular attention must be paid to certain women who are at higher risk for nutritional deficits. This category includes women who take antiseizure medication, have used combination oral contraceptives for a number of years, are food faddists, have had three or more pregnancies in the past 2 years, are smokers, chronically use weight loss or therapeutic diets for systemic medical illnesses, and athletes who engage in sports requiring prolonged aerobic expenditures (38). These patients will be better prepared for conception with purposeful attempts to achieve normal body mass index combined with the prophylactic daily use of vitamin and mineral supplementation.

Prenatal Care

A primary goal of prenatal care is to deliver a baby of appropriate weight for gestational age at term. This is more likely to happen in the normal body mass index woman who gains a total of 25 to 35 lb with an increment of about 4 lb a month after the first trimester. This can be accomplished with a diet of 35 Cal per kilogram body weight. The daily diet of the pregnant woman should contain 1 g of protein per kilogram body weight and at least 250 g of complex carbohydrates.

Vitamin Supplementation

An appropriate and balanced diet is sufficient to supply the daily needs of normal women for the fat-soluble vitamins A, E, and K as well as the water-soluble vitamins B_1, B_2, B_{12}, niacin, and C. Prenatal vitamins should be considered a supplement, rather than a substitute, for such a diet.

There is an increased need for vitamin D. This can be met from sunlight and the use of fortified milk products. There is also an increased need for folic acid secondary to the increase in DNA synthesis and the increased erythropoiesis. Because this vitamin is easily destroyed by cooking, routine supplementation is recommended. Supplementation should also be given to women taking antiseizure medications and those with hemoglobinopathies. Complete vegetarians should take a B_{12} supplement.

Mineral Supplementation

Iron supplementation during pregnancy and the postpartum period is considered standard practice. Approximately 20% of low-income white women and 40% of low-income African-American women have iron deficiency anemia during the third trimester (39). Maternal iron deficiency anemia during pregnancy is associated with premature labor, low birth weight newborns, urinary tract infection, and fetal death (40). There is no direct effect of maternal iron deficiency on fetal hemoglobin concentration.

An additional 1,000 mg of iron is needed during pregnancy. Although there is a diminished loss of daily iron because of amenorrhea and improved gastrointestinal absorption, the deficit emanates from the increase in circulating maternal red blood cell mass and fetal requirements. The use of low-dose iron supplements daily will correct this relative net deficit (9).

The fetal need for about 30 g of calcium is met from increased maternal calcium stores absorbed by the mother via the gastrointestinal tract (41). Maternal needs can be satisfied by the daily consumption of dairy products. The question of the relationship between calcium deficiency and hypertension has influenced the use of calcium supplementation as an attempt to reduce the incidence of pregnancy-induced hypertension and preeclampsia. Preliminary clinical data suggest that such reduction can occur with calcium supplementation without apparent associated risk (42).

Similar improved pregnancy outcome from routine supplementation of zinc, magnesium, copper, selenium, and chromium as well as other minerals has not been consistently demonstrated. However, because of the relatively low zinc content of vegetables, vegetarians should receive zinc supplementation. The normal use of iodized salt will fulfill the requirements for iodine during the pregnancy. There is no recommended dietary allowance for fluorine.

Sodium is an essential mineral. It is required in pregnancy to retain the additional water necessary for the expanded blood volume. It is the main ion that helps preserve osmotic equilibrium between the intravascular and extravascular spaces. There is no benefit in the restriction of sodium in pregnancy and there may be the potential for harm. Specifically, restricted sodium intake does not prevent pregnancy induced hypertension nor decrease its severity when it occurs (43).

Weight Gain

To decrease the risk of a low birth weight baby, an underweight woman should be counseled to gain 30 to 40 lb during pregnancy. This should be accomplished with a linear increment of 5 lb a month in the second half of pregnancy (9).

Obesity is a health hazard. It is associated with an increased incidence of medical illness and decreased life span. Dietary advice during pregnancy may facilitate changes in eating habits that may result in eventual achievement of optimal weight.

There is a decreased incidence of low birth weight infants in women with high prepregnant weight independent of subsequent weight gain during pregnancy. In the markedly obese woman, there does not appear to be any effect of weight gain on birth weight. Caloric restriction in the obese woman that results in a total weight gain of between 15 and 20 lb will result in no net weight gain after pregnancy and no increase in the incidence of low birth weight newborns. This can be accomplished with a balanced diet that results in an incremental weight gain of approximately 3 lb per month in the second half of pregnancy. Consultation with a nutritionist is important since obesity is often associated with malnutrition (44,45).

Assessment of Maternal Weight

Weights should be recorded carefully during the prenatal examination. This sets the stage for the accurate design of nutritional counseling. The accuracy of collection and recording techniques cannot be overemphasized. Scales should be standardized at preset, regular intervals. The procedure for weighing should be identical each time. Patients should be weighed wearing only underclothing and/or an examining robe. Bladders should be emptied, shoes and purses removed. Variables will include differences in the time of day, lower extremity edema, and/or a full bowel.

The weight should be plotted on a weight-gain versus gestational-age grid so that trends and relationships can be identified (46). The degree of incremental change and trends in rate gain data can then be compared. This information, when compared to the baseline weight data, can help the health team give accurate advice and counseling for the remaining gestational period.

Assessment of Fetal Growth

The pregnant uterus becomes an abdominal organ after the 12th week of gestation. Measurement of the height of the fundus is performed using a tape measure that follows the contour of the maternal abdominal wall. The height of a singleton pregnancy with normal growth is equivalent, in centimeters, to the weeks' gestation. When there is doubt about fetal growth, diagnostic ultrasound is used. Formulas have been compiled that use some combination of the fetal head and abdominal circumferences, biparietal diameter and femur length. The fetal weight estimated by ultrasound is more accurate before 28 weeks' gestation. After this time, there is an approximate 15% error in the estimate.

Postpartum Care

The goals for the postpartum mother include a return to her prepregnant state of health and lactation adequate for successful breast-feeding. A weight loss of up to 20 lb can be expected during the first 3 weeks postpartum.

Preparation for breast-feeding is the focus of a number of physiological changes during pregnancy. During lactation, an additional 500 to 700 Cal per day are required to support the energy requirement of milk production. Approximately 150 Cal per day can be provided by maternal fat stores (47).

There is a potential problem when a mother who must consume sufficient calories to support breast-feeding tries to return too soon to her prepregnant or desired weight. A clinical guideline suggests a loss of maternal weight of no greater than half a pound a week after the initial 3-week postpartum period. After weaning, with appropriate exercise and reduction in diet, the remainder of excess pregnancy weight will be lost. The average woman, however, will gain about 2 lb of permanent weight after each birth.

SUMMARY

The measurable and observed changes during pregnancy can be used to construct plausible explanations for various clinical phenomena. These explanations, however, may merely reflect perceptions limited by the incompleteness of our knowledge. Changes that do occur may be compensatory, primary, or secondary. The possibility that some of these changes are of primal origin with no contemporary, easily recognized, purpose must be considered. Live, healthy births occur in women with disease, malnutrition, and disability states within which some of these physiologic changes do not and cannot occur. This, of course, raises questions as to the impact and import on pregnancy outcome of any one nutritional observation, guideline, or recommendation.

There are, however, consistent, reproducible statistical associations between maternal prepregnant weight, incremental weight gain, total weight gain, vitamin and mineral supplementation, and perinatal outcome. For clinical decision-making oriented toward a goal of optimal maternal and fetal-newborn health, these associations serve as the basis for prophylactic and therapeutic interventions. Given appropriate guidance and instruction, the mother's responsibility is to achieve the best nutritional state prior to pregnancy, during pregnancy, and during lactation that her socioeconomic resources and any coexisting medical condition allow (48).

REFERENCES

1. Public Health Service. *Caring for our future: the content of prenatal care.* Washington, DC: U.S. Department Health and Human Services, 1989.
2. Nagey DA. The content of prenatal care. *Obstet Gynecol* 1989;74:516–527.
3. Hytten FE, Thomson AM, Taggart N. Total body water in normal pregnancy. *J Obstet Gynecol Br Comm* 1966;73:553–561.
4. Hytten FE, Leitch I. *The physiology of human pregnancy,* 2nd ed. Oxford: Blackwell, 1971.
5. Hytten F, Chamberlain G. *Clinical physiology in obstetrics.* Oxford: Blackwell, 1980.
6. Forsum E, Sadurskis A, Wager J. Resting metabolic rate and body composition of healthy Swedish women during pregnancy. *Am J Clin Nutr* 1988;47:942–947.
7. Emerson Jr K, Poindexter EL, Kothar IM. Changes in total body composition during normal and diabetic pregnancy. *Obstet Gynecol* 1975;45:505–511.
8. Clapp JF, Seaward BL, Sleamaker RH, Hiser J. Maternal physiologic adaptations to early human pregnancy. *Am J Obstet Gynecol* 1988;159:1456–1460.
9. Institute of Medicine. *Nutrition during pregnancy.* Committee on Nutritional Status During Pregnancy. Food and Nutrition Board, National Academy of Science. Washington, DC: National Academy Press, 1990.
10. Taggart NR, Holliday RM, Billewicz WZ, Hytten FE, Thomson AM. Changes in skin folds during pregnancy. *Br J Nutr* 1967;21:439–451.
11. Durnin JVGA. Energy requirements of pregnancy: an integration of the longitudinal data from the five-country study. *Lancet* 1987;1:1131–1133.
12. Kleinman JC. *Maternal weight gain during pregnancy: determinants and consequences.* Working Paper Series 33. Hyattsville, MD: U.S. Department of Health and Human Services, National Center for Health Statistics, 1990.
13. Eastman NJ, Jackson E. Weight relationships in pregnancy. I. The bearing of maternal weight gain and prepregnancy weight on birth weights in full term pregnancies. *Obstet Gynecol Surv* 1968;23:1003–1025.
14. Taffel SM. *Maternal weight gain and the outcome of pregnancy:*

15. Singer JE, Westphal M, Niswander K. Relationship of weight gain during pregnancy to birth weight and infant growth and development in the first year of life: a report from the collaborative study of cerebral palsy. *Obstet Gynecol* 1968;31:417–423.
16. Naeye RL. Weight gain and the outcome of pregnancy. *Am J Obstet Gynecol* 1979;135:3–9.
17. McCormick M. The contribution of low birth weight to infant mortality and childhood morbidity. *N Engl J Med* 1985;312:82–90.
18. Meyer J, Joans BS, Tonascia JA. Perinatal events associated with maternal smoking during pregnancy. *Am J Epidemiol* 1976;103:464–476.
19. Kramer MS. Intrauterine growth and gestational duration determinants. *Pediatrics* 1987;80:502–511.
20. Scholl TO, Salmon RW, Miller LK, Vasilenko P, Furey CH, Christine SM. Weight gain during adolescent pregnancy. *J Adolesc Health Care* 1988;9:286–290.
21. Abrams B, Newman V, Key T, Parker J. Maternal weight gain and preterm delivery. *Obstet Gynecol* 1989;74:577.
22. Susser M. Prenatal nutrition, birth weight, and psychological development: an overview of experiments, quasiexperiments, and natural experiments in the past decade. *Am J Clin Nutr* 1981;34:784–803.
23. Rush D, Horvitz DG, Seaver WB, Alvir JM, Garbowski GC, Leighton J, Sloan NL, Johnson SS, Kulka RA, Shanklin DS. The national WIC evaluation: evaluation of the special supplemental food program for women, infants, and children. I. Background and introduction. *Am J Clin Nutr* 1988;48:389–393.
24. Rush D, Stein Z, Susser M. A randomized controlled trial of prenatal nutritional supplementation in New York City. *Pediatrics* 1980;14:613–625.
25. Ruge S, Andersen T. Obstetric risks in obesity. An analysis of the literature. *Obstet Gynecol Surv* 1985;40:57–60.
26. Pedersen J. Weight and length at birth of infants of diabetic mothers. *Acta Endocrinol (Copenh)* 1954;16:330–339.
27. Brown JE, Schloesser PT. Prepregnancy weight status, prenatal weight gain, and the outcome of term twin gestations. *Am J Obstet Gynecol* 1990;162:182–186.
28. Skukla R, Bornschein RL, Dietrick KN. Fetal and infant lead exposure: effects on growth in stature. *Pediatrics* 1989;84:604–612.
29. Bellinger D, Leviton A, Warternaux C, Needlemen H, Rabinowitz M. Longitudinal analysis of prenatal and postnatal lead exposure and early cognitive development. *N Engl J Med* 1987;316:1037–1043.
30. Matsumoto H. "Fetal minimata disease." *J Neuropathol Exp Neurol* 1965;24:563–574.
31. Swanson CA, King JC. Zinc and pregnancy outcome. *Am J Clin Nutr* 1987;46:763–771.
32. Milunksy A, Jack H, Jack SS, Bruell CL, MacLaughlin DS, Rothman KJ, Willett W. Multivitamin/folic acid supplementation in early pregnancy reduces the prevalence of neural tube defects. *JAMA* 1989;262:2847–2852.
33. Reece EA, Hobbins JC. Diabetic embryopathy: pathogenesis, prenatal diagnosis and prevention. *Obstet Gynecol Surv* 1986;41:325–335.
34. Freinkel N. Of pregnancy and progeny. *Diabetes* 1980;29:1023–1035.
35. Churchill JA, Berendes HW. *Intelligence of children whose mothers had acetonuria during pregnancy.* Perinatal Factors Affecting Human Development. Pan American Health Organization Scientific Publication No. 185, Washington D.C.
36. Naeye RL, Chez RA. Effects of maternal acetonuria and low pregnancy weight gain on children's psychomotor development. *Am J Obstet Gynecol* 1981;139:189–194.
37. Chez RA, Curcio FD. Ketonuria in normal pregnancy. *Obstet Gynecol* 1987;69:272–274.
38. American Academy of Pediatrics/American College of Obstetricians and Gynecologists. *Guidelines for perinatal care,* 2nd ed. Elk Grove IL: American Academy of Pediatrics, 1988.
39. Center for Disease Control. Anemia during pregnancy in low-income women—United States, 1987. *MMWR* 1990;39:73–76.
40. Garn SM, Ridella SA, Petzold AS, Falkner F. Maternal hematologic values and pregnancy outcomes. *Semin Perinatol* 1981;5:155–162.
41. Pitkin RM. Calcium metabolism in pregnancy and the perinatal period. A review. *Am J Obstet Gynecol* 1985;151:99–109.
42. Belizan JM, Villar J, Repke JT. The relationship between calcium intake and pregnancy induced hypertension. Up to date evidence. *Am J Obstet Gynecol* 1988;158:898–902.
43. Lindheimer MD, Katz AI. Sodium and diuretics in pregnancy. *Obstet Gynecol* 1974;44:434–440.
44. Borgberg C, Gillmer MDG, Brunner EJ. Obesity in pregnancy: the effect of dietary advice. *Diabetes Care* 1980;3:476–481.
45. Abrams B. Maternal weight gain and pregnancy outcome in overweight women. *Clin Nutr* 1988;7:197–204.
46. Dimperio D. *Prenatal nutrition: clinical guidelines for nurses.* White Plains, NY: March of Dimes Birth Defects Foundation, 1988.
47. Worthington-Roberts BS. Lactation and human milk: nutritional considerations. In: Worthington-Roberts BS, Vermeersch J, Williams SR, eds. *Nutrition in pregnancy and lactation,* 3rd ed. St. Louis: C. V. Mosby, 1985;236–296.
48. Taffel SM, Keppel KG. Advice about weight gain during pregnancy and actual weight gain. *Am J Public Health* 1986;76:1396–1399.

CHAPTER 2

Nutritional Requirements of the Term Newborn

Fernando R. Moya

CHARACTERISTICS OF THE TERM NEWBORN

In the United States the average weight of male and female newborns at term is 3.27 kg and 3.23 kg, respectively; the weight range accepted as "normal" (10th to 90th percentiles) is 2.78 to 3.82 kg (1). Standards used for normal weight at birth vary according to race, socioeconomic status, altitude, and other biodemographic factors (2–4).

Body composition changes drastically with advancing gestation. Total body water, which amounts to over 85% of body weight in the early third trimester fetus, decreases to about 75% at term. During the first postnatal week, it drops further, to 65% to 68% of body weight (Fig. 1). Most of this loss is accounted for by modifications of the extracellular compartment and takes place mainly through the skin and renal system. The possibility of racial influences on these changes has been raised (5).

The term infant has about 11% to 12% of body weight as protein, and a slightly higher proportion as fat. Premature infants differ in composition, particularly in fat, which can be as low as 1% at about 28 weeks of gestation. The energy reserve is, therefore, much higher in the term newborn, oscillating around 6,800 kilocalories (Cal) of which 75% is in the form of fat and 1% as glycogen (6).

At term, the kidneys have their full number of nephrons, but their function is somewhat limited compared to the adult. Renal blood flow and glomerular filtration rate are lower than adult values (7). Tubular function, also less than in the adult, is evidenced by a higher fractional excretion of Na and a limited ability for tubular reabsorption of substances like glucose and bicarbonate. The capability to excrete an acid load is also limited.

Urine-diluting capacity during the neonatal period is similar to the adult, although excretion takes substantially longer. The ability to concentrate urine is, however, limited in term newborns; water deprivation leads to concentrations of only 600 to 700 mOsm/l.

The characteristics of the neonatal kidney impose certain limitations on water and nutrient intake by the newborn, especially of nutrients that determine the renal solute load, i.e., protein, sodium (Na), potassium (K), chloride (Cl), phosphorus (P).

Gastrointestinal tract status of the term newborn includes mature coordinated sucking and swallowing mechanisms, an initially limited gastric volume (about 10 ml/kg), and delayed gastric emptying. Gastric acid secretion is less than in the adult despite high serum gastrin concentrations (8). Although this lower gastric acidity may limit protein and carbohydrate acid hydrolysis, it may also allow certain key proteins, i.e., hormones, enzymes, immunoglobulins, to cross the gastric acid barrier intact. Developmental changes of enzymes and hormones involved in the digestion of specific nutrients are briefly discussed in their corresponding sections.

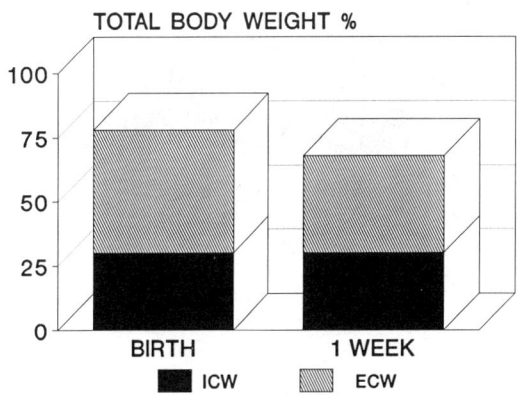

FIG. 1. Changes in body water in the term newborn. ECW, extracellular water; ICW, intracellular water.

F. R. Moya: Department of Pediatrics, Obstetrics, and Gynecology, University of Texas Southwestern Medical Center, Dallas, Texas 75235.

ENERGY REQUIREMENTS

Each vital function of the body has an energy demand that must be met, either by nutritional intake, utilization of stored energy, or both. In the term neonate, part of the energy stored in the form of glycogen and fat is rapidly utilized during the transition from fetal to extrauterine existence. The neonate is, therefore, almost immediately dependent on exogenous energy sources. About 5% of this intake will be lost, from either lack of absorption, or excretion (Fig. 2).

Most of the available energy supplies basal metabolic needs. Estimations of basal metabolic needs of newborns are actually more reflective of a resting metabolic rate (RMR) since they are not performed in the fasted and basal state. The range of RMR in term newborns is approximately 48 to 55 Cal/kg/day (9). Determinations of the RMR are done in a neutral thermal environment. This is the environmental temperature at which oxygen consumption and energy expenditure for maintenance of a stable and normal body temperature is minimal. If the newborn infant is placed in an environment that is above or below the neutral thermal environment, energy expenditure and oxygen consumption for thermoregulation will increase.

Term newborns are definitely better suited than prematures to withstand lower and more variable environmental temperatures. They have a thicker subcutaneous fat layer, a larger amount of brown fat necessary for chemical thermogenesis, and a relatively smaller surface area for heat loss. However, even in term newborns, heat loss must be minimized, to avoid losing precious energy, which should be utilized for growth, to thermogenesis.

Brain, heart, liver, and kidneys account for over 60% of the RMR. At term, the brain is proportionally larger than in later life and its weight is about 10% of total body weight. Its relatively high metabolic rate, large mass, and the lack of stored energy explain why this organ utilizes the highest portion of the basal metabolic needs. The brain is solely dependent on glucose and ketone bodies delivered by the circulation for its energy demands. Most of the energy utilized in the first hours after birth derives from glucose oxidation. In subsequent hours and days, this changes to a mixture of energy derived from carbohydrate and fat (10). Thus, fatty acid oxidation and ketone utilization are additional important metabolic pathways during the perinatal and neonatal periods.

Soon after birth, oxygen consumption, which is directly related to energy expenditure, is about 4.8 ml/kg/min. By the end of the first week after birth, it rises to about 7 ml/kg/min, remaining stable throughout the first year of life (11). In the early neonatal period, the respiratory quotient changes from close to 1.0 at birth to about 0.8 at 1 week of age. This denotes a change from energy derived essentially from carbohydrate utilization to that of lipid oxidation (6).

The energy remaining after losses are accounted for and resting metabolic needs are met is utilized for physical activity, the thermic effect of feeding (TEF), and for growth. During the neonatal period energy expenditure for physical activity is limited since many hours are spent at rest, and motor activity is not weight-bearing or prolonged. Actual values for this component of energy needs are somewhat scarce and are usually derived from data obtained in infants above 2 to 3 months of age. Nonetheless, energy estimates for activity during the neonatal period are approximately 15% to 25% of RMR or 10 to 15 Cal/kg/day.

Although crying may substantially increase metabolism, overall it is a minor determinant of total energy needs. After a feeding, energy is spent in digestion, transport, and conversion of nutrients to either storage forms or easily metabolizable compounds. This energy cost represents the TEF and has been estimated at about 10% of the daily energy expenditure. However, this estimate can be quite variable from infant to infant. In addition, it can vary in the same infant at different times (12). Furthermore, the composition of a feeding also influences TEF. For example, the energy dissipated after protein ingestion can be several times higher than that observed after fat or carbohydrate ingestion.

Besides RMR, growth is the other major determinant of energy requirements during the neonatal period and early infancy. In normal newborns, growth does not really occur during the first 4 to 5 days after birth; any increases in weight observed during this early period are generally secondary to changes in the state of hydration. This lack of early growth is not only a function of an initially limited availability of substrates and energy, but also a reflection of the hormonal milieu. This status is characterized by high levels of catecholamines, cortisol, and glucagon, which are not promoters of growth but rather serve to acutely mobilize stored energy. Most term newborns, if healthy and given adequate amounts of fluids and calories, will recover birth weight by 7 to 10

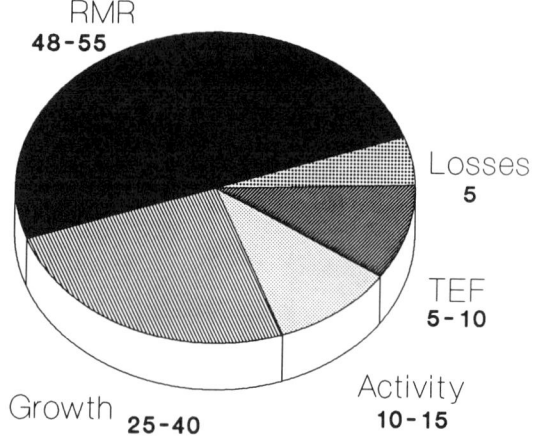

FIG. 2. Partition of energy intake in the term newborn. RMR, resting metabolic rate; TEF, thermic effect of feeding.

days after birth. Subsequent growth during the neonatal period is highly variable and depends on energy availability, type of feeding, and composition of the tissue deposited.

At about 1 week of age, most healthy newborns are ingesting about 140 to 150 ml/kg/day of either breast milk or a commercially available infant formula. The energy provided (~100 Cal/kg/day) is generally sufficient to promote adequate growth. Although different infants grow at different rates, an adequate daily weight gain in term newborns has been estimated at about 10 to 12 g/kg/day. In smaller, more premature infants, the rate of weight gain can be two- to three-fold higher. Weight gain on a per kilogram basis decelerates considerably after 2 to 3 months of age in term infants.

Term newborns with special circumstances that limit either the volume per feeding or nutrient absorption, e.g., gastroesophageal reflux or malabsorption, may not receive adequate energy intakes with regular feedings. The same is true for those rare occasions when energy expenditure is higher than expected, e.g., congestive heart failure or hyperthyroidism. Energy needs for maintenance will always take precedence over growth and protein synthesis.

The type of feeding is also a significant variable. Breast milk is superior to formulas in digestibility and efficiency of energy utilization (13). Infants who are breast-fed exclusively gain weight at adequate rates although intakes are lower than that of infants fed infant formulas (14,15). Nutrient absorption only partially explains this difference since absorption of breast milk and infant formulas is quite good. A more likely explanation is the presence of growth factors, enzymes, hormones, or other selective components in breast milk.

The composition of tissue accretion also varies with the type of feeding. Although there is no consensus on why, formula-fed term infants appear to lay down tissue with a higher fat content than those who are breast-fed (16). Since the cost of deposition of fat is about 11.5 Cal/g, more energy is required for tissue deposition with formula feeding (17).

The energy cost of growth is comprised of what is needed for tissue synthesis and what remains in the tissue as energy storage. Values for energy requirements per gram of tissue deposited are generally around 4 to 5 Cal/g, assuming about 30% to 35% fat and 10% to 11% protein in the new tissue. This is just a gross estimate, however, because of the factors previously discussed. In fact, with minimal fat deposition, growth can occur at a cost of less than 3 Cal/g (14). Overall energy needs for the term infant are approximately 95 to 120 Cal/kg/day, although this may vary in some infants. Current estimates are lower than had been previously reported (18). Newborns receiving parenteral nutrition exclusively may grow well on energy intakes below those of orally fed infants, since certain components of energy requirements, including fecal losses and TEF, are minimized.

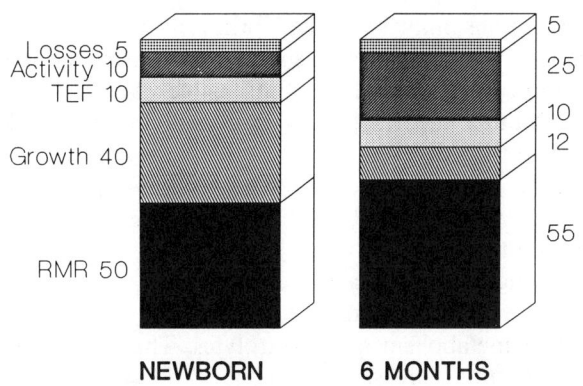

FIG. 3. Age-related changes in energy needs between the neonatal period and 6 months of age.

In spite of increased energy needs for physical activity, an infant's total energy needs decrease in the months after birth as growth rate decelerates (Fig. 3).

COMPONENTS OF NUTRITION

Water

As previously described, there are significant changes in total body water, mainly in the extracellular compartment, that occur during the first week after birth (Fig. 1). The proportion of total body water and its distribution between intra- and extracellular compartments continue to change during the first year of life (19). In a well-hydrated infant, water requirements are regulated by the need to compensate for insensible or measurable (urine, stools) losses, and for growth (Fig. 4). Also important is the need to supply nutrients and minerals in such concentrations that they will be well tolerated and absorbed. Although thirst is an important determinant of water intake at any age, its role in the newborn is limited since infants cannot regulate intake at will.

Insensible water losses in the term newborn have been estimated at less than 1.0 ml/kg/hr or 20 ml/kg/day (20).

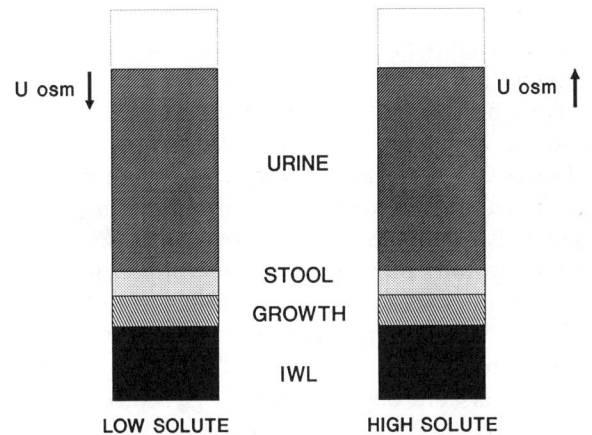

FIG. 4. Water requirements in the term newborn. IWL, insensible waterloss.

Fluctuations may be related primarily to changes in health status, activity, and shifts of environmental temperature. About one-third of insensible water losses occur through the respiratory tract and the remainder through the skin.

Stools generally account for less than 5 ml/kg/day of water loss even in exclusively breast-fed newborns with their more frequent stooling patterns. Urinary losses are much higher, influenced essentially by the need to excrete the daily renal solute load, mainly nitrogen from protein metabolism and electrolytes. The renal solute load of human breast milk is about 8 mOsm/100 ml or 10 mOsm/100 Cal. This is less than that of standard infant formulas [20 calories (cal) per ounce] since the mineral content of breast milk is lower and the protein composition different. With an intake of about 150 ml/kg/day of breast milk or of a standard commercial formula (20 cal per ounce), the renal solute load oscillates between 12 and 15 mOsm/100 ml or 15 and 22 mOsm/100 Cal. At this level, urine will be produced without stressing the term kidney to significantly dilute or concentrate it. If the solute load or water intake varies, changes in urine volume and osmolarity should be expected (Fig. 4). This is the case when more concentrated formulas are used. Formulas with greater than 350 mOsm/100 ml should be avoided.

After all losses are accounted for, the remaining component of water requirement is growth. For every gram of tissue accrued, a proportionate amount of water will be utilized. A very small part of this need is supplied by endogenous water production; most is supplied by the diet. Water requirements for growth drop several months after birth, when the proportion of body water is less than in the neonatal period.

Carbohydrate Requirements

The functions of carbohydrates in the human are primarily those of an energy source for both fuel and storage and a precursor for nucleic acid synthesis. Glucose is the main carbohydrate utilized during fetal life and the early neonatal period. Once feedings have begun, other monosaccharides start to play a role. Except in newborns receiving parenteral fluids, for whom glucose is the only carbohydrate source, carbohydrates are usually provided as disaccharides (lactose, sucrose) or larger monosaccharide chains (glucose polymers and maltodextrins). Starch is generally introduced in subsequent months.

Carbohydrates provide approximately 39% to 43% of the calories in breast milk or cow's milk formulas (Table 1). Lactose, the main carbohydrate of breast milk, is usually found in concentrations of about 7 g/dl. Other minor sugars are oligosaccharides, glycoproteins, and traces of glucose. These components are found in concentrations up to 1.3 g/dl and may play a role in the

TABLE 1. *Primary carbohydrate sources in breast milk and infant formulas[a]*

Formula	Carbohydrate	% of total calories
Breast milk	Lactose	39–43
Enfamil 20	Lactose	41
Similac 20	Lactose	43
SMA	Lactose	43
Good Start	Lactose, maltodextrin	44
Prosobee	Glucose polymers	40
Isomil	Sucrose, glucose polymers	40
Nursoy	Sucrose	41
Nutramigen	Glucose polymers, corn starch	54
Pregestimil	Glucose polymers, glucose	41
Alimentum	Sucrose, modified tapioca starch	41

[a] Infant formula compositions as of October 1990.

pattern of bacterial colonization of the gut as well as local host defense mechanisms of the gastrointestinal tract (21,22). Lactose, in concentrations similar to breast milk, is also the main carbohydrate source in cow's milk formulas. Most soy-based formulas, however, contain either sucrose or glucose polymers.

Lactose is metabolized to glucose and galactose by the enzyme lactase, which is located at the upper end of the intestinal villi. Glucose then crosses into the portal circulation by either simple diffusion, facilitated diffusion, or active transport. Glucose transport across the intestinal wall is the rate-limiting step in carbohydrate absorption. There is debate as to whether glucose absorption at term is less completely developed than in older children.

Galactose is absorbed in a similar fashion to glucose and is metabolized by the liver. In early postnatal life there is still a certain degree of dependency on gluconeogenesis despite efficient conversion of dietary galactose to glucose. The development of lactase activity occurs later than that of other disaccharidases, but lactase levels at term are more than adequate to handle the lactose load provided by routine feeding.

This is not the case in small premature infants in whom lactose malabsorption may occur. Lactose still present in the lumen of the colon is fermented by bacterial flora to lactic acid.

The hydrolysis of sucrose carried out by the enzyme sucrase produces glucose and fructose. Fructose is absorbed by facilitated diffusion and metabolized by the liver. Sucrase is also located near the tip and lateral aspects of the intestinal villi. Sucrase levels are detectable throughout the third trimester of pregnancy in amounts comparable to those found at term.

Glucose polymers have become common in many formulas, either as a substitute for lactose or as an additional source of carbohydrate. They consist of chains of 5 to 10 units of glucose joined by 1 to 4 alpha linkages. These bonds can be hydrolyzed by α-glucosidases like amylase, glucoamylase, and maltase. The latter two enzymes are present at midgestation, and by the end of pregnancy are at 50% to 100% of the adult level of activity (23). They are also more resistant to injury than other disaccharidases. Pancreatic amylase, on the other hand, is present in very low levels at birth and is not responsive to hormonal stimulation by pancreozymin or secretin (24). This lack of enzymatic activity is partially circumvented by the presence of amylase in breast milk. Salivary amylase, albeit found in smaller quantities than in the adult, also contributes to carbohydrate hydrolysis. Glucose polymers are less osmotically active than glucose because of their larger size and molecular weight. Since gastric emptying is delayed with increasing caloric content and osmolality, an isocaloric amount of glucose polymers would be preferable to glucose (25).

The term newborn needs carbohydrates primarily as a steady source of energy at a time when gluconeogenesis may be somewhat limited (26). A carbohydrate intake of less than 4 mg/kg/min leads to gluconeogenesis (27). Since gluconeogenesis is even less active in preterm infants, such infants are much more dependent on an exogenous source of carbohydrates. Fatty acid oxidation and generation of ketone bodies may serve as alternative fuels. An estimated 40% to 45% of caloric intake must be supplied as carbohydrates. This translates into a carbohydrate requirement of 10 to 14 g/kg/day. Higher proportions of carbohydrate in the diet may interfere with gastric emptying and may also surpass the absorptive capacity of the digestive system.

The role of carbohydrates, particularly lactose, in the absorption of calcium and phosphorus is still not fully understood.

Protein Requirements

Proteins are diverse in structure, function, and role. They include structural and transport proteins, enzymes, hormones, and neurotransmitters, as well as coagulation and immune proteins. Proteins may also be a source of energy but, because protein metabolism leads to a substantial renal solute load, other energy sources are preferentially utilized in the human except in situations of energy deprivation. High-quality protein's importance lies in the essential amino acids and nitrogen (N) that it supplies. These nutrients must be replenished constantly since they cannot be stored and essential amino acids cannot be synthesized.

Placental transfer of amino acids during late gestation has been estimated at about 2.0 to 2.5 g/kg/day, whereas body protein accretion during this period and in early postnatal life is between 0.8 and 1.5 g/kg/day (6). This results in a change in body protein content from 9% at 28 weeks of gestation to approximately 11% to 12% at term.

The first step in dietary protein digestion is acid and enzymatic hydrolysis in the stomach. The term newborn has a limited gastric secretion of HCl despite high levels of gastrin (8). Pepsins also are found in smaller quantities in the stomach and their activity is lower in the less acid gastric pH of the term neonate. Between 6 months and 2 years of age, these steps of protein digestion mature to adult levels. Further steps in protein digestion involve the action of pancreatic and intestinal enzymes. The activities of enterokinase and chymotrypsin are less than in adults, but very early trypsin activity is relatively comparable to that found in older infants.

Despite these limitations, between 80% and 90% of the dietary N is absorbed by the action of specific transport systems for amino acids, dipeptides, and tripeptides. Absorption and utilization of dipeptides and tripeptides is more efficient than that of pure amino acids. After absorption, the degradation of most essential amino acids occurs in the liver except that of branched amino acids, which takes place primarily in skeletal muscle. Metabolism of nonessential amino acids takes place both in liver and peripherally (28).

Hepatic metabolism of certain amino acids such as methionine, phenylalanine, and tyrosine is limited, particularly in preterm infants. At term, the generation of cysteine from methionine through the action of cystathionase is poor. Thus, cysteine is considered an essential amino acid in the human newborn. Taurine, a β–amino acid further derived from cysteine, has also been considered conditionally essential for the neonate, especially prematures (29,30). Breast milk contains considerable amounts of taurine (3.5 to 4 mg/dl). Presently, taurine is added to infant formulas for term and preterm infants in comparable amounts, even though its absolute necessity has not been established (31).

Other hepatic enzymatic systems, such as those that participate in the urea cycle and gluconeogenesis through alanine, also have a lower activity at birth. Their functions, however, appear to mature rapidly in the early neonatal period.

About 4 mOsm of renal solute load are derived per gram of protein metabolized.

The type of protein intake is dependent on whether breast milk or formula is given (Table 2). Whey proteins predominate in breast milk and certain formulas. Casein is found in breast milk in concentrations not exceeding 30% of total protein (32). Most proteins in breast milk exhibit changes with lactational age; total protein content is significantly less than in commercial formulas.

Recent evidence suggests that 90% of the N in breast milk is absorbed in term and some preterm infants (33,34). Earlier studies had reported that a sizable proportion of the whey protein fraction of breast milk was lost in the stool (35). Protein absorption from commercial formulas is above 80%.

Nonprotein N is proportionately much higher in breast milk than in cow's milk–based formulas. It constitutes about 35% to 40% of the total N of mature breast milk. Urea, small peptides, and free amino acids account

TABLE 2. *Approximate protein composition of breast milk and selected infant formulas[a]*

	Breast milk[b]	Enfamil	Similac	SMA	Good Start
Total protein (g/dl)	0.85–1.30	1.5	1.5	1.5	1.6
Casein (%)	20–30	40	82	40	—
Whey (%)	70–80	60	18	60	100
α-Lactalbumin (g/dl)	0.22–0.46	—	—	—	—
Immunoglobulin (g/dl)	0.1–0.2	—	—	—	—
Lactoferrin (g/dl)	0.1–0.5	—	—	—	—
Lysozyme (g/dl)	0.05	—	—	—	—
Albumin (g/dl)	0.05	—	—	—	—
Nonprotein N (mg N/dl)	45–50	—	—	—	—

[a] Infant formula composition as of October 1990.
[b] Estimated values from refs. 13, 32, and 44.

for most of the nonprotein N. A variable percentage of the nonprotein N of breast milk must be available for absorption and metabolism, otherwise normal rates of growth and protein accretion would not be possible in exclusively breast-fed infants. For instance, ammonia resulting from bacterial hydrolysis of urea can be used for glutamine synthesis. It has been postulated that low levels of glycine ingestion during exclusive breast-feeding would promote the activity of glutamine synthetase (13). Glycine exerts a negative feedback effect on the activity of this enzyme.

At similar volume and energy intakes, breast-fed infants receive considerably less protein than those fed infant formulas. Despite this, normal rates of growth and protein accretion in breast-fed infants during the first several months of age have been documented (13,14,36). On the other hand, some reports in the literature have suggested that the rate of growth of breast-fed infants may be less than that of bottle-fed infants, although most of the differences observed are evident only after 2 to 3 months of age (37,38). However, if one accepts the concept that growth and indices of protein metabolism of exclusively breast-fed healthy newborns and small infants constitute the standard by which other infant formulas should be judged, then several other factors must be taken into consideration. Utilization of nonprotein N from breast milk has already been mentioned. Differences in amino acid composition and interaction with other nutrients of breast milk should also be considered. Moreover, growth factors and hormones, some of which are abundant in breast milk, may also be crucial in the regulation of growth and metabolism (39).

The pros and cons of breast milk versus infant formulas have been reviewed extensively (32). Current concern is focused on the optimum protein content for infant formulas and whether recommendations for protein intake in term newborns and small infants are excessive (28,36,40). Indeed, protein and amino acid metabolism are markedly influenced by protein intake. The newborn may, however, lack the ability to accommodate a high protein intake. As a result, the renal solute load will be higher and abnormal amino acid accumulations may occur.

Higher blood levels of urea and various amino acids have been demonstrated in term newborns subjected to protein intakes above 2.5 g/kg/day (41). Part of this metabolic constraint during the neonatal period may relate to a lower muscle mass compared to the adult. Protein needs are also a function of energy intake; when energy intake is insufficient protein synthesis will cease. Conversely, at high growth rates, the requirement for protein increases.

As mentioned previously, dietary protein's importance lies in its ability to provide essential amino acids and N. Breast milk and infant formulas differ in their amino acid compositions. Plasma amino acid concentrations change quickly to reflect respective intake. Although the use of plasma amino acid levels to evaluate adequacy of infant formulas has been questioned, comparisons between plasma amino acid profiles of breast-fed and formula-fed infants are constantly being reported.

The plasma amino acid profiles of term infants fed a whey-based formula (casein to whey ratio 40:60) or a casein-predominant preparation (casein to whey ratio 82:18) are different from those of exclusively breast-fed infants (41–43). Furthermore, differences in plasma amino acid patterns also exist between these formulas. Elevated plasma levels of total essential amino acids, valine, threonine, phenylalanine, methionine, and branched amino acids are commonly observed with formula versus breast milk intake. Infants receiving parenteral nutrition have plasma amino acid patterns quite different from enterally fed infants. In spite of these variations, the use of either breast milk or currently available infant formulas meets the estimated requirements for essential amino acids (Table 3). The significance of the generally mild elevations of certain amino acids in plasma observed at acceptable volumes of formula feeding is not clear.

Recent recommendations for protein intake during the first month of life in term infants are 2.0 to 2.5 g/kg/

TABLE 3. *Essential amino acids during the neonatal period*

Amino acid	Requirements (mg/kg/day)
Isoleucine	111
Leucine	153
Lysine	96
Methionine + cysteine[a]	50
Phenylalanine + tyrosine	90
Threonine	66
Tryptophan	19
Valine	95
Histidine	25
Taurine[a]	?

Modified from ref. 44.
[a] Conditionally essential because of temporary limitations in endogenous synthesis.

day (43,44). It is clear, however, that newborns breast-fed exclusively grow well with lesser amounts of protein intake during the neonatal period and the first few months after birth (15,36,45).

Fat Requirements

Lipids have very diverse functions in humans. They constitute a major energy source and an almost unlimited form of energy storage. They also act as vehicles for absorption and transport of important compounds such as fat-soluble vitamins. Phospholipids are integral parts of cell membranes and pulmonary surfactant. Other members of the lipid family, such as the essential fatty acids, are critical for normal growth and development, especially of brain and retina (46). Fatty acids are also the precursors of prostaglandins and serve as a major energy source.

During the third trimester of pregnancy, the fetus rapidly accumulates fat. Percent body fat increases from 1% at 28 weeks of gestation to 12% to 16% at term. Most of this is deposited as white fat, a form of energy storage. In fact, more than 90% of the calories accumulated by the term fetus are in the form of fat (47). A small proportion of body fat becomes a more specialized tissue called brown fat. This is the site of chemical thermogenesis, critical for temperature control during the neonatal period.

Placental transfer of lipids occurs primarily at the level of fatty acids and ketones (48). Triglycerides do not seem to cross the placenta but are subjected to breakdown by placental lipoprotein lipase to release fatty acids into the fetal circulation (48). Despite the predominant use of glucose as fuel during fetal life, oxidation of fatty acids and ketone bodies is also important, particularly for the fetal brain.

Soon after birth, there is a rapid increase in fatty acid oxidation and ketogenesis (26). This metabolic adaptation is in part due to the effect of hormones like glucagon and catecholamines. Changes in oxidative metabolism during the perinatal period have been extensively reviewed (26).

The absorption of lipids from the diet involves several steps. Initial breakdown of triglycerides takes place in the stomach by the actions of lingual and gastric lipases (49). This step is extremely important to the newborn infant who lacks adequate amounts of pancreatic lipase. Moreover, since milk fat globules are relatively resistant to the action of this enzyme, prior hydrolysis by lingual lipase, which is able to penetrate the core of the milk-fat particle, is necessary. The slower gastric emptying and less acid gastric pH of the newborn contribute to the optimal functioning of lingual and gastric lipases. Some short- and middle-chain fatty acids released by gastric hydrolysis of triglycerides are absorbed directly across the mucosa of the stomach.

The remaining glycerides (mono-, di-, and triglycerides) are subjected to further intraluminal hydrolysis in the small intestine. Biliary and pancreatic secretions participate in this phase. The activity of pancreatic lipase is decreased at term. In addition, bile salt levels are low and the response to hormonal stimulation is attenuated.

In this phase of fat absorption, diglycerides, triglycerides, and phospholipids are incorporated into micelles along with bile salts and calcium. These last two components are necessary for hydrolysis of long-chain phospholipids by pancreatic phospholipase A_2. Pancreatic lipase requires the presence of a colipase to have higher affinity for attachment to the micelle. In human milk there is a bile salt–stimulated lipase which also contributes to intraluminal hydrolysis of fat globules (50).

After intraluminal hydrolysis, absorption of monoglycerides and free fatty acids takes place mainly by passive diffusion, although the presence of a specific carrier protein for fatty acids located in the membrane of the enterocyte has been suggested. Within the mucosal cells, triglycerides are synthesized again by reesterification. Afterward, transport into the lymphatics occurs in the form of chylomicrons. Short- and middle-chain fatty acids can be absorbed into the portal circulation directly. Once in the circulation, polar lipids bind to albumin and nonpolar lipids are transported by lipoproteins. An updated review of lipoprotein metabolism in early postnatal life has recently been published (51).

Catabolism of circulating lipids occurs primarily through the actions of lecithin-cholesterol acyltransferase in plasma, or lipoprotein lipase in the capillary endothelium. After tissue uptake of lipids, oxidation of fatty acids takes place within the mitochondria. Transport across the inner mitochondrial membrane requires the presence of carnitine. Carnitine is synthesized in the liver and kidney from lysine and methionine. Biosynthesis of carnitine may not be fully developed at birth, and plasma and tissue levels are low, particularly in neonates exclusively receiving parenteral nutrition (52). The

TABLE 4. *Fat composition of breast milk and selected infant formulas*[a]

Fat	Breast milk	Enfamil	Similac	SMA	Good Start
Total (g/dl)	3.5–4.5	3.8	3.6	3.5	3.4
Triglycerides (%)	98–99	99	99	99	99
Cholesterol (mg/dl)	10–15	1.0	1.1	3.3	0.6
Phospholipids (mg/dl)	15–20	30	—	—	66
Fatty acids (% of total fatty acids)					
Linoleic (18:2 ω-6)	16	25	33	13	12.5
α-Linolenic (18:3 ω-3)	1	2.5	4.5	1.0	0.3
Docosahexanoic (22:6 ω-3)	0.4–0.6	—	—	—	—

[a] Infant formula compositions as of October 1990.

amount of carnitine in most infant formulas is similar to that found in breast milk (60 to 100 nmol/ml). Soy-based formulas currently available in the United States are also being supplemented with comparable amounts.

Fat is the most variable component of breast milk and accounts for about 50% to 55% of its energy, varying in mature breast milk from 3.5 to 4.5 g/dl (Table 4). The fat content of colostrum is lower (53,54). Close to 98% to 99% of the fat content of breast milk and infant formulas is in the form of triglycerides. Cholesterol and phospholipids exist in smaller quantities in breast milk; both are found in higher quantities in colostrum. Infant formulas, with the exception of Good Start (Carnation) and SMA (Wyeth), contain little cholesterol. Although breast-fed infants of both sexes have higher serum cholesterol than formula-fed infants, the significance of this finding is unknown (55,56). More than 90% to 95% of dietary fat is absorbed by the term newborn; a lower percentage may be absorbed by prematures.

Although the fat content of breast milk is markedly influenced by lactational age, fat composition remains relatively constant throughout lactation. Breast milk contains primarily fatty acids of 10 to 20 carbon (C) chains. Middle-chain fatty acids (C < 12) constitute only 10% of the total in mature breast milk at term and close to twice that amount in milk of mothers of premature infants. Oleic (18:1), palmitic (16:0), and linoleic (18:2 ω-6) acids are the most abundant in mature breast milk. α-Linolenic acid (18:3 ω-3) represents only about 1% of the total fatty acids in breast milk. The latter two are considered essential fatty acids because of the inability of animal tissues to introduce double bonds in positions prior to carbon 9 from the omega terminus side (57). Through further elongation and desaturation of ω-3 and ω-6 fatty acids, several biologically significant compounds are generated. Among these are the prostaglandins and eicosapentaenoic (EPA) (20:5 ω-3) and docosahexanoic (DHA) (22:6 ω-3) acids. These long-chain polyunsaturated fatty acids (LCPUFA) are present in breast milk in amounts of less than 0.6% of total fatty acids; colostrum and preterm breast milk contain higher amounts (58,59).

During fetal life there is substantial accretion of ω-6– and ω-3–derived fatty acids (Fig. 5). This amounts to 400 and 50 mg/kg/day of ω-6 and ω-3 fatty acids, respectively (60). The majority of the fatty acids are accumulated in white fat but the highest relative concentration of ω-3 LCPUFA, particularly DHA, is localized in the retina and brain (46).

Accumulation continues after birth, at which time the fatty acid composition of brain and other tissues is quite vulnerable to dietary modifications. Numerous studies have demonstrated biochemical and functional changes secondary to ω-3 fatty acid deficiency in animals and, more recently, humans (46,61). Premature infants, either breast-fed or on infant formulas deficient in DHA, have demonstrated significant decreases of this fatty acid in red blood cell membranes. More importantly, visual acuity, as determined by electroretinograms and pattern reversal visual-evoked responses, was superior among

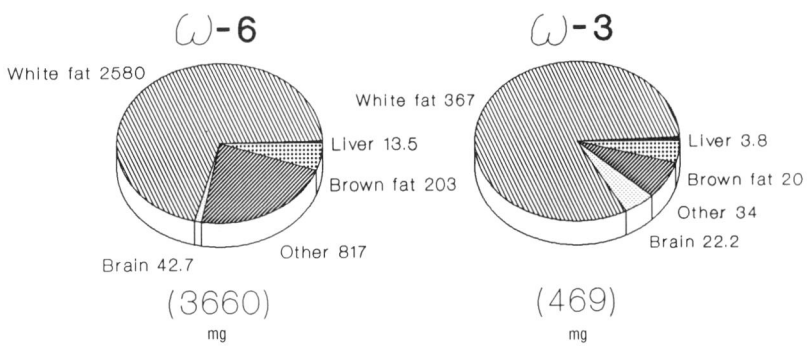

FIG. 5. Intrauterine accretion and distribution of essential fatty acids during the third trimester of pregnancy in milligrams of fatty acids per week. (From ref. 60, with permission.)

premature infants either breast-fed or on a formula supplemented with DHA (61,62). Biochemical differences in red blood cell membranes between term infants who are breast-fed versus those on formula have also been documented (Fig. 6) (63). The functional significance of these changes in the term newborn remains to be determined. However, since human brain and retinal development continues to take place for several months after birth, a finding that has been corroborated by studies in rhesus monkeys, the necessity for ω-6 and ω-3 LCPUFAs can no longer be ignored (61,64,65).

The current recommendation for the term infant is, therefore, a fat intake of between 3.5 and 6.0 g/kg/day or 30% to 55% of total daily calories (49). The recommendation for total ω-6 and ω-3 fatty acids oscillates between 4% and 12% of total energy or 0.5 to 0.7 g/kg/day of linoleic acid (18:2 ω-6) and 70 to 150 mg/kg/day of α-linolenic acid (18:3 ω-3) (49,61). Amounts of linoleic acid above 12% of total energy may actually interfere with desaturation and elongation processes thereby potentially decreasing synthesis of ω-3 and ω-6 long-chain derivatives. Because of the transient limitation in desaturation and elongation enzymatic activities, approximately half of the ω-3 fatty acids should be supplied as derivatives above the 18-carbon chain length (61).

Since the role of dietary cholesterol and phospholipids in the first month after birth is still not fully defined, an intake similar to that obtained through breast-feeding is assumed acceptable. Whether both of these components should be present in infant formulas in amounts similar to breast milk cannot be ascertained at this time (31).

Nucleotides

The presence of nucleotides in human and animal milk has been known for some time. They, together with nucleic acids, account for a substantial proportion of the nonprotein N content in breast milk. Appreciation of their importance as dietary components is more recent (66). Nucleotides derive from the bases purine and pyrimidine and can be acquired through the diet or synthesized *de novo* from amino acid precursors. Also, reconstitution of bases generated by salvage of nucleic acid catabolism is an important source of intracellular nucleotides.

Nucleotides are involved in many biologic functions. Cellular immunity in mice and other laboratory animals is influenced by dietary nucleotides. Deficiency of these compounds in the diet of mice results in abnormal function of helper/inducer T lymphocytes and decreased production of interleukin-2 (67). In the same animal species, supplementation of the diet with nucleotides during weaning increases natural killer cell activity (68). Decreased macrophage phagocytic activity and lower resistance to bacterial and fungal challenges have also been shown in mice (69). Preliminary evidence in a controlled study indicates that healthy neonates either breast-fed or fed formula (SMA) with nucleotide supplementation showed an enhancement of natural killer cell activity and lymphocyte proliferation (70). However, *de novo* synthesis of nucleotides seems to be sufficient for human lymphocyte proliferation (71).

Nucleotides also exert an effect on the type of bacterial flora in the gut. The percentage of bifidobacteria, a species thought to be "protective" by competing for substrate with other more pathogenic organisms, is higher in stools of breast-fed versus formula-fed infants. The differences decrease when a nucleotide-supplemented formula is used (72). This may be explained by enhanced growth of bifidobacteria cultured *in vitro* with media containing nucleotides. The availability of iron for bacterial growth within the intestine may also be a factor. Nucleotides such as inosine that seem to facilitate intestinal iron absorption may explain the better absorption of iron in breast-fed infants (73,74). Thus, some nucleotides of breast milk could act in a fashion similar to lactoferrin in restricting available iron to the gut microflora, a possibility that needs to be explored.

Dietary nucleotides appear to play a role in the synthesis of long-chain polyunsaturated derivatives of ω-3 and ω-6 fatty acids. The fatty acid composition of the membrane of red blood cells shows a higher proportion of polyunsaturated ω-3 and ω-6 fatty acids in infants either breast-fed or fed a formula supplemented with nucleotides, compared to the pattern observed in infants fed an unsupplemented formula (63). Lipoprotein synthesis may also be influenced by dietary nucleotides. At 1 month, infants fed breast milk or a nucleotide-supplemented formula have lower very-low-density lipoprotein cholesterol and higher high-density lipoprotein cholesterol than those receiving unsupplemented formula (75). The long-term significance of these findings is unknown.

Studies have not shown a relationship between nu-

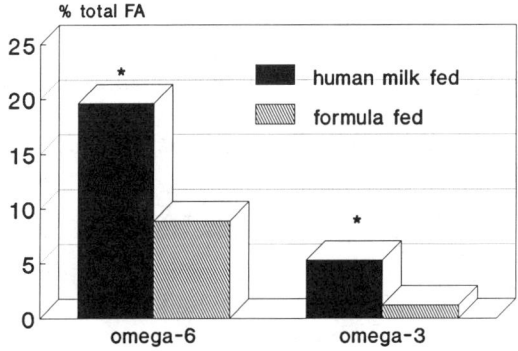

FIG. 6. Comparison of long-chain polyunsaturated fatty acid (LCPUFA) composition of red blood count phospholipids at 30 days postnatal age in term neonates fed breast milk or formula. (From ref. 46, with permission.)

cleotide intake and improved growth (63,76). Unresolved issues remain regarding growth in premature infants in whom *de novo* synthesis of nucleotides may be limited, and among infants receiving parenteral nutrition with solutions not containing nucleotides.

The nucleotides present in higher quantities in breast milk are cytidine, uridine, adenosine, inosine, and guanosine. They are found primarily in their monophosphate form and in concentrations oscillating between 150 and 1,500 µg/dl (66). Variations with lactational age have been reported (74). Ribonucleic and deoxyribonucleic acids are additional dietary nucleotides present in much larger concentrations than free nucleotides (77).

Nucleotide requirements for normal growth and replacement of urinary losses in term newborns have been estimated at about 160 mg/kg/day (66). Nucleotides do not seem to be essential for term infants in early life because *de novo* generation of these compounds is usually sufficient under conditions of dietary restriction. For the very immature neonate or those on prolonged exclusive parenteral nutrition, some investigators feel that nucleotides should be considered essential or conditionally essential nutrients.

Sodium, Potassium, Chloride

The requirements for sodium (Na), potassium (K), and chloride (Cl) for term newborns are lower than for premature infants (Table 5). This reflects the more advanced renal maturation of the term neonate, as well as changes in total body water and its compartments.

Sodium is the primary electrolyte of extracellular fluid. The Na content of mature breast milk is about 17 to 20 mg/dl or 8 to 10 mEq/l. Colostrum and transitional milk have a higher concentration of Na. Cow's milk has a substantially higher Na content than breast milk; most infant formulas have amounts similar to, or up to 40% higher than, breast milk. At average intakes, breast-fed neonates receive less Na than those who are formula-fed. Na renal excretion is higher in formula-fed neonates, reflecting the higher intake. Both feeding methods supply Na adequate for healthy term newborns. Not yet established is the relationship between Na intake during infancy and the risk of hypertension later in life.

Potassium is the main cation of the intracellular compartment. The requirements for K are influenced primarily by the rate of growth and urinary losses. Mature breast milk and infant formula contain more K than Na; average intake of either is sufficient to meet the K requirement of healthy term newborns. Colostrum contains a slightly higher amount of K than mature breast milk.

Chloride is also supplied in sufficient amounts by breast milk and infant formulas. In the past, metabolic alkalosis and hypochloremia, as a result of deficient dietary chloride from formula, has occurred. This can lead to significant developmental consequences (78).

Calcium, Phosphorus, Magnesium

Calcium (Ca) and phosphorus (P) are the main minerals of bone. Magnesium (Mg) is also part of bone structure as well as a critical cation of intracellular fluid. Despite the abundance of these minerals in the human body, only a very small fraction is found in the circulation. Therefore, the serum concentration of these elements is not a good reflection of tissue content. The regulation of absorption, metabolism, and excretion of these minerals involves a series of hormones, vitamin D, and other dietary components (79,80).

Ca is absorbed primarily in the upper small intestine by active transport and, to a lesser degree, by passive diffusion. Vitamin D and larger amounts of Ca, P, and medium-chain triglycerides in the diet increase Ca absorption to a certain degree. The role of lactose in Ca absorption is still debated. Calcium in breast milk, estimated at 30 to 40 mg/dl, is better absorbed than Ca from infant formulas. Formulas have a higher Ca content than breast milk, and soy-based formulas have even more. In the latter, absorption is limited because of the presence of phytates. Breast-fed infants have higher serum Ca and lower P concentrations than formula-fed infants. This is largely reflective of the higher P content of formulas. The estimated Ca needs for healthy, growing, term neonates are about 60 mg/kg/day (79).

Phosphorus is absorbed in the small intestine by active and passive mechanisms involving vitamin D. Increases in P intake from milk decreases the percent absorption of P, whereas urinary P excretion increases. However, overall P retention is higher if the milk source contains more P, e.g., cow's milk–based formulas compared to breast milk. An excess of Ca decreases P absorption by precipitating it in the intestinal lumen.

The P content of breast milk varies between 10 and 15 mg/dl. Cow's milk–based formulas have about twice this quantity; soy-based formulas have even more. The daily needs of P for term neonates have been estimated at about 40 mg/kg (79). The ratio of Ca to P in bone is 2:1, approximately that of breast milk. Adequate skeletal

TABLE 5. *Approximate mineral requirements of term newborns*

Mineral	Requirement (kg/day)
Sodium (Na)	1–1.5 mEq
Potassium (K)	1–2.0 mEq
Chloride (Cl)	1–2.0 mEq
Calcium (Ca)	60 mg
Phosphorus (P)	40 mg
Magnesium (Mg)	8 mg
Iron (Fe)	1 mg

growth can occur at ratios below this. Recently, upper limits of 45 to 50 mg/dl for Ca and 30 to 40 mg/dl for P have been recommended for infant formulas (81).

Magnesium is absorbed throughout the small intestine at rates of 50% to 75%. A dietary increase in medium-chain triglycerides enhances Mg absorption. Dietary modifications of Mg intake probably have no effect on Ca and P absorption (82). However, hypomagnesemia has profound effects on parathyroid hormone homeostasis. Hypocalcemia observed concomitantly with hypomagnesemia is thought to be secondary to decreased parathyroid hormone secretion (83). The Mg content of mature breast milk, usually between 2 and 5 mg/dl, is lower than that of infant formulas. An intake of 8 mg/kg/day has been suggested for term infants (79). An upper limit of 12 mg/dl in infant formulas has been recommended (81).

Iron

The term infant is born with adequate iron (Fe) stores even if the mother has mild to moderate Fe deficiency (84). Exceptions are newborns with anemia due to external hemorrhage, either evident (cord rupture) or occult (fetomaternal hemorrhage). During the first several months of age, iron stores remain essentially unchanged (85). Iron nutrition from birth to 2 years has recently been reviewed (86).

Iron is absorbed in the small intestine. Although breast milk contains only a small amount of Fe, 0.3 to 0.5 mg/l, about 50% of it is absorbed. This is in contrast with a much lower absorption of Fe from infant formulas or cow's milk. Possible explanations for the enhanced breast milk absorption include the presence of lactoferrin, a lower phosphate and protein content, and the presence of inosine and other nucleotides. As Fe in formulas increases, its percent absorption decreases. Currently, iron-fortified infant formulas have about 12 mg/l of which 4% to 5% is absorbed. The Fe content of soy-based formula varies.

Iron stores usually last more than 4 to 6 months in breast-fed infants (87). In infants receiving a low-iron infant formula (1.5 mg/l), Fe stores may be depleted much sooner. Based on this, and the lack of side effects, iron-fortified formulas are recommended for all formula-fed infants (88). Whether the amount of Fe fortification should be decreased is still controversial (89).

Trace Minerals

Although recommended daily intakes of trace minerals have been reported, it is difficult to define requirements for these elements based on current knowledge (Table 6) (90,91). Most of the recommended amounts derive from concentrations of trace minerals in breast milk and the lack of signs of deficiencies and/or depletion in breast-fed infants. Extrapolations from adult data are also occasionally used.

During the third trimester of pregnancy, the human fetus accumulates a large amount of zinc (Zn) and copper (Cu). Infants born prematurely, before substantial accumulation of these trace elements has occurred, are at higher risk of deficiency during the first few months after birth. In addition, infants receiving parenteral nutrition can rapidly develop trace mineral deficiencies when these elements are not supplied in the infusions.

Human breast milk contains Zn, Cu, selenium (Se), chromium (Cr), manganese (Mn), fluoride (F), iodine (I), and molybdenum (Mo) as well as trace elements found in even lower concentrations, such as nickel and cobalt (32; Table 6). Reported variability may reflect population differences as well as variance in methodologies. Furthermore, several of these trace minerals vary according to lactational age. Higher levels of Zn, Cu, and Mn have been reported in colostrum than in mature breast milk, whereas Cr remains essentially the same (92). The absorption of most of these elements from breast milk is good (93). Since many trace elements share absorptive pathways, changes in their relative concentrations in infant formulas may alter their bioavailability.

TABLE 6. *Approximate breast milk content of trace minerals and their recommended daily allowances (RDA) for infants 0–6 months*

Trace mineral	Amount in mature breast milk[a]	Increase in breast milk content with supplementation	RDA 1990
Zinc (Zn)	100–300 µg/dl	No	2–3 mg
Copper (Cu)	20–60 µg/dl	No	0.4–0.6 mg
Selenium (Se)	1.5–2 µg/dl	Yes	10 µg
Chromium (Cr)	10–40 ng/dl	Uncertain	10–40 µg
Manganese (Mn)	0.3–0.6 µg/dl	Uncertain	0.3–0.6 mg
Fluoride (F)	10 µg/dl	No	0.1–0.5 mg
Iodine (I)	6 µg/dl	Yes	100 µg × kg
Molybdenum (Mo)	1–2 ng/dl	Uncertain	15–30 µg

[a] Data from refs. 90, 91, and 95.

With few exceptions, trace elements are increased in infant formulas compared to breast milk; absorption is, however, decreased. Phytates and other proteins in soy-based formulas may impose a further constraint. Considering these and other factors, upper limits for trace elements in infants formulas have been suggested recently (94–97).

Fluoride, while no longer present in infant formulas in the United States, is nonetheless found in breast milk. Maternal fluoride supplementation does not increase its amount in breast milk. The American Academy of Pediatrics has recommended supplementation with 250 µg/day of F for infants 2 weeks to 2 years old living in areas where the water content of F is less than 0.3 parts per million (98).

Vitamins

With the exception of vitamin D, the vitamin requirements of the term infant are satisfied by an adequate intake of breast milk. Formula-fed newborns also get adequate vitamin supplies, including vitamin D, which is usually added in amounts of 60 IU per 100 Cal.

The amount of vitamin D in breast milk is less than 40 IU per liter; between 30% and 75% is 25-OHD. A very small amount of $1,25(OH)_2$-D is also present (56). The concentrations of vitamin D in breast milk vary according to race, exposure to sunlight, and lactational age. Its concentration is also lower if the mother is deficient (99). Maternal supplementation increases vitamin D levels in breast milk, but not enough to satisfy the infant's requirement (100).

The current recommendation is for 400 IU/day for infants with limited sun exposure (101,102). Infants fed standard infant formula (400 IU/l of vitamin D) maintain adequate status of this vitamin. Although supplementation of breast-fed infants during summer months may not be necessary, adequate sun exposure needs to be ensured (103). Furthermore, when sun exposure is limited or there is a strong racial influence, i.e., darker skin, supplementation is essential (104).

SUMMARY

The approximate nutrient needs of the healthy term newborn and young infant have been reviewed. Many estimates of requirements are derived from analysis of the breast milk content of specific nutrients and subsequent growth of exclusively breast-fed infants. Infant formulas attempt to mimic human breast milk, which remains the ideal form of feeding for the term infant except when contraindications, e.g., drugs, infections, are present. Even if formulas could duplicate exactly the components of breast milk, the benefits of breast-feeding, including maternal-infant bonding and uterine contractility postpartum, could never be duplicated. Breast-feeding for infants is, in fact, one of the finer designs of nature.

REFERENCES

1. Hamill PVV, Drizd TA, Johnson CL, Reed RB, Roche AF, Moore WM. Physical growth: National Center for Health Statistics percentiles. *Am J Clin Nutr* 1979;32:607–629.
2. Babson SG, Behrman RT, Lessel R. Liveborn birth weights for gestational age of white middle class infants. *Pediatrics* 1970;45:937–944.
3. Arbuckle T, Sherman G. An analysis of birth weight by gestational age in Canada. *Can Med Assoc J* 1989;140:157–165.
4. Wilcox A, Russell I. Why small black infants have a lower mortality rate than small white infants: the case for population-specific standards for birth weight. *J Pediatr* 1990;116:7–10.
5. Offringa PJ, Boersma ER, Brunsting JR, Meeuwsen WP, Velvis H. Weight loss in full-term negroid infants: relationship to body water compartments at birth? *Early Hum Dev* 1990;21:73–81.
6. Uauy R, Mayfield SR, Warshaw JB. Growth and metabolic adaptation of the fetus and newborn. In: Oski F, DeAngelis C, Feigin R, Warshaw J, eds. *Principles and practice of pediatrics.* Philadelphia: JB Lippincott, 1990;261–268.
7. Lorenz JM, Kleinman LI. Ontogeny of the kidney. In: Tsang R, Nichols B, eds. *Nutrition during infancy.* Philadelphia: Hanley & Belfus, 1988;58–85.
8. Euler AR, Byrne WJ, Cousins LM, et al. Increased serum gastrin concentrations and gastric acid hyposecretion in the immediate newborn period. *Gastroenterology* 1977;72:1271–1273.
9. Schofield WN, Schofield C, James WPT. Basal metabolic rate—review and prediction, together with an annotated bibliography of source material. *Hum Nutr Clin Nutr* 1985;39C(Suppl 1):5–41.
10. Cowett RM, Stern L. Carbohydrate homeostasis in the fetus and newborn. In: Avery GB, ed. *Neonatology: pathophysiology and management of the newborn,* 3rd ed. Philadelphia: JB Lippincott, 1987;691–709.
11. Widdowson EM. Nutrition. In: Davis JA, Dobbing J, eds. *Scientific foundations of pediatrics.* Philadelphia: WB Saunders, 1974;44–55.
12. Schulze K. A model of variability in metabolic rate of neonates. In: Fomon SJ, Heird WC, eds. *Energy and protein needs during infancy.* Orlando: Academic Press, 1986;19–40.
13. Garza C, Schanler RJ, Butte NF, Motil KJ. Special properties of human milk. *Clin Perinatol* 1987;14:11–32.
14. Butte NF, Garza C, O'Brian Smith E, Nichols BL. Human milk intake and growth in exclusively breast-fed infants. *J Pediatr* 1984;104:187–195.
15. Garza C, Butte NF. Energy intakes of human milk-fed infants during the first year. *J Pediatr* 1990;117:S124–131.
16. Harrison GG, Graver EJ, Vargas M, Churella HR, Paule CL. Growth and adiposity of term infants fed whey-predominant or casein-predominant formulas or human milk. *J Pediatr Gastroenterol Nutr* 1987;6:739–747.
17. Pullar JD, Webster AJF. The energy cost of fat and protein deposition in the rat. *Br J Nutr* 1977;37:355–363.
18. Davies PSW, Lucas A. Energy expenditure in early infancy. *Br J Nutr* 1989;62:621–629.
19. Friis-Hansen B. Body water compartments in children: changes during growth and related changes in body composition. *Pediatrics* 1961;28:169–181.
20. Nash MA. Provision of water and electrolytes. In: Fanaroff AA, Martin RJ, eds. *Neonatal-perinatal medicine.* St. Louis: CV Mosby, 1987;460–466.
21. Roberts AK, Van Biervliet JP, Harzer G. Factors of human milk influencing the bacterial flora of infant feces. In: Schaub J, ed. *Composition and physiological properties of human milk.* New York: Elsevier, 1985;259–270.
22. Goldman AS, Thorpe LW, Goldblum RM, Hanson LA. Anti-inflammatory properties of human milk. *Acta Paediatr Scand* 1986;75:689–695.

23. Lifschitz CH. Carbohydrate needs in preterm and term newborn infants. In: Tsang R, Nichols, eds. *Nutrition during infancy*. Philadelphia: Hanley & Belfus, 1988;122–132.
24. Hadorn B, Zoppi G, Shmerling DH, et al. Quantitative assessment of exocrine pancreatic function in infants and children. *J Pediatr* 1968;73:39–50.
25. Siegel M, Lebenthal E, Krantz B. Effect of caloric density on gastric emptying in premature infants. *J Pediatr* 1984;104: 118–122.
26. Kimura RE, Warshaw JB. Metabolism during development. In: Lebenthal E, ed. *Textbook of gastroenterology and nutrition in infancy*. New York: Raven Press, 1989;13–26.
27. Kalhan SC, Savin SM, Adam PAJ. Measurement of glucose turnover in the human newborn with glucose-1-13C. *J Endocrinol Metab* 1976;43:704–707.
28. Young VR, Pelletier VA. Adaptation to high protein intakes, with particular reference to formula feeding and the healthy, term infant. *J Nutr* 1989;119:1799–1809.
29. Chesney RW. Taurine: is it required for infant nutrition? *Am J Nutr* 1988;118:6–10.
30. Tyson JE, Laskey R, Flood D, et al. Randomized trial of taurine supplementation for infants < 1300 gram birth weight: effect on auditory brainstem-evoked responses. *Pediatrics* 1989;83: 406–415.
31. Rassin DK, Raihä NCR, Minoli I, Moro G. Taurine and cholesterol supplementation in the term infant: responses of growth and metabolism. *J Parenter Ent Nutr* 1990;14:392–397.
32. George DE, DeFrancesca BA. Human milk in comparison to cow milk. In: Lebenthal E, ed. *Textbook of gastroenterology and nutrition in infancy*. New York: Raven Press, 1989;239–261.
33. Davidson LA, Lonnerdal B. Effect of development on the fecal excretion of lactoferrin and secretory IgA in breast-fed infants. *Am J Clin Nutr* 1986;43:699.
34. Schanler R, Goldman R, Garza C, et al. Enhanced fecal excretion of selected immune factors in very low birth weight infants fed fortified human milk. *Pediatr Res* 1986;20:711–715.
35. Spik G, Brunet G, Mazurdier-Dehaine C, et al. Characterization and properties of the human and bovine lactotransferrins extracted from the faeces of newborn infants. *Acta Paediatr Scand* 1982;71:979–985.
36. Raihä N, Minoli I, Moro G. Milk protein intake in the term infant: 1. Metabolic responses and effects on growth. *Acta Paediatr Scand* 1986;75:881–886.
37. Salmenperä L, Perheentupa J, Siimes MA. Exclusively breast-fed healthy infants grow slower than reference infants. *Pediatr Res* 1985;19:307–312.
38. Nelson SE, Rogers RR, Ziegler EE, Fomon S. Gain in weight and length during early infancy. *Early Hum Dev* 1989;19:223–239.
39. Koldovsky O. Hormones in milk: their possible physiological significance for the neonate. In: Lebenthal E, ed. *Textbook of gastroenterology and nutrition in infancy*. New York: Raven Press, 1989;97–119.
40. Beaton GH, Chery A. Protein requirements of infants: a reexamination of concepts and approaches. *Am J Clin Nutr* 1988; 48:1403–1412.
41. Raihä N, Minoli I, Moro G, Bremer HJ. Milk protein intake in the term infant. II. Effects on plasma aminoacid concentrations. *Acta Paediatr Scand* 1986;75:887–892.
42. Janas LM, Picciano MF, Hatch TF. Indices of protein metabolism in term infants fed human milk, whey-predominant formula, or cow's milk formula. *Pediatrics* 1985;75:775–784.
43. Rassin DK. Protein requirements in the neonate. In: Lebenthal E, ed. *Textbook of gastroenterology and nutrition in infancy*. New York: Raven Press, 1989;281–292.
44. Motil KJ. Protein needs for term and preterm infants. In: Tsang R, Nichols B, eds. *Nutrition during infancy*. Philadelphia: Hanley & Belfus, 1988;100–121.
45. Janas LM, Picciano MF, Hatch TF. Indices of protein metabolism in term infants fed either human milk or formulas with reduced protein concentration and various whey/casein ratios. *J Pediatr* 1987;110:838–848.
46. Uauy R, Treen M, Hoffman DR. Essential fatty acid metabolism and requirements during development. *Semin Perinatol* 1989;13:118–130.
47. Heim T. Energy and lipid requirements of the fetus and preterm infant. *J Pediatr Gastroenterol Nutr* 1983;2:16–41.
48. Coleman RA. The role of the placenta in lipid metabolism and transport. *Semin Perinatol* 1989;13:180–191.
49. Hamosh M. Fat needs for term and preterm infants. In: Tsang R, Nichols B, eds. *Nutrition during infancy*. Philadelphia: Hanley & Belfus, 1988;133–159.
50. Hernell O, Bläckberg L, Lindberg T. Human milk enzymes with emphasis on the lipases. In: Lebenthal E, ed. *Textbook of gastroenterology and nutrition during infancy*. New York: Raven Press, 1989;209–217.
51. Franklin FA. The effects of infant feeding practices on lipid and lipoprotein levels and metabolism. In: Lebenthal E, ed. *Textbook of gastroenterology and nutrition during infancy*. New York: Raven Press, 1989;503–514.
52. Shenai JP, Borum PR, Mohan P, et al. Carnitine status at birth of newborn infants of varying gestation. *Pediatr Res* 1983;17: 579–582.
53. Saint L, Smith M, Hartman PE. The yield and nutrient content of colostrum and milk of women from giving birth to 1 month postpartum. *Br J Nutr* 1984;52:87–95.
54. Dewey KG, Finley DA, Lonnerdal B. Breast milk volume and composition during late lactation. *J Pediatr Gastroenterol Nutr* 1984;3:713–720.
55. Fomon SJ, Rogers RR, Ziegler EE, Nelson SE, Thomas LN. Indices of fatness and serum cholesterol at eight years in relation to feeding and growth during early infancy. *Pediatr Res* 1984;18:1233–1238.
56. Jensen RG. Lipids in human milk-composition and fat-soluble vitamins. In: Lebenthal E, ed. *Textbook of gastroenterology and nutrition during infancy*. New York: Raven Press, 1989;157–208.
57. Willis AL. Essential fatty acids, prostaglandins, and related eicosanoids. In: *Present knowledge in nutrition*. Washington, DC: Nutrition Foundation, 1984;90–113.
58. Gibson RA, Kneebone GM. Fatty acid composition of human colostrum and mature human milk. *Am J Clin Nutr* 1981;34:252–257.
59. Bitman J, Wood DL, Hamosh M, et al. Comparison of the lipid composition of breast milk from mothers of term and preterm infants. *Am J Clin Nutr* 1983;38:300–312.
60. Clandinin MT, Chappell JE, Leong S, et al. Intrauterine fatty acid accretion rates in human brain: implications for fatty acid requirements. *Early Hum Dev* 1980;4:121–129.
61. Uauy R. Are omega-3 fatty acids required for normal eye and brain development in the human? *J Pediatr Gastroenterol Nutr* 1990;11:296–302.
62. Carlson SE, Cooke RJ, Peeples JM, Werkman SH, Tolley EA. Docosahexaenoate (DHA) and eicosapentaenoate (EPA) status of preterm infants: relationship to visual acuity in n-3 supplemented and unsupplemented infants. *Pediatr Res* 1989;25:285A.
63. DeLucchi C, Pita ML, Faus MJ, et al. Effects of dietary nucleotides on the fatty acid composition of erythrocyte membrane lipids in term infants. *J Pediatr Gastroenterol Nutr* 1987;6:568–574.
64. Neuringer M, Connor WE, Van Petten C, et al. Dietary omega-3 fatty acid deficiency and visual loss in infant rhesus monkeys. *J Clin Invest* 1984;73:272–276.
65. Carroll KK. Upper limits of nutrients in infant formulas: polyunsaturated fatty acids and trans fatty acids. *J Nutr* 1989; 119:1810–1813.
66. Uauy R. Dietary nucleotides and requirements in early life. In: Lebenthal E, ed. *Textbook of gastroenterology and nutrition in infancy*. New York: Raven Press, 1989;265–280.
67. Van Buren CT, Kulkarni AD, Fanslow WC, Rudolph FB. Dietary nucleotides: a requirement for helper/inducer T lymphocytes. *Transplantation* 1985;40:694–697.
68. Carver JD, Cox WI, Barness LA. Dietary nucleotide effects upon murine natural killer cell activity and macrophage activation. *J Parenter Enter Nutr* 1990;14:18–22.
69. Kulkarni AD, Fanslow WC, Drath DB, Rudolph FB, Van Buren CT. Influence of dietary nucleotide restriction on bacterial sepsis and phagocytic cell function in mice. *Arch Surg* 1986;121: 169–172.
70. Carver JD, Pimentel B, Barness LA. Nucleotide effects in formula-fed infants. *Pediatr Res* 1989;25:286A.

71. Wasserman RL, Molto R, Uauy R. De novo nucleotide (N) synthesis is sufficient to support human lymphocyte (L) proliferation. *Pediatr Res* 1988;23:495A.
72. Gil A, Corral E, Martinez A, Molina JA. Effects of dietary nucleotides on the microbial pattern of feces of at term newborn infants. *J Clin Nutr Gastroenterol* 1986;1:34–38.
73. McMillan JA, Oski FA, Lourie G, Tomarelli RM, Landau SA. Iron absorption from milk, simulated human milk and proprietary formulas. *Pediatrics* 1977;60:896–900.
74. Janas LM, Picciano MF. The nucleotide profile of human milk. *Pediatr Res* 1982;16:659–662.
75. Sanchez-Pozo A, Pita ML, Martinez A, Molina JA, Sanchez-Medina F, Gil A. Effects of dietary nucleotides upon lipoprotein pattern of newborn infants. *Nutr Res* 1986;6:763–771.
76. Pita ML, Fernandez MR, DeLucchi C, et al. Changes in fatty acids pattern of red blood cell phospholipids induced by type of milk, dietary nucleotide supplementation and postnatal age in preterm infants. *J Pediatr Gastroenterol Nutr* 1988;7:740–747.
77. Sanguansermsri J, Gyorgy P, Zilliken F. Polyamines in human and cow's milk. *Am J Clin Nutr* 1974;27:859–865.
78. Willoughby A, Moss HB, Hubbard VS, et al. Developmental outcome in children exposed to a chloride-deficient formula. *Pediatrics* 1987;79:851–857.
79. Koo WWK, Tsang RC. Calcium, magnesium and phosphorus. In: Tsang R, Nichols B, eds. *Nutrition during infancy.* Philadelphia: Hanley & Belfus, 1988;175–189.
80. Chan G. Calcium and bone mineral status in infant's and children's nutrition. In: Lebenthal E, ed. *Textbook of gastroenterology and nutrition in infancy.* New York: Raven Press, 1989;403–411.
81. Greer FR. Calcium, phosphorus, and magnesium: how much is too much for infant formulas? *J Nutr* 1989;119:1846–1851.
82. O'dell BL. Mineral interactions relevant to nutrient requirements. *J Nutr* 1989;119:1832–1838.
83. Shaul P, Mimouni F, Tsang RC, Specker BL. The role of magnesium in neonatal calcium homeostasis: effects of magnesium infusion on calciotropic hormones and calcium. *Pediatr Res* 1987;22:319–323.
84. Agrawal RMD, Tripathi AM, Agarwal KN. Cord blood hemoglobin, iron and ferritin status in maternal anemia. *Acta Paediatr Scand* 1983;72:545–548.
85. Dallman PR. Iron deficiency in the weanling: a nutritional problem on the way to resolution. *Acta Paediatr Scand* 1986;323:59–67.
86. Filer Jr, LJ. *Dietary iron. Birth to two years.* New York: Raven Press, 1989.
87. Siimes MA, Salmenperä L, Perheentupa J. Exclusive breast-feeding for 9 months: risk of iron deficiency. *J Pediatr* 1984;104:196–199.
88. American Academy of Pediatrics. Committee on Nutrition. Iron-fortified infant formulas. *Pediatrics* 1989;84:1114–1115.
89. Dallman PR. Upper limits of iron in infant formulas. *J Nutr* 1989;119:1852–1855.
90. Food and Nutrition Board, National Research Council. *Recommended dietary allowances,* 10th ed. Washington, DC: National Academy Press, 1989.
91. Milner JA. Trace minerals in the nutrition of children. *J Pediatr* 1990;117:S147–155.
92. Casey CE, Hambidge KM, Neville MC. Studies in human lactation: zinc, copper, manganese and chromium in human milk in the first month of lactation. *Am J Clin Nutr* 1985;41:1193–1200.
93. Casey CE, Walravens PA. Trace elements. In: Tsang R, Nichols B, eds. *Nutrition during infancy.* Philadelphia: Hanley & Belfus, 1988;190–215.
94. Lönnerdal B. Trace element absorption in infants as a foundation to setting upper limits for trace elements in infant formulas. *J Nutr* 1989;119:1839–1845.
95. Fisher DA. Upper limit of iodine in infant formulas. *J Nutr* 1989;119:1865–1868.
96. Hambidge KM, Krebs NF. Upper limits of zinc, copper and manganese in infant formulas. *J Nutr* 1989;119:1861–1864.
97. Levander OA. Upper limit of selenium in infant formulas. *J Nutr* 1989;119:1869–1873.
98. American Academy of Pediatrics. Committee on Nutrition. Fluoride supplementation. *Pediatrics* 1986;77:758–761.
99. Hollis BW, Lambert PW, Herst RL. Factors affecting the antirachitic sterol content of native milk. In: Holick MF, Gray TK, and Anast CS, eds. *Perinatal calcium and phosphorus metabolism.* New York: Elsevier, 1983;157–182.
100. Hollis BW. Individual quantitation of vitamin D-2, vitamin D-3, 25-hydroxyvitamin D-2, and 25-hydroxyvitamin D-3 in human milk. *Anal Biochem* 1983;131:211–219.
101. American Academy of Pediatrics. Committee on Nutrition. The prophylactic requirements and the toxicity of vitamin D. *Pediatrics* 1963;31:512.
102. Specker BL, Greer F, Tsang RC. Vitamin D. In: Tsang R, Nichols B, eds. *Nutrition during infancy.* Philadelphia: Hanley & Belfus, 1988;264–276.
103. Ala-Houhala M. 25-Hydroxyvitamin D levels during breast feeding with or without maternal or infantile supplementation of vitamin D. *J Pediatr Gastroenterol Nutr* 1985;4:220–226.
104. American Academy of Pediatrics. Committee on Nutrition. Vitamin and mineral supplement needs of normal children in the United States. In: Forbes GB, Woodruff KW, eds. *Pediatric nutrition handbook.* Elk Grove, IL: American Academy of Pediatrics, 1985.

CHAPTER 3

Nutritional Requirements of the Premature and Small for Gestational Age Infant

David A. Clark

The nutritional requirements of premature and growth-retarded infants are similar to those of the full-term infant. There are also many differences, however, especially related to developmental and maturational aspects of the gastrointestinal tract, renal function, and cutaneous permeability.

The body composition of the premature infant is significantly different from that of the infant who is full term (1). The tripling in weight that occurs in the last 12 weeks of gestation is largely due to increased caloric reserve in the form of glycogen and fat, both subcutaneous and brown. A premature infant at 28 weeks' gestation may have as little as 1% body weight as fat compared to the 15% to 16% fat content of a full-term healthy infant. The energy reserve in the term newborn is nearly 7,000 kilocalories (Cal) with approximately 75% as fat (1). Thus, the term newborn is more capable of handling perinatal stress and has the caloric reserve to maintain body temperature without severe metabolic consequences.

DEVELOPMENTAL ASPECTS

The primary function of the stomach and small intestine is to provide a very large surface area for efficient digestion and absorption. The increase in absorptive surface area results from both formation of villi from stratified epithelium and subsequently dense microvilli on those cells (2). Intestinal crypts and villi can be found in the human intestine by 10 to 12 weeks of gestation with a progressive development from proximal to distal intestine. Morphological development is nearly complete in humans by 20 to 22 weeks of gestation (2,3). The microvillus membrane of the columnar epithelial cells becomes the primary locus of digestion and absorption with progressive maturation of intestinal enzymes from fetal through postnatal life.

By 22 weeks' gestation most of the peptidases are present to allow efficient digestion of the whey-like proteins swallowed from amniotic fluid (4). Well-developed active amino acid transport has been demonstrated in fetal intestine. The digestion of lipid is inefficient in newborns because of low bile salt pools and immature ileal reabsorption in combination with low levels of lipase. Active transport of monosaccharides occurs as early as 11 to 12 weeks of gestation and reaches 60% of adult value by 21 weeks (5).

The coordination of the mature sucking reflex to swallowing mechanisms occurs at approximately 34 weeks' gestation (6). Since it involves neurologic maturation of the intestinal tract, it cannot be induced in a more immature infant. Premature infants have limited gastric volumes (approximately 10 ml/kg) and delayed gastric emptying (7). Gastric acid secretion is low in response to a protein meal and may limit initial digestion of protein and carbohydrate.

The ability of the kidneys to eliminate waste products and to regulate electrolyte, acid-base, and water balance reaches a mature level at approximately 1 year of age (8). The final differentiation of renal tubular cells occurs postterm and involves reorganization and structural development, increased transport proteins in the membrane, and an increase in sensitivity to hormonal influences. Postnatal growth of the kidneys is based on both cell division and cell hypertrophy. Renal blood flow and glomerular filtration rates are lower than in term infants. The premature infant has decreased capability of excreting an acid load. Such infants are also less capable of diluting and concentrating urine, which may result in

---

D. A. Clark: Department of Pediatrics, Louisiana State University School of Medicine, New Orleans, Louisiana 70112.

dehydration or fluid excess if total daily fluid balance is not maintained (9).

WEIGHT GAIN AND ENERGY REQUIREMENTS

There are many obstacles to appropriate weight gain in the premature and small for gestational age infant. Inefficient digestion, especially of fats and carbohydrates, may result in less available calories than presumed by oral intake. Limited excretory function, both renal and hepatic, may limit utilization, either intravenously or enterally, of the caloric intake required for optimal growth (10). In addition, calories that might be used for growth must often be used to maintain body temperature in infants with the poor insulation that has resulted from decreased subcutaneous fat content (11). This stress response includes an increased metabolic rate from the release of catecholamines (12). Growth may also be limited when calories are used for other excess activities such as seizures and/or drug withdrawal.

Although most premature infants are genetically healthy, many severely growth-retarded infants have relatively poor protoplasm. In addition, infants with various chromosomal anomalies such as trisomy 18 and trisomy 13 tend to grow poorly because of a poor suck and swallow. This problem also exists in other developmental syndromes where neurologic dysfunction is prominent.

Illnesses that interfere with caloric intake and caloric utilization disproportionately afflict the premature and growth-retarded populations. The respiratory distress of surfactant deficiency, which increases the work of breathing, increases caloric expenditure (13) and limits the ability to feed. In such cases, parenteral glucose solutions may be the only significant caloric intake for the first several days; lipid infusion is contraindicated since it limits oxygenation of hemoglobin, may displace bilirubin from albumin, and interferes with neutrophil function in infants who may be infected. Transplacental viral and parasitic infections such as cytomegalovirus and toxoplasmosis, which result in significant tissue disruption, may also retard growth. Infected infants show central nervous system and hepatic involvement with resulting limitations on caloric intake, decreased ability to clear metabolic waste, and excess caloric expenditure. Premature infants are also susceptible to many intestinal dysfunctions including gastroesophageal reflux and malabsorption. They are at great risk for developing necrotizing enterocolitis which, in the short term, decreases total caloric intake, and, when severe, may require intestinal resection with resulting short bowel syndrome and its nutritional limitations.

Weight gain is relatively easy to document. It is difficult, however, to determine clinically whether weight gain is the result of fluid retention due to limited renal function or true tissue growth (9). Extrauterine growth of the premature infant will not match expected intrauterine fetal growth since all babies lose weight in the first several days after birth. The healthy full-term infant, adequately nourished, will recover birth weight approximately 7 to 10 days after birth. Premature infants return to birth weight more slowly, due to the limitations of caloric intake, excess fluid loss, and increased caloric expenditure (11). In a healthy pregnancy, at no time does the fetus lose weight.

The caloric requirements for premature and growth-retarded infants are poorly defined, ranging from 60 Cal/kg/day to 150 Cal/kg/day. The calories available for growth are those remaining after the subclasses of caloric expenditure have been subtracted: food digestion (specific dynamic action), basal metabolism, and superimposed spontaneous activity (13). The response to intake also varies widely. Some premature infants show true growth with an intake as low as 60 Cal/kg/day, whereas very active newborns, perhaps those undergoing drug withdrawal, may not grow on as much as 150 Cal/kg/day.

Optimum nutrition for the care of the premature and small for gestational age infants includes water, carbohydrates, fats, proteins, and vitamins.

WATER

Dehydration is a common problem in the more premature infant because of the very high insensible water loss. It is essential, therefore, that sufficient available free water be administered to maintain adequate hydration and urine output. The transepidermal water loss in appropriately grown babies on the first day of life is minimal by approximately 34 weeks' gestation (greater than 2,000 g) (Fig. 1) (14). Transepidermal water loss increases with decreasing gestational age; a 1-kg baby has two to three times the water loss of a term infant (15). The kidney in the preterm infant also has limited capabilities for both dilution and concentration (9). A fluid intake of less than 80 ml/kg/day will almost invariably lead to hypernatremic dehydration with metabolic acidosis, especially in the very low birth weight babies of less than 1,000 g (16,17). On the other hand, premature infants between 1 and 2 kg are often unable to handle excess fluid intake. Fluids given in excess of 200 ml/kg/day will commonly result in fluid overload and congestive heart failure. In the more preterm infants (<1000 g) a total fluid intake of greater than 200 ml/kg/day is not uncommon to compensate for the severe transepidermal water loss (17).

These infants require extra fluid for other reasons, including the unusual transcutaneous water loss from radiant warmers and phototherapy (18), and the extrarenal fluid loss in the recovering phase of acute tubular necro-

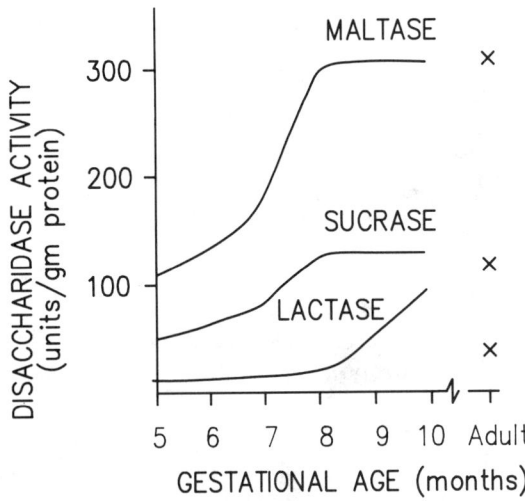

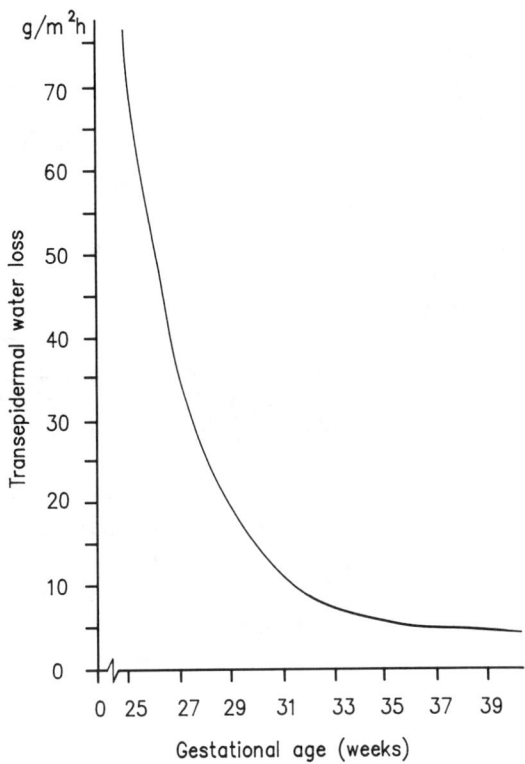

FIG. 1. Transepidermal water loss in relation to gestational age (completed weeks) in appropriate for gestational age (AGA) newborn babies on the first day of life. (From ref. 14.)

FIG. 2. Disaccharidase activity of jejunal mucosa of human fetus in relation to lunar months of gestational age. (Modified from ref. 20.)

sis and from loose watery stools. Water replacement must be accompanied by the appropriate electrolytes.

Fluid restriction with appropriate monitoring of the serum electrolytes is important in babies with congestive heart failure and a patent ductus arteriosus. This is also true when there is inappropriate antidiuretic hormone (ADH) secretion and in the anuric phase of renal damage secondary to asphyxia.

CARBOHYDRATE

Carbohydrates are the primary energy source and a precursor for many metabolites such as nucleic acids and bilirubin conjugation (19). The primary carbohydrate utilized in fetal life is D-glucose (dextrose). The primary carbohydrate in breast milk or infant formula is the disaccharide lactose (glucose and galactose) (20). Infants are exposed to disaccharides when feedings are initiated. Intestinal lactase activity increases at approximately 34 weeks' gestation; in the term infant it is maximal shortly after birth (Fig. 2). The activities of sucrase and maltase, in contrast, reach adult levels by 30 weeks of gestation. Intestinal lactase activity cannot be prematurely induced by oral lactose feeding.

In formulas for premature infants, polymers of glucose have been substituted for a portion of the carbohydrate content to allow for better digestion and absorption (21). Generally these formulas contain no more than 50% lactose. The glucose polymers, which are readily hydrolyzed by maltase and glucoamylase, are present on the microvillus and are resistant to ischemic or mucosal injury.

Undigested carbohydrates have been detected in the stools of premature and growth-retarded infants. If these carbohydrates reach the lower intestinal tract, the various colonic flora are able to ferment them to produce organic acids, carbon dioxide, and hydrogen. Breath hydrogen levels are commonly elevated in premature infants. The organic acids, if absorbed, may be further metabolized and provide a recovery mechanism for some of the calories lost by inefficient digestion in the small intestine. However, an accumulation of organic acids in the distal small intestine and colon, which lowers the intraluminal pH, is one of the prime factors in the induction of late onset, feeding-associated necrotizing enterocolitis (22).

Specific carbohydrate requirements for infants are not well defined (23). A nearly carbohydrate-free formula has relatively little impact on the newborn (23,24); hypoglycemia is rare once feedings have been established. Most formulas contain a balance of fat, proteins, and carbohydrate, providing for caloric options other than glucose alone. In a complete formula the carbohydrate provides approximately 40% of the total caloric intake.

FAT REQUIREMENTS

Lipids have multiple functions in mammals. They are vital for normal growth and development. Fat is the primary energy source of the newborn and is essential for brain development (25). Lipids and proteins are the primary components of all cell membranes. Vitamins A, D, and E are dependent on fat for adequate ileal absorption.

The body fat of a 28-week, 1,000-g fetus is only 1%. By term birth, 12 weeks later, body fat has increased to about 15% to 16% (1). Approximately 10% of this is brown fat, which is found in the mediastinum, axillae, between the scapulae, and surrounding the adrenal glands. Brown fat is more vascular than yellow fat with a high density of mitochondria. It is responsive to the adrenal catecholamines, especially norepinephrine, allowing for rapid mobilization of the stored fatty acid energy source.

Lipases are critical to fat digestion. They are found in human milk but not in proprietary formula (26,27). Present in the mouth, stomach, and small intestine, lipases are produced by both the pancreas and the intestinal microflora (28). Primary fat digestion requires that lipase strip the fatty acids from the glycerol molecule. The short- and medium-chain fatty acids are better absorbed than the more complex fatty acids. The relatively higher pH in the stomach of the newborn, accompanied by slower gastric emptying, allows for limited digestion and absorption of fat in the stomach. Once the meal has been passed into the small intestine, bile salts and intestinal and pancreatic lipases continue the process. The relative fat malabsorption of the premature infant is due primarily to decreased intraluminal bile salts and inadequate amounts of secreted pancreatic lipase (25). Glycerol, monoglycerides, and free fatty acids are absorbed primarily by passive diffusion. Within the mucosa, triglycerides are again formed by the reattachment of the fatty acids to glycerol. These triglycerides, along with the phospholipid proteins and cholesterol, are assembled into lipoproteins called chylomicrons and low-density lipoproteins (29). Polar lipids, such as the free fatty acids, are bound to plasma proteins, primarily albumin, whereas the nonpolar lipids are transported in complexes as the core of the lipoproteins.

The catabolism of long-chain fatty acids in the mitochondria releases energy and produces water and carbon dioxide. These fatty acids can only cross the mitochondrial membranes bound to carnitine, a dipeptide synthesized from lysine and methionine in the kidney and liver (30). Carnitine is, therefore, critical for newborn fat metabolism. It is added to all standard and preterm formulas to supplement the low plasma and tissue concentrations that result from immature biosynthesis in the full-term newborn (31).

Most medium chain fatty acids are metabolized without the carnitine cofactor. Breast milk of mothers of premature infants contains nearly twice as much fat in the form of medium-chain fatty acids as the milk of mothers delivering at term. Because of these observations, premature formulas now contain approximately 50% of the fat content as medium-chain triglycerides.

Fat requirements are approximately 30% to 55% of the total caloric intake (3.3 to 6 g/100 Cal) (32). The essential fatty acids $C_{18:2}$ should provide approximately 0.3 g/100 Cal, primarily as linoleic acid (33). The N-3 fatty acids are important for neonatal brain development and normal nerve function. The long-chain polyunsaturated fatty acids C-20 and C-22 should be included because the preterm newborn is unable to desaturate linolenic acid or elongate the chain (33). These fatty acids are important in cell proliferation, myelinization of the central nervous system, and retinal development (34).

Phospholipids are critical components of all cell membranes. Pulmonary surfactant, which is comprised of dipalmatoylphosphatidylcholine (DPPC) and phosphatidylglycerol (PG), lowers surface tension and allows alveolar expansion. Fats are also the precursors of many major metabolic intermediates. Arachidonic acid (20:4), present in the membrane phospholipids, can be metabolized to the eicosanoids, i.e., the prostaglandins and leukotrienes (35). The prostaglandins and leukotrienes are very important in modulating blood flow at the tissue level. Prostaglandins and their metabolites are important in regulation of hemostasis. Leukotrienes are potent mediators of inflammation and activation of granulocytes, whether tissue bound or freely circulating.

Excess polyunsaturated fatty acids may act as oxidants especially disrupting the red cell membrane. Adequate vitamin E levels are important in premature infants to protect the red blood cells from hemolysis.

PROTEIN REQUIREMENTS

Protein is the most limiting nutrient for growth and development of the premature infant. Nitrogen and amino acids, supplied exclusively by dietary protein, are synthesized into membrane and transport proteins, intracellular and circulating enzymes, peptide hormones, immunoglobulins, coagulation factors, neurotransmitters, and hormones. The physiology and metabolic immaturity of the premature infant, especially with respect to hepatic and renal function, have special implications for protein needs in premature infants. Mature digestion and absorption of proteins are dependent on a series of proteolytic enzymes found in the duodenal enterocyte and released in pancreatic secretions (36). The enzymes trypsin, chymotrypsin, and elastase, and the carboxypeptidases A and B hydrolyze peptides at various specific sites to release amino acids. The amino acids and peptides are actively transported via carrier systems through the mucosal cells and then transported to the liver via the portal vein (37).

By 3 months' gestation the fetal intestine has established carrier-mediated, active transport systems for amino acids and dipeptides (4,36). By this time the liver is capable of synthesizing all the major plasma proteins with increasing concentrations of these proteins up to term gestation. By 28 weeks' gestation the premature infant has partially developed gastric, intestinal, and pancreatic function for protein digestion and absorption (38). Enzymatic function, however, may not be fully developed. Cystathionase, the enzyme responsible for metabolism of methionine to cysteine, is undetectable in the premature infant. Cysteine is, therefore, considered an essential amino acid in the preterm infant. Phenylalanine and tyrosine are also poorly metabolized in premature infants.

Total protein intake is limited by immature renal function (9). Although approximately 90% of protein nitrogen is incorporated into tissue protein, the kidney of a premature infant has a limited ability to handle a solute load. Premature infants fed 6 g/kg/day of protein have much higher blood nitrogen levels than premature infants fed 2 g/kg/day of protein (39). These differences persist beyond the time the infants would have reached term.

The digestion of milk proteins is complex. The caseins, which are found only in milk, are less easily digested than the whey or more-soluble proteins (40,41). They have no analogous systemic proteins. In addition, the caseins have been associated with delayed gastric emptying and lactobezoars. They bind the divalent cations calcium, manganese, magnesium, zinc, iron, and copper, reducing their bioavailability. They are proinflammatory, both promoting chemotaxis and stimulating the phospholipase A_2 and 5-lipoxygenase pathways. A pancreatic digest of casein found in tryptone agar induces accelerated carbohydrate fermentation. Casein impairs phagocytosis by milk leukocytes. It has also been associated with intestinal allergy and inflammation and has been implicated in the intraluminal pathogenesis of neonatal necrotizing enterocolitis (22).

Utilization of the whey protein fraction approximates 95% as compared to approximately 80% of the casein protein fraction. Studies indicate that caseins tend to promote higher tyrosine, phenylalanine, urea, and ammonia blood levels (40). Although metabolic acidosis is linked, in part, to total protein consumption, there is a correlation between casein consumption and metabolic acidosis, especially in the premature infant.

Protein requirements for the preterm and growth-retarded infants are considered to be approximately 2.5 to 4.0 g/kg/day (39,42,43). Current premature formulas have been adjusted to a casein fraction of no greater than 40% of the total protein content. However, since the cow's milk protein in the premature formula is not fully utilized, the total protein concentration has been adjusted to 1.5 g/100 ml, which is greater than in human milk. Knowledge of which amino acids are essential in the newborn is increasing (Table 1) (42). Taurine, which is derived from cysteine, another essential amino acid in the newborn, is of particular concern. Taurine is a soft hydroxy-β–amino acid, found in large amounts in breast milk (44). It is critical to development of the central nervous system (45), and taurine deficiency in newborn kittens promotes a retinopathy with some similarities to the retinopathy of prematurity. All standard formulas for term and premature infants as well as parenteral amino acid solutions contain taurine.

TABLE 1. *Essential and possibly essential amino acids in the premature infant*

Essential	Possibly essential
Leucine	Cysteine
Isoleucine	Taurine
Valine	Tyrosine
Threonine	Histidine
Methionine	
Phenylalanine	
Tryptophan	
Lysine	

MINERALS

The mineral requirements for premature infants are considerably higher than for full-term infants. This is due to excess mineral loss via the immature newborn kidneys and also because fetal mineral accretion is greatest in the last trimester, especially with respect to the divalent cations.

Sodium Chloride

Sodium chloride and water are intimately related. Over 90% of sodium chloride is extracellular, including the bone, connective tissue, plasma, and interstitial fluid. Extracellular fluid is approximately 40% of the body weight of a term infant, increasing with decreasing maturity. The extracellular fluid is 50% of the body weight of a 30-week fetus and 70% of the body weight of a 23-week fetus (46). The distribution and requirements for sodium chloride are, therefore, intimately linked to distribution and physiology of body water. With excessive insensible water loss, premature infants are prone to hypernatremia (47). On the other hand, excessive urinary excretion of sodium, along with retention of water relative to solute, may result in hyponatremia.

The sodium chloride requirement of a preterm infant weighing between 1,500 and 2,000 g is similar to that of a full-term infant: approximately 1 to 1.5 mM/kg/day (48). Low birth weight infants (<1500 g) frequently have hyponatremia and poor growth on an intake of 1.5 mM/kg/day. The current recommendation for sodium chloride intake in premature infants is 2 to 4 mM/kg/day for the first several weeks decreasing to about 2 mM/kg/day until an adjusted age of 35 weeks (46,47).

Potassium

Potassium is the principal cation within the cell. For very low birth weight infants, who may gain up to 15 g/kg/day, the requirement for growth is 1 mM/kg/day (49).

Hyperkalemia in premature infants is often indicative of a catabolic state, with the breakdown of glycogen and protein leading to the release of potassium into the extracellular fluid, and its subsequent urinary loss (50). Hyperkalemia may also occur with metabolic acidosis or excessive potassium intake.

Calcium, Phosphorus, and Magnesium

These three elements are intimately linked in their physiology and metabolism. They are essential for skeletal formation and enzymatic function in tissues.

Calcium is the most abundant mineral in the body, increasing most rapidly during the third trimester. In fact, 75% of the total body calcium of a full-term baby has accrued from 24 weeks' gestation until term (51). Premature infants fed a formula supplemented with additional calcium and phosphorus acquire a bone mineral content similar to that seen with intrauterine growth (52) (Fig. 3).

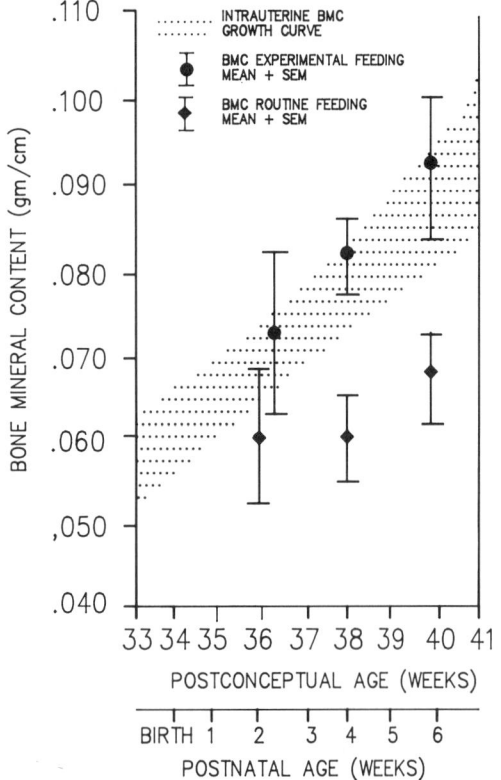

FIG. 3. Bone mineral content of preterm appropriate for gestational age (AGA) infants of gestational age 33 to 35 weeks.

The intestinal absorption of calcium is primarily by active transport in the duodenum (53). Premature infants fed their own mothers' milk absorb approximately 90% of the calcium. Calcium absorption increases with phosphate supplementation and when there is no vitamin D deficiency. The recommendations for higher calcium intake for premature infants is based on the need to improve bone mineralization. Elemental calcium intake should be approximately 150 to 200 mg/kg/day (51), easily attained by the use of any standard calcium and phosphorus fortified formulas for premature infants. Excess calcium loss may occur in infants with chronic acidosis such as in the hypercarbia of children with chronic bronchopulmonary dysplasia.

Phosphorus is critical for skeletal growth as well as a crucial component of the high-energy compounds within the body, adenosine diphosphate (ADP) and adenosine triphosphate (ATP) (51). It is absorbed in the proximal small intestine by both active and passive mechanisms (53). An excess of dietary divalent cations tends to decrease phosphorus absorption by complexing it within the intestinal lumen. Premature infants absorb approximately 90% of the phosphorus content of their mothers' milk. The oral requirement for phosphorus ranges from 100 to 125 mg/kg/day, approximately half of that of calcium (51). The premature kidney retains phosphorus within several weeks, primarily by reabsorption in the proximal convoluted tubule.

Magnesium is absorbed throughout the entire small intestine with similar rates in the jejunum and ileum. Absorption is thought to occur by simple diffusion with some evidence for facilitated diffusion (53). It is the second most common intracellular electrolyte in the body. Renal absorption in magnesium occurs primarily in the loop of Henle (50% to 60%), with less being absorbed in the proximal convoluted tubule (20% to 30%). Recommended intake for premature infants is approximately 8 mg/kg/day, similar to that of the full-term infant (51). For infants tolerating feedings, both human milk and premature formula provide adequate amounts of magnesium. Although uncommon, hypocalcemia that is resistant to replacement therapy may be secondary to decreased parathyroid hormone secretion and corrected by identifying a concurrent hypomagnesemia.

Iron

Iron is present in the body primarily complexed either to storage compounds, ferritin and hemosiderin, or constitutively in metabolic compounds such as hemoglobin, myoglobin, and the cytochromes. It is absorbed primarily in the small intestine. Approximately 50% of the iron from breast milk is absorbed, which is ten times the absorption of iron from iron-fortified formulas. The reasons for the 50% absorption of breast milk iron includes the presence, in human milk, of an iron-binding protein, lactoferrin, which may enhance the transfer of iron and the presence, in breast milk, of more digestible protein with a lower total protein content and lower phosphate concentration.

All newborns, including the premature infant, have sufficient body iron at birth to supply needs to approximately double their birth weight (54). Sick premature infants frequently develop iron excess as a result of receiving more iron in the packed red blood cells than is being lost from frequent blood sampling.

Breast-fed, low birth weight infants will develop iron deficiency anemia without iron supplementation (55). Recommended doses, as a ferrous sulfate of iron, are as follows: less than 1,000 g birth weight, 4 mg/kg/day; 1,000 to 1,500 g birth weight, 3 mg/kg/day; 1,500 to 2,500 g birth weight, 2 mg/kg/day (54,56). Appropriate iron supplementation may predispose to vitamin E deficiency.

TRACE MINERALS

The need for supplemental trace minerals in premature and growth-retarded infants is well recognized (Table 2) (57,58). Zinc deficiency, more common than previously thought, may present with decreased growth velocity, failure to thrive, diarrhea, hair loss, and, in its more chronic form, perioral and perianal skin lesions (59). Copper deficiency has been demonstrated in premature infants with poor weight gain, diarrhea, edema and, occasionally, hypotonia and apnea (59). These infants may be anemic, leukopenic [total white blood count (WBC) less than 5,000/mm^3, polymorphonuclear neutrophil leukocytes (PMN) less than 1,500/mm^3], and with decreased ceruloplasmin.

Other trace elements including selenium, iodine, chromium, fluorine, molybdenum, manganese, and cobalt have been studied in term infants, but relatively little information is available to define the subtleties of deficiencies or clearly determine supplementation of the premature infant.

TABLE 2. *Trace elements: recommended daily oral intakes for premature infants*

Zinc	0.3–0.6 mg
Copper	80 μg/kg
Selenium	10–40 μg
Manganese	2–5 μg/kg
Chromium	0.2–0.5 μg/kg
Molybdenum	0.2–0.5 μg/kg
Iodine	40 μg
Fluorine	0.25 mg

VITAMINS

Vitamin metabolism of premature infants has been a major area of study during the last 20 years (60,61). Few deficiencies have been demonstrated in the water-soluble vitamins such as vitamin C, the B-complex vitamins, niacin, biotin, and pantothenic acid (62). Virtually all parenteral solutions are vitamin supplemented, probably to excess. There are also adequate amounts of vitamins in human milk and in the formulas designed for premature infants.

In contrast, the recommendations for supplementation of the fat-soluble vitamins have ranged from replacement levels to pharmacologic doses. Vitamin A or its dimer, carotene, has been suggested as a preventive therapy for bronchopulmonary dysplasia (BPD) (63,64). Vitamin D has been used effectively to improve bone mineral content primarily by calcium absorption and for the treatment of osteopenia of prematurity and rickets in more mature newborns (65,66). Vitamin E (α-tocopherol), alcohol vitamin has been used as a drug to reduce the severity of retinopathy of prematurity by the scavenging of free radicals (67). It may also be useful in reducing the severity of bronchopulmonary dysplasia and intraventricular hemorrhage (68,69).

Finally, vitamin K has long been recognized as critical in preventing hemorrhagic disease to the newborn (70). This hemorrhage characteristically occurs in approximately 1% to 2% of babies on the 3rd to 5th day of life and may involve the central nervous system, lungs, or adrenal glands. Recently, it has been demonstrated that giving the mother vitamin K more than 12 hr prior to delivery may provide sufficient vitamin K to the newborn. Vitamin K may also be given orally to the newborn. It is well absorbed, will effectively prevent hemorrhagic disease of the newborn, and will also avoid the trauma of an intramuscular injection.

SUMMARY

The nutritional requirements of the healthy full-term newborn are relatively well defined. In contrast, preexisting factors and the variability of illnesses of the premature and growth-retarded infants have complicated assessment of their nutritional status. Nutritional studies of prematures usually have relatively small numbers of patients. In addition, the variability of water loss, gastrointestinal function, and hepatic and renal function, along with peripheral alimentation and frequent blood sampling, are confounding variables in these studies. The survival of the extremely low birth weight baby under 1000 g has improved dramatically within the last 5 years but, other than those regarding insensible water loss and glucose metabolism, few randomized, well-controlled comprehensive studies are available on this population.

REFERENCES

1. Widdowson EM, Southgate DAT, Hay EN. Body composition of the fetus and infant. In: Vissar HKA, ed. *Nutrition and metabolism of the fetus and infant.* The Hague: Martinus Nijhoff, 1979;169–174.
2. Grand RJ, Watkins JB, Torti FM. Development of the human gastrointestinal tract. *Gastroenterology* 1976;70:790–810.
3. Montgomery RK. Functional development of the gastrointestinal tract: the small intestine. In: Heird WC, ed. *Nutrition during the second six months of life.* Glendale: Carnation Company, 1989;21–23.
4. Henning S. Functional development of the gastrointestinal tract. In: Johnson LR, ed. *Physiology of the gastrointestinal tract,* 2nd ed. New York: Raven Press, 1987;285–300.
5. Lebenthal E, Lee PC, Heitlinger LA. Impact of development of the gastrointestinal tract on infant feeding. *J Pediatr* 1983;102:1–9.
6. Lebenthal E, Leung YK. Feeding the premature and compromised infant: gastrointestinal considerations. *Pediatr Clin North Am* 1988;35(2):215–238.
7. Siegel M, Lebenthal E, Krantz B. Effect of caloric density on gastric emptying in premature infants. *J Pediatr* 1984;104:118–122.
8. Lorenz JM, Kleinman LI. Ontogeny of the kidney. In: Tsang R, Nichols B, eds. *Nutrition during infancy.* Philadelphia: Hanley & Belfus, 1985;58–85.
9. El-Dahr SS, Chevalier RL. Special needs of the newborn infant in fluid therapy. *Pediatr Clin North Am* 1990;37(2):323–336.
10. Whyte RK, Bayley HS, Sinclair JC. Energy intake and the nature of growth in low birth weight infants. *Can J Physiol Pharmacol* 1985;63:565–570.
11. Sauer PJJ, Dane HJ, Visser HKA. Longitudinal studies on metabolic rate, heat loss, and energy cost of growth in low birth weight infants. *Pediatr Res* 1984;18:709–713.
12. Schofield WN, Schofield C, James WPT. Basal metabolic rate—review and prediction, together with an annotated bibliography of source material. *Hum Nutr Clin Nutr* 1985;39C(Suppl 1):5–41.
13. Davies PSW, Lucas A. Energy expenditure in early infancy. *Br J Nutr* 1989;62:621–629.
14. Hammarlund K, Sedin G. Transepidermal water loss in newborn infants. III. Relation to gestational age. *Acta Paediatr Scand* 1979;68:799–803.
15. Friis-Hansen B. Body water compartments in children: changes during growth and related changes in body composition. *Pediatrics* 1961;28:169–181.
16. Nash MA. Provision of water and electrolytes. In: Fanaroff AA, Martin RJ, eds. *Neonatal-perinatal medicine.* St. Louis: CV Mosby, 1987;460–466.
17. Arant BS Jr. Fluid therapy in the neonate: concepts in transition. *J Pediatr* 1982;101:387–391.
18. Bell EF, Neidich GA, Cashore WJ, Oh W. Combined effect of radiant warmer and phototherapy on insensible water loss in low-birth-weight infants. *J Pediatr* 1979;94:810.
19. Gray GM. Carbohydrate absorption and malabsorption. In: Johnson LR, ed. *Physiology of the gastrointestinal tract.* New York: Raven Press, 1981;1063–1072.
20. Aurricchio S, Rubino A, Murset G. Intestinal glycosidase activities in the human embryo, fetus and newborn. *Pediatrics* 1965;35:944–954.
21. Cicco R, Holzman IR, Brown DR, Becker DJ. Glucose polymer tolerance in premature infants. *Pediatrics* 1981;67:498–501.
22. Clark DA, Miller MJS. The intraluminal pathogenesis of necrotizing enterocolitis. *J Pediatr* 1990;117:S64–S67.
23. Cowett RM, Stern L. Carbohydrate homeostasis in the fetus and newborn. In: Avery GB, ed. *Neonatology: pathophysiology and management of the newborn,* 3rd ed. Philadelphia: JB Lippincott, 1987;691–709.
24. Lifschitz CH. Carbohydrate needs in preterm and term newborn infants. In: Tsang R, Nichols B, eds. *Nutrition during infancy.* Philadelphia: Hanley & Belfus, 1988;122–132.
25. Hamosh M. Fat needs for term and preterm infants. In: Tsang R, Nichols B, eds. *Nutrition during infancy.* Philadelphia: Hanley & Belfus, 1988;133–159.
26. Hamosh M, Bitman J, Wood DL. Lipids in milk and the first steps in their digestion. *Pediatrics* 1985;75(suppl):146.
27. Hernell O, Bläckberg L, Lindberg T. Human milk enzymes with emphasis on the lipases. In: Lebenthal E, ed. *Textbook of gastroenterology and nutrition during infancy.* New York: Raven Press, 1989;209–217.
28. Hamosh M. Lingual and breast milk lipases. *Adv Pediatr* 1982;29:33–67.
29. Franklin FA. The effects of infant feeding practices on lipid and lipoprotein levels and metabolism. In: Lebenthal E, ed. *Textbook of gastroenterology and nutrition during infancy.* New York: Raven Press, 1989;503–514.
30. Brennan J. Carnitine metabolism and function. *Physiol Rev* 1983;63:1420–1434.
31. Shenai JP, Borum PR, Mohan P, et al. Carnitine status at birth of newborn infants of varying gestation. *Pediatr Res* 1983;17:579–582.
32. Heim T. Energy and lipid requirements of the fetus and preterm infant. *J Pediatr Gastroenterol Nutr* 1983;2:16–41.
33. Uauy R, Treen M, Hoffman DR. Essential fatty acid metabolism and requirements during development. *Semin Perinatol* 1989;3:118–130.
34. Carlson SE, Cooke RJ, Peeples JM, Werkman SH, Tolley EA. Docosahexaenoate (DHA) and eicosapentaenoate (EPA) status of preterm infants: relationship to visual acuity in n-3 supplemented and unsupplemented infants. *Pediatr Res* 1989;25:285A.
35. Willis AL. Essential fatty acids, prostaglandins, and related eicosanoids. In: *Present knowledge in nutrition.* Washington, DC: Nutrition Foundation, 1984;90–113.
36. Gray GM, Cooper HL. Protein digestion and absorption. *Gastroenterology* 1971;61:535–544.
37. Matthews DM, Adibi SA. Peptide absorption. *Gastroenterology* 1976;71:151–161.
38. Motil KJ. Protein needs for term and preterm infants. In: Tsang R, Nichols B, eds. *Nutrition during infancy.* Philadelphia: Hanley & Belfus, 1988;100–121.
39. Rassin DK. Protein requirements in the neonate. In: Lebenthal E, ed. *Textbook of gastroenterology and nutrition in infancy.* New York: Raven Press, 1989;281–292.
40. Miller MJS, Witherly S, Clark DA. Casein: a milk protein with diverse biologic consequences. *Proc Soc Exp Biol Med* 1990;195:143–159.
41. Hirata Y, Matsuo P, Kobuhu H. Digestion and absorption of milk proteins in infants' intestine. *Kobe J Med Sci* 1965;11:103–108.
42. Millward DJ, Rivers JPW. The nutritional role of indispensable amino acids and the metabolic basis for their requirements. *Eur J Clin Nutr* 1988;42:367–393.
43. Beaton GH, Chery A. Protein requirements of infants: a reexamination of concepts and approaches. *Am J Clin Nutr* 1988;48:1403–1412.
44. Chesney RW. Taurine: is it required for infant nutrition? *Am J Nutr* 1988;118:6–10.
45. Tyson JE, Laskey R, Flood D, et al. Randomized trial of taurine supplementation for infants < 1300 gram birth weight: effect on auditory brainstem-evoked responses. *Pediatrics* 1989;83:406–415.
46. Engelke SC, Shah BL, Vasan U. Sodium balance in very low birth weight infants. *J Pediatr* 1978;93:837–844.
47. Al Duhhan J, Haycock GB, Nichol B. Sodium homeostasis in term and preterm infants. *Arch Dis Child* 1984;59:945–950.
48. Haycock GB. Sodium and water. In: Holliday MA, Barratt TM, Vernier R, eds. *Pediatric nephrology,* 2nd ed. Baltimore: Williams and Wilkins, 1987;84–89.
49. Schwartz GJ, Feld LG. Potassium. In: Holliday MA, Barratt TM, Vernier R, eds. *Pediatric nephrology,* 2nd ed. Baltimore: Williams and Wilkins 1987;114–127.
50. Engle WD, Arant BS Jr. Urinary potassium excretion in the critically ill neonate. *Pediatrics* 1984;74:259.
51. Koo WWK, Tsang RC. Calcium, magnesium and phosphorus. In: Tsang R, Nichols B, eds. *Nutrition during infancy.* Philadelphia: Hanley & Belfus, 1988;175–189.
52. Steichen JJ, Gratton TL, Tsang RC. Osteopenia of prematurity: the cause and possible treatment. *J Pediatr* 1980;96:528–534.

53. Wilkinson R. Absorption of calcium, phosphorus and magnesium. In: Nordin BEC, ed. *Calcium, phosphorus and magnesium metabolism.* New York: Churchill Livingstone, 1976;36–112.
54. Siimes MA. Iron nutrition in low-birth-weight infants. In: Stekel A, ed. *Iron nutrition in infancy and childhood.* New York: Raven Press, 1984;75–91.
55. Dallman PR. Anemia of prematurity. *Annu Rev Med* 1981;32:143–160.
56. Lundstrom U, Siimes MA, Dallman PR. At what age does iron supplementation become necessary in low-birth-weight infants? *J Pediatr* 1977;91:878–883.
57. Casey CE, Walravens PA. Trace elements. In: Tsang R, Nichols B, eds. *Nutrition during infancy.* Philadelphia: Hanley & Belfus, 1988;190–215.
58. Milner JA. Trace minerals in the nutrition of children. *J Pediatr* 1990;117:S147–155.
59. Tyrala EE. Zinc and copper balances in preterm infants. *Pediatrics* 1986;77:513–517.
60. Orzalesi M. Vitamins and the premature. *Biol Neonate* 1987;52(Suppl 1):97–112.
61. Committee on Nutrition. American Academy of Pediatrics. Nutritional needs of low-birth-weight infants. *Pediatrics* 1985;75:976–986.
62. Schanler RJ. Water-soluble vitamins: C, B_1, B_2, B_6, niacin, biotin, and pantothenic acid: In: Tsang R, Nichols B, eds. *Nutrition during infancy.* Philadelphia: Hanley & Belfus, 1988;236–252.
63. Zachman RD. Vitamin A. In: Tsang R, Nichols B, eds. *Nutrition during infancy.* Philadelphia: Hanley & Belfus, 1988;253–263.
64. Shenai JP, Chytil F, Stahlman MT. Vitamin A status of neonates with chronic lung disease. *Pediatr Res* 1985;19:185–189.
65. American Academy of Pediatrics. Committee on Nutrition. The prophylactic requirements and the toxicity of vitamin D. *Pediatrics* 1963;31:512.
66. Specker BL, Greer F, Tsang RC. Vitamin D. In: Tsang R, Nichols B, eds. *Nutrition during infancy.* Philadelphia: Hanley & Belfus, 1988;264–276.
67. Phelps DL. Vitamin E and retinopathy of prematurity. In: Silverman W, Flynn J, eds. *Contemporary issues in fetal and neonatal medicine: retinopathy of prematurity.* Boston: Blackwell, 1985;181–205.
68. Bell EF. Prevention of bronchopulmonary dysplasia: vitamin E and other antioxidants. In: Farrell PM, Taussig LM, eds. *Bronchopulmonary dysplasia and related chronic respiratory disorders.* Report of the Ninetieth Ross Conference on Pediatric Research, 1986;77–82.
69. Chiswick ML, Johnson M, Woohhall C, et al. Protective effect of vitamin E against intraventricular hemorrhage in premature babies. *Br Med J* 1983;287:81–84.
70. Greer FR, Suttie JW. Vitamin K and the newborn. In: Tsang R, Nichols B, eds. *Nutrition during infancy.* Philadelphia: Hanley & Belfus, 1988;289–297.

CHAPTER 4

Human Milk and Infant Formula

Cutberto Garza, Nancy F. Butte, and Armond S. Goldman

The Surgeon General's Report on Nutrition and Health and the most recent report of the Dietary Guidelines Advisory Committee on the Dietary Guidelines for Americans identify the special nutrient needs of infants and recognize human milk as the best food for that group. Human milk's nutrient balance, its content of other growth-promoting substances, and the immunological protection it provides against infectious diseases form the essential rationale for the recommendation of human milk as the food of choice for infants (1,2). Human milk's physical complexity also merits special consideration. Constituents are compartmentalized in a water-soluble phase, in complex fat globules, and in multiple cells with immunoprotective characteristics. In this regard it is "tissue-like" in composition. The second choice for normal term infants is bovine milk–based formula. The contents of selected nutrients in human milk, bovine milk–based formulas, as well as other milks are summarized in Table 1.

The major compositional similarities between human milk and infant formulas are the concentrations and generally high bioavailabilities of total fat and carbohydrate. The fat composition of each differs, however; artificial formulas generally contain higher levels of polyunsaturated fat and lower levels of monounsaturated fat.

Lactose is the major carbohydrate in human milk and most bovine milk–based infant formulas. Formulas, however, lack the complex range of carbohydrates found in human milk. In addition, the concentrations of other nutrients, except possibly chloride, tend to be significantly higher in most bovine milk–based formulas, whereas nutrient bioavailabilities tend to be lower. This chapter focuses on human milk and examines the biological significance of compositional differences between human milk and bovine milk–based infant formulas. Emphasis is given to the compositional changes human milk undergoes at various stages of lactation, functional components of human milk, and selected physiological responses of breast- and formula-fed infants.

DUAL ROLES OF HUMAN MILK COMPONENTS

Human milk constituents play dual roles: (a) the classically recognized role that is associated with most nutrients, i.e., the provision of energy substrates, enzymatic cofactors and components for the synthesis of body tissues, enzymes, and other functional components necessary for normal metabolism; and (b) functional roles that complement immunological and other metabolic abilities of maturing infants (3). The organic macronutrients are found in both artificial formulas and human milk but, whereas those in artificial formulas fulfill only classically recognized nutritional roles, those in human milk commonly have other functions. Human milk proteins provide amino acids for growth as well as aiding digestion, host defense, and, possibly, tissue maturation. Human milk fat provides energy; some of the shorter chain fats commonly found in human milk have antiviral properties and some of the longer chain, unsaturated fats may act to enhance maturing membrane functions in diverse cell types. Lactose is also a primary source of energy in human milk, but human milk complex carbohydrates and lactose modulate bacterial growth in the infant's colon and prevent the attachment of selected bacteria to the infant's respiratory and gastrointestinal epithelial cells.

C. Garza: Division of Nutritional Sciences, Cornell University, Ithaca, New York 14853.
N. F. Butte: USDA/ARS Children's Nutrition Research Center, Houston, Texas 77030.
A. S. Goldman: Department of Pediatrics, University of Texas Medical Branch, Galveston, Texas 77350.

TABLE 1. *Content of selected nutrients in human milk, commercial formulas, and other milks used for feeding normal full-term infants*

Nutrient	Per liter	Mature human milk[a] (21.6 ± 1.5 Cal/oz)	Milk-based formulas[b] (20 Cal/oz)	Soy protein–based formulas (20 Cal/oz)	Whole cow milk (20 Cal/oz)	Skimmed milk (11 Cal/oz)	Goat milk (21 Cal/oz)
Protein	g	10.5 ± 0.2	15	18–21	34	35	37
Fat	g	39.0 ± 0.4	36–38	36–39	37	2	43
Carbohydrate	g	72.0 ± 0.25	69–72.3	66–69	48	50	46
Calcium	mg	280 ± 26	400–510	630–700	1,219	1,270	1,380
Phosphorus	mg	140 ± 22	300–390	420–500	959	1,050	1,140
Sodium	mEq	7.8 ± 1.7	7–10	9–15	22	23	23
Potassium	mEq	13.4 ± 0.9	14–21	19–24	38	44	54
Chloride	mEq	11.8 ± 1.7	11–14	11–15	27	31	44
Iron	mg	0.3 ± 0.1	1.1–1.5	12–12.7	0.4	0.4	0.5
Estimated renal solute load	mOsm	73	(12–12.7)[c] 92–105	122–138	226	240	269

Data from ref. 1.
[a] Average values with standard deviations for comparison.
[b] Values listed are subject to change. Refer to product label or packaging for current information. Milk-based formulas contain lactose, and soy protein–based formulas do not.
[c] Iron content of iron-fortified formulas.

COMPOSITION OF HUMAN MILK: NUTRITIONAL FACTORS

Human milk composition undergoes well-regulated, predictable changes independent of maternal diet or other factors that modulate its contents (4). Although the physiological significance to the infant is not completely understood, the functional roles of the specific constituents suggest that the changes are beneficial.

Carbohydrates

Generally, nutrient concentrations either remain unchanged or fall after lactation is established. Lactose concentrations are maintained at approximately 7 g% throughout lactation, after the transition from colostrum to mature milk, and account for approximately 40% to 50% of human milk's gross energy content. Lactose concentration is probably the most tightly regulated of all nutrient levels in human milk. Normal lactose concentrations are maintained even under conditions of the severe nutritional stress associated with reductions in milk volume (5). These observations suggest that lactose synthesis and total milk production are affected similarly (6). Statistically significant inverse relationships have been reported between lactose and fat concentrations in milk, but the changes in lactose concentrations are small and probably of little biological consequence (7). Little is known about the changes that occur in the content of other milk carbohydrates as lactation progresses.

The high level of lactose in human milk presents an interesting problem in the management of gastrointestinal infections in breast-fed infants. Unlike formula-fed infants, who often become clinically intolerant to lactose during acute phases of gastrointestinal infections, breast-fed infants appear to tolerate the high level of lactose in human milk during similar periods of illness. Possible explanations include differences in the groups' bacterial flora, amelioration of the severity of infection by immune components in the milk, the increased potential for hyperosmolar dehydration in affected formula-fed infants, or other unidentified mechanisms that influence lactose absorption or the utilization of fermented products of unabsorbed lactose. Although a temporary change to a nonlactose formula is effective in the management of lactose intolerance secondary to a gastrointestinal infection, a cessation of breast-feeding is not recommended for infants with diarrhea (8).

Fat

The total content (3.5 g/dl) of human milk fat is also fairly stable in individual women throughout the period of established lactation and accounts for approximately 50% of human milk's gross energy content. The level of fat, however, varies significantly among women. The reported range of concentrations is from 1 to over 7 g/dl. These extreme values probably reflect the mechanism of fat secretion as well as inappropriate collection procedures for milk analysis rather than the actual physiologic range of fat concentrations of "complete" feedings. Nonetheless, the mechanisms responsible for the less extreme and more common range in fat concentrations, approximately 2.5 to 5 g/dl, have not been described.

Human milk's fat composition is influenced significantly by maternal diet and the stage of lactation (9). In Western societies, long-chain fats (carbon length ≥16) account for approximately 95% of fatty acids in human milk; the remaining 5% are of shorter chain lengths (fats of 12 to 14 carbons in length). Palmitic and oleic acids account for approximately 20% and 38%, respectively, of the total fatty acids in human milk. Of the fatty acids usually found in human milk, linoleic acid is among the most variable. The level of linoleic acid in human milk is influenced significantly by the mother's consumption of vegetable fat. Usually, however, among Western women, linoleic acid accounts for approximately 15% of the total fatty acids in human milk.

The major differences in the fat composition of human milk and representative artificial formulas are the contents of the longer chain fats (≥ 20) and the proportions and absolute levels of mono- and polyunsaturated fats (Table 2). The significance of those differences is not completely understood. Although the fatty acid composition of cellular membranes is affected by dietary fats, the functional consequences of those compositional differences remain unclear. The recent negative association between the proportion of dihomo-gamma-linolenic acid in human milk and the occurrence of atopic dermatitis in breast-fed infants supports early observations that related atopic eczema to serum lipid patterns and the functional significance of specific fatty acid intakes in infancy (10). The digestibility of the various fat blends in formulas appears comparable to that of human milk fat. The digestibility of human milk fat has not been studied systematically in infants affected by clinical conditions associated with fat intolerance.

Cholesterol is the other human milk lipid of interest. The concentration of human milk cholesterol is approximately 100 to 200 mg/l. Those levels appear to be independent of the mother's cholesterol intake or her general status. The functional significance of its presence in human milk and absence from bovine milk–based formulas is not known.

Protein

The concentration of total protein falls as lactation progresses. It is approximately 1.3 g% by the second postpartum week. By the end of the second to third month, the concentration falls by 30% to approximately 0.9 g%. Concentrations remain close to this level until weaning is initiated, rising to approximately 1.2 g% during the weaning process, when milk production is reduced substantially. Maternal diets do not appear to influence net protein concentrations in milk, although there is controversy as to whether the concentrations of specific proteins are influenced by significant degrees of undernutrition.

Whey proteins account for approximately 80% of the total protein content. The major whey proteins are α-lactalbumin, lactoferrin, and secretory IgA (SIgA). α-Lactalbumin catalyzes specific reactions in the biosynthesis of lactose. Its concentration falls as lactation progresses, but its levels at distinct stages of lactation have not been as well described as those of lactoferrin and SIgA. Lactoferrin binds iron avidly and presumably limits the availability of iron to potentially pathogenic enteric flora. Human milk lactoferrin is not saturated with iron when it is secreted. Growth-promoting and other immune-modulating functions also have been described for lactoferrin, but it is not clear if human milk lactoferrin fulfills those functions in the infant. Lactoferrin concentrations fall during the first 12 weeks of lactation (from 0.5 g% at week 1 to 0.08 g% at week 12) and remain stable for as long as 2 years.

SIgA shows a similar pattern. Its concentrations fall from 0.2 g% at week 1 to 0.05 g% at week 12. Those levels also remain stable for as long as 2 years and apply to the total amount of SIgA that is secreted. SIgA titers against specific pathogens rise and fall in apparent response to maternal exposure to specific antigens. SIgA has the abil-

TABLE 2. *Fatty acid composition of human milk, SMA, and Enfamil, expressed as weight percent of total fatty acid methyl esters*

Fatty acid	Human milk[a] (mean ± SEM)	SMA (mean)	Enfamil (mean)
8:0	0.3	2.6	2.1
10:0	1.4	1.4	1.1
12:0	6.2	13.5	10.1
14:0	7.6	5.9	4.0
16:0	20.5 ± 0.70	14.7	11.0
18:0	9.0 ± 0.46	7.2	4.0
18:1	37.6 ± 0.75	43.3	19.9
18:2n6	15.8 ± 0.61	14.0	45.1
20:0	0.3 ± 0.02	Trace	Trace
18:3n3	0.8 ± 0.09	1.2	5.0
20:1	0.9 ± 0.7	Trace	Trace
20:2n6	0.4 ± 0.03		
20:4n6	0.6 ± 0.03		
22:1	0.0 ± 0.02		
20:5n3	0.1 ± 0.03		
24:0	0.5 ± 0.01	Trace	Trace
22:5n6	0.1 ± 0.02		
22:5n3	0.1 ± 0.01		
22:6n3	0.1 ± 0.01		
UI[b]	79.6 ± 1.13	74.9	125.1
% PUFA 18C	1.9 ± 0.09	ND	ND
%:0	38.6 ± 0.72	43.3	19.9
%n3 PUFA	1.1 ± 0.09	1.2	5.0
%n6 PUFA	17.4 ± 0.62	14.0	45.1
%n3 PUFA 18C	0.3 ± 0.02	ND	ND
%n6 PUFA 18C	1.6 ± 0.09	ND	ND
12:2n6/18:3m3	18.8 ± 1.2	11.7	9.0

Adapted from ref. 9.
PUFA, polyunsaturated fatty acid; ND, none detectable.
[a] The mean value of individual milk samples; one sample was taken from each mother at approximately 8 weeks of lactation.
[b] Unsaturation index: [(% each fatty acid) (no. double bonds/fatty acid)].

ity to bind specific antigens in the infant's gastrointestinal tract, thereby preventing clinical infection.

The availability of some whey proteins, particularly lactoferrin and SIgA, to the infant has been questioned because of the resistance of these proteins to *in vitro* hydrolysis. Digestion may be delayed sufficiently to permit them to exert a biological effect before hydrolysis. Fecal SIgA appears to fall with age, but detailed balance studies have not been performed to determine if that decrease parallels changes in SIgA intakes from human milk. The nitrogen (N) balance studies performed in normal term breast-fed infants suggest, however, that approximately 95% of human milk nitrogen is eventually absorbed. No supportive data are available for the absorption of large quantities of whole proteins by the infant; it is likely, therefore, that most of the whey proteins are digested and that the constituent amino acids and small peptides are absorbed by the infant.

Not all human milk protein concentrations fall as lactation progresses. Lysozyme, after an initial nadir in the first 3 months, increases substantially during the first year of lactation. The concentrations of lysozyme are too low to be considered of nutritional importance although they may play a significant role in host protection. Lysozyme can kill potential pathogens by the lysis of cell walls.

Caseins make up the remaining 20% of human milk proteins. They make significant contributions to the total amino acid pattern of human milk and are highly digestible. Their most significant functional property appears to be the ability to form stable aggregates that include calcium (Ca) and phosphorus (P). This characteristic permits greater concentrations of Ca and P in milk than is allowed by the simple solubility of either mineral.

Vitamins

As lactation progresses, the concentrations of vitamins in human milk show distinct patterns. Some, such as riboflavin, vitamin A, and vitamin K, are higher in colostrum than in mature milk, their levels usually stabilizing by 3 to 4 months. The concentrations of other vitamins, including thiamin, niacin, and vitamin B_6, are lower in colostrum than in mature milk. Although the concentrations of most vitamins appear to remain stable after 3 to 4 months, folate is reported to increase and riboflavin to decrease as lactation progresses. The significance of these distinct compositional patterns to infant nutrition merits further study.

Generally, vitamin levels in human milk are more responsive to maternal diet than are the levels of human milk fat, carbohydrate, and protein. However, this responsiveness to diet is more apparent when intake is marginal; it is less likely to occur from a balanced diet and when intake is sufficient to meet energy requirements.

Vitamins that warrant special attention are vitamins D, K, B_{12}, and B_6. Vitamin D levels in milk partially reflect maternal vitamin D status. However, even in women with an adequate vitamin D status, the vitamin D content of human milk may be low relative to the need of infants whose exposure to sunlight is limited. The amount of sunlight exposure necessary to ensure normal serum 25-hydroxycholecalciferol levels is approximately 30 min per week when infants wear only a diaper or 2 hr per week when fully clothed (11). Infants with pigmented skin or those living in climates that limit sun exposure are most at risk (12). A daily supplement of 400 IU of vitamin D is safe, but of no known benefit unless sun exposure is limited (13).

All infants, regardless of the mothers' vitamin K status, or whether they are breast-fed or fed artificial formulas, should be supplemented with vitamin K at birth. The most dependable method of preventing vitamin K deficiency and its serious manifestation, hemorrhagic disease of the newborn, is to inject 0.5 to 1.0 mg of vitamin K_1 at birth (14). Vitamin K levels in milk are insufficient to prevent this condition in all newborns. In the later stages of infancy, however, the levels of vitamin K_1 in human milk and the normal production of vitamin K_2 (menaquinone) by normal bacterial flora in the infant's gastrointestinal tract are sufficient to maintain normal vitamin K status.

The frequency of vitamin B_{12} deficiency in breast-fed infants of vegetarian women warrants supplementation of mothers (2.6 µg/d) and infants (0.1 to 0.3 µg/d) (13). The deficiency usually appears in infants between 6 months and 1 year old and is often observed before any maternal signs or symptoms of B_{12} deficiency are noted. The deficiency is not seen in breast-fed infants of women eating diets adequate in B_{12}.

The need to supplement lactating women and/or their infants with vitamin B_6 remains highly controversial (15). The concern stems from unconfirmed reports of convulsions related to vitamin B_6 status in infants of women who had been on hormonal birth control over 4 years. The difficulty in ascribing the convulsions to the infants' vitamin B_6 status, the apparently rare occurrence of these convulsions, the currently reduced estrogen levels in contraceptives, the relatively high vitamin intakes required to reach near-maximum concentrations of B_6 in human milk, as well as the problems involved in assessing B_6 status in infants have made this issue particularly difficult to resolve.

Minerals and Electrolytes

The concentrations of calcium (Ca), phosphorus (P), magnesium (Mg), sodium (Na), chloride (Cl), and potassium (K) in human milk are independent of the mothers' diets and do not appear to limit the term infant's normal growth and development. The supply of Ca and P may not be adequate, however, for the repletion of deficits found in premature infants or those with deficiencies resulting from poor early nutritional management. Generally, the concentrations of Ca, P, Mg, Na, Cl, and K are much lower in human milk than in bovine milk–based formulas. The disparities are, however, either the result of attempts to adjust for lower bioavailabilities of specific minerals, for example, Ca and P, in formulas, or are due to technical requirements associated with processing. The functional significance of those differences remains controversial, particularly concerns related to the putative adverse effects of higher Na intakes in early life on the predisposition to adult-onset hypertension (16,17).

The trace minerals of most concern are iron (Fe), copper (Cu), and zinc (Zn); less is known about selenium (Se), manganese (Mn), and iodine (I) in human milk. The iron content of human milk is much less than that of iron-fortified bovine milk–based formulas, but the bioavailability of human milk iron is much higher. The medium value of human milk iron is approximately 0.3 mg/l. The medium may be more useful than the mean because of a distribution skewed toward higher values in Western study populations. Iron deficiency among exclusively breast-fed infants is rare before 4 to 6 months (14). Similar data for infants breast-fed exclusively for longer periods are not available. The relatively high iron stores of normal term infants and the high bioavailability of human milk iron probably protect the infant against iron deficiency. Because supplementary foods may interfere with the bioavailability of human milk iron, supplementation to exclusively breast-fed infants should be with iron-fortified foods or foods with highly bioavailable iron (18). No differences are observed through 4 to 6 months in the iron status of exclusively breast-fed infants and infants fed iron-fortified bovine milk–based formulas.

Potential adverse effects of high iron concentrations on the gastrointestinal tract's bacterial flora remain controversial. The low iron concentrations of human milk and its high bioavailability combine to produce very low levels of iron in the gastrointestinal lumen. Those low concentrations are viewed as limiting the growth of potential bacterial pathogens.

Human milk zinc is also highly bioavailable. Its concentrations are highest in colostrum, falling progressively throughout lactation (3 mg/l at month 1 to 0.5 mg/l at month 12) (19). Maternal Zn supplementation does not appear to influence milk Zn levels among Western women (20) although some investigators report a positive effect of supplementation in late lactation (21). Plasma zinc levels in breast-fed infants are similar to adult levels and to those of infants fed artificial formulas with much higher concentrations of Zn (22).

Milk Cu concentrations are highest in colostrum. These levels decline over the first 4 months of lactation and either remain stable or continue to decline, at a more gradual rate, as lactation progresses. The concentration of human milk Cu is 0.1 to 0.6 mg/l by the third or fourth month; values are skewed toward the lower part of the range. In contrast to human milk Cu, serum Cu and ceruloplasmin levels appear to rise for as long as 12 months in exclusively breast-fed infants (23). Maternal Cu status does not appear to affect significantly the concentrations in human milk.

HUMAN MILK COMPOSITION: OTHER FUNCTIONAL FACTORS

Various constituents of human milk have been associated with immunoprotective, digestive, growth promoting, and bioavailability-enhancing properties. The significance of those properties to the infant is not fully understood; the prevailing consensus is that they promote the infant's well-being, particularly under conditions associated with a high risk of malnutrition and infection.

Protective properties are found in the protein, lipid, carbohydrate, and leukocyte fractions of human milk. Most comparisons of morbidity between breast- and formula-fed infants have demonstrated significantly fewer or less severe illnesses in breast-fed infants. Human milk has been demonstrated to ameliorate or protect against infections with shigella, rotavirus, cholera, *Giardia lamblia,* and respiratory syncytial virus. A few studies have found no differences between feeding groups. None, however, has reported increases in morbidity among breast-fed infants. Disputes regarding human milk's efficacy in reducing the risk to infection stem from the difficulty in controlling for the potentially confounding or modifying environmental and demographic variables that play a part in outcome, such as possible contamination of artificial formula, number of caretakers with whom each child has contact, and behavioral characteristics of principal caretakers (24).

Three nonexclusive mechanisms have been proposed to explain human milk's protective properties: (a) the interaction of specific human milk constituents with potential pathogens in the infant's gastrointestinal lumen and the lumen's resident bacterial flora; (b) the direct modulation of the infant's immune system by these constituents through anti-inflammatory and other mechanisms; and (c) the promotion of the infant's nutritional well-being through human milk's high nutrient bioavailability and biological value.

The first mechanism results in the killing of potential pathogens, the prevention of invasion by pathogens of the gastrointestinal tract, and/or impairment of pathogen proliferation. One especially attractive feature of this mechanism is that it is responsive to pathogens encountered by the mother and infant in their common environments when the infant's mucosal immune response is not completely developed. Sensitized plasma cells are transported from the gastrointestinal and bronchotracheal-associated lymphatic tissues to the mammary gland during lactation (25,26). Specific antibodies provided by those cells are secreted in milk. The infant, therefore, has access to maternal antibodies directed specifically against potential pathogens. This provides human milk with a composition that can be viewed as environmentally specific. The second mechanism is postulated to result in the enhanced functioning of the immune system, either through the enhanced production of specific immunoproteins by the infant or a more rapid response to specified challenges. The postulated third mechanism is based on the association between poor nutritional status and impaired immune functions.

Goldman and Goldblum (27,28) described the constituents of human milk's immune complex: (a) it is biochemically heterogeneous; (b) it is present throughout all stages of lactation, i.e., from the production of colostrum through weaning; (c) its factors are resistant to digestion; (d) individual components interact in the inhibition or killing of microbial pathogens; (e) constituents are common to mucosal sites and are primarily protective of the gastrointestinal and respiratory systems; and (f) many appear to protect through noninflammatory mechanisms (Table 3). Anti-inflammatory agents in human milk include factors that double as direct protective agents, antioxidants, enzymes that degrade inflammatory mediators, antienzymes, cytoprotective agents, and modulators of leukocyte activation (29).

The presence of immune components in milk throughout lactation merits further consideration. The highest concentrations of most immunoproteins are found in colostrum; these levels usually fall for the first 3 to 4 months and then remain stable through the early stages of weaning. In the latter phases of weaning, however, the concentration of some factors may increase. Importantly, however, not all immune factors demonstrate the same pattern: lysozyme falls for the first 2 to 4 months and then increases tenfold at 6 months, a level at which it remains fairly consistently. For those factors whose concentrations remain at the lower levels observed at 2 to 4 months, increased volume between early and established periods of lactation partially offset decreases in concentration so that the quantities of immune proteins delivered to the infant remain significant.

The digestive, growth-promoting, and bioavailability-enhancing properties of human milk have been studied less well. Among the digestive properties of human milk, those that promote fat digestion are probably best studied (30). Bile salt–stimulated lipase activity in human milk complements the normally low level of pancreatic lipase activity of young infants. Its activity is stable at a pH of 3.5 at 37°C for 1 hr. The inactivation produced *in vitro* by trypsin and chymotrypsin, at pH 6.5, is prevented by bile salts. This stability and its normal activity in human milk should suffice to digest the amounts of fat usually consumed by breast-fed infants.

The other notable aspect of fat digestibility relates to the positional distribution of fatty acids in human milk triglycerides. In contrast to the equal distribution of the fatty acids in most dietary and depot fat triglycerides, fully saturated human milk triglycerides usually contain stearate in position 1, palmitate in position 2, and fatty acids of 14 to 18 carbon chain length in position 3. The 2-monoglyceride of palmitic acid is better absorbed than is free palmitic acid. Bile salt–stimulated lipase has no positional specificity; pancreatic lipase acts preferentially on the first and second position.

Significant fat malabsorption is reported in normal infants fed fats with palmitic acid in positions 1 and 2 and in premature infants fed human milk heated sufficiently to inactivate the milk's bile salt–stimulated lipase. Therefore, both features are potentially important to the infant.

The functional significance *in vivo* of growth-promoting and bioavailability-enhancing properties of human milk is less well described. Growth-promoting properties have been attributed to hormones, various immunologic proteins, and growth factors found in human milk (31–34). Their *in vivo* significance, however, has not been evaluated satisfactorily. Iron and zinc are excellent examples of nutrients with high bioavailability. The bioavailability of both trace elements is several times greater than that found in commercial formulas. The basis for their increased bioavailability is unclear. Folate is another example; it is secreted bound to a whey protein that may account for its high bioavailability. Increased bioavailability of nutrients is partially responsible for the very efficient utilization of many key nutrients in human milk.

TABLE 3. *Examples of immunoprotective factors in human milk*

Direct-acting antimicrobial agents
    Lactoferrin
    Lysozyme
    Secretory IgA
    Fibronectin
    Oligosaccharides—glycoconjugates
    Leukocytes
Protective factors produced by limited enzymatic digestion of substrates from human milk
    Fatty acids
    Monoglycerides
    B-casomorphins
Promoters of protective microflora
    Oligosaccharides

From ref. 28.

TABLE 4. *Energy intake, energy expenditure, and growth of breast-fed and formula-fed infants*

	Breast-fed infants		Formula-fed infants	
	1 month (n = 27)	4 months (n = 25)	1 month (n = 27)	4 months (n = 26)
Energy intake (Cal/kg/day)	99.9 (16.6)[a]	73.2 (11.1)	111.7 (18.0)	95.2 (11.9)
SMR (Cal/kg/day)	51.5 (4.1)	50.0 (6.0)	53.7 (5.5)	52.3 (4.4)
MOEE (Cal/kg/day)	45.2 (3.9)	44.1 (4.9)	48.0 (4.9)	47.1 (4.4)
Weight gain (g/day)	35.3 (10.7)	16.1 (7.7)	36.9 (12.7)	22.4 (7.9)
Weight gain (g/kg/day)	8.2 (2.5)	2.5 (1.2)	8.6 (2.9)	3.5 (1.2)

Adapted from ref. 37.
MOEE, minimal observable energy expenditure; SMR, sleeping metabolic rate.
[a] Mean (SD).

ENERGY INTAKE AND GROWTH OF BREAST-FED INFANTS

The average energy allowance for infants 0 to 6 months of age is estimated at 108 kilocalories per kilogram (Cal/kg) (13). That estimate is significantly greater than the observed intakes of exclusively breast-fed infants the first 4 months of life and during the subsequent period of mixed feeding, i.e., human milk and solid foods. Studies that have measured the energy content of milk by direct calorimetry estimate the energy intakes of exclusively breast-fed infants at approximately 100 Cal/kg at 1 month of age and approximately 70 to 80 Cal/kg by month 4. Studies that have used Atwater factors to convert the results of macronutrient analysis to energy or that assume energy densities of human milk (69 to 75 Cal/dl) usually estimate intakes of above 110 Cal/kg at 1 month and 80 to 90 Cal/kg at 4 months (35). In longitudinal studies with low attrition rates, absolute volumes of milk ingested by infants do not appear to change substantially during the first 4 months of lactation after the transition from colostrum to mature milk; milk volume remains at approximately 750 ml/day.

The addition of solid foods after the fourth month to previously exclusive human milk diets does not appear to alter the infant's energy intake adjusted for body size (36). Increased intakes of solid foods by breast-fed infants are accompanied by a decreased consumption of human milk, i.e., the absolute volume of milk consumed falls. This observation suggests that the lower energy intakes noted after the first month are physiologically regulated and are not the consequence of limited milk production by the mother.

Although comparable systematic longitudinal studies of infants fed bovine milk–based formulas have not been published, cross-sectional studies of formula-fed infants suggest that this group's energy intakes are close to 110 Cal/kg the first month and fall to between 90 and 100 Cal/kg by month 4. Higher rates of absorption of energy from human milk cannot fully explain the differences in energy intake (37). Southgate and Barret (38) measured equivalent losses of energy in urine and stool of infants fed human milk or bovine milk–based formula. Studies of formula intake during the transitional period from exclusive formula feeding to mixed diets are underway.

The long-term consequences, if any, of differences in

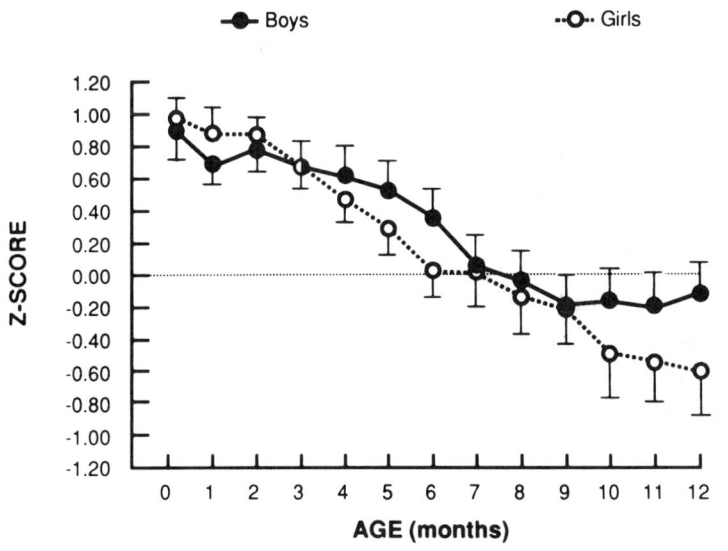

FIG. 1. Weight-for-age Z scores for boys and girls (mean ± SEM). (From ref. 39.)

energy intakes of breast- and formula-fed infants during the first year of life are not known. Over the short term, differences in growth rate and differences in the patterns of energy expenditure have been noted between feeding groups. Cross-sectional comparisons of breast- and formula-fed infants indicate mean weight gains of 8 to 9 g/kg/day for both groups at 1 month. By 4 months, however, formula-fed infants appear to gain weight faster (3.5 g/kg/day) than infants who are breast-fed (2.5 g/kg/day) (Table 4). Differences in body composition between groups, however, have not been demonstrated.

Longitudinal studies of breast-fed infants document significant deviations from NCHS (National Center for Health Statistics) growth patterns (39). Breast-fed infants do not appear to track weight/age percentiles established in early infancy. Weight-for-age Z scores for male and female breast-fed infants fall in the first year; length-for-age Z scores also fall, but the decrease is less (Fig. 1). Neither the timing of the introduction of solid foods nor the relatively large birth weight of the infants studied appears to explain this decline. The major clinical implication illustrated in Fig. 1 is that declining Z scores, even of this magnitude, are not necessarily indicative of inadequate human milk intake when breast-feeding is managed appropriately.

PATTERNS OF ENERGY EXPENDITURE IN BREAST- AND FORMULA-FED INFANTS

Differences in the energy consumption between breast-fed and formula-fed infants, "deviations" in growth patterns of breast-fed infants from NCHS references, and decreased rates and/or severity of infectious illness in breast-fed compared with formula-fed infants raise the possibility of other functional differences between the two groups. Ideally, long- and short-term consequences of infant feeding practices should be examined.

Among the short-term outcomes that have been studied are patterns of energy expenditure. These cross-sectional studies have examined sleeping metabolic rates (SMR), i.e., energy expenditure of sleeping infants between 3 and 4 hr postprandial; minimal observed rates of energy expenditure (MOEE), i.e., the lowest rate of energy expenditure sustained at least 5 min during the measurement of SMR; the thermic effect of food (TEF), i.e., percentage rise in energy expenditure at 0 to 2 hr postprandial above either SMR or MOEE; total energy expenditure (TEE); and energy available for discretionary activities, i.e., TEE − SMR (35,37). Measurements of metabolic rates and TEF have been obtained by classical calorimetry; TEE has been estimated by studies of the kinetics of water-bound ^{2}H and ^{18}O following the bolus administration of both isotopes (40).

SMR (Cal/kg/day) is approximately 4% lower in breast-fed than formula-fed infants at both 1 and 4 months of age. MOEE (Cal/kg/day) is 89% to 90% of SMR. MOEE is approximately 6% lower in breast-fed infants at 1 and 4 months. TEF is estimated at 6% to 8% in both feeding groups, at both ages. Because energy intake has been found to be a significant predictor of TEF, it is likely that large individual and experimental variability has precluded the detection of statistically significant differences between feeding groups. The physiological significance of differences in the groups' SMR and MOEE is not clear. Three possibilities merit careful consideration. Differences may reflect (a) adjustments in expenditure to dissipate excess energy consumption to lower the positive energy balance of formula-fed infants, (b) metabolic rates imposed by distinct nutrient balances in the respective diets, (c) disparities in time-related residuals in TEF. No physiologic mechanisms have been demonstrated that support either of the first two possible explanations. However, the positive relationships among energy intakes, SMR, MOEE, 24-hr heart rates, and rectal temperature suggest that feeding choice in infancy affects several basic parameters of energy expenditure.

Total daily energy expenditure (TDEE) also appears to differ between feeding groups. The mean rate of TDEE is approximately 64 Cal/kg/day in breast-fed infants at 1 and 4 months of age; corresponding values for formula-fed infants are 67 and 73 Cal/kg/day. The difference between TDEE and SMR may well reflect the amount of energy expended on activity—this discounts transient increases in SMR in response to feeding. These calculations indicate no statistically significant differences in activity between feeding groups. Approximately 13 Cal/kg/day are expended for activity by infants at 1 month of age and approximately 18 Cal/kg/day at 4 months of age. These values represent 13% and 25% of gross energy intakes or 20% and 28% of total daily energy expenditure of breast-fed infants at 1 and 4 months of age, respectively. Formula-fed infants spend approximately 12% and 20% of gross energy intakes on activity at 1 and 4 months of age, respectively; corresponding values expressed as percent of total daily energy expenditure are 19% and 25%. Age-related differences in the absolute and relative amounts of energy expended for activity underscore the potential importance of normal activity patterns in the regulation of energy balance in infants.

LONG-TERM CONSEQUENCES OF INFANT FEEDING CHOICE

Long-term consequences of infant feeding choice are difficult to examine retrospectively because of a lack of accurate documentation of degree and duration of breast-feeding and long-term follow-up. In addition, intervening events between infancy and adulthood are expected to diminish the consistency, strength, and specificity of potential interrelationships among diet, genetic endowment, environmental factors, and targeted outcomes. Although the incidence and severity of atopic disease appear to be less in breast-fed children through, at least, the fifth year (41), early feeding practices have not been demonstrated conclusively as a causal factor (24). The development of type I diabetes (42), lymphoma (43), and Crohn's disease (44) is also reported to be less frequent among children who were breast-fed. These reports, however, require both confirmation and the identification of mechanisms that mediate the putative protection.

Longer-term associations between breast-feeding and health outcomes, for example obesity and cardiovascular disease, are more speculative. To date, studies that have attempted to relate infant feeding practices to these outcomes have been severely limited by obstacles including inadequate definitions of the duration and degree of breast-feeding, the lack of characterization of fats in bovine milk–based diets, as well as the lack of information on the composition of supplementary foods and the timing of their introduction.

SUMMARY

The compositional differences between human milk and bovine milk–based formulas remain large and significant. These differences, however, do not appear to influence the ability of normal infants to digest and absorb adequate amounts of nutrients to maintain growth and development within normal limits. Decreased bioavailability of key nutrients, for example Fe and Zn, in formulas, is compensated by increased concentrations in the formulations. Vitamin K supplements at birth are recommended for both breast- and formula-fed infants. Supplementation of breast-fed infants with vitamins D and B_{12} is indicated under specified conditions.

Differences in various functional characteristics occur, however, between feeding groups. The rate and severity of gastrointestinal disease are less among breast-fed infants. Controversy remains regarding differences in the rates of respiratory infections between groups, but severity appears to be less among infants who are breast-fed. Immunoprotective constituents in human milk and child care practices related to breast-feeding appear to be important in protecting the child against infections.

Differences also have been noted in the amounts of energy, protein, and other nutrients consumed by breast- and formula-fed infants. Growth patterns of breast-fed infants deviate from NCHS references. Declines in weight-for-age and length-for-age Z scores are observed in breast-fed infants of mothers with normal lactation. Energy intakes and declines in anthropometric Z scores persist during periods of mixed feeding, i.e., human milk and solid foods. Therefore, it is likely that the decline in Z scores does not represent growth faltering. Comparable longitudinal studies of formula-fed infants are in progress.

Patterns of energy expenditure also differ among breast- and bottle-fed infants. Breast-fed infants have lower sleeping metabolic rates and lower rates of total energy expenditure than formula-fed infants. The physiological significance of these observations to energy regulation and dietary nutrient balance remains unresolved.

Longer-term consequences of infant feeding choice remain key areas of study. Breast-feeding is a factor in the reduced incidence and severity of atopic disease through at least 5 years of age. Preliminary reports suggest that breast-feeding may lead to a reduced risk for the development of type I diabetes, lymphoma, and Crohn's disease during childhood. Those reports require confirmation. Relationships between early feeding practices and longer-term outcomes, such as obesity and cardiovascular disease, remain highly speculative and are the subject of current research.

ACKNOWLEDGMENTS

This work was funded in part by grant no. 5R01HD21049 from the National Institute of Child Health and Human Development and in part by Hatch project no. 199408.

REFERENCES

1. *The Surgeon General's Report on Nutrition and Health.* Washington, DC: U.S. Department of Health and Human Services, 1988.
2. *Report of the Dietary Guidelines Advisory Committee on the Dietary Guidelines for Americans, 1990.* Hyattsville, MD: United States Department of Agriculture.
3. Garza C, Schanler RJ, Butte NF, Motil KJ. Special properties of human milk. *Clin Perinatol* 1987;14:104–128.
4. Garza C, Hopkinson J. Human milk synthesis and secretion. In: Grand R, Sutphen JL, eds. *Perinatal nutrition: theory and practice.* Boston: Butterworth, 1987;279–292.
5. Garza C, Butte NF. The effect of maternal nutrition on lactational performance. In: Kretchmer N, ed. *Frontiers in clinical nutrition.* Rockville, MD: Aspen Press, 1985;15–36.
6. Kronfeld DS. Major metabolic determinations of milk volume, mammary efficiency, and spontaneous ketosis in dairy cows. *J Dairy Sci* 1982;65:2204–2212.
7. Butte NF, Garza C, Smith EO, Nichols BL. Human milk intake and growth performance of exclusively breast-fed infants. *J Pediatr* 1984;104:187–195.
8. National Research Council, Food and Nutrition Board. Subcommittee on Nutrition and Diarrheal Diseases Control. *Nutritional Management of Acute Diarrhea in Infants and Children,* Washington, DC: National Academy Press, 1985.
9. Jensen RG. *The lipids of human milk.* Boca Raton, FL: CRC Press, 1989.
10. Wright S, Bolton C. Breast milk fatty acids in mothers of children with atopic eczema. *Br J Nutr* 1989;62:693–697.
11. Specker BL, Tsang RC, Hollis BW. Effect of race and diet on human-milk vitamin D and 25-hydroxyvitamin D. *Am J Dis Child* 1985;139:1134–1137.
12. Specker BL, Valanis B, Hertzberg V, Edward N, Tsang RC. Sunshine exposure and serum 25-hydroxyvitamin D concentrations in exclusively breast-fed infants. *J Pediatr* 1985;107:372–376.

13. National Research Council, Food and Nutrition Board. Subcommittee on the Tenth Edition of the RDAs. *Recommended dietary allowances,* 10th ed. Washington, DC: National Academy Press, 1989.
14. Committee on Nutrition, American Academy of Pediatrics. *Pediatric nutrition handbook.* Elk Grove Village, IL, 1985;39–45.
15. Chang SJ, Kirksey A. Pyridoxine supplementation of lactating mothers: relation to maternal nutrition status and vitamin B-6 concentrations in milk. *Am J Clin Nutr* 1990;51:826–831.
16. Hoffman A, Hazebroek MD, Valkenburg HA. A randomized trial of sodium intake and blood pressure in newborn infants. *JAMA* 1983;250:370–373.
17. Miller JZ, Weinberger MH, Christian JC, Daugherty SA. Familial resemblance in the blood pressure response to sodium restriction. *Am J Epidemiol* 1987;126(5):822–830.
18. Oski FA, Landaw SA. Inhibition of iron absorption from human milk by baby food. *Am J Dis Child* 1980;134:459–460.
19. Casey CE, Neville MC, Hambidge KM. Studies in human lactation: secretion of zinc, copper, and manganese in human milk. *Am J Clin Nutr* 1989;49:773–785.
20. Lonnerdal B, Keen CL, Hurley LS. Iron, copper, zinc, and manganese in milk. *Annu Rev Nutr* 1981;1:149–174.
21. Krebs NF, Hambidge KM, Jacobs MA, Rasbach JO. The effects of dietary zinc supplement during lactation on longitudinal changes in maternal zinc status and milk zinc concentrations. *Am J Clin Nutr* 1985;41:560–570.
22. Hambidge KM, Walravens PA, Casey CE, Brown RM, Bender C. Plasma zinc concentrations of breast-fed infants. *J Pediatr* 1979;94:607–608.
23. Salmenpera L, Perheentupa J, Pakarinen P, Siimes MA. Cu nutrition in infants during prolonged exclusive breast-feeding: low intake but rising serum concentrations of Cu and ceruloplasmin. *Am J Clin Nutr* 1986;43:251–257.
24. Kramer MS. Breast feeding and child health: methodologic issues in epidemiologic research. In: Goldman AS, Atkinson SA, Hanson LA, eds. *Human lactation 3: the effects of human milk on the recipient infant.* New York: Plenum Press, 1987;339–360.
25. Fishuat M, Murphy D, Neifert M, et al. Bronchomammary axis in the immune response to respiratory syncytial virus. *J Pediatr* 1981;99:186–191.
26. Goldblum RM, Ahlstedt S, Carlsson B, et al. Antibody-forming cells in human colostrum after oral immunization. *Nature (London)* 1975;257:797–799.
27. Goldman AS, Goldblum RM. Immunological system in human milk: characteristics and effects. In: Lebenthal E, ed. *Textbook of gastroenterology and nutrition in early childhood,* 2nd ed. New York: Raven Press, 1989;135–142.
28. Goldman AS, Goldblum RM. Human milk: immunologic-nutritional relationships. *Ann NY Acad Sci* 1990(May 15);236–245.
29. Goldman AS, Thorpe LW, Goldblum RM, Hanson LA. Anti-inflammatory properties of human milk. *Acta Paediatr Scand* 1986;75:689–695.
30. Jensen RG, Clark RM, DeJong FA, Hamosh M, Liao TH, Mehta NR. The lipolytic triad: breast milk and pancreatic lipases; physiologic implications of their characteristics in digestion of dietary fats. *J Pediatr Gastroenterol Nutr* 1982;1:243–255.
31. Koldovsky O, Bedrick A, Pollack P, Rao RK, Thornburg W. Possible physiological role of hormones and hormone-related substances present in milk. In: Hanson LA, ed. *Biology of human milk,* vol 15. New York: Raven Press, 1988;123–139.
32. Mushtaha AA, Schmalstieg FC, Hughes TK Jr, Rajaraman S, Rudloff HE, Goldman AS. Chemokinetic agents for monocytes in human milk: possible role of tumor necrosis factor-α. *Pediatr Res* 1989;25:629–633.
33. Zimecki M, Pierce-Cretel A, Spik G, Wieczorek Z. Immunoregulatory properties of the proteins present in human milk. *Arch Immunol Ther Exp* 1987;35:351–360.
34. Klagsbrun M. Human milk stimulates DNA synthesis and cellular proliferation in cultured fibroblasts. *Proc Natl Acad Sci USA* 1978;75:5057–5061.
35. Butte NF, Smith ED, Garza C. Energy utilization of breast-fed and formula-fed infants. *Am J Clin Nutr* 1990;51:350–358.
36. Garza C, Stuff J, Butte N. Growth of the breast-fed infant. In: Goldman AS, Atkinson SA, Hanson LA, eds. *Human lactation 3: the effects of human milk upon the recipient infant.* New York: Plenum Press, 1989;109–121.
37. Butte N, Wong W, Garza C, Klein P. Adequacy of human milk for meeting energy requirements during early infancy. In: Atkinson SA, Hanson LA, Chandra RK, eds. *Breastfeeding, nutrition, infection and infant growth in developed and emerging countries.* St John's, Newfoundland, Canada: ARTS Biomedical, 1990;359–368.
38. Southgate DAT, Barret IM. The intake and excretion of calorific constituents of milk by babies. *Br J Nutr* 1966;20:363–372.
39. Dewey KG, Heinig MJ, Mommsen LA, Lonnerdal B. Growth patterns of breast-fed infants during the first year of life: the Darling study. In: Atkinson SA, Hanson LA, Chandra RK, eds. *Breastfeeding, nutrition, infection and infant growth in developed and emerging countries.* St. John's, Newfoundland, Canada: ARTS Biomedical, 1990;273.
40. Lifson N, McClintock R. Theory of use of the turnover rates of body water for measuring energy and material balance. *J Theor Biol* 1966;12:46–74.
41. Chandra RK. Long-term health consequences of early infant feeding. In: Atkinson SA, Hanson LA, Chandra RK, eds. *Breastfeeding, nutrition, infection and infant growth in developed and emerging countries.* St John's, Newfoundland, Canada: ARTS Biomedical, 1990;47–54.
42. Mayer EJ, Hamman RF, Gay EC, Lezotte DC, Savitz DA, Klingensimth GJ. Reduced risk of insulin dependent diabetes mellitus (IDMM) among breast fed children: a case control study. *Diabetes* 1988;47:1625–1632.
43. Davis MK, Savitz DA, Graubard BI. Infant feeding and childhood cancer. *Lancet* 1988;2:365–368.
44. Koletzko S, Sherman P, Corey M, Griffiths A, Smith C. Role of infant feeding practices in development of Crohn's disease in childhood. *Br Med J* 1989;298:1617–1618.

CHAPTER 5

Mother-Infant Interaction

Relationship to Early Infant Nutrition and Feeding

Helen Britton

Although nutritional status and mother-infant interaction appear to be unrelated topics, they share an important common ground, the feeding environment. Furthermore, success in each is measured by similar standards: physical growth, cognitive performance, and child behavior.

The process of infant feeding is a complex relationship involving both the acquisition of nutrients by the infant as well as the interaction between the infant and the mother (Fig. 1). This interaction may, itself, be influenced by current and past nutritional status, medical and developmental factors, patterns of cue-giving and response unique to each mother-infant pair, and the synchronous adjustment of the dyad to specific behavioral states. Not only do these factors influence the initial feeding interaction, but the results of that initial interaction have a continuing, compounding effect on the mother-infant relationship, either negatively or positively.

A positive outcome results when the process of feeding provides both physical comfort, by satisfying hunger, as well as a pleasurable social experience. In those instances the infant maintains interest, and is more socially responsive during feedings, using less energy because the caregiver is more attuned to his/her cues. The long-term results include a better nutritional outcome and continued positive feeding experiences.

A negative feeding experience, on the other hand, may have both short-term effects on an infant's nutritional and development status as well as serious long-term effects, as a result of the compounding characteristic of the factors determining the delicate mother-infant relationship.

HISTORICAL PERSPECTIVE

Throughout history, it has been recognized that infant feeding fulfills not only an important nutritional need but also facilitates critical early social interaction. This significant interaction has been analyzed in psychological, educational, social, and medical literatures.

In the 1940s, Freud's secondary drive theory was based on the hypothesis that infant-adult relationships have their roots in the infant's need for the provision of food by the caregiver (1). Harlow (2) redefined the infant-food-caregiver relationship in the late 1950s by demonstrating, with baby monkeys, that physical contact was as important as the hunger drive in the mother-infant relationship.

In the 1970s, Bowlby further expounded on the work of Harlow by placing it into the framework of evolutionary biology (3). He theorized that infant behavior is adapted to complement caregiver behavior when the caregiver's behavior is appropriate and responsive to infant cues. Since human infants are altricial, i.e., physically dependent on their caregivers, Bowlby postulated that, in order to survive, they develop behaviors that effectively elicit and maintain maternal proximity. Examples of such behavior are crying, sucking, making eye contact, smiling, and cuddling. These proximity-seeking behaviors may be cues to fulfill either a physical need, such as hunger, or an emotional need, such as contact, thus creating the necessary association of physical and social needs. Bowlby's theory laid the foundation for

---

H. Britton: Department of Pediatrics, University of Utah School of Medicine, Salt Lake City, Utah 84132.

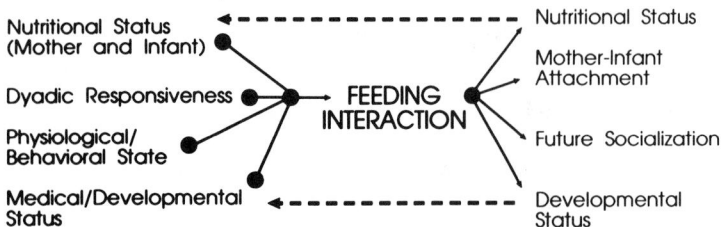

FIG. 1. Diagrammatic model showing the multifactorial nature of the feeding interaction.

current thought, which suggests that when a caregiver does not respond appropriately to proximity-seeking cues demanding feeding and contact, both nutritional and social consequences may result.

Today, one of the most reliable and consistent methods of evaluating mother-infant interaction is the observational scale developed by Dr. Kathryn Barnard (4), which analyzes the dyadic behavior occurring between mother and infant in the feeding situation. High reciprocity scores for a mother-infant pair not only correlate significantly with other measures of mother-infant interaction, but also with later cognitive development as measured by the Bayley Scales (4). This framework, which relates developmental outcome to early dyadic feeding interactions, is now being applied to high-risk populations such as premature infants and infants born to drug-using mothers (5,6).

NUTRITIONAL STATUS OF MOTHER AND INFANT

The nutritional status of mother and infant, both pre- and postnatally, may affect the feeding interaction. The effect of prenatal maternal malnutrition on the developing infant depends on the duration of the malnutrition and the gestational age of the fetus when it occurs.

Fetal malnutrition may result from maternal malnutrition as well as from placental insufficiency or fetal disease processes. Long-term fetal malnutrition may lead to reduced head size and abnormal neurobehavioral performance (Fig. 2). Lipper et al. (7), in a study of small-for-dates infants, observed that only infants with reduced head size showed definable neurodevelopmental delays. Other studies, however, such as those of Brazelton et al. (8) and Vuori et al. (9), indicate that infants malnourished *in utero* have decreased capacity to respond to appropriate cues. Small-for-gestational-age infants studied shortly after birth were found to have poor muscle tone and to be less capable of responsive and focused interactive behavior (10). The inferior proximity-seeking behaviors in these infants, such as decreased sucking and responsive smiling, increase the likelihood of both social and nutritional deprivation with inherent long-term consequences.

Postnatal malnutrition also results in negative social and nutritional consequences. Dodge et al. (11) found that malnourished infants exhibited increased lethargic behavior, decreased attentional ability, an inability to motivate social response, as well as nonspecific electroencephalographic changes. More recently, early human malnutrition has been shown to alter sleep-wake states, decreasing the period of sustained quiet sleep and interfering with normal diurnal cycles (12). Nutritional rehabilitation may reverse some of these effects, although long-term studies suggest persistence of abnormalities in intellectual functioning (13).

The effects of chronic marginal nutrition, a level of deprivation not uncommon in sections of the United States today, appear to result in behavioral characteristics similar to what might be expected with more severe nutritional deprivation. Cravioto and Delacardie (14) found that poorly nourished infants tended to have increased frequency of illness and, thus, less time for interactional learning; they tended to appear apathetic and inattentive, and were generally less responsive to environmental stimuli. This supports the theory that infant malnutrition results in behavioral changes that first decrease the infant's capacity for positive interaction and the resultant learning experience and, second, elicit negative interaction, compounding the initial deficits.

In addition to infant malnutrition, postpartum maternal malnutrition may also have a negative impact on both physical and behavioral development of the infant. In a breast-feeding mother, malnutrition may produce diminished milk volume and maternal fatigue, reducing both the food supply and the maternal energy available for emotional nurturing of the infant (Fig. 3).

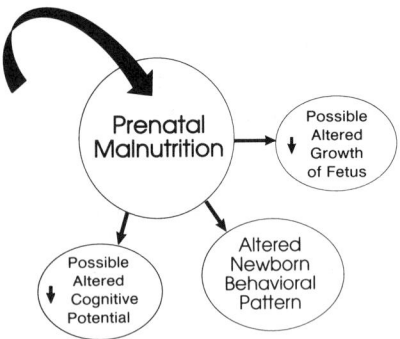

FIG. 2. Illustration of the threefold effect of prenatal malnutrition.

DYADIC RESPONSIVENESS AND FEEDING

Brody (15), in one of the earliest studies investigating infant feeding patterns and maternal behavior, concluded that maternal behavior during feeding is representative of a mother's overall behavior toward her infant. A very specific example of maternal responsiveness to early infant cues is the suck-pause phenomenon that occurs during feeding. Kaye (16) found that infants suck in 8- to 10-sec bursts separated by 2- to 5-sec pauses. The pauses appear to have no physiologic basis, such as the need to swallow or breathe. During the pause, most mothers talk, smile, or make eye contact with their infants. This led Kaye to hypothesize that the suck-pause sequence in infant feeding is one of the earliest examples of mother-infant dialogue.

If successful feeding interaction is defined as the process by which infants acquire optimal nutritional and social nurturing, one of the most important determinants is dyadic responsiveness of mother and infant. Barnard et al. (17) describe this relationship as a mutually adaptive dance between partners. They continue the analogy by explaining that each partner must have certain skills including the skill to read each other's signals, and should one partner lack the skills the dance goes less smoothly. With practice, as in dancing, the feeding interaction becomes smoother and requires decreasing effort from each partner. Barnard's Nursing Child Assessment Feeding Scales (NCAFS), developed to assess this synchronous interaction, have been used to follow a large population of children through the second grade. Scores on the feeding scales have correlated with Bayley scores at 2 years, and with other behavioral patterns, such as expressive and receptive language, at 3 years (18).

Barnard's feeding scales assess maternal feeding behavior within the categories of sensitivity to cues, response to distress, and cognitive and social-emotional growth fostering (19). "Sensitivity to cues" behaviors include comfortable positioning of the baby for feeding and socialization, responses to infant gaze or verbalization, and maternal response to infant signals, allowing for pauses in feeding and social interaction. "Response to distress" includes appropriate maternal response to obvious and subtle signs of infant stress such as when the infant cries, averts gaze, or makes an "unhappy" face. "Social-emotional growth fostering" behavior may be maternal singing, touching, or finger play, whereas cognitive-fostering activities involve maternal verbalizations or facilitation of the infant's exploratory behavior.

Many studies have evaluated infant positioning during feeding as an important type of body language. Clearly, the mother who fails to have body contact with her infant while loosely holding the bottle and watching television, provides a much different feeding experience from the mother who cradles her infant close to her body, quietly attentive to her infant's needs.

Certainly the infant's behavior also affects the delicate feeding interaction. In 1937, Gesell and Ilg (20) concluded that an infant's feeding behavior is the most inclusive and informative indicator of the infant's personality. Barnard (19), acknowledging this factor, evaluates two major areas of infant behavior in the feeding situation: clarity of cues and responsiveness to the parent. "Clarity of cues" involves the infant's skill in signaling his sense of hunger and satisfaction, as well as his desire for social interaction. "Responsiveness to cues" includes infant responses, such as smiling or direct gaze, which have been elicited by parental cues such as touch or verbalization.

The studies done, therefore, on the relationship between maternal and infant behavior during feeding indicate strongly that behavioral responses of both the mother and the infant during feeding are indicative of social responses seen on a broader scale in other social instances. There also seems to be a clear relationship between interactional behaviors during feeding, mother-infant attachment, and cognitive and social development of the infant (Fig. 4).

PHYSIOLOGIC AND BEHAVIORAL STATE AND FEEDING

A third important variable in feeding interaction is the infant's physiological and behavioral state. Studies by Brazelton (21) on the relationship between an infant's behavioral state and its capacity to interact have provided an exciting framework for many studies of synchrony in caregiver-infant relationships. Behaviors identified during the Brazelton examination can be categorized into several clusters: habituation, orientation, motor performance and tone, range and regulation of state, autonomic response, and reflex response. The elicitation of these responses will vary depending upon the

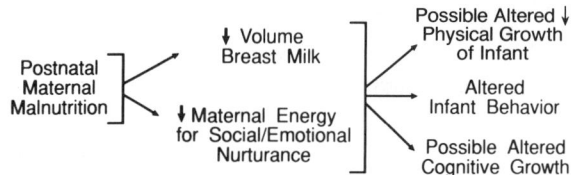

FIG. 3. Illustration of the escalating effect of postnatal maternal malnutrition on the developing infant.

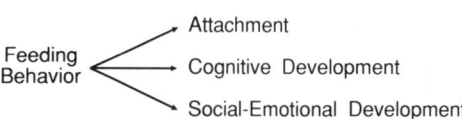

FIG. 4. Three major developmental outcomes related to early infant feeding interactions.

behavioral state of the infant, which may range from deep sleep through the quiet-alert state to the state of irritable crying. The infant provides additional cues through its repertoire of behaviors that are meant to communicate needs to his caregivers. Orienting and alerting responses indicate a desire to maintain interaction, whereas gaze aversion and habituation signal the need to reduce external stimulation.

Poor state regulation in early infancy may lead to both poor intake and increased energy utilization. This is frequently a problem in babies of substance-abusing mothers and in premature infants. One example of poor state regulation is the habituation response to an aversive auditory stimulus. Most sleeping babies initially respond to an external stimulus, such as a ringing bell, with some form of body movement. If the disturbing stimulus continues, the baby responds in one of two ways, either gradually "tuning out" the disturbance, and continuing in a deeper sleep, or changing to an awake state (22). In infants with poor state regulation, the auditory stimulus may provoke a sudden change from deep sleep to tremulous crying. Infants with poor state regulation may also be difficult to bring to the appropriate state of arousal, "quiet alert," for optimal feeding and caregiver-infant interaction to take place. Furthermore, the level of arousal of an infant during feeding will affect the simultaneous reception of visual, auditory, tactile, and kinesthetic cues. Problems, therefore, with state regulation can affect the synchrony of the mother-infant interaction, decrease the intake of nutrients, and decrease available energy for cognitive stimulation (Fig. 5). Subsequent consequences may include a long-term effect on the ability to interact.

MEDICAL/DEVELOPMENTAL FACTORS AND THE FEEDING INTERACTION

Current research has focused on medical and developmental factors and how they relate to the feeding interaction. Of particular interest is the large population of premature infants and the growing population of infants affected by maternal drug abuse. These infants bring a new set of physical problems to the question of feeding interaction, including oral-motor dysfunction. In addition, these infants are likely to have disorders that directly alter their ability to regulate their behavioral state and to send or respond to cues.

Compared to the term infant, the premature infant provides a different set of feeding and socialization cues to its parents (23,24). Optimal feeding behavior and nutritional intake may depend on the ability of the caregiver to help the infant regulate his state, enhance his level of arousal at feeding time, and modify patterns of contingent response (25). Appropriately and continually modifying the surrounding environment for these infants appears to further enhance both physical and cognitive growth. Als and her associates (26) have demonstrated that individualized behavioral and environmental care for very low birth weight preterm infants improves both their medical and behavioral status as measured by oxygen requirements, length of time on a ventilator, onset of normalized feeding patterns, and improved scores on both the mental and psychomotor Bayley scales at 3, 6, and 9 months of age. Individualized care implies that caregivers are taught to recognize each infant's behavioral cues, which may be discerned through measures such as the Newborn Behavioral Assessment Scale, in order to develop individualized caregiving techniques.

Other studies have investigated methods of improving state regulation and interactional capabilities of premature and other medically at-risk infants during feeding. Nonnutritive sucking is one feeding-related behavior that appears to enhance both physical growth and weaning from gavage feeds, by increasing nutrient absorption from the gut, as well as helping infants achieve and maintain states of alertness prior to routine feeding (27,28). State regulation, as well as other interactional abilities, may be adversely influenced by both obstetric medications (29) and medications given in the neonatal intensive care setting. When possible, type and dosage schedule used in intensive care need to be adjusted to feeding schedules and opportunities for social interaction.

Other medical conditions, such as blindness, deafness, and cleft palate, may also adversely affect mother-infant interactions during feeding unless caregivers are trained in appropriate alterations of cue giving and contingent response.

OTHER CONSIDERATIONS AND CONTROVERSIES

Of Breast and Bonding

Controversy exists regarding the developmental and social advantages of breast-feeding, especially with respect to its effect on the improved cognitive outcomes observed in some studies of breast-fed infants (30). It is

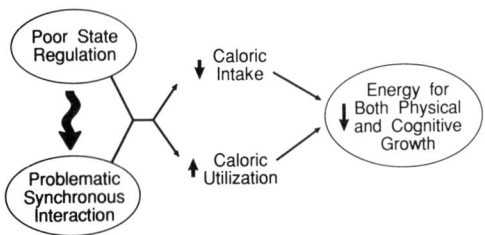

FIG. 5. Relationship of state regulation, synchronous interaction, nutritional status, and developmental outcome.

unclear, however, whether the breast-feeding itself, or the interactional exchange that it facilitates, is responsible for these observations. Certainly, breast-feeding necessitates holding the infant in close skin-to-skin contact with the mother's body, and allows for maternal detection of sensitive physical cues communicated via the infant's suck directly on the mother's breast. A bottle-feeding mother must, of course, make a more conscious effort to provide this type of infant contact and to sense, as easily, the infant's sucking cues. Using the Barnard scales, breast-feeding mothers do not show a significant difference in feeding interactions when compared to bottle-feeding mothers (4). Cunningham et al. (31), however, indicates that holding an infant close to the body does facilitate secure mother-infant attachment. Perhaps this closeness, as well as other subtle interactional behaviors necessitated by the act of breast-feeding, are responsible for the improved developmental scores reported in older children who had been breast-fed.

Kangaroo Care

Kangaroo care is a new method of caring for very low birth weight infants which involves skin-to-skin contact and breast-feeding as soon as the infants are medically stable. The infant is clothed only in a diaper and held upright and prone between the mothers breasts, allowing for self-regulatory breast-feeding. Appropriate use of kangaroo care appears to provide adequate temperature regulation, improve oxygenation, reduce apnea and bradycardia, improve the infant's ability to regulate his state, and enhance the volume of breast milk and duration of breast-feeding (32,33). Kangaroo care is, thus, an example of a social and medical intervention that may provide more optimal outcomes for infants at risk.

Obesity and Failure to Thrive

The role of the infant-caregiver feeding-behavior relationship on the nutritional state of the older child cannot be overlooked. Often problems, such as obesity and failure to thrive, reflect long-standing disturbances in the infant-caregiver relationship that may have stemmed from a lack of attention to, or misreading of, infant cues. Behavioral and developmental difficulties that frequently accompany these nutritional problems may be further indications that the food-infant-caregiver relationship is not in harmony.

SUMMARY

Recognition of the important interaction that occurs between the mother and infant during feeding may assist in the production of a positive outcome on both the infant's nutritional as well as developmental status. Lack of recognition of this important interaction may have negative short-term, as well as long-term, effects on both of these parameters.

REFERENCES

1. Freud S. *An outline of psychoanalysis.* New York: Norton, 1940.
2. Harlow HF. The development of affectional patterns in infant monkeys. In: Foss BM, ed. *Determinants of infant behavior,* vol 1. London: Methven, 1961.
3. Lamb ME, Thompson RA, Gardner W, Charnov E. The development of attachment theory. In: *Infant-mother attachment: the origins and developmental significance of individual differences in strange situation behavior.* Hillsdale, New Jersey: Lawrence Erlbaum, 1985;8–26.
4. Barnard KE, Eyres SS. *Child health assessment, part 2: the first year of life.* (Publication Number DHEW No. HRA 79-25). Washington, DC: U.S. Government Printing Office, 1979.
5. Barnard KE, Bee HL, Hammond MA. Developmental changes in maternal interactions with terms and preterm infants. *Infant Behav Dev* 1984;7:101–113.
6. Beckwith L, Cohen SE, Kopp CB, Parmelee AH, Marcy TG. Caregiver-infant interaction and early cognitive development in preterm infants. *Child Dev* 1976;47:579–587.
7. Lipper E, Lee K, Gartner LM, Grellong B. Determinants of neurobehavioral outcome in low-birth-weight infants. *Pediatrics* 1981;67:505.
8. Brazelton TB, Tronick E, Lechtig A, Lasky KE, Klein RE. The behavior of nutritionally deprived Guatemalan infants. *Dev Med Child Neurol* 1977;19:364–372.
9. Vuori L, Christiansen N, Clement J, Mora JO, Wagner M, Herrera MG. Nutritional supplementation and the outcome of pregnancy. II. Visual habituation at 15 days. *Am J Clin Nutr* 1979;32:463–469.
10. Als H, Tronick E, Adamon L, Brazelton TB. The behavior of the full-term but underweight infant. *Dev Med Child Neurol* 1976;18:590–602.
11. Dodge PR, Prensky AL, Feigin RD. In: Holmes S *Nutrition and the developing nervous system.* St. Louis: CV Mosby, 1975.
12. Peirano P, Fagioli I, Singh BB, Salzarulo P. Effect of early human malnutrition on waking and sleep organization. *Early Hum Dev* 1989;20:67–76.
13. Stoch MA, Smythe PM. Fifteen year developmental study of severe undernutrition during infancy on subsequent physical growth and intellectual functioning. *Arch Dis Child* 1976;51:327.
14. Cravioto J, Delacardie ER. Nutrition, mental development and learning. In: Falkner F, Tanner JM, eds. *Human growth. III.* New York: Plenum Press, 1978.
15. Brody S. *Patterns of mothering.* New York: International Universities Press, 1956.
16. Kaye K. Toward the origin of dialogue. In: Schaffer HR, ed. *Studies in mother-infant interaction.* New York: Academic Press, 1977.
17. Barnard KE, Hammond MA, Booth CL, Bee HL, Mitchell SK, Spieker SJ. Measurement and meaning of parent-child interaction. In: Morrison F, Lord C, Keating D, eds. *Applied developmental psychology,* vol III. Orlando, Florida: Academic Press, 1985.
18. Eyres SJ, Barnard KE, Gray CA. *Child health assessment part III; 2–4 years.* Final report of project supported by grant number RO2-NU-00559, Division of Nursing, Bureau of Health Manpower, Health Resources Administration, Department of Health, Education, and Welfare, 1979.
19. Barnard KE. *Nursing Child Assessment Feeding Scale* (instruction manual). Seattle: Maternal and Child Nursing Department, School of Nursing, University of Washington, 1978.
20. Gesell A, Ilg F. *Feeding behaviors of infants.* Philadelphia: JB Lippincott, 1937.
21. Nugent K. *Using the Neonatal Behavioral Assessment Scale with infants and their families.* White Plains, New York: March of Dimes Birth Defects Foundation, 1985.

22. Brazelton TB. *Neonatal Behavioral Assessment Scale.* Philadelphia: JB Lippincott, 1973.
23. Lester BM, Hoffman J, Brazelton TB. The rhythmic structure of mother-infant interaction in term and preterm infants. *Child Dev* 1985;56:15–27.
24. Caesar P, Daniels H, Devlieger H, et al. Feeding behavior in preterm neonates. *Early Hum Dev* 1982;7:331–346.
25. Behnke M, Gill NE, Conlon M, Anderson GC. Determining optimal behavioral states for feeding premature infants. *Infant Behavior and Development* 1989;11(Special ICIS Issue):23.
26. Als H, Lawhon G, Brown E, Giber R, Duffy F, McAnulty G, Blickman JG. Individualized behavioral and environmental care for the very low birth weight preterm infant at high risk for bronchopulmonary dysplasia: neonatal intensive care unit and developmental outcome. *Pediatrics* 1986;78(6):1123–1132.
27. Bernbaum J, Pereira G, Watkins J. Nonnutritive sucking during gavage feeding enhance growth and maturation in premature infants. *Pediatrics* 1983;71:41–45.
28. Woodson R, Hamilton C. The effect of nonnutritive sucking on heart rate in preterm infants. *Dev Psychobiol* 1988;21:207–213.
29. Sanders-Phillips K, Strauss ME, Gutberlet RL. The effect of obstetric medication on newborn infant feeding behavior. *Infant Behav Dev* 1988;11:251–263.
30. Morley R, Cole TJ, Powell R, Lucas A. Mother's choice to provide breast milk and developmental outcome. *Arch Dis Child* 1988;63:1382–1385.
31. Cunningham N, Anisfeld E, Casper V, Noyzce M. Infant carrying, breast feeding, and mother-infant relations. *Lancet* 1987;1:379.
32. Acolet D, Sleth K, Whitelaw A. Oxygenation, heart rate and temperature in very low birthweight infants during skin-to-skin contact with their mothers. *Acta Paediatr Scand* 1989;78:193–198.
33. Whitelaw A, Heisterkamp G, Sheath K, Acolet D, Richards M. Skin-to-skin contact for very low birthweight infants and their mothers: a randomized trial of "Kangaroo Care". *Arch Dis Child* 63:1377–1381.

CHAPTER 6

Disorders of the Fat-Soluble Vitamins A, D, E, and K

Robert E. Olson

Vitamins A, D, E, and K are fat-soluble vitamins. They were discovered between 1917 and 1929, subsequently isolated, characterized chemically, and synthesized. Their chemical names, precursors and biologically active forms are shown in Table 1. Much has been learned about the mode of action of these vitamins during the past two decades.

Fat- and water-soluble vitamins differ beyond simple solubility. Fat-soluble vitamins, as a class, deal with the regulation of protein synthesis. This is in contrast to the B-complex vitamins, which form coenzymes that catalyze the oxidation of small molecules and the production of energy. The active forms of vitamins A and D are now identified as ligands for receptors belonging to a superfamily of steroid and thyroid hormone receptors that interact with DNA and control gene expression. Vitamin E is an antioxidant but, in addition, controls the synthesis of some biologically significant proteins. Tocopherol may be, like vitamin A, a double-threat vitamin, providing both epigenetic and genetic regulatory activities. Vitamin K controls the synthesis of a number of coagulation factors at the posttranslational level.

In addition to being soluble in fats and oils, these lipid vitamins have interesting chemical properties. They resemble the steroid hormones because of their isoprenoid structure and because each has a set of active homologues, called *vitamers*. These vitamins also require carrier proteins for transport, which is true of all lipids in the body. Vitamins A and D are carried by specific plasma proteins; vitamins E and K are carried by plasma lipoproteins, principally the low-density lipoproteins (LDL).

All of the fat-soluble vitamins are converted to active forms. Retinal, which is not concerned with protein synthesis, is an oxidation product of vitamin A (retinol) and functions as a photosensitive pigment in the eye. Retinoic acid is a further oxidation product of vitamin A and is the active form for interaction with a DNA receptor. Even α-tocopherol must be ionized before its electrons become available for antioxidation; vitamin K must be reduced to the hydroquinone in order to participate in the production of γ-carboxyglutamic acid.

Although these vitamins are not required by lower forms such as bacteria and other unicellular organisms, they are needed by higher organisms to regulate the synthesis of proteins concerned with differentiation, bone and mineral metabolism, reproduction, and the proliferation of various cell types.

Fat-soluble vitamins are absorbed and distributed via a common pathway (Fig. 1). They are absorbed with other lipids and incorporated into chylomicrons in the gut. Most of the chylomicron triglyceride is cleared by lipoprotein lipase and the free fatty acids are taken up, primarily, by adipose tissue. The chylomicron remnant, a smaller spherical lipoprotein that remains after triglyceride clearance, contains cholesterol and other nonsaponifiable materials including all the fat-soluble vitamins. It is taken up by an apo-E lipoprotein receptor–mediated event in the liver. Two fat-soluble vitamins, E and K, are repackaged and incorporated into very low-density lipoprotein (VLDL), which is the secretory lipoprotein of the liver, and follow the fate of VLDL and LDL and probably enter tissues by means of the LDL receptor. Vitamins A and D, on the other hand, have specific transporters. Vitamin A is reprocessed in the liver and secreted as a complex with retinol-binding protein (RBP). Vitamin D is hydroxylated to 25-OH-vitamin D in the liver and then secreted with a specific α_2-globulin. Only vitamins A and E are stored exten-

---

R. E. Olson: Departments of Medicine and Pharmacology, Health Sciences Center, State University of New York at Stony Brook, Stony Brook, New York 11794-8651.

TABLE 1. *Characteristics of the fat-soluble vitamins*

Vitamin	Date of discovery	Chemical name	Precursor	Active form
Vitamin A	1917	Retinol	β-Carotene	Retinal, retinoic acid
Vitamin D	1920	Cholecalciferol	7-Dehydrocholesterol	1,25–Dihydroxycholecalciferol
Vitamin E	1925	α-Tocopherol	None	α-Tocopherol anion
Vitamin K	1929	Phylloquinone	Menadione	Dihydrophylloquinone

sively in the body; vitamins D and K are present in comparatively small amounts.

Xerophthalmia, rickets, and neonatal hemorrhage, all caused by dietary deficiencies of fat-soluble vitamins in children, have been recognized since the turn of the century. The spinocerebellar syndrome, due to vitamin E deficiency, is relatively rare and is a more recent discovery. Frequency of the more common fat-soluble vitamin deficiency diseases has declined in recent years with the development of better preventive medicine and definitive therapies, although recurrence in malnourished children secondary to physiological immaturity, child abuse, or malnutrition of genetic origin, has been noted. Very low birth weight infants are particularly at risk, and full-term newborns are more susceptible than older infants. Premature infants are particularly at risk because of biochemical immaturity and failure of the placenta to transport lipids effectively until the middle of the third trimester.

In this chapter, each fat-soluble vitamin will be discussed under the following topics: (a) history, (b) chemistry, (c) absorption and transport, (d) metabolism, (e)

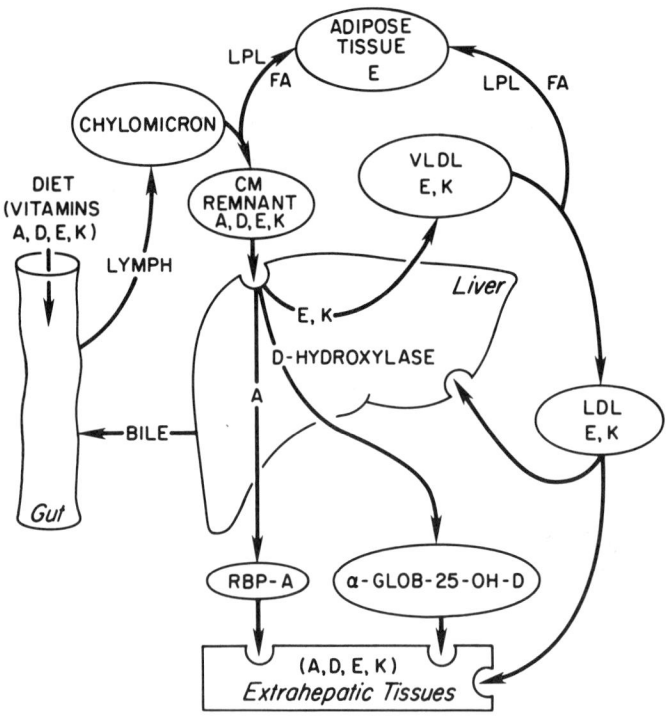

FIG. 1. Absorption and transport of the fat-soluble vitamins. Monoglycerides, fatty acids, and fat-soluble vitamins are absorbed in the gut, which leads to the formation of chylomicrons rich in triglycerides and containing vitamins A, D, E, and K. This very low-density particle is altered by lipoprotein lipase (LPL) in the capillary endothelium to hydrolyze triglycerides to glycerol and free fatty acids (FA), which are taken up by adipose and other tissue cells. The resulting smaller and higher density remnants containing nonsaponifiable components of the chylomicron (CM), including fat-soluble vitamins and cholesterol, are then taken up rapidly by the liver through a receptor-mediated pathway. The liver also secretes a very low-density lipoprotein (VLDL) whose components include vitamins E and K. VLDL is also a substrate for lipoprotein lipase and is converted to low-density lipoproteins (LDL). Some vitamin E may enter fat cells at this stage. LDL, which contains vitamins E and K, is taken up by LDL receptors in both liver and peripheral tissues. Vitamin A and 25-hydroxyvitamin D_3 are secreted by the liver with their respective specific carrier proteins and are delivered to peripheral tissues by receptor-mediated endocytosis. Average normal postabsorption concentrations in human plasma are as follows: vitamin A, 0.5 μg/ml; 25-hydroxyvitamin D_3, 30 ng/ml; vitamin E, 10 μg/ml; and vitamin K, 1 ng/ml. RBP = retinol-binding protein; α-glob = α-globulin.

physiological function, (f) nutritional requirements, (g) deficiency disease, (h) illustrative cases, and (i) hypervitaminosis.

VITAMIN A

History

Vitamin A was discovered in 1913 by McCollum and Davis (1) in experiments that showed that butterfat and egg yolk promoted growth in rats not achieved by lard and olive oil. In 1917, McCollum (2) suggested that xerophthalmia, which had been observed in humans on poor diets for centuries, was related to vitamin A as a deficiency disease. Carotene was identified as a precursor of vitamin A *in vivo* by Moore (3) in 1930 and the isolation, structure and synthesis of vitamin A was accomplished by Karrer, Morf, and Schopp (4) in 1931. In 1934, while working with Karrer, Wald (5) discovered the involvement of vitamin A in the visual cycle.

Chemistry

Vitamin A refers generically to all compounds structurally related to retinol that have biological activity (Fig. 2). Six isomers of retinol are known. In addition to the common all-trans retinol, there are 13-cis, 11-cis, 9-cis, 7-cis, and 9,13-cis retinols. Vitamin A_2 is dehydrovitamin A derived from freshwater fish. In addition, the oxidation products of retinol, such as all-trans retinal, and all-trans retinoic acid are active forms of vitamin A. Of the 400 carotenoids isolated from natural sources only 50 are precursors of vitamin A. All-trans β-carotene is the most effective precursor of vitamin A and the most widely distributed.

Absorption

Vitamin A is present in food mainly as the palmitate ester. It is hydrolyzed in the small intestine by a pancreatic esterase and an intestinal brush border hydrolase. Bile salts are required for activation of these enzymes and the formation of a micelle conductive to absorption. Retinol is absorbed as the free alcohol by an active transport system containing a cellular retinol binding protein CRBPII (6). The yellow β-carotene also requires bile salts for absorption and is converted to vitamin A in the intestinal tract.

Metabolism

The enzymatic cleavage of β-carotene to vitamin A was originally visualized as being a central fission of carotene to provide two molecules of retinal (7). Since this enzyme (15,15 carotene/dioxygenase) has never been isolated and fully characterized, and since the original stoichiometry has not been confirmed, there is now a question as to whether the enzyme actually generates two moles of retinal per mole of β-carotene (8,9). Furthermore, this enzyme has been recognized as fairly nonspecific since it also cleaves β-apo-carotenals to retinal. The retinal produced as a result of carotene cleavage is reduced by an alcohol dehydrogenase in the gut to retinol which is esterified with palmitic acid and enters the chylomicron as the palmitate ester (Fig. 3).

Retinol, whether derived from retinol esters in food or

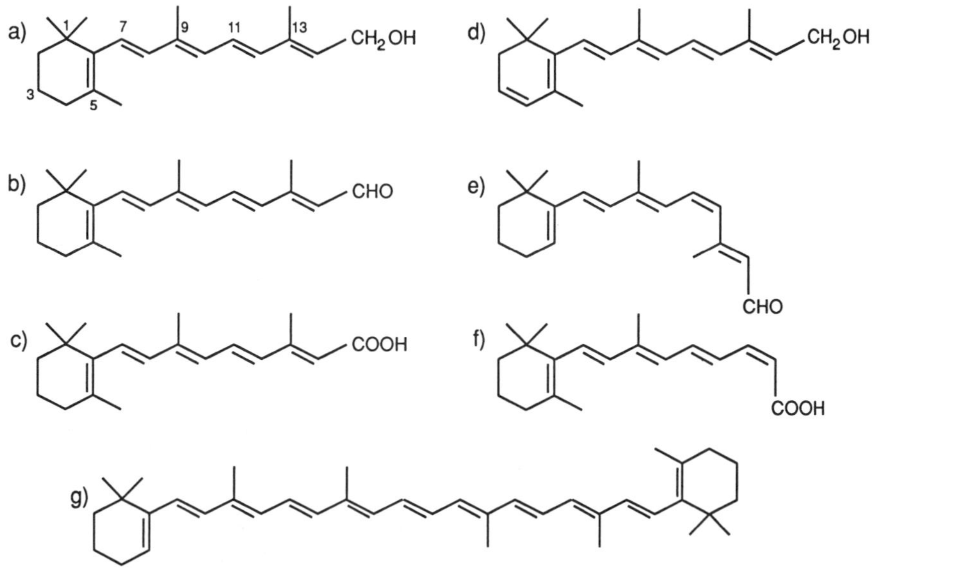

FIG. 2. Structures of selected retinoids and β-carotene: a) all-trans retinol; b) all-trans retinal; c) all trans retinoic acid; d) all-trans dehydroretinol (vitamin A_2); 3) 11-cis retinol; f) 13-cis retinoic acid (isotretinoin); and g) all-trans β-carotene.

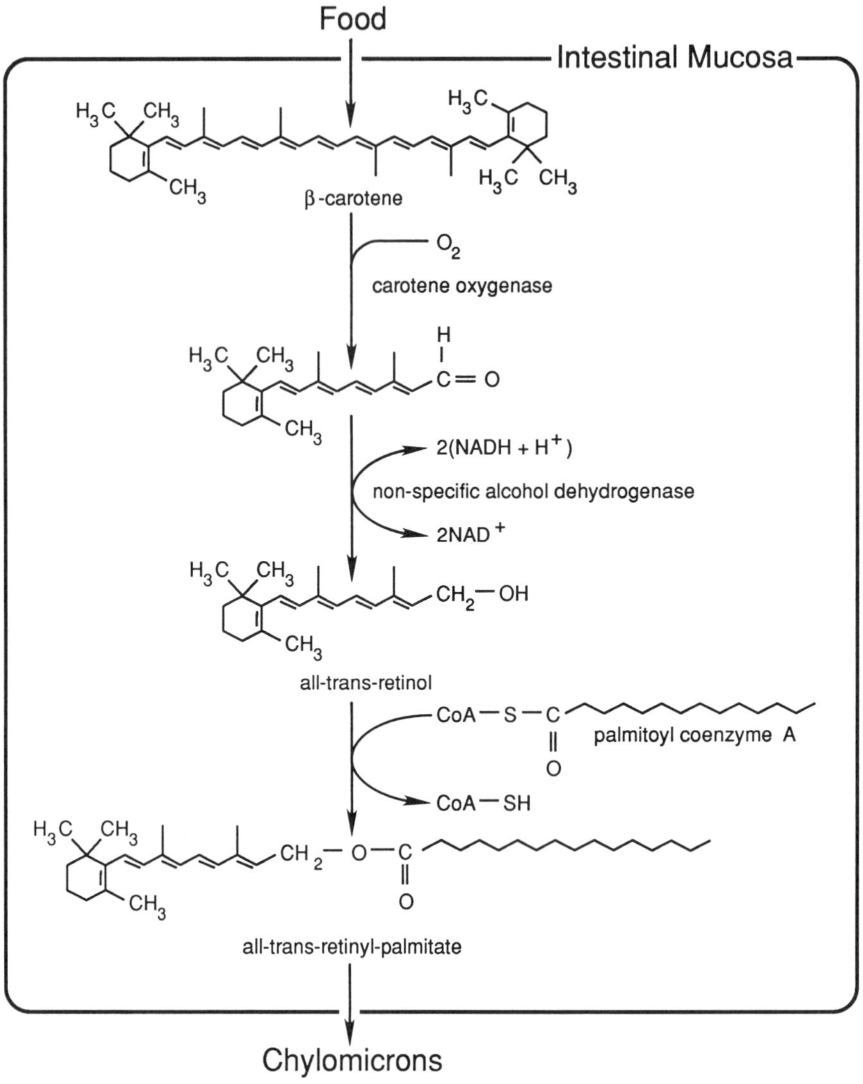

FIG. 3. Metabolism of β-carotene in the intestinal mucosa. Carotene is oxidized to retinaldehyde, which is reduced to retinol and esterified with palmitate via its coenzyme A (CoA) thioester.

β-carotene, is taken up by liver parenchymal cells via the chylomicron remnant. After uptake from the chylomicron, retinol ester is hydrolyzed to free retinol, incorporated into retinol-binding protein (RBP) (MW 21,000) and secreted as a complex into the plasma where it combines with transthyretin (MW 55,000) to form a ternary complex (MW 76,000) resistant to glomerular filtration in the kidney (Fig. 4). Vitamin A in plasma is distributed to peripheral cells and taken up by them via a cell-surface RBP receptor.

In animals with normal vitamin A status, hepatocytes transfer most of the retinol acquired from the diet, via RBP, to the perisinusoidal stellate cells that occupy the space of Disse (also called Ito cells, lipocytes, or interstitial cells) (10). This accounts for 60% to 80% of the vitamin A stored in the liver (Fig. 4). Large amounts of cellular retinol-binding protein (MW 15,000) are found in both hepatic parenchymal cells and stellate cells, with stellate cells having a concentration of this binding protein 20 times that of hepatocytes. On the other hand, the other two nonparenchymal cells in the liver (Kupffer cells and endothelial cells) contain neither vitamin A nor its binding proteins. In vitamin A deficiency, very little retinol is transferred to stellate cells, whereas in hypervitaminosis A, the stellate cells are packed with retinol. The body pool of vitamin A in humans is normally about 10 mg/kg body weight with 90% in the liver, mostly in stellate cells. In the steady state, the daily intake of about 1.0 mg of retinol equivalents is oxidized to retinoic acid and other chain-shortened acids and excreted as the glucuronides in the bile via the stool and free acids via the urine.

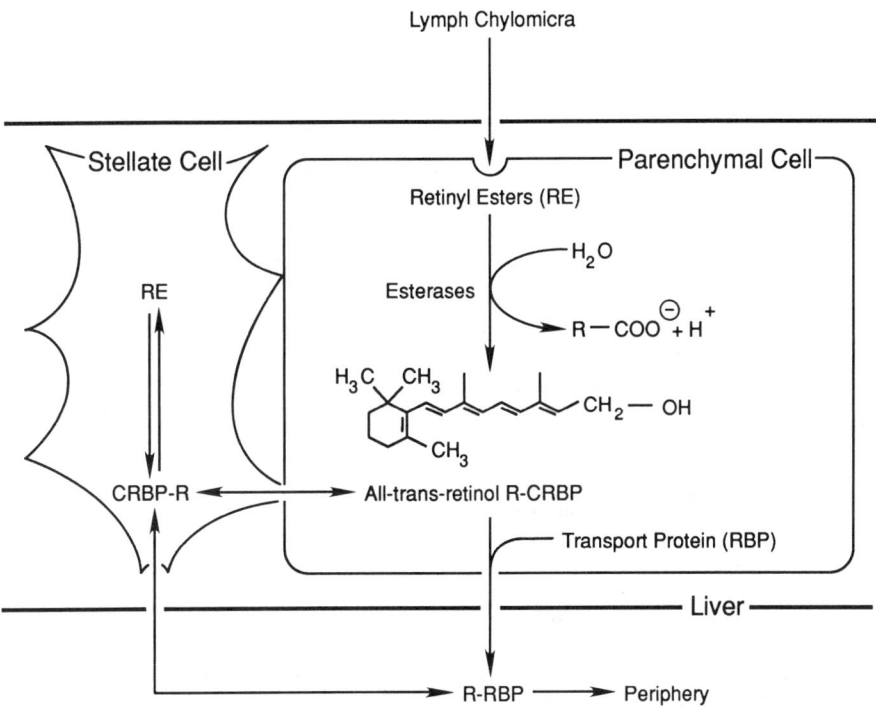

FIG. 4. Metabolism of retinol esters in the liver. Retinol palmitate is delivered to the hepatocyte via the chylomicron remnant. The ester is hydrolyzed and the free retinol is taken up by a cellular retinol-binding protein (CRBP). If retinol is in excess of hepatocyte needs for secretion to the plasma, the retinol is transferred to the stellate cell for storage, which can return retinol to the hepatocyte as needed. The hepatocyte, and possibly the stellate cell, secrete plasma retinol-binding protein (RBP) complexed with retinol for delivery to peripheral tissues. RBP-specific receptors exist on the membranes of most cells.

Physiological Functions

There are two main functions of vitamin A: (a) maintenance of vision, particularly night vision; and (b) maintenance of epithelial tissues and differentiation of many other tissues, particularly during reproduction and gestation. In vision, all-trans retinol is taken up by an RBP receptor in the eye, the retinol is endocytosed, oxidized to retinal, and isomerized to the 11-cis derivative (Fig. 5). Then, 11-cis retinal condenses with opsin, which is the apopeptide of rhodopsin (transmembrane protein of MW 40,000). When light strikes rhodopsin in rods, it causes an isomerization of the 11-cis retinal, and a conformational change in opsin to produce metarhodopsin II. This photoexcited rhodopsin (R*) then triggers an enzymatic cascade that results in the hydrolysis of cyclic guanosine monophosphate (cGMP). The linkage between R* and cGMP involves a G-protein, transducin (T) and a transducin subunit, T_x, that activates a phosphodiesterase (PDE) that, in turn, splits cGMP and closes the Na^+ channels in the plasma membrane of the rod cell. The hyperpolarization that results produces a nervous impulse that travels to the brain and is registered as light (11).

Vitamin A's other function is to maintain epithelial tissues and to stimulate differentiation of a number of tissues by controlling gene expression. Retinol, bound to RBP, is endocytosed via the cell-surface RBP receptor, and the intracellular retinol is quickly bound to a cellular retinol-binding protein CRBP (MW 15,000). When retinol is oxidized to retinoic acid, it is quickly bound to another cellular-binding protein for retinoic acid (CRABP) that may be part of the shuttle system for delivering retinol to its final DNA-binding receptor (6). Figure 6 illustrates the structures of four of the receptor molecules that mediate the action of steroids, thyroid, and fat-soluble vitamins on the genome (12). This group of hormone receptors also includes those for aldosterone, progesterone, and estrogen. Three structural domains of these receptors are discernible: an enhancer region, a DNA-binding region, and a hormone-binding region. In the cortisol receptor, there is a fairly elongated enhancer region, which also gives immunospecificity to the protein. The cortisol receptor is the largest (MW 86,000) and the vitamin D hormone receptor is the smallest (MW 47,000). Each of these receptors has been cloned and the sequences determined. The x-ray configuration of each protein is being studied. Present in the DNA-binding domain are zinc fingers that involve cysteine residues coordinated with zinc. They play an important role in the function of the receptor protein and explain why zinc is so important in DNA metabolism.

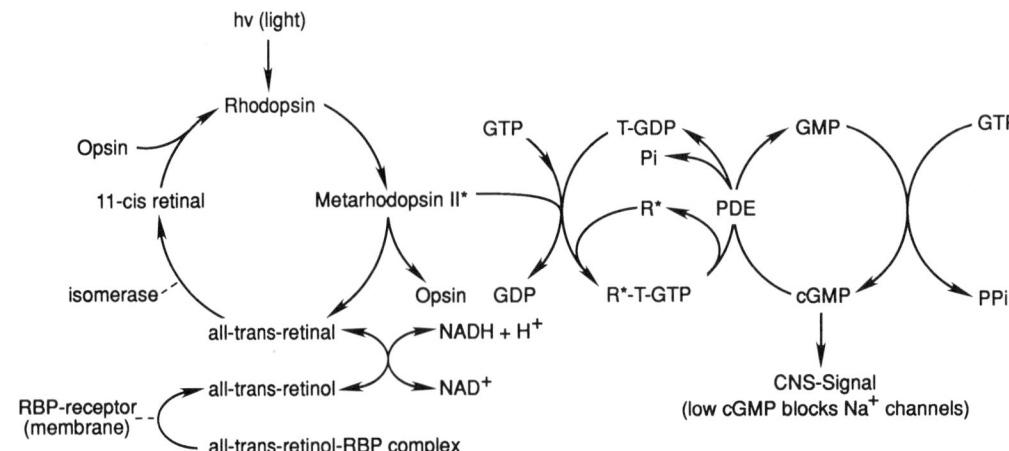

FIG. 5. Rhodopsin and the visual cycle. All-trans retinol is delivered to the eye via the RBP receptor. It is oxidized to all-trans retinal in the rod cell and isomerized to 11-cis retinal, the chromophore of rhodopsin. When light strikes rhodopsin, 11-cis retinal is isomerized to all-trans retinal and the product is metarhodopsin II, also called photoexcited rhodopsin (R*). This triggers an enzymatic cascade that results in amplification of the light signal and produces a neural impulse to the brain. The photoexcited rhodopsin (R*) catalyzes an exchange of guanosine triphosphate (GTP) for guanosine diphosphate (GDP) attached to transducin (a G-protein), which, in turn, activates a phosphodiesterase (PDE) that splits cyclic guanosine monophosphate (cGMP) to guanosine monophosphate (GMP) and blocks Na^+ channels in the outer segment of the rod cell. This abrupt charge in Na^+ ion flux causes hyperpolarization of the cell membrane and sends a signal via the optic nerve to the occipital cortex of the brain where it is perceived as light. In the dark, PDE is deactivated by the hydrolysis of GTP to GDP and cGMP is restored by guanylate cyclase (11).

Finally, there is the hydrophobic steroid-binding area that extends to the C-terminal portion of the protein. The retinoic acid receptor (RAR), which contains 462 amino acids, has the same domains but a short enhancer region. The RAR activates genes that control glycoprotein synthesis, epithelial cell integrity, and a variety of proteins essential for normal reproduction and differentiation of the fetus.

Requirements

Requirements for vitamin A intake are based upon studies of dark adaptation, electroretinograms, and the ability of dietary vitamin A to maintain a plasma concentration of 20 µg/dl in the plasma. The vitamin A requirement of humans ranges from 10 to 30 µg retinol/kg body weight, although infants have higher requirements.

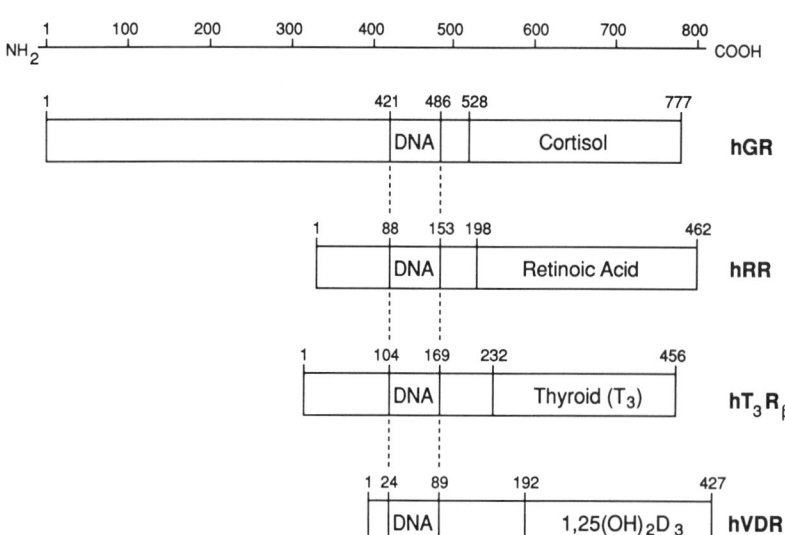

FIG. 6. Structures of human genomic receptors for glucocorticoids (hGR), retinoic acid (hRR), thyroid hormones (hT_3R_β) and $1,25(OH)_2$-vitamin D_3 (hVDR). The amino acid content of each receptor is shown by numbers at the right of each bar. The receptors are aligned to show the constancy of the highly conserved DNA-binding domain. The enhancer domain, which provides immunologic specific and maximum activity, is at the N-terminal portion of the receptor and is highly variable. The hormone- or vitamin-binding domain averages about 250 amino acids in length and is at the C-terminal end of the receptor. When the hormone or vitamin combines with the receptor it alters its confirmation, promotes DNA binding, and affects gene expression (12).

The recommended dietary allowances (RDA) of the National Academy of Sciences National Research Council (NAS/NRC) Food and Nutrition Board, which are designed to satisfy the needs of healthy infants, children, and adults, are shown in Table 2 in retinol equivalents (13). For the purpose of setting public health standards, 6 µg of β-carotene is considered equal to 1 µg of retinol because of the poor absorption of β-carotene and its inefficient conversion to retinol.

Vitamin A Deficiency

New developments in the understanding of the somatic function of vitamin A have improved our understanding of the clinical manifestations of vitamin A deficiency. The syndrome of vitamin A deficiency in infants consists of night blindness, Bitot spots, xerophthalmia, keratomalacia, corneal opacities, hyperkeratosis, growth failure, and death. The deficiency disease in humans was called xerophthalmia (dry eyes) because of the prominence of the eye signs. Other findings include infertility, metaplastic bones, and general keratinization of epithelial tissue particularly in the skin, genitourinary system, and the lung. Urinary calculi are common and fetal abnormalities are seen in pregnancy. Diets consisting of polished rice with little or no vegetables or fruits increase the risk of xerophthalmia. Thirty percent of children admitted with protein-energy malnutrition to our clinic in Chiang Mai, Thailand, had xerophthalmia. Protective foods are liver, green leafy vegetables, and milk and dairy products.

Laboratory tests show a mild leukopenia occurring in vitamin A deficiency, including a serum retinol level of 15 µg/dl or less (normal = 20 to 80 µg/dl). Clouding of the cornea in a child with vitamin A deficiency is a medical emergency and requires parenteral administration of 50,000 to 100,000 IU (15 to 30 mg retinol). The following two cases illustrate relevant clinical and laboratory findings (14–16).

Illustrative Cases

Case 1

A pale 5-month-old boy with severe marasmus was admitted to Luzmilla Hospital in Amman, Jordan, for the study treatment. Physical examination revealed extreme wasting, apathy, and ocular changes that included, in the left eye, Bitot spots as well as conjunctive and corneal xeroses. In the right eye, corneal liquefaction and keratomalacia had occurred with subsequent prolapse of the iris, extrusion of the lens, and loss of vitreous humor. His height was 65 cm (26 in) and his weight 4.5 kg (9.9 lb). His malnutrition had begun after cessation of breast-feeding at 4 months of age, with subsequent weight loss and diarrhea. Laboratory studies showed that his hemoglobin was 10.7 g/dl (normal: 12 to 16 g/dl), hematocrit 36 ml/dl (normal: 35 to 47 ml/dl), white blood count 15,000/1 (normal: 5,000 to 9,000/1), serum protein 5.6 g/dl (normal: 6 to 8 g/dl), serum albumin 2.49 g/dl (normal: 3.5 to 5.5 g/dl). Plasma electrolytes included a sodium of 139 mEq/1 (normal: 136 to 145 mEq/1), potassium 3.5 mEq/1 (normal: 3.5 to 5.0 mEq/1), blood glucose 70 mg/dl (normal: 60 to 100 mg/dl), total bilirubin 1.1 mg/dl (normal: less than 1 mg/dl), serum vitamin A 5.5 µg/dl (normal: 20 to 80 g/dl). In addition, β-carotene was 10.7 µg/dl (normal: 50 to 250 µg/dl) and vitamin E 220 µg/dl (normal: 500 to 1,500 µg/dl). The child was infected, as evidenced by otitis media and salmonella septicemia; both responded to antibiotic treatment in the first week.

TABLE 2. *Recommended daily dietary allowances for vitamins A, D, E, and K*

Group	Age (yr)	Vitamin A (µg RE)[a]	Vitamin D (µg)[b]	Vitamin E (mg α-TE)[c]	Vitamin K (µg)
Infants	0–0.5	375	7.5	3	5
	0.5–1.0	375	10.0	4	10
Children	1–3	400	10.0	6	15
	4–6	500	10.0	7	20
	7–10	700	10.0	7	30
Males	11–24	1,000	10.0	10	65
	25–51+	1,000	5.0	10	80
Females	11–24	800	10.0	8	55
	25–51+	800	5.0	8	65
Pregnant		800	10.0	10	65
Lactating		1,300	10.0	12	65

From ref. 13.
[a] Retinol equivalents. 1 retinol equivalent = 1 µg retinol or 6 µg β-carotene of vitamin A activity of diets as retinol equivalents.
[b] As cholecalciferol. 10 µg cholecalciferol = 400 IU of vitamin D.
[c] α-Tocopherol equivalents. 1 mg d-α-tocopherol = 1 α-TE.

After diagnostic blood samples were obtained, the patient was given a water dispersion of 3,000/μg/kg per day of retinol palmitate with Tween 80-R, by nasogastric tube, for 4 days. His plasma vitamin A level of 5 μg/dl increased to 35 μg/dl on the second day and was maintained at about that level for the next 12 days. The child responded to general nutritional rehabilitation first with a high-calorie formula and then with a combination of whole milk supplement and solid foods. At 12 weeks the child was totally blind in the right eye with a residual corneal opacity in the left. After 12 weeks, he attained proper weight-for-height but remained dwarfed.

Case 2

A 41-year-old man, along with seven other volunteers, took part in a 2-year, in-hospital, clinical investigation of vitamin A deficiency at the University of Iowa School of Medicine. The subject weighed 77.3 kg (170 lb) and was healthy by the usual criteria of history, physical examination, and laboratory studies. He was fed a casein formula containing less than 10 μg of vitamin A per day for 505 days. The initial plasma vitamin A level was 58/μg/dl and his body pool of vitamin A, determined by isotope dilution, was 766 mg (about 10 mg/kg body weight). At the end of 1 year on the low vitamin A diet, his plasma vitamin A had declined to about 25 μg/dl, at which time he began to show follicular hyperkeratosis, a classic sign of vitamin A deficiency (Fig. 7). A mild anemia developed on the 300th day (hemoglobin 12.6 mg/dl), when plasma vitamin A was 20 μg/dl. Two months later, at which time his plasma vitamin A level was 10 μg/dl, he developed night blindness as evidenced by changes in dark adaptation and electroretinogram. Finally, when his plasma vitamin A level reached 3 μg/dl, repletion with vitamin A was begun. He received increasing doses of vitamin A starting with 150 μg which was increased gradually to 1,200 μg retinol per day for 145 days. After receiving 150 μg per day of retinol for 82 days, his night blindness was partially repaired, but not his skin keratinization. Furthermore, this dose did not elevate his plasma retinol beyond 8 μg/dl. On 300 μg oral retinol for 42 days, the follicular hyperkeratosis resolved and plasma levels rose to about 20 μg/dl. On 600 μg retinol per day, plasma vitamin A was in the subnormal range but all other signs of vitamin A deficiency disappeared. It appears, therefore, that the requirement for vitamin A in adult males, based on a curative dose, is between 600 and 1,200 μg of retinol per day.

Hypervitaminosis A

Hypervitaminosis A has been observed in children and adults ingesting more than 50,000 IU/day of vitamin A for several months. Pediatric toxicity is commonly related to excessive doses of fish liver oil or thera-

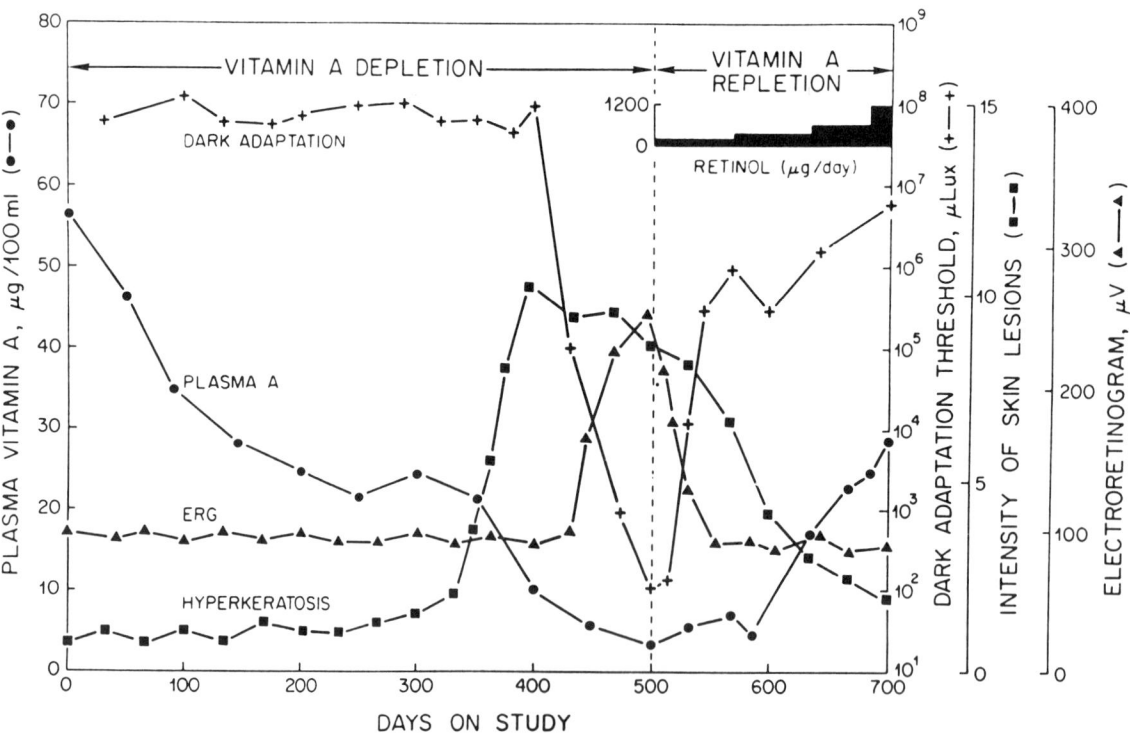

FIG. 7. The induction and remission of vitamin A deficiency in a healthy volunteer. Changes in dark adaptation, plasma vitamin A concentration, electroretinogram (ERG), and hyperkeratosis are followed during the onset of vitamin A deficiency (first 500 days) and its treatment with retinol in the range of 300 to 1,200 μg per day (16).

peutic vitamin preparations. In adults, its occurrence is related to excessive use of retinol or retinoic acid for various skin disorders, particularly globular acne. The presenting symptoms are fatigue, malaise, anorexia, vomiting, headache, and diplopia related to elevated cerebral spinal fluid pressure. Other findings are bone pain, dermatitis, hepatomegaly with liver abnormalities, hypercalcemia, hypoprothrombinosis, and fetal abnormalities.

VITAMIN D

History

Vitamin D was discovered by Mellanby (17) in 1919. He produced rickets in dogs by feeding them low-fat diets and then cured the disease with cod liver oil. Although rickets had been recognized in children for centuries, its cause remained unknown until then. In 1924, Steenbock and Black (18) discovered that ultraviolet irradiation could produce vitamin D activity from various sterols. In 1932, the structure of vitamin D was determined by Windaus et al. (19) in Germany and Askew et al. (20) in England.

Vitamin D is required for the prevention of rickets in children and osteomalacia in adults. It is now known that vitamin D is a precursor of a hormone that is the active form of vitamin D (1,25-dihydroxycholecalciferol), synthesized in the kidney and secreted by the kidney under the control of parathyroid hormone and tissue phosphate concentrations (21). Vitamin D is a facultative vitamin that is required in the diet when there is insufficient vitamin D_3 made from 7-dehydrocholesterol in the skin by irradiation with ultraviolet light. In Northern and Western countries where sunlight is less available due to cloudiness or the poor angle of radiation, dietary vitamin D is essential. In the tropics, however, dietary vitamin D is not necessary when there is sufficient exposure to sunlight.

Chemistry

Vitamin D is the generic term for a family of secosteroids with antirachitic activity. In the secosteroid rings, A, C, and D are intact whereas the opened ring B is converted into a conjugated system of double bonds (Fig. 8). All molecules with vitamin D activity have the same interrupted ring system but vary in their side chains. For example, ergosterol, the sterol of yeast, has an additional double bond at position 22 and an additional methyl group at position 24. The vitamin D arising from irradiation of ergosterol is known as vitamin D_2, or ergocalciferol, which is the principal source of vitamin D for fortification of foods.

The biological availability of given vitamers of D vary. For example, cholecalciferol, vitamin D_3, which is the animal vitamin D, is not active in the chick, whereas vitamin D_2, from irradiated yeast, is. Both vitamins D_2 and D_3 are active in animals.

Absorption and Transport

Vitamin D is absorbed in the small intestine, mainly in the duodenum, by an active transport system that delivers vitamin D to the enterocyte; there it is incorporated into chylomicrons for delivery to the liver. In the liver, vitamin D is hydroxylated to 25-OH-vitamin D_3 and secreted in association with an α-2 globulin (MW 60,000). This carrier transports all three forms of vitamin D, of which 25-OH-vitamin D_3 is in the highest concentration, in plasma (20 to 40 ng/ml) whereas vitamin D itself is present in a concentration of 2 to 4 ng/ml and the hormone $1,25(OH)_2D_3$ is present in very small amounts, normally 20 to 40 pg/ml.

Metabolism

Is vitamin D a vitamin or a hormone? A vitamin is defined as a trace organic substance required for the health of organisms. A hormone, on the other hand, is a substance, secreted from one tissue, which travels through the blood to another tissue where it exerts its biological effect. There is nothing in the rules of biochemistry that prevents a vitamin derivative from being a hormone, coenzyme, or any other biologically active substance. Hydroxylations significantly alter the properties of endogenously synthesized steroid hormones (e.g., corticosterone vs 11-hydroxycorticosterone). Vitamin D is hydroxylated twice, once in the liver, and then again in the kidney, to produce the hormone 1,25-dihydroxycholecalciferol. This hormone, which is secreted by the kidney, travels to the gut where it increases calcium absorption and to the bones where it alters calcium turnover (22).

Thus, vitamin D is a vitamin when sunlight is limiting, and its hydroxylated derivative, $1,25(OH)_2D_3$, is a hormone. The formation of vitamin D, and its conversion into active and inactive forms, are shown in Fig. 9. As noted, the small amount of vitamin D in the plasma is 25-hydroxyvitamin D (20 to 40 ng/ml). Vitamin D is 10% of that (2 to 4 ng/ml), and the hormonal derivative 1,25-dihydroxyvitamin D is present in 20 to 40 pg/ml, 1,000 times less concentrated. The kidney is the endocrine organ synthesizing $1,25(OH)_2$-vitamin D_3 from $25(OH)$-vitamin D_3 under control of parathormone (PTH) and inorganic phosphate concentrations. The hydroxylations are catalyzed by a cytochrome P-450 aided by a flavoprotein and an iron-S protein. The 1-α-hydroxylase in kidney is stimulated by PTH and inhibited by its product $1,25(OH)_2$-vitamin D_3. The 24-

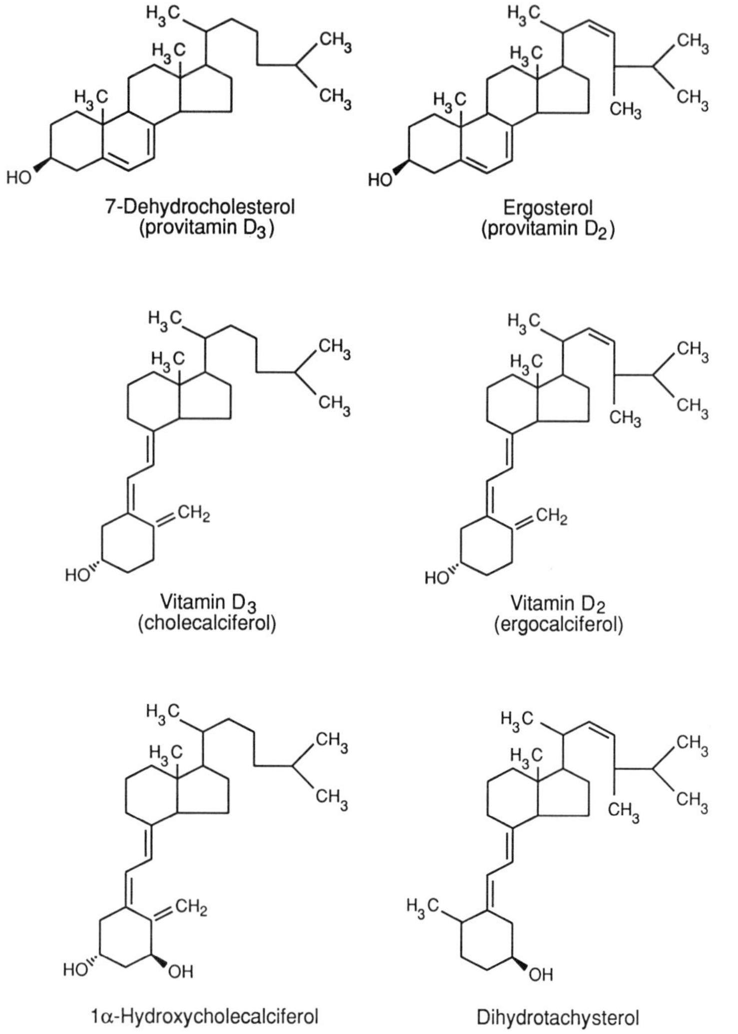

FIG. 8. Structures of compounds related to vitamin D. Provitamins D₂ and D₃, vitamins D₂ and D₃, and the synthetic compounds, 1-α-hydroxycholecalciferol and dihydrotachysterol, formed as a by-product of ergosterol irradiation are shown.

hydroxylase, which is an inactivating enzyme, is stimulated by vitamin D hormone and inhibited by PTH.

The body pool of vitamin D secosteroids is small, about 5 µg/kg of which 90% is 25-OH-D₃. Vitamin D and 1,25(OH)₂D₃ make up less than 10% of the total.

Physiological Function

The actions of vitamin D in various systems are the actions of its 1,25-dihydroxy derivative, the vitamin D hormone. These relate to maintenance of calcium homeostasis and bone metabolism. They are the result of changes in gene expression that are under the control of vitamin D hormone and mediated by a vitamin D receptor protein present in a variety of tissues that bind to DNA (23). The vitamin D receptor gene has been cloned and its product characterized with respect to amino acid sequence and three domains: an enhancer region, a DNA-binding domain, and a 1,25(OH)₂D₃–binding domain. It contains 427 amino acids and has a molecular weight of 47,000 (24) (Fig. 6).

The organs affected by vitamin D hormone in its control of calcium homeostasis are the intestine, kidney, and bones. In the intestine, the hormone induces a calcium transport system involving transport proteins and an intracellular calcium-binding protein (CBP) called calbindin, which aids in the transport of calcium across the enterocyte (Fig. 10). In the kidney, vitamin D hormone enhances calcium reabsorption in the tubule by a mechanism similar to that in the gut. It also inhibits the synthesis of 1-α-hydroxylase activity (to diminish hormone synthesis) and stimulates 25(OH)D₃ 24-hydroxylase activity which inactivates both the substrate and the product of 1-α-hydroxylase; 1-α-hydroxylase activity is also stimulated by parathormone (PTH) and low tissue phosphate concentrations (Fig. 9).

In hypoparathyroidism, 1-α-hydroxylation is depressed and requires 1-α-(OH)D₃ or 1,25(OH)₂D₃ for normalization of calcium metabolism (25). 1-α-(OH)D₃

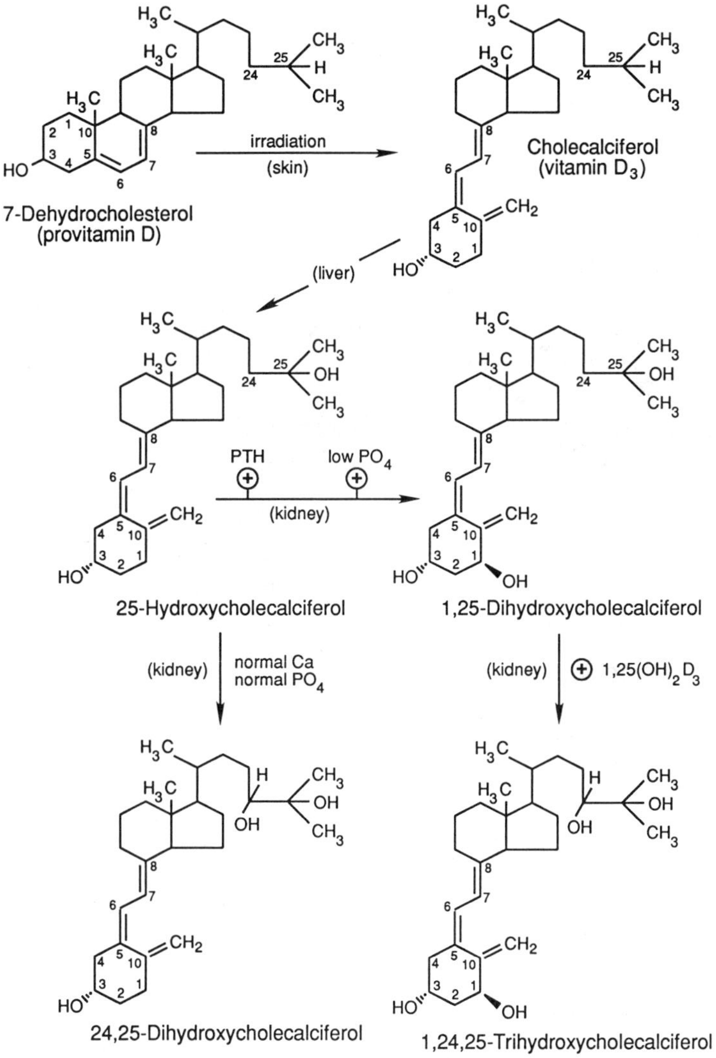

FIG. 9. The formation of vitamin D_3 and its metabolism. The hydroxylation of vitamin D_3 to 25-OH-vitamin D_3 occurs in the liver and is nearly quantitative. The hydroxylation of 25-OH-vitamin D_3 to the hormone, $1,25(OH)_2$-vitamin D_3 in the kidney is highly regulated by parathormone (PTH) and inorganic phosphate. The inactivation of 25-OH-vitamin D_3 and $1,25(OH)_2$-vitamin D_3 by 24-hydroxylation occurs in the kidney as a final step in the regulation of hormone levels.

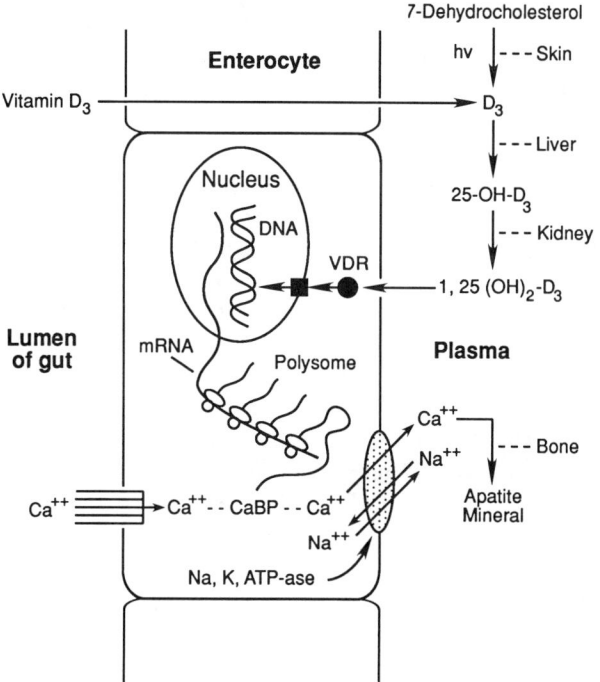

FIG. 10. The production of $1,25(OH)_2$-vitamin D_3 and its action in stimulating calbindin (CaBP) synthesis in the intestinal mucosa. VDR is a vitamin D receptor protein (●) whose conformation is changed by the uptake of $1,25(OH)_2$-vitamin D_3 (■). The holoprotein migrates to the nucleus and combines with the hormone receptor element of the genome, which initiates transcription of the calbindin gene. The resulting mRNA is translated into a protein by interaction with ribosomes.

is hydroxylated in the 25 position in the liver to make it an active hormone.

When vitamin D intake is inadequate, vitamin D hormone levels and calcium absorption fall. This reduces plasma calcium concentrations which increases PTH output, thereby causing a fall in plasma phosphate and an increase in 1-α-hydroxylase activity in the kidney. These events collectively increase $1,25(OH)_2D_3$ synthesis, and attempt to restore calcium homeostasis. Unless vitamin D becomes available, rickets results.

There is evidence that vitamin D hormones stimulate bone-forming cells (osteoblasts) to produce more alkaline phosphatase and osteocalcin and less collagen, all of which favor bone formation. At higher doses, the vitamin D hormone stimulates mononuclear cells (including HL-60 leukemic cells) to differentiate into macrophages. Macrophages then fuse with osteoclasts and stimulate bone turnover and calcium mobilization. Calcitonin, a hormone of the thyroid clear cells, is secreted when plasma calcium levels are too high and blocks the actions of vitamin D hormone and PTH on calcium mobilization from bone.

Recent studies indicate that the vitamin D endocrine system has many other effects on the body than the control of calcium homeostasis (26). Vitamin D hormone receptors have been found in skin, muscle, most endocrine tissues, thymus, lymphocytes, and monocytes, as well as in intestine, bone, and kidney. Clear effects of vitamin D deficiency upon endocrine secretion, immunity, and oncogene expression have been demonstrated in animals.

Vitamin D Requirements

Since vitamin D_3 is produced endogenously in the skin through the action of sunlight on 7-dehydrocholesterol, there is no nutritional requirement for vitamin D when sufficient sunlight is available. However, when shielded from sunlight, breast-fed infants will develop rickets unless supplemented with vitamin D (27).

In 1970, from a review of the literature, the Expert Committee of the Food and Agricultural Organization/World Health Organization (FAO/WHO) concluded that full-term infants showed greater absorption of calcium and greater growth rates when given 400 IU (1 international unit = 0.025 μg vitamin D) per day compared to infants given 100 IU/day, although 100 IU is enough to prevent rickets. A dosage of 400 IU may be considered an allowance rather than a requirement. Since rickets is more prevalent in preschool-age children, the FAO/WHO committee recommended 10 μg/day until the age of 6, and, thereafter, 5.0 μg daily. Current recommendations by the United States Food and Nutrition Board of the National Research Council are 7.5 μg for infants up to 6 months of age, and 10 μg for children, adolescents, pregnant women, and lactating mothers. For adults 25 years and older, the recommendation is 200 IU or 5 μg vitamin D per day.

Vitamin D Deficiency

Clinical manifestations of rickets include skeletal deformities with bone pain, muscle weakness, failure to grow, hypocalcemia, and hypophosphatemia (28). The failure to mineralize osteoid tissue at the epiphyseal-diaphyseal junction of bones causes a variety of deformities, e.g., craniotabes, enlargement of joints, "rachitic rosary" at the costochondral junctions, "bow legs," and "knock knees." X-ray examination of long bones in rickets shows rarefied shafts and uneven, blurred ends that brighten with vitamin D treatment. Fractures are not uncommon. Laboratory data reveal hypocalcemia, hypophosphatemia, and elevated alkaline phosphatase. The 25-$(OH)D_3$ levels in plasma are reduced to below normal. These features are also seen in osteomalacia, the adult form of vitamin D deficiency.

Human milk is deficient in vitamin D and contains only 22 IU (0.55 μg) per liter, mostly from 25-$(OH)D_3$. Breast-fed infants must receive an additional source of vitamin D. Cow's milk and most formulas are enriched to the level of 400 IU (10 μg) per liter. Treatment of rickets should begin with a dose of 100 μg of vitamin D daily (4,000 IU), roughly 10 times the RDA.

Vitamin D–Resistant Rickets

There are several types of vitamin D–resistant rickets (VDRR). One results from familial hypophosphatemia due to a hereditary defect in renal resorption of phosphate associated with low calcium absorption. This disorder can be treated with oral $1,25(OH)_2D_3$ plus phosphate supplements.

Other types are due to abnormalities in the metabolism of vitamin D. In type I disease, the defect is in the activity of the 1-α-hydroxylase in the kidney with resulting elevated levels of 25-$(OH)D_3$ and reduced levels of $1,25(OH)_2D_3$ in plasma. Physiological doses (0.05 μg/kg) of $1,25(OH)_2D_3$ are curative.

Type II VDRR is due to a defect in the vitamin D receptor (VDR) protein. Children have high levels of $1,25(OH)_2D_3$ in plasma and do not respond to massive doses of vitamin D hormone. Partial management results from high calcium and phosphate intake. Molecular biological studies of persons with type II VDRR have identified defects in all three parts of the VDR, i.e., the enhancer region, the DNA-binding region, and the vitamin D binding region (24).

Illustrative Cases of Rickets in Infancy (27,28)

Case 1

A 20-month-old African-American boy was admitted to the emergency room with progressive swelling and tenderness over the left thigh that began following a fall from a bed 1 week before admission. Radiographs revealed a nondisplaced proximal femoral fracture. The patient's mother refused treatment and took the child to a "nature healer." Police retrieved the child, and his left leg was placed in a cast. Follow-up films of the left femur revealed progressive healing. Comparison films of the opposite femur, however, also demonstrated a healing fracture, and the question of child abuse was raised. Skeletal survey revealed diffuse demineralization of bone with a trabecular pattern in multiple vertebral bodies and epiphyseal plate changes including widening and fraying. The patient was admitted for medical evaluation.

The patient was born at term to a gravida 4, para 1 mother; birth weight was 3.9 kg (8.6 lb). He was breast-fed for 9 months without vitamin supplementation, after which he received only home-prepared unsupplemented soy milk, fruits, and vegetables until the time of admission. The parents were strict vegetarians.

On physical examination, the child was an active toddler with prominent bowing of the legs, rachitic rosary, and flaring of both wrists and ankles. His weight was 11.5 kg (25 lb, 25th percentile), height was 79 cm (31 in, third percentile), hemoglobin was 10.9 g/dl (normal: 10 to 15 g/dl), and the hematocrit was 33% (normal: 30% to 40%). Serum calcium was 9.6 mg/dl (normal: 9.0 to 11.0 mg/dl), phosphorus 3.2 mg/dl (normal: 4.5 to 6.7 mg/dl) and alkaline phosphatase 21.8 Bodansky units/ml (normal: 4 to 8 units/ml). The 25-hydroxyvitamin D value in plasma was 7 ng/ml (normal: 20 to 40 ng/ml). Vitamin D, in a dose of 250 µg (10,000 IU), was given daily, and clinical and radiographic evidence of healing was present 2 weeks later (27).

Case 2

Seventeen children, most under 26 months of age, with clinical rickets, were evaluated for serum 25-(OH)D$_3$, 24,25-dihydroxy-D$_3$, and 1,25(OH)$_2$D$_3$ as well as serum calcium, phosphorous, and alkaline phosphatase. They were treated with 50 µg of vitamin D per day for 66 days; biochemical values were measured during recovery (Fig. 11). The level of 25-(OH)D, the most reliable indicator of vitamin D deficiency on admission, usually normalized during the treatment period (28).

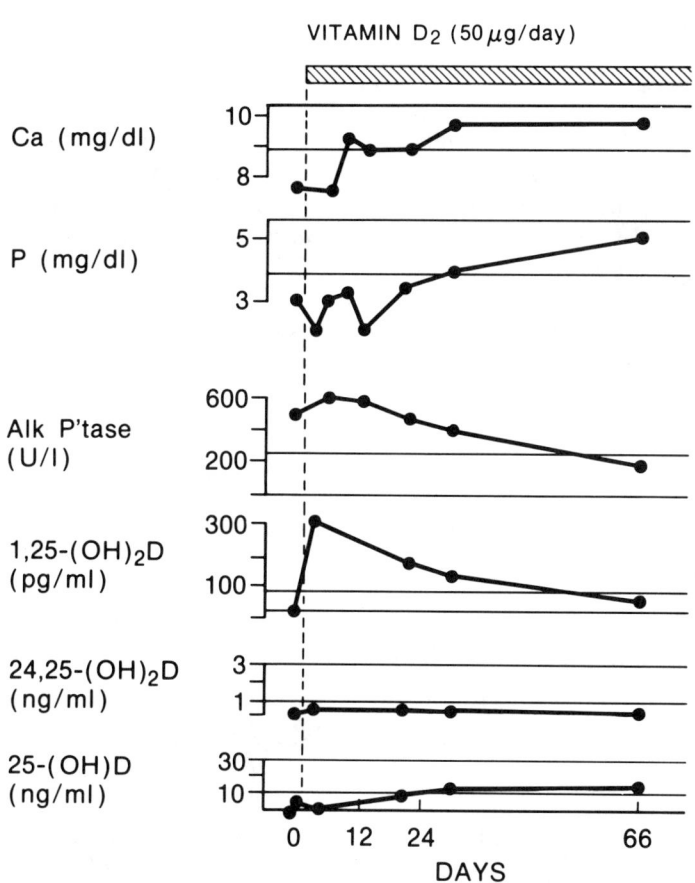

FIG. 11. The effect of vitamin D$_2$ on plasma values for calcium (Ca), phosphorus (P), alkaline phosphatase (Alk P'tase), and vitamin D metabolites during the treatment of a child with rickets (28). Normal values shown.

Hypervitaminosis D

Vitamin D is the most likely vitamin to cause overt toxic reactions in small multiples of the United States RDA. An epidemic of "idiopathic hypercalcemia" in infants, with anorexia, vomiting, hypertension, renal insufficiency, and failure to thrive, occurred in England in the 1950s. It was traced to an intake of vitamin D between 2,000 and 3,000 IU/day. In adults, dosages of 10,000 IU/day of vitamin D for several months have resulted in marked disturbances in calcium metabolism with hypercalcemia, hyperphosphatemia, hypertension, anorexia, nausea, vomiting, weakness, polyuria, polydypsia, azotemia, nephrolithiasis, ectopic calcification, renal failure, and, in some cases, death (29).

VITAMIN E

History

Vitamin E was discovered in 1922 by Evans and Bishop (30) as essential for reproduction in the rat. They later named the vitamin tocopherol, from the Greek *tokos* (childbirth) and *pherein* (to bring forth). Vitamin E was isolated by Evans et al. (31) in 1936 and synthesized by Karrer et al. (32) in 1938.

The diseases caused by tocopherol deficiency vary widely according to the affected species. Disorders of reproduction, abnormalities of muscle, liver, bone marrow, and brain function, defective embryogenesis, and exudative diathesis, a disorder of capillary permeability, have been observed. Skeletal muscle dystrophy has been noted as well and, in certain species, is accompanied by cardiomyopathy. In ruminants, the cardiac disease is severe, but is mild in rabbits and nonexistent in primates. Hemopoiesis is affected only in monkeys and pigs; hepatic necrosis occurs only in rats and pigs. This bewildering and unpredictable array of manifestations has impeded an in-depth understanding of the vitamin's function at the cellular and molecular level. A number of enzymes are controlled by α-tocopherol in animals. These include xanthine oxidase, creatine kinase, cytochrome oxidase, lipoxygenase, glutathione reductase, aldolase, and arylsulfatase (33).

In humans, the main manifestations of vitamin E deficiency are (a) a mild hemolytic anemia associated with increased erythrocyte hemolysis, and (b) spinocerebellar disease, mostly observed in children who have fat-malabsorption due to abetalipoproteinemia, chronic biliary disease with cholestasis, or other types of malabsorption.

Chemistry

Vitamin E is a generic term for compounds that have a 6-chromanol ring structure, an isoprenoid side chain, and the biological activity of α-tocopherol. The tocols have a phytyl side chain, and the trienols have a classical isoprenoid side chain with double bonds at the 3', 7', and 11' positions (Fig. 12). Both tocols and trienols occur as a variety of isomers that differ by the number and location of methyl groups on the chromanol ring. α-Tocopherol is the most active form of vitamin E (Table 3).

The only naturally occurring stereoisomer of α-tocopherol, formerly known as d-α-tocopherol should be designated RRR-α-tocopherol. The totally synthetic α-tocopherol, formerly known as dl-α-tocopherol, should be designated *all-rac*-α-tocopherol (for all racemic α-tocopherol). Esters of tocopherols should be designated as esters (e.g., α-tocopherol acetate) (34).

α-Tocopherol, which is practically insoluble in water, is completely soluble in oils, fats, and fat solvents. Tocopherols are stable to heat and alkali in the absence of oxygen and are unaffected by acids up to 100°C. They are, however, slowly oxidized by atmospheric oxygen. Oxidation is accelerated by exposure to light, heat, and alkali, and the presence of iron and copper salts. Oxidation products include tocopheroxide, tocopherol quinone, and tocopherol hydroquinone, as well as dimers and trimers (Fig. 13). Since the esters of the free phenolic hydroxyl group are much more stable in the presence of oxygen, tocopherol is usually provided commercially as the acetate ester. The esters, however, cannot function as antioxidants.

Absorption and Transport

Only 20% to 40% of orally ingested tocopherol and/or its esters are absorbed. Tocopherol esters are almost completely hydrolyzed by a duodenal mucosal esterase prior to absorption. As the dose increases, the percentage of absorption decreases. The efficiency of absorption is enhanced by the simultaneous digestion and absorption of dietary lipids. Medium-chain triglycerides enhance absorption, whereas polyunsaturated fatty acids are some-

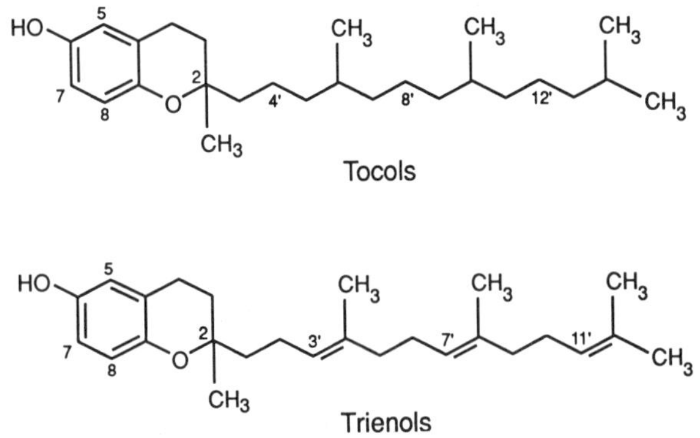

FIG. 12. Basic structures of molecules with vitamin E activity. The tocols have a phytol side chain, whereas the tocotrienoids have a classical isoprenoid side chain.

TABLE 3. *Relationship of biopotency of tocopherols to their structures*

Name	Structure	Bioassay activity		
		Fetal resorption (rat) %	RBC hemolysis (rat) %	Muscle dystrophy (chicken) %
α-T[a]	5, 7, 8 Trimethyl tocol[b]	100	100	100
β-T	5, 8 Dimethyl tocol	37	21	12
γ-T	7, 8 Dimethyl tocol	6	12	5
α-T	8 Methyl tocol	1	1	—
α-T-3[a]	5, 7, 8 Trimethyl tocotrienol	29	21	—
β-T-3	5, 8 Dimethyl tocotrienol	5	3	—

[a] α-T, alpha-tocopherol; α-T-3, alpha tocotrienol.
[b] Because tocopherols contain three asymmetric carbon atoms, there are eight possible diastereoisomers. Only one of these configurations is found in nature and is termed RRR. Thus, the most commonly occurring and also the most active tocopherol, α, is designated RRR-α-tocopherol (formerly d-α-tocopherol). When this vitamin is synthesized, a mixture of the eight isomers is obtained and the product is designated all-rac-α-tocopherol (formerly dl-α-tocopherol). The international unit of α-tocopherol is equivalent to the biological activity 1.0 mg of all-rac-α-tocopheryl-acetate. The corresponding unitage/mg of related compounds is RRR-α-tocopherol, 1.49; RRR-α-tocopherol-acetate, 1.36; all-rac-α-tocopherol, 1.10; RRR-α-tocotrienol, 0.37 (33).

what inhibitory. Both bile and pancreatic juice are necessary for maximal absorption of vitamin E.

Vitamin E is absorbed as a lipid-bile micelle together with free fatty acids, monoglycerides, and other fat-soluble vitamins by penetrating the epithelial cells through the apical plasma membrane. Absorption of vitamin E is maximal in the median portion of the small intestine; none is absorbed in the large intestine. Unlike cholesterol or vitamin A, α-tocopherol is not reesterified prior to its incorporation into the chylomicron and its delivery to the liver in the chylomicron remnant. From the liver it is secreted with VLDL and delivered to LDL [and high-density lipoproteins (HDL) via lipid exchange] and most likely is delivered to peripheral tissues via the LDL receptor. Plasma tocopherol levels in children range from 3 to 10 μg/ml with an average of 6 μg/ml. The ratio of tocopherol to total lipid in plasma of children is 1.2 mg/g (36). Values for tocopherol in the plasma of adults is about 50% higher than in children. Red blood cells, which contain about 20% of the vitamin E in plasma, also participate in the transport of the vitamins.

Free tocopherol is concentrated in the membranes of cells including those of the mitochondria and reticulum. Isomers of RRR-α-tocopherol are not retained well in tissue membranes (36). Distribution of α-tocopherol within cells may be facilitated by a specific cytosol-binding protein. Adipose tissue, adrenal, testes, and pituitary contain the highest concentration of α-tocopherol. The human body stores about 40 mg/kg of vitamin E, the greatest amount of any fat-soluble vitamin. About 77% of stored vitamin E is in adipose tissue, 20% in muscle, and only 1% in liver.

Metabolism

Vitamin E is metabolized to oxidized and chain-shortened products. Less than 1% of orally ingested vitamin E is excreted in the urine as metabolites; most is

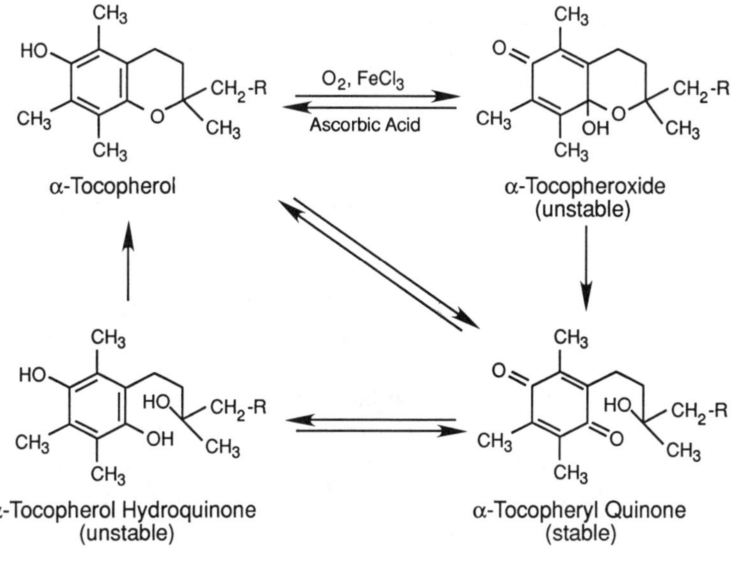

FIG. 13. Oxidation products of α-tocopherol (35).

found in the gut where excretion occurs by the hepatobiliary system. In addition, as an antioxidant, vitamin E is oxidized to a variety of products, including tocopherol quinone and chain-shortened compounds, such as Simon's lactone, usually excreted in the urine as the glucuronide (37).

Physiological Function

The principal function of vitamin E is to serve as a physiological membrane-bound antioxidant. Since free radical–catalyzed lipid peroxidation seems to be a continual biologic process that damages cellular and intracellular structures, vitamin E appears to promote health by inhibiting this process and terminating radical chain reactions (Table 4).

This mode of action of vitamin E is supported by seven lines of evidence: (a) α-tocopherol *in vitro* is a lipid antioxidant; (b) a high intake of polyunsaturated fat increases the vitamin E requirement; (c) tissues of vitamin E–deficient animals are more easily peroxidized than those of normal animals; (d) ceroid pigments, which are products of peroxidation, accumulate in vitamin E deficiency; (e) several labile polyunsaturated lipids like vitamin A and carotene are protected by vitamin E; (f) synthetic antioxidants can protect against certain signs of vitamin E deficiency in certain species; and (g) the metabolic products of tocopherol are consistent with its antioxidant function.

Lipid peroxidation is a chain reaction that occurs in three stages; initiation, propagation, and termination. Antioxidants in general and α-tocopherol in particular inhibit propagation by inducing termination early in the process (38).

TABLE 4. *Radical catalyzed lipid peroxidation and the action of antioxidants*

1. Initiation (formation of free radical)
   Initiators
   $$RH \xrightarrow{H^\bullet} R^\bullet$$
2. Propagation
   1) $R^\bullet + O_2 \rightarrow RO_2^\bullet$
   2) $RO_2^\bullet + RH \rightarrow R^\bullet + ROOH$
3. Termination
   $2 RO_2^\bullet \rightarrow$ inactive products
4. Antioxidant reaction
   $RO_2^\bullet + ArOH \rightarrow ArO^\bullet + ROOH$
5. Regeneration of antioxidant
   $ArO^\bullet + GSH \rightarrow ArOH + GS^\bullet$
   $2GS^\bullet \rightarrow GSSG$
   $GSSG + NADPH + H^+ \rightarrow 2GSH + NADP^+$

RH, polyunsaturated fatty acid; $R^\bullet$, carbon-centered fatty acid radical; $RO_2^\bullet$, peroxyradical; ArOH, α-tocopherol; $GS^\bullet$, glutathione radical; GSSG, oxidized glutathione; GSH, reduced glutathione.

Initiators are reactants (often other radicals) that abstract an H atom from a substrate, in this case a polyunsaturated fatty acid. In the propagation stage, the fatty acid radical reacts with oxygen to form a peroxy radical and then with another polyunsaturated fatty acid to form another fatty acid radical that recycles to form more peroxy radicals. It can easily become a runaway process.

Vitamin E terminates this chain reaction by reacting with peroxy radicals. In fact, α-tocopherol reacts with peroxy radicals faster than they can react with other fatty acids and 200 times faster than the rate at which a commercial antioxidant, butylated hydroxytoluene (BHT), reacts with peroxy radicals. Some of the α-tocopherol is regenerated by glutathione and glutathione reductase. Vitamin C may also accomplish this. Some of the ArO$^\bullet$ is dimerized to inactive products. Because vitamin E is gradually used during antioxidation, daily replacement from the diet is necessary. Since vitamin E stores are ample in all but infants, the incubation period for vitamin E deficiency is relatively long.

There are some features of vitamin E deficiency, however, that are not consistent with the antioxidant hypothesis and have led to the view that, like vitamins A and D, vitamin E may affect the expression of some genes (37,39–42). Evidence in favor of a genetic regulatory function for vitamin E is the following: (a) defects in embryogenesis are observed in the absence of vitamin E; (b) alteration in sexuality and morphology has been induced by vitamin E in the rotifer *Asplanchna*, a carnivorous metazoan; (c) the synthesis of the enzyme creatine kinase and xanthine oxidase is increased four to eight times in vitamin E–deficient animals; (d) a cytoplasmic binding protein for α-tocopherol has been identified; and (e) DNA and RNA turnover are altered in dystrophic muscle of vitamin E–deficient rabbits.

Karl Mason, in 1944, voiced the sentiments of many investigators (39–42). "The antioxidant function of the tocopherols, important as it may be, cannot represent the prime role of vitamin E in the animal body" (43). Like insulin, vitamin A and vitamin B_6, vitamin E may have several actions at the molecular level.

Nutritional Requirements

The vitamin E requirement of normal infants, estimated from the amount needed to prevent peroxidative hemolysis, is approximately 0.4 μg/kg body weight/day. For premature infants, 15 to 20 mg/day may be required to maintain normal plasma values. The RDA for vitamin E for both infants and adults are presented in Table 2. The RDA for infants increases from 3 to 6 mg of RRR-α-tocopherol from birth to 2 years of age.

Vitamin E allowances for adults are 8 mg of RRR-α-tocopherol/day for women and 10 mg/day for men. These allowances are based on diets containing 7% of calories from polyunsaturated fatty acid (PUFA). If the PUFA content of the diet varies, a guideline for healthy persons is 0.4 mg α-TE (tocopherol equivalents) per gram of dietary polyunsaturated fat (13).

Vitamin E Deficiency

Infants are born in a state of relative tocopherol deficiency with plasma α-tocopherol levels below 5 µg/ml. The smaller the infant, the greater the degree of deficiency. Term infants who are breast-fed quickly attain adult blood tocopherol values. The vitamin E–deficient state of premature infants during the first few weeks of life can be attributed to limited placental transfer of vitamin E, low tissue levels at birth, relative dietary deficiency in infancy, intestinal malabsorption, and rapid growth. As the digestive system matures, tocopherol absorption improves and blood vitamin E levels rise. Infants weighing less than 1,500 g at birth may, however, have tocopherol malabsorption until 2 to 3 months of age.

Hemolytic anemia in premature infants may be a manifestation of vitamin E deficiency. The anemia presents with hemoglobin levels in the range of 7 to 9 g/dl, and is accompanied by low plasma vitamin E levels, reticulocytosis and hyperbilirubinemia. In these children administration of iron may exacerbate red blood cell destruction unless vitamin E is also administered. This anemia has been associated with ingestion of formulas high in PUFA and low in α-tocopherol. Parenteral vitamin E improves the anemia and corrects the hemolysis (34).

In children and adults, fat malabsorption generally underlies vitamin E deficiency. Abetalipoproteinemia, caused by the genetic absence of apolipoprotein B, causes serious fat malabsorption and steatorrhea, with progressive neuropathy and retinopathy in the first two decades of life. Plasma vitamin E levels are sometimes undetectable. High-dose vitamin E has improved symptoms in young patients and arrested the neurological disorder in older patients (43).

In 1981, a similar neurological disorder was linked to vitamin E deficiency in children with chronic cholestatic hepatobiliary disease (45). Plasma vitamin E levels below 3 µg/ml, elevated hydrogen peroxide hemolysis of red blood cells, and marked depletion of tissue vitamin E stores were found in these children. Children with cystic fibrosis also manifest this disease. The neurologic syndrome is that of spinocerebellar ataxia with loss of deep tendon reflexes, truncal and limb ataxia, loss of vibration and position sense, ophthalmoplegia, muscle weakness, ptosis, and dysarthria (Table 5) (45,46). A pigmented retinopathy may also occur.

A rare, isolated form of vitamin E deficiency without general fat malabsorption has been reported. Most of these malabsorption syndromes respond to massive doses of oral vitamin E (100 to 200 mg/kg/day) with amelioration of the deficiency and prevention of the neurological sequelae (47).

In adults, spinocerebellar ataxia due to vitamin E deficiency is much rarer, probably because depletion of vitamin E stores to a critical level would require severe malabsorption for more than 20 years. Enhanced peroxidation of red cells and isolated instances of muscle atrophy with creatinuria responsive to vitamin E have been reported.

Clinical Case

A severely crippled 8-year-old boy with biliary atresia and growth failure (height and weight below the third percentile) was referred to the Children's Hospital Research Foundation, University of Cincinnati, for treatment of his progressive neurological disease (47–49). The patient was a thin, jaundiced, dwarfed boy with prominent forehead and widely spaced eyes who needed a walker for ambulation. He had the murmur of pulmonic stenosis and exhibited massive hepatosplenomeg-

TABLE 5. *Clinical features of vitamin E deficiency disorders (46)*

	Abetalipoproteinemia	Chronic childhood cholestasis	Other fat malabsorption disorders	Isolated vitamin E deficiency
Hypo/areflexia	++	++	++	±
Cerebellar ataxia	++	++	++	++
Loss of position sense	++	++	+	±
Loss of vibratory sense	++	++	++	++
Loss of touch, pain	+	±	+	−
Ophthalmoplegia	+	+	+	−
Ptosis	+	+	±	−
Muscle weakness	+	+	+	+
Pigmented retinopathy	++	±	+	−
Dysarthria	+	±	+	±

++, always present; +, commonly present; ±, inconsistently present; −, absent.

aly. Neurological examination showed severe areflexia and severe truncal ataxia, severe dysmetria and markedly decreased vibration sense, decreased proprioception, and ophthalmoplegia. Sural nerve biopsy showed moderate axonal degeneration and mild axonal loss. Muscle biopsy showed moderate neuropathy and severe myopathy. Laboratory studies found total plasma proteins to be 7.3 g/dl (normal: 5.5 to 7.5 g/dl), albumin 3.9 g/dl (normal: 3.8 to 5.4 g/dl), total bilirubin 21.6 mg/dl (normal: less than 1.0 mg/dl), and direct bilirubin 14.8 mg/dl (normal: less than 0.4 mg/dl). Total plasma lipids were 1,070 mg/dl (normal: 320 to 570 mg/dl), serum cholesterol was 316 mg/dl (normal: 120 to 230 mg/dl), and triglycerides were 206 mg/dl (normal: 20 to 120 mg/dl). Fecal fat was normal at 14.5% of the administered dose (normal: less than 5%). A liver biopsy showed atresia of intrahepatic biliary ducts and cirrhosis.

A vitamin E absorption test was carried out by administering 100 IU of dl-α-tocopherol per kilogram body weight, with 150 ml of milk. Following this, serum vitamin E was measured at 0 time and at 6, 12, 24, and 48 hr. The maximum change in plasma α-tocopherol was recorded and expressed as the rise in serum vitamin E concentration divided by the total serum lipid concentration (Δ vitamin E in milligrams/total lipids in grams), a ratio that identifies children with vitamin E malabsorption. In this patient, the vitamin E absorption test revealed a coefficient of 0.05 (normal: 1.9 to 9.2). The patient had a serum vitamin E level of less than 1 μg/ml (normal: 3.8 to 15.5 μg/dl) on an intake of 50 mg α-tocopherol per day. His serum E/cholesterol ratio was 0.16 (normal: 0.9 to 5.9). The red cell hemolysis test showed 38% hemolysis (normal: 0%). He was treated with 1 to 2 mg of intramuscular vitamin E per kilogram per day, which arrested progression of the disease.

Hypervitaminosis E

Relatively large amounts of vitamin E, in the range of 400 to 800 mg of l-α-tocopherol, have been taken daily by adults for months to years without causing any apparent harm. Occasionally, muscle weakness, fatigue, nausea, and diarrhea have been reported in persons taking 800 to 3,200 mg/day. The most significant toxic effect of vitamin E at dosages exceeding 1,000 mg/day is the antagonism to vitamin K action and the enhancement of the effect of oral coumarin anticoagulant drugs, with overt hemorrhage (50).

VITAMIN K

In 1929, Dam observed subcutaneous and intraperitoneal hemorrhages in chicks fed a fat-free diet (51). He then demonstrated the cause to be a dietary deficiency of a previously unrecognized fat-soluble substance. This factor, the absence of which caused delayed coagulation of the blood, was not identical to any known lipid including the fat-soluble vitamins A, D, and E. Further investigation found it to be broadly distributed in the plant kingdom, particularly in green leafy vegetables. Dam named the new substance "vitamin K" for its "koagulation" activity (52).

In 1939, Doisy and his colleagues (53) and Dam and coworkers (54) announced independently the isolation of vitamin K from alfalfa. In addition, Doisy's group reported the isolation of a related, but not identical, vitamin K from putrefied fish meal (55). They named these compounds vitamins K_1 and K_2.

Chemistry

Vitamin K is a generic term for derivatives of 2-methyl-1,4-naphthoquinone with procoagulation activity. The natural forms are substituted in position 3 with an alkyl side chain. Vitamin K_1, called phylloquinone, has a phytol side chain in position 3 and is the only homologue of vitamin K in plants. Vitamin K_2 is a family of homologues of 2-methyl-1,4-naphthoquinone substituted in position 3 with isoprenyl side chains containing from 4 to 13 isoprenyl units. These are called menaquinones, with a suffix denoting the chain length (Fig. 14). For example, menaquinone-7 was the first member of the vitamin K_2 family isolated from fermented fish meal. The menaquinones synthesized by bacteria in the intestinal tract of humans can contribute to vitamin K requirements. Vitamin K is essential for humans because the 1,4-naphthoquinone moiety cannot be synthesized in animal cells.

Menaquinone-4 is synthesized in animals and birds from the provitamin menadione (2-methyl-1,4-naphthoquinone), formerly known as vitamin K_3 (Fig. 14), by enzymatic alkylation with digeranyl pyrophosphate (56).

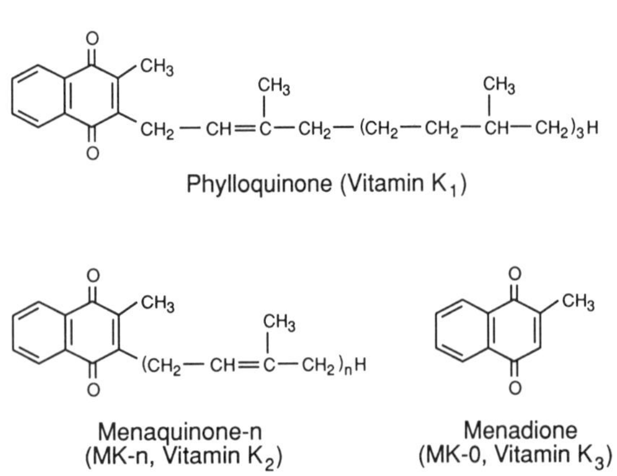

FIG. 14. Structures of vitamin K homologues, which are derivatives of 1,4-naphthoquinone. Phylloquinone (vitamin K_1), menaquinone (vitamin K_2), and menadione (vitamin K_3) are shown.

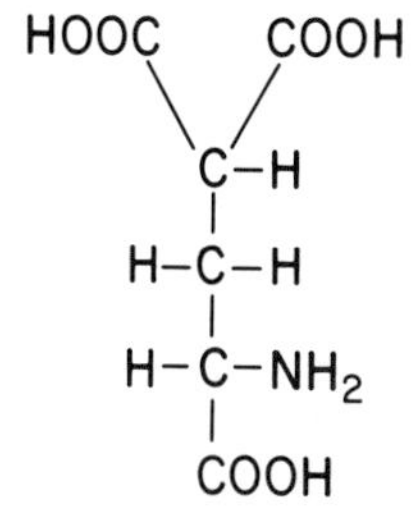

```
HOOC    COOH
    \  /
     C-H
      |
    H-C-H
      |
    H-C-NH₂
      |
     COOH
```

FIG. 15. Structure of α-carboxyglutamic acid (Gla). Gla is a tricarboxylic acid that is stable in strong base but decomposes with γ-decarboxylation in strong acid. Its isoelectric point is pH 3.0.

The enzyme has been partially purified and characterized from chick and rat liver microsomes (57,58). The other menaquinones are products of bacterial biosynthesis and range from menaquinone-6 to menaquinone-13. Partially saturated menaquinones, menaquinone-9-H and menaquinone-8-H, are known.

Absorption and Transport

The absorption of phylloquinone and the menaquinones requires bile and pancreatic juice for maximum effectiveness. Dietary vitamin K is absorbed in the small bowel, incorporated into chylomicrons, and delivered to the circulation via the lymph. The efficiency of absorption has been measured from 40% to 80%, depending on the vehicle in which the vitamin is administered and the extent of the enterohepatic circulation generally characteristic of isoprenoid lipids. When isotopically labeled phylloquinone was administered to animals and humans by mouth, in doses ranging from physiologic to pharmacologic, the vitamin appeared in the plasma within 20 min, peaked at 2 hr, and then declined exponentially to low values over 48 to 72 hr, reaching fasting levels of 1 to 3 ng/ml. During this period, vitamin K in the chylomicron remnant is taken up by the liver and resecreted into the plasma as VLDL and ultimately introduced into cells via the LDL receptor. No specific carrier protein for vitamin K in plasma has been identified (59). Both phylloquinone and menaquinone are present in human plasma. Phylloquinone is present in the range of 0.5 ng to 3.0 ng/ml, with an average of 1.5 ng/ml, in healthy persons. Menaquinone is present in much lower amounts.

Metabolism

The liver appears to be the primary target of administered vitamin K in animals and humans. As much as 50% of a parenterally administered dose of vitamin K_1 may appear in the liver of rats within 1 hr. After oral administration, the liver may contain as much as 20% of the administered dose at 2 hr, which then declines to low values after 24 hr. The principal sites of uptake, after liver, are skin and muscle. The total body pool of vitamin K, in animals and humans, is surprisingly small, approximately 1 to 3 μg/kg, of which 80% is in the liver with 65% present in the hepatic endoplasmic reticulum. In omnivorous animals like humans, both phylloquinone and the higher molecular weight menaquinones (MK-7 to MK-13) of bacterial origin are found in the liver (60). Haroon and Hauschka (61) have found phylloquinone levels in rat liver to vary between 8 and 44 ng/g fresh weight (20 to 100 pmol/g) and Shearer (62) has found somewhat lower levels in human liver, i.e., 1 to 21 ng/g. Taggart and Matschiner (63) estimated that 10 pmol/g (4.5 ng/g) of vitamin K is the minimum hepatic concentration to sustain normal prothrombin levels in the rat.

The terminal oxidation of vitamin K and its epoxides involves chain shortening and excretion in urine and stool mainly as glucuronides of vitamin K lactones (57).

Physiological Function

The physiological function of vitamin K is to carboxylate selected glutamic acids in the translation products of vitamin K–dependent proteins to produce γ-carboxyglutamates (64) (Fig. 15). The number of γ-carboxyglutamic acid (Gla) per mole of coagulant protein ranges from 10 to 12. Factors II (prothrombin), VII, IX, and X are procoagulant proenzymes whereas proteins C, S, and M are anticoagulant proenzymes (Table 6). The function of Gla in these proteins is to facilitate the chelation of calcium ions to Gla and platelet phosphatide, which is essential for the coagulation cascade to operate (65) (Fig. 16).

TABLE 6. *Characteristics of the vitamin K-dependent proenzymes*

Characteristic	Factor				Protein		
	II	X	IX	VII	C	S	Z
Plasma concentration (μg/ml)	100	20	3	1	10	1	<1
Molecular weight	72,000	55,000	55,000	46,000	57,000	69,000	55,000
Carbohydrate percentage	8	15	17	13	11	8	(+)
Number of chains	1	2	1	1	2	1	1
Number of Gla residues	10	12	12	10	11	10	13

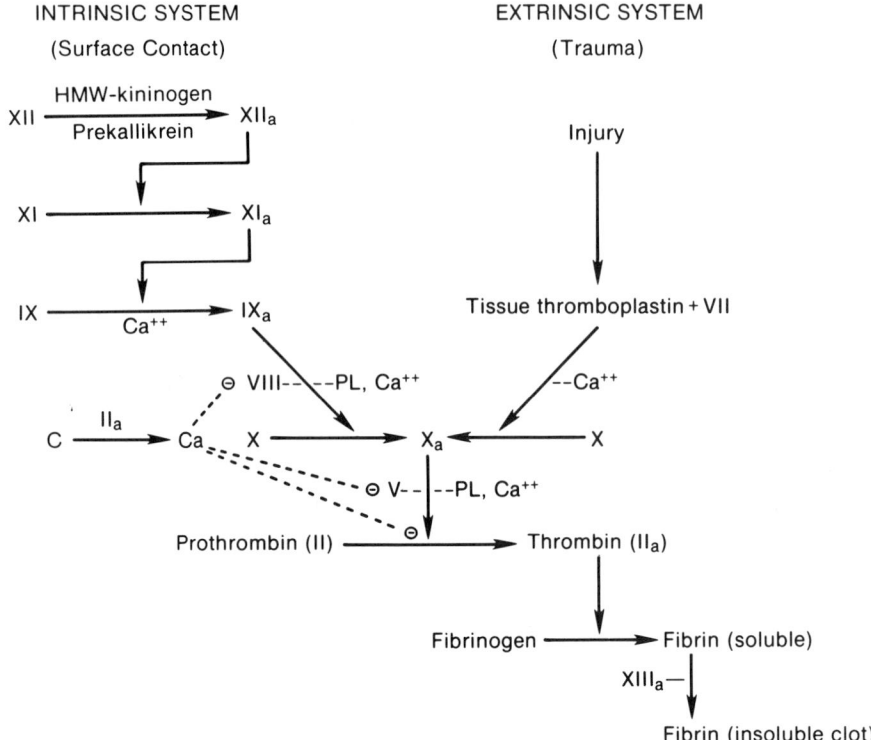

FIG. 16. The clotting factor cascade. Factors II, VII, IX, and X, and protein C contain Gla and are vitamin K–dependent. The first four factors occupy the core of the clotting scheme, whereas protein C is an anticoagulant protein that inactivates Factors V_a and VIII_a. Protein S is a cofactor for protein C and enhances its rate of activation by thrombin. Ca^{2+} is required to activate Gla-containing factors. Factor V (accelerator globulin) and Factor VIII (antihemophilic globulin) are cofactors. Factor XIII is a transpeptidase (65).

The vitamin K–dependent carboxylase system is a membrane-bound component of the reticulum. It has been solubilized from microsomes and, in the soluble form, retains most of the properties of the microsomal system. The system requires a peptide substrate, O_2, CO_2, and either vitamin K plus nicotinamide-adenine dinucleotide, reduced (NADH) or vitamin K hydroquinone; adenosine triphosphate (ATP) is not required. The active form of the vitamin is the hydroquinone (the reduced form) and constitutes the electron donor for a microsomal electron transport system for which oxygen is the terminal acceptor. This electron transport system is coupled to a CO_2-fixation reaction converting peptide-bound glutamate to γ-carboxyglutamate. Artificial substrates initiating partial sequences of prothrombin precursor such as Phe-Leu-Glu-Glu-Leu have proved to be active in this system.

The mechanism of the vitamin K–dependent carboxylation is still obscure. Figure 17 presents a hypothesis that attempts to explain the overall reaction:

$$KH_2 + Glu_p + CO_2 + O_2 \xrightarrow[\text{carboxylase}]{Mn^{2+}} KO + Gla_p + H_2O.$$

It is visualized that this is an ordered reaction in which O_2 can bind with reduced vitamin K to produce a hydroperoxide anion. This, or a derivative, in turn, removes a proton from the γ-carbon of glutamate to generate a carbanion which can attack CO_2 and produce Gla. Both the glutamic acid reactant and the γ-carboxyglutamate product are peptide bound (66).

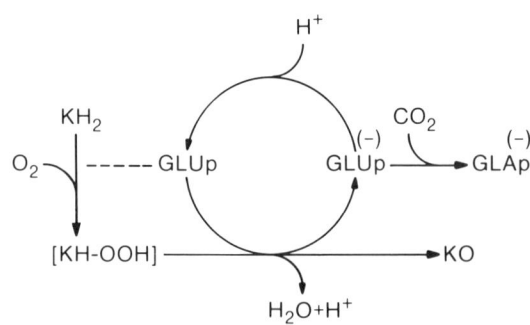

FIG. 17. Hypothetical mechanism for the coupling of carboxylation and epoxidation in vitamin K–dependent Gla synthesis. Vitamin K hydroquinone is KH_2; vitamin K hydroperoxide is KH-OOH; vitamin K-2,3-epoxide is KO; peptide-bound glutamate is GLUp; peptide-bound γ-carboxyglutamate is GLAp (65).

Vitamin K Cycle

In 1970, Matschiner et al. (67) reported the isolation and characterization of phylloquinone 2,3-epoxide as a new metabolite of phylloquinone in the rat. Normally found in small amounts, marked accumulations of the epoxide were demonstrated in the presence of warfarin. Approximately 30 years earlier, Fieser and his colleagues (68) had synthesized the 2,3-epoxide of phylloquinone and shown that it was rapidly converted to vitamin K in normal animals and humans. The vitamin K cycle is a salvage pathway for vitamin K, a vitamin present in only nanomolar quantities in liver and other tissues (Fig. 18). The cycle postulates that the vitamin K–dependent carboxylase converts vitamin K to its 2,3-epoxide, usually in excess of the carboxylation rate. The epoxide is then reduced to the quinone by a dithiol-dependent epoxide reductase, and the vitamin K formed is reduced to the vitamin K hydroquinone by several possible enzymes, at least one driven by a dithiol and others by nicotinamide-adenine dinucleotide phosphate, reduced (NADPH). The dithiol-dependent epoxide reductase and quinone reductase are strongly inhibited by warfarin, whereas the NADPH-dependent dehydrogenases are relatively insensitive (69).

Nutritional Requirements

The vitamin K requirement of mammals is met by a combination of dietary intake and microbiological biosynthesis in the gut. Genetic factors play a role as shown by the higher requirements for vitamin K by males than females. In conventional rats the vitamin K requirement is about 10 μg/kg body weight, whereas, in germ-free rats, the requirement is more than doubled.

The vitamin K–dependent coagulation factors are depressed to 30% of normal at birth in full-term infants and even lower in premature newborns. The vitamin K requirement for the normalization of prothrombin and other factor levels in newborns is 3 to 5 μg/day. Since breast milk contains only 2 μg phylloquinone per liter, breast-fed infants must be fortified with vitamin K in order to prevent the hemorrhagic disease of the newborn. In adults, studies in volunteers have shown that prothrombin levels can be maintained on intakes of 10 to 30 μg of phylloquinone per day for 8 weeks. From these data, it may be concluded that the requirement for adults is in the range of 10 to 30 μg/day or 0.2 to 0.5 μg/kg/day. Usual diets in the United States contain between 100 and 500 μg phylloquinone per day. Green leafy vegetables are rich in phylloquinone, animal foods intermediate, and cereals low in this vitamin (70).

The RDA for vitamin K is shown in Table 2. The allowance for infants increases from 5 μg/day at birth to 10 μg/day at 2 years. For adults, the recommended amounts are 50 μg/day for women and 60 μg/day for men.

Vitamin K Deficiency

The vitamin K nutrition of newborn infants warrants special attention because (a) the placenta is a relatively poor organ for the maternal-fetal transmission of lipids, (b) the neonatal liver is immature with respect to

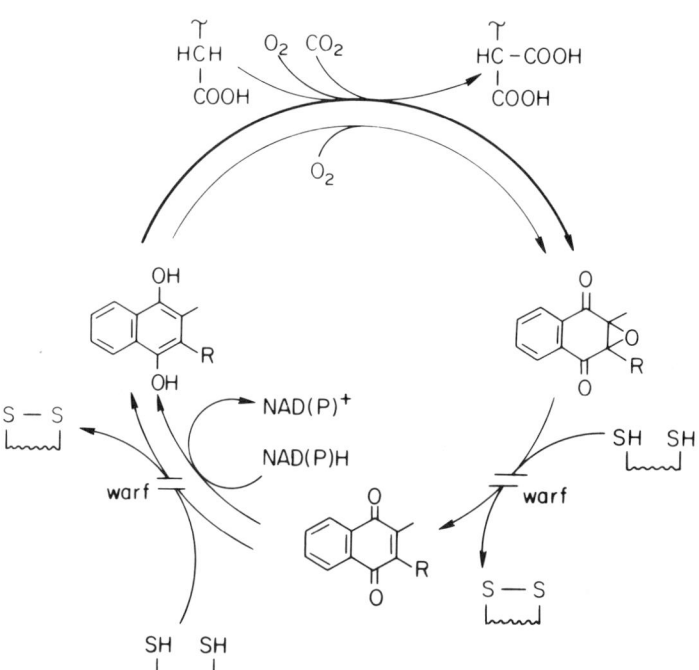

FIG. 18. The vitamin K cycle occurs in the hepatic endoplasmic reticulum. The carboxylation and epoxidation activities are catalyzed by the same enzyme. The dithiol-dependent reductions of the vitamin K epoxide and of vitamin K are extremely sensitive to the action of coumarin anticoagulants such as warfarin (warf). NADPH-dependent dehydrogenases, however, are not inhibited by warfarin (68).

prothrombin synthesis, and (c) the gut is sterile during the first few days. In normal newborns, the plasma prothrombin concentration and that of the other vitamin K–dependent factors may be as low as 30% of adults, gradually climbing, as food adequate in vitamin K is taken, to normal adult values over a period of weeks (71). If prothrombin and other vitamin K–dependent protein values fall below 10%, hemorrhagic disease of the newborn may appear (72). Reduced vitamin K levels in plasma and the appearance of des-γ-carboxyprothrombin (abnormal prothrombin) appears in plasma in deficient patients. Premature infants are even more susceptible to vitamin K deficiency than are full-term infants (Fig. 19) (71).

In 1937, it was recognized that breast-fed infants were at higher risk of hemorrhage than were formula-fed babies (72). Recent high-pressure liquid chromatographic studies of the vitamin K content of human and cow's milk have shown that human milk contains only 1 to 2 μg/l, whereas cow's milk contains 5 to 17 μg/l. Since the requirement for vitamin K in the newborn is estimated to be 0.5 μg/kg/day, the very low content of vitamin K in human milk accounts for the greater predisposition of breast-fed infants to develop the hemorrhagic syndrome. Since breast milk is sterile and delays colonization of the gut with bacteria, Seeler (73) recommends that breast-fed babies receive 1 mg phylloquinone intramuscularly at birth.

Infants of mothers on hydantoin anticonvulsants should have prophylactic vitamin K because diphenylhydantoin is an antagonist to vitamin K. Patients receiving anticonvulsant drugs show increased levels of abnormal prothrombin in their plasma. Neonatal complications such as diarrhea, malabsorption, cystic fibrosis, idiopathic cholestasis, atresia of the bile duct, and prolonged parenteral nutrition are all indications for intramuscular vitamin K administration.

Adults are relatively resistant to vitamin K deficiency unless they have biliary obstruction, malabsorption, liver disease, or receive total parenteral nutrition or coumarin anticoagulant drugs (70).

Clinical Case

A 3,100 g (6.8 lb) full-term male infant, the child of a 22-year-old primigravida, was delivered naturally from the cephalic position after a labor of 7 hr and 13 min at the Cincinnati General Hospital. The infant was breast-fed and appeared normal in all respects during the first 3 days. On the fourth day he was circumcised and bled abnormally from the wound, requiring resuturing. On that day he also passed a bloody stool. A study of his coagulation profile showed a prothrombin time of 47 sec (normal 12 sec) and a thromboplastin generation time of 36 sec (normal: 10 sec). Factor VII was 6% of normal, Factor X 29% of normal. He was switched to a cow's milk formula and within 8 hr his prothrombin time was 15 sec and the bleeding had stopped (Fig. 20). Equally dramatic results were obtained in other children with hemorrhagic disease of the newborn with 100 μg of menadione sodium bisulfite (74).

Hypervitaminosis K

Menadione unsubstituted in the 3 position causes toxicity in children expressed by jaundice, hemolysis, and kernicterus. Phylloquinone is essentially nontoxic (29).

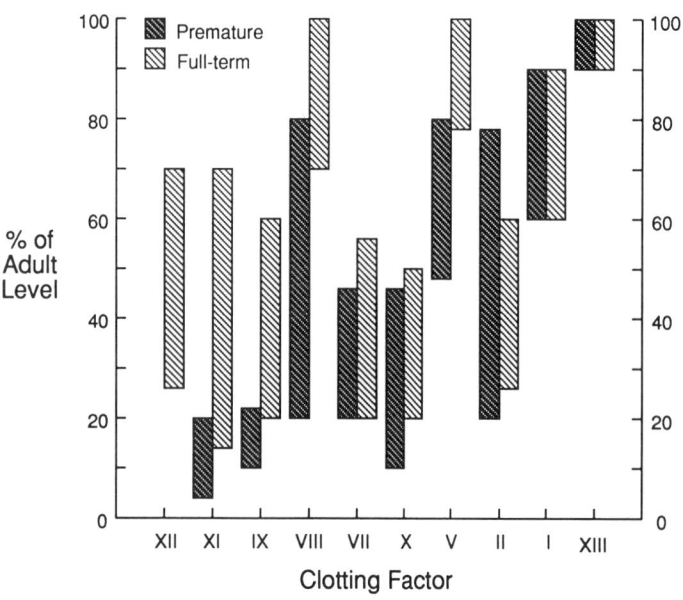

FIG. 19. Comparison of coagulation factor activities of full-term and premature newborn infants with those of adults (71).

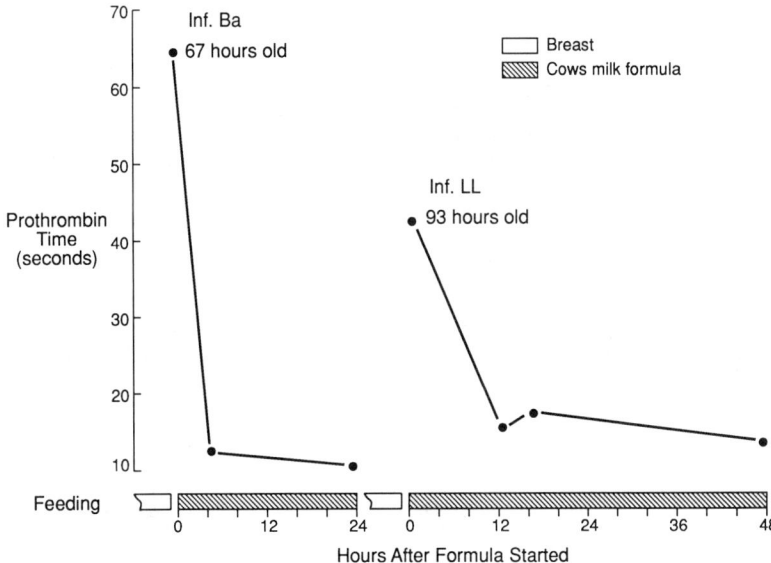

FIG. 20. Effect of changing diet from breast milk to cow's milk formula on the prothrombin time of two infants with hemorrhagic disease of the newborn. Infant LL is described in the case presentation (74).

SUMMARY

The fat-soluble vitamins, A, D, E, and K, control protein synthesis at either the transcriptional or posttranscriptional level. All of them are converted to active forms in the body, by oxidation, hydroxylation, reduction, or simple ionization. The active forms of vitamins A and D are ligands for receptors that interact with DNA and control gene expression. In addition, vitamins A and E exercise epigenetic effect in vision and antioxidation. Both normal and particularly premature newborn infants are at risk for fat-soluble vitamin deficiency disease because the placenta is a poor organ for the transmission of lipids to the fetus. Older children subsisting on low-fat rice-based diets are at continuing risk for vitamin A deficiency. Breast milk, usually considered an "ideal" food, is deficient in both vitamins D and K, and must be supplemented with these vitamins to protect breast-fed infants.

REFERENCES

1. McCollum EV, Davis M. The necessity of certain lipids in the diet during growth. *J Biol Chem* 1913;15:167–175.
2. McCollum EV. The supplementary dietary relationship among our natural foodstuffs. *Harvey Lect* 1917;12:151–180.
3. Moore T. The conversion of carotene to vitamin A *in vivo*. *Biochem J* 1930;24:682–702.
4. Karrer P, Morf R. The constitution of β-carotene. *Helv Chim Acta* 1931;14:1033–1040.
5. Wald G. Carotenoids and vitamin A cycle in vision. *Nature* 1934;134:65.
6. Ong DE. Vitamin A-binding proteins. *Nutr Rev* 1985;43:225–232.
7. Goodman DS, Olson JA. Enzymatic conversion of all-trans-β-carotene into retinal. *Methods Enzymol* 1969;15:462–475.
8. On the mechanism of β-carotene cleavage to vitamin A. *Nutr Rev* 1988;46:327–329.
9. Lakshman MR, Mychkovsky I, Attlesey M. Enzymatic conversion of all-trans-β-carotene to retinal by a cytosolic enzyme from rabbit and rat intestinal mucosa. *Proc Natl Acad Sci USA* 1989;86:9124–9128.
10. Blomhoff R, Green H, Berg T, Norum KR. Transport and storage of vitamin A. *Science* 1990;250:399–403.
11. Stryer L. Cyclic GMP cascade of vision. *Annu Rev Neurosci* 1986;9:87–119.
12. Evans RM. The steroid and thyroid hormone receptor superfamily. *Science* 1988;240:889–894.
13. Food and Nutrition Board. *Recommended dietary allowances*, 10th ed. Washington, DC: National Research Council/National Academy Press, 1989.
14. Vitamin A deficiency—a global disease. *Nutr Rev* 1985;43:240–243.
15. McClaren DS, Shirajian E, Tchalian M, Khoury G. Xerophthalmia in Jordan. *Am J Clin Nutr* 1965;17:117–130.
16. Sauberlich HE, Hodges RE, Wallace H, et al. Vitamin A metabolism and requirements studied with the use of labeled retinol. *Vitam Horm* 1974;32:251–275.
17. Mellanby E. An experimental investigation on rickets. *Lancet* 1919;i:407–412.
18. Steenbock H, Black A. Fat-soluble vitamins. *J Biol Chem* 1924;61:405–422.
19. Windaus A, Linsert O, Luttringhaus A, Weidlich A. Crystalline vitamin D_2. *Ann Chemie* 1932;492:226–241.
20. Askew F, Bourdillon RG, Bruce HM, Callow RK, Philpot J, Webster TA. Crystalline vitamin D. *Proc R Soc Lond* 1932;109:448–506.
21. Holick MF, Schnoes HK, De Luca HF. Identification of 1,25-$(OH)_2D_3$, a form of vitamin D_3 metabolically active in the intestine. *Proc Natl Acad Sci USA* 1971;68:803–804.
22. DeLuca HF. Vitamin D and its metabolites. In: Shils ME, Young VR, eds. *Modern nutrition in health and disease*, 7th Ed. Philadelphia: Lea & Febiger, 1988; 313–327.
23. Haussler MR. Vitamin D receptors: nature and function. *Annu Rev Nutr* 1986;6:527–562.
24. Pike JW. Vitamin D_3 receptors: structure and function in transcription. *Annu Rev Nutr* 1991;11:189–216.
25. Neer RM, Holick MF, DeLuca HF, Potts JT. Effect of 1-α-hydroxyvitamin D_3 and 1,25-dihydroxyvitamin D_3 on calcium and phosphorous metabolism in hypoparathyrodism. *Metabolism* 1975;24:1403–1413.
26. Minghetti PP, Norman AW. 1,25$(OH)_2$vitamin D_3 receptors: gene regulation and genetic circuitry. *FASEB J* 1988;2:3043–3053.
27. Rickets in a breast-fed infant. *Nutr Rev* 1984;42:380–382.
28. Garabedian M, Vainsel M, Mallet E, et al. Circulating vitamin D metabolite concentrations in children with nutritional rickets. *J Pediatr* 1983;103:381–386.
29. Council on Scientific Affairs. Vitamin preparations as dietary supplements and as therapeutic agents. *JAMA* 1987;257:1929–1936.

30. Evans HM, Bishop K. On the relation between fertility and nutrition. *Am J Physiol* 1922;63:396–402.
31. Evans HM, Emerson OH, Emerson GA. Isolation from wheat germ oil of alcohol, α-tocopherol, having properties of vitamin E. *J Biol Chem* 1936;113:319–332.
32. Karrer P, Fritzsche H, Ringier BH, Salomon H. α-Tocopherol. *Helv Chim Acta* 1938;21:520–525.
33. Olson RE. Vitamin E and its relation to heart disease. *Circulation* 1973;48:179–184.
34. Machlin LJ. Vitamin E. In: Machlin LJ, ed. *Handbook of vitamins.* New York: Marcel Dekker, 1984;99–145.
35. Scott ML, Nesheim MC, Young RJ. *Nutrition of the chicken.* Ithaca, NY: M. Scott, 1969.
36. Farrell PM, Levine SL, Murphy MD, Adams AJ. Plasma tocopherol levels and tocopherol-lipid relationships in a normal population of children as compared to healthy adults. *Am J Clin Nutr* 1978;31:1720–1726.
37. Simon EJ, Eisengart A, Sundheim L, Milhorat AT. Purification and characterization of urinary metabolites of α-tocopherol. *J Biol Chem* 1956;221:807–817.
38. Burton GW, Traber MG. Vitamin E: antioxidant activity, biokinetics and bioavailability. *Annu Rev Nutr* 1990;10:357–382.
39. Olson RE. Are we looking at the right enzyme systems? *Am J Clin Nutr* 1967;20:604–611.
40. Olson RE. Creatine kinase and myofibrillar proteins in hereditary muscular dystrophy and in vitamin E deficiency. *Am J Clin Nutr* 1974;27:1117–1129.
41. Cantignani GL. Vitamin E: its role in nucleic acid and protein metabolism. In: Machlin LJ, ed. *Vitamin E: a comprehensive treatise.* New York: Marcel Dekker, 1980;318–332.
42. Wasserman RH, Taylor AN. Fat-soluble vitamins. *Annu Rev Biochem* 1972;41:179–202.
43. Mason K. Physiological action of vitamin E and its homologues. *Vitam Horm* 1944;2:107–159.
44. Kayden HJ, Silben R, Kossman CE. The role of vitamin E deficiency in the abnormal autohemolysis and acanthocytosis. *Trans Assoc Am Physicians* 1965;78:334–342.
45. Rosenblum JL, Keating JP, Prensky AL, Nelson JS. Progressive neurological syndrome in children with chronic liver disease. *N Engl J Med* 1981;304:503–508.
46. Sokol RJ. Vitamin E deficiency and neurologic function. *Annu Rev Nutr* 1988;8:351–373.
47. Harding AE, Muller DPR, Thomas PK, Willison JH. Spinocerebellar degeneration associated with a selective defect in vitamin E absorption. *N Engl J Med* 1985;313:32–35.
48. Sokol RJ, Henbi JE, Iannoccane ST, Bove RE, Balistreri WF. Vitamin E deficiency with normal serum vitamin E concentrations in children with chronic cholestasis. *N Engl J Med* 1984;310:1209–1212.
49. Vitamin E deficiency in children with chronic cholestasis. *Nutr Rev* 1984;42:284–286.
50. Corrigan JJ, Marcus FI. Coagulopathy associated with vitamin E ingestion. *JAMA* 1974;230:1300–1301.
51. Dam H. Cholesterinstoffwechsel in Huhnereiern und Hugnchen. *Biochem Zeitschr* 1929;215:475–492.
52. Dam H. The antihemorrhagic vitamin of the chick. *Biochem J* 1935;29:1273–1285.
53. Binkley SB, MacCorquodale D, Thayer SA, Doisy EA. The isolation of vitamin K$_1$. *J Biol Chem* 1939;130:219–234.
54. Dam H, Geiger A, Glavind J, et al. Isolierung des vitamins K in hochgereinigter form. *Helv Chim Acta* 1939;22:310.
55. McKee RW, Binkley SB, Thayer SA, MacCorquodale DW, Doisy EA. The isolation of vitamin K$_2$. *J Biol Chem* 1939;131:327–344.
56. Dialameh GH, Taggart WV, Matschiner JT, Olson RE. Isolation and characterization of menaquinone-4 as a product of menadione metabolism in chicks and rats. *Int J Vitam Nutr Res* 1971;41:391–400.
57. Dialameh GH, Yekundi KG, Olson RE. Enzymatic alkylation of menaquinone-O to menaquinones by microsomes from chick liver. *Biochim Biophys Acta* 1970;223:332–338.
58. Lee FC, Olson RE. Localization of the menaquinone-O alkylating enzyme in the smooth reticulum of chicken liver microsomes. *Biochim Biophys Acta* 1984;799:166–170.
59. Olson RE. The function and metabolism of vitamin K. *Annu Rev Nutr* 1984;4:281–337.
60. Matschiner JT, Amelotti JM. Characterization of vitamin K from bovine liver. *J Lipid Res* 1968;9:176–179.
61. Haroon Y, Hawschka PV. Application of high pressure liquid chromatography to the assay of phylloquinone in rat liver. *J Lipid Res* 1983;24:481–484.
62. Shearer MJ. Vitamin K and vitamin K–dependent proteins. *Br J Haematol* 1990;75:156–162.
63. Taggart WV, Matschiner JT. Metabolism of menadione-6,7-^{3}H in the rat. *Biochem J* 1969;8:1141–1146.
64. Stenflo J, Fernlund P, Egan W, Roepstorff P. Vitamin K–dependent modification of glutamic acid residues in prothrombin. *Proc Natl Acad Sci USA* 1974;71:2730–2733.
65. Davie EW, Ratnoff OD. Waterfall sequence for intrinsic blood clotting. *Science* 1964;145:1310–1312.
66. Olson RE, Hall AL, Lee FC, Kappel WK. Properties of vitamin K–dependent γ-glutamyl carboxylase for rat liver. *Chemica Scripta* 1987;27A:187–192.
67. Matschiner JT, Bell RG, Sinelotti JM, Knaner JM. Isolation and characterization of a new metabolite of phylloquinone in the rat. *Biochim Biophys Acta* 1970;201:309–315.
68. Fieser LF, Tishler M, Sampson WL. Vitamin K activity and structure. *J Biol Chem* 1941;137:659–692.
69. Wallin R, Hatson S. Vitamin K–dependent carboxylation. Evidence that at least two microsomal dehydrogenases reduce vitamin K to support carboxylation. *J Biol Chem* 1982;257:1583–1586.
70. Olson RE. Vitamin K. In: *Modern nutrition in health and disease,* 7th ed. Shils M, Young V, eds. Philadelphia: Lea & Febiger, 1988;328–338.
71. Bleyer WA, Hakami N, Shepard TH. The development of hemostasis in the human fetus and newborn infant. *J Pediatr* 1971;79:838–853.
72. Brinkhous KM, Smith HP, Warner ED. Plasma prothrombin level in normal infancy and in hemorraghic diseases of the newborn. *Am J Med Sci* 1937;193:475–480.
73. Seeler RA. Vitamin K—revisited. *Illinois Med J* 1975;147:59–61.
74. Sutherland JM, Glueck HI, Gleser G. Hemorrhagic disease of the newborn: breast-feeding as a necessary factor in pathogenesis. *Am J Dis Child* 1967;113:524–533.

Textbook of Pediatric Nutrition, Second Edition,
edited by R.M. Suskind and L. Lewinter-Suskind.
Raven Press, Ltd., New York © 1993.

CHAPTER 7

Disorders of the Water-Soluble Vitamin B-Complex and Vitamin C

Harry L. Greene

The compounds considered to be the class of B-complex vitamins are water-soluble and include thiamine (B_1), riboflavin (B_2), niacin (B_3, nicotinic acid and nicotinamide), pyridoxine (B_6), folate, vitamin B_{12} (cyanocobalamin), pantothenic acid and biotin (Table 1). Each of these vitamins acts as a cofactor for a variety of biochemical reactions. Compared to the fat-soluble vitamins A, D, and E, depletion of water-soluble vitamins may more easily occur. Daily losses in urine, as well as the normal rate of catabolism, dictate frequent dietary intake in order to avoid deficiency. In addition, deficiencies may occur because of increased requirements due to such factors as hypermetabolic states (severe injury, pregnancy, hyperthyroidism), malabsorption, and rapid rates of growth. Symptoms may become clinically overt if increased requirements from any cause are superimposed on borderline deficiency states. Thus, acute or chronic infection often leads to overt clinical manifestations of vitamin deficiency and is commonly a major component of the manifestations of protein-energy malnutrition.

Several members of the vitamin B complex are utilized in the metabolism of a common substrate and, therefore, a deficiency of one vitamin will affect utilization of another. For example, oxidation of ketoacids involves nicotinamide-adenine dinucleotide (NAD) derived from niacin, thiamine, and coenzyme A (which contains pantothenate). In addition, since several vitamins are common to single foods, dietary deficiency of one vitamin is commonly associated with deficiencies of other vitamins, as well as with protein-energy deficiency. Thus, the classic clinical manifestations of a single vitamin deficiency that can be experimentally produced is generally caused only by unusual diets, specific disease (for example, liver or ileal diseases), or drugs that interfere with absorption or metabolism of a vitamin.

H. L. Greene: Bristol Meyers Squibb Company, Mead Johnson Nutritional Group, Evansville, Indiana 47721.

Although a number of compounds will not be discussed, such as carnitine and choline, lipoic acid, inositol para-aminobenzoic acid, pteridines, and ubiquinone, because they are not considered vitamins but act as cofactors for many important enzymatic reactions, they may be useful in management of certain disease entities, for example, lipoate for subacute necrotizing encephalitis or mushroom poisoning. Several of these compounds, which may be synthesized to some degree in man, and are generally not considered as dietary essentials, have been referred to as "conditional vitamins."

This chapter is concerned primarily with the cofactor functions, the deficiency states, and their treatment, as well as the recommended dietary and intravenous intake of the B vitamins (with the exception of B_{12}) and ascorbic acid.

Several clinical states related to abnormal vitamin metabolism are peculiar to children (1). These include a number of inborn errors of metabolism that may respond to pharmacologic doses of vitamins, and certain conditions resulting in inadequate vitamin intake or increased vitamin requirements (Table 2).

CHILDHOOD CONDITIONS AFFECTING VITAMIN STATUS

Vitamin Intake

Breast Milk

If taken in adequate quantity, human milk usually provides daily requirements of vitamin C and all the B vitamins except preformed niacin (Table 3). However,

TABLE 1. Recommended daily allowances of fat-soluble and water-soluble vitamins

Age (yr) and sex group	Fat-soluble vitamins					Water-soluble vitamins								
	Vitamin A (µg R.E.)	Vitamin D (µg)	Vitamin E (mg α-T.E.)	Vitamin K (µg)		Vitamin C (mg)	Thiamine (mg)	Riboflavin (mg)	Niacin (mg N.E.)	Vitamin B_6 (mg)	Folacin (µg)	Vitamin B_{12} (µg)	Biotin (µg)	Pantothenic acid (mg)
Infants														
0–0.5	375	7.5	3	5		30	0.3	0.4	5	0.3	25	0.3	35	2
0.5–1.0	375	10	4	10		35	0.4	0.5	6	0.6	35	0.5	50	3
Children														
1–3	400	10	6	15		40	0.7	0.8	9	1.0	50	0.7	65	3
4–6	500	10	7	20		45	0.9	1.1	12	1.1	75	1.0	85	3–4
7–10	700	10	7	30		45	1.0	1.2	13	1.4	100	1.4	120	4–5
Males														
11–14	1,000	10	10	45		50	1.3	1.5	17	1.7	150	2.0	100–200	4–7
15–18	1,000	10	10	65		60	1.5	1.8	20	2.0	200	2.0	100–200	4–7
Females														
11–14	800	10	8	45		50	1.1	1.3	15	1.4	180	2.0	100–200	4–7
15–18	800	10	8	55		60	1.1	1.3	15	1.5	180	2.0	100–200	4–7

N.E., Niacin equivalents; R.E., Retinol equivalents; T.E., Tocopherol equivalents. Biotin and pantothenate represent safe and adequate intakes.

human milk is rich in tryptophan so that the intake of niacin equivalents (preformed niacin plus niacin precursors) is more than adequate. Breast milk vitamin content is considerably below cow's milk and proprietary formulas (Table 2). In addition, because vitamin nutriture in the mother may adversely affect breast milk vitamin levels, maternal vitamin deficiency may reduce the maternal milk levels to a degree that causes deficiency in the infant. For example, infants breast-fed by thiamine-deficient mothers (as a result of dietary deficiency or, often, alcoholism) may develop infantile beriberi characterized by aphonia, a weak, high-pitched cry, and congestive failure during the second to fourth week of life. Treatment with thiamine, 10 to 50 mg/day, reverses the symptoms.

Cow's Milk

The concentration of B vitamins is higher in cow's milk than in breast milk, whereas the concentration of vitamin C in cow's milk is only one-quarter of that in human milk. In addition, vitamin C content decreases with processing and storage. For this reason, cow's milk has been commercially supplemented with vitamin C in order to provide the child with the recommended daily requirement of vitamin C.

Low Birth Weight Infants

Breast milk and commercially prepared formulas may supply inadequate amounts of vitamins for low birth weight infants because of decreased consumption. In the absence of specific information on the vitamin requirement of such infants, it seems reasonable to insure intakes comparable with amounts of vitamins recommended for full-term infants (2).

Vegetarian and Health Food Diets

A number of fad diets may fail to provide the nutrient requirements for the growing child (3,4). Pure vegetarian and vegan diets, if varied and supplemented with legumes and nuts or dairy products and eggs, tend to be nutritionally similar to diets containing meats. Vegetarian diets may also supply the requirements of vitamin C and the B vitamins with the exception of vitamin B_{12}, which is found in animal products. Most vegetarians either take B_{12} supplements or consume B_{12}-fortified soy or nut milks available in health-food stores. The Zen macrobiotic diet is currently the potentially most dangerous diet for growing children because of the severe protein-energy restriction that has caused some children to become emaciated, anemic, and scorbutic.

TABLE 2. *Metabolic defects that may improve with pharmacologic doses of B vitamins and vitamin C*

Vitamin	Disease	Biochemical defects	Usual dose (mg/day)	Comment
Thiamine (B₁)	Chronic lactic acidosis	Pyruvate carboxylase	25–50	The vitamin cofactor for this enzyme is biotin and one patient has improved with biotin therapy
	Hyperalaninemia and lactic acidosis	Pyruvate dehydrogenase	25–50	
	Leigh's subacute necrotizing encephalopathy	Defective thiamine triphosphate formation due to presence of inhibitor	25–50	Thiamine propyl disulfide or tetrafurfuryl disulfide are better able to increase CSF B₁
	Rare form of maple syrup urine disease (MSUD)	?	10	Clinical forms of MSUD unresponsive to B₁
	Unusual form of megaloblastic anemia	?	10–20	Rare condition, and unresponsive to B₁₂ or folate
Riboflavin (B₂)	None known	—	—	—
	Boric acid poisoning	—	20–200	Animal studies suggest potential use in boric acid poisoning
	?Glutathione reductase deficiency causing nonspherocytic hemolytic anemia	—	—	Possibly useful
Niacin (B₃)	Hartnup disease	Tryptophan and neutral amino acid active transport	40–200	Apparently results from poor absorption of tryptophan plus increased renal losses of indoles
	Congenital tryptophanuria	Defective conversion of tryptophan to kynurenine	40–200	Transient improvement; no data on long-term effect
Pyridoxine (B₆)	B₆-dependent infantile convulsions	?Defective glutamic acid decarboxylase	5–10 IV; maintenance 10–25 p.o.	Mental retardation may occur unless treated promptly
	B₆-responsive anemia (sideroblastic anemia)	?Defective δ-aminolevulinic acid synthetase	25–75	—
	Cystathioninuria	Cystathionase	100–500	—
	Xanthurenic aciduria	Binding of pyridoxal phosphate to kynureninase	100–500	—
	Xanthurenic aciduria (hydroxykynureninuria)	Kynureninase	100–500	—
	Homocystinuria	Cystathionine synthase	25–500	—
	Vitamin B₆–dependent infantile convulsions, cystathioninuria, and xanthurenic aciduria after tryptophan load	Possible defect of phosphorylation of vitamin B₆	50–100	—
	Hyperoxaluria	—	100–500	—
Biotin	Propionic acidemia	Propionyl-CoA carboxylase	1–4	—
	β-Methylcrotonylglycinuria	β-Methylcrotonyl-CoA-carboxylase	5–10	—
	Chronic lactic acidosis of infancy with hyperalaninemia	Pyruvate carboxylase	1–4	May also improve with thiamine
Pantothenate	None known	—	—	—
Ascorbic acid	None known; conceivably of benefit in treatment of alkaptonuria	—	—	Large doses may interfere with B₁₂ absorption; scurvy has developed in infants of mothers treated with mega-C during pregnancy. Megadoses of ascorbic acid have been useful in the treatment of Chediak-Higashi syndrome

TABLE 3. *Vitamins in milk (quantity per liter)*

Vitamin	Human milk	Cow's milk	Standard formula	Premature formula
Vitamin A (IU)	2,500	1,030	2,000–2,500	2,440
Vitamin D (IU)	22	34	400–500	490
Vitamin E (mg)	1.8	0.4	9.5–25	24
Vitamin K (g)	20	60	55–70	65
Thiamine (B_1) (mcg)	140	440	635–810	1,020
Riboflavin (B_2) (mcg)	370	1,750	1,000–1,265	1,220
Vitamin B_6 (mcg)	110		420–500	490
Vitamin B_{12} (mcg)	0.4	4.2	1.3–2.0	2.0
Niacin (mcg)	1,830	930	5,000–10,125	8,530
Folic acid (folacin) (mcg)	50		50–130	120
Pantothenic acid (mcg)	2,300	3,520	2,100–3,800	3,650
Biotin (mcg)	7	40	15–36	36
Vitamin C (ascorbic acid) (mcg)	50	12	55–70	100
Choline (mg)	0.07	200	100–130	130
Inositol (mg)	0.4	170	32–38	38

Source: Courtesy of Ross Laboratories, Columbus, Ohio.

Total Parenteral Nutrition

Vitamin C and the B vitamins are often added to parenteral fluids in amounts that provide two to three times the recommended intake (Table 4). When this has been done in term infants and children, no vitamin deficiencies or extreme excesses have been observed. Preterm infants, however, may show marked elevation in blood levels of several vitamins.

Radiographic features of scurvy have been seen in

TABLE 4. *Suggested intakes of parenteral vitamins in infants and children*

Vitamin	Term infants and children: dose per day[a]	Preterm infants: dose/kg body wt (maximum not to exceed term infant dose)	
		Current suggestions[b]	Best estimate for new formulation[c]
Lipid-soluble			
A (μg)[d]	700	280	500
E (mg)[d]	7	2.8	2.8
K (μg)	200	80	80
D (μg)[d]	10	4	4
(IU)	400	160	160
Water-soluble			
Ascorbic acid (mg)	80	32.0	25
Thiamin (mg)	1.2	0.48	0.35
Riboflavin (mg)	1.4	0.56	0.15
Pyridoxine (mg)	1.0	0.4	0.18
Niacin (mg)	17	6.8	6.8
Pantothenate (mg)	5	2.0	2.0
Biotin (μg)	20	8.0	6.0
Folate (μg)	140	56	56.0
Vitamin B-12 (μg)	1.0	0.4	0.3

[a] These guidelines for term infants and children are identical to those of the AMA (NAG). MVI-Pediatric (Armour) meets these guidelines. Recent data indicate that 40 IU·kg^{-1}·d^{-1} of vitamin D (maximum of 400 IU/day) is adequate for term and preterm infants (Koo et al, JPEN 1987;11:172–7) (68). The higher dose of 160 IU·kg^{-1}·d^{-1} has not been associated with complications and maintains blood levels within the reference range for term infants fed orally. This dosage therefore appears acceptable until further studies using the lower dose formulation indicates its superiority.

[b] These represent a practical guide [40% of the currently available single dose vial MVI-Pediatric (Armour) formulation per kg body weight], which will provide adequate levels of vitamins E, D, and K but low levels of retinol and excess levels of most of the B vitamins. The maximum daily dose is one single dose vial for any infant.

[c] Because of elevated levels of the water-soluble vitamins, the current proposal is to reduce the intake of water-soluble vitamins and increase retinol as indicated in the text.

[d] 700 μg RE = 2,300 international units (IU); 7 mg α-tocopherol = 7 IU; 10 μg vitamin D = 400 IU.

children receiving total parenteral nutrition (TPN) for long periods. These changes have more recently been recognized to be secondary to copper deficiency.

Conditions Increasing Vitamin Requirements

Liver Disease

Most vitamin deficiencies seen in liver disease are ascribed to fat-soluble vitamins. However, patients with chronic liver disease have been found to have low circulating levels of pyridoxine and pyridoxal-5'-phosphate (PLP), thiamine pyrophosphate, and riboflavin. Whether this represents an abnormality in intake, metabolism, or conservation is not generally defined. However, supplemental vitamins are usually corrective.

Pregnancy

Requirements for all vitamins are increased during pregnancy. Some patients with gestational diabetes mellitus may improve glucose tolerance after 100 mg pyridoxine daily for 2 weeks (5).

Drugs

Agents such as isonicotinic acid hydrazide (INH), cycloserine, hydralazine, and penicillamine are B_6 agonists and increase pyridoxine requirements. Thus, with chronic intake of these agents, B_6 deficiency may occur. Sulfasalazine (Azulfidine) interferes with folate absorption and chronic use of amitriptyline, chlorpromazine, and imipramine may interfere with riboflavin metabolism. Conceivably, other drugs may antagonize absorption or metabolism of vitamins or vitamin cofactors. The most commonly associated agent resulting in both impaired absorption and metabolism of thiamine and riboflavin is ethanol.

Hypermetabolism

Severe trauma, burns, and chronic or acute infection are often associated with an increased excretion of several of the B vitamins. The degree to which supplemental vitamins are needed in extreme exercise has not been clearly defined, although increased excretion of several water-soluble vitamins occurs in marathon runners.

THE B VITAMINS
THIAMINE

Recommended Daily Intake

Infants	Children 1–11	Children 12–18	Pregnancy
0.3 mg	0.9–1.0 mg	1.3 mg	1.5 mg

Thiamine (vitamin B_1 aneurine) is water-soluble; most commercial preparations contain about 4% water by weight. It is stable on heating to 100°C in the dry form, or in aqueous solution, provided the pH is kept below 5.5. Sterilization of solutions at physiologic pH results in destruction of thiamine. Some destruction also occurs in the presence of alkaline drugs, such as sodium phenobarbital, or by the tannins found in wine and tea.

Thiamine is absorbed both actively and passively from the gastrointestinal tract. It is dependent on the sodium ion for active absorption (6). Active absorption can be inhibited by ethanol and, unless higher doses are administered, the usually physiologic dose is insufficient to maintain normal levels in the chronic alcoholic.

Cocarboxylase (thiamine pyrophosphate), the phosphorylated, active form of thiamine, is an integral component of two general enzymatic sequences: (a) decarboxylation of α-ketoglutaric and branched-chain α-ketoacids, and (b) transketolase reactions involving a direct pathway for metabolism of glucose (7). Although less than 10% of glucose is utilized in the transketolase pathway, it is the only way the body can produce ribose for RNA synthesis (8). Thiamine also occurs as the triphosphate form in nerve tissue, but the precise physiologic significance of this compound is unclear, although some patients with subacute necrotizing encephalomyelopathy lack the triphosphate derivative (9) and have improved with pharmacologic doses of thiamine (10).

Dietary Sources of Thiamine

Dietary sources of thiamine are multiple and include rice husks, cereal grains, yeast, liver, eggs, milk, green leaves, and roots. Human milk is relatively low in thiamine (16 μg/ml) compared to cow's milk, which contains 42 μg/ml. Freezing foods results in little loss.

Although isolated thiamine deficiency may occur, it is often associated with riboflavin and niacin deficiency. Chronic alcoholism is generally associated with thiamine and folate deficiency and occasionally with B_{12} deficiency, since ethanol decreases absorption of the three vitamins.

Most nonlipid tissues contain about a microgram of thiamine per gram of tissue. Excess thiamine intake results in its excretion in the urine. Thus, determination of urinary thiamine excretion has been used to estimate thiamine status. Measurement of activity of erythrocyte transketolase, a thiamine-requiring enzyme, has been used to screen for thiamine deficiency.

Thiamine Deficiency

Thiamine deficiency, or beriberi, occurs in adults when the level of intake drops below 1 mg/day. The biologic half-life of ^{14}C-labeled thiamine is 9 to 18 days and deficiency symptoms usually develop within 2 to 3 months on a thiamine-deficient diet. Deficiency may result from nutritional ignorance among individuals who subsist largely on rice, wheat, or corn, or among those unable to obtain thiamine-containing foods. A combination of low intake plus increased requirements (increased growth, lactation, heavy physical labor, and conditions giving rise to increased catabolic states) may also cause symptomatic thiamine deficiency. In the United States, beriberi is most commonly associated with alcoholism. Ethanol inhibits the active transport of thiamine for 2 to 3 months (11). Passive transport of thiamine continues, however, and larger doses of thiamine should prevent thiamine deficiency under these conditions. Certain foods, such as shellfish and raw carp or herring, contain thiamine-destroying enzymes (thiaminases) which may decrease the thiamine content of food by as much as 50%. If a diet containing these foods is already low in thiamine, and is continued for a sufficient period of time, thiamine deficiency may result.

The neurologic symptoms of beriberi may not occur for several months after tissue levels of thiamine are deficient because of the slow degeneration of affected nervous tissue. Reactions involving decarboxylation of α-ketoacids are more affected and accumulation of pyruvate, lactate, α-ketoglutarate, and glutamate occur in the serum and urine before neurologic symptoms develop.

Clinical Features of Thiamine Deficiency

Three forms of beriberi have been described: dry, wet, and acute. The dry and wet (edematous) forms are different manifestations of a polyneuritis. The pathogenesis of the edema in wet beriberi is unclear. Infantile beriberi may be more subtle than that found in adults. Children may present with a polyneuritis (pseudomeningitic type), cardiopathy, and/or aphonia. The disease may be slowly progressive or wax and wane and, left untreated, may result in death after a few weeks, in the infantile form, or years, in the adult form, where the diet may not be totally devoid of thiamine (12).

Diagnosis of Thiamine Deficiency

Thiamine deficiency should be suspected whenever there is a history, or findings of, starvation and/or malnutrition (13). The differential diagnosis should also include chronic poisoning (arsenic, triorthocresol phosphate, gamma-hexochlorobenzene, etc.), infection, porphyria, mononeuritis complex, Guillain-Barré syndrome, pernicious anemia, and pellagra. A number of clinical states may result in congestive heart failure in children. However, with associated lactic and pyruvic acidemia and a burning sensory neuropathy, the diagnosis strongly favors beriberi. The diagnosis may be confirmed by measurement of 24-hr urinary thiamine excretion or by computing the urinary thiamine-to-creatine ratio from a single urine sample. The normal 24-hr urinary thiamine output in children is 40 to 100 μg/day or 176 μg/g creatinine. Values less than 15 μg/24-hr and less than 120 μg/g creatinine are in the deficient range. If red blood cell transketolase activity increases by 20% or more with thiamine added to the reaction mixture, thiamine deficiency must be considered. However, transketolase activity may be abnormal in acute febrile states.

Treatment of Beriberi

Treatment of beriberi with thiamine usually leads to resolution of neurologic symptoms within 24 hr, cardiac symptoms in 24 to 48 hr, and edema in 48 to 72 hr. Motor weakness, however, may require 1 to 3 months before being completely resolved. Occasionally, treatment will apparently be progressing satisfactorily when the patient will die suddenly in congestive heart failure. The precise reason for this phenomenon is unclear, but may be related to inadequate treatment or severe degeneration of cardiac muscles.

Treatment of children with mild beriberi with an oral dose of 5 mg thiamine per day is usually satisfactory. Severely ill children should receive 10 mg intravenously twice daily. Adults with mild beriberi respond to 10 mg orally three times daily and in severe cases to 25 mg intravenously twice daily. In the management of fulminate heart disease, 100 mg thiamine hydrochloride plus vigorous treatment of congestive heart failure is necessary (12).

Thiamine Requirements

Requirements are generally based on carbohydrate intake since thiamine functions primarily in the metabolism of carbohydrates. From nutritional surveys and measurement of biologic half-life, individuals should receive at least 0.4 mg/1,000 cal or a total of 0.3 to 1.2 mg for children and 1.3 to 2.1 mg of thiamine daily for adults.

Thiamine Dependency Syndromes

Thiamine dependency syndromes that involve specific metabolic defects are rare. Those that may respond to large doses of thiamine (12) include the following: (a) A rare form of maple syrup urine disease (MSUD) corrected by 10 mg thiamine hydrochloride a day. This form of MSUD is benign as compared to the other forms of MSUD and has been described in only one child. The other more classical types of MSUD are not responsive to thiamine. (b) A megoblastic anemia unresponsive to vitamin B_{12} or folate but responsive to thiamine (14). The nature of the defect is unknown. (c) Some patients with subacute necrotizing encephalopathy (Leigh's encephalopathy) of infants and children have responded transiently with 25 to 50 mg thiamine daily (9). The pathologic features resemble Wernicke's encephalopathy (8,10) and although there is no clinical evidence of beriberi, the blood lactate and pyruvate are elevated. The precise defect in these patients is unclear but apparently is related to decreased levels of thiamine triphosphate. Patients with the illness show a decrease in the rate of conversion of thiamine pyrophosphate to thiamine triphosphate as a result of an inhibitor present in the spinal fluid of the patients. Treatment has been with thiamine propyldisulfide, and thiamine tetrafurfuryl disulfide, which are better able to maintain high spinal fluid thiamine levels. (d) Chronic lactic acidosis of infancy. There are patients who appear to have a defect in the pyruvate dehydrogenase system. Presumably, those responding to high doses of thiamine have a defect in thiamine metabolism, whereas those unresponsive to thiamine would most likely be deficient in pyruvate decarboxylase enzyme (15). Two infants with lactic acidosis, hyperalaninemia, and hypoglycemia had pyruvate carboxylase deficiency. Although the cofactor for pyruvate carboxylase is biotin rather than thiamine, the patients improved with high doses of thiamine.

Thiamine Toxicity

Doses of 500 mg given intravenously to thiamine-deficient individuals have been well tolerated. In mice, the LD_{50} is 3 g/kg orally. Rapid, intravenous injection of 50 mg/kg thiamine in dogs causes respiratory paralysis, hypotension, bradycardia, and vasodilation. However, if adequate ventilation is maintained, these effects are transient. In rare instances, 100 mg thiamine or less has caused an anaphylactic-type reaction (16). Hypersensitivity has also been demonstrated by passive transfer. The nature of this toxicity or so-called thiamine shock is not understood.

RIBOFLAVIN

Recommended Daily Intake

Infant	Children 1–10	Children 11–18	Pregnancy
0.4 mg	0.8–1.2 mg	1.5–1.7 mg	1.6 mg

Riboflavin (vitamin B_2) is water-soluble, has a yellow or orange-yellow color, and a characteristic green fluorescence under ultraviolet (UV) radiation. It is relatively stable in the dry state and in the dark at acid pH is resistant to heat and oxidation. However, it deteriorates rapidly in an alkaline solution, a reaction accelerated by visible or UV light. It is present in all cells only as functioning compounds and not as stored material. The liver (with 16 µg/g) and kidney (with 25 µg/g) usually contain more than other tissues, which average about 2.3 µg/g.

Riboflavin is absorbed in the small intestine by a site-specific, saturable, specialized transport process. In the liver it is transformed by riboflavin kinase (flavokinase) and adenosine triphosphate (ATP) into flavin mononucleotide (FMN), a reaction that may also occur in intestinal epithelium. FMN is further phosphorylated by flavinadenine dinucleotide (FAD) pyrophosphorylase and ATP in the liver to form FAD. Both FAD and FMN serve as cofactors for several enzymes, the majority of which are oxidases (17).

Flavoproteins are relatively unstable, especially when tissue protein is depleted by physiologic stress, dietary deficiency, or disease. Under these conditions, increased levels of riboflavin are excreted in the urine (18).

Dietary Sources of Riboflavin

Dietary sources of riboflavin are milk products, eggs, meat, fruits, and green leafy vegetables. It is not destroyed by ordinary cooking unless alkali is added, although prolonged exposure to sunlight may degrade it.

Riboflavin Deficiency

Riboflavin deficiency may occur from inadequate intake or malabsorption. In adults, 3 to 8 months may be required before deficiency develops and often, by that time, other vitamin deficiencies have become manifest. In infants and children, dietary deficiency, which is most common in spring and summer, may lead to symptoms within 1 to 2 months. During pregnancy and the rapid growth of children, there is an increased need for riboflavin. Similarly, acute and chronic infection or trauma may increase excretion as well as increase riboflavin requirements. Structural similarities between riboflavin and amitriptyline, imipramine, and chlorpromazine have been noted. When taking these drugs on a chronic basis, tissue depletion of flavins, increased urinary riboflavin excretion, and reduced erythrocyte glutathione reductase activity have been noted (19). Riboflavin absorption is decreased in hepatitis, cirrhosis, and probenecid treatment.

Clinical Features of Riboflavin Deficiency

Clinical features are manifest by photophobia, a burning ocular sensation, dim vision, and sore mouth and tongue. Nonspecific symptoms of anorexia, weight loss, weakness, headache, dizziness, and confusion may precede overt symptoms of stomatitis, pharyngitis, glossitis, seborrheic dermatitis, normochromic normocytic anemia, and corneal vascularization. Skin lesions may improve and recur irregularly. Late complications of ariboflavinosis are unusual with prompt therapy. Corneal opacities usually resolve with additional vitamin A often increasing the rate of response. Rarely, evidence of brain damage may persist in infants.

Diagnosis of Riboflavin Deficiency

Diagnosis should be considered with a history of dietary deficiency and clinical manifestations. The diagnosis can be confirmed by a decreased 24-hr urinary excretion of riboflavin. Normal values for adults are greater than 100 μg/24-hr and excretion of less than 50 μg/24-hr is indicative of deficiency. Measurement of erythrocyte glutathione reductase activity has also been used to evaluate riboflavin status (20). Enzyme activity is measured without added FAD and again after preincubation with FAD. An increase in enzyme activity of more than 20% with the addition of FAD (activity coefficient of 1.20) is indicative of riboflavin deficiency (21). This latter test is particularly useful in diagnosing deficient riboflavin intake before development of overt disease. Urinary riboflavin is usually measured microbiologically with *Lactobacillus casei* or by a fluorescent technique, the former being more sensitive. More recently, high-performance liquid chromatography (HPLC), with fluorescent detection, has been used to measure riboflavin in plasma and its active cofactors in red cells. Using this technique, plasma concentrations below 10 μg/dl suggest inadequate riboflavin intake.

Treatment of Riboflavin Deficiency

Children may be successfully treated with 1 mg riboflavin three times daily for several weeks, and infants usually respond to 0.5 mg twice daily. Increased strength and sense of well-being usually occurs within 24 hr. Often, therapeutic doses of vitamin A will improve the corneal lesions more rapidly. If oral administration is precluded, intramuscular or intravenous injection of a multiple-vitamin preparation may be necessary three times daily until oral administration is possible.

Requirements of Riboflavin

Requirements are often based on caloric intake. The recommended dietary intake of riboflavin for adults is 1.8 mg daily and expressed in terms of caloric intake is 0.5 to 0.6 mg/1,000 kilocalories (Cal).

Riboflavin Dependency Syndrome

Although theoretically possible, riboflavin dependency syndromes have not been described. Patients with glutathione reductase deficiency and nonspherocytic hemolytic anemia conceivably might be helped by pharmacologic doses of riboflavin if the syndromes were due to defective FAD binding of the enzyme (22).

In animals, large doses of riboflavin have prevented the toxicity associated with boric acid poisoning. Riboflavin appears to bind boric acid. The riboflavin-boric acid complex is stable and excreted in the urine. Massive riboflavinuria, a condition known to occur after accidental poisoning in humans, occurs after administration of boric acid to animals. These observations raise the possibility that pharmacologic doses of riboflavin may be therapeutically useful in boric acid poisoning in humans (23). Studies suggest that the superoxide-forming enzyme from human neutrophils is a FAD-requiring enzyme; thus, granulomatous disease, in which superoxide forming activity in the neutrophils is lacking, might improve from riboflavin administration.

Riboflavin Toxicity

Riboflavin toxicity has not been clearly demonstrated in humans. Large doses of riboflavin (600 mg/kg body weight) given intraperitoneally caused riboflavin crystals to develop in the renal collecting system of experimental animals. No other pathology was observed. Even with large doses of riboflavin, tissue levels of riboflavin and of the flavin coenzymes were not substantially increased, suggesting that there is an upper limit above which riboflavin cannot be increased (18). Preterm infants have shown more than a 100-fold increase in plasma riboflavin with little change in red cell riboflavin and FAD content (24). Riboflavin may enhance the reduction of serum bilirubin in newborns receiving phototherapy (25). *In vitro* studies indicate that riboflavin in the presence of light alters the DNA structure of HeLa cells. These results imply a carcinogenic potential when large doses of riboflavin are given in conjunction with phototherapy. Although no actual relationship has been demonstrated in humans, the administration of pharmacologic amounts of the vitamin to infants requiring phototherapy is not routinely recommended (25). The finding of extremely elevated levels of riboflavin in very low birth weight (VLBW) infants receiving TPN indicates that further experiments are needed to provide more meaningful data concerning the potential carcinogenic relationship between riboflavin and phototherapy.

PYRIDOXINE

Recommended Daily Intake			
	Children		
Infant	1–10	11–18	Pregnancy
0.3 mg	1.0–1.4 mg	1.7–2.0 mg	2.2 mg

Pyridoxine (vitamin B_6) occurs in nature as three closely related compounds: pyridoxine, most abundant in plants, and pyridoxal and pyridoxamine, which predominate in animal tissues. All three forms, and their respective phosphates, can be interconverted to the enzymatically active form, PLP (26). They, and their phosphate derivatives, are all water-soluble, stable to air and light, and relatively resistant to heat.

The active form, PLP, acts as a coenzyme for a number of biologically important reactions mostly involving nitrogen metabolism. These reactions include transamination, decarboxylation, racemization, amine oxidation (monoamine oxidase and diamine oxidase), aldol reactions, and desulfhydration. Synthetases, phosphorylase b kinase, and phosphorylase phosphatase are also B_6-requiring enzymes. Approximately one-half the B_6 content of the body can be accounted for in the phosphorylase of skeletal muscle (27).

Pyridoxine is absorbed almost completely from the upper gastrointestinal tract. Little or none is absorbed from the action of microorganisms in the colon.

Most ordinary diets contain adequate levels of B_6. Excellent sources are liver, vegetables, fruits, whole-grain cereals, and meats. Milling of wheat may reduce B_6 content by 80% to 90% and cooking frozen vegetables may reduce the B_6 content by 25%.

Pyridoxine Requirements

Requirements vary with age, protein intake, and state of health. There is virtually no storage of pyridoxine in humans; about 0.4 mg is excreted in the urine daily. The half-life of pyridoxine is about 15 to 20 days judging by tracer studies in two volunteers receiving 1.75 to 2 g pyridoxine daily. On a B_6-deficient diet, encephalographic abnormalities appeared in less than 3 weeks. Requirements of pyridoxine are based on protein intake because of the important role played by pyridoxine in protein metabolism. Between 15 and 25 μg B_6/g protein is recommended. In the infant, this usually amounts to 0.1 to 0.5 mg/day; in the child, 0.5 to 1.5 mg/day; in the adolescent and adult, 1.5 to 2.0 mg/day; and in the pregnant woman, 5.0 to 10.0 mg/day (28).

Pyridoxine Deficiency

Pyridoxine deficiency, due to an inadequate intake of B_6, generally occurs only with deficiencies of other B vitamins. B_6 deficiency may result from inadequate intake of pyridoxine. However, such an isolated deficiency is rare in the United States. In the early 1950s, a formula containing only 60 μg/l vitamin B_6 (one-third to one-half the recommended dose) was inadvertently given to a number of infants. After several weeks, symptoms of hyperactivity, hyperacusis, and convulsive seizures developed. Symptoms were aggravated by increases in protein intake and corrected by 5 or 10 mg pyridoxine. These observations suggest that a decreased B_6 intake could produce symptoms primarily manifest by abnormal CNS function. One possible explanation for this disturbance is the lowering of CNS levels of α-aminobutyric acid in B_6 deficiency, which may decrease the irritability threshold of the brain (29).

Pyridoxine deficiency in the United States most commonly occurs in individuals who are genetically "slow-inactivators" of isonicotine hydrazine (INH), a potent antagonist of B_6. These individuals are particularly susceptible to developing a B_6-responsive peripheral neuropathy. In addition, INH may precipitate a B_6-responsive anemia. Contraceptive steroids, penicillamine, hydrazine (used in rocket fuels), and hydralazine (an antihypertensive agent) may precipitate B_6 deficiency (29).

Clinical Features of Pyridoxine Deficiency

Although deficient adults may present initially with a peripheral neuritis, children, who seem to be resistant to developing neuritis, may present with diarrhea, instead. Other clinical features are nonspecific and include insomnia, weakness, mental depression, cheilosis, stomatitis, nasolabial seborrhea, and dermatitis. Later symptoms usually include peripheral neuropathy and convulsive seizures (30).

Diagnosis of Pyridoxine Deficiency

Diagnosis may be difficult in areas of the world where malnutrition is not endemic. It should be considered in infants with convulsive disorders, microcytic-hypochromic anemias unresponsive to iron, poor nutrition, severe catabolic states, and in persons with anorexia nervosa or food faddism. Confirmation of the diagnosis is dependent on several laboratory measurements (31). Normally urinary excretion of 4-pyridoxic acid is greater than 0.8 mg/day and of pyridoxine greater than 20 μg/g creatinine. Urinary excretion of less than 0.2 mg 4-pyridoxic acid or less than 10 μg pyridoxine per mg creatinine is indicative of deficiency. Accepted values for children have not been determined. Indirect evaluation of pyridoxine status can be assessed by determining the glutamic-pyruvic or glutamic-oxaloacetic transaminase activities in red cells with or without preincubation with PLP. Increased activity of greater than 20% with PLP preincubation suggests pyridoxine deficiency. Urinary excretion of xanthurenic and kynurenic acid following an L-tryptophan load (50 mg/kg to a maximum of 2 g) may also be used to determine pyridoxine status. Normal subjects excrete less than 50 mg xanthurenic acid and usually less than 30 mg kynurenic acid in 24 hr. Increased xanthurenic acid excretion is seen in children with leukemia, infection, diabetes, porphyria, and other illnesses. As a result, urinary excretion of tryptophan should not be used as the sole determinant of B_6 status (32). Newer methods of pyridoxine measurement in blood by HPLC have not defined clear-cut levels at which deficiency is established.

Treatment of Pyridoxine Deficiency

Treatment is generally the same as that outlined under the treatment of the various pyridoxine dependency syndromes. The convulsive disorder and other symptoms of B_6 deficiency in infants are usually promptly relieved by administration of 10 mg pyridoxine intravenously and of 10 mg p.o. daily for 1 to 2 weeks or until the clinical manifestations of the illness have been corrected.

Pyridoxine Dependency Syndromes

Pyridoxine dependency syndromes, essentially inborn errors of metabolism, are favorably influenced by supplements several times the usual requirement, occasionally as much as 200 to 600 mg pyridoxine/day (33).

Pyridoxine-dependent convulsions in the neonate appear to result from a defect in the γ-aminobutyric acid (GABA) system. Convulsions occurring within the first 2 weeks of life usually respond to 5 to 10 mg pyridoxine intravenously, followed by 10 to 25 mg p.o. daily. Mental retardation may occur unless therapy is promptly instituted (30,34).

Pyridoxine-responsive, microcytic-hypochromic anemia has been described in patients with elevated serum iron levels, increased saturation of iron-binding protein, and hemosiderin deposits in bone marrow and liver (35,36). Therapy with 0.1 to 1.0 g/day pyridoxine causes a prompt reticulocytosis on the third or fourth day of therapy. A megaloblastic anemia, unresponsive to the usual therapy, has also responded to B_6 (36).

Administration of large doses of B_6 also effects improvement in (37) xanthurenic aciduria, which is characterized by abnormal excretion of kynurenine, 3-hydroxykynurenine, and xanthurenic acid following a tryptophan tolerance test and cystathioninuria, which presents with a variety of clinical features including mental retardation, acromegaly, thrombocytopenia, renal calculi, nephrogenic diabetes insipidus, and severe anemia (32).

Although large doses of B_6 effected treatment in one group of patients with homocystinuria by abolishing the homocystinuria and normalizing the plasma methionine levels, other patients have not been helped.

Toxicity to Pyridoxine

Toxicity in humans has been seen with 1,000 to 2,700 times the RDA (2 to 6 g/day) being used for treatment of carpel tunnel syndrome. These patients developed a peripheral neuropathy similar to that seen with B_6 deficiency. The synthetic analogue, desoxypyridoxine, is highly poisonous.

Other Therapeutic Uses of Vitamin B_6

Other therapeutic uses have included the treatment of anemia, cardiac decompensation, the side effects of radiation therapy, skin grafting, isoniazid toxicity, atherosclerosis, and alcoholism. In general, there does not appear to be any specific requirement for B_6 other than the prevention of pyridoxine deficiency, ameliorating various dependency syndromes, and as an adjunct to INH therapy. Oral pyridoxal in doses of 50 to 100 mg three times weekly reportedly aids in moderating vomiting during pregnancy. However, controlled studies have failed to support this impression. Pyridoxine has been used in some patients with hereditary or primarily acquired sideroblastic anemia (sideroachrestic anemia). Some responded to relatively small doses (0.5 to 1.0 mg/day), whereas others required much larger doses. These conditions must be distinguished from the pyridoxine-responsive anemia.

NIACIN

Recommended Daily Intake

Infant	Children		Pregnancy
	1–10	11–18	
5 mg	9–13 mg	17–20 mg	17 mg

Nicotinic acid and nicotinamide, which are biologically equivalent vitamins, are both referred to as niacin (vitamin B_3). Biosynthesis of this vitamin occurs in almost all organisms; and in humans the conversion ratio of tryptophan to nicotinic acid is only about 60 to 1, making it possible for large amounts of tryptophan to meet niacin requirements. Niacin is absorbed in the proximal small bowel and incorporated into nicotinamide adenine dinucleotide (NAD) and nicotinamide adenine dinucleotide phosphate (NADP). These two compounds are coenzymes for oxidation-reduction reactions (including synthesis of high-energy phosphate compounds, glycolysis, pyruvate metabolism, pentose biosynthesis, glycerol, and fatty acid metabolism), for obtaining energy from protein, and in excision-repair mechanisms of DNA. With adequate dietary niacin, free nicotinic acid, nicotinamide, N^1-methylnicotinamide from 1.3 to 6.1 mg/day on a diet providing about 6.6 mg niacin/1,000 Cal/day.

Niacin is stable in boiling water but is incompatible with sodium nitrite, the substance used to maintain normal meat coloring.

Dietary Sources of Niacin

Dietary sources of niacin include liver, yeast, white meat, poultry, peanuts, and legumes; some niacin is present in potatoes, vegetables, and wheat. Because of their high tryptophan content, milk and eggs are also good sources of niacin. Roasting of coffee converts trigonelline to nicotinic acid so that one cup of coffee may contain 1 to 2 mg of nicotinic acid. An excess of dietary leucine, which is found, for example, in corn, interferes with conversion of tryptophan to niacin and accounts for the high prevalence of niacin deficiency in individuals who subsist almost entirely on corn (38,39). Nicotinic acid is not totally absent in corn, but it is present in an unbound form (niacytin). When corn is lime-treated, however, as is the practice when making tortillas in Central America, or when sweet corn is roasted, e.g., by the Hopi Indians of Arizona, then the niacin is made available.

Niacin Deficiency

Niacin deficiency leads to pellagra, named after the pathognomonic skin changes that result: *pelle,* skin; *agro,* rough. Pellagra is prone to occur in individuals subsisting predominantly on corn, corn products, or millet (sorghum) because of the high leucine content (40). Pellagra resulting from millet ingestion can be reversed by isoleucine. In the United States, pellagra may be seen in alcoholics (41) or, rarely, in food faddists during pregnancy. By and large, pellagra occurs in low-income groups and in patients with anorexia or gastrointestinal disease associated with severe malabsorption. Since vitamin B_6 is required for transformation of tryptophan to niacin, pellagra is occasionally seen in individuals treated with INH who develop B_6 deficiency. It is also common in patients with malignant carcinoid tumors, and in infants with Hartnup disease, an inborn error of tryptophan metabolism.

Clinical Features of Niacin Deficiency

Clinical features of niacin deficiency are chronic, relapsing, and popularly characterized by three (or four) *D*s: dermatitis, diarrhea, dementia, and, if untreated, death. The cutaneous lesions, usually noted first, appear as an erythema resembling sunburn on those parts of the body exposed to sunlight, heat, and other forms of mild trauma. These areas are erythematous and infiltrated, and they itch and burn. More acute cases may progress to vesiculation, ulceration, and secondary infection. Classically, the erythema progresses to roughening and keratosis with scaling. In most cases, a brownish pigmentation develops and, in the process of healing, peels off, leaving pink skin underneath. Oral lesions with angular stomatitis are often present but may reflect associated vitamin deficiencies. The rectum and anus are often inflamed as well, with an extension to the small bowel to produce varying degrees of villus effacement and infiltration. This involvement accounts for the diarrhea and malabsorption frequently accompanying the dermatitis. Dietary intakes of less than 7.5 mg niacin without tryptophan have been associated with the development of pellagra.

Although neurologic manifestations may appear without skin manifestations, they usually follow development of skin lesions. Neurological signs may be mild to moderate, presenting with some weakness, malaise, anxiety, and/or short attention span, or, when severe, with delirium. In most chronic forms, amentia, posterolateral cord degeneration, and peripheral nerve lesions are present. Only in the most severe and chronic cases do the neurologic lesions persist after adequate treatment with niacin (42).

Diagnosis of Niacin Deficiency

Diagnosis may be suspected by a history of inadequate diet, INH treatment, or chronic ethanol ingestion when the typical skin lesions, diarrhea, and mental symptoms are present. Determination of urinary excretion of niacin or one of its products (N^1-methylnicotinamide) is most helpful in confirmation of the clinical impression (31).

Normal excretion of N^1-methylnicotinamide is usually between 4 and 6 mg/day and values less than 3 mg/day suggest deficient niacin intake; in pellagra, urinary N^1-methylnicotinamide is 0.5 to 0.8 mg/day. With a niacin intake of 5.5 mg/day, urinary niacin excretion was between 0.5 and 1 mg/day. One study showed that the pyridone derivative of N^1-methylnicotinamide was not excreted unless niacin intake was sufficient. However, measurement of this compound is difficult, and few laboratories are equipped to determine it on a routine basis.

Treatment of Pellagra

Treatment is usually more effective with oral niacin than with parenteral administration, since blood levels remain elevated longer following oral treatment. The usual daily dose is about 10 times the recommended dietary intake or about 50 to 100 mg for adults. Nicotinamide is usually preferred over nicotinic acid in order to avoid certain unpleasant side effects (flushing, tachycardia, etc.) seen with large doses of nicotinic acid. Parenteral therapy may be preferable when gastrointestinal absorption is deficient and a dose of 25 mg five times a day is recommended. In infants, 50 to 100 mg nicotinamide can be dissolved in the daily milk allotment. Parenteral nicotinamide may also be given at 5 mg three or five times a day. Prevention of pellagra can be achieved by eating an adequate protein diet containing tryptophan and foods containing niacin.

Requirements of Niacin

Requirements are expressed in terms of niacin equivalents and calculated from the sum of niacin intake plus 0.017 times the tryptophan intake. A diet providing 4.0 mg niacin equivalents/1,000 Cal is generally pellagragenic, whereas one providing 4.4 equivalents/1,000 Cal is protective. Human milk provides about 8 equivalents/1,000 Cal and the recommended intake is 6.4 to 8.0 equivalents/1,000 Cal.

Niacin Dependency Syndromes

Niacin dependency syndromes have been described in some patients with Hartnup disease and congenital tryptophanuria. Pharmacologic doses of nicotinic acid (not nicotinamide) have been used to treat patients with types II, IV, and V hyperlipoproteinemia, generally 1.5 to 3 g, but as much as 9 g/day. Abnormal liver function tests may develop, but no consistent histologic abnormality has been demonstrated. Nicotinic acid has no favorable effect on any types of psychosis or mental illness other than that seen in pellagra. Nicotinic acid, 300 to 500 mg/day, has also been recommended for treatment of livedoid vasculitis, although not all patients respond (43).

Toxicity to Nicotinic Acid

Toxicity has been reported in some patients taking large doses for hypercholesterolemia. Atypical cystoid macular edema with loss of central vision has been the most potentially serious toxic manifestation. However, vision improved and the macular edema resolved with discontinuation of nicotinic acid. Nicotinic acid, but not nicotinamide, will cause dilatation of skin capillaries, a reaction most severe with systemic injection.

PANTOTHENIC ACID

Safe and Adequate Daily Intake

Infant	Children 1–10	Children 11–18	Pregnancy
2–3 mg	3–5 mg	4–7 mg	10 mg

Pantothenic acid (vitamin B_5) is an unstable, pale yellow, viscous oil that is difficult to purify. It is easily destroyed by acids, bases, and heat, and is commercially available as the water-soluble calcium salt. Pantothenate is absorbed in the proximal small intestine; in the liver it becomes an integral part of coenzyme A. Coenzyme A plays a fundamental role in many metabolic reactions. Its active form, acetylcoenzyme A, is involved primarily in the Krebs cycle, the transfer of two-carbon units, and the synthesis of fats, steroids, and porphyrins.

Dietary Sources of Pantothenate

Dietary sources include virtually all naturally occurring foods.

Pantothenate Deficiency

As an isolated entity, pantothenate deficiency rarely occurs. Under extreme circumstances, e.g., famine, prolonged anorectic illness, imprisonment during wartime, or alcoholism, deficiency of pantothenate probably only exists with other vitamin deficiencies to which the symptoms may be ascribed. Isolated deficiency of pantothenate has been experimentally produced in humans on a "pantothenate-free" diet together with a pantothenic acid antagonist, ω-methylpantothenic acid (44,45).

Clinical Features of Experimental Pantothenate Deficiency

Clinical features of experimental pantothenate deficiency consist of apathy, lethargy, irritability, depression, insomnia, burning paresthesia, numbness, muscle cramping, incoordination, and occasional vomiting and diarrhea. Fatigue, headache, and weakness were the most persistent and annoying symptoms. Evidence that humans suffer from naturally occurring pantothenate deficiency is primarily suggestive. The "burning foot" syndrome observed in Japanese war prisoners was reported to respond to administration of pantothenic acid (46,47). No evidence has been presented that infants and young children have developed pantothenic acid deficiency.

Diagnosis of Isolated Pantothenate Deficiency

Diagnosis is based on symptoms produced during experimental studies (44,45,48). These symptoms, plus a blood pantothenate level of less than 100 µg/100 ml, is suggestive of a deficient intake. However, pantothenate measurements in naturally occurring deficiency have not been measured. The reliability of acetylation of a test dose of sulfanilamide or para-aminobenzoic acid to detect deficiency in humans has not been tested. Urinary excretion of pantothenate normally ranges between 0.78 and 7.4 mg/day and deficiency is suggestive with urinary levels less than 0.7 mg/24-hr.

Requirements of Pantothenate

Requirements are based on a few isolated studies and the suggested daily intake is 10 mg for adults.

Vitamin Dependency Syndromes

Vitamin dependency syndromes for pantothenate have not been described.

Toxicity to Pantothenate

Toxicity has not been demonstrated, even with daily doses of 50 to 100 mg/day for a month. A single dose of 100 mg intravenously had no apparent toxic effect.

BIOTIN

Recommended Daily Intake
(as included in vitamin supplements)

Infant	Children	Adult	Pregnancy
0.15 mg	0.15 mg	0.3 mg	0.3 mg

Biotin is a coenzyme for carbon dioxide fixation (carboxylation reactions). Six such reactions have been found to require biotin as an essential cofactor in mammals: acetyl coenzyme A carboxylase, β-methylcrotonyl-CoA carboxylase, propionyl-CoA carboxylase, geraniol-CoA carboxylase, and pyruvate carboxylase. Avidin, a specific protein in egg albumin *in vitro,* markedly inhibits each of these enzymes because of its great affinity for biotin. Biotin deficiency may not occur naturally, since gastrointestinal bacteria produce biotin (49–51).

Dietary Sources of Biotin

Dietary sources include liver, egg yolk, milk, yeast extracts, and meat. Nuts, chocolate, and some vegetables (especially cauliflower), have lesser amounts present. Cereals are relatively poor sources.

Biotin Deficiency

Biotin deficiency can be produced experimentally with a biotin-deficient diet by giving large doses of antibiotics for long periods of time, thereby destroying gastrointestinal flora, or by giving large amounts of avidin for a long period of time. Biotin deficiency has been observed in individuals who consume large numbers of raw eggs (rich in avidin) for several months. The avidin in raw eggs is not hydrolyzed by gastrointestinal enzymes; it binds biotin, and prevents its absorption. Cooking of eggs destroys avidin (51–53). Before biotin was routinely added to TPN solutions, several children developed biotin deficiency with the typical skin and biochemical changes seen in adults (54).

Clinical Features of Biotin Deficiency

Clinical features of biotin deficiency include a fine, nonpruritic dermatitis; after 5 weeks, lassitude, muscular pain, and hypesthesias appear. After 10 weeks, anorexia, nausea, anemia, and hypercholesterolemia develop (55). In infants, the skin rash is said to be a seborrheic dermatitis and resembles Leiner's disease. The rash is characterized by scaling of inflamed skin, particularly on the scalp, cheeks, and neck, in the gluteal region, and sometimes around the umbilicus and groin.

Diagnosis of Biotin Deficiency

Diagnosis is difficult since it is seldom suspected clinically. The symptoms are relatively nonspecific and definitive laboratory tests are usually unavailable. An assay of blood and urine may reveal biotin deficiency. Whole blood biotin levels usually range between 820 and 2,700 pg/ml and urinary excretion of biotin between 14 and 100 µg/day (56).

Treatment of Biotin Deficiency

A parenteral biotin dose of 200 µg daily for 2 to 5 days effectively treated deficiency secondary to the ingestion of raw egg whites. Oral administration of 2 to 5 mg daily for 2 to 3 weeks is recommended for mild cases.

Requirements of Biotin

Requirements are difficult to determine since biotin is produced by bacteria in the gastrointestinal tract (1). No recommended intake has been determined, although the RDA permits inclusion of 0.15 mg biotin in the multivitamin supplements for infants and children and 0.3 mg in supplements for adults.

Biotin Dependency Syndromes

Propionic acidemia ("ketotic hyperglycinemia"), has, in some cases, been successfully treated with 1 to 4 mg/day. In some patients with β-methylcrotonyl glycinuria (deficient β-methylcrotonyl-CoA carboxylase), biotin (the enzyme cofactor) administered in the range of 10 mg/day corrected the metabolic acidosis. One patient with pyruvate carboxylase deficiency responded to pharmacologic doses of biotin.

Toxicity to Biotin

Toxicity to biotin has not been described (33,57).

VITAMIN C

Recommended Daily Intake

Infant	Children	Adult	Pregnancy
35 mg	40 mg	40 mg	60 mg

Most animals synthesize ascorbate from glucose via glucuronic acid and gluconic acid. Humans and other primates, the guinea pig, the elephant, the red-breasted bulbul bird, and the fruit-eating bat do not, however, synthesize vitamin C.

Vitamin C appears to function primarily in the capacity of a strong reducing agent or in reactions involved in electron transport within biologic systems. Although it appears to have multiple functions in humans, its specific biochemistry is not clearly defined. Its most striking property is its capacity for reversible oxidation-reduction.

Ascorbic acid is absorbed in the upper small intestine. An average dietary intake of 50 to 150 mg/day maintains a plasma level of about 1.2 mg/100 ml. The renal threshold of ascorbate is about 1.4 mg/100 ml. Vitamin C appears unchanged in the urine or as the sulfate when the renal threshold is exceeded. It is metabolized to 2,3-diketogulonic acid and oxylate, both of which are excreted in urine (58).

Dietary Sources of Vitamin C

Dietary sources include raw liver, fruits, and vegetables. Much of the vitamin C in foods may be lost in cooking and storage since it is destroyed by both heat and oxidation. Ascorbate is relatively stable in canned and frozen foods.

Vitamin C Deficiency

Vitamin C deficiency is manifest by formation of abnormal collagen fibers. After proline is inserted into a precollagen protein unit by the cellular ribosomes, ascorbate and oxygen are necessary for hydroxylation of carbon-4 proline to form normal collagen. The enzyme collagen proline hydroxylase catalyzes this reaction. Ascorbate also is involved in the hydroxylation of other compounds, such as norepinephrine, tryptophan, and certain steroids. All hydroxylations presumably involve ascorbate-dependent electron-transfer mechanisms at the microsomal level.

Other reactions involving ascorbate include the oxidation of phenylalanine and tyrosine, hydroxylation of tryptophan, utilization of iron (59), conversion of folic to folinic acid, maintenance of normal activity of serum complement, and conversion of cholesterol to bile acids (60). Ascorbate also spares or protects several of the B vitamins including B_1, B_2, folate, and pantothenate. However, ascorbate will destroy vitamin B_{12} in serum (61).

Prolonged vitamin C deficiency results in scurvy. The more common associations leading to scurvy are food faddism, alcoholism, famine, or other reasons for marginal subsistence such as deficiencies suffered by prisoners of war. Infantile scurvy has occurred most commonly in infants fed exclusively cow's milk for the first 6 to 12 months of life. At present, most commercial distributors in the United States supplement their milk with vitamin C, making scurvy uncommon in this country. However, losses of vitamin C may increase substantially following severe trauma, and more than the usual recommended doses of vitamin C may be necessary to facilitate healing of extensive burns.

Clinical Features of Scurvy

In infancy, clinical features of scurvy (Barlow's disease) occur between 8 and 13 months of age and begin with anorexia, intermittent diarrhea, failure to gain weight, pallor, irritability, apathy, and increased susceptibility to infection. As the illness progresses, long-bone tenderness and failure of spontaneous leg movement may occur. Hemorrhage under the periosteum of long bones, mucus membranes, and skin is common. Advanced stages of scurvy are characterized by hematuria, hematemesis, bloody diarrhea, epistaxis, ecchymosis of the eyelids, and proptosis from orbital hemorrhage.

The scorbutic infant is often febrile with tachycardia and tachypnea out of proportion to the degree of fever. A rounded type of costochondral beading (scorbutic rosary) may be confused with rickets. This phenomenon is due to costochondral separation which causes the sternum to sink slightly inward, leaving a sharp edge on the rib side of the junction.

Radiographic changes are seen at the cartilage shaft junction and appear earliest at sites of most active growth, e.g., sternal ends of ribs, distal femur, proximal humerus, both ends of tibia and fibula, and distal radius and ulna (62). There is broadening of the zone of divisional calcification at the epiphyseal end of the shaft causing a thickened white line (of Fraenkel) which results from accumulation of calcified cartilage. If there is a zone of rarefaction under the white line at the metaphysis, the x-ray is said to be diagnostic of scurvy. The cortex of the bone is thinned, giving a ground glass appearance and causing the white line to be more prominent. After several days of treatment with ascorbate, areas of subperiosteal hemorrhage become clearly outlined by bone formation in the periphery. The zone of rarefaction, called the scurvy line, gradually becomes filled with normal bone trabeculae which form a dense shadow that fuses with the epiphyseal line. Following a year of treatment, normal bone architecture is usually restored.

The radiographic features of copper deficiency may be identical to those features resulting from ascorbate deficiency, since both ascorbate and copper are required for mature collagen formation. The use of total parenteral feedings without copper supplements has caused an increase in the prevalence of copper deficiency during infancy, which may be confused radiographically with the scurvy of ascorbate deficiency (63).

Diagnosis of Scurvy

Diagnosis can often be made by the presence of characteristic physical findings and a history of dietary inadequacy of vitamin C. Roentgenograms of the bones may be diagnostic in infantile scurvy. Low plasma ascorbate may not be diagnostic since the level may be near zero for as long as 3 months before scurvy develops. The vitamin C content of leukocytes may be a valuable aid in diagnosis. However, levels may be depressed by tetracycline, which lowers leukocyte ascorbate content and increases urinary losses (64). Long-term hemodialysis, chronic inflammatory diseases, heavy cigarette smoking, and contraceptive steroids are also associated with low serum ascorbate levels. Serum levels of less than 0.10 mg/100 ml are considered deficient, and a level of 0.20 mg/100 ml is generally considered the lower limit of normal.

Treatment of Infantile Scurvy

Treatment is often dramatic, with improvement in appetite and disposition within 24 to 48 hr. Tenderness of extremities, fever, and hemorrhagic phenomena disappear within a few days. The usual treatment dose for infantile scurvy is 25 mg four times daily (usually given with feedings) for 4 to 5 days, then decreased to 25 mg twice daily until complete healing occurs. Prevention of scurvy in areas where milk is not fortified with vitamin C can be accomplished by administering 1 to 2 oz of orange or tomato juice or an intake of 25 mg of vitamin C, daily. Although limes have relatively small amounts of vitamin C, when taken in sufficient quantity they are also effective in prevention.

Requirements for Vitamin C

Requirements vary with age. Recommendations of daily ascorbate intake from the Food and Nutrition Board of the National Academy of Sciences, National Research Council are as follows: normal adults, 40 to 70 mg; nursing mothers, 60 to 100 mg; infants, 30 to 40 mg.

Pharmacologic Doses of Vitamin C

In controlled trials, pharmacologic doses of vitamin C have failed to prevent upper respiratory infections (65). However, a relationship has been demonstrated between the level of dietary ascorbate and strength of wound healing. Because of the decrease in plasma ascorbate following severe trauma or surgical procedures, it has been suggested that the daily dose of vitamin C be increased to 100 to 300 mg. Since vitamin C is a cofactor in the *in vitro* reaction of homogentisic acid oxidase, it is conceivable that pharmacologic doses could be of benefit in the treatment of homogentisic aciduria (alkaptonuria).

Vitamin C Toxicity

Daily administration of 12 g ascorbate for several months has caused no detrimental effects, although changes in lipid levels may occur. Large doses may cause diarrhea in children and may precipitate hemolysis in individuals with glucose-6-phosphate dehydrogenase deficiency (66). Large doses of vitamin C can interfere with vitamin B_{12} absorption and metabolism in humans, and this interference may be overcome by supplemental vitamin B_{12} (61). Healthy adults can become conditioned to high doses of ascorbate (0.5 to 1.6 g/day) over a 2-week period, resulting in a lower-than-normal serum and leukocyte ascorbate level on returning to a normal vitamin C intake (67). Such a phenomenon in the fetus may explain the development of scurvy in normally fed offspring of mothers who ingested 400 mg ascorbate daily throughout pregnancy (13).

Since ascorbate is an acidifying agent, large doses may be contraindicated in gout, renal tubular acidosis, cirrhosis, paroxysmal nocturnal hemoglobinuria, and other conditions aggravated by acid loading (67).

REFERENCES

1. American Academy of Pediatrics Committee on Nutrition. Vitamin deficiencies. *Pediatrics* 1977;61:230.
2. American Academy of Pediatrics Committee on Nutrition. Nutritional needs of low-birth-weight infants. *Pediatrics* 1977;60:519–530.
3. American Academy of Pediatrics Committee on Nutrition. Nutritional aspects of vegetarianism, health foods and fad diets. *Pediatrics* 1977;59:460–464.
4. Robson JRK. Food fadism. *Pediatr Clin North Am* 1977;24:189–201.
5. Spellacy WN, Buhi WC, Birk SA. Vitamin B_6 treatment of gestational diabetes mellitus: Studies of blood glucose and plasma insulin. *Am J Gynecol* 1977;127:599–602.
6. Rindi G, Ventura U. Thiamine intestinal transport. *Physiol Rev* 1963;52:821–827.
7. Krampitz LO. *Annu Rev Biochem* 1969;38:213–240.
8. Drenick EJ, Joven CB, Swendseid ME. Occurrence of acute Wernicke's encephalopathy during prolonged starvation for the treatment of obesity. *N Engl J Med* 1966;274:937–939.
9. Pincus JH, Copper JR, Murphy JV, Rabe EF, Lonsdale D, Dunn HG. Thiamine derivatives in subacute necrotizing encephalomyelopathy. *Pediatrics* 1973;51:716–721.
10. Shah N, Wolff JA. Thiamine deficiency: probable Wernicke's encephalopathy successfully treated in a child with acute lymphocytic leukemia. *Pediatrics* 1973;51:750–751.
11. Hoyumpa AM Jr, Nichols S, Henderson GI, et al. Intestinal thiamine transport: effect of chronic ethanol administration in rats. *Am J Clin Nutr* 1978;31:938–945.
12. Herman RH, Stifel FB, Greene HL. Vitamins. In: Dietschy JM, ed. *Disorders of the gastrointestinal tract, disorders of the liver, nutritional disorders,* vol I. New York: Grune & Stratton, 1976;364–400.
13. Phornphutkul C, Gamble WJ, Monsoe RG. Ventricular performance, coronary flow and myocardial consumption in rate with advanced thiamine deficiency. *Am J Clin Nutr* 1974;27:136–143.
14. Porter FS, Rogers LE, Sidbury JB Jr. Thiamine-responsive megaloblastic anemia. *J Pediatr* 1969;74:494–504.
15. Brunette MG, Delvin E, Hazel R, Scriver CR. Thiamine-responsive lactic acidosis in a patient with deficient low-KM pyruvate carboxylase activity in liver. *Pediatrics* 1972;50:702–711.
16. Tetreault AF, Beck IA. Anaphylactic shock following intramuscular thiamine chloride. *Ann Intern Med* 1956;45:134–138.
17. Rivlin RS. Riboflavin metabolism. *N Engl J Med* 1970;283:463–472.
18. Rivlin RS. Riboflavin. In: Recheigl M, ed. *Handbook of nutrition and food.* Cleveland: CRC Press, 1977;88–101.
19. Pinto J, Haung YP, Rivlin RS. Inhibition of riboflavin metabolism rat tissues by chlorpromazine, imipramine, and amitriptyline. *J Clin Invest* 1981;67:1500–1508.
20. Beutler E. Effect of flavin compounds on glutathione reductase activity: *in vivo* and *in vitro* studies. *J Clin Invest* 1970;48:1957.
21. Tillotson JA, Baker EM. An enzymatic measurement of the riboflavin status in man. *Am J Clin Nutr* 1972;25:425–429.
22. Loos H, Roos D. Familial deficiency of glutathione reductase in human blood cells. *Blood* 1976;48:53–69.
23. Rivlin RS, Huang YP, Pinto J, McConnell RJ. Increased excretion of riboflavin due to boric acid intoxication. *Clin Res* 1978;24:424A.
24. Baeckert PA, Greene HL, Fritz I, Oelberg DG, Adcock EW III. Vitamin concentrations in very low birth weight infants given vitamins intravenously in a lipid emulsion: measurement of vitamins A, D, and E and riboflavin. *J Pediatr* 1988;113(6):1057–1065.
25. Greene HL, Hambidge MK, Schanler R, Tsang RC. Guidelines for the use of vitamins, trace elements, calcium, magnesium, and phosphorus in infants and children receiving total parenteral nutrition: Report of the Subcommittee on Pediatric Parenteral Nutrient Requirements from the Committee on Clinical Practice Issues of the American Society for Clinical Nutrition. *Am J Clin Nutr* 1988;48(5):1324–1342.
26. Lumeng L, Brashear RE, Li TK. Pyridoxal 5′-phosphate in plasma: source protein binding and cellular transport. *J Lab Clin Med* 1974;84:334–343.
27. Sebrell WM Jr, Harris RS, eds. *The vitamins,* vol 2. New York: Academic Press, 1968;1–117.
28. Brown RR. Normal and pathological conditions which may alter the human requirement for vitamin B_6. *J Agric Food Chem* 1972;20:498–505.
29. Kelsall MA. Clinical pyridoxine deficiency. *Ann NY Acad Sci* 1969;166:1–56.
30. Lott IT, Coulombe BA, DiPado RV. Vitamin B_6-dependent seizures: pathology and chemical findings in brain. *Neurology* 1978;28:47–54.
31. Sauberlich HE, Canhan JE, Baker EM, Raica N, Herman YF. Biochemical assessment of the nutritional status of vitamin B_6 in the human. *Am J Clin Nutr* 1972;25:629–642.
32. Longhi RC, Fleisher LD, Tallan HH, Gaull GE. Cystathionine β-synthase deficiency: a qualitative abnormality of the deficient enzyme modified by vitamin B_6 therapy. *Pediatr Res* 1977;11:100–103.
33. Gompertz D. Inborn errors of organic acid metabolism. *Clin Endocrinol Metabol* 1974;3:107–130.
34. McKenzie SA, MacNab AJ, Katz G. Neonatal pyridoxine responsive convulsions due to isoniazid therapy. *Arch Dis Child* 1976;51:567–568.
35. Beaupre EM, Gorwney PM. Pyridoxine-responsive anemia with neuropathy. *Ann Intern Med* 1963;59:724–730.
36. Harris JW, Horrigan DL. Pyridoxine-responsive anemia—prototype and variations on the theme. *Vitam Horm* 1964;22:721–753.
37. Scriber ER, Rosenberg LE. *Amino acid metabolism and its derivatives.* Philadelphia: WB Saunders, 1973.
38. Anonymous. Retinitis pigmentosa and vitamin A. *Nutr Rev* 1976;21:334–336.
39. Nakagawa I, Ohguri S, Takahashi T. Effects of excess intake of leucine and valine deficiency on tryptophan and niacin metabolites in humans. *J Nutr* 1975;105:1241–1252.
40. Goldsmith GA, Sarett MP, Register R, Gibbens J. Studies of niacin requirements in man. I. Experimental pellagra in subjects on corn diets low in niacin and tryptophan. *J Clin Invest* 1952;31:533–542.
41. Spivak JA, Jackson DL. Pellagra: an analysis of 18 patients and a review of the literature. *Johns Hopkins Med J* 1977;140:295–309.
42. Jolliffe N, Bowman KM, Rosenblum LA, Fein HD. Nicotinic acid deficiency encephalopathy. *JAMA* 1940;114:304–312.
43. Winkelman RK, Schroeter AL, Kierland RR, Ryan TM. Clinical studies of livedoid vasculitis (segmenting hyalinizing vasculitis). *Mayo Clin Proc* 1974;49:746–750.
44. Bean WB, Hodges RE. Pantothenic acid deficiency induced in human subjects. *Proc Soc Exp Biol Med* 1954;86:693–698.
45. Hodges ER, Ohlson MA, Bean WB. Pantothenic acid deficiency in man. *J Clin Invest* 1958;37:1642–1657.
46. Glusman M. Syndrome of "burning feet" (nutritional malalgia) as manifestation of nutritional deficiency. *Am J Med* 1947;3:211–223.
47. Gopalan C. Etiology of "phrynoderma." *Ind M Gaz* 1947;82:16–20.

48. Gross P, Harvalik Z, Runne E. Role of unsaturated fatty acids in acrodynia (vitamin B_6 deficiency) of albino rat. *J Invest Dermatol* 1941;4:385–398.
49. Bonjour JP. Biotin in man's nutrition and therapy—a review. *Int J Vitam Nutr Res* 1977;47:107–118.
50. Knappe J. Mechanism of biotin action. *Annu Rev Biochem* 1970;39:757–776.
51. Oppel TW. *Am J Med Sci* 1942;204:856–875.
52. Baugh CM, Malone HJ, Butterworth CE Jr. Human biotin deficiency: a case history of biotin deficiency induced by raw egg consumption in a cirrhotic patient. *Am J Clin Nutr* 1968;21:173–182.
53. Sydenstricker VP, Singal SA, Briggs AP, DeVaughn NM, Isabel H. Observations on "egg white injury" in man and its cure with biotin concentrate. *JAMA* 1942;118:1199–1200.
54. Mock DM, DeLorimer AA, Liebman WM, Sweetman L, Baker H. Biotin deficiency—an unusual complication of parenteral alimentation. *N Engl J Med* 1981;304:820–823.
55. Williams RH. Clinical biotin deficiency. *N Engl J Med* 1943;288:247–252.
56. Baker H, Frank O, Matovitch VB, Pasher MI, Aaronson S, Hutner SH, Sobotka H. A new assay method for biotin in blood, serum, urine and tissues. *Ann Biochem* 1962;3:31–39.
57. Hillman RE, Keating JP, Williams JC. Biotin-responsive propionic acidemia presenting as the rumination syndrome. *J Pediatr* 1978;92:439–441.
58. Stein HBA, Hasan A, Fox IH. Ascorbic acid-induced uricosuria a consequence of megavitamin therapy. *Ann Intern Med* 1976;84:385–388.
59. Cook JD, Monsen ER. Vitamin C, the common cold, and iron absorption. *Am J Clin Nutr* 1977;30:235–244.
60. Ginter E. Cholesterol: vitamin C controls its transformation to bile acids. *Science* 1973;179:702–704.
61. Herbert V, Jacob E. Destruction of vitamin B_{12} by ascorbic acid. *JAMA* 1974;230:241–242.
62. Hood J, Burns CA, Hodges RE. SjöGren's syndrome in scurvy. *N Engl J Med* 1970;282:1120–1124.
63. Ashkenazi A, Levin S, Djaldetti M, Fishel E, Benvensti SD. The syndrome of neonatal copper deficiency. *Pediatrics* 1977;52:525–533.
64. Boxer LA, Watanabe AM, Rister M, Besch HR Jr, Allen J, Baenner R. Correction of leukocyte function in Chediak-Higashi syndrome by ascorbate. *N Engl J Med* 1976;295:1041–1045.
65. Pauling L. Are recommended daily allowances for vitamin C adequate? *Proc Natl Acad Sci USA* 1974;71:4442–4446.
66. Campbell GD, Steinberg MH, Bower JD. Ascorbic acid-induced hemolysis in G-6 PD deficiency. *Ann Intern Med* 1975;82:810.
67. Rhead WJ, Schrauzer GN. Risks of long-term ascorbic acid overdosage. *Nutr Rev* 1971;29:262–263.
68. Koo WK, Tsang RC, Succo PP. Vitamin D requirements in infants receiving parenteral nutrition. *JPEN* 1987;11:172–177.

CHAPTER 8

Nutritional Anemias in Childhood

Iron, Folate, and Vitamin B_{12}

Peter R. Dallman

Iron, folic acid, and vitamin B_{12} play important roles in the production of red blood cells. Hemoglobin, of which iron is a constituent, contains about 75% of the iron found in the body. Folic acid and vitamin B_{12} are essential for the cell proliferation that proceeds at a rapid rate in the body as a whole during very early development and in the hematopoietic tissue throughout life. Deficiencies of vitamin B_{12} and folic acid, which occur rarely as a result of nutritional deficits, may result from inborn errors of metabolism. It is important that these errors are recognized in infancy, since they have serious neurological consequences and usually require lifelong treatment. Iron, folic acid, and vitamin B_{12} are appropriately discussed in the same chapter because a deficiency of any of them will eventually lead to anemia. Iron deficiency is very common (1), especially among infants and adolescents, and is easily prevented by appropriate diets.

DEFINITION OF ANEMIA

Anemia is defined as a hemoglobin concentration (or hematocrit) below the 95% range for healthy subjects of the same age and sex. Before 10 years of age, there is no difference according to sex (2,3). Because of the marked age-related changes that normally occur in hemoglobin concentration, it is essential to compare the patient's values to age-specific reference standards. The current reference values are based on healthy populations in whom laboratory studies and/or nutritional management excluded iron deficiency and other recognized causes of anemia (Fig. 1; Table 1) (2–6).

P. R. Dallman: Department of Pediatrics, University of California, San Francisco, California 94143.

In a healthy term infant, the mean concentration of hemoglobin declines by approximately 30%, from about 170 to 110 g/l, within the first 6 to 8 postnatal weeks. In the premature infant, the postnatal fall in hemoglobin concentration is more marked, even with what is considered optimal nutrition, as described in the sections on iron and vitamin E. At 2 months of age, values fall to a mean of about 95 g/l in infants with birth weights between 1,500 and 2,000 g, and to 90 g/l in those with birth weights between 1,000 and 1,500 g (Fig. 1) (6).

These extremes represent highest and lowest values in any period of development. Subsequently, there is a rise to a mean of 125 g/l at about 4 months of age, followed

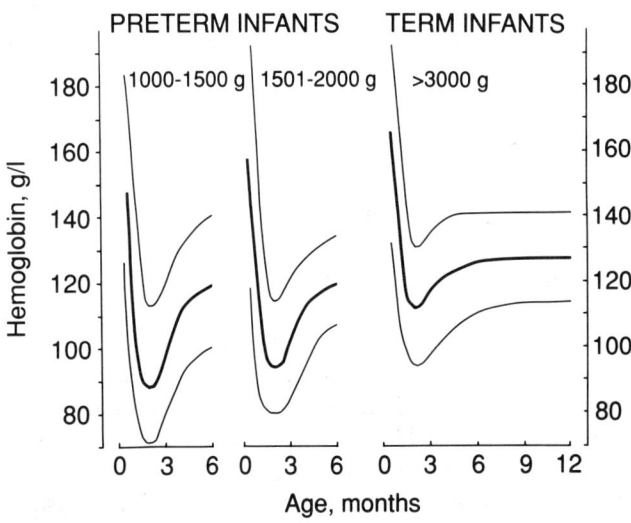

FIG. 1. Hemoglobin concentration in term and preterm infants: median values and 95% ranges. (Data from refs. 47 and 66.)

TABLE 1. *Hemoglobin, hematocrit and mean corpuscular volume (MCV): mean values and lower limits of 95% range (24, 44, 83)*

Age (yr) and sex	Hemoglobin (g/l)		Hematocrit (%)		MCV (fl)	
	Mean	Lower limit	Mean	Lower limit	Mean	Lower limit
0.5–4	125	110	36	32	80	72
5–10	130	115	38	33	83	75
11–14 F	135	120	39	34	85	77
11–14 M	140	120	41	35	85	77
15–19 F	135	120	40	34	88	79
15–19 M	150	130	43	37	88	79
20–44 F	135	120	40	35	90	80
20–44 M	160	135	45	39	90	80

by a very gradual increase to 135 g/l in preadolescents. In adolescent boys, there is another period of rapid change from a mean hemoglobin of 135 g/l at age 11 to 150 g/l at 16. Values in females remain fairly stable at about 135 g/l throughout adulthood.

Age-related changes in hemoglobin concentration are primarily attributable to corresponding alterations in the rate of red blood cell production. The rate of division and differentiation of nucleated red blood cells in bone marrow is controlled by a humoral substance, erythropoietin, that is produced primarily in the kidney in response to tissue hypoxia (7). The resulting increase in concentration of hemoglobin restores tissue oxygenation to normal. The high hemoglobin concentration of the newborn is attributable to a relatively hypoxic intrauterine environment that stimulates erythropoietin production in the fetus and results in a high rate of erythropoiesis. At birth, oxygen tension suddenly rises and the rate of erythropoiesis decreases. A marked depression in the rate of red blood cell production continues for 6 to 8 weeks after birth, resulting in a low point of hemoglobin values. After 6 to 8 weeks, red cell production increases to keep pace with growth as well as to result in an increase in hemoglobin concentration.

IRON DEFICIENCY

Normal Iron Homeostasis

Essential and Storage Iron

The iron-containing compounds of the body fall into two categories: the essential compounds that serve metabolic or enzymatic functions and those associated with iron storage (8,9). The essential compounds function in the transport and utilization of oxygen for the production of cellular energy; they include hemoglobin, myoglobin, the cytochromes, and iron-sulfur proteins. Hemoglobin accounts for most of the essential iron and about two-thirds of total body iron. The storage compounds, ferritin and hemosiderin, are involved in the maintenance of iron homeostasis. When the supply of dietary iron becomes inadequate, iron is mobilized from the storage compounds to maintain the production of hemoglobin and other essential iron compounds. Not until the production of hemoglobin (the most easily measured essential iron compound) becomes restricted does impairment of body function become apparent.

Definitions of Deficiency (8)

The general term *iron deficiency* refers to a deficit that is sufficiently severe to restrict the production of hemoglobin. *Iron deficiency anemia* is the advanced condition that occurs only when the concentration of hemoglobin has fallen sufficiently to fulfill the laboratory definition of anemia, i.e., when it is below the 95% reference range for age. *Iron deficiency without anemia,* or impaired hemoglobin production, refers to the milder form of iron deficiency in which the hemoglobin concentration has decreased, but not sufficiently to meet the definition of anemia. It is typically recognized on the basis of other laboratory abnormalities that indicate impaired hemoglobin production and is characterized by a low-normal hemoglobin concentration that increases in response to iron treatment.

Iron deficiency anemia and iron deficiency without anemia both have a potential for causing impairment of body function since they affect the production of essential iron compounds. In contrast, the presence of low iron stores is physiological during most of infancy and childhood. This may explain some common conceptual difficulties, since the term *depletion of iron stores* implies that there is an abnormality. Depletion of iron stores is usually defined in terms of a low serum ferritin concentration, reflecting low tissue iron stores; cutoff values of anywhere from 10 to 20 µg/l have been suggested. Depletion of iron stores, without other laboratory evidence of iron deficiency, is relatively common among healthy children (2) and is not known to result in any impairment of body function. It does, however, indicate a greater vulnerability or potential for developing iron deficiency.

Iron Balance

A distinctive feature of iron metabolism is the remarkable extent to which the body conserves and reutilizes iron once it has been absorbed. The amount of body iron is regulated primarily through modulation of iron absorption over a more than 20-fold range. Iron absorption depends on the abundance of body iron stores, on the form and amount of iron in foods, and on the combination of foods in the diet (10,11). Absorption increases as storage iron becomes decreased. Iron excretion occurs mainly by loss with desquamation of the intestinal mucosa. The amount of iron lost in this manner varies only over a fourfold range, decreasing in iron deficiency and increasing in iron overload (12). Consequently, the major determining factor in maintaining iron homeostasis is absorption.

Iron Absorption

The proportion of iron absorbed from food is determined both by the nature of the diet and by a homeostatic regulatory mechanism in the intestinal mucosa that is responsive to the abundance of storage iron (10).

Dietary Iron (10,11)

There are two broad categories of iron in food. *Heme iron,* which is present in hemoglobin and myoglobin, is supplied mainly by meat and accounts for about 10% of the iron in the average diet of children and adults, although less in infants. Heme iron is relatively well absorbed; its absorption is little influenced by other constituents of the diet. Most of the remaining iron is present in the form of iron salts and is called *nonheme iron.* Infant diets, which include little meat, contain iron almost entirely in the nonheme form.

The absorption of nonheme iron depends on how soluble the iron becomes in the intestine, which, in turn, is determined by the composition of foods that are consumed (10,11). Absorption of nonheme iron from a mixed meal is about four times greater when the major protein source is meat, fish, or chicken, as opposed to dairy products or eggs (13). The beverage consumed with the meal plays an equally important role (14). Orange juice, when compared to water, will double the absorption of nonheme iron from a breakfast, whereas tea decreases absorption by about 75% and cow's milk to a lesser degree (Fig. 2).

The most important enhancers of nonheme iron absorption are ascorbic acid, meat, fish, and poultry (Table 2) (10,11,15). Major inhibitors are bran, polyphenols, including the tannates in tea, calcium, and phosphate. The basis for the excellent absorption of iron from human milk (16,17) is not known. The lower calcium and phosphate content of human milk compared to cow's milk, and the high concentration of the iron-binding protein, lactoferrin, have been postulated to play a role (18) but cannot explain this phenomenon entirely. Some evidence suggests that ingestion of human milk per se may influence the intestinal mucosa in a way that facilitates iron absorption (17).

TABLE 2. *Nonheme iron absorption: enhancers and inhibitors*

Enhancers	Inhibitors
Ascorbic acid (orange juice)	Phosphates (cow milk, egg yolk)
Citric acid	Bran (whole grain cereals)
	Oxalates (spinach)
Meat	Polyphenols (tannate in tea)

Homeostatic Regulation of Body Iron by the Intestinal Mucosa

The basis for the homeostatic regulation of iron absorption by the intestinal mucosa remains unclear (19). Iron absorption, however, is increased when iron stores are low, as is normally the case in late infancy (20) and in iron-deficient individuals of any age (10,11). This response protects the body against iron deficiency to the extent that the diet supplies potentially absorbable iron. Conversely, when iron stores are abundant, for example, in the first postnatal month, iron absorption is decreased (Fig. 3) (20).

Although little is understood about the mechanism of intestinal iron absorption, great progress has been made in defining the regulation of iron uptake by individual cells from the circulation (21,22). This process involves the control of cell surface receptors for transferrin, so that the number of receptors corresponds to the changing iron needs of the cell. This knowledge is pertinent to the recently proposed measurement of circulating transferrin receptor in the diagnosis of iron deficiency.

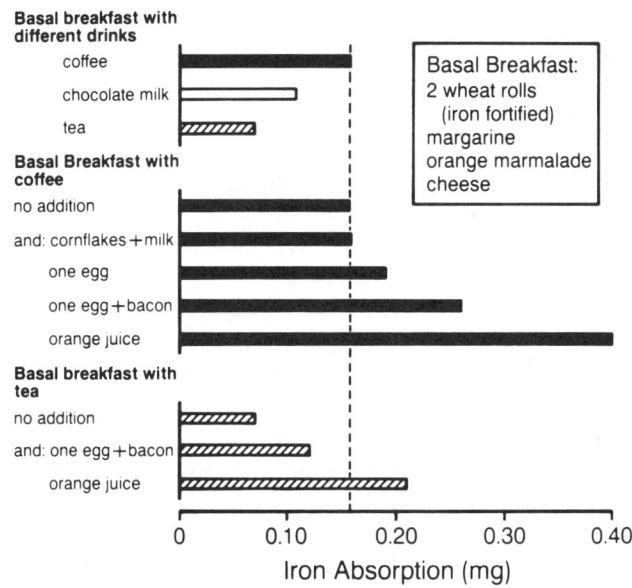

FIG. 2. Iron absorption from breakfast meals. The *dashed vertical line* represents the amount of nonheme iron absorbed from the basal breakfast with coffee. (Redrawn with permission from ref. 63.)

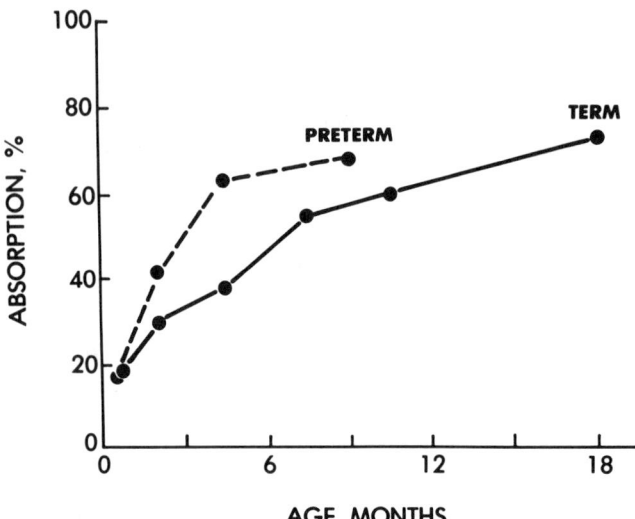

FIG. 3. Increasing iron absorption during infancy as iron stores decrease. A test dose of 0.56 mg ferrous iron was administered under fasting conditions.

Causes of Iron Deficiency

Iron deficiency may be caused by insufficient intake or assimilation of iron from the diet, dilution of body iron as a result of rapid growth, blood loss, or a combination of these factors (23). During the periods of most rapid weight gain in infancy and adolescence, the diet is often low in iron or contains iron in poorly absorbable forms. Anemia, particularly in young infants under 6 months of age, may also result from intestinal blood loss resulting from the ingestion of large amounts of cow's milk (24).

Changing Iron Needs During Development (23)

During pregnancy, iron is efficiently transported from the maternal circulation to the fetus. This transport is scarcely impaired even when the mother has mild iron deficiency anemia. At birth, the hemoglobin concentration is normally high and the liver reserves of storage iron are relatively generous. Consequently, most newborn infants are well supplied with iron. However, low neonatal iron stores may occur in cases of uteroplacental insufficiency associated with maternal diabetes and preeclampsia (25). Despite the usual preservation of the newborn's hemoglobin production and liver iron stores, there is epidemiological evidence that maternal iron deficiency anemia is associated with prematurity, low birth weight, and increased perinatal mortality (26,27). Although these findings are intriguing, a cause and effect relationship has not been established.

In the normal term infant, there is little change in total body iron and little need for exogenous iron between birth and 4 months of age (Fig. 4). The usually abundant neonatal iron stores gradually decline during this period

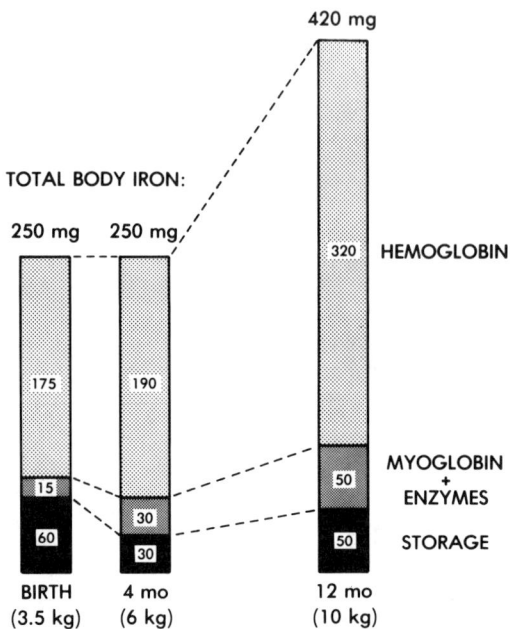

FIG. 4. Changes in body iron during infancy. From birth to 4 months, total body iron remains stable and little exogenous iron is needed. Subsequently, large amounts of iron are assimilated to meet the needs of rapid growth and an expanding blood volume (18).

to provide for the synthesis of hemoglobin, myoglobin, and enzyme iron. Despite rapid growth and a substantial rise in blood volume, total hemoglobin iron scarcely increases because of the marked decline in concentration of hemoglobin. For this reason, iron deficiency is rare within the first few postnatal months except when there has been substantial loss of iron through perinatal or subsequent blood loss or in cases of uteroplacental insufficiency associated with maternal diabetes and preeclampsia (25).

After about 4 months of age, there is a gradual shift from an abundance of iron to the marginal iron reserves that characterize the period of continued rapid growth during the remainder of infancy (Fig. 4). This transition is primarily due to the large amount of iron required to maintain the hemoglobin concentration during a period of rapid growth and corresponding increase in blood volume. Between 4 and 12 months, an average of 0.8 mg of iron/day must be absorbed from the diet to provide 0.6 mg/day for growth and 0.2 mg/day to balance basal losses (Fig. 5) (28). The rate and extent to which storage iron becomes depleted during this period depend on the magnitude of iron storage at birth as well as on the postnatal diet.

Iron needs are also unusually high during adolescence due to rapid growth, as well as a rise in hemoglobin in males and menstrual blood loss in females. Boys gain an average of 10 kg, or 22 lb, during the peak year of their growth spurt, some time between about 12 and 15 years of age. During this period, the concentration of hemoglobin increases toward values that are characteristic of

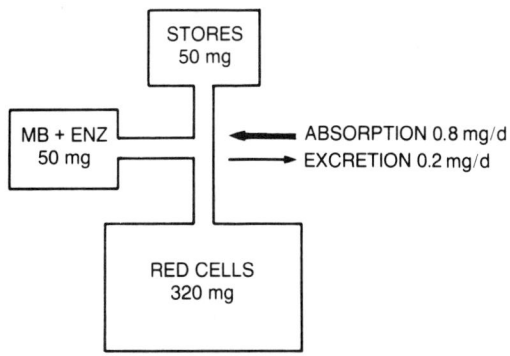

FIG. 5. Iron balance at 12 months of age. In contrast to adults, in whom iron absorption balances iron losses, in growing infants, iron absorption is about four times greater than iron losses.

adult men. The double burden of increased red cell mass and increased hemoglobin concentration requires an increase of about 25% in total body iron that must be supplied by the diet during the year of peak growth. The iron needs of adolescent girls also increase. Female weight gain averages 9 kg during the peak year of the growth spurt, which usually occurs between 10 and 12 years of age. Although the concentration of hemoglobin changes little, the onset of menstruation imposes additional iron needs.

In contrast to very early childhood and adolescence, the period between 3 and 10 years of age is marked by slower growth and lower iron needs. In the United States, iron deficiency anemia is rare during this period (2,29), even though iron stores, as reflected by the serum ferritin, are typically low (2).

Manifestations of Iron Deficiency (9,30)

The symptoms of iron deficiency in individual patients are nonspecific. Mild iron deficiency is usually diagnosed on the basis of laboratory screening. The findings in severe iron-deficiency anemia are usually similar to those of other anemias. Fatigue, decreased exercise tolerance, irritability, loss of appetite, and pallor may be noted, but the gradual onset of the anemia, which is characteristic of nutritional iron lack, may escape notice even when the concentration of hemoglobin is below 60 g/l. Tachycardia and cardiomegaly are present only when anemia is severe.

Recent studies have revealed more subtle manifestations of iron deficiency.

Decreased Work Performance

Both human and rat studies demonstrate that anemia causes a substantial reduction in work capacity, particularly when the concentration of hemoglobin falls below 100 g/l. Studies in humans indicate that even milder anemia can decrease performance in brief, hard exercise (31). The practical significance of these findings (32) is reflected in the decreased productivity of manual laborers in developing countries who suffer from iron deficiency (32–35). Iron-deficient children and adolescents in industrialized countries may have impaired athletic performance or fitness.

Behavior and Intellectual Performance

Increasing evidence suggests that changes in behavior, impaired psychomotor development (36,37), and intellectual performance (36,38) may result from iron deficiency. Most studies have evaluated infants between 6 months and 2 years of age using the Bayley Scale of Infant Development, which tests sensory development, fine and gross motor skills, and language development (36,37). The results have indicated that even infants with relatively mild iron deficiency anemia have a decrease in responsiveness, physical activity, and attentiveness with a concomitant increase in body tension, fearfulness, and tendency to fatigue. Of particular concern are preliminary data suggesting that infants who were treated for iron deficiency at about 1 year of age had persistent deficits in cognitive function at 5 years (37). This concern is reinforced by the results of experiments in the iron-deficient rat (39,40).

Resistance to Infection (41)

Iron-deficient children have functional abnormalities of lymphocytes and neutrophils, both of which play important roles in the host defense against infections. Despite numerous studies that show impaired cellular immunity, there is no conclusive proof of an increased rate of infections that is attributable to iron deficiency. However, persistent or repeated infection can predispose to iron deficiency by decreasing iron absorption (42). This provides, at least in theory, a basis for a vicious cycle of infection leading to iron deficiency which then predisposes to further infection.

Lead Poisoning

Iron deficiency is associated with a substantially increased risk of lead poisoning, particularly in young children. Iron-deficient individuals absorb increased amounts of lead (43), and are at increased risk of having elevated blood lead concentrations (44).

Prevention of Iron Deficiency

There is general agreement about most aspects of preventing iron deficiency (45). Only some relatively minor issues of timing remain controversial. Recommendations differ for term and preterm infants and according

TABLE 3. *Ways to improve iron nutrition (and overall nutrition)*

Unfortified foods
   Maintain breast-feeding for at least 6 months
   No cow's milk until after 9 to 12 months
   Include ascorbic acid–rich foods and/or meat in meals of solid food after about 6 months
Iron- and ascorbic acid–fortified foods
   If formula is used, use a cow's milk–based formula fortified with iron
   Use infant cereal or milk-cereal products that are fortified with iron or iron and ascorbic acid
   Use ascorbic acid–fortified fruit juice with meals of solid foods
Iron supplementation (ferrous sulfate or similarly bioavailable compounds)
   In low birth weight infants start prophylactic iron at about 1 month of age and continue through 6 to 12 months of age to provide the following *total* amounts according to birth weight: 1,500 to 2,500 g, 2 mg/kg/day; 1,000 to 1,500 g, 3 mg/kg/day; and <1000 g, 4 mg/kg/day. Iron-fortified formula in the United States provides about 2 mg/kg/day
   For established iron deficiency: 3 mg/kg/day

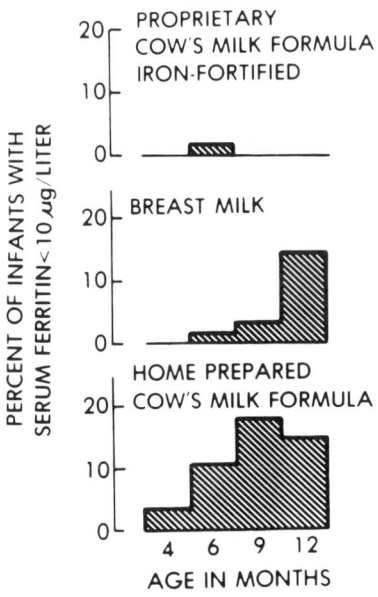

FIG. 6. Depletion of iron stores (serum ferritin < 10 μg/l) as a function of milk feeding. The percentage of infants with depleted iron stores increases markedly during the latter part of infancy in those fed unfortified formula. Some breast-fed infants also become iron depleted after 6 months of age. (From ref. 64.)

to whether infants are breast-fed or formula-fed (Table 3).

The iron needs of infants are more appropriately discussed in terms of the types of diet that prevent iron deficiency than in relation to milligrams of dietary iron required per day. Because of the marked variations in the bioavailability of dietary iron from various kinds of food, a diet may contain a substantial amount of iron and still result in iron deficiency if the iron is largely present in poorly absorbable forms (16).

Term Breast-Fed Infants

Term breast-fed infants do not routinely require iron supplementation, since their iron stores rarely become depleted before 6 months of age (Fig. 6) (46). Subsequently, an appropriate selection of solid foods will provide adequate dietary iron. Cereal and fruit juice are usually among the first non-milk foods given to infants. Iron-fortified dry infant cereal is generously fortified with iron (4.5 mg in a typical 10 gm serving). The absorption of iron from cereal (15,47) can be enhanced if it is also fortified with ascorbic acid (16) or by feeding an ascorbic acid–rich food, such as orange juice or ascorbic acid–fortified juice, at the same meal (15). Ready-to-serve cereals in jars and Cream of Wheat are less generously fortified with iron.

The absorption of iron from an entire meal can be enhanced by the inclusion of a small amount of meat. Egg yolk and spinach, although rich in iron, are now recognized to inhibit iron absorption (10,11). It also seems best not to feed solid foods near the time of breast-feeding, as this may reduce the excellent bioavailability of the small amount of iron in human milk (48).

If breast-feeding is discontinued before 4 to 9 months, it is advisable to substitute iron-fortified infant formula rather than fresh cow's milk which commonly results in occult intestinal blood loss, especially before 6 months of age (24). Early use of fresh cow's milk is the most common dietary characteristic shared by infants who are later found to have iron deficiency anemia when "screened" at about 1 year of age (49).

Term Formula-Fed Infants

Cow's milk formula is available in the United States in "unfortified" or iron-fortified forms. "Unfortified" formula supplies at least 1.5 mg of iron per reconstituted liter, whereas the iron-fortified formula has at least 12 mg of iron as ferrous sulfate added per reconstituted liter. Since term infants who are fed "unfortified" formula may deplete their iron stores as early as 6 months of age (46), it is advisable to change to iron-fortified formula before about 3 months of age.

Whether iron-fortified formula is preferable right from birth is uncertain. On one hand, it is more convenient to give a single formula throughout infancy. Alternatively, it may be argued that additional iron is not yet needed, and is poorly absorbed, before 3 or 4 months of age when iron stores are still abundant (20). Another argument involves the animal and *in vitro* evidence of increased infections (50,51). Transferrin and lactoferrin are iron-binding proteins present in milk. Both have bacteriostatic properties that disappear when they become saturated with iron. Despite animal and *in vitro* evidence that iron-fortified formula or oral iron medication might predispose to infections, epidemiologic support for this hypothesis in infants remains scant. This issue remains widely debated and is discussed in several reviews (41,50,51).

The use of iron-fortified formula is, in any case, a reliable way of preventing iron deficiency (52). The use of iron-fortified formula in the Federal Special Supplementary Food Program for Women, Infants, and Children (WIC) has contributed to a decline in prevalence of iron deficiency among infants in the United States (53,54). The Committee on Nutrition of the American Academy of Pediatrics has recommended that the change from breast milk or formula to fresh cow's milk can take place at any time between 6 and 12 months (45). I believe it is preferable to make the change to regular milk closer to 12 months in order to provide a convenient and effective vehicle for fortification iron and to avoid the risk that parents will use skim milk or low fat milk, which provide an inadequate caloric-density food for infants (55).

There is good evidence that fortifying cow's milk formula with 12 mg iron/l as ferrous sulfate is effective in preventing iron deficiency (45). In much of Europe, cow's milk formula is fortified with about 6 mg iron/l. Because the percentage of iron absorbed increases as the concentration is decreased, this is probably adequate (56). About 6% of the iron is absorbed from the formula fortified with 6 mg iron/l compared with 4% from the 12 mg iron/l formula.

Low Birth Weight Infants

Low birth weight (LBW) infants fed human milk almost invariably develop iron deficiency anemia unless they are given iron supplements (57). The Committee on Nutrition of the American Academy of Pediatrics recommends 2 mg of iron/kg/day to a maximum of 15 mg iron/day for low birth weight infants (45). This can be begun at 1 month of age as a single daily dose in the form of a liquid ferrous sulfate preparation. The iron is best absorbed when given before or between feedings. Intestinal intolerance to iron is rarely a problem at these dosages (58). A recent study showed no difference in prevalence of side effects between infants fed iron at a dose of 3 mg/kg/day and placebo-treated infants. The dose should be increased for very low birth weight (VLBW) infants during the first 6 months to accommodate their greater iron needs for growth (Table 3) (57). Medication should be continued at a dose of 2 mg/kg/day until at least 12 months of age.

Opinions vary regarding the exact age at which iron medication should be started in preterm, breast-fed infants. There is no urgency to administer iron before iron stores become depleted at about 1 or 2 months of age (see Iron Excess, below). A starting age of 1 month seems appropriate. There is no benefit of earlier initiation of iron unless there has been substantial blood loss for laboratory studies or in association with the delivery because iron stores normally become augmented in the first postnatal weeks as the fall in hemoglobin concentration releases more iron than can be reutilized for the production of new red blood cells.

In formula-fed preterm infants it is reasonable to begin iron-fortified formula no later than about 1 or 2 months of age. Iron-fortified formula (containing 12 mg iron/l) is adequate as the sole source of iron in infants with a birth weight > 1500 g and supplies the equivalent of 2 mg/kg of iron (5,57). Infants of lower birth weight may need an additional 1 or 2 mg/kg as ferrous sulfate, starting at about 1 month of age, to bring them up to the totals tabulated above. As in the case of the breast-fed preterm infant, exactly when to provide an additional source of iron is unresolved, but this does not appear to be of critical importance. Evidence of vitamin E deficiency has been reported among <1,500 g birth weight infants fed iron-fortified formula at 2 weeks of age (59). However, changes in formula composition, including decreased unsaturated fatty acids and increased vitamin E, have resulted in at least partial resolution of this problem (60).

Among older children and adults, fortification of cereal and grain products is a relatively inexpensive means of increasing iron intake (16,61). However, field studies are badly needed to determine the impact of the fortification iron in cereal products on overall iron nutrition.

Supplementation, in contrast to fortification, has the disadvantages of requiring extra effort and expense, as well as uncertain compliance. Iron supplements are also less available to the poor and other groups most likely to be iron deficient. It is not surprising, therefore, that the WIC program, which supplies fortified formula to infants below the poverty line, has contributed to a major decline in prevalence of anemia over the past 15 years (53).

Developing Countries

Prevention of iron deficiency is a more complex and urgent problem in underdeveloped countries, where parasitic infestation and the predominance of cereals and starches in the diet are responsible for a high prevalence of iron deficiency (1). Vehicles for fortification are limited, since most food products do not go through commercial processing. Cereal staples, such as rice and wheat, and such products as sugar and salt, have been used as vehicles when they form a relatively constant and predictable fraction of the diet (16). Even when some foods are fortified, however, absorption often remains low because the diet is poor in meat or ascorbic acid–rich foods that facilitate iron assimilation.

Diagnosis (62)

Iron deficiency is usually suspected on the basis of history or detected by routine "screening" for anemia. Screening for anemia is generally included as part of a routine health maintenance visit between about 9 and 12 months of age for term infants and between 2 and 6 months for preterm infants. It is also useful to check for anemia in adolescents because of their increased iron needs for rapid growth. The prevalence of iron deficiency at these ages is about 5% to 10% in the United States (2), with higher values among the poor and lower ones where good medical care and nutritional counseling are more available (54,63). Iron deficiency anemia is far less common than iron deficiency (2).

It is best to delay screening for anemia if there has been a recent illness. This is because acute infection is the most common cause of anemia other than iron deficiency, and the laboratory abnormalities that mimic iron deficiency can persist for several weeks, even after recovery from a mild upper respiratory infection (51,64,65).

The measurement of hemoglobin concentration is the most useful laboratory test in screening for iron deficiency anemia, since it directly reflects the quantity of the most abundant essential iron compound in the body. A microhematocrit may be more convenient in an office or clinic and is a close second choice. However, the hematocrit does not exactly parallel the hemoglobin concentration and is apt to be normal despite a slightly subnormal hemoglobin value. This is because the microcytic, hypochromic cells of iron deficiency have slightly less hemoglobin than normal for any given packed cell volume. In addition, some degree of stiffness of the red cell membranes in iron deficiency probably results in more trapped plasma when red cells are packed by centrifugation.

Two values to remember when screening for anemia in infants are hemoglobin <110 g/l and hematocrit <33%. These values apply from 6 months to 4 years of age, when iron deficiency anemia is most common. For other ages, it is helpful to refer to published standards (Table 1; Fig. 1).

Since venipuncture is often difficult in infants, skin puncture blood samples are more commonly used. Although this is a justifiable sacrifice of accuracy (62) for the sake of practicality, it is necessary to be aware of the large sampling error involved (a 2-SD sampling error of more than 1.0 g/dl compared to 0.3 g/dl for venipuncture blood), even when appropriate care is taken to warm the extremity and avoid squeezing to obtain the sample. The practical implication of the large sampling error is that many infants who are mildly anemic by skin puncture sampling prove not to be anemic when a repeat analysis is obtained on venipuncture blood (62,66). Not surprisingly, there are differences of opinion about how to proceed when a skin puncture result suggests mild anemia. Some reasonable options are as follows:

1. A trial of iron therapy (see Treatment, below) if the history is suggestive: low birth weight and/or prolonged use of cow's milk or unfortified formula.
2. A recheck on skin-puncture blood after about 1 month where there is reasonable doubt on the basis of history or if there has been a recent infection.
3. A repeat hemoglobin analysis of venipuncture blood if the history is suggestive, with or without an additional laboratory test such as mean corpuscular volume (MCV), serum ferritin, or erythrocyte protoporphyrin.

If anemia is moderate or severe (hemoglobin <100 g/l), it is less commonly due to simple dietary iron deficiency alone. Other causes must then be considered.

The hemoglobin analysis is often part of a routine blood count done on an electronic counter. Such blood counts provide red cell indices, of which the mean red cell volume (MCV) and mean red cell hemoglobin (MCH) are the earliest to become abnormal in iron deficiency. If the indices are available, they are helpful in making a diagnosis, e.g., between 6 months and 4 years of age an MCV < 72 fl or an MCH < 24 pg will support the diagnosis of iron deficiency if it accompanies anemia or a low-normal hemoglobin. Very few other causes of anemia are characterized by microcytosis. These include thalassemia minor in Mediterranean and Southeast Asian populations and hemoglobin E trait in the latter. In these conditions, erythrocyte protoporphyrin (EP), serum ferritin, and transferrin saturation are normal.

Some electronic counters provide a quantitative measure of anisocytosis or the variation in red cell size, termed the red cell distribution width (RDW). Although the RDW appears on many laboratory reports, its role remains uncertain. A few years ago, reports indicated that an elevated RDW was evidence of iron deficiency whereas a normal RDW was typical of thalassemia minor and infection (67), but there is now considerable doubt about the diagnostic reliability of the RDW.

Confirmatory tests for iron deficiency include the serum ferritin, MCV, serum iron/iron binding capacity (transferrin saturation), and the EP. Only rarely is it practical or cost-effective to use more than one of these tests in evaluating a mild anemia (62). The selection of a confirmatory test depends on availability, cost, and the most likely differential diagnosis in the particular clinical setting. The MCV and EP are less likely to yield false-positive results during an acute infection than the serum ferritin and transferrin saturation.

The serum ferritin currently appears to be the most reliable test, since it is depressed only in iron deficiency. It is most useful in infants who have been entirely well in the previous 2 weeks, since the result may be in the normal range despite iron deficiency if there has been a recent infection or inflammation; infection or inflammation raises serum ferritin concentrations. Although the small amount of blood required can easily be obtained from a skin puncture sample, the results are often not available as promptly as they are for other laboratory studies.

The erythrocyte protoporphyrin, done with a drop of fresh blood, can provide an immediate result. However, the test is less well standardized. Elevated values reflect depressed hemoglobin production and are characteristic not only of iron deficiency but also of concurrent or recent infection and lead toxicity.

The serum iron/iron-binding capacity (transferrin saturation) is the most widely available of the three confirmatory tests but requires a venipuncture to obtain a larger volume of blood. Results fluctuate considerably with time of day, the nature of recent meals, and other factors. Typically the serum iron is depressed and the iron-binding capacity elevated in iron deficiency, but the latter is not a consistent finding and its absence by no means excludes the diagnosis. A low transferrin saturation and serum iron are characteristics of both iron deficiency and a recent concurrent infection.

A promising new test for the evaluation of iron status is the measurement of transferrin receptor (68). Its concentration in the circulation is elevated with increased red blood cell production and depressed in all conditions of decreased red cell production with the exception of iron deficiency, in which it is also elevated. From limited observations, the combination of a low hemoglobin, a low serum ferritin, and an elevated transferrin receptor is diagnostic of iron deficiency anemia, with the latter two abnormalities alone being characteristic of iron deficiency without anemia.

The following values are consistent with iron deficiency in infancy:

Serum ferritin <10 μg/l
Erythrocyte protoporphyrin >2.5 μg/g Hb
30 μg/dl whole blood, or 70 μg/100 ml packed RBC
MCV <72 (from 6 months to 4 years).

Treatment

Treatment of established iron deficiency anemia generally involves changes in the diet (see Prevention, below) as well as the administration of iron, usually as ferrous sulfate. The most widely used preparations for infants are in liquid form and are administered by a dropper marked to deliver 0.6 or 1.2 ml (15 and 30 mg of iron, respectively). A dose of 3 mg/kg/day represents about 30 mg/day for the average 1-year-old infant. This dose is well tolerated as a single, before-breakfast dose in infants (58). If there are gastrointestinal symptoms, the dose can be divided or decreased. However, one dose per day has the advantage of favoring compliance. Older children can be given iron divided into two daily doses, ideally on an empty stomach with water or fruit juice (not milk) to enhance absorption.

In regard to iron dose, it is important to distinguish between the iron compound and the equivalent in terms of elemental iron. For example, hydrated ferrous sulfate [USP] contains 20% of iron by weight; therefore a 300 mg tablet of ferrous sulfate contains 60 mg elemental iron. Doses of elemental iron in excess of 3 mg/kg/day unnecessarily risk side effects and do not result in a more rapid response. Indeed, the lower the dose of iron, the higher the percentage absorbed (69). Iron absorption is markedly enhanced in iron deficiency, allowing small doses to be efficiently utilized. Parents should be alerted to the danger of toxicity due to accidental ingestion but reassured about the dark color of the stool with iron treatment. Staining of teeth may occur with liquid iron preparations, but this is not permanent and can be removed by gentle brushing.

The rate of response to iron treatment is relatively rapid during the first few weeks of treatment, although complete correction of the anemia may require more than 2 or 3 months. A repeat hemoglobin (or hematocrit) determination to check for a therapeutic response can therefore be done after about 4 weeks of treatment. Treatment should be maintained for 3 to 4 months to allow some accumulation of storage iron.

A lack of response usually indicates that the medication has not been administered. Only rarely is there a failure to absorb iron; this can be detected by measuring a fasting serum iron concentration and repeating the determination 2 to 4 hr after a test dose of 3 mg/kg iron as ferrous sulfate (70). The increase in serum iron should be greater than 30 μg/dl.

When iron deficiency anemia recurs, after it has been corrected by treatment, the possibility of occult blood loss should be investigated.

Iron Excess

Two important issues regarding iron excess involve the predisposition to vitamin E deficiency that may result from administration of iron or iron-fortified formula to preterm infants during the first postnatal month (59) and iron poisoning as a result of accidental ingestion (71). Preterm infants weighing less than 1,500 g at birth have marginal supplies of vitamin E due to low placental transfer of the vitamin, decreased tissue stores, and impaired absorption. Their vitamin E needs generally can be satisfied either by breast milk or by infant formulas that are not iron-fortified. However, even a dose of 2 mg/kg/day of iron at 2 weeks of age (an amount that can be supplied by iron-fortified formula) can predispose to vitamin E deficiency (36). For this reason, it seems advisable to delay giving iron-fortified formula until about 1 month of age to preterm infants weighing less than 1,500 g at birth.

Accidental ingestion of iron remains one of the most common causes of fatal poisoning in children (71). It is important to caution parents to keep the medications out of reach, particularly of children between the ages of 1 and 5 years. Patients with accidental ingestion of iron who are found to have a serum iron concentration in excess of 300 µg/dl commonly have diarrhea, vomiting, leukocytosis, hyperglycemia, and radiographic evidence of iron ingestion. Management involves prompt removal of iron by induction of emesis or by lavage with a 1% to 5% bicarbonate solution and chelation of absorbed iron by administration of deferoxamine.

NUTRITIONAL MEGALOBLASTIC ANEMIAS

Megaloblastic anemias are rare in children. The causes in order of frequency are folate deficiency, vitamin B_{12} deficiency, and inborn errors of metabolism including hereditary orotic aciduria. Many of the laboratory manifestations of megaloblastic anemias are related to impaired DNA synthesis, particularly in rapidly proliferating hematopoietic cells (55,72–75).

Hypersegmentation of the nucleus in circulating neutrophils is a useful aid to early diagnosis, since it is easy to detect on a routine blood smear. Hypersegmentation should be suspected when a quick examination of the blood smear shows numerous neutrophils with four, five, or more distinct lobes. This impression can then be confirmed by a lobe count in 100 neutrophils; an average of more than 3.4 lobes per cell is considered abnormal. However, lobe counting is not a routine procedure in most laboratories. For this reason, depending on the history, the subjective impression of hypersegmentation will typically lead to analyses of serum and red cell folate and serum vitamin B_{12} concentrations. About 1% of healthy individuals have hypersegmented neutrophils. Consequently, if hypersegmentation is used as a basis for diagnosis, its disappearance should be verified after treatment.

Increased red cell size is believed to result from a skipped cell division due to impaired DNA synthesis during red cell maturation. It is not as early a finding as hypersegmentation. In clinical practice, an elevated MCV for age is often the first evidence of a megaloblastic disorder because it is part of a routine blood count by electronic counter. However, blood loss and hemolytic anemia are far more common causes of an elevated MCV; these two conditions are associated with polychromatophilia and reticulocytosis attributable to the large cell volume of young erythrocytes from increased red cell production. The elevated MCV of increased red cell production can be distinguished from that of megaloblastic disorders, since only the latter is associated with hypersegmented neutrophils and macroovalocytes (large oval red cells). A marked variation in size of red cells (anisocytosis) is also evident on the blood smear and is reflected in an elevated red cell distribution width (RDW). Megaloblasts, nucleated red blood cells that are larger than normal and in which the nucleus appears immature for the stage of cytoplasmic development, are noted in the peripheral blood and bone marrow in severe or advanced cases. The megaloblastic disorders may also be associated with mild neutropenia and/or thrombocytopenia.

Other laboratory abnormalities common to megaloblastic anemias are an elevated lactate dehydrogenase and occasionally a mild increase in unconjugated bilirubin, both reflecting destruction of immature red cells before release from the bone marrow.

FOLATE DEFICIENCY

Folate deficiency may result from a low dietary intake or malabsorption of folate, from folate-drug interactions or from an increased folate requirement, as in hemolytic anemias (Table 4). It can develop within a few weeks of birth in low birth weight infants fed an evaporated milk formula because of the scant storage of folate in the newborn, in contrast to the large, long-lasting stores of vitamin B_{12}.

Dietary Lack of Folate

A dietary lack of folate is most common under circumstances that increase its requirement (75–77), such as rapid cell proliferation in the preterm infant and in severe hemolytic disease of the newborn. Rare inborn errors of folate metabolism may also present with megaloblastic anemia in infancy.

Infants require about 10 times as much folate as adults on the basis of body weight. The recommended intake of folate for infants is between 22 (78) and 65 µg/day (79). Folate is abundant in green vegetables and liver. Breast milk and cow's milk contain about 50 µg/l. Breast-fed term infants have far higher serum and red cell folate values than adults. Term infants fed proprietary formulas have even higher folate levels (80), probably because of the very high level of folate fortification now used in the United States, about 160 µg of folate/l. The current

TABLE 4. *Causes of folate and vitamin B_{12} deficiencies*

	Folate	Vitamin B_{12}
Inadequate intake	Evaporated milk formulas, goat milk, prolonged heating of formula	Breast milk of vegetarians who consume no eggs or dairy products
Inadequate absorption	Chronic diarrhea, broad spectrum antibiotics, congenital malabsorption, inflammatory bowel disease, sprue, gluten enteropathy	Pernicious anemia, disease, or absence of terminal ileum
Inadequate transport or utilization	Drugs	Congenital deficiencies of transcobalamin I or II
Increased requirement	Hemolytic disease, deficiencies in enzymes of folate metabolism	Deficiencies in enzymes of vitamin B_{12} metabolism

folate content of United States formulas should, therefore, be more than adequate, even for low birth weight infants, once formula consumption reaches about 300 ml/day. Some European formulas, however, may be less adequate, e.g., a formula containing 20 µg/l of folate resulted in much lower serum folate levels in preterm than in term, breast-fed infants (79,80). Folate deficiency has been reported in a breast-fed infant whose mother took oral contraceptives (81).

Heat treatment lowers the folate content of milk. Thus, heat sterilizing a home-prepared formula can decrease its folate content by about half. Evaporated milk has less than 20 µg of folate per reconstituted liter. The widespread use of heat-sterilized, evaporated milk formulas in the 1940s and 1950s probably accounted for the folate deficiency common at that time. More recently, folate deficiency has been reported primarily in low birth weight infants who were fed formulas based on heated or boiled evaporated milk or regular cow's milk (77). Goat milk is an even poorer source of folate than evaporated milk, with less than 6 µg/l, and severe megaloblastic anemia may result if it is the main source of calories.

Very low birth weight infants probably should be given supplemental folate, as well as other vitamins, to support their very rapid growth, especially until their human milk or formula intake increases sufficiently to provide adequate folate (about 300 ml/day, or at a body weight of 2,000 g). Until that time, about 0.05 to 0.1 mg/day of supplemental folic acid seems reasonable (82). The same dose for a period of 2 or 3 months also seems appropriate for the increased needs of infants with hemolytic disease of the newborn. Liquid vitamins containing folate are not commercially available because of the instability of folate in solution. A pharmacy-prepared "premie vitamin mix" that contains folate added to a proprietary vitamin preparation has a shelf life of about 1 month.

Malabsorption of Folate

Chronic diarrhea that results in a deficiency in intestinal conjugase may lead to folate deficiency due to malabsorption. In such cases, the conjugated polyglutamate forms of folate that predominate in the diet may not be broken down to the monoglutamate form that can be absorbed. A small dose of unconjugated folate, the usual therapeutic form, can produce a prompt response, whereas large amounts of dietary polyglutamic folate might have no effect. Diarrhea may also interfere with the normal enterohepatic circulation of folate by resulting in excessive losses due to rapid intestinal transit.

There are, in addition, rare cases, typically detected in early infancy, of congenital malabsorption of folate associated with mental retardation and seizures (83). Also, because intestinal bacteria may normally supplement the dietary folate supply, partial elimination of intestinal bacteria by prolonged use of broad-spectrum antibiotics may also be associated with folate deficiency.

Drug Interactions

Folate analogues such as methotrexate and certain antibiotics such as trimethoprim (Septra, Bactrim) inhibit dihydrofolate reductase, an enzyme required for the production of the active form of the vitamin. Megaloblastic changes in bone marrow and peripheral blood are common with methotrexate therapy. A different mechanism is responsible for the folate deficiency associated with the use of phenytoin and other anticonvulsants. These drugs interact with polyglutamates in the intestinal lumen and interfere with their digestion to the absorbable monoglutamate form.

Diagnosis

As a deficiency of folate progresses, laboratory abnormalities develop in the following sequence: low serum folate, hypersegmentation of neutrophil nuclei, low red cell folate, megaloblastic bone marrow, and macrocytic anemia. Initial laboratory findings are likely to include hypersegmentation of neutrophils and megaloblastic changes on the blood smear. In low birth weight infants, these are most likely to be noted between 6 and 12 weeks of age in association with poor growth. Macrocytic anemia and neurologic manifestations such as hypotonia are only evident in severe or advanced cases. Macrocytosis (an elevated MCV) is more difficult to detect in low birth weight infants since, in these infants, MCV is normally elevated to widely varying degrees and because many of them will have had a blood transfusion. When folate deficiency is suspected, confirmation of the diagnosis is obtained by a determination of serum and red cell folate, and serum vitamin B_{12} concentration. Because serum folate reflects recent dietary changes, it may be too sensitive to dietary fluctuations to be an ideal test of chronic folate status. The red cell folate level is a more stable and reliable index. A serum folate below 3 ng/ml is subnormal; the lower limit for red cell folate is 140 ng/ml. Serum vitamin B_{12} levels are normal in folic acid deficiency. However, a potential source of confusion is the low red cell folate that can occur in vitamin B_{12} deficiency. Folate deficiency is likely to coexist with iron deficiency in infants fed only an evaporated milk formula or goat's milk. With this combination of deficiencies, the MCV and some of the other laboratory tests give unpredictable results. However, hypersegmentation of the neutrophil nuclei is still likely to be a helpful test, unless the folate supply from the diet or from medication was increased a few days prior to the test.

Treatment

A therapeutic dose of folate, 0.5 to 1.0 mg/day of pteroylglutamic acid (ten or more times the daily allowance), may be given when the diagnosis of folate deficiency is firmly established. Large doses of folate mistakenly given to a patient with vitamin B_{12} deficiency can worsen the clinical manifestations. A safe maintenance dose to prevent deficiency or to correct it slowly is 0.1 mg/day.

Folic acid is available in scored tablets of 0.1, 0.4, 0.8, and 1.0 mg. Folate in liquid multivitamin preparations for oral use is not available commercially because of its lability under the pH conditions used in such formulations. However, a pharmacist can use vials of injectable folate to formulate a liquid preparation that can be kept refrigerated for about 1 month. If anemia is present, treatment can be monitored by the reticulocyte response and by the rate of rise in hemoglobin and hematocrit, which are similar to the response during the iron treatment of iron deficiency anemia.

VITAMIN B_{12} DEFICIENCY

Vitamin B_{12} deficiency, although rare, is clinically important because of the danger of irreversible neurologic damage occurring if the deficiency is not diagnosed and treated early. Most causes of vitamin B_{12} deficiency require continuing therapy throughout life. Dietary vitamin B_{12} is usually present in considerable excess over requirements. Exclusively breast-fed infants typically ingest about 0.3 μg/day of vitamin B_{12}, an amount that is considered more than adequate. An exception is breast milk from strictly vegetarian mothers who consume no meat, eggs, or dairy products. Prolonged consumption of such a diet leads to a markedly subnormal concentration of vitamin B_{12} in maternal milk and eventually to megaloblastic anemia with neurologic changes in the nursing infant.

The absorption of a physiologic amount of vitamin B_{12} is dependent upon the formation of a complex between the vitamin and a mucoprotein (intrinsic factor) produced by the parietal cells of the stomach. The complex is taken up by the distal ileum. Vitamin B_{12} is bound to a specific serum transport protein (transcobalamin II) in the blood. The vitamin is stored in the liver. These stores are large in the newborn, averaging about 25 μg, and are rarely depleted before 1 year of age.

Pathogenesis

In addition to dietary deficiency in breast-fed infants of vegetarian mothers, vitamin B_{12} deficiency may result from the absence of intrinsic factor or from a failure to absorb the vitamin–intrinsic factor complex. The term *pernicious anemia* is reserved for those conditions in which there is a deficiency of intrinsic factor. Two types of pernicious anemia are distinguished in children; in both of them, malabsorption of vitamin B_{12} can be corrected if intrinsic factor is supplied. Juvenile pernicious anemia occurs in older children and is similar to pernicious anemia in the adult. Gastric atrophy and decreased secretion of acid and pepsin commonly are associated with antibodies to intrinsic factor or to parietal cells. Concurrent endocrinopathies and manifestations of immune deficiency also may be present. In contrast, congenital pernicious anemia usually is evident during late infancy. Although secretion of normally active intrinsic factor is lacking, the morphology and secretory function of the gastric mucosa are normal. There are no demonstrable antibodies or associated endocrinopathies, and long-term follow-up examination does not show progression to the typical adult form of pernicious anemia. An autosomal recessive inheritance pattern is suggested by a high incidence of consanguinity and the occurrence in siblings.

Other causes of deficiency are not properly called pernicious anemia, since there is no lack of intrinsic factor. These include removal of the vitamin from the intestinal lumen by parasites or bacteria, as with heavy infestations of fish tapeworm, *Diphyllobothrium latum*. Bacterial consumption of vitamin B_{12} in intestinal diverticuli or blind loops also can result in the removal of the vitamin before it is absorbed.

Since vitamin B_{12} is selectively absorbed by the distal half of the ileum, surgical removal of this section of bowel for treatment of intussusception, regional enteritis, or congenital malformation results in a lifelong deficiency. Chronic disease of the ileum, most commonly regional enteritis, can also produce a deficiency of vitamin B_{12} but usually one that is mild and manifested primarily by a low serum concentration of the vitamin.

Inherited defects of vitamin B_{12} metabolism have been described (84). Absorption and transport of vitamin B_{12} are decreased in a rare inherited deficiency or abnormality of transcobalamin II. Presumably the transport protein is necessary as an acceptor in the transport of the vitamin across the ileal mucosa. There are also numerous rare disorders of vitamin B_{12} metabolism that may present with neurological abnormalities and megaloblastic anemia.

Diagnosis

Most forms of vitamin B_{12} deficiency do not become evident in early infancy, since neonatal liver stores are normally very abundant. Exceptions are the development of megaloblastic anemia in the breast-fed infant of a mother with vitamin B_{12} deficiency and in some of the inherited disorders of vitamin B_{12} metabolism, e.g., the deficiency of transcobalamin II.

Depression of serum vitamin B_{12} below 100 pg/ml (75 pmol/l) and the appearance of hypersegmented neutrophils are the earliest manifestations of vitamin B_{12} deficiency. Late findings include megaloblastic anemia, megaloblastic changes in the bone marrow, leukopenia, thrombocytopenia, and mild jaundice, similar to the findings of folate deficiency. However, neurologic manifestations generally are quite distinct from those of folate lack. They include posterior and lateral column demyelinization in the spinal cord and associated paresthesias, sensory deficits, loss of deep tendon reflexes, slowing of mental processes, confusion, and memory defects. Neurologic changes may precede anemia. Inappropriate administration of large doses of folate, in excess of 0.1 mg/day in an adult, to vitamin B_{12}-deficient individuals can aggravate the neurologic manifestations.

The serum folate concentration is usually normal or elevated in vitamin B_{12} deficiency, but the red cell folate can be a source of confusion since it is often decreased. Consequently, all three tests, serum B_{12}, serum folate, and red cell folate, are helpful in the differential diagnosis of vitamin B_{12} and folate deficiency. If the dietary history is unremarkable, absorption of ^{57}Co-vitamin B_{12} may be determined by the Schilling test. A standard dose of the labeled vitamin is given orally after a fast; 2 hr later a flushing dose of vitamin B_{12} is given parenterally. This allows the excretion of labeled vitamin B_{12} into the urine in readily detectable amounts. Less than 7% of the administered label is recovered in the urine in 24 hr if there is a lack of intrinsic factor or a defective absorption of vitamin B_{12} for other reasons. If absorption is impaired, the Schilling test is repeated with oral intrinsic factor. Enhancement of urinary excretion of the radiolabel with intrinsic factor confirms the diagnosis of intrinsic factor deficiency. The availability of assays for intrinsic factor in gastric juice provides an alternative diagnostic tool.

Treatment

Most cases of vitamin B_{12} deficiency that are not of dietary origin require treatment throughout life. Optimal doses for infants and children are not as well defined as those for adults. If the diagnosis is firmly established, an intramuscular dose of 50 to 100 μg may be used to initiate therapy. Maintenance therapy then consists of monthly intramuscular injections in the same dosage range.

Cancer Chemotherapy and Inborn Errors

Chemotherapeutic agents, such as methotrexate, cytosine arabinoside, and 5-fluorouracil commonly result in megaloblastic anemia. Very rarely, megaloblastic anemias are unresponsive to folic acid and vitamin B_{12} treatment. These rare causes include inborn errors of pyrimidine metabolism (hereditary orotic aciduria) and purine metabolism (Lesch-Nyhan syndrome).

SUMMARY

A deficiency of iron, folate, or vitamin B_{12} will eventually lead to anemia. Iron deficiency is important because it is common and easily prevented. Although deficiencies of folate or vitamin B_{12} are less frequently encountered, their early detection can prevent serious neurological consequences.

REFERENCES

1. DeMaeyer E, Adiels-Tegman M, Rayston E. The prevalence of anemia in the world. *World Health Stat Q* 1985;38:302–316.
2. Life Science Research Office, Federation of American Societies for Experimental Biology. Expert Scientific Working Group. Senti FR, Pilch SM, eds. *Assessment of the folate nutritional status of the U.S. population based on data collected in the Second National Health and Nutrition Survey, 1976–1980*. Bethesda, MD: FASEB, 1984.
3. Yip R, Johnson C, Dallman PR. Age-related changes in laboratory values used in the diagnosis of anemia and iron deficiency. *Am J Clin Nutr* 1984;39:427–436.
4. Dallman PR, Siimes MA. Percentile curves for hemoglobin and red cell volume in infancy and childhood. *J Pediatr* 1979;94:26–31.
5. Lundström U, Siimes MA, Dallman PR. At what age does iron supplementation become necessary in low-birth-weight infants? *J Pediatr* 1977;91:878–883.
6. Saarinen UM, Siimes MA. Developmental changes in red blood

counts and indices of infants after exclusion of iron deficiency by laboratory criteria and continuous iron supplementation. *J Pediatr* 1978;92:412–416.
7. Dallman PR. Anemia of prematurity. *Annu Rev Med* 1981;32:143–160.
8. Bothwell TH, Charlton RW, Cook JD, Finch CA. *Iron metabolism in man.* Oxford: Blackwell Scientific Publications, 1979.
9. Dallman PR. Biochemical basis for manifestations of iron deficiency. *Annu Rev Nutr* 1986;6:13–40.
10. Charlton RW, Bothwell TH. Iron absorption. *Annu Rev Med* 1983;34:55–68.
11. Hallberg L. Bioavailability of dietary iron in man. *Annu Rev Nutr* 1981;1:123–147.
12. Green R, Charlton RW, Seftel H, et al. Body iron excretion in man. A collaborative study. *Am J Med* 1968;45:336–353.
13. Cook JD, Monsen ER. Food iron absorption in human subjects. III. Comparison of the effect of animal proteins on non-heme iron absorption. *Am J Clin Nutr* 1976;29:859–867.
14. Rossander L, Hallberg L, Björn-Rasmussen E. Absorption of iron from breakfast meals. *Am J Clin Nutr* 1979;32:2484–2489.
15. Monsen ER, Hallberg L, Layrisse M, Klegsted DM, Cook JD, Mertz W, Finch CA. Estimation of available dietary iron. *Am J Clin Nutr* 1978;31:134–141.
16. Cook JD, Bothwell TH. Availability of iron from infant food. In: Stekel A, ed. *Nutrition in infancy and childhood.* New York: Raven Press, 1984;119–143.
17. Saarinen UM, Siimes MA, Dallman PR. Iron absorption in infants: high bioavailability of breast milk iron as indicated by the extrinsic tag method of iron absorption and by the concentration of serum ferritin. *J Pediatr* 1977;91:36–39.
18. Davidson LA, Lonnerdal B. Specific binding of lactoferrin to brush-border membrane: ontogeny and effect of glycon chain. *Am J Physiol* 1988;254:G580–585.
19. Peters TJ, Raja KB, Simpson RJ, Snape S. Mechanisms and regulation of iron absorption. *Ann NY Acad Sci* 1988;526:141–147.
20. Götze C, Schäfer KH, Heinrich HC, Bartels H. Eisenstoffwechselstudien an Frühgeborenen und gesunden Reifgeborenen während des ersten Lebensjahres in dem Ganzkörperzähler und anderen Methoden. *Mschr Kinderheilk* 1970;118:210–213.
21. Casey JL, Hentze MW, Koeller DM, et al. Iron-responsive elements: regulatory RNA sequences that control mRNA levels and translation. *Science* 1988;240:924–928.
22. Casey JL, DiJeso B, Rao K, Rouault TA, Klausner RD, Harford JB. The promoter region of the human transferrin receptor gene. *Ann NY Acad Sci* 1988;526:54–64.
23. Dallman PR, Siimes MA, Stekel A. Iron deficiency in infancy and childhood. *Am J Clin Nutr* 1980;33:86–118.
24. Fomon SJ, Ziegler EE, Nelson SE, Edwards BB. Cow's milk feeding in infancy: gastrointestinal blood loss and iron nutritional status. *J Pediatr* 1981;98:540–545.
25. Chockalingam UM, Murphy E, Ophoven JC, Weisdorf SA, Georgieff MK. Cord transferrin and ferritin values in newborn infants at risk for prenatal uteroplacental insufficiency and chronic hypoxia. *J Pediatr* 1987;111:283–286.
26. Garn SM, Ridella SA, Tetzold AS, Falkner F. Maternal hematological levels and pregnancy outcomes. *Semin Perinatol* 1981;5:155–162.
27. Murphy JF, O'Riordan J, Newcombe RG, Coles EC. Relation of haemoglobin levels in first and second trimesters to outcome of pregnancy. *Lancet* 1986;1:992–994.
28. Dallman PR. Iron deficiency in the weanling: a nutritional problem on the way to resolution. *Acta Paediatr Scand* 1986;323:59–67.
29. Dallman PR, Yip R, Johnson C. Prevalence and causes of anemia in the United States. 1976–80. *Am J Clin Nutr* 1984;39:437–435.
30. Dallman PR. Manifestations of iron deficiency. *Semin Hematol* 1982;19:19–30.
31. Viteri FE, Torun B. Anemia and physical work capacity. *Clin Hematol* 1974;3:609–626.
32. Levin HM. A benefit-cost analysis of nutritional programs for anemia reduction. *Research Observer* 1986;1:219–245.
33. Basta SS, Soekirman MS, Karyadi D, Scrimshaw NS. Iron deficiency anemia and the productivity of adult males in Indonesia. *Am J Clin Nutr* 1979;32:916–925.
34. Edgerton VR, Gardner GW, Ohira Y, Gunawardena KA, Senewiratne B. Iron-deficiency anemia and its effect on worker productivity and activity patterns. *Br Med J* 1979;2:1546–1549.
35. Gardner GW, Edgerton VR, Senewiratne B, Barnard RJ, Ohira Y. Physical work capacity and metabolic stress in subjects with iron deficiency anemia. *Am J Clin Nutr* 1977;30:910–917.
36. Lozoff B. Behavioral alterations in iron deficiency. *Adv Pediatr* 1988;35:331–359.
37. Walter T, de Andraca I, Chadud P, Perales CG. Iron deficiency anemia: adverse effects on infant psychomotor development. *Pediatrics* 1989;84:7–17.
38. Pollitt E, Hathirat P, Kotchabharkdi NJ, Missel L, Valyasevi A. Iron deficiency and educational achievement in Thailand. *Am J Clin Nutr* 1989;50:687–697.
39. Weinberg J, Levine S, Dallman PR. Long term consequences of early iron deficiency in the rat. *Pharmacol Biochem Behav* 1979;11:631–638.
40. Yehuda S, Youdim MBH. Brain iron deficiency: biochemistry and behaviour. In: Youdim MBH, ed. *Brain iron. Neurochemical and behavioral aspects.* London: Taylor and Francis, 1988.
41. Dallman PR. Iron deficiency and the immune response. *Am J Clin Nutr* 1987;46:329–334.
42. Götze C, Ludwig U, Schäfer KH, Heinrich HC, Oppitz KH. Cytochemische Knochenmarksbefunde und diagnostische $^{59}Fe^{2+}$-Absorption während des akuten und chronischen Infectes im Kindesalter. *Mschr Kinderheilk* 1976;124:305–307.
43. Watson WS, Morrison J, Bethel MIF, et al. Food iron and lead absorption in humans. *Am J Clin Nutr* 1986;44:248–256.
44. Yip R, Dallman PR. Developmental changes in erythrocyte protoporphyrin: roles of iron deficiency and lead toxicity. *J Pediatr* 1984;104:710–713.
45. Committee on Nutrition. American Academy of Pediatrics. Iron balance and requirements in infancy. *Pediatrics* 1969;43:134–142.
46. Saarinen UM. Need for iron supplementation in infants on prolonged breast feeding. *J Pediatr* 1978;93:177–180.
47. Rios E, Hunter RE, Cook JD, et al. The absorption of iron as supplements in infant cereal and infant formulas. *Pediatrics* 1975;55:686–693.
48. Oski FA, Landaw SA. Inhibition of iron absorption from human milk by baby food. *Am J Dis Child* 1980;134:459–460.
49. Sadowitz PD, Oski FA. Iron status and infant feeding practices in an urban ambulatory center. *Pediatrics* 1983;72:33–36.
50. Committee on Nutrition. American Academy of Pediatrics. Relationship between iron status and incidence of infection in infancy. *Pediatrics* 1978;62:246–250.
51. Weinberg ED. Iron withholding: a defense against infection and neoplasia. *Physiol Rev* 1984;64:65–102.
52. Martinez GA, Krieger FW. 1984 milk feeding patterns in the United States. *Pediatrics* 1985;76:1004–1008.
53. Yip R, Binkin NJ, Fleshood L, Trowbridge FL. Declining prevalence of anemia among low-income children in the United States. *JAMA* 1987;258:1619–1623.
54. Yip R, Walsh KM, Goldfarb MG, Binkin NJ. Declining prevalence of anemia in childhood in a middle class setting: a pediatric success story? *Pediatrics* 1987;80:330–334.
55. Meyers PA, Miller DR. Megaloblastic anemias. In: Miller DR, Baehner RL, McMillan CW, eds. *Blood diseases of infancy and childhood.* St. Louis: CV Mosby, 1984;147–170.
56. Saarinen UM, Siimes MA. Iron absorption from infant formula and the optimal level of iron supplementation. *Acta Paediatr Scand* 1977;66:719–722.
57. Siimes MA. Iron nutrition in low-birth-weight infants. In: Stekel A, ed. *Iron nutrition in infancy and childhood.* New York, Raven Press, 1984;75–91.
58. Reeves JD, Yip R. Lack of adverse side effects of oral ferrous sulfate therapy in 1-year-old infants. *Pediatrics* 1985;75:352–355.
59. Gross SJ, Gabriel E. Vitamin E status in preterm infants fed human milk or infant formula. *J Pediatr* 1985;106:635–640.
60. Zipurski A, Brown EJ, Watts J, et al. Oral vitamin E supplementation for the prevention of anemia in premature infants: a controlled trial. *Pediatrics* 1987;79:61–68.
61. Clydesdale FM, Wiemer KL, eds. *Iron fortification of foods.* Orlando, FL: Academic Press, 1985.
62. Dallman PR, Reeves JD. Laboratory diagnosis of iron deficiency.

In: Stekel A, ed. *Nutrition in infancy and childhood.* New York: Raven Press, 1984;11–44.
63. Dallman PR, Yip R. Changing characteristics of childhood anemia. *J Pediatr* 1989;114:161–164.
64. Jansson LT, Kling S, Dallman PR. Anemia in children with acute infections seen in a primary care pediatric outpatient clinic. *Pediatr Infect Dis* 1986;5:424–427.
65. Reeves JD, Yip R, Kiley V, Dallman PR. Iron deficiency in infants, the influence of antecedent infection. *J Pediatr* 1984;105:874–879.
66. Reeves JD, Driggers DA, Lo EYT, Dallman PR. Iron deficiency in one-year-old infants: hemoglobin alone or hemoglobin and mean corpuscular volume as predictors of response to iron treatment. *J Pediatr* 1981;98:894–898.
67. Bessman JD, Gilmer PR Jr, Gardner FH. Improved classification of anemias by MCV and RDW. *Am J Clin Pathol* 1983;80:322–326.
68. Kohgo Y, Nishisato T, Kondo H, Tsushima N, Niitsu Y, Urushizaki I. Circulating transferrin receptor in human serum. *Br J Haematol* 1986;64:277–281.
69. Hahn PF, Bale WF, Ross JF, Balfour WM, Whipple GH. Radioactive iron absorption in gastrointestinal tract: influence of anemia, anoxia, and antecedent feeding distribution in growing dogs. *J Exp Med* 1943;78:169–188.
70. Massa E, MacLean WC Jr, Lopez de Romana G, et al. Oral iron absorption in infantile protein-energy malnutrition. *J Pediatr* 1978;93:1045–1049.
71. Banner W Jr, Tong TG. Iron poisoning. *Pediatr Clin North Am* 1986;33:393–409.
72. Chanarin I. *The megaloblastic anaemias,* 2nd ed. Oxford: Blackwell, 1979.
73. Hillman RS. Vitamin B_{12}, folic acid, and the treatment of megaloblastic anemias. In: Gilman AG, Goodman LS, Rall TW, Murad F, eds. *The pharmacologic basis of therapeutics,* 7th ed. New York: Macmillan, 1985;1323–1337.
74. Lindenbaum J. Status of laboratory testing in the diagnosis of megaloblastic anemia. *Blood* 1983;61:624–627.
75. Shojania AM. Folic acid and vitamin B12 deficiency in pregnancy and in the neonatal period. *Clin Perinatol* 1984;11:433–459.
76. Gandy G, Jacobson W. Influence of folic acid on birthweight and growth of the erythroblastic infant. *Arch Dis Child* 1977;52:1–21.
77. Strelling MK, Blackledge DG, Goodall HB. Diagnosis and management of folate deficiency in low birthweight infants. *Arch Dis Child* 1979;54:271–277.
79. Ek J, Behncke L, Halvorsen KS, Magnus E. Plasma and red cell folate values and folate requirements in formula-fed premature infants. *Eur J Pediatr* 1984;142:78–82.
80. Smith AM, Picciano MF, Deering RH. Folate intake and blood concentrations of term infants. *Am J Clin Nutr* 1985;41:590–598.
81. Mandel H, Berant H. Oral contraceptives and breastfeeding: haematological effects on the infant. *Arch Dis Child* 1985;60:971–980.
82. Herbert V. Recommended dietary intakes (RDI) of folate in humans. *Am J Clin Nutr* 1987;45:661–670.
83. Urbach J, Abrahamov A, Grossowicz N. Congenital isolated folic acid malabsorption. *Arch Dis Child* 1987;62:78–80.
84. Cooper BA, Rosenblatt DS. Inherited defects of vitamin B12 metabolism. *Annu Rev Nutr* 1987;7:291–320.

CHAPTER 9

The Effects of Iron Deficiency, Food Additives, and Other Nutrients on Behavior

David A. Levitsky and Barbara J. Strupp

The effect of nutrition on the behavior of children has, in recent times, become a popular concern and a serious consideration within the scientific community. Unfortunately, the poor and/or unstandardized methodology of early studies often resulted in unconvincing or seemingly conflicting data. More recent studies have improved experimental design. In addition, close scrutiny of past and present research does reveal a fairly consistent pattern of observations. This chapter attempts to establish the apparent consistencies in these studies as well as to articulate the remaining questions concerning the relationship between nutrition and the behavior of children.

IRON DEFICIENCY

There is strong evidence that iron deficiency may seriously affect the behavior and cognitive development of children. Iron is involved in almost all the oxygen transporting mechanisms of the body (1); the brain is particularly sensitive to any disruption in oxygen transport. Within the brain, iron plays an integral role as part of the enzymes controlling the rate of metabolism of neurotransmitters (2). Animal studies have shown that severe iron deficiency causes profound alterations in neurotransmitter systems (3-7). Further animal research indicates that brain iron stores of previously iron-deficient animals may never fully recover to their predeficiency levels (8,9) and the cognitive and behavioral effects resulting from early iron deficiency may never be completely reversed with subsequent iron treatment (10-14).

D. A. Levitsky, B. J. Strupp: Division of Nutritional Sciences and Department of Psychology, Cornell University, Ithaca, New York 14853.

Early Observations of Humans

Cantwell (15) described long-term cognitive deficits resulting from iron deficiency. He observed that children who had low iron status (hemoglobin between 6.1 and 9.5 g/dl) at 6 to 18 months of age displayed signs of inattentiveness and hyperactivity 6 to 7 years later. Since that study, several pediatricians have reported anecdotally on observed infant apathy, distractibility, and irritability, which they have related to iron deficiency (16-19). In addition, Oski and Honig (20) demonstrated that 9- to 26-month-old infants with hemoglobins less than or equal to 10.5 g/dl displayed significantly depressed scores on the Bayley Mental Scale, a well-accepted test of infant behavioral development. Depressed Bayley scores have since been reported by many investigators (21-26).

Long-Term Behavioral Effects of Early Iron Deficiency

Recent research has not substantiated earlier studies indicating that the long-term effects of iron deficiency on infants are totally reversible. In 1978, Oski and his associates (20) reported that infants with low hemoglobins had significantly higher Bayley scores 1 week following an intramuscular injection of iron. Similarly in 1983 Palti et al. (27) reported significantly improved developmental and IQ scores in 24-month-old children who had been given iron therapy at 9 months of age. Subsequent research, however, has not been as optimistic. More recent studies have indicated that the negative effects of iron deficiency on behavior are not totally reversible with iron therapy (24-26,28).

The reason for these apparently conflicting conclusions may actually be in the difference in the behaviors being assessed. Lozoff et al. (24), in an excellent series of behavioral analyses, showed that motor responses are considerably more responsive to iron rehabilitation than are those that are primarily cognitive and emotional. Since the Bayley test essentially assesses motor skills, positive results from early studies may actually be reflecting the effect of supplemental iron on the rapid recovery of motor, as opposed to other, behavioral skills.

Other, more subtle, aspects of behavior have not seemed as responsive to iron rehabilitation. Lozoff et al. (29) observed that children with a history of iron deficiency initiated significantly more body contact with their mothers during testing than controls. Such responses were interpreted as reflecting increased fearfulness of the testing situation. Similarly, the mothers of previously iron-deficient infants remained in closer proximity to their children than did mothers of control children. Although, earlier, Johnson and McGrowan (30) had failed to find such differences in attachment, their measures of iron status were considerably less sensitive than those of the Lozoff group.

Although further studies are warranted, the long-term effects of iron deficiency on motor skills appear to be reversed with iron therapy. The ability to reverse long-term effects of iron deficiency on emotionality or cognitive processing with iron therapy appears to be poor.

Effects of Iron Deficiency on Attentional Processes in Infancy

Attentional processes are also affected by iron deficiency. Heywood et al. (31) examined infants in Papua, New Guinea, an area of prevalent iron deficiency. In a well-designed study, infants with low hemoglobins were given either a therapeutic injection of iron or a placebo. Attention was then assessed by measuring the length of time infants remained visually fixated on characters in a short puppet show. Heywood found that supplemented children had higher total fixation times, indicating a relationship between iron deficiency and a child's ability to sustain attention.

Cognitive Effects of Iron Deficiency in Schoolchildren

To assess the role of iron deficiency on cognitive processes in older children, Pollitt et al. (32) analyzed intelligence, math, and language scores of over 2,000 Thai schoolchildren. They found a significant, positive correlation between IQ and language scores and the child's iron status. Subjects were then given iron supplementation in order to evaluate the possible reversibility of the cognitive deficits. After 16 weeks, there was no apparent improvement. These findings may, however, simply reflect an insufficient period of supplementation. Kashyap and Gopaldas (33) observed that cognitive test scores of iron-deficient, anemic Indian schoolgirls were not affected by 16 weeks of iron suppplementation, but were significantly improved after 32 weeks of treatment. It is interesting, however, that the advantage of the supplemented group over the placebo-treated group disappeared 4 months after the cessation of the iron treatment.

Other studies demonstrating an improvement in intelligence scores with iron supplementation of anemic schoolchildren (34–36), suffer from weak methodology (37).

Perhaps the most detailed study of the kinds of cognitive processes disrupted by iron deficiency was reported by Soewondo et al. (37a). Three independent processes were examined: attention acquisition, attention extinction, and conceptual learning. Consistent with other reports, iron-deficient anemic children performed more poorly on tasks than children with normal iron stores, and showed greatest improvement following 8 weeks of oral iron supplementation. These results, supporting two earlier studies (38,39), strongly suggest that attentional processes appear to be extremely sensitive to iron deficiency and considerably more reversible, in response to iron repletion, than are IQ measurements.

Summary

There is strong evidence that iron deficiency produces significant motor, attentional, emotional, and cognitive impairments in children. Although motor and attentional effects appear to be reversible with iron therapy, emotional and cognitive effects appear much more resistant to iron supplementation or may not be reversible.

FOOD ADDITIVES AND ATTENTIONAL DISORDERS

Reports of the effect of food additives on attentional disturbances in children have been in the literature since 1947 (41–45). It was, however, the book, *Why Your Child is Hyperkinetic* by the allergist, Benjamin Feingold (45), that opened the floodgates of alarm by nutritionists, food scientists, psychologists, pediatricians, educators, and thousands of parents that food additives might cause, or at least exacerbate, attentional disorders in children. Fifteen years of research have given us knowledge, not just about food additives and behavior, but also about the problems involved in trying to relate diet to behavior in humans.

Early Correlational Studies

If a relationship exists between food additives and behavioral or attentional disorders, then a statistically significant relationship should exist between the amount of additives a child consumes and either the incidence of behavioral disruptions or the intensity of the behavioral disturbances. Despite various attempts to find such a relationship, none has been observed (46–48). The Kaplan study (48), particularly notable for its use of the most sensitive dietary methodology, found no difference in the amount of food additives consumed by hyperkinetic children versus controls.

It may be argued, however, that it is not the quantity of consumption that is the issue, but the presence of the additive, itself, to an additive-sensitive child, that is responsible for the phenomenon. Finding no difference in the consumption of additives, therefore, does not invalidate the hypothesis that food additives exacerbate, or cause, behavioral problems in certain children.

Open Clinical Trials

Feingold (45) claimed that 50% of hyperactive children benefited when all additives were removed from their diet. This figure was rejected by most of the scientific community until other studies, conducted in open clinical trials, confirmed this finding (49–57).

The problem involves the strength of data acquired from open clinical trials. In such studies, everyone concerned—the subject, physician, nutritionist, parents, siblings of the subject, and in most instances, the subject's teacher—is aware that the subject is being treated with a special diet in order to correct behavioral problems. The possible change in attitude and behavior toward the child is obvious, as is the possibility of spontaneous improvement in the child because of a change in attention as well as expectations about the effect of the diet. This has encouraged experimenters to design more sophisticated "double-blind" studies.

Double-Blind Studies

Results of the double-blind studies did not corroborate the positive effects of additive-free diets on hyperactive children. In each study, a control diet was designed that was identical both nutritionally and in appearance to the additive-free diet, except that it would contain the additives suspected of causing the behavioral disturbances (51,58). In addition to the two diets, the studies used a crossover design, each child receiving both diets during the course of each study: During the first period of the study, one-half of the subjects received the placebo diet, the other half received the diet containing additives. During the second period the groups were reversed. Teachers and parents maintained behavioral rating scales that had been standardized and validated to measure hyperactive behavior.

Other researchers, using similar designs, have also found no relationship between additives and behavior (55,59), although Williams et al. (60) found a very slight improvement when additive-free diets were combined with medication. Both Conners et al. (51) and Harley et al. (58) reported a curious effect of the order of diet presentation. They observed a significant improvement in hyperactivity from the additive-free diet only in children receiving the additive-free diet after the control diet. The results suggested that a weak effect of additives on hyperactivity may exist that was obscured by other variables less well understood.

Challenge Studies

The double-blind crossover studies did not definitively answer the question as to whether certain children respond to food additives with an increase in hyperactivity. A more direct test of this question involves food challenge studies. Subjects for such studies are usually children who respond favorably to additive-free diets or whose reported behavior worsened when additives were consumed and improved on an additive-free diet.

Food challenge studies involve the administration of an additive-free diet with a single challenge food, such as a cookie or drink. The challenge food contains a suspected additive in concentrations equivalent to the usual daily consumption by an American child, and prepared so that it is undetectable as a test food. Only one or two additives were tested in each study.

In one of the first such studies, Goyette et al. (61) examined the behavior of 16 additive "responders" for 4 hr after the subjects were challenged with food additives. They observed a small but statistically significant deterioration in visual tracking, a task that measures attention, compared to results after a placebo challenge. Several subsequent studies, measuring other responses, have yielded similar results: following a challenge with food additives, some children display a slight worsening of behavioral symptoms (55,62–68).

Not every study, however, has reported positive effects (69,70). Results of the challenge studies seem to indicate that only a very small number of hyperactive children, about 5%, demonstrate a worsening of behavior in response to an additive challenge. This is in contrast to parental assertions of improvement, with an additive-free diet, in their children and the 50% improvement claimed by Feingold (45). Why should such a great disparity exist between clinical observations and double-blind crossover studies using food challenges?

Failure to Find an Exacerbation of Hyperactivity with Food Additives

The more general reaction observed in hyperactive children to any kind of challenge may obscure any difference in behavior that the additives may impose. Salamy et al. (71) reported that hyperactive children not only exhibit a greater behavioral and physiological reaction to a food-additive challenge than controls, but they also showed an exaggerated response to the placebo.

Results are also hindered by the inadequacy of our measuring devices. Although the behavioral scales typically used in these studies are well accepted, their ability to reliably detect a worsening or improvement in symptoms is less than perfect. This, combined with the problem of increased variability of responding, indicates that the figure of 5% may well be an underestimate of the number of hyperactive children who respond to food additives with a worsening of symptoms.

The experimental design of food challenge studies may also have limited their ability to identify the full numbers of affected children. Unlike clinical trials, food challenges involve only one or two additives. This may have the double effect of either missing the real additive culprit or eluding the fact that, ultimately, it is a synergistic relationship among several additives or additives combined with chemicals within the environment, that is responsible for aggravating hyperactive behavior.

Kaplan and her associates (72) recently published a very well controlled, double-blind, crossover study in which a large number of additives and common household chemicals were eliminated from the diet and the environment of hyperactive children. Behavioral assessment was done daily by parents and day-care workers using the Abbreviated Symptom Questionnaire (ASQ), a ten-item version of the Conners Rating Scale. This scale assesses restlessness, impulsiveness, tendency to disturb other children, short attention span, fidgeting, distractibility, frustration, crying, mood changes, and temper outbursts. Parents also kept daily records of physical symptoms such as skin rashes, red cheeks, dry skin, stomach bloat or cramps, leg cramps, stuffy/runny nose, headache, earaches, and bad breath.

During the first 3 weeks of the study, the parents kept a daily diet diary in order to establish baseline data. During the next 3 weeks, the children were divided into two groups. One-half of the children was given the additive-free Alberta Children's Hospital (ACH) diet, the other half a control "equivalent diet." During the last 3 weeks, the two groups were reversed.

The equivalent diet was identical to that consumed by the family during the baseline period but prepared and provided to the household by the experimenters. The ACH diet consisted of similar foods, but devoid of all food dyes, food flavors, preservatives, monosodium glutamate, chocolate, and caffeine. In addition, the amount of simple sugars was reduced and any substance that the parents suspected of aggravating hyperactivity was eliminated.

The results of the Kaplan study were impressive. Ten of the 24 children (42%) showed significant improvement in behavioral ratings when given the additive-free ACH diet. The mean ASQ scores for the last 14 days of each treatment were as follows: baseline = 14.5 (SD 4.1); equivalent diet = 13.1 (SD 4.2); and ACH diet = 10.8 (SD 4.2). The overall effect of treatment was highly significant ($p < .0001$). Scores taken during the baseline period did not differ from those during the equivalent diet, indicating that there was no placebo effect.

Physical symptoms were also shown to improve. Halitosis ($p < .01$) and headache ($p < .05$) were significantly affected by diet. The effect for rhinitis, however, was only marginal ($p = .07$). The finding relating additives to physical symptoms supports earlier work indicating that hyperactive children seem to be sensitive, not only to food additives, but to many kinds of antigens (73). In a previous study, Kaplan et al. (74) found that hyperactive children display significantly more physical symptoms, such as skin rashes and red cheeks, stomach bloating and cramps, leg cramps, stuffy and runny nose, and headaches than do nonhyperactive children.

Summary

Although further research is needed to define more clearly the relationship between additive intake and hyperactivity, recent research seems to corroborate the Feingold hypothesis that such a relationship does indeed exist. Certainly, pediatricians should seriously consider parental concerns that a child's behavior is worsened by certain foods or chemicals.

BREAKFAST AND SCHOOL PERFORMANCE

Between 5% and 20% of children in well-developed countries begin school without having eaten breakfast. This is significant in light of the numerous studies indicating the importance of breakfast as a factor in both good health and achievement in children (75–78).

Early Studies

Early studies indicating the importance of a good breakfast or a midmorning snack were totally observational. These studies were critically reviewed by Pollitt et al. (79) in 1978. The methodology was poor and consequently the conclusions that could be drawn from these studies were tenuous.

Iowa Breakfast Studies

Tuttle et al. (80) studied the effects of omitting breakfast, calculated at 25% of daily caloric intake, on behavior and cognition in seven boys, 12 to 14 years of age. Known collectively as the "Iowa Breakfast Studies," these studies focused primarily on physical performance in adults, but also included studies relating breakfast to schoolroom and laboratory performance of school-age children. The generally positive conclusions reached by observation are, at best, tenuous, as a result of the lack of verifiable measurements and double-blind methodology.

Other studies have also failed to find quantitative evidence that eating breakfast significantly improves cognition or school performance (81–87). However, just as it is difficult to conclude from the Tuttle study that consumption of breakfast improves school performance, it is equally difficult to conclude from these later studies that it does not. The problem lies, as it does in almost all field research, in the difficulty in constructing standardized measuring tools that accurately assess changes in cognitive function while controlling for an almost endless number of variables such as individual cognitive potential, socioeconomic factors, pretesting nutritional-health status, and pretesting performance.

More Recent Studies

Aware of the important methodological limitations of the previous research, Pollitt (39,88) designed a series of studies that included more sensitive response measures than those previously used. These studies indicated that when breakfast was not given, children performed more poorly on a test of matching familiar figures but had relatively higher recall of incidental information in the Hagen Central Incidental Test. The "better" recall was not attributed to an improved memory with omitted breakfasts but, rather, was interpreted as indicating that children may pay closer attention to incidental information when fasting. Conners and Blouin (89), using the Continuous Performance Test, a technique for measuring attention, also found that children made fewer "attentional" errors on days in which breakfast was given.

Simeon and Grantham-McGregor (90) recently investigated the cognitive effects of eating breakfast on previously malnourished schoolchildren, and matched controls, in Jamaica. The first group had been hospitalized for malnutrition during the first 2 years of life; control children were matched for social class, gender, and area of residence. Children were given cognitive tests after consuming either a standard breakfast or only tea, a standard morning drink for children in that region.

Results indicated a strong association between the effects of omitting breakfast and previous nutritional status. Although the omission of breakfast had no adverse cognitive effect in the control children, it produced significant deficits in performance in those children with a previous history of malnutrition. This corroborates animal studies that have shown that animals subjected to malnutrition early in life, then rehabilitated, continue to be more disrupted by food deprivation than their well-nourished controls (91).

Summary

Although there is indication that breakfast is an important factor in the cognitive performance of schoolchildren, the effects are subtle and not easily measured. Attentional processes seem to be particularly sensitive. In addition, the effect may be related to the nutritional history of the child. Children recovered from severe malnutrition appear to be more deleteriously affected by the absence of breakfast than those who have a history of good nutrition. This may explain the greater positive effects of school breakfast programs on school performance in poorer (92), rather than the more developed (87,93), countries.

SUGAR AND BEHAVIOR

Refined sugar, sucrose, has historically been blamed by lay writers, healers, and parents as a major cause of behavioral and physical illness (94). Sugar has been accused of being the cause for anxiety and depression (95,96), juvenile delinquency (97), and learning disabilities in children (98,99). Pediatricians and family practitioners may prescribe a low-sugar diet for treating children with behavioral problems (100). The question is, how much of the assertion about sugar is fact and how much is traditional "feeling", an important consideration to the pediatrician who has to solve a medical problem. In this case, scientific data does not support "intuition."

Correlation Studies

Many of the studies that investigate the relationship of sugar to behavior must be interpreted with care.

Prinz et al. (101) correlated a 7-day intake diary, provided by parents of hyperkinetic and control children, to several indices of behavior measured in the laboratory. Their study indicated a significant correlation between the amount of sugar consumed at home and a measure of "restlessness." Lester et al. (102) found a negative correlation between the percentage of carbohydrate consumed as sugar, scores on intelligence tests, and school achievement. Thatcher and Lester (103) also found a negative correlation between sugar consumption and several measures of IQ. Kruesi et al. (104), however, found no relationship between sugar intake and behavior.

The problem in interpreting these studies lies in the problem of knowing exactly what is being tested. Although an active, or hyperactive, child may consume more sugar, such consumption may actually be reflecting the need for fast energy, rather than the cause of it. Is intelligence lowered by the consumption of sugar, or do intelligent children generally come from homes where a smaller percentage of the total daily nutrient intake is from sugar? Fortunately, several well-controlled sugar challenge studies have been reported.

Causative Studies

Goldman et al. (105) examined eight preschool children who had no history of hyperactivity or major physical or psychological pathology. Following an overnight fast, the children were given an orange drink sweetened with either sugar (2 g/kg) or aspartame, a nonnutritive sweetener. Cognitive tests were begun 15 min before the drink and continued for 90 min after. Each subject was tested twice, once after a sugared drink, once after a nonsugared drink.

Performance on the Continuous Performance Task, which measures sustained attention, was significantly worse following the intake of sucrose. In addition, the number of "inappropriate behaviors" during free play was significantly increased. There was also an increase in locomotor behavior and a decrease in "task orientation."

The Goldman et al. (105) observations of clear behavioral response to sugar-containing foods, however, stands in stark contrast to the results of other studies published in this area. Conners and Blouin (89) observed a very subtle effect of a sugar challenge on the behavior of children institutionalized for severe behavior disorders. Even these slight effects were not detectable to either teachers or nurses on the ward. Rosen et al. (106) observed inconsistent effects of high- or low-sucrose breakfasts on the behavior of 30 preschoolers and 15 elementary school children. All other studies that have examined the effect of a sugar challenge on behavior have universally failed to find any statistically significant deterioration in behavior (107–112).

Roshon and Hagen (113) recently attempted to replicate the findings of Goldman et al. (105) by duplicating the conditions and methodology that the study employed. Their study, as well, failed to find any evidence that a high sugar intake causes disruption in the behavior of children.

The study by Mahan et al. (112) is particularly significant for its precise methodology and design. Subjects were children whose parents attested that their child's behavior clearly worsened after the child consumed high sugar-containing foods. Behavioral measurements included actometers for detecting movement and the Stony Brook Scale, which had been designed to detect an effect of medication on hyperactivity.

During phase one, each child was tested before and after an open challenge with candy, in the presence of the observer and one or both of the parents. Following the candy challenge, 7 of the 16 children (44%) were observed to display a 15% increase in three of the four behavior measures of hyperactivity. Five of those seven children (two subjects refused to continue) were asked to return for the second phase of the study.

During the second phase the routine measures were identical to those in phase one. In this phase, however, placebo and double-blind techniques were used. Under these conditions, three of the five children showed no consistent response to the sugar challenge compared to the placebo. The two children who did respond with some change in behavior in response to the sugar load were retested with the sugar and placebo challenge, but upon retesting failed to show any difference.

These results are instructive for several reasons. First, parents' claims that the behavior of their children is affected by sugar intake were documented. Second, these claims were clearly refuted by careful study design. There is some indication, however, that some children may either be sensitive to other ingredients in candy, or that some children react to the psychological value of certain foods by displaying alterations in their behavior. Candy, ice cream, cookies, and other high sucrose-containing foods are likely to be associated with active behavioral states such as parties, rewards, holiday celebrations, etc. The behavioral disruption witnessed by parents may be more the result of psychological context in which the food is eaten than the effect of the food itself.

CONCLUSION

Although sugar is frequently thought to adversely affect the behavior of children, there is little scientific evidence to support such an assertion.

REFERENCES

1. Fairbanks VF, Beutler E. Iron. In: Shils ME, Young VR, eds. *Modern nutrition in health and disease.* Philadelphia: Lea and Febiger, 1988.
2. Leibel RL, Greenfield D, Pollitt E. Iron deficiency: behavior and brain biochemistry. In: Winick M, ed. *Nutrition: pre- and postnatal development.* New York: Plenum Press, 1978.
3. Youdim MB, Green AR. Biogenic monoamine metabolism and function activity in iron-deficient rats. Behavioral correlates. *Ciba Found Symp* 1977;5:201–225.
4. Mackler B, Person R, Miller LR, et al. Iron deficiency in the rat: biochemical studies of brain metabolism. *Pediatr Res* 1978;12:217–220.
5. Sourkes TL. Transition elements and the nervous system. In: Pollitt E, Leibel RL, eds. *Iron deficiency: brain biochemistry and behavior.* New York: Raven Press, 1982;1–29.
6. Kaladhar M, Narasinga Rao BS. Effect of maternal iron deficiency in rat on serotonin uptake in vitro by brain synaptic vesicles in the offspring. *J Neurochem* 1983;40:1768–1770.
7. Vorhess ML, Stuart MJ, Stockman JA, et al. Iron deficiency anemia and increased urinary norepinephrine excretion. *J Pediatr* 1975;86:542–547.
8. Dallman PR, Spirito RA. Brain iron in the rat: extremely slow

turnover in normal rats may explain long-lasting effects of early iron deficiency. *Am J Clin Nutr* 1976;26:1075.
9. Dallman PR, Shimes MA, Manies EC. Brain iron: persistent deficiency following short-term iron deprivation in the young rat. *Br J Haematol* 1975;31:209–215.
10. Glover J, Jacobs A. Activity pattern of iron-deficient rats. *Br Med J* 1972;2:627–628.
11. Findlay E, Ng KT, Reid RL. The effect of iron deficiency during development on passive avoidance learning in the adult rat. *Physiol Behav* 1981;27:1089–1096.
12. Massaro TF, Widayer P. The effect of iron deficiency on cognitive performance in the rat. *Am J Clin Nutr* 1981;34:864–870.
13. Weinberg J, Levine S, Dallman PR. Long-term consequences of early iron deficiency in the rat. *Pharmacol Biochem Behav* 1979;11:631.
14. Weinberg J, Dallman PR, Levine S. Iron deficiency during early development in the rat: behavioral and physiological consequences. *Pharmacol Biochem Behav* 1980;12:493.
15. Cantwell RJ. The long term neurological sequelae of anemia in infancy (abstr). *Pediatr Res* 1974;8:342.
16. Harris JW, Kellermeyer RW. *The red cell.* Cambridge: Harvard University Press, 1970.
17. Miller DR, Pearson HA, Baehjner RL, et al., eds. *Smith's blood diseases of infancy and childhood,* 4th ed. St. Louis: CV Mosby, 1978.
18. Werkman S, Shifman L, Skelly T. Psychosocial correlates of iron deficiency anemia in early childhood. *Psychosom Med* 1964;26:125–134.
19. Lingam S. Severe nutritional iron deficiency and behavior disorder in an infant. *J Human Nutr* 1980;34:41–42.
20. Oski FA, Honig AS. The effects of therapy on the developmental scores of iron-deficient infants. *J Pediatr* 1978;92:21.
21. Lozoff B, Brittenham G, Viteri FE, Wolf AW, Urrutia JJ. The effects of short-term oral iron therapy on developmental deficits in iron-deficient anemic infants. *J Pediatr* 1982;100:351–357.
22. Oski FA, Honig AS, Helu B, et al. Effect of iron therapy on behavior performance in nonanemic, iron-deficient infants. *Pediatrics* 1983;71:877–880.
23. Lozoff B, Wolf AW, Urrutia JJ, Viteri FE. Abnormal behavior and low developmental test scores in iron-deficient anemic infants. *Dev Behav Pediatr* 1985;6:69–75.
24. Lozoff BL, Brittenham GM, Wolf AW, et al. Iron deficiency anemia and iron therapy effects on infant developmental test performance. *Pediatrics* 1987;79:981–994.
25. Walter T, Kovalskys J, Stekel A. Effect of mild iron deficiency on infant mental development scores. *J Pediatr* 1983;102:519–522.
26. Walter T. Infancy: mental and motor development. *Am J Clin Nutr* 1989;50(suppl):655–666.
27. Palti H, Pevsner B, Adler B. Does anemia in infancy affect achievement on developmental and intelligence test? *Hum Biol* 1983;55:183–193.
28. Lozoff B, Brittenham GM, Biteri FE, et al. Developmental deficits in iron-deficient infants: effects of age and severity on iron lack. *J Pediatr* 1982;101:948–952.
29. Lozoff B, Klein NK, Probucki KM. Iron-deficient anemic infants at play. *Dev Behav Pediatr* 1986;7:152–158.
30. Johnson DL, McGrowan TJ. Anemia and infant behavior. *Nutr Behav* 1983;1:185–192.
31. Heywood A, Oppenheimer S, Heywood P, Jolley D. Behavioral effects of iron supplementation in infants in Madang, Papua New Guinea. *Am J Clin Nutr* 1989;50(suppl):630–640.
32. Pollitt E, Hathirat P, Kotchabhakdi NJ, Missel L, Valyasevi A. Iron deficiency and educational achievement in Thailand. *Am J Clin Nutr* 1989;50:687–697(suppl).
33. Kashyap P, Gopaldas T. Impact of hematinic supplementation on cognitive function in underprivileged school girls. *Nutr Res* 1987;7:1117–1126.
34. Seshadri S, Gopaldas T. Impact of iron supplementation on cognitive function in preschool and school aged children: the Indian experience. *Am J Clin Nutr* 1989;50(suppl):675–686.
35. Seshadri S, Hirode K, Naik P, Malhtra S. Behavioral responses of young anaemic Indian children in iron-folic acid supplements. *Br J Nutr* 1982;48:233–240.
36. Gopaldas T, Kale M, Bhardwaj P. Prophylactic iron supplementation for underprivileged school boys. II: Impact on selected tests of cognitive function. *Indian Pediatr* 1985;22:737–743.
37. Pollitt E, Metallinos-Katsaras E. Iron deficiency and behavior: constructs, methods and validity of the findings. In: Wurtman R, Wurtman J, eds. *Nutrition and the brain,* vol 8. New York: Raven Press, 1990.
37a. Soewondo S, Husanini M, Pollitt E. Effects of iron deficiency on attention and learning processes in preschool children: Bandung, Indonesia. *Am J Clin Nutr* 1989;50:667–674(suppl).
38. Pollitt E, Lewis N, Leibel RL, Greenfield DB. Iron deficiency and play behavior in preschool children. In: Garry PJ, ed. *Human nutrition: clinical and biochemical aspects.* Washington, DC: American Association of Clinical Chemistry, 1981;290–301.
39. Pollitt E. Behavioral effects of iron deficiency anemia in children. In: Pollitt E, Leibel RL, eds. *Iron deficiency, brain biochemistry and behavior.* New York: Raven Press, 1982.
40. Crook WG, Harnson WW, Crawford SE, Emerson BS. Systemic manifestation due to allergy. *Pediatrics* 1961;27:790.
41. Randolph TG. Allergy as a causative factor in fatigue, irritability and behavior problems of children. *J Pediatr* 1947;31:560.
42. Rinkle HJ, Randolph TG, Zeller M. *Food allergy.* Springfield, IL: Charles C Thomas, 1951.
43. Rowe AH. Allergic toxemia and fatigue. *Ann Allergy* 1950;8:72.
44. Speer F. Allergic tension-fatigue in children. *Ann Allergy* 1954;12:168.
45. Feingold BF. *Why your child is hyperkinetic.* New York: Random House, 1975.
46. Palmer S, Rapaport JL, Quinn PO. Food additive and hyperactivity: a comparison of food additive in the diets of normal and hyperactive boys. *Clin Pediatr* 1975;14:756.
47. Prinz RJ, Roberts WA, Hantman E. Dietary correlates of hyperactive behavior in children. *J Consult Clin* 1980;48:760.
48. Kaplan BJ, McNicol J, Conte RA, Moghadam HK. Overall nutrient intake of preschool hyperactive and normal boys. *J Abnorm Child Psychol* 1989;17:127–132.
49. Brenner A. A study of the efficacy of the Feingold diet on hyperkinetic children. *Clin Pediatr* 1977;16:652.
50. Burlton-Bennett JA, Robinson VMJ. A single subject evaluation of the K-P diet for hyperkinesis. *J Learn Disabil* 1987;20:331–346.
51. Conners CK, Goyett CH, Southwick DA, et al. Food additives and hyperkinesis: a controlled double-blind experiment. *Pediatrics* 1976;58:154–166.
52. Conners CK, Goyette CH, Southwick DA. Food additives and hyperkinesis: preliminary report of a double-blind crossover experiment. *Psychopharmacol Bull* 1976;12:10.
53. Hindle RC, Priest J. The management of hyperkinetic children: a trial of dietary therapy. *NZ Med J* 1978;88:43.
54. Rose TL. The functional relationship between artificial food colors and hyperactivity. *J Appl Behav Anal* 1978;11:439.
55. Rowe KS. Synthetic food colourings and "hyperactivity": a double-blind crossover study. *Aust Paediatr J* 1988;24:143–147.
56. Saltzman LK. Allergy testing, psychological assessment and dietary treatment of the hyperactive child syndrome. *Med J Aust* 1976;2:248.
57. Stine JJ. Symptom alleviation in the hyperactive child by dietary modification: a report of two cases. *Am J Orthopsychiatry* 1972;44:639.
58. Harley JP, Mathews CG, Eichman P. Synthetic food colors and hyperactivity in children: a double-blind challenge experiment. *Pediatrics* 1978;62:975–983.
59. Gross MD, Tofanelli RA, Butzirus SM, Snodgrass EW. The effect of diets rich in and free from additives on the behavior of children and hyperkinetic and learning disorders. *J Am Acad Child Adolesce Psychiatry* 1987;26:153–155.
60. Williams JI, Cram DM, Tausig FT, Webster E. Relative effects of drugs and diet on hyperactive behaviors: an experimental study. *Pediatrics* 1978;61:811.
61. Goyette CH, Conners CK, Petti PA, et al. Effects of artificial colors on hyperkinetic children: a double-blind challenge study. *Psychopharmacol Bull* 1978;14:39–40.
62. Egger J, Carter CM, Graham PJ, Gumley D, Soothill JF. Controlled trial of oligoantigenic treatment in the hyperkinetic syndrome. *Lancet* 1985;1:540–545.

63. Harley JP, Mathews CG. Food additives and hyperactivity in children. In: Knight R, Bakker DJ, eds. *Treatment of hyperactive and learning disordered children.* Baltimore: University Park Press, 1980.
64. Mattes JA, Gittelman R. A cross-over study of artificial food colorings in a hyperkinetic child. *Am J Psychol* 1978;135:987.
65. Levy G, Hobbes G. Hyperkinesis and diet: a replication study. *Am J Psychiatry* 1978;135:1559.
66. Swanson JM, Kinsborne M. Food dyes impair performance of hyperactive children on a laboratory learning test. *Science* 1980;207:1485–1487.
67. Weiss B et al. Behavioral responses to artificial food colors. *Science* 1980;207:1487–1489.
68. Williams JI, Cram DM, Tausig FT, Webster E. Relative effects of drugs and diet on hyperactive behaviors: an experimental study. *Pediatrics* 1978;61:811–817.
69. Mattes JA, Gittelman R. Effects of artificial food colorings in children with hyperactive syndromes. *Arch Gen Psychiatry* 1981;388:714.
70. David TJ. Reactions to dietary tartrazine. *Arch Dis Child* 1987;62:119–122.
71. Salamy J, Schucard D, Alexander H, Peterson D, Braud L. Physiological changes in hyperactive children following the ingestion of food additives. *Int J Neurosci* 1982;16:241–246.
72. Kaplan BJ, McNicol J, Conte RA, Moghadam HK. Dietary replacement in preschool-aged hyperactive boys. *Pediatrics* 1989;83:7–17.
73. Trites RL, Dugas E, Lynch G, et al. Prevalence of "hyperactivity." *J Pediatr Psychol* 1979;4:179.
74. Kaplan BJ, McNicol J, Conte RA, Moghadam HK. Physical signs and symptoms in preschool-age hyperactive and normal children. *Dev Behav Pediatr* 1987;8:305–310.
75. Bender AE, Magee P, Nash AH. Surveys of school meals. *Br Med J* 1972;2:383.
76. Steller W. Results of the follow-up of the Mainz school breakfast test. *Nutr Abst Rev* 1967;37:1162.
77. Story M, Rosen GM. Diet and adolescent behavior. *Psychiatr Ann* 1987;17:811–817.
78. Wirth W. School catering tests in the light of nutritional physiology. *Nutr Abst Rev* 1976;46:554.
79. Pollitt E, Gersovitz M, Gargiulo M. Educational benefits of the United States school feeding program: a critical review of the literature. *Am J Public Health* 1978;68:477–481.
80. Tuttle WW, Daum K, Larsen R, Salzano J, Roloff L. Effect on school boys of omitting breakfast. *J Am Diet Assoc* 1954;30:674.
81. Laird DA, Levitan M, Wilson VA. Nervousness in school children as related to hunger and diet. *Med J Rec* 1931;134:494–499.
82. Keister M. Relationship of mid-morning feeding to behavior of nursery school children. *J Am Diet Assoc* 1950;26:25–29.
83. Galloway ME, Robertson EE. Types of breakfast eaten and other effects on blood sugar. *J Can Diet Assoc* 1948;10:53.
84. Anonymous. *A complete summary of the Iowa Breakfast Studies.* Chicago: Cereal Institute, 1962.
85. Koonce TM. Does breakfast help? *School Food Svc J* 1972;26:51–54.
86. Tisdall FF, Robertson EC, Drake GH, et al. Canadian Red Cross school meal study. *Can Med Assoc J* 1951;64:477–489.
87. Dickie N, Bender A. Breakfast and performance in school children. *Br J Nutr* 1982;48:483–496.
88. Pollitt E, Leibel R, Greenfield D. Brief fasting, stress and cognition in children. *Am J Clin Nutr* 1981;34:1526–1533.
89. Conners CK, Blouin AG. Nutritional effects on behavior of children. *J Psychiatr Res* 1982/1983;17:193–201.
90. Simeon DT, Grantham-McGregor S. Effects of missing breakfast on the cognitive functions of school children of differing nutritional status. *Am J Clin Nutr* 1989;49:646–653.
91. Levitsky DA, ed. *Malnutrition, environment, and behavior: new perspectives.* Ithaca, NY: Cornell University Press, 1975.
92. Powell C, Grantham-McGregor S, Elston M. An evaluation of giving the Jamaican school meal to a class of children. *Hum Nutr Clin Nutr* 1983;37C:381–388.
93. Pollitt E, Gersovitz M, Gargiulo M. Educational benefits of the United States school feeding program: a critical review of the literature. *Am J Public Health* 1978;68:477.
94. Deutsch RM. *The nuts among the berries.* New York: Ballantine Books, 1961.
95. Cheraskin E, Ringsdorf WH, Brecher A. *Psychodietetics: food as the key to emotional health.* New York: Stein and Day, 1974.
96. Passwater RA. *Supernutrition.* New York: Dial Press, 1975;94.
97. Schoenthaler SJ. The effect of sugar on the treatment and control of antisocial behavior on an incarcerated juvenile population. *Int J Biosoc Res* 1982;1:1–118.
98. Fishbein D. The contribution of refined carbohydrate consumption to maladaptive behavior. *J Orthomolec Psychiatr* 1982; 11:17.
99. Green G. Diagnosis and treatment of perceptual dysfunctions, hyperactivity, and learning disabilities. *J Orthomolec Psychiatr* 1961;10:161.
100. Bennett FC, Sherman R. Management of childhood "hyperactivity" by primary care physicians. *J Dev Behav Pediatr* 1983;4:88–93.
101. Prinz RJ, Roberts WA, Hantman E. Dietary correlates of hyperactive behavior in children. *J Consult Clin Psychol* 1980;48: 760–769.
102. Lester MB, Thatcher RW, Monroe-Lord L. Refined carbohydrate intake, hair cadmium levels, and cognitive functioning in children. *Nutr Behav* 1982;1:3.
103. Thatcher RW, Lester NL. Nutrition, environmental toxins and computerized EEG: a mini-max approach to learning disability. *J Learn Dis* 1985;8:287–297.
104. Kruesi MJP, Rapoport JL, Berg C, Stables G, Bou E. Seven-day carbohydrate and other nutrient intakes of preschool boys alleged to be behavior responsive to sugar intake and their peers. In: Essman WB, ed. *Nutrients and brain function.* Basal, New York: Karger, 1987;127–133.
105. Goldman JA, Lerman RH, Contois JG, Udall JN. Behavioral effects of sucrose on preschool children. *J Abnorm Child Psychol* 1986;14:565–577.
106. Rosen LA, Booth SR, Bender ME, McGrath MI, Sorrel S, Drabman RS. Effects of sugar (sucrose) on children's behavior. *J Consult Clin Psychol* 1988;56:583–589.
107. Behar D, Rapoport JL, Adams AJ, Berg CJ, Cornelath M. Sugar challenge testing with children considered behaviorally "sugar reactive." *Nutr Behav* 1984;1:277–288.
108. Ferguyson HB, Stoddart C, Simeon JG. Double-blind challenge studies of behavioral and cognitive effects of sucrose-aspartame ingestion in normal children. *Nutr Rev* 1986;(Suppl):144–150.
109. Gross MD. Effect of sucrose on hyperkinetic children. *Pediatrics* 1984;74:876–878.
110. Wolraich M, Milich R, Stumbo P, Schultz F. The effects of sucrose ingestion on the behavior of hyperactive boys. *Pediatrics* 1985;106:675–692.
111. Milich R, Pelham WE. Effects of sugar ingestion on the classroom and playgroup behavior of attention deficit disordered boys. *J Consult Clin Psychol* 1986;54:714–718.
112. Mahan LK, Chase M, Furukawa CT, et al. Sugar "allergy" and children's behavior. *Ann Allergy* 1988;61:453–457.
113. Roshon MS, Hagen RI. Sugar consumption, locomotion, task orientation, and learning in preschool children. *J Abnorm Child Psychol* 1989;17:349–357.

CHAPTER 10

Trace Element Deficiencies in Childhood

Michael Hambidge

Eleven "major" elements constitute 99% of human body weight. These essential-for-life elements are hydrogen, carbon, nitrogen, oxygen, sodium, potassium, chlorine, calcium, phosphorus, sulfur, and magnesium. In addition, the body is composed of numerous "trace" elements (1,2). Each of these contributes less than 0.01% of total body weight. Their concentrations range from less than one part per billion to several hundred parts per million depending on the element and on the particular tissue or subcellular fraction. Although definitive minimum requirements have yet to be established, a growing number are considered to be of biological importance in humans (Table 1) (3,4).

This chapter provides an overview of all trace elements of established importance in human nutrition, with special attention to zinc and copper. Food sources for the various trace elements are given in Table 2. More detailed information for zinc and copper is given in Table 3.

M. Hambidge: Department of Pediatrics, University of Colorado Health Sciences Center, Denver, Colorado 80262.

TABLE 1. *Trace elements that have a generally recognized role in human nutrition*

Element	Recommended allowance [FNB, NRC]	Added to IV infusate	Deficiency reported in children
Iron	a	±	+
Iodide	a	±	+
Zinc	a	+	+
Copper	b	+	+
Selenium	a	+	+
Molybdenum	b	+	−
Manganese	b	+	−
Chromium	b	+	±
Fluoride	b	−	+

a, RDA (10th ed.); b, Estimated safe and adequate intake; +, yes; −, no; ±, sometimes.

BIOLOGICAL FUNCTIONS OF THE TRACE ELEMENTS

Each trace element has at least one and, in some instances, many specific physiological roles. Biological functions for some of the "new" trace elements (5), tin,

TABLE 2. *Overview of food sources of trace elements*

Food source	Iron	Zinc	Copper	Selenium	Manganese	Chromium	Iodine
Animal meats	+++	++	++	++	+	+	
Shellfish	++	+++	+++				
Fish				++			
Legumes	++[b]	++[b]	+		++		
Nuts	++[b]	++[b]	++		++		
Whole grain cereals[c]	++[a,b]	++[b]	+	++[d]	+++		
Green leafy vegetables	++		+		+		+
Water			±				
Milk							+

[a] Especially when fortified.
[b] Relatively poor absorption.
[c] Majority of trace elements lost during milling.
[d] Very dependent on levels in soil.

TABLE 3. Trace element content of various foods

Item	Zinc (mg/100 g)	Copper (mg/100 g)
Meat group		
Regular ground beef	4.0	0.061
Round steak	5.8	0.045
Beef liver	5.1	4.6
Chicken—drumstick, fried	2.5	0.02
Pork chop	3.8	0.011
Bologna	1.8	0.02
Hot dog	1.6	0.08
Fish group		
Oyster	74.7	3.62
Perch fillet	1.0	0.21
Tuna	1.1	0.011
Milk and egg group		
Whole milk	0.43	0.005
Nonfat dry milk	4.5	<0.05
Cheddar cheese	4.0	0.11
American cheese	3.0	0.11
Ice cream	0.5	0.05
Eggs	1.0	0.053
Infant formulas	0.4	0.04
Nuts and legumes		
Cooked common beans		
(red, kidney, pinto)	1.0	0.17
Peanut butter	2.9	0.61
Roasted peanuts	3.0	0.43
Bread and cereal group		
White bread	0.6	0.11
Whole wheat bread	1.8	0.17
Pancakes	0.82	0.05
Crackers		
Graham	1.1	0.04
Saltines	0.5	0.09
Corn flakes	0.3	0.023
Rice Krispies	1.4	0.085
Shredded wheat	2.8	0.17
Oatmeal, cooked	0.5	0.03
Macaroni, cooked	0.5	0.02
Popcorn, popped	3.0	0.37
Rice	0.4	0.02
Granola	2.1	0.85
Vegetable and fruit group		
Green beans, canned	0.3	0.02–0.10
Potatoes		
Boiled	0.3	0.10
Mashed	0.37	0.10
Chips	0.81	0.29
French fries	0.28	0.27
Corn	0.4	0.011
Carrots, raw	0.4	0.011–0.10
Tomatoes	0.2	<0.01–0.11
Lettuce	0.4	0.037
Orange	0.2	0.004–0.08

for example, have not yet been identified. The "essentiality" of others becomes apparent only when a specific physiological role is identified, such as the atom of cobalt at the center of the vitamin B_{12} molecule and the requirement for molybdenum as a component of xanthine oxidase. The major functions of the trace elements are related to enzyme systems where they may act either as cofactors for metal-ion–activated enzymes or as specific constituents of metalloenzymes. Molybdenum, iron, copper, zinc, selenium, and manganese are known to be specific constituents of metalloenzymes. Trace elements are also constituents of other proteins and hormones such as iodine in thyroxine and chromium as a cofactor for insulin. Thus, the trace elements are necessary for the normal function of several crucial metabolic pathways (Table 4).

Zinc

Zinc participates exclusively in many biological processes. Most attention has been directed to its catalytic role. It is, for example, a component of over 100 zinc metalloenzymes, including at least one of every major enzyme classification. There is growing evidence to support a structural role for zinc in biological membranes. In addition, its role as an intracellular regulatory ion analogous to the role of calcium, although rarely studied, is of great potential importance (6). It has been hypothesized, for example, that zinc may function as an intracellular hormone contributing to the regulation of cellular growth. Zinc also impacts on nucleic acid metabolism and protein synthesis. For example, the enzymes thymidine kinase, DNA polymerase, and RNA polymerase have each been reported to be zinc dependent. Zinc is a component of a range of transcription proteins in which it has a crucial role in the confirmation of the "zinc fingers" that allows them to bind with DNA to initiate the transcription process (7). Zinc may also have a structural role in nucleic acid metabolism.

TABLE 4. Major biological roles of the trace elements

Element	Biological role(s)
Iron	Oxygen transport in blood and muscle
	Electron transfer enzymes
Iodine	Thyroxine; triiodothyronine
Zinc	Gene expression
	Zinc metalloenzymes (catalytic, regulatory, and structural)
	Cell membrane structure and function
	Induction of metallothioneine synthesis (antioxidant; protects against metal toxicity)
Copper	Oxidative enzymes (e.g., cytochrome oxidase, ferroxidases, amine oxidases, dopamine betahydroxylase)
Selenium	Glutathione peroxidase (GSHX) role of other selenoproteins not yet established
Molybdenum	Xanthine oxidase; sulfite oxidase
Manganese	Mitochondrial SOD; pyruvate carboxylase
	Mucopolysaccharide synthesis
	Carbohydrate metabolism
Chromium	?Facilitates binding of insulin to receptors
Fluorine	Integrity of teeth and skeleton
Cobalt	Structure of cobalamin

Metallothioneins, an unusual, very high sulfur amino acid–containing low molecular weight group of proteins of approximately 6,000 daltons, have a major role in the intracellular metabolism of zinc and copper (8). In addition to other physiological roles, zinc thionein protects against heavy metal toxicity. *In vitro,* zinc thioneine exhibits very strong antioxidant activity, which may be of substantial physiologic importance.

Copper

Copper is a component of several metalloenzymes that are required for oxidative metabolism, including cytochrome oxidase, ferroxidases, amine oxidases, superoxide dismutase, ascorbic acid oxidase, and tyrosinase. Cytochrome oxidase, the terminal enzyme in the electron transport chain, catalyzes the oxidation of reduced cytochrome-c and, in this process, reduces molecular oxygen to water. This key enzyme is necessary for the production of most of the energy of metabolism in aerobic cells. Copper amine oxidases are essential for the cross-linking of elastin and collagen. Mammalian superoxide dismutase, which removes superoxide–free radical anions, is a zinc and copper metalloenzyme. Ceruloplasmin, a glycoprotein that contains eight copper atoms per molecule, accounts for more than 95% of the copper present in the blood plasma. The physiological role of this cuproprotein is still unclear. It appears, however, that ceruloplasmin may also have important ferroxidase activity. It has been reported to be necessary for the optimal rate of oxidation of Fe^{2+} from body stores in the liver and bone marrow to Fe^{3+} (9). This is a necessary step before iron can attach to transferrin for transport to and uptake by the erythrocyte precursors in the bone marrow. Ceruloplasmin may also have a role in the oxidative metabolism of biogenic amines.

BODY CONTENT

The body content of zinc is approximately equal to that of iron and is more than one and two orders of magnitude greater than that of copper and chromium, respectively (Table 5). Highest concentrations of zinc, exceeding 100 µg/g wet weight, occur in hair, nails, the prostate, semen, spermatozoa, and the choroid of the eye and bone, whereas muscles, liver, and kidney contain about 50 µg/g wet weight of this cation. Approximately 90% of total body zinc is in muscle and bone from which exchange with plasma zinc is relatively slow. The liver, brain, heart, and kidneys contain the highest concentrations of copper. Half of the copper in the term newborn is located in the liver; this is an important copper store for infants.

Intestinal Absorption, Metabolism, and Excretion

Trace element absorption varies from less than 1% to nearly 100% (Table 6). Total body content of iron is efficiently regulated at the site of intestinal iron absorption. Regulation also plays a key role in the homeostasis of zinc and manganese. Absorption of trace elements may be affected by dietary factors (10) as well as several abnormal host factors (Table 7). Because of the remarkably high absorption of iron, copper, and especially zinc from human milk, dietary requirements are substantially lower for young, fully breast-fed infants compared with formula-fed infants.

Zinc is absorbed throughout the small intestine probably by a process of facilitated diffusion. The quantity that crosses the brush border membrane is controlled as in transport across the enterocyte to the basolateral membrane (11).

Absorbed zinc is transported in the portal system attached to albumin or transferrin. In the systemic circulation, the major fraction of plasma zinc is loosely bound to albumin, which is in equilibrium with a small amino acid–bound fraction involving histidine and cysteine. The amino acid–bound fraction is available for uptake by cells, and zinc, excreted in the urine, is also derived primarily from this fraction. Part of the plasma zinc is also bound to an α_2-macroglobulin, the function of which is unknown.

Most of the absorbed zinc is taken up temporarily by the liver, which plays a central role in zinc metabolism. Uptake of zinc by the liver leads to an increase in hepatic metallothionein messenger RNA. Hepatic zinc exchanges readily with plasma zinc, and the half-life of zinc in the liver is only about 13 hr.

The major excretory route for endogenous zinc is via the feces. Endogenous zinc enters the lumen of the gastrointestinal tract via the pancreatic fluids and, to a lesser extent, the bile. There is also substantial secretion of zinc directly through the enterocyte. The majority of the se-

TABLE 5. *Approximate values for zinc, copper, and chromium in adults*

	Body content (mg)	Daily intake (mg)	Plasma level (µg/dl)	Urine excretion (µg/day)
Zinc	2,000	10–15	80	500
Copper	100	1.5–2	100	<50
Chromium	10	0.05–0.2	0.1–0.5	5–10

TABLE 6. *Trace element metabolism*

Element	Intestinal absorption from mixed diet	Excretion of endogenous element	Homeostasis
Iron	10%	Limited	Intestinal absorption
Iodine	>90%	Urine	Thyroid
Zinc	25%	Feces > urine & sweat	Intestinal absorption
Copper	30–40%	Bile	Liver (excretion + storage)
Selenium	60–80%	Urine	Kidney
Molybdenum	High (decreased by sulfur)	Urine	Kidney
Manganese	1–10%	Bile	Intestinal absorption; liver (excretion)
Chromium	<1–10%	Urine	?
Fluorine	60–100%	Urine	?

creted zinc is reabsorbed, making this the second important site of homeostatic control of total body zinc. The quantity excreted in the feces depends on the quantity of dietary zinc absorbed and on zinc nutritional status (12).

In normal circumstances, of course, the majority of the zinc appearing in the feces is unabsorbed dietary zinc. In adults, approximately 0.5 mg is excreted each day in the urine. Children excrete a comparable amount on a body weight basis. A similar quantity of zinc is excreted in the sweat.

Approximately 40% of ingested copper is absorbed in the stomach and small intestine. Ionic copper probably enters the mucosal cells by a process of simple diffusion. Copper may also be actively transported attached to amino acids.

Absorbed copper is transported attached to albumin to the liver. In the liver it is utilized by the hepatocytes in the synthesis of ceruloplasmin, which is subsequently released into the systemic circulation. More than 80% of absorbed copper is excreted by the liver into the bile. The intestinal mucosa is a minor excretory route and less than 50 µg per day is excreted in the urine. Abnormal retention of both copper and manganese occurs in cholestatic liver disease.

TABLE 7. *Factors affecting absorption of trace elements*

Quantity of trace elements in diet
Dietary factors that form insoluble complexes (phytate, fiber, phosphate, oxalate)
Factors affecting oxidation state (ascorbate)
Dietary factors that facilitate absorption [lactose (Cu); amino acids (Zn); ascorbate (Fe)]
Chemical form (heme vs inorganic iron)
Competitive inhibition at mucosal cell (iron-zinc-copper; molybdenum-copper)
Host factors (nutritional status, diarrhea, inherited and acquired defects of intestinal mucosa)

Absorption of several trace elements, including iron (Fe), zinc (Zn), and copper (Cu), is especially favorable from human milk. Hence, dietary requirements for these nutrients are notably lower for the fully breast-fed infant.

The major excretory route for iodine, selenium, molybdenum, chromium, and fluorine is via the kidneys. Although the kidneys regulate the body content of selenium and molybdenum, regulation of chromium and fluorine is unclear.

ETIOLOGY OF TRACE ELEMENT DEFICIENCY STATES

Many factors responsible for human trace element deficiency states have been documented since these deficiencies were first suspected (Table 8).

Isolated Nutritional Deficiency States

Iron deficiency is the most common nutrient deficiency in the United States, despite the favorable impact of iron-fortified infant formulas and the Women, Infants, and Children (WIC) program. Zinc deficiency also occurs. Copper deficiency has been reported in term infants fed unprocessed cow's milk, which is a poor source of copper, since early infancy (13).

The increased consumption of mineral supplements and fortified foods has increased the potential for interactions between trace elements, notably iron, zinc, and copper (14). The effect of moderate doses of zinc on copper absorption is sufficient for zinc to be used as an effective supplement to, and possible alternative therapy for, Wilson's disease. Although geochemical deficiencies of trace elements, notably iodine and selenium, continue to afflict much of the world, neither is a problem in North America today. In China, however, selenium deficiency in the soil is a major factor in the etiology of Keshan disease, a frequently fatal cardiomyopathy that strikes young children and women of childbearing age (15).

Deficiencies of zinc, copper, selenium, and possibly of chromium may each have a significant impact on the course of more generalized malnutrition. Iron deficiencies may as well, although there is concern that excessive

TABLE 8. Etiology of trace deficiencies

Element	Dietary deficiency	Interactions	Geochemical deficiency	Generalized malnutrition	Prematurity	Intravenous nutrition	Inborn metabolic diseases	Acquired diseases	Chelators
Iron	+	+		+[a]	+	+		+	+
Iodine			+						
Zinc	+	+		+	+	+	+	+	+
Copper	±	+		+	+	+	+	+	+
Selenium			+	+	+[b]	+			
Molybdenum						+	+		
Manganese									
Chromium				±		+			
Fluorine	+				?	?			

[a] Low laboratory values, clinical significance not determined.
[b] Biochemical evidence only, at this time.

iron may, in some cases, increase mortality from protein-energy malnutrition (16).

Prematurity

The premature infant is at increased risk for all nutrient deficiencies. This applies in particular to elements, such as copper, that are accumulated extensively during the last 2 to 3 months of gestation. Severe symptomatic copper deficiency has been reported in formula-fed premature infants by 2 to 3 months of age (17). This problem has been ameliorated by copper supplementation of infant milk formulas. Chromium is another element that appears to be accumulated quite extensively in late fetal life. Unlike copper and iron, there is no particular storage of zinc by the fetus in late pregnancy. Nevertheless, the marked increase in the total body zinc at this time is commensurate with a rapid rate of fetal growth (18). Positive zinc balance is difficult to achieve in the premature infant in early postnatal life.

Although low circulating selenium concentrations in the premature infant have been suggested to indicate selenium deficiency with putative adverse effects on antioxidant capacity, these low levels are not influenced by increasing selenium intake.

Multinutritional Deficiency States

Copper deficiency described in malnourished Peruvian infants is associated with milk-based rehabilitation diets (19). Chromium deficiency has been found to complicate protein-energy malnutrition in Turkey (20), Nigeria, and Jordan. It has not, however, been described in areas where dietary sources of chromium are adequate (21). Although further studies are needed, there is evidence that zinc and selenium (16) depletion may complicate recovery from PEM (protein energy malnutrition). Zinc is more likely to be inadequate in vegetarian diets.

Synthetic Diets

Severe zinc (22), copper, and selenium (23) deficiency syndromes have occurred in patients maintained on prolonged total intravenous feeding without adequate trace element supplements. Molybdenum (24) and chromium (25) deficiencies have also been described. Oral synthetic diets may also result in trace element deficiencies. Selenium deficiency may occur in children with metabolic diseases who receive specially formulated diets that are low in selenium (26).

Impaired Intestinal Absorption

Intestinal malabsorption syndromes may impair the absorption of many nutrients, including zinc (27) and copper (28). In the presence of steatorrhea, zinc can form insoluble complexes with fat and phosphates (27). Secondary zinc deficiency has been reported as an important clinical complication in regional enteritis (29) and celiac disease (30). Studies are presently investigating the role of zinc in persistent diarrhea in developing countries. Low zinc levels have been associated with cystic fibrosis (31) and disaccharide intolerance (32). Zinc and copper deficiency syndromes can also result from inherited defects in the intestinal absorption of these micronutrients (see Inborn Errors of Trace Metal Metabolism, page 120).

Excessive Excretion

Abnormal zinc losses resulting from chronic hemorrhage and diaphoresis are considered to be contributory factors in the zinc depletion of adolescents in the Middle East (33). Excessive zinc losses may also occur via other routes including jejunostomy fluids or burn exudates (34). Hyperzincuria may lead to both acute (35) and chronic zinc deficiency syndromes. Urinary zinc excretion is increased in various liver diseases (36), including alcoholic cirrhosis (37), acute infectious hepatitis (38), in catabolic states (39), and in patients fed intravenously (40). Zinc deficiency, as a complication of sickle-cell disease, is attributed to a chronic mild hyperzincuria resulting from the zinc released from hemolyzed red cells (41).

Copper deficiency in malnourished Peruvian infants may have resulted from an associated diarrhea. Excessive chromium excretion has been observed in juvenile-onset diabetics (42). Excessive excretion of trace elements has also been observed as a side effect of drug therapy, for example the severe chronic zinc deficiency reported in a patient on penicillamine therapy (43).

Altered Metabolism

In certain circumstances trace element metabolism can be altered with redistribution of specific trace elements within the body causing some body fluids or tissues to contain unusually low levels of certain elements (44). It is not yet known whether this is entirely a physiological adaptation to abnormal circumstances or an undesirable effect that justifies therapeutic intervention. For example, in rheumatoid arthritis, both zinc and manganese metabolism are disturbed (45,46). Zinc therapy has been beneficial in adult rheumatoid arthritis (46), and, possibly, in burn patients (47), although it has not been established as beneficial in juvenile rheumatoid arthritis.

Inborn Errors of Trace Metal Metabolism

Menkes's steely-hair syndrome and acrodermatitis enteropathica are two recently identified inborn errors of trace metal metabolism. Menkes's steely-hair syndrome is attributable to a complex and multiorgan disturbance of copper metabolism (48,49). One location of the inherited defect is the mucosa of the small intestine where disrupted copper transport across the mucosal cells results in a severe state of copper deficiency. In acrodermatitis enteropathica there is a partial block in the intestinal absorption (50) of zinc leading to a profound and, if untreated, fatal state of zinc deficiency (51,52).

CLINICAL FEATURES

Each trace element deficiency state displays specific clinical features (Table 9). In copper deficiency, many of these features are correlated with the impaired activity of specific cuproproteins. The clinical features of zinc deficiency are not as clearly associated to biochemical correlates.

TABLE 9. *Clinical features of trace element deficiencies*

Element	Severe deficiency only	Mild deficiency	Deficiency in fetus
Iron	Heart failure	Anemia	
	?Anorexia	Impaired cognitive development	
	?Failure to thrive	Decreased exercise tolerance	
Iodine	Hypothyroidism	Goiter	Cretinism
			Deafness
			Milder impairment of brain function
Zinc	Acroorificial	Growth retardation	?Intrauterine growth retardation (IUGR)
	Skin lesions	Anorexia	Congenital malformations
	Diarrhea	?Hypogeusia	
	Alopecia	?Immune dysfunction	
	Increased incidence of infections		
	Immune dysfunction		
	Delayed wound healing		
	Personality changes		
	Hypogonadism		
Copper	Mental retardation	Anemia	?Connective tissue defects
	Convulsions	Neutropenia	
	Connective tissue defects	Osteoporosis	
	Fractures	Seborrheic skin lesions	
Selenium	Cardiomyopathy	?Macrocytosis	
	Skeletal myopathy	?Loss of hair pigment	
Molybdenum	Coma		
	Central scotomas		
	Vomiting		
Chromium	Peripheral neuropathy	?Impaired glucose tolerance	
Fluorine	Increased incidence of dental caries		

Zinc

One of the earliest and most prominent features of zinc deficiency in infants and children is impairment of physical growth velocity. This was first noted in zinc-deficient adolescents in Iran and Egypt in whom zinc supplementation was followed by a period of accelerated growth (53). A study of zinc supplementation of infant formula has clearly demonstrated the importance of zinc for the growth of infants (54). Zinc deficiency should be a consideration in the differential diagnosis of infants who fail to thrive.

Poor physical growth is also a documented feature of zinc depletion in preschool and school-age children in the United States (55–57), and elsewhere (58,59). Zinc supplementation has been reported to accelerate growth in adolescents suffering from intestinal malabsorption (29) and sickle-cell disease (60). Delayed sexual maturation is also a prominent feature of zinc deficiency in adolescents. Catch-up growth has followed the introduction of zinc therapy in patients with acrodermatitis enteropathica (61).

In zinc-deficient animals, growth retardation is preceded by, and at least partly attributable to, severe anorexia (62). Impaired appetite or reduced food intake has also been documented in human zinc deficiency (63,64). Anorexia is also a feature of untreated acrodermatitis enteropathica. Pica may also be present in some cases (65). Impaired taste perception has been demonstrated in zinc-depleted children (66,67), although it is not a problem of which the child is usually aware.

Zinc is necessary for normal brain growth (68) and function (35). However, there is no evidence that acquired zinc deficiency is a cause of mental retardation, learning disability, or behavioral disorders in infants and children. The mental development of children with acrodermatitis enteropathica, in whom severe deficiency has its onset in early infancy, is not grossly abnormal, although improvement in IQ in one case has been reported following zinc therapy (69). On the other hand, lethargy, irritability, and depression are often prominent features of zinc deficiency states, with very rapid and dramatic improvement following the institution of zinc therapy (35).

Wound healing is delayed in zinc-deficient animals (70). Accelerated healing of surgical wounds and decubitus ulcers has been reported in adults receiving zinc therapy (71,72). Not unexpectedly, such improvement has been found to be limited to those patients who have low plasma levels (73). Epithelialization of burns may also be improved with zinc therapy (47). Similar pediatric studies have not been reported.

More severe deficiency states, both acute and chronic, manifest a number of other characteristic clinical features. These features have been documented in acquired zinc deficiency, particularly in patients maintained on intravenous feeding without zinc supplementation, and in acrodermatitis enteropathica, the phenotypic expression of which is attributable to a severe zinc deficiency state. The cardinal features of acrodermatitis enteropathica are skin lesions, diarrhea, and alopecia. The skin lesions have a typical distribution, primarily adjacent to the body orifices and at the extremities. They usually present as an acute dermatitis, but chronic hyperkeratotic plaques may also occur. In formula-fed infants, symptoms commence in early infancy and, if untreated, the disease is progressive with severe failure to thrive, frequent monilial and bacterial infections, with a fatal outcome in later infancy or early childhood. The marked susceptibility to infections suggest that immune defense mechanisms may be compromised. One defect that has been clearly demonstrated is in monocytic and neutrophil chemotaxis, which can be corrected *in vitro* and *in vivo* with zinc supplementation (74).

Eye lesions that occur in some untreated or partially treated patients include severe photophobia, blepharitis, and corneal opacities (75). These improve with zinc therapy. Similar ocular manifestations exist in acquired zinc deficiency states (43). Of three women who have survived to adulthood without zinc therapy, two have delivered offspring with lethal congenital malformations, one of the skeletal system, the other an anencephalic stillbirth (76). These malformations are similar to those that occur in the offspring of zinc-deficient rats.

Copper

The earliest and most consistent features of human copper deficiency are related to the hematopoietic and skeletal systems. Specifically, the patient develops a microcytic hypochromic anemia unresponsive to iron therapy, neutropenia, and osteoporosis (77). The anemia is thought to result initially from a deficiency of copper ferroxidases, including ceruloplasmin, which have a role in the oxidation of Fe^{2+} in the intestinal mucosa and body stores to Fe^{3+} (9). Later, iron metabolism within the normoblast is also disrupted. Examination of the bone marrow reveals marked vacuolization of the erythroid series with megaloblastic changes. Ferritin deposits are present in many of the vacuoles. In addition, there is maturation arrest of the granulocytic series.

Skeletal lesions in a more severe copper deficiency state include periosteal elevation, cupping and flaring of long-bone metaphyses with spur formation, and, in some cases, submetaphyseal fractures, flaring of the anterior ribs, and spontaneous fractures of the ribs. The abnormalities may resemble those of scurvy and have been mistaken for nonaccidental trauma. These defects result from a deficiency of copper monoamine oxidases, which are required for the cross-linking of collagen, and of ascorbic acid oxidase, another copper metalloenzyme.

Other physical findings associated with copper deficiency in premature infants include pallor, depigmentation of skin and hair, prominent dilated superficial veins, skin lesions resembling seborrheic dermatitis, anorexia, diarrhea, and failure to thrive. Central nervous system involvement is suggested by the occurrence of hypotonia, psychomotor retardation, lack of visual responses, and apneic episodes, all of which improve with copper supplementation. In Menkes's steely-hair syndrome there is severe neurological degeneration leading to a fatal outcome by early childhood. This probably results from deficiencies of several copper metalloenzymes, including cytochrome oxidase, to which the hypothermia that occurs can also be attributed. As with copper-deficient animals, the tortuosity of arteries, demonstrable with arteriograms, probably results from impaired elastin synthesis due to lack of amine oxidases.

Selenium

Severe selenium deficiency is the major etiological factor in Keshan disease, which presents primarily as a cardiomyopathy in young children (15). Skeletal myopathies have also been reported (78). Mild selenium deficiency, often complicated by other factors, is associated with macrocytosis and loss of hair pigment (79).

Chromium

Glucose intolerance, which complicates malnutrition in young children, has, in some countries, been attributed in part to chromium deficiency (20). Chromium deficiency in one adult was deemed responsible for glucose intolerance, an abnormal respiratory quotient, the necessity for exogenous insulin, weight loss despite high caloric intake, abnormal nerve conduction with peripheral neuropathy, and evidence of disturbed nitrogen and lipid metabolism (25). Many reports of chromium deficiencies, however, require further confirmation.

DIAGNOSIS (Table 10)

Trace element deficiencies are discovered by way of suggestive symptomatology and predisposing circumstances. This may be relatively simple as, for example, in a patient with the typical features of acrodermatitis or in a premature infant with anemia, neutropenia, and osteoporosis. In other situations clinical features may be entirely nonspecific, for example, mild nutritional zinc deficiency in an infant with evidence of growth retardation.

Laboratory assays can confirm some deficiency states but are not always easy to interpret. Sample contamination is a major problem. Contaminant-free collection tubes, rather than vacutainers, are essential for fluid samples.

TABLE 10. *Laboratory diagnosis of trace element deficiencies*

Element	Test	Usefulness of test
Iron	CBC	+++
	Serum ferritin	+++
	Serum iron	+++
Iodine	Urine iodide	Epidemiological studies
	Thyroid function	++
Zinc	Plasma zinc	Mild deficiency: +
		Severe deficiency: +++[a]
	Other tests	Further validation needed
Copper	Serum copper	+
	Serum ceruloplasmin	+
	Erythrocyte SOD	Further validation needed
Selenium	Plasma/whole blood SE	+++
	Serum/whole blood GSHX	+++

GSHX, glutathione peroxidase; SE, selenium; SOD, superoxide dismutase.

[a] Severe zinc deficiency can occur in early postnatal life (typically in premature infants) who are breast-fed and whose mothers have a metabolic defect that prevents normal secretion of zinc by the mammary gland.

Because laboratory standards differ, results must be evaluated in the context of the laboratory performing the analysis. In some instances normal values are age-dependent, e.g., plasma copper concentrations, urine zinc excretion rates, and probably hair zinc concentrations. Low plasma and possibly hair zinc concentrations are supportive of a diagnosis of zinc deficiency. However, plasma zinc concentrations can be moderately depressed without zinc depletion in certain circumstances, including any acute infection. Urinary zinc excretion rates are depressed in severe, chronic zinc deficiency states, but measurement of these rates is more important in circumstances where hyperzincuria is suspected of contributing to zinc depletion. Serum alkaline phosphatase activity may be depressed, but this is not a sensitive index of zinc depletion. Hypocupremia and low serum ceruloplasmin levels are found in copper deficiency syndromes. However, many other factors may depress these levels, including nephrosis, protein-losing enteropathy, protein-energy malnutrition, and Wilson's disease. Levels are normally low during the first 3 months of life. Acceptable nominal ranges for premature infants urgently require better definition. Low circulating levels of selenium and glutathione peroxidase accompany selenium deficiency.

TREATMENT (Tables 11 and 12)

Zinc Deficiency

Acquired zinc (Zn) deficiency states can be treated with 0.5 to 1.0 mg Zn^{2+}/kg body weight/day for a period

TABLE 11. *Treatment of trace element deficiencies*

Element	Treatment
Iodine	Iodized salt or water; iodized oil by mouth or intramuscularly (2–4 ml)
Zinc	1 mg Zn^{2+}/kg/day Acrodermatitis enteropathica: 25–150 mg Zn^{2+}
Copper	0.2–0.6 mg Cu/day as 1% solution of copper sulfate for infants; <1–2 mg Cu/day for children.
Selenium	0.1 mg sodium selenite/day
Molybdenum	Ammonium molybdate < 0.5 mg/day
Chromium	0.1 mg trivalent chromium
Fluorine	0.25 mg/day at age 2 weeks–2 years 0.5 mg/day at age 2–3 years 1.0 mg/day at age 3–16 years (if concentration in drinking water < 0.3 ppm)

of several weeks or months. If factors contributing to malabsorption or excessive losses of zinc are a continuing problem, it may be necessary to consider a modest increase in this quantity. Rapid and sustained clinical and biochemical improvement in acrodermatitis enteropathica is uniformly achieved with 20 to 45 mg Zn^{2+} orally per day; even smaller quantities are adequate in some infants. Oral Zn^{2+} can be administered as the sulfate (heptahydrate), acetate, or other salts. One milligram Zn^{2+} is equivalent to approximately 4.5 mg zinc sulfate or 3 mg zinc acetate. Intravenous requirements for patients maintained on prolonged intravenous feeding approximate 50 μg Zn^{2+}/kg body weight/day. However, these requirements can be considerably higher in the presence of excessive zinc losses.

Zinc therapy should be monitored with determinations of both plasma zinc and copper concentrations. Excessive zinc therapy can lead to a copper deficiency syndrome (80). Other side effects of zinc therapy have not been reported, although zinc sulfate may produce gastrointestinal irritation in a small percentage of subjects.

Copper Deficiency

Effective treatment of acquired copper deficiency syndromes in infants is achieved with a 1% solution of copper sulfate, 0.1 ml (containing 200 μg Cu^{2+}) orally 2 to 3 times daily. Intravenous requirements approximate 20 to 30 μg/kg body weight/day. Intravenous copper supplements are probably not necessary unless total intravenous feeding has to be continued for several weeks, or the underlying disease state has already predisposed to depletion of copper stores. No side effects of copper therapy have been detected. However, both acute and chronic copper toxicity have been reported due to excessive environmental exposure or to an inborn error of copper metabolism (Wilson's disease). Etiological factors have included the prolonged consumption of drinking water containing excessive quantities of copper, hemodialysis, the application of copper salts to skin lesions, and the accidental or deliberate ingestion of copper salts in quantities of more than 1 g. Both acute and chronic copper toxicity can be fatal. Cirrhosis and erythroderma polyneuropathy have been reported as complications of chronic copper toxicity (81). Symptoms of acute toxicity from ingestion include a metallic taste, nausea, vomiting, diarrhea, hemoglobinuria, and jaundice due to hepatic necrosis.

Nutritional Requirements and Dietary Sources

The 10th edition of the *Recommended Dietary Allowances* published by the Food and Nutrition Board, National Academy of Sciences (82), contains recommendations for iron, zinc, iodine, and selenium (Table 13) as well as copper, manganese, fluorine, chromium, and molybdenum (Table 14). Premature infants require 100 μg copper/kg body weight/day (77). There is increasing evidence that zinc requirements, like those of iron, are dependent on the source. The bioavailability from meats is higher than from many vegetable products, including unrefined grains. More important to the infant is the

TABLE 12. *Recommended intravenous intakes of trace elements*

	Infants (μg/kg/day)		Children (μg/kg/day) [maximum μg/day]
	Preterm	Term	
Zinc	400	250 < 3 mo 100 > 3 mo	50 [5,000]
Copper[a]	20	20	20 [300]
Selenium	2.0	2.0	2.0 [30]
Chromium	0.2	0.2	0.20 [5.0]
Manganese[a]	1.0	1.0	1.0 [50]
Molybdenum	0.25	0.25	0.25 [5.0]
Iodine	2.0	2.0	2.0 [5.0]

[a] Omit in patients with obstructive jaundice.

TABLE 13. *Recommended dietary allowances (revised 1989)*[a]

Category	Age	Iron (mg)	Zinc (mg)	Iodine (μg)	Selenium (μg)
Infants	0.0–0.5	6	5	40	10
	0.5–1.0	10	5	50	15
Children	1–3	10	10	70	20
	4–6	10	10	90	20
	7–10	10	10	120	30
Males	11–14	12	15	150	40
	15–18	12	15	150	50
Females	11–14	15	12	150	45
	15–18	15	12	150	50

[a] Food and Nutrition Board, National Academy of Sciences, National Research Council, 10th edition, 1989.

TABLE 14. *Estimated safe and adequate daily dietary intakes of selected trace elements (revised 1989)*

Category	Age	Copper	Manganese	Fluorine	Chromium	Molybdenum
Infants	0–0.5	0.4–0.6	0.3–0.6	0.1–0.5	10–40	15–30
	0.5–1	0.6–0.7	0.2–1.0	0.2–1.0	20–60	20–40
Children and adolescents	1–3	0.7–1.0	1.0–1.5	0.5–1.5	20–80	25–50
	4–6	1.0–1.5	1.5–2.0	1.0–2.5	30–120	30–75
	7–10	1.0–2.0	2.0–3.0	1.5–2.5	50–200	75–250
	11+	1.5–2.5	2.0–5.0	1.5–2.5	50–200	75–250

Since the toxic levels for many trace elements may be only several times usual intakes, the upper levels for the trace elements given in this table should not be habitually exceeded.

TABLE 15. *Toxicity of trace elements*

Element	Effect	Dose
Iodine	Thyrotoxicosis Goiter	1,000 μg I/day (children)
Zinc	Copper deficiency	50 mg Zn/day (adults) 30 mg Zn/day (infants)
	Depressed HDL-cholesterol	150 mg Zn/day (adults)
	Diarrhea, nausea, vomiting, irritability, headache, lethargy	Acute ingestion of several grams of zinc
Copper	Chronic: ? cirrhosis ?recurrent diarrhea and vomiting ?pro-oxidant mediated CNS damage	0.4 mg Cu/kg/day (infants) 8 mg Cu/liter water
	Acute: gastrointestinal disturbance; hepatic centrilobular necrosis; intravascular hemolysis; renal tubular damage; cardiotoxicity	Excess quantities administered orally absorbed via the skin or administered in dialysis fluids
Selenium	Chronic: loss of hair; roughening of nails; fatigue; discoloration of skin	>1 mg/day
	Acute: vomiting and diarrhea; paresthesias; irritability; garlicky breath	>25 mg/day
Molybdenum	Interferes with copper metabolism	
Manganese	Extrapyramidal central nervous system dysfunction ?Hepatic damage	
Chromium	None recognized for Cr^{3+}	
Fluorine	Fluorosis (mottling of teeth)	>4 mg/day (adults)

type of milk feeding. The bioavailability of zinc from human milk may be considerably higher than from cow's milk and cow's milk products.

The effects of trace elements are dose-dependent and all are potentially toxic if given in excess (Table 15).

ACKNOWLEDGMENTS

The points of view expressed in this chapter are based in part on studies supported by United States Public Health Service grant ROI-AM-12432 from National Institute of Arthritis and Metabolic Diseases, and by grant RR-69 from the General Clinical Research Centers Program of the Division of Research Resources, National Institutes of Health.

REFERENCES

1. Mertz W, ed. *Trace elements in human and animal nutrition,* vol 1, 5th ed. San Diego: Academic Press, 1987.
2. Mertz W, ed. *Trace elements in human and animal nutrition,* vol 2, 5th ed. San Diego: Academic Press, 1987.
3. National Research Council. *Recommended dietary allowances,* 10th ed. Washington, DC: National Academy Press, 1989.
4. Greene HL, Hambidge KM, Schanler R, Tsang R. *Guidelines for the use of vitamins, trace elements, calcium, magnesium and phosphorus in infants and children receiving total parenteral nutrition.* Report of subcommittee. Committee on Clinical Practice Issues of the American Society for Clinical Nutrition. *Am J Clin Nutr* 1988;48:1324–1342.
5. Nielsen FH. Nutritional significance of the ultratrace elements. *Nutr Rev* 1988;46:337–341.
6. Williams RJP. An introduction to the biochemistry of zinc. In: Mills DF, ed. *Zinc in human biology.* Springer Verlag: London 1989:15–31.
7. Lee MS, Gippert GP, Soman KV, Case DA, Wright PE. Three dimensional solution structure of a single zinc finger DNA-binding domain. *Science* 1989;245:635–643.
8. Cousins RJ. Metallothionein-aspects related to copper and zinc metabolism. *J Inherited Metab Dis* 1983;6:15–21.
9. Frieden E, Hsieh HS. Ceruloplasmin, a multifunctional metalloprotein. In: Kirchgessner M, ed. *Trace element metabolism in man and animals,* vol 3. Germany: Arbeitskreis fier Tierernahrungsforschung, Weihenstephan, 1977:36–39.
10. Navert B, Sandstrom B. Reduction of the phytate content of bran by leavening in bread and its effect on zinc absorption in man. *Br J Nutr* 1985;53:47–53.
11. Lonnerdal B. Intestinal absorption of zinc. In: Mills DF, ed. *Zinc in human biology.* Springer Verlag: London 1989:33–41.

12. Jackson MJ, Jones DA, Edwards RHT, Swainbank IG, Coleman ML. Zinc homeostasis in man: studies using a new stable isotope-dilution technique. *Br J Nutr* 1984;51:199–208.
13. Levy Y, Zaharia A, Grunebaum M, Nitzan M, Steinherz R. Copper deficiency in infants fed cow milk. *J Pediatr* 1985;786–788.
14. Yadrick MK, Kenny AM, Wintefeldt EA. Iron, copper and zinc status: response to supplementation with zinc or zinc and iron in adult females. *Am J Clin Nutr* 1989;49:145–150.
15. Keshan Disease Research Group. Observations on effect of sodium selenite in prevention of Keshan disease. *Chin Med J* 1979;92:471–476.
16. Golden MHN, Ramdath D. Free radicals in the pathogenesis of kwashiorkor. In: Taylor TG, Jenkins NK, eds. *Proceedings of the XIII International Congress of Nutrition.* London: John Libbey, 1986:597–598.
17. Sutton AM, Harvie A, Cockburn F, et al. Copper deficiency in the preterm infant of very low birthweight. *Arch Dis Child* 1985;60:644–651.
18. Hambidge KM. Zinc deficiency in the premature infant. *Pediatr Rev* 1985;6:209–216.
19. Cardano A, Baertl JM, Graham GG. Copper deficiency in infancy. *Pediatrics* 1964;34:324.
20. Gurson CT, Saner G. Effects of chromium supplementation on growth in marasmic protein-calorie malnutrition. *Am J Clin Nutr* 1971;24:1313–1319.
21. Golden MHN, Golden BE. Effect of zinc supplementation on the dietary intake, rate of weight, gain and energy cost of tissue deposition in children recovering from severe malnutrition. *Am J Clin Nutr* 1981;34:900–908.
22. Arlette JP, Johnston MM. Zinc deficiency dermatosis in premature infants receiving prolonged parenteral alimentation. *J Am Acad Dermatol* 1981;5:37–42.
23. Kien CL, Ganther HE. Manifestations of chronic selenium deficiency in a child receiving total parenteral nutrition. *Am J Clin Nutr* 1983;37:319–328.
24. Abumrad NN, Schneider AJ, Steele D, Rogers LS. Amino acid intolerance during prolonged total parenteral nutrition reversed by molybdate therapy. *Am J Clin Nutr* 1981;34:2551–2559.
25. Jeejeeboy KN. Zinc and chromium in parenteral nutrition. *Bull NY Acad Med* 1984;60(2):118–124.
26. Yannicelli S, Hambidge KM. Evidence of selenium deficiency in a child with propionic acidemia. *J Inherited Metab Dis* 1992 (in press).
27. Sandstead HH, Vo-Khactu KP, Solomons N. Conditioned zinc deficiencies. In: Prasad AS, Oberleas D, eds. *Trace elements in human health and disease,* vol 1. New York: Academic Press, 1976:33–46.
28. Cordano A, Baertl JM, Graham GG. Copper deficiency in infancy. *Pediatrics* 1964;34:324–336.
29. Sandstead HH. Zinc nutrition in the United States. *Am J Clin Nutr* 1973;26:1251–1260.
30. Love AHG, Elmes M, Golden MK, McMaster K. Zinc deficiency and coeliac disease. In: Kirchgessner M, ed. *Trace element metabolism in man and animals,* vol 3. Germany: Arbeitskreis fier Tierernahrungs-forschung, Weihenstephan, 1977:357–358.
31. Halsted JA, Smith JC Jr. Plasma zinc in health and disease. *Lancet* 1970;1:322–324.
32. McMahan RA, Parker MLM, McKinnon MC. Zinc treatment in malabsorption. *Med J Aust* 1968;2:210–212.
33. Prasad AS, Miale A Jr, Farid Z, Sandstead HH, Schulert AR. Zinc metabolism in patients with the syndrome of iron deficiency anemia, hepatosplenomegaly, dwarfism and hypogonadism. *J Lab Clin Med* 1963;61:537–549.
34. Cohen IK, Schechter PJ, Henkin RI. Hypogeusia, anorexia and altered zinc metabolism following thermal burn. *JAMA* 1973;223:914–916.
35. Henkin RI, Graziadei PPG, Bradley DF. The molecular basis of taste and its disorders. *Ann Intern Med* 1969;7:791–821.
36. Cassidy WA, Brown ED, Smith JC, Jr. In: Hambidge KM, Nichols BL, eds. *Zinc and copper in clinical medicine.* New York: Spectrum, 1977:59–79.
37. Vallee BL, Wacker WEC, Bartholomay AF, Hoch FL. Zinc metabolism in hepatic dysfunction. II. Correlation of metabolic patterns with biochemical findings. *N Engl J Med* 1957;257:1055–1065.
38. Henkin RI, Smith FR. Zinc and copper metabolism in acute viral hepatitis. *Am J Med Sci* 1972;264:401–409.
39. Evans GW. Copper homeostasis in the mammalian system. *Physiol Rev* 1973;53:535–570.
40. Freeman JB, Stegink LD, Meyer PD, Fry LK, Denbesten L. Excessive urinary zinc losses during parenteral alimentation. *J Surg Res* 1974;18:463–469.
41. Prasad AS, Oberleas D. Thymidine kinase activity and incorporation of thymidine into DNA in zinc deficient tissue. *J Lab Clin Med* 1974;61:537–549.
42. Hambidge KM. Chromium nutrition in the mother and growing child. In: Mertz W, Cornatzer WC, eds. *Newer trace elements in nutrition.* New York: Marcel Dekker, 1971:169–194.
43. Klingberg WG, Prasad AS, Oberleas D. Zinc deficiency following penicillamine therapy. In: Prasad AS, ed. *Trace elements in human health and disease,* vol 1. New York: Academic Press, 1976:51–64.
44. Beisel WR, Pekarek RS, Wannemacher RW. Homeostatic mechanisms affecting plasma zinc levels in acute stress. In: Prasad AS, ed. *Trace elements in human health and disease,* vol 1. New York: Academic Press, 1976:87–102.
45. Cotzias MD. In: Hemphill DD, ed. *Proceedings of 1st annual conference on trace substances in environmental health.* Columbia, MO: University of Missouri, 1967:5–19.
46. Simkin PA. Oral zinc sulphate in rheumatoid arthritis. *Lancet* 1976;2:539–542.
47. Larson DL. Oral zinc sulfate in the management of severely burned patients. In: Pories WJ, Strain WH, Hsu JM, Woosley RL, eds. *Clinical applications of zinc metabolism.* Springfield, IL: Charles C Thomas, 1974:229–236.
48. Danks DM, Camakaris J, Stevens BJ. The cellular defect in Menkes' syndrome and in mottled mice. In: Kirchgessner M, ed. *Trace element metabolism in man and animals,* vol 3. Germany: Arbeitskreis fier Tierernahrungs-forschung, Weihenstephan, 1977;401–404.
49. Danks DM, Campbell PE, Stevens BJ, Mayne V, Cartwright E. Menkes' kinky hair syndrome: an inherited defect in copper absorption with widespread effects. *Pediatrics* 1972;50:188–201.
50. Lombeck I, Schnippering HG, Kasperek K, Ritzl F, Kaster H, Feinendegen LE, Bremer JH. Akrodermatitis enteropathica—eine zinckstoffwechselstorung mit zinkmalabsorption. *Z Kinderheilkd* 1975;120:181–189.
51. Moynahan EM. Acrodermatitis enteropathica. A lethal inherited human zinc deficiency disorder. *Lancet* 1974;2:399–400.
52. Neldner KH, Hambidge KM. Zinc therapy of acrodermatitis enteropathica. *N Engl J Med* 1975;292:879–882.
53. O'Dell BL. Dietary factors that affect biological availability of trace elements. *Ann NY Acad Sci* 1972;199:70–81.
54. Walravens PA, Hambidge KM. Growth of infants fed a zinc-supplemented formula. *Am J Clin Nutr* 1976;29:1114–1121.
55. Walravens PA, Krebs NF, Hambidge KM. Linear growth of low income preschool children receiving a zinc supplement. *Am J Clin Nutr* 1983;38:195–201.
56. Hambidge KM, Krebs NF, Walravens PA. Growth velocity of young children receiving a dietary zinc supplement. *Nutr Res* 1985;1:306–316.
57. Walravens PA, Hambidge KM, Koepfer DM. Zinc supplementation in infants with a nutritional pattern of failure to thrive: a double-blind, controlled study. *Pediatrics* 1989;83(4):532–538.
58. Gibson RS, Vanderkooy S, MacDonald AC, et al. A growth-limiting mild zinc-deficiency syndrome in some Southern Ontario boys with low weight percentiles. *Am J Clin Nutr* 1989;49(6);1266–1273.
59. Hong Z, et al. Observation on the therapeutic effect of zinc on underweight children. *Natl Med J China* 1982;62(7):415–419.
60. Prasad AS, Abbasi A, Ortega J. In: Brewer GJ, Prassad AS, eds. *Zinc metabolism: current aspects in health and disease.* New York: Alan R Liss, 1977:211–236.
61. Hambidge KM, Neldner KM, Walravens PA, Weston WL, Silverman A, Sabol JL, Brown RM. Zinc and acrodermatitis enteropathica. In: Hambidge KM, Nichols BL, eds. *Zinc and copper in clinical medicine.* New York: Spectrum, 1977;81–98.
62. Underwood EJ., ed. *Trace elements in human and animal nutrition.* New York: Academic Press, 1971.
63. Krebs NF, Hambidge KM, Walravens PA. Increased food intake of young children receiving a zinc supplement. *Am J Dis Child* 1984;138:270–273.

64. Prasad AS. *Manifestations of zinc abnormalities in human beings.* Nriagu J. ed. *Zinc in the environment, part II.* John Wiley & Sons: New York 1980;29–59.
65. Hambidge KM, Silverman A. Pica with rapid improvement after dietary zinc supplementation. *Arch Dis Child* 1973;48:567–568.
66. Hambidge KM, Hambidge C, Jacobs M. Low levels of zinc in hair, anorexia, poor growth and hypoguesia in children. *Pediatr Res* 1972;6:868–874.
67. Solomons NW, Rosenfield RL, Jacob RA, Sandstead HH. Growth retardation and zinc nutrition. *Pediatr Res* 1976;10:923–927.
68. Hambidge KM, Walravens PA, Brown RM, Webster J, White S, Anthony M, Roth ML. Zinc nutrition of preschool children in the Denver Headstart program. *Am J Clin Nutr* 1976;29:734–738.
69. Hambidge KM, Walravens PA, Neldner KH. The role of zinc in the pathogenesis and treatment of acrodermatitis enteropathica. In: Brewer GJ, Prasad AS, eds. *Zinc metabolism: current aspects in health and disease.* New York: Alan R Liss, 1977;329–340.
70. Wacker WEC. Role of zinc in wound healing: a critical review. In: Prasad AS, ed. *Trace elements in human health and disease,* vol 1. New York: Academic Press, 1976;107–113.
71. Pories WJ, Henzel JH, Rob CG, Strain WH. Acceleration of wound healing in man with zinc sulfate given by mouth. *Lancet* 1967;1:121–124.
72. Pories WJ, Mansour EG, Plecha FR, Flynn A, Strain WH. Metabolic factors affecting zinc metabolism in the surgical patient. In: Prasad AS, ed. *Trace elements in human health and disease,* vol 1. New York: Academic Press, 1976;115–141.
73. Hallbook T, Lanner E. Serum zinc and healing of venous leg ulcers. *Lancet* 1972;2:780–782.
74. Weston WL, et al. Zinc correction of defective chemotaxis in acrodermatitis enteropathica. *Arch Dermatol* 1977;113:422–425.
75. Hambidge KM, Casey CE, Krebs NF. Zinc. In: Mertz W, ed. *Trace elements in human and animal nutrition,* vol 2, 5th ed. Florida: Academic Press, 1986;1–137.
76. Hambidge KM, Neldner KH, Walravens PA. Zinc, acrodermatitis enteropathica and congenital malformations. *Lancet* 1975;1:577.
77. Cordano A. In: Hambidge KM, Nichols BL, eds. *Zinc and copper in clinical medicine.* New York: Spectrum, 1977;119–126.
78. Kien CL, Ganther HE. Manifestations of chronic selenium deficiency in a child receiving total parental nutrition. *Am J Clin Nutr* 1983;37:319–328.
79. Vinton NE, Dahlstrom KA, Strobel CT, Ament ME. Macrocytosis and pseudoalbinism; manifestations of selenium deficiency. *J Pediatr* 1987;111:711–717.
80. Hambidge KM, Walravens PA, Neldner KH, Daugherty NA. Zinc, copper and fatty acids in acrodermatitis enteropathica. In: Kirchgessner M, ed. *Trace element metabolism in man and animals,* vol 3. Germany: Arbeitskreis fier Tierernahrungs-forschung, Weihenstephan, 1978;413–417.
81. Walker-Smith J, Blomfield J. Wilson's disease or chronic copper poisoning? *Arch Dis Child* 1973;48:476–479.
82. National Research Council. *Recommended dietary allowances,* 10th ed. Washington, DC: National Academy Press, 1989.

CHAPTER 11

The Malnourished Child

Leslie Lewinter-Suskind, Dana Suskind, Krishna K. Murthy, and Robert M. Suskind

---

Over 14 million of the world's preschool children die each year, 40,000 each day. Most of these children are malnourished (1). These deaths represent, however, only a fraction of the children in developing countries who suffer from malnutrition, many of whom survive (2–4). For those who do survive, early malnutrition generates a long-term insult to their adult potential and, consequently, to the community and world in which they must participate.

The basis of childhood malnutrition, in much of the world, is poverty (5–10), often exacerbated by natural and political disasters (8,11,12). In the United States, primary protein-energy malnutrition (PEM) is less commonly seen (13). There is, however, an increasing awareness of the occurrence of malnutrition secondary to disease states (14) such as diarrhea (15) AIDS (16), cancer (17), intrauterine growth retardation (18), and child abuse (19). Also evident is the importance of nutritional status in the overall prognosis of a disease state (20). This observation, together with recognition of the long-term effects of malnutrition on growth and development, has highlighted the need for accurately determining deficiencies, for methods to discern their impact on disease states, and for effective programs for their prevention and treatment (21–26).

L. Lewinter-Suskind: Departments of Psychiatry and Pediatrics, Louisiana State University School of Medicine, New Orleans, Louisiana 70112.

D. Suskind: Department of Otolaryngology, University of Pennsylvania School of Medicine, Philadelphia, Pennsylvania 19104.

K. K. Murthy: Department of Virology and Immunology, Southwest Foundation for Biomedical Research, San Antonio, Texas 78227.

R. M. Suskind: Department of Pediatrics, Louisiana State University School of Medicine, New Orleans, Louisiana 70112.

ANTHROPOMETRIC CLASSIFICATION OF PROTEIN-ENERGY MALNUTRITION

In 1956, Gomez et al. (27) used local standards to define malnutrition in terms of weight-for-age. Current classifications use internationally accepted standards derived from the weights and heights of healthy children from North America or Europe. Several studies support the use of such standards for all children. Habicht et al. (28) reviewed anthropometric data taken from several racial-ethnic groups and concluded that the differences among diverse well-nourished populations were small compared to the differences between socioeconomic classes of the same populations. They concluded that data drawn from studies of well-to-do populations could, therefore, be used as standards. Martorell et al. (29) in Honduras, showed a clear association between socioeconomic status and "stunting," that is, severe growth retardation, as well as correlations even within gradations of poverty to eventual height deficits.

Height-for-age and weight-for-height are basic indices for defining a child's nutritional status. A decreased weight-for-height indicates an acute state of malnutrition; a decreased height-for-age, on the other hand, indicates that the child has, at some period, been chronically malnourished (30). Combined deficits of height-for-age and weight-for-height indicate long-term malnutrition as well as the existence of current nutritional deficits. The effect of malnutrition on linear growth may not in fact be apparent until approximately 4 months after its effect on weight velocity (31).

Weight-for-height is classified as grades I, II, and III of 80% to 90%, 70% to 80%, and less than 70% of ideal weight-for-height, respectively (32). Height-for-age classifications are grades I, II, and III of 90% to 95%, 85% to 90%, and less than 85% of height-for-age, respectively.

Children in developing countries commonly become wasted between 1 and 2 years of age. By 3 to 4 years of age, when they are better able to procure their own food, wasting may be replaced by stunting (32). The result is a short child with a normal weight-for-height.

Other anthropometric methods, such as arm circumference and triceps skin fold, are also used for determining the presence of malnutrition. Anderson et al. (33), however, in a study of over 5,000 Indian children, found arm circumference measurements unreliable for determining severe malnutrition. They concluded that, because of the possibility of misclassification of moderately to severely malnourished children, use of weight was preferable in determining nutritional status. Ross et al. (34) in Sudan found that weight-for-height measurements and mid-upper-arm circumference measurements did not always identify the same individual children as malnourished. Keet et al. (35), in an investigation of triceps skin-fold measurements, found that marasmic children had skin-fold values below the 3rd percentile for normal children of the same sex. Children with marasmus-kwashiorkor and kwashiorkor ranged from below the 3rd percentile to the 50th percentile. Koskelo et al. (36) used ultrasonography to assess muscle and fat in the arms and legs of malnourished children and reported that this, combined with anthropometric measurements, was a useful tool in assessing children suspected of being malnourished.

CLINICAL CLASSIFICATION OF PROTEIN-ENERGY MALNUTRITION

The three states of protein-energy malnutrition are marasmus, marasmic-kwashiorkor, and kwashiorkor. They are compounded by a whole spectrum of nutritional disorders that include deficiencies of one or more vitamins, minerals, and trace minerals. The three states of protein-energy malnutrition can be differentiated most clearly on the basis of clinical findings.

Marasmus, which predominates in infancy, is characterized by severe weight reduction, gross wasting of muscle and subcutaneous tissue, no detectable edema and, if prolonged, marked stunting (Fig. 1). Marasmus results from a severe deprivation, or impaired absorption, of protein, energy, vitamins, and minerals. The hair and skin changes and hepatomegaly resulting from fatty infiltration of the liver, which are seen in kwashiorkor, are not usually found in marasmus. The marasmic child, characteristically irritable and apathetic, is the skin-and-bones portrait of starvation. The term for this is *wasting*. When such malnutrition continues on a long-term basis in a young child, it results in *stunting*, a term introduced by Waterlow (30) to describe the profound effect of nutritional deprivation on linear growth.

Marasmic-kwashiorkor presents with the clinical findings of both marasmus and kwashiorkor (Fig. 2). The

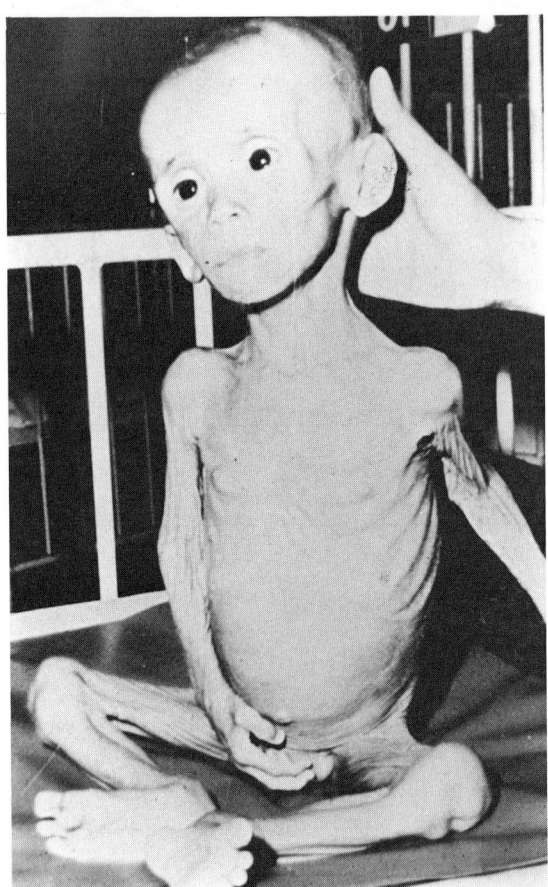

FIG. 1. Marasmic child (2 years old) with characteristic growth retardation, weight loss, muscular atrophy, and loss of subcutaneous tissue.

child with marasmic-kwashiorkor has edema, gross wasting, and is usually stunted. There may also be mild hair and skin changes and a palpable fatty-infiltrated liver. The child with marasmus-kwashiorkor is one who demonstrates the combined effects of an inadequate intake of nutrients to meet requirements plus superimposed infection.

Kwashiorkor results from either inadequate protein intake or, more commonly, from an acute or chronic infection. It appears predominantly in older infants and young children. Clinically, it is characterized by edema, skin lesions, hair changes, apathy, anorexia, a large fatty liver, and decreased serum albumin (Fig. 3). Weight loss is also usual, even without a decrease in energy intake. The edema of kwashiorkor can only partially be explained by the low serum albumin; other contributing factors include increased capillary permeability, increased cortisol, and antidiuretic hormone levels (37).

Prognosis and Mortality

Although mortality in the presence of severe PEM varies with the level of care, a study of over 2,400 cases

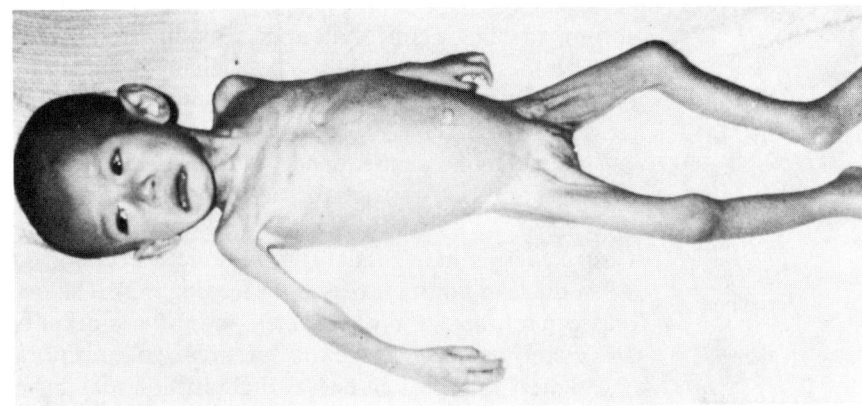

FIG. 2. Child (1.5 years old) with marasmic-kwashiorkor, with wasting, stunting, edema, and mild hepatomegaly.

concluded that the worst prognostic factors were infection and water and electrolyte disturbances (38). Garrow and Pike (39) found that a decreased serum sodium and increased serum bilirubin were negative prognostic signs. Waterlow et al. (40) reported an increased mortality among children with gross hepatomegaly. Poor prognosis was also attributed to hypothermia, when the rectal temperature was less than 35°C, especially when accompanied by profound hypoglycemia (41).

Pathogenesis

Marasmus results from inadequate energy intake, kwashiorkor from the catabolic stress of infection and/or a deficiency of dietary protein. Gopalan (42), in 1968, found that there was no essential difference between the protein/energy ratios in the diets of children with marasmus and those with kwashiorkor; that each of the clinical syndromes appeared in different children for whom there was no demonstrable difference in diet. Instead, Gopalan suggested that kwashiorkor was essentially a failure of adaptation occurring when sufficient food was consumed for energy maintenance but without sufficient dietary protein available for the synthesis of visceral proteins (42). More recently, Keusch (43) described the mechanism by which infection, as a result of the production of tumor necrosis factor IL-1 by macrophages, inhibited the production of visceral proteins and stimulated the release of acute-phase reactants. Amino acids, for the most part, are diverted into the production of acute-phase reactants at the expense of visceral protein synthesis. As a result, the production of albumin and lipoproteins is decreased, leading to the development of hypoalbuminemia, edema, and fatty infiltration of the liver.

Marasmus, on the other hand, results from a lack of both energy and protein. The resulting "adaptation" produces increased cortisol levels and decreased insulin levels. Muscle provides the essential amino acids for the maintenance of visceral protein synthesis, which leads, in turn, to the production of adequate amounts of serum albumin and lipoproteins, avoiding the occurrence of edema and fatty infiltration of the liver.

When infection is superimposed on the marasmic state, essential amino acids are diverted to the production of acute-phase reactants, rather than to visceral proteins. Cortisol and growth hormone, rather than insulin, become the major contributors to the metabolic status of the patient. Growth hormone further contributes to the amino acid deficit by driving amino acids into the lean body mass so that they are no longer available for visceral protein synthesis.

Scrimshaw and Behar (44) developed a triangular model to describe the development of a spectrum of protein-energy deficiency states (Fig. 4). Time is represented on the horizontal axis. The vertical axis demonstrates the rapid development of metabolic disorders, leading to edema and fatty infiltration of the liver, seen in kwashior-

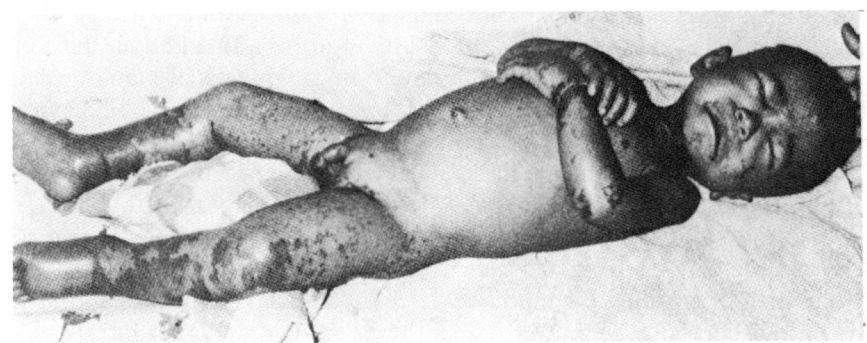

FIG. 3. Child (2.5 years old) with kwashiorkor, with evidence of edema, skin lesions, muscular atrophy, and enlarged liver.

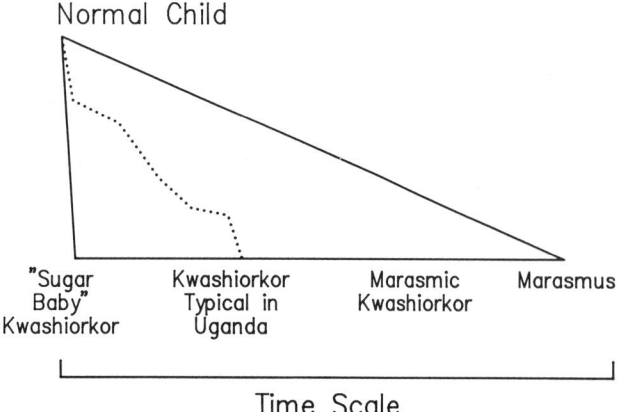

FIG. 4. The development of protein-energy malnutrition spectrum of diseases. (Adapted from ref. 44.)

kor; the hypotenuse reflects the overall slower process of wasting seen in marasmus. The typical patient falls somewhere in between.

INTERACTION OF INFECTION AND NUTRITION

Malnourished children are clearly more susceptible to infection (45). The consequent interaction of infection with malnutrition is, unquestionably, one of the major factors in the increased morbidity and mortality associated with PEM. In 1973, Puffer and Serrano (46) demonstrated that nutritional deficiency was associated with 60.9% of the deaths from infectious disease. Diarrhea and measles were the diseases with the greatest morbidity and mortality in which malnutrition was a factor (47).

The mechanisms by which infection leads to a malnourished state include (a) anorexia; (b) replacement of solid foods with a low-energy, low-protein diet; (c) decreased nutrient absorption resulting from diarrhea and intestinal parasites; and (d) increased urinary losses of nitrogen, potassium, magnesium, zinc, phosphate, sulfur, and vitamins A, C, and B_2 (48). Increased urinary nitrogen excretion, which exists in the mildest of infectious diseases, results from an increased mobilization of amino acids from peripheral muscle for gluconeogenesis in the liver with deamination and excretion of nitrogen in the form of urea. Without an increased dietary intake to compensate for losses, a kwashiorkor-like syndrome results. In addition, with infection, there is sequestration or diversion of iron, copper, and zinc from normal metabolic pathways. Despite the mobilization of amino acids from peripheral muscle, there is also a decrease in whole blood amino acids after exposure to an infectious agent (49). An increased synthesis of acute-phase reactants, including haptoglobin, C-reactive protein, α_1-antitrypsin, and α_2-macroglobulin, also occurs, accompanied by a concomitant decrease in visceral protein synthesis (50). Each of these changes is felt to be mediated by tumor necrosis factor and interleukin-1 (IL-1) (20).

The metabolic consequence of infectious diseases such as severe gastroenteritis or measles is often the development of marasmic-kwashiorkor or kwashiorkor (51). Gastroenteritis may result from seasonal infections or when unclean bottles are used for feeding (52). The decrease in serum albumin characteristic of kwashiorkor is also closely associated with the appearance of infection.

Children with protein-energy malnutrition may have either hypochromic microcytic or normochromic normocytic anemia (53,54). In chronic infections, anemia may occur as a result of defective hemoglobin synthesis accompanied by inadequate bone marrow stores of iron (55). Infection also affects the endocrine system. Changes in hormone levels occur simultaneously with infection and precede the changes in amino acids and serum albumin levels (37). With infection, there is a decrease in serum albumin and insulin levels as well as an increase in cortisol levels. In addition, decreased food intake results in negative nitrogen balance secondary to increased tissue catabolism.

During infectious episodes, diarrhea results in a significant loss of potassium and magnesium in the stools, leading to a decrease in serum electrolytes (56). There is also urinary loss of electrolytes as a result of increased muscle breakdown (57). Iron absorption and metabolism are also affected by infection (55,58). Infections such as malaria and typhoid may cause increased hemolysis and resultant acute hemolytic anemia.

NUTRITION AND IMMUNITY

The Cellular Immune Response

The cell-mediated immune response is compromised in malnourished children. This is illustrated by the fact that the mortality rate for measles among malnourished children is four times that of well-nourished children (59). In addition, individuals given supplemental protein have a significantly lower incidence of tuberculosis than nonsupplemented, poorly nourished individuals (60).

Atrophy of the thymus was the first indication that malnutrition could affect cellular immunity in children who died from kwashiorkor (61). In addition, the concentration of thymulin in the thymus of malnourished children has been found to be decreased (62). Thymic atrophy, which occurs as a result of protein, energy, vitamin, and mineral deficiencies, especially zinc (63), is associated with a decreased production of thymic hormone, an underlying T-cell deficiency (64), and an increased susceptibility to disseminated infections (65).

Lymph nodes, tonsils (66), and spleen also appear to be smaller in malnourished children (67). Children who are malnourished have a significantly higher percentage of false negative skin tests than well-nourished children (68). Further studies have confirmed this defective skin test responsiveness to antigens such as *Monilia* (69), streptococcal antigen (70), *Trichophyton* (71), and mumps virus (72). There is also a correlation between the degree of immune impairment and the degree of weight loss, with alterations in cellular immunity being normalized as nutritional status improves (72,73).

Edelman et al. (74) performed a series of in vivo and in vitro experiments designed to evaluate the inflammatory, sensitizing, and recall limbs of the cell-mediated immune system, as well as the responsiveness of isolated lymphocytes. To evaluate T-lymphocyte function in vivo, there must be intact circulating thymus-derived T lymphocytes, which are capable of being sensitized to a foreign antigen. Sensitized lymphocytes must be able to identify the foreign antigen and release lymphokines, which, in turn, produce a localized inflammatory response. In this study, dinitrofluorobenzene (DNFB) was applied to the forearms of 30 malnourished children. Only 4 (13%) had positive inflammatory responses, indicating that the inflammatory response is depressed in children with PEM.

Other investigators have found that isolated peripheral lymphocytes from malnourished children react poorly to stimulation with mitogens such as phytohemagglutinin (PHA) (66,71) and pokeweed (72). The depression in lymphocyte transformation improved with nutritional recovery (66,72). Sellmeyer et al. (75) also reported a profound depression of lymphocyte transformation in well-nourished children who had measles and gastroenteritis. Decreased T-cell response to mitogen or antigen stimulation has been attributed to an increase in cell cycle duration (76), deficiency of a humoral factor required for optimum response of T cells (77), an inhibitory substance in the serum (78), or increased levels of α-fetoprotein (79). In addition to the depressed in vitro responsiveness of isolated lymphocytes to antigenic and mitogenic stimulation (80), circulating lymphocytes are numerically decreased in malnourished children (80), particularly the helper phenotype (81), which is replaced by a proportionate increase in "null" lymphoid cells (81). Keusch et al. (82), however, found that not all malnourished patients had decreased circulating T cells, although all were clinically similar. This suggests that specific nutrient defects associated with PEM may be important etiologic factors in the depressed cellular immune response.

Natural Killer Cells

Natural killer (NK) cells are non-T, non-B large granular lymphoid cells that play a vital role in immune surveillance against virus-infected and cancer cells. Unlike cytotoxic T cells, which are antigen-specific and major histocompatibility complex (MHC)-restricted, NK cells act nonspecifically and in an unrestricted manner (83). Depressed NK cell activity in children with PEM returned to normal levels with improved nutritional status (84). Addition of exogenous interferon, a potent stimulator of NK cells in vitro, had variable effects on NK activity depending on the degree of malnutrition. In well-nourished and nutritionally recovered children, interferon-enhanced NK activity, although it had no effect on cells from marasmic children, had a suppressive effect on cells from kwashiorkor patients.

Interleukins

Interleukins (IL), a family of peptide/glycoprotein hormones or factors produced by activated leukocytes, act as autoparacrine signals for activation, differentiation, and proliferation of a variety of cell types participating in the immune response. A number of these factors have been studied extensively; genes for some have been cloned. Recombinant products are undergoing clinical trials.

The most extensively characterized interleukins are interleukin-1 (IL-1) and interleukin-2 (IL-2), products primarily of macrophages and T cells, respectively. Macrophages also produce tumor necrosis factor (TNF) or cachectin. Interleukin-1 acts as an activation signal for T- and B-cell proliferation and participates in inflammatory responses as well. IL-2 is synthesized and secreted by activated helper T cells with T4 or CD4 phenotype and acts as a potent stimulator of cytotoxic/suppressor T cells, NK cells, B cells, and lymphokine-activated killer cells. Helper T cells also produce interferon-α, which has potent stimulatory effects on macrophages and NK cells.

The effect of malnutrition on synthesis and secretion of interleukins is not well defined. A significant decrease in IL-1 activity was observed following in vitro stimulation of macrophages from children with severe malnutrition (85). In addition, macrophages from children with kwashiorkor produced a suppressor factor(s) that inhibits the proliferation of murine thymocytes. The investigators suggest that a significant impairment of macrophage function may result in suppression of cell-mediated immunity in the malnourished child. Zinc has also been shown to enhance the activation and response of thymocytes to IL-1 (86). Addition of zinc to in vitro cultures of human peripheral blood T cells (87) or murine splenic T cells (88) resulted in the induction of interferon-α and interleukin-4 (IL-4) production, respectively. The other macrophage products, cachectin and TNF (89,90), have been shown to be identical molecules based on bioactivity, on immunologic studies, and on amino acid sequence homology (91–93). Increased serum cachectin levels have been reported in human patients with gram-negative septic shock (94), parasitism, and severe malnutrition (95,96). Cachectin also appears to play an important role in the pathogenesis of the cerebral form of murine malaria (97,98) and in the early stages of graft-versus-host disease (99).

Earlier studies suggested that severe malnutrition has a markedly suppressive and long-lasting effect on cell-mediated immunity, as reflected by defective T-cell function. Since T cells play a central role in the regulation of the duration and the magnitude of the immune response, one can expect a wide-ranging effect on different cell types participating in a protective immune response (100). One study suggests that cell-mediated immunity may remain depressed for several years in small for gestation, low birth weight infants (101). Paradoxically, overnutrition or obesity can also result in variable impairment of cell-mediated immune responses (102,103). Although there is little information available describing the relationship between IL-2 levels and human malnutrition, a single-nutrient deficiency, such as vitamin A (104,105), or iron (106), has been shown to result in decreased T-cell proliferation and IL-2 production in animals. Murthy et al. (104) evaluated the effect of vitamin A deficiency in rats with regard to T-cell numbers and function. A decrease in the absolute number and percentage of T cells was observed, primarily reflecting the helper T-cell subset, which in turn resulted in altered helper/suppressor T cell ratio. Furthermore, T cells from vitamin A–deficient rats had a significantly decreased proliferative response to PHA and produced significantly decreased levels of IL-2 when compared with pair-fed and normal control rats. These observations have been extended to in vitro studies by Murthy et al. (107). Rat splenic T cells cultured with PHA, or a combination of PHA and various concentrations of retinoic acid, were evaluated for proliferative response and IL-2 production by the T cells. Retinoic acid enhanced the level of PHA-induced T-cell proliferation and IL-2 production. Severe iron deficiency in mice resulted in a decreased proliferative response of T-cell to mitogens, such as concanavalin A, as well as suppressed levels of IL-2 production. Mild to moderate iron deficiency, on the other hand, does not appear to affect IL-2 production (106).

These observations suggest that synthesis and secretion of various interleukins produced by macrophages and T cells may be adversely affected by single-nutrient deficiencies. Severe PEM and/or deficiencies of essential vitamins and minerals are most likely to result in defective T-cell functions and, in turn, in a poor cell-mediated immune response to infections and vaccines.

One must also consider the possibility that certain factors such as α_1-globulin and C-reactive protein, which are elevated in response to infection (66), may interfere with in vivo and in vitro cell-mediated immune response in malnourished children. All these influences may play roles of varying importance in the depressed cell-mediated immunity, which often improves long before the malnourished child has completely recovered nutritionally (80).

The Humoral Immune Response

The B lymphocyte is responsible for immunoglobulin production. Determining if the humoral immune system has been altered is accomplished by measuring various aspects of the humoral system, such as serum immunoglobulins, secretory immunoglobulins, the number of circulating B cells, and the antibody response to antigens.

In malnutrition, the number of B cells and the circulating immunoglobulin levels are normal or elevated (108). These levels may be secondary to either a depressed suppressor T-cell population or an increased exposure to various antigens (108). Although there are normal or increased levels of circulating immunoglobulins and B cells, one cannot assume competency of the humoral immune response to foreign antigens. Antibody response to antigens appears to vary, depending on the specific antigen, in malnourished children. Antibody response to antigens such as yellow fever (109) and typhoid vaccines (110), for example, is markedly impaired, whereas the response to measles, polio virus, tetanus, and diphtheria toxoid antigens is adequate (111). There is also a decreased affinity of antibodies to tetanus toxoid and an increased incidence of circulating immune complexes (112,113). The response to an antigenic stimulus constitutes a much more sensitive and reliable evaluation of the humoral immune system than does the level of circulating immunoglobulins. Although malnourished children have normal or elevated immunoglobulins, the fact that their antibody responses to several vaccines are depressed suggests that nutritional status does affect the humoral immune system.

The increased incidence of respiratory and gastrointestinal (GI) tract infections common to malnourished children may reflect a deficient secretory IgA system. A significant decrease in secretory IgA (sIgA) and secretory component levels associated with malnutrition has been reported (114,115). Appropriate renutrition results in restoration of sIgA to normal levels. It is significant that, as the malnourished child's nutritional status improves, his antibody response to certain antigens also improves.

Polymorphonuclear Leukocyte Response

The polymorphonuclear (PMN) leukocyte, which is important in controlling bacterial infections, derives its energy for the phagocytosis and killing of bacteria from glycolysis. Malnourished and normally nourished children have the same total white cell count and the same proportion of PMNs. In malnourished children, however, there is impairment of leukocyte metabolism (116) that affects the activity of key enzymes needed for the completion of bactericidal action of the leukocyte (117). There is, however, no defect in the phagocytosing ability of PMNs in the malnourished child, although the glycolytic phagocytosing ability of PMN as judged by lactate production is impaired (118,119). There is also no apparent abnormality either in vacuole formation or in degranulation after phagocytosis by PMNs (120). Studies of bactericidal activity of PMNs have produced conflicting results (121,122). The PMNs in malnourished children respond appropriately to dermal injury, are able to phagocytose bacteria adequately, and are able to kill bacteria adequately in the majority of patients. The PMN appears to be the least-affected component of the immune system in PEM.

Complement System

Defects in the complement system have been associated with increased susceptibility to bacterial infection. Activation of the complement system leads to production of complement fragments that are involved in viral neutralization, chemotaxis of PMN leukocytes, monocytes, eosinophils, opsonization of fungi, endotoxin inactivation, lysis of virus-infected cells, and bacteriolysis (123). Coovadia and his colleagues (124) were the first to report reduced hemolytic activity in the serum of children with PEM. Many of the children they studied had C3 and C4 on the surface of the red blood cell as a result of activation of the complement system. Other investigators have found decreased complement values for malnourished children compared with those for well-nourished controls (125,126). Suskind et al. (127) found that the hemolytic complement activity of children with malnutrition was significantly depressed, with a significant percentage of the children having anticomplementary activity in their serum. With recovery, the hemolytic activity of the patients' serum improved and the anticomplementary activity disappeared. In addition, about 40% of children had, at the time of admission, circulating endotoxin which disappeared with treatment (128).

The increased morbidity-mortality associated with infection and malnutrition is most likely a result of the effect of malnutrition on the immune response. Malnourished children also have an increased susceptibility to infectious agents. It is well established that this increased susceptibility to infection is secondary to the effect of severe PEM on the cell-mediated immune system, humoral immune system, and complement system, and is reversed with improvement in nutritional status. Studies also confirm that the PMN leukocyte system is relatively intact. In order to combat potentially lethal infections in undernourished children, both antibiotic and nutritional therapy are essential.

TREATMENT OF THE MALNOURISHED CHILD

Diagnostic Studies

It is important to document the deficiencies that are present in the newly admitted, severely malnourished, child. These may include any one or a combination of deficits, including deficits of protein, energy, vitamins, and minerals. Since nearly all seriously malnourished children are infected, it is essential to determine the site, etiologic agent, and antibiotic sensitivities to all identified pathogens. In addition to a thorough history and physical examination, each child requires a complete blood count and cultures of nasopharynx, throat, ear exudate, blood, urine (by suprapubic aspiration), and stool. Cerebrospinal fluid is obtained when clinically indicated. An electrocardiogram and chest film are routine. Serum electrolytes are measured on admission and throughout recovery. Plasma vitamin A and E levels and the plasma proteins, including serum albumin, should be measured on admission.

The prevalence of infection in malnourished children is significant (129). Of greatest concern is the septic patient with a life-threatening infection. Signs that have been helpful in diagnosing the septic patient include hypothermia (rectal temperature, <36°C), hypotension (blood pressure, <60/40), leukocytosis with a marked shift to the left, petechiae, and a positive blood culture.

Fluid and Electrolyte Therapy

Children with PEM have a significant increase in total body water. Active and passive transport of sodium and potassium is severely affected in malnourished children (130). Normally, the patient presents with normal or low serum Na^+, low K^+, low Mg^{2+}, and trace minerals (131). The use of Mg^{2+} in the treatment of children with PEM is based on the work of Caddell et al. in Thailand (132) and in East and West Africa (133).

The initial rehydrating fluid is ½ N saline/5% glucose or a 1:2:3 solution of lactate/normal saline/glucose, with 50 ml of 50% dextrose/water (D/W) added to each 500 ml of either solution to make a 10% glucose solution. This solution supplies 75 mEq of Na^+ per liter. Patients showing evidence of severe K^+ depletion may be given up to 6 to 7 mEq/kg of K^+ through oral supplementation. The intravenous solution may contain up to 40 mEq/l of K^+.

Although these children have an increase in their total body water, they often show evidence of intravascular dehydration. This is especially true of children with a history of severe diarrhea. If there is evidence of intravascular dehydration, the water deficit is replaced in the first 8 to 12 hr of therapy. This means that a 5-kg child who is 10% dehydrated receives a total of 500 ml of fluid over the first 8 to 12 hr of treatment. A severely dehydrated child may receive as much as 20 ml/kg of intravenous solution (2% of body weight) during the first hour of therapy to increase his intravascular volume and therefore his renal blood flow. B-complex vitamins are given parenterally for the first several days of hospitalization (Table 1).

Initial rehydration is followed by maintenance intravenous therapy using ¼ N saline/5% glucose or 1:2:6 lactate/normal saline/glucose solution with 50 ml of 50% D/W added to each 500 ml until oral therapy is initiated. Because of the marked decrease in total body K^+, the patient is given supplemental intravenous and oral K^+ at a maintenance dose of 5 mEq/kg daily. Magnesium is given at a dose of 0.4 mEq/kg intramuscularly for 7 days followed by oral Mg^{2+} in dosage of 1.4 mEq/kg/day. Once a patient has reached an oral intake of 175 kilocalories (Cal) and 4 g/kg/day of protein, his requirement for Mg^{2+} at doses of 1.4 mEq/kg/day and K^+ at 5 mEq/kg/day is met by the formula alone. No further oral supplementation is usually required.

Dietary Therapy

During the famine in Ethiopia, Lindtjorn (134) found that although malnutrition did not increase the incidence of diarrheal disease, nutritional rehabilitation reduced the problem of diarrhea and led to a decreased mortality. When diarrhea is severe, oral intake may be withheld for up to 24 hr. Hypoglycemia is lessened when the intravenous infusion includes 10% D/W. After the first 24 to 48 hr, patients may be placed on gradually increasing protein and energy intakes. Graham et al. (135), Waterlow (136), and others have demonstrated that the ultimate dietary intake required for optimum recovery from PEM is 175 Cal and 3 to 4 g/kg/day of protein. Fjeld et al. (137) have suggested a method, using doubly labeled water, in which energy for maintenance, activity, tissue synthesis, and storage are measured in patients to predict energy requirements necessary to achieve catch-up. Dietary intake is initiated at 50 Cal/kg and 1 g/kg of protein.

Children with PEM who are offered ad libitum solid food and formula reach an intake of 160 to 180 Cal/kg and 4 g/kg of protein by the second week of hospital treatment. This intake is maintained until the children have attained optimum weight-for-height, when energy intake falls to 110 to 120 Cal/kg. Monitored care is essential until a patient has reached at least 90% of weight-for-height.

In early stages of PEM, feeding is more efficiently accomplished via a milk-based formula given by tube. Formulas supplemented with dextromaltose and corn oil do not seem to result in the prolonged diarrhea associated with lactose or monosaccharide intolerance. Formulas should also contain appropriate supplementation of essential vitamins and minerals (Table 1).

It is important to consider iron supplementation. Lynch et al. (138) have shown that iron absorption in PEM is decreased. Without supplementation, the decreased bone marrow iron stores seen in PEM patients on admission disappear completely within 4 to 6 weeks. Intramuscular iron produces an immediate increase in bone marrow stores. Because of the poor absorption of oral iron in PEM, parenteral iron or high doses of oral iron in the range of 6 mg/kg/day of elemental iron is recommended. Iron therapy should be initiated, how-

TABLE 1. *Diet composition*

Macronutrient composition of formula (per kg body weight)

Energy (Cal)	Protein (g)	Fat (g)	Carbohydrate (g)
175	4	9.5	18.3

Vitamin supplementation

Vitamin	Unit	Daily initial therapy IM or IV for 3 days beginning on day 2	Daily maintenance therapy from the 5th day until the end of week 10
Thiamine	(mg)	5.0	0.7
Riboflavin	(mg)	5.0	1.0
Pyridoxine	(mg)	2.5	1.0
Nicotinamide	(mg)	37.5	11.0
Pantothenate	(mg)	5	5.0
Ascorbic acid	(mg)	200	45.0
Folic acid	(mg)	1.5	0.1
Vitamin B_{12}	(μg)	7.5	5.0
Vitamin A	(IU)[a]	5,000	2,500
Vitamin D	(IU)[a]	400	400
Vitamin E	(IU)	50	10
Vitamin K	(μg)[a]	300	100

Mineral requirements/day (formula plus supplement)

Mineral	Unit	Dose
Sodium (Na)	mEq/kg	2–3
Potassium (K)	mEq/kg	5
Magnesium (Mg)	mEq/kg	1.4
Zinc (Zn)	mg/kg	1–2.0
Iron (Fe)	mg/kg	6.0
Calcium (Ca)	mg	800.0
Phosphorus (P)	mg	800.0
Fluorine (F)	mg	0.5–1.5
Manganese (Mn)	mg	1.0–1.5
Copper (Cu)	mg	1.0–1.5
Molybdenum (Mo)	mg	0.05–0.1
Chromium (Cr)	mg	0.02–0.08
Selenium (Se)	mg	0.02–0.08
Iodine (I)	mg	0.07

[a] Therapeutic doses of the fat-soluble vitamins are given as indicated to combat overt deficiency disease.

ever, only when the patient is on antibiotics and/or when the threat of infection has passed, usually after about 1 to 2 weeks of hospitalization.

Zinc supplementation should also be considered. Investigators in Chile found that 2 mg/kg of elemental zinc as zinc acetate given to marasmic infants had significant positive effects on weight gain and host defense mechanisms (139). Investigators in Bangladesh have also found zinc supplementation to be important in the recovery of malnourished children (140,141).

In addition to nutritional supplementation, several investigators have found that psychostimulation improves developmental catch-up in malnourished children (24,142,143).

Antibiotic Therapy

Because several of the host defenses against infection are affected in PEM, survival is dependent on the immediate identification and treatment of infection. The use of antibiotics is associated with decreased morbidity and mortality in PEM, especially in the septic child (Table 2). For septic children, a regimen of ampicillin and gentamicin, or a cephalosporin, is standard. Gentamicin is often used because of the common occurrence of *Pseudomonas* sepsis.

Two drugs may be used for intestinal antisepsis against aerobic and anaerobic organisms (Table 2). They are considered because of the occurrence of small bowel overgrowth (129). The GI tract is one of the major sources of endotoxin production and an increased incidence of endotoxemia has been described in children with protein-energy malnutrition (144). If the GI tract is sterilized, a potential source of gram-negative sepsis and endotoxic shock may be eliminated for the few days needed to regenerate an intact GI mucosa. Gastrointestinal antisepsis plus one broad-spectrum antibiotic is considerably less expensive than the traditional systemic antibiotics used for 7 to 10 days.

LONG-TERM CONSEQUENCES OF PEM

Growth

Children who survive malnutrition are generally stunted (3,145). In one squatter colony in Cape Town, South Africa, 47.2% of preschool children were below the 3rd percentile for height-for-age—significant evidence of chronic malnutrition (2). An estimated 32% to 52% of preschool Ethiopian children in Sudanese refugee camps were less than 80% of reference standards for height and weight (12). The mortality rate for these children was 22 per 10,000 per day.

The severity of the effects of malnutrition is correlated with the age of onset and duration; the most profound damage results when the period of deprivation occurs during the first 2 years of life (146–150). Korean children who were adopted in the United States before 2 years of age had better catch-up than those adopted later (151). Animal studies confirm the negative effects of early and prolonged nutritional deprivation (152,153). In addition, there is some indication that this influence may begin as early as the first weeks after birth (154).

As increasing numbers of children survive episodes of malnutrition, investigators have attempted to ascertain the potential for improving or reversing the deleterious effects (152,155). Results of these studies generally indicate that, even under optimal circumstances, "catch-up", that is, attaining the growth and development of children who have not had early nutritional deprivation, is never complete. Malnourished rats demonstrated limited catch-up in height and weight when compared with controls (156). Prolonged malnutrition in pigs during the suckling period produced long-term stunting even when rehabilitation included *ad libitum* food intake (153). In Hyderabad, India, previously malnourished boys who were studied through adulthood demonstrated significant stunting of ultimate stature (157). In addition, the severity of their stunting was proportional to

TABLE 2. *Antibiotics used in treating the malnourished child*

Indications	Antibiotic	Dose (mg/kg · day)
Pneumonia or otitis media	Ampicillin	50–100
	Penicillin	50–100
	Bactrim (TMP-SMZ)	8–10 mg/k TMP
Staph pneumonia	Oxacillin	100–200
Genitourinary infection	Ampicillin	100
	Gantrisin	150–200
Sepsis	Systemic antibiotics	
	Ampicillin and	200–300
	Gentamycin, or	3–7.5
	Cefuroxime, or	75–150
	Ceftriaxone	50–100
Gastrointestinal antisepsis	Colistin (for aerobic organisms)	5–10
	Flagyl (for anaerobic organisms)	35–50

the severity of the childhood malnutrition. The 240 malnourished Korean orphans adopted in the United States surpassed the standards of Korean children but were still significantly shorter and weighed less than well-nourished controls (151). Bone age, an indicator of height potential, is also affected. Delayed bone maturation was seen in 17 of 20 kwashiorkor patients studied by Belli et al. (158). Alvear et al. (149) also correlated bone age to nutritional status. All studies on catch-up in humans do not reach the same conclusions, but these differences may well reflect differences in study design (159,160).

Although ultimate catch-up is usually limited, recovering malnourished children often have accelerated growth compared to healthy controls (161). In northern Thailand, infants between 6 and 18 months fed a high-protein diet grew at or above reference standards in height and weight, although they were not able to attain complete catch-up for age (162).

The onset of puberty is also affected as a result of early malnutrition (163). Cameron et al. (164) found that boys who had experienced kwashiorkor had significant delays to all pubertal stages. Galler et al. (161) reported that girls with histories of marasmus had significant delays in the onset of menarche compared to healthy controls.

Development

Less easily measurable, but perhaps more important, is the effect of early malnutrition on psychological and behavioral development. Head circumference, because of its relationship to brain development, is an important growth parameter. Househam and de Villiers (165) performed computed tomography on the brain of eight kwashiorkor patients 4 years of age and under and found severe cerebral atrophy in all children. Stoch and Smythe (166), studying the effects of early malnutrition on intellectual development, reported that previously malnourished children were not able to catch up in head circumference. They concluded that since there was little growth in head circumference after 10 years of age, that this effect was likely to be permanent. Chase and Martin (147) reported that a malnourished child who began renourishment at 5 months of age achieved the 50th percentile in height and weight after 3 years of age, but remained below the 3rd percentile in head circumference. A study of 150 preterm and full-term infants also found that catch-up growth of head circumference lagged behind that of height (167). Graham and Adrianzen (168), on the other hand, found that head circumference paralleled the increase in stature in 13 malnourished Peruvian children.

Investigators have attempted to ascertain the extent of the effect of malnutrition on intellectual development (166,169–171). Grantham-McGregor et al. (150) reported that the developmental delays found in severely malnourished children were associated with stunting, indicating a relationship with chronic deprivation rather than acute malnutrition. Agarwal et al. (172), using the Wechsler Intelligence Scale for Indian Children and a series of Piagetian tasks, demonstrated a relationship between cognitive development and malnutrition in 1,300 children between 6 and 8 years of age that was not influenced by other environmental factors. Galler et al. (169,170,173) found a significant impact of early malnutrition on later intellectual performance, fine motor skills, and classroom attention.

There is evidence, however, that by adding psychostimulation to a dietary rehabilitative program, the prognosis of these children greatly improves (24,142,143). In addition, Carughi et al. (174) found, in studies on rats, that stimulation during nutritional rehabilitation enhanced dendritic branching and thickness of the occipital cortex.

SUMMARY

Prognosis for the child with severe protein-energy malnutrition is optimal with hospital treatment. Careful clinical and laboratory diagnosis must be complemented by an adequate hospital stay. Considerations include careful diagnosis of the type of deficiency disease, the extent of fluid and electrolyte imbalance, and the kind, site, and antibiotic sensitivity of existing infection(s). When the malnutrition is secondary to another disease state, consideration must be given to the impact of the disease state and its therapy on nutritional status as well as on nutritional interventions.

Immediate management of malnutrition includes fluid and electrolyte therapy, nutritional support and antibiotic therapy. Ultimately, nutritional intake should provide at least 175 Cal/kg/day and 4 g protein/kg/day, plus appropriate vitamin and mineral supplementation. The problem of sepsis must be combated with vigorous antibiotic therapy.

Because of its relationship to eventual prognosis, it is important to recognize the prevalence of malnutrition secondary to other disease states. For most of the world's children, however, the main cause of malnutrition is poverty and deprivation. Some of these children suffer severely enough to be hospitalized, but the majority survive with critical physical and developmental stunting. Improving the mortality from malnutrition is, of course, an important objective. It is, however, the long-term ramifications of malnutrition, especially those that may prevent a child from developing intellectually and behaviorally, that accentuate the need for innovative and creative solutions to this critical problem.

REFERENCES

1. U.S. Agency for International Development. *Child survival: a third report to congress on the USAID program.* Washington, DC: 1987;19–20.
2. Hugo-Hamman CT, Kibel MA, Michie CA, Yach D. Nutrition status of pre-school children in a Cape Town Township. *S Afr Med J* 1987;72:353–355.
3. Bagenholm G, Nasher AA, Kristiansson B. Stunting and tissue depletion in Yemeni Children. *Eur J Clin Nutr* 1990;44:425–433.
4. Leichsenring M, Doehring-Schwerdtfeger E, Bremer HJ, et al. Investigation of the nutritional state of children in a Congolese village. I. Anthropometrical data, plasma prealbumin, albumin, immunoglobulins, ferritin, C-reactive protein, circulating immune complexes. *Eur J Pediatr* 1988;148:155–158.
5. Coulter JB, Omer MI, Suliman GI, et al. Protein-energy malnutrition in northern Sudan: prevalence, socio-economic factors and family background. *Ann Trop Paediatr* 1988;8:96–102.
6. Victora CG, Barros FC, Vaughan JP, et al. Birthweight, socioeconomic status and growth of Brazilian infants. *Ann Hum Biol* 1987;14:49–57.
7. Brown KH, Solomons NW. Nutritional problems of developing countries. *Infect Dis Clin North Am* 1991;5:297–317.
8. Lindtjorn B. Famine in southern Ethiopia 1985-6: population structure, nutritional state, and incidence of death among children. *Br Med J* 1990;301:1123–1127.
9. Gillam SJ. Mortality risk factors in acute protein-energy malnutrition. *Trop Doct* 1989;19:82–85.
10. Lima M, Figueira F, Ebrahim GJ. Malnutrition among children of adolescent mothers in a squatter community of Recife, Brazil. *J Trop Pediatr* 1990;36:14–19.
11. Lindtjorn B. Famine in Ethiopia 1983-1985: kwashiorkor and marasmus in four regions. *Ann Trop Paediatr* 1987;7:1–5.
12. Shears P, Berry AM, Murphy R, Nabil MA. Epidemiological assessment of the health and nutrition of Ethiopian refugees in emergency camps in Sudan, 1985. *Br Med J (Clin Res)* 1987;295:314–318.
13. Avery ME, Rotch TM. The care of infants and children. *Acta Paediatr Hung* 1991;31:149–158.
14. Fuchs GJ. Secondary malnutrition in children. In: Suskind R, Lewinter-Suskind L, eds. *The malnourished child.* Nestlé Nutrition Workshop Series, vol 19. New York: Raven Press, 1990;23–36.
15. Sallon S, Deckelbaum RJ, Schmid II, et al. Cyptosporidium, malnutrition, and chronic diarrhea in children. *Am J Dis Child* 1988;142:312–315.
16. Warrier RP, Kuvibidila S, Wulfe K, et al. Nutritional evaluation of children with hemophilia. *Clin Res* 1988;36:62A.
17. Smith DE, Stevens MC, Booth IW. Malnutrition at diagnosis of malignancy in childhood: common but mostly missed. *Eur J Pediatr* 1991;150:318–322.
18. Gayle HD, Dibley MJ, Marks JAS, Trowbridge FL. Malnutrition in the first two years of life. The contribution of low birth weight to population estimates in the United States. *Am J Dis Child* 1987;14:531–534.
19. Karp RJ, Scholl TO, Decker E, Ebert E. Growth of abused children. Contrasted with the non-abused in an urban poor community. *Clin Pediatr (Phila)* 1989;28:317–320.
20. Keusch G. Malnutrition, infection, and immune function. In: Suskind R, Lewinter-Suskind L, eds. *The malnourished child.* Nestlé Nutrition Workshop Series, vol 19. New York: Raven Press, 1990;37–59.
21. Monqueberg F. Treatment of the malnourished child. In: Suskind R, Lewinter-Suskind L, eds. *The malnourished child.* Nestlé Nutrition Workshop Series, vol 19. New York: Raven Press, 1990;339–358.
22. Soekirman. Prevention of protein-energy malnutrition through socioeconomic development and community participation. In: Suskind R, Lewinter-Suskind L, eds. *The malnourished child.* Nestlé Nutrition Workshop Series, vol 19. New York: Raven Press, 1990;359–370.
23. Conclusions: proposed areas of research during the next decade. In: Suskind R, Lewinter-Suskind L, eds. *The malnourished child.* Nestlé Nutrition Workshop Series, vol 19. New York: Raven Press, 1990;395–400.
24. Super CM, Herrera MG, Mora JO. Long-term effects of food supplementation and psychosocial intervention on the physical growth of Colombian infants at risk of malnutrition. *Child Dev* 1990;61:29–49.
25. Rivera JA, Habicht JP, Robson DS. Effect of supplementary feeding on recovery from mild to moderate wasting in preschool children. *Am J Clin Nutr* 1991;54:62–68.
26. Latham MC. Protein-energy malnutrition—its epidemiology and control. *J Environ Pathol Toxicol Oncol* 1990;10:168–180.
27. Gomez F, Galvan RR, Frenk S, et al. Mortality in second and third degree malnutrition. *J Trop Pediatr* 1956;2:77–83.
28. Habicht JP, Martorell R, Yarbrough C, et al. Height and weight standards for preschool children: how relevant are ethnic differences in growth potential? *Lancet* 1974;i:611–615.
29. Martorell R, et al. Poverty and stature in children. In: Waterlow JC, ed. *Linear growth retardation in less developed countries.* Nestlé Nutrition Workshop Series, vol 14. New York: Raven Press, 1988;57–73.
30. Waterlow JC. Observations on the natural history of stunting. In: Waterlow JC, ed. *Linear growth retardation in less developed countries.* Nestlé Nutrition Workshop Series, vol 14. New York: Raven Press, 1988;1–6.
31. Bairagi R. A comparison of five anthropometric indices for identifying factors of malnutrition. *Am J Epidemiol* 1987;126:258–267.
32. Waterlow JC. Note on the assessment and classification of protein-energy malnutrition in children. *Lancet* 1973;2:87–89.
33. Anderson MA, Gopaldes T, Abbi R, Gujral S. Agreement between arm circumference, weight for age and weight for height measures of malnutrition in children. *Indian Pediatr* 1990;27:247–254.
34. Ross DA, Taylor N, Hayes R, McLean M. Measuring malnutrition in famines: are weight-for-height and arm circumference interchangeable? *Int J Epidemiol* 1990;19:636–645.
35. Keet MP, Hansen JDL, Truswell AS. Are skinfold measurements of value in the assessment of suboptimal nutrition in young children? *Pediatrics* 1970;45:965–972.
36. Koskelo EK, Kivisaari LM, Saarinen UM, Siimes MA. Quantitation of muscles and fat by ultrasonography: a useful method in the assessment of malnutrition in children. *Acta Paediatr Scand* 1991;80:682–687.
37. Gardner LI, Amacher P. *Endocrine aspects of malnutrition: marasmus, kwashiorkor and psychosocial deprivation.* Kroc Foundation symposia number 1. California: The Kroc Foundation, 1973.
38. Ramos Galván R, Miranda Calderon J. Deaths among children with third degree malnutrition; influence of the clinical type of the condition. *Am J Clin Nutr* 1965;16:351–355.
39. Garrow JS, Pike MC. The short term prognosis of severe primary infantile malnutrition. *Br J Nutr* 1967;21:155–165.
40. Waterlow JC, Cravioto J, Stephen JML. Protein malnutrition in man. *Adv Protein Chem* 1960;15:131–238.
41. Kahn E, Falcke HC. Syndrome simulating encephalitis affecting children recovering from malnutrition (kwashiorkor). *J Pediatr* 1956;49:37–45.
42. Gopalan C. Kwashiorkor and marasmus: evolution and distinguishing features. In: McCance RA, Widdowson EM, eds. *Calorie deficiencies and protein deficiencies.* Boston: Little, Brown, 1968;49–58.
43. Keusch GT. Malnutrition, infection, and immune function. In: Suskind RM, Lewinter-Suskind L, eds. *The malnourished child.* Nestlé Nutrition Workshop Series, vol 19. New York: Raven Press, 1989;37–60.
44. Scrimshaw NS, Behar M. Protein malnutrition in young children. *Science* 1961;133:2039–2047.
45. Scrimshaw NS, Taylor CE, Gordon JE. Interaction of nutrition and infection. *World Health Organization Monograph Series*, No. 57, 1968.

46. Puffer RR, Serrano CV. Nutritional deficiency and mortality in childhood. *Bol Of Sanit Panam* 1973;75:1–30.
47. Coovadia HM, Parent MA, Loening WE, et al. An evaluation of factors associated with the depression of immunity in malnutrition and in measles. *Am J Clin Nutr* 1974;27:665–669.
48. Beisel WR. Malnutrition as a consequence of stress. In: Suskind RM, ed. *Malnutrition and the immune response.* New York: Raven Press, 1977;21–26.
49. Feigin RD, Klainer AS, Beisel WR, et al. Whole-blood amino acids in experimentally induced typhoid fever in man. *N Engl J Med* 1968;278:293–298.
50. Beisel WR, Cockerell GL, Janssen WA. Nutritional effects on the responsiveness of plasma acute phase reactant glycoproteins. In: Suskind RM, ed. *Malnutrition and the immune response.* New York: Raven Press, 1977;395–402.
51. Morley DC. Measles in Nigeria. *Am J Dis Child* 1962;103:230–233.
52. Alleyne GAO, Hay RW, Picou DI, et al. *Protein energy malnutrition.* London: Edward Arnold, 1977;17.
53. Warrier RP, Dole MG, Warrier J, Suskind RM. The anemia of malnutrition. In: Suskind R, Lewinter-Suskind L, eds. *The malnourished child.* Nestlé Nutrition Workshop Series, vol 19. New York: Raven Press, 1990;395–400.
54. Wickramasinghe SN, Akinyanju OO, Grange A. Ultrastructure and cell cycle distribution of bone marrow cells in protein-energy malnutrition. *Clin Lab Haematol* 1988;10:135–147.
55. Alleyne GAO, Hay RW, Picou DI, et al. Effect of infection on nutrition. In: *Protein-energy malnutrition.* Alleyne GAO, ed. London: Edward Arnold, 1977;95–96.
56. Alleyne GAO. Study on total body potassium in malnourished infants. Factors affecting potassium repletion. *Br J Nutr* 1970;24:205–212.
57. Alleyne GAO, Millward DJ, Scullard GH. Total body potassium, muscle electrolytes, and glycogen in malnourished children. *J Pediatr* 1970;76:75–81.
58. Beresford R, Neale RJ, Brooke OG. Iron absorption and pyrexia. *Lancet* 1971;1:568–572.
59. Gordon JE, Jansen AA, Ascoli W. Measles in rural Guatemala. *J Pediatr* 1965;66:779–786.
60. Leyton GB. Effects of slow starvation. *Lancet* 1946;2:73–79.
61. Vint FW. Post-mortem findings in natives of Kenya. *East Afr Med J* 1937;13:352.
62. Jambon B, Ziegler O, Maire B, et al. Thymulin (facteur thymique serique) and zinc contents of the thymus glands of malnourished children. *Am J Clin Nutr* 1988;48:335–342.
63. Golden MH, Jackson AA, Golden BE. Effect of zinc on thymus of recently malnourished children. *Lancet* 1977;2:1057–1059.
64. Chandra RK. Serum thymic hormone activity protein-energy malnutrition. *Clin Exp Immunol* 1979;38:228–230.
65. Purtillo DT, Conner DA. Fatal infections in protein-calorie malnourished children with thymolymphatic atrophy. *Arch Dis Child* 1975;50:149–152.
66. Smythe PM, Brereton-Stiles GG, Grace HJ, et al. Thymolymphatic deficiency and depression of cell-mediated immunity in protein-calorie malnutrition. *Lancet* 1971;2:939–943.
67. Mugerwa JW. The lymphoreticular system in kwashiorkor. *J Pathol* 1971;105:105–109.
68. Jayalakshmi VT, Gopalan C. Nutrition and tuberculosis. I. An epidemiological study. *Indian J Med Res* 1958;46:87–92.
69. Feldman G, Gianantonio CA. Immunologic aspects of malnutrition in children. *Medicina (Firenze)* 1972;32:1–9.
70. Work TH, Infekwunigwe A, Jelliffe DB, et al. Tropical problems in nutrition. *Ann Intern Med* 1973;79:701–711.
71. Chandra RK. Immunocompetence in undernutrition. *J Pediatr* 1972;81:1194–1200.
72. Abbassy AS, El-Din MK, Hassan AI, et al. Studies of cell-mediated immunity and allergy in protein energy malnutrition. I. Cell-mediated delayed hypersensitivity. *J Trop Med Hyg* 1974;77:13–17.
73. Law DK, Kudrick SJ, Abdou NI. Immunocompetence of patients with protein-calorie malnutrition. The effects of nutritional repletion. *Ann Intern Med* 1973;79:545–550.
74. Edelman R, Suskind R, Olson RE, Sirisinha S. Mechanisms of defective delayed cutaneous hypersensitivity in children with protein calorie malnutrition. *Lancet* 1973;1:506–509.
75. Sellmeyer E, Bhettay E, Truswell AS, et al. Lymphocyte transformation in malnourished children. *Arch Dis Child* 1972;47:429–435.
76. Murthy PB, Rahiman MA, Tulpule PG. Lymphocyte proliferation kinetics in malnourished children measured by differential chromatoid staining. *Br J Nutr* 1982;47:445–450.
77. Beatty DW, Dowdle EB. The effects of kwashiorkor serum on lymphocyte transformation *in vitro*. *Clin Exp Immunol* 1978;32:134–143.
78. Salimonu LS, Johnson AO, Williams AI, et al. The occurrence and properties of E-rosette inhibitory substance in the sera of malnourished children. *Clin Exp Immunol* 1982;47:626–634.
79. Chandra RK, Bhujwala MA. Elevated serum alpha-fetoprotein and impaired immune response in malnutrition. *Int Arch Allergy Appl Immunol* 1977;53:180–185.
80. Kulapongs P, Suskind R, Vithayasai V, Olson RE. In vitro cell-mediated immune response in Thai children with protein-calorie malnutrition. In: Suskind RM, ed. *Malnutrition and the immune response.* New York: Raven Press, 1977;99–104.
81. Chandra RK. T and B lymphocyte subpopulations and leukocyte terminal deoxynucleotidyl-transferase in energy-protein undernutrition. *Acta Paediatr Scand* 1979;68:842–845.
82. Keusch GT, Cruz JR, Torun B, et al. Immature circulating lymphocytes in severely malnourished Guatemalan children. *J Pediatr Gastroenterol Nutr* 1987;6:265–270.
83. Ritz J, Schmidt RE, Michan J, et al. Characterization of functional surface structures on human natural killer cells. *Adv Immunol* 1988;42:181–211.
84. Salimonu LS, Johnson AO, Laditan AA, et al. Depressed natural killer cell activity in children with protein-calorie malnutrition. II. Correction of the impaired activity after nutritional recovery. *Cell Immunol* 1983;82:210–215.
85. Bhaskaram P, Sivakumar B. Interleukin-1 in malnutrition. *Arch Dis Child* 1986;61:182–185.
86. Winchurch RA. Activation of thymocyte responses to interleukin-1 by zinc. *Clin Immunol Immunopathol* 1988;47:174–180.
87. Salas M, Kirchner H. Induction of interferon gamma in human leukocyte cultures stimulated by Zn^{2+}. *Clin Immunol Immunopathol* 1987;45:139–142.
88. Winchurch RA, Togo J, Adler WH. Supplemental zinc (Zn^{2+}) restores antibody formation in cultures of aged spleen cells. II. Effects on mediator production. *Eur J Immunol* 1987;17:127–132.
89. Kawakami M, Cerami A. Studies of endotoxin-induced decrease in lipoprotein lipase activity. *J Exp Med* 1981;154:631–648.
90. Craswell EA, Old LJ, Kassel RL, et al. An endotoxin-induced serum factor that causes necrosis of tumors. *Proc Natl Acad Sci USA* 1975;72:3666–3670.
91. Beutler B, Mahoney J, LeTrang N, et al. Purification of cachectin, a lipoprotein lipase-suppressing hormone secreted by endotoxin-induced RAW 264.7 cells. *J Exp Med* 1985;161:984–995.
92. Pennica D, Hayflick JS, Pzringman TS, et al. Cloning and expression in *Escherichia coli* of the cDNA for murine tumor necrosis factor. *Proc Natl Acad Sci USA* 1985;82:6060–6064.
93. Caput D, Beutler B, Hartog K, et al. Identification of a common nucleotide sequence in the 3′-untranslated region of mRNA molecules specifying inflammatory mediators. *Proc Natl Acad Sci USA* 1986;83:1670–1674.
94. Waage A, Halstensen A, Espevik T. Association between tumor necrosis factor in serum and fatal outcome in patients with meningococcal disease. *Lancet* 1987;1:335.
95. Scuderi P, Lam KS, Ryan KJ, et al. Raised serum levels of tumor necrosis factor in parasitic infections. *Lancet* 1986;2:1364–1366.
96. Cerami A, Ikeda Y, LeTrang N, et al. Weight loss associated with an endotoxin-induced mediator from peritoneal macrophages: the role of cachectin (tumor necrosis factor). *Immunol Lett* 1985;11:173–175.
97. Clark IA, Cowden WB, Butcher GA, Hunt NH. Possible roles of tumor necrosis factor in the pathology of malaria. *Am J Pathol* 1987;129:192–199.
98. Grau GE, Fajardo LF, Piguet PF, et al. Tumor necrosis factor

cachectin as an essential mediator in murine cerebral malaria. *Science* 1987;237:1210–1212.
99. Piguet PF, Grau G, Allet B, Bassalli P. Tumor necrosis factor/cachectin has an effect on skin and gut lesions of the acute phase of graft-vs-host disease. *Immunobiology* 1987;175:27–38.
100. Chandra RK. Interactions of nutrition, infection and immune response. Immunocompetence in nutritional deficiency, methodological considerations and intervention strategies. *Acta Paediatr Scand* 1979;68:137–144.
101. Xanthou M. Immunologic deficiencies in small-for-dates neonates. *Acta Paediatr Scand* 1985;319:143–149.
102. Chandra RK, Kutty KM. Immunocompetence in obesity. *Acta Paediatr Scand* 1980;69:25–30.
103. Chandra RK. Immune response in overnutrition. *Cancer Res* 1981;41:3795–3801.
104. Murthy KK, Suskind SA L, Venkatash V, et al. Decreased T lymphocyte function and interleukin-2 production associated with vitamin A deficiency (abstract and resumé). 6th International Congress of Immunology 1986;86.
105. Murthy KK, Suskind RM. Vitamin A deficiency and T-lymphocyte function (abstract). 11th Clinical Congress, ASPEN, New Orleans 1987;339.
106. Kuvibidila S, Murthy KK, Suskind RM. Alteration of interleukin-2 production in iron deficiency anemia. *J Nutr Immunol* 1992;1:81–98.
107. Murthy KK, Bhandaru S, Pethe S, Sharina S. Effect of vitamin A analogs on interleukin-2 production by splenic T-lymphocytes. (Unpublished.)
108. Suskind RM, Sirisinha S, Edelman R, et al. Immunoglobulins and antibody response in Thai children with protein calorie malnutrition. In: Suskind RM, ed. *Malnutrition and the immune response.* New York: Raven Press, 1977;185–190.
109. Brown RE, Katz M. Failure of antibody production to yellow fever vaccine in children with kwashiorkor. *Trop Geogr Med* 1966;19:125–128.
110. Jose DG, Welch JS, Doherty RL. Humoral and cellular immune responses to streptococci, influenza and other antigens in Australian Aboriginal school children. *Aust Paediatr J* 1970;6:192–202.
111. Brown RE, Katz M. Antigenic stimulation in undernourished children. *East Afr Med J* 1965;42:221–232.
112. Chandra RK, Chandra S, Gupta S. Antibody affinity and immune complexes after immunization with tetanus toxoid in protein-energy malnutrition. *Am J Clin Nutr* 1984;40:131–134.
113. Spurr GB, Reina JC, Barac-Nieto M. Marginal malnutrition in school-aged Colombian boys: anthropometry. *Am J Clin Nutr* 1984;39:452–459.
114. Sirisinha S, Suskind R, Edelman R, et al. Secretory and serum IgA in children with protein-calorie malnutrition. *Pediatrics* 1975;55:166–170.
115. Watson RR, McMurray DN, Martin P, Reyes MA. Effect of age, malnutrition and renutrition on free secretory component and IgA in secretions. *Am J Clin Nutr* 1985;42:281–288.
116. Selvaraj RJ, Bhat KS. Metabolic and bactericidal activities of leukocytes in protein-calorie malnutrition. *Am J Clin Nutr* 1972;25:166–174.
117. Selvaraj RJ, Bhat KS. Phagocytosis and leukocyte enzymes in protein-calorie malnutrition. *Biochem J* 1972;127:255–259.
118. Yosida T, Metcoffe J. Intermediary metabolites and adenine nucleotides in leukocytes of children with protein-calorie malnutrition. *Nature* 1967;214:525–526.
119. Seth V, Chandra RK. Opsonic activity, phagocytosis, and bactericidal capacity of polymorphs in undernutrition. *Arch Dis Child* 1972;47:282–284.
120. Douglas SD, Schopfer K. The phagocyte in protein-calorie malnutrition—a review. In: Suskind RM, ed. *Malnutrition and the immune response.* New York: Raven Press, 1977;231–243.
121. Patrick J, Golden M. Leukocyte electrolytes and sodium transport in protein energy malnutrition. *Am J Clin Nutr* 1977;30:1478–1481.
122. Tuck R, Burke V, Gracey M, et al. Defective *Candida* killing in childhood malnutrition. *Arch Dis Child* 1979;54:445–447.
123. Sirisinha S, Suskind R, Edelman R, et al. The complement system in protein-calorie malnutrition—a review. In: Suskind RM, ed. *Malnutrition and the immune response.* New York: Raven Press, 1977;309–320.
124. Coovadia HM, Parent MA, Loaning WE, et al. An evaluation of factors associated with the depression of immunity in malnutrition and in measles. *Am J Clin Nutr* 1974;27:665–669.
125. Neumann CG, Lawlor GJ, Stiehm ER, et al. Immunologic responses in malnourished children. *Am J Clin Nutr* 1975;28:89–104.
126. Sirisinha S, Edelman R, Suskind R, et al. Complement and C3-proactivator levels in children with protein-calorie malnutrition and effect of dietary treatment. *Lancet* 1973;1:1016–1020.
127. Suskind R, Edelman R, Kulapongs P, et al. Complement activity in children with protein-calorie malnutrition. *Am J Clin Nutr* 1976;29:1089–1092.
128. Klein K, Suskind RM, Kulapongs P, et al. Endotoxemia, a possible cause of decreased complement activity in malnourished children. In: Suskind RM, ed. *Malnutrition and the immune response.* New York: Raven Press, 1977;321–328.
129. Suskind R. The in-patient and out-patient treatment of the child with severe protein-calorie malnutrition. In: Olson RE, ed. *Protein-calorie malnutrition.* New York: Academic Press, 1975;403–410.
130. Willis JS, Golden MH. Active and passive transport of sodium and potassium ions in erythrocytes of severely malnourished Jamaican children. *Eur J Clin Nutr* 1988;42:635–645.
131. Garrow JS, Smith R, Ward EE. *Electrolyte metabolism in severe infantile malnutrition.* Oxford: Pergamon, 1968.
132. Caddell JL, Suskind R, Sillup H, Olson RE. Parenteral magnesium load evaluation of malnourished Thai children. *J Pediatr* 1973;83:129–135.
133. Caddell JL, Goddard DR. Studies in protein-calorie malnutrition. I. Chemical evidence for magnesium deficiency. *N Engl J Med* 1967;276:533–555.
134. Lindtjorn B. Famine in southern Ethiopia 1985–1986. Malnutrition, diarrhoea and death. *Trop Geogr Med* 1990;42:365–369.
135. Graham GG, Cordano A, Baertl JM. Studies on infantile malnutrition. II. Effect of protein and calorie intake on weight gain. *J Nutr* 1963;81:249–254.
136. Waterlow JC. The rate of recovery of malnourished infants in relation to the protein and calorie levels of the diet. *J Trop Pediatr* 1961;7:16–22.
137. Fjeld CR, Schoeller DA, Brown KH. A new model for predicting energy requirements of children during catch-up growth using doubly labeled water. *Pediatr Res* 1989;25:503–508.
138. Lynch SR, Becker D, Seftel H, et al. Iron absorption in kwashiorkor. *Am J Clin Nutr* 1970;23:792–797.
139. Castillo-Duran C, Heresi G, Fisburg M, Uauy R. Controlled trial of zinc supplementation during recovery from malnutrition: effects on growth and immune function. *Am J Clin Nutr* 1987;45:602–608.
140. Khanum S, Alam AN, Anwar I, et al. Effect of zinc supplementation on the dietary intake and weight gain of Bangladeshi children recovering from protein-energy malnutrition. *Eur J Clin Nutr* 1988;42:709–714.
141. Simmer K, Khanum S, Carlsson L, Thompson RP. Nutritional rehabilitation in Bangladesh—the importance of zinc. *Am J Clin Nutr* 1988;47:1036–1040.
142. Grantham-McGregor S, Shofield W, Powell C. Development of severely malnourished children who received psychosocial stimulation: six-year follow-up. *Pediatrics* 1987;79:247–254.
143. Puentes-Rojos R, Winter-Elizalde A, Mateluna-Garate E et al. Intensive psychosensorial stimulation of malnourished children. I. Effects on psychomotor development and physical growth. *Bol Med Hosp Infant Mex* 1989;46:308–315.
144. Klein K, Fuchs GJ, Kulapongs P, et al. Endotoxemia in protein-energy malnutrition. *J Pediatr Gastoenterol Nutr* 1988;7:225–228.
145. Keller W, Filmore CM. Prevalence of protein-energy malnutrition. *World Health Stat Q* 1983;36:129–166.
146. Waterlow JC. Observations on the natural history of stunting. In: Waterlow JC, ed. *Linear growth retardation in less developed countries.* Nestlé Nutrition Workshop Series, vol 14. New York: Raven Press, 1988;1–6.

147. Chase H, Martin P. Undernutrition and child development. *N Engl J Med* 1970;282(17):933–939.
148. Briers PJ, Hoorweg J, Stanfield JP. The long-term effects of protein energy malnutrition in early childhood on bone age, bone cortical thickness and height. *Acta Paediatr Scand* 1975;64:853–858.
149. Alvear J, Artaza C, Vial M, et al. Physical growth and bone age of survivors of protein energy malnutrition. *Arch Dis Child* 1986;61:257–262.
150. Grantham-McGregor S, Powell C, Fletcher P. Stunting, severe malnutrition and mental development in young children. *Eur J Clin Nutr* 1989;43:403–409.
151. Lien NM, Meyer KK, Winick M. Early malnutrition and "late" adoption: a study of their effects on the development of Korean orphans adopted into American families. *Am J Clin Nutr* 1977;30:1734–1739.
152. Eberhardt J, Halas S. Developmental delays in offspring of rats undernourished or zinc deprived during lactation. *Physiol Behav* 1987;41:309–314.
153. Widdowson EM. Changes in pigs due to undernutrition before birth, and for one, two, and three years afterwards, and the effects of rehabilitation. In: Roche AF, Falkner F, eds. *Nutrition and malnutrition, identification and measurement.* New York: Plenum Press, 1974;165–181.
154. Lucas A. Does early diet program future outcome? *Acta Paediatr Scand Suppl* 1990;365:58–67.
155. Alleyne GAO, et al. The effects of protein energy malnutrition on growth. In: Alleyne GAO, ed. *Protein energy malnutrition.* London: Edward Arnold, 1977;124–126.
156. Smart JL, Massey RF, Nash SC, et al. Effects of early-life undernutrition in artificially reared rats: subsequent body and organ growth. *Br J Nutr* 1987;58:245–255.
157. Satyanarayana K, Prasanna-Krishna T, Narasinga-Rao BS. Effect of early childhood undernutrition and child labour on growth and adult nutritional status of rural Indian boys around Hyderabad. *Hum Clin Nutr* 1985;40C:131–139.
158. Belli L, Andreatta M, Reggiori A, Tragni C. Evaluation of bone age in patients with kwashiorkor. *Radiol Med (Torino)* 1990;79:568–570.
159. Waterlow JC, Buzina R, Keller W, et al. The presentation and use of height and weight data for comparing the nutritional status of groups of children under the age of 10 years. *Bull WHO* 1977;55:489–498.
160. Sutphen L. Growth as a measure of nutritional status. *J Pediatr Gastroenterol Nutr* 1985;4:169–181.
161. Galler JR, Ramsey FC, Salt P, et al. Long-term effects of early kwashiorkor compared with marasmus. I. Physical growth and sexual maturation. *J Pediatr Gastroenterol Nutr* 1987;6:841–846.
162. Lewinter-Suskind L. Study on the effects of high protein supplement diets on children in northern Thailand. International Conference on Nutrition, Chiang Mai, Thailand, 1974.
163. Kulin HE, Bwibo N, Mutie D, Santner SJ. The effect of chronic childhood malnutrition on pubertal growth and development. *Am J Clin Nutr* 1982;36:527–536.
164. Cameron N, Mitchell J, Meyer X, et al. Secondary sexual development of Cape coloured boys following kwashiorkor. *Ann Hum Biol* 1990;17:217–228.
165. Househam KC, de Villiers JF. Computed tomography in severe protein energy malnutrition. *Arch Dis Child* 1987;62:589–592.
166. Stoch MB, Smythe PM. Does undernutrition during infancy inhibit brain growth and subsequent intellectual development? *Arch Dis Child* 1963;38:546–552.
167. Brandt I. Growth in head circumference: parent-child correlation and secular trend. (German). *Arztl Jugendkd* 1990;81:321–326.
168. Graham GG, Adrianzen B. Growth, inheritance and environment. *Pediatr Res* 1971;5:691–697.
169. Galler JR, Ramsey FC, Forde V, et al. Long-term effects of early kwashiorkor compared with marasmus. II. Intellectual performance. *J Pediatr Gastroenterol Nutr* 1987;6:847–854.
170. Galler JR, Ramsey FC, Salt P, Archer E. Long-term effects of early kwashiorkor compared with marasmus. III. Fine motor skills. *J Pediatr Gastroenterol Nutr* 1987;6:855–859.
171. Grantham-McGregor SM. Malnutrition, mental function, and development. In: Suskind R, Lewinter-Suskind L, eds. *The malnourished child.* Nestlé Nutrition Workshop Series, vol 19. New York: Raven Press, 1990;197–212.
172. Agarwal D, Upedhyay SK, Agarwal KN. Influence of malnutrition on cognitive development assessed by Piagetian tasks. *Acta Paediatr Scand* 1989;78:115–122.
173. Galler JR, Ramsey FC, Morley DS et al. The long-term effects of early kwashiorkor compared with marasmus. IV. Performance on the national high school entrance examination. *Pediatr Res* 1990;28:253–259.
174. Carughi A, Carpenter KJ, Diamond MC. Effect of environmental enrichment during nutritional rehabilitation on body growth, blood parameters and cerebral cortical development of rats. *J Nutr* 1989;119:2005–2016.

CHAPTER 12

Malnutrition and the Immune Response

Ricardo U. Sorensen, Lily E. Leiva, and Solo Kuvibidila

HOST DEFENSE MECHANISMS

Despite the outstanding progress made during this century in food science and technology, malnutrition still affects millions of children in the world. The association between malnutrition and infectious morbidity/mortality has been recognized for many decades. Evidence for the role of malnutrition in the impairment of the immune defense, however, has accumulated only in recent years. Understanding host defense mechanisms and their interaction is important for understanding their derangement in patients with malnutrition.

Host defense mechanisms include nonspecific and specific mechanisms. Nonspecific mechanisms include the complement system and the phagocytic system. These two mechanisms develop independently of the presence of infections, and are not specific for given infectious agents. Specific mechanisms include antibody-mediated immunity and cell-mediated immunity. These host defenses mature independently of antigen stimulation. They become fully functional, however, only after interaction with an infectious agent. The relative importance and efficiency of these defense mechanisms against different infectious agents is summarized in Table 1.

The interaction of these different mechanisms of defense to prevent or clear infections is depicted in Fig. 1. The first mechanism that clears microorganisms breaking the epithelial surface integrity is phagocytosis by polymorphonuclear (PMN) and mononuclear (MO) phagocytes (monocytes and macrophages). In the initial absence of antibodies, bacterial surface polysaccharides activate the alternative pathway of complement resulting in the attachment of C3b. C3b, in turn, activates the membrane attack components of complement (C5 to C9) which will lyse susceptible bacteria. For resistant, encapsulated bacteria, C3b provides the necessary opsonization for PMN and MO phagocytosis. Furthermore, complement-derived factors will open the vascular bed and attract additional phagocytic cells to the site of infection. Minor bacterial infections are terminated by these mechanisms without causing disease. These subclinical infections may be sufficient, however, to trigger the development of protective antibodies and/or cell-mediated immunity. Viruses generally do not activate the alternative pathway of complement and will always cause disease in the unimmunized host. Only after specific immunity develops is the viral infection terminated and protective immunity established.

Specific immunity develops after presentation of antigenic microbial components by antigen-presenting cells, usually MOs, to T and B lymphocytes. B lymphocytes have small amounts of immunoglobulins on their surface which serve as antigen receptors. The interaction of bacterial antigen with selected B cell clones triggers proliferation and differentiation into plasma cells, cells which secrete large amounts of specific antibodies. These antibodies attach to the remaining bacteria producing further opsonization for PMN and MO phagocytosis. Furthermore, IgM and IgG activate complement through the classic pathway, leading to lysis of susceptible bacteria and opsonization by C3b. Three to six days after the initial infection, the nonspecific host defenses are directed and amplified by specific antibodies and normally terminate any extracellular bacterial infections that survived the early, nonspecific clearance mechanisms. If infections are not effectively cleared, the continued activation of phagocytic cells may cause tissue damage through the release of oxygen radicals, proteases, and other inflammatory mediators.

Cell-mediated immunity plays an important role against intracellular pathogens, which are able to survive within host cells. In response to stimulation by bacterial antigens, helper T cells (CD4$^+$ cells) proliferate and se-

---

R. U. Sorensen, L. E. Leiva, S. Kuvibidila: Department of Pediatrics, Louisiana State University School of Medicine, New Orleans, Louisiana 70112.

TABLE 1. *Host defense mechanisms effective against different infectious agents*

Extracellular bacteria and viruses
Complement, antibodies, phagocytosis
Intracellular bacteria, fungi, and parasites
T lymphocytes (lymphokines), monocytes and macrophages
Intracellular viruses
Natural killer cells, cytotoxic T cells
Toxins
Antibodies

TABLE 2. *Functional classification of immunodeficiencies according to the host defense mechanism affected*

Complement deficiencies
Single complement deficiencies
Multiple complement deficiencies
Inhibitor deficiencies
Deficiencies of phagocytosis
Chemotaxis abnormalities
Adherence abnormalities
Ingestion abnormalities
Intracellular killing abnormalities
T-cell deficiencies
Lymphopenia; decreased helper T cells and/or suppressor T cells
Abnormal proliferation
Abnormal lymphokine secretion
Antibody deficiencies
Decreased immunoglobulin(s)
Decreased specific antibodies with normal or elevated total immunoglobulins
Combined cellular and antibody deficiencies

crete lymphokines, e.g., interferon-γ, which activates MO phagocytes. MO activation by T lymphocyte products is an essential step in clearing the intracellular pathogens that have resisted killing by nonactivated MO phagocytes. However, MO activation may also lead to the release of inflammatory mediators and tumor necrosis factor, which in excess have a detrimental effect on the host. Upon interaction with antigens, T suppressor cells ($CD8^+$ cells) develop into cytotoxic cells capable of killing virally infected cells in absence of opsonizing antibody. This helps terminate a viral infection since it exposes viruses liberated by lysed cells to the action of antibodies, complement, and phagocytic cells.

Enhanced susceptibility to infectious disease occurs in hosts with anatomic, metabolic, or immunologic abnormalities. Undernutrition is the cause of various immunologic abnormalities and these immunodeficiencies themselves affect specific host defense mechanisms (Table 2) (1). Understanding the molecular basis through which nutritional abnormalities may cause immunodeficiencies or contribute to increased inflammation is enhanced when the specific pathways of maturation of immune cells and activation of immunity and inflammation are understood.

T and B Cell Maturation Pathways

Both T and B lymphocytes have a common precursor in the bone marrow. T cells undergo further antigen-independent development in the thymus gland and B cells differentiate in the fetal liver, spleen, and in the bone marrow of adult mammals. The immense T cell antigen receptor diversity and the B cell immunoglobulin diversity, which are the bases of specificity, are generated through rearrangement of variable gene segments (2).

The maturation of immature T cells (thymocytes) into $CD4^+$ and $CD8^+$ effector cells occurs within the thymus under the influence of thymic hormones and self major histocompatibility antigens, which positively select non–self-reacting lymphocytes (3,4). Zinc is an essential cofactor of the hormone thymulin. A deficiency of this trace element negatively impacts on T cell maturation.

The first identifiable B cells are found in the fetal liver. They are characterized by the presence of immunoglobulin heavy chains in the cytoplasm without a light-chain component. Subsequent differentiation gives rise to immature B cells. These cells synthesize complete surface IgM molecules. As they proliferate, some of their progeny begin to produce other surface immunoglobulin classes on their membranes including IgD, IgG, and IgA (5). This maturation process occurs in the absence of

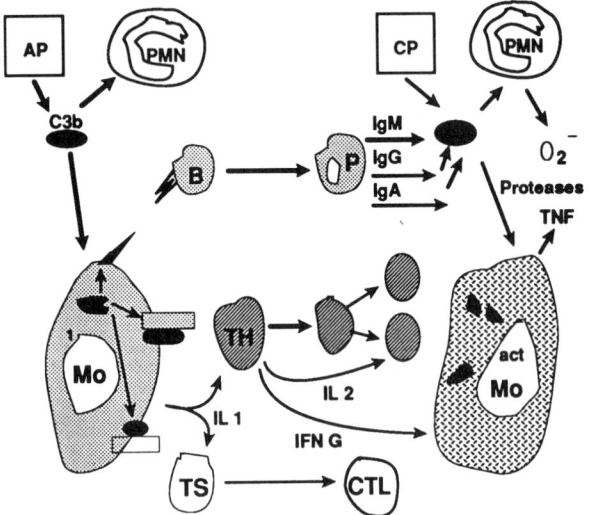

FIG. 1. Interaction of host defense mechanisms. AP, alternative pathway of complement activation; CP, classic pathway of complement activation; C3b, a fragment of the third complement component; PMN, polymorphonuclear cell; Mo, monocyte/macrophage; B, B lymphocyte; TH, helper T cell; TS, suppressor T cell; IL, interleukin; IFN G, interferon gamma; CTL, cytotoxic T lymphocyte; Ig, immunoglobulins; TNF, tumor necrosis factor. See text for further explanation.

antigen and appears to be resistant to the effect of malnutrition.

Lymphocyte Activation Pathways

T Lymphocytes

T lymphocytes can be activated to produce lymphokines, to express new cell surface molecules, and to proliferate through ligand-receptor interactions occurring at the plasma membrane (6). The T-cell receptor (TCR) on most mature T cells is composed of two covalently linked polypeptides, designated alpha and beta, which are extremely diverse and confer antigen specificity. A group of five nonpolymorphic peptide chains, designated CD3, is associated with the alpha/beta TCR on the plasma membrane of all T cells (6). T-cell activation by antigen-presenting cells involves the ligation of the processed antigen with the TCR-CD3 complex plus CD4 (on helper cells) or CD8 (on cytotoxic cells), and presumably with other adhesion molecules.

The triggering of the T-cell antigen receptor results in hydrolysis by phospholipase of membrane phosphatidyl inositol biphosphate (PIP_2) to generate two second messengers, inositol-1,4,5-triphosphate (IP_3), which releases Ca^{2+} from intracellular stores, and diacylglycerol (DG), which activates protein kinase C. A sustained increase of intracellular Ca^{2+} from the extracellular medium also occurs and appears to be required for complete activation (6,7). In addition, a guanine nucleotide–binding protein (G protein), a member of a family of membrane proteins associated with the transduction of various signals, has been implicated in this activation process (8). These signals and biochemical events lead to the eventual transcription of lymphokine genes and subsequent production and secretion of lymphokines, some of which act as growth factors.

The generation and expression of receptors for these lymphokines are essential requirements for lymphocyte proliferation. Resting lymphocytes do not express growth-factor receptors on their surface. The induction of growth-factor receptor expression appears to require two signals, one of which is delivered by the TCR-antigen interaction and the other by interleukin-1 (IL-1), a cytokine produced by the antigen-presenting macrophages (9).

Interleukin-2 (IL-2), a growth factor for lymphocytes produced mainly by helper T cells, plays a major role in T-cell proliferation. Once released, IL-2 promotes the proliferation of any T cell expressing surface IL-2 receptors, regardless of its antigenic specificity. The specificity of the immune system is maintained, however, at the level of induction of IL-2 receptor expression. Only a small fraction of cells specific to the particular antigen introduced into the system will produce and express IL-2 receptors. The effect of IL-2 binding to its receptor causes the cell to progress from the late G1 (preparatory) phase of the cell cycle into the S (DNA replication) phase. In addition, IL-2 appears to stimulate T cells to secrete a variety of other lymphokines (10). The activated T cell will then either fulfill its role as effector cell or become a memory cell.

An important rate-limiting step in the proliferation of activated lymphocytes is the production of deoxynucleotides from ribonucleosides. This production is accomplished by the enzyme ribonucleotide reductase, a nonheme iron–containing enzyme which is decreased in iron deficiency states.

Recently, evidence has accumulated that activation pathways of different T-cell subsets may differ, thus differing as well in susceptibility to malfunction in nutritional deficiencies. Suppressor/cytotoxic T cells bind antigen in association with class I major histocompatibility complex (MHC)-encoded proteins; helper T cells bind antigen in association with class II MHC-encoded proteins (3). Helper T cells have been subdivided into two distinct subsets, designated TH1 and TH2, on the basis of the types of lymphokines they secrete (11). TH1 cells produce IL-2 and interferon (IFN)-γ but not interleukin-4 (IL-4), whereas TH2 cells produce IL-4 and interleukin-5 (IL-5) but not IFN-γ or IL-2. TH1 and TH2 clones utilize different TCR-associated signal transduction mechanisms (7). At least four regulatory phenomena appear to differentially regulate the activation of these two subsets of helper T cells (12).

Antibody Production by B Cells

Binding of an antigen to a B-cell receptor leads to cell division and differentiation of the mature B cell into a clone of antibody-producing plasma cells. The production of specific antibodies to many microbial antigens is dependent on help by $CD4^+$ helper T cells. Although immunoglobulin secretion is preserved even in severe forms of malnutrition, specific antibody production is sometimes impaired.

Inflammation and Hypersensitivity Pathways

Activation of PMNs

PMNs are the phagocytic cells of major importance during the early phase of an inflammatory response. Products present at a site of infection or inflammation such as the chemotactic peptide formyl-methionine-leucine-phenylalanine (FMLP), complement fragments, bacterial lipopolysaccharide and leukotriene B4 are known to stimulate PMN function (13). In addition, several cytokines are strong stimulators of PMN function. For example, IL-1 stimulates endothelial adhesion and PMN activity; granulocyte-monocyte colony-stimulating factor (GM-CSF) modulates PMN function; and tumor necrosis factor (TNF) induces PMN chemotaxis, phagocytosis, respiratory burst, and C3b receptor expression (13). Stimulation of PMNs releases Ca^{2+} from intracellular stores and activates protein kinase C after its translocation from the cytosol to the cell membrane. Protein kinase C plays an important role as a regulatory enzyme for PMN degranulation and activation of the respiratory burst and production of superoxide anion (14). Superoxide anion formed as a result of nicotinamide-adenine dinucleotide phosphate, reduced (NADPH) activation is converted to H_2O_2 by superoxide dismutase. The seleno-enzyme glutathione peroxidase produces oxidized glutathione which is the substrate for glutathione reductase, an enzyme necessary for the generation of NADPH. This is step sensitive to selenium deficiency, which decreases H_2O_2 production. The interaction among H_2O_2, myeloperoxidase released from primary granules, and a chloride ion produces hypochlorous acid, a potent microbicidal agent. In anaerobic environments, oxygen-independent mechanisms kill bacteria using lysozyme, lactoferrin, and cationic proteins (14).

Arachidonic Acid Metabolism

Arachidonic acid is an important source of potent inflammatory mediators including prostaglandins, thromboxane, and leukotrienes. There are two main pathways by which arachidonic acid can be metabolized: via the cyclooxygenase enzyme to form prostaglandins and thromboxanes, and via the lipoxygenase enzyme to produce leukotrienes and hydroxy acids. Leukotriene B4 has chemotactic, edema- and pain-inducing properties, and immunomodulatory properties. The cysteinyl-containing leukotrienes, LTC4, LTD4, LTE4, and LTF4, induce edema and affect vascular tone and permeability. All these mediators act on phagocytic cells by stimulating adherence to endothelial surfaces, chemotaxis, phagocytosis, and intracellular killing of bacteria (15). However, they also mediate many harmful inflammatory reactions that need to be considered in the complex interactions among nutrition, immunity, and inflammation.

INTERACTIONS BETWEEN NUTRITION AND IMMUNITY

The interactions between immunity and nutrition are manifold, affecting both host defense mechanisms and nutritional status. The immunological consequences of malnutrition involve secondary immunodeficiency, reduced clearing of infections, and sometimes increased inflammatory responses and tissue damage. The nutritional consequences of the immune response include wasting, which may be initiated by the secretion of cachectin or tumor necrosis factor (TNF).

Immunoregulatory Effects of Diet Components

There are several possible mechanisms for the regulation of immune responses by nutrients (Fig. 2). Some nutrients bind to cellular receptors and may have direct immunoregulatory functions affecting DNA replication or RNA transcription. In addition, nutrients are necessary building blocks for immune cell proliferation, differentiation, and secretion of cytokines and other mediators. Obviously, both immunity and nutrition have an equally important interaction with infections, an interaction that may trigger immune and inflammatory responses and may cause severe changes in caloric uptake and requirements.

The immunoregulatory role of diet components is exemplified by 1,25(OH)$_2$-vitamin D$_3$ which serves as an immunoregulatory hormone in addition to its classic role in mineral homeostasis (16). It inhibits DNA synthesis possibly through the inhibition of IL-2 in activated T lymphocytes (17). Concomitantly, 1,25(OH)$_2$-vitamin D$_3$ upregulates cell surface differentiation antigens such as Fc and complement receptors and human leukocyte antigens HLA-DR in myelomonocytic leukemia cells (18). Thus, vitamin D may influence the function of both key players in cellular immunity: T lymphocytes and monocyte macrophages.

The role of iron and trace metals in the composition and activity of thymic hormones (zinc) and enzymes (e.g., iron in ribonucleotide reductase, selenium in glutathione peroxidase) is another example of the regulation of immune responses by nutrients.

The Role of Tumor Necrosis Factor (TNF) in Nutrition and Immunity

Cytokines, hormone-like molecules, constitute essential transmitters of intercellular communication in inflammation, immunity and in several pathophysiologic processes. Few cytokines have been found to exert activities on cells outside the immune system. One of them, TNF, initially discovered because of its cancer-killing activity, has numerous immunologic and metabolic functions (Table 3) (19–23). Two different types of TNF have been described, TNF-α or cachectin, produced by monocyte macrophages, and TNF-β or lymphotoxin, produced by lymphocytes. Although both TNF-α and TNF-β have similar tumoricidal activities and bind to the same cell receptors, they are distinct molecules that share about 45% homology on the nucleotide level (21,23).

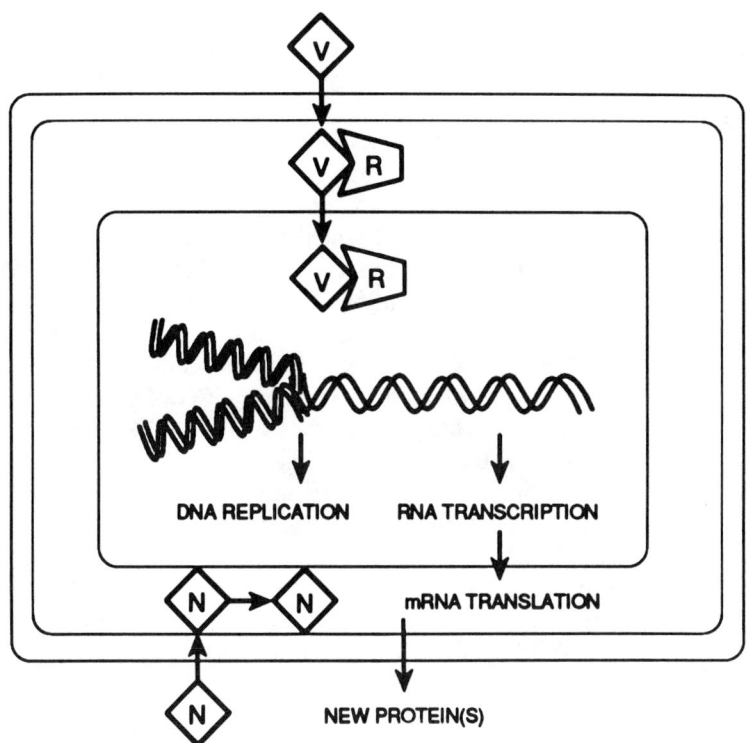

FIG. 2. Effect of nutrients on immune responses. V, vitamin (or other nutrients with immunoregulatory properties); R, cell receptor for V; N, nutrient used as a building block for products of the immune response. See text for further explanation.

In vivo production of TNF activity was originally demonstrated after endotoxin injection in animals that had been primed with BCG or other microbes. Blood from these animals induced hemorrhagic necrosis in tumors of other animals and killed cancer cells *in vitro* (19). It

TABLE 3. *Activation, metabolic, immunologic, and inflammatory activities of tumor necrosis factor (TNF)*

Inducers of TNF
  Bacterial lipopolysaccharide
  Viral infections
  Parasitic infections
Metabolic activities of TNF
  Anorexia and weight loss
  Decreased skeletal protein synthesis
  Loss of body protein content
  Decrease in albumin synthesis
  Inhibition of lipoprotein lipase
  Decrease in fatty acid biosynthesis
  Stimulation of lipolysis
  Alteration of the distribution of zinc, iron, and copper
Immunologic activities of TNF
  Increased adhesion of granulocytes to blood vessels
  Increased chemotaxis and microbiocidal activities of granulocytes
  Regulation of B and T lymphocyte activity
  Enhanced cytotoxicity against tumor cells
  Enhanced delayed-type hypersensitivity (DTH)
  Increased *in vivo* antibody responses to sheep red blood cells
Inflammatory activities of TNF
  Increased acute-phase protein production
  Excessive production of free oxygen radicals
  Excessive production of PGE_2, thromboxane B_2

was later demonstrated that high levels of TNF could not only be induced by bacterial lipopolysaccharide (LPS), but also during cancer, inflammation, and viral and parasitic infections (21,23).

The study of the role of TNF in inflammation and immunity has been facilitated by the recent availability of recombinant TNF (rTNF) and monoclonal antibodies specific to TNF. TNF starts to exert its many effects once macrophages, which also release IL-1 and colony-stimulating factors, are activated. rTNF-α stimulates the adherence of PMN phagocytes to human umbilical endothelium (24), increases complement and FMLP receptors on PMNs and enhances the production of superoxide (13,25,26). rTNF-β, on the other hand, induces phagocytosis of latex particles (27). The immunoregulatory activity of TNF has been demonstrated by its ability to augment *in vivo* antibody responses to sheep red blood cells (28), to enhance T cell–mediated responses (22,29), and to regulate the production of other cytokines (30). TNF has also been demonstrated to have antiparasitic activity (23).

In addition to its beneficial immune properties, TNF has been demonstrated to be a potent mediator of systemic metabolic changes which are potentially deleterious to the host (19,21,23,31). Among the several cytokines released during an immune response, IL-1, TNF-α, and IL-6 are the major mediators of intermediary metabolism (21,23). Certain systemic effects of the inflammatory and immune responses, for example induction of fever, anorexia, and cachexia, are attributed in part to TNF and IL-1 (19,21,32). Cachexia, a nutritionally important condition seen during uncontrolled chronic infections and in cancer patients, is characterized by a profound weight loss that results from the disappearance of fat deposits and the atrophy of muscles.

TNF and IL-1 have also been implicated in the acute-phase response, which is a reaction produced by the systemic and clinical changes induced during the early stages of an infection or after trauma (31). In addition, an increased TNF production by peripheral blood mononuclear cells *in vitro* has been reported in patients during acute starvation (33) and in patients with anorexia nervosa (34). Undoubtedly, a better understanding of the role of cytokines in general, and of TNF in particular, in the regulation of nutrition of patients with cancer and chronic infections will lead to improved nutritional management of these conditions.

IMMUNOLOGICAL ABNORMALITIES IN DIFFERENT FORMS OF MALNUTRITION

Numerous epidemiologic studies conducted in Latin America and many countries in Africa and Asia have established malnutrition as a determinant of morbidity and mortality of infection in children (35,36). It is not always easy to establish, however, whether malnutrition is the cause or the effect of the existing pathology. Diarrhea, for example, may often be the precipitating factor of malnutrition resulting, as it does, in reduced caloric intake, poor absorption of nutrients caused by alteration of the GI tract, loss of nitrogen and other essential nutrients, and increased catabolism. The deficiency of specific nutrients may, in turn, condition the type of immune deficit and the outcome of infections. In Africa, for instance, measles infection causes death in many children, especially those with malnutrition (37). However, the high mortality rate due to measles infection observed in African children may not always be explained in terms of protein-energy malnutrition (PEM) alone since malnourished Indian children do not show any greater complications of measles infection than well-nourished children (38). This leads to speculation that other factors, including genetic, environmental, as well as deficiencies of vitamins and trace elements, might also contribute to the mortality associated with measles infection in malnourished African children.

Complex Nutrient Deficiencies

Primary protein-energy malnutrition (PEM) results in either marasmus and/or kwashiorkor. Marasmus, caused by inadequate intake of calories and protein, leads to loss of body fat and muscle tissue (i.e., wasting) and, eventually, to severe linear growth retardation (i.e., stunting) (39). Biochemical indicators of malnutrition, such as total serum proteins, albumin, prealbumin (transthyrenin), transferrin, retinol-binding protein, and hemoglobin, may be in the normal range of values.

Kwashiorkor results from protein deficiency with adequate caloric intake. It often occurs in infected children where the metabolic response to TNF leads to a decreased production of such visceral proteins as albumin, transferrin, and retinol-binding protein. Children suffering from kwashiorkor, which is an acute illness, show less deficit in anthropometric measurements (height-for-age, weight-for-age, and weight-for-height) than children with marasmus. Signs of kwashiorkor include edema, skin lesions and depigmentation, hair color and texture changes, and enlarged fatty liver due to decreased levels of lipoproteins required for the transport of fatty acids in blood (39). Biochemical indicators of malnutrition as well as some enzymes (lipase, amylase) are decreased to lower levels than those found in marasmic children. Many children present the characteristics of both kwashiorkor and marasmus (marasmus-kwashiorkor).

Within the groups of children suffering from either form of PEM, the severity of malnutrition is determined by the degree of deficits in anthropometric measurements (40,41). It is likely that the different degrees of malnutrition also determine the type and severity of immunological abnormalities.

PROTEIN ENERGY MALNUTRITION (PEM)

Anatomic Barriers

Alteration of anatomic barriers such as skin and mucosal lesions found in children with kwashiorkor, favors the penetration of microorganisms in an already compromised host. Alteration of the gastrointestinal mucosa by PEM favors the invasion and colonization by pathogens. This in turn may impair the absorption of essential nutrients and lead to more alterations in the immune response.

Phagocytic System

In malnourished children circulating PMN numbers are either normal or elevated (42), whereas the bone marrow reserves are reduced (43). PMNs from malnourished children show cytologic abnormalities such as cytoplasmic vacuolization. Malnourished children have normal migration of PMN to skin abrasion sites compared to well-nourished children (42). However, in untreated children with kwashiorkor, the mobilization and migration of monocytes is significantly delayed resulting in a higher ratio of PMN/monocytes. PMN chemotaxis *in vitro* is either normal (44) or reduced (45) in infected malnourished children. Although energy production by activated PMN via the glycolytic pathway is reduced in malnutrition, phagocytosis is normal (43). Nitroblue tetrazolium (NBT) reduction, a measure of PMN NADPH oxidase activation and superoxide generation, is either normal or reduced in PEM. However, microbial killing is reduced (43,45). The reduced bactericidal capacity may be related to specific nutrient deficiencies such as iron deficiency, in addition to PEM.

The Complement System

Most studies suggest that malnutrition reduces the levels of complement components, especially C3, factor B, and total hemolytic activity (46–48). The C4 component, however, is not decreased. C3 levels are lower in kwashiorkor than in marasmus or marasmus-kwashiorkor. The reduced complement levels may be due to either increased consumption as a result of infections or to a decrease in the rate of biosynthesis. Only 1 month of renutrition leads to correction of C3 levels (48).

Cell-Mediated Immunity

The effect of PEM on the cellular immune response was first reported in 1925 (49). At autopsy, children who have died of malnutrition usually show thymus atrophy (50,51), lymphocyte depletion in the corticomedullary regions of the thymus, and depletion of lymphocytes in spleen, lymph nodes, and tonsils (50,52). The pathogenesis of lymphoid atrophy is multifactorial. It may be due to cell death, decreased rate of cell division due to lack of certain nutrients, reduced protein, RNA and DNA synthesis, an imbalance in hormones, or high levels of free cortisol (52). Malnourished children also show reduced levels of thymic hormones, such as thymulin, required for the maturation of thymocytes (51,53). The decreased thymulin levels, a hormone produced by the thymus epithelial cells, suggest that the thymic epithelium is not spared by malnutrition.

Total white blood counts (WBC) may be either normal or increased, especially in the presence of infection. Increased WBC is due to increased polymorphonuclear leukocytes but not lymphocytes. In fact, the absolute as well as relative total blood lymphocytes, helper T (CD4) cells, suppressor T cells (CD8), and the ratio of CD4/CD8 cells, are decreased in malnourished children compared to well-nourished children (54–57). The decrease in helper T cells is, in general, more important than that of suppressor T cells. Malnourished children have elevated levels of null cells, lymphocytes which are neither T nor B cells, but have a normal range of B cells (52,54). Nutritional rehabilitation for a few weeks restores normal T cell number and T4/T8 ratio.

Malnourished children usually show a poor or reduced skin response *in vivo* to antigens and other sensitizing agents (delayed type hypersensitivity, DTH). Skin response to antigens is a complex process that involves different types of cells including T lymphocytes, macrophages, polymorphonuclear neutrophils, and basophils. In order for an adequate inflammatory process to take place, circulating lymphocytes must be sensitized against the foreign antigen and become memory cells. When these cells make contact with the same antigen, as in the tuberculin test, they become activated and release soluble mediators that attract different cell types to the sensitized site. The activation of these cells results in the inflammatory response. Impairment in skin response to antigens may therefore be the result of a defect in either T cell sensitization, lymphokine production, or migration of different cells to the skin. DTH to antigens like tuberculin, candida, diphtheria, and tetanus toxoids is a measure of the hosts immunological memory and the capability of generating an inflammatory response. DTH to sensitizing agents and mitogens such as dinitrochlorobenzene (DNCB) and phytohemagglutinin (PHA) measures the ability of the host to process and respond nonspecifically to a new activator of cell-mediated immunity. DTH to antigens is reduced in children with PEM (48,58). Skin responses to DNCB and PHA are also decreased (58). This implies that both the recall immunological responses and responses to new antigens are impaired by malnutrition.

Lymphocytes from malnourished children show a reduced proliferative response to mitogens and antigens *in vitro* (54,55,59). The reasons for impaired lymphocyte proliferative responses to mitogens and antigens are multifactorial, including reduced proportions of immunocompetent T cells in blood cell preparations and an increase in the proportion of null cells that have been shown to be inhibitory for lymphocyte proliferation (52,54–57). Other factors that may contribute to impaired lymphocyte proliferation are high levels of cortisol sometimes found in sera from malnourished children (52) and decreased production of IL-1 by macrophages (60,61).

There are conflicting reports on the secretion of lymphokines in PEM. Gamma-interferon has been found to be either reduced (62) or unaltered (37). Single nutrient deficiencies such as zinc, iron, folic acid, and vitamin A may also contribute to these differences.

Antibody-Mediated Immunity

In contrast to cell-mediated immunity, antibody-mediated immunity is generally unaltered by PEM and single nutrient deficiencies. The absolute and relative (percent) circulating B cell numbers are within normal range (55,59). Immunoglobulin levels are either normal (63) or slightly elevated, especially in infected malnourished children (46). Rarely, slightly decreased immunoglobulin levels have been reported (64). Unaltered specific antibody production to diphtheria and tetanus toxoids (46), and pneumococcal polysaccharides and keyhole-limpet hemocyanin (58) have also been documented in PEM.

Secretory IgA, required for the protection of mucosal cells from infections and parasites, is decreased in malnourished children (65,66). Reduced levels of IgA in tears and saliva, but increased levels of IgG in tears, have been reported in malnourished Colombian children (67). Malnutrition does not seem to affect lysozyme and aminopeptidase activity in serum, tears, and saliva.

Serum IgE levels are usually high in malnutrition. This may be due to the increased incidence of intestinal parasites and/or to deficient T cell control of IgE production. As in intestinal parasitoses, high IgE levels in malnutrition are not associated with increased allergic manifestations (64).

Children with PEM usually have multiple nutritional deficiencies including vitamin A, iron, and zinc deficiency. These deficiencies as well as concomitant infections are known to alter the immune response. To determine the effects of either protein or caloric deficiency on the immune response, several investigators have utilized laboratory animals (mice, rats, guinea pigs, rabbits) that have received synthetic diets. The synthetic diets given were adequate in all nutrients except protein and/or calories. These studies confirm the deleterious effects of PEM on absolute and/or relative numbers of splenic T lymphocytes, skin responses to DNCB, lymphocyte proliferation, IL-2 production (68–70), and specific antibody production in response to rotavirus infection (71). In certain strains of mice such as C3H/He, reduced dietary protein has been shown to enhance splenic lymphocyte proliferation (72).

SINGLE NUTRIENT DEFICIENCIES

Vitamin A

Besides the well established role of vitamin A for vision, vitamin A deficiency in humans and laboratory animals is known to affect reproduction, growth and development, and mucus secreting cells, and to increase susceptibility to bacterial, viral, and parasitic infections (73–75). The increased susceptibility to infections is related to the function of vitamin A on differentiation of lymphocytes and hence lymphocyte functions. The effect of vitamin A deficiency on the immune responses in humans has been difficult to evaluate due, in part, to the rarity of pure vitamin A deficiency. Some studies have suggested low percentages of circulating T lymphocytes and reduced skin response to PHA, and a normal *in vitro* proliferative response of T cells to PHA (76,77).

The role of vitamin A deficiency in the immune response is corroborated in animal studies. In rats, vitamin A deficiency depletes thymocytes from the thymus cortex and reduces the number of germinal centers in the spleen (78–80) but has no effect on the biological activity of thymulin (79). Splenic lymphocytes from vitamin A–deficient rats show poor proliferative responses to all doses of concanavalin A (ConA), PHA, and LPS (78–81) as well as reduced IL-2 production (82,83). However, mesenteric lymph node lymphocytes have significantly increased (67%) proliferative responses compared to pairfed and *ad libitum* control animals (84), suggesting relocation of immunocompetent T lymphocytes as the principal cause of immune abnormalities in vitamin A deficiency. Splenic lymphocyte proliferative responses return to normal after *in vitro* or after 3 days of *in vivo* repletion of vitamin A in deficient animals (80). Antibody responses to sheep red cells, pneumococcal polysaccharides, and diphtheria and tetanus toxoids are also impaired in these animals (80,83).

Vitamin E

Vitamin E is an antioxidant considered very useful in retarding or preventing aging and certain degenerative diseases by maintaining a normal cell membrane structure and composition. Its metabolism is closely related to that of selenium. Vitamin E deficiency in humans is rare except in premature infants and elderly patients. Both these population groups have many other nutrient deficiencies, as well as abnormalities, in the immune system per se.

Most vitamin E studies on immunity have involved patients who were not necessarily vitamin E–deficient. In elderly subjects (>60 years old), administration of 800 IU of vitamin E once per day for 30 days increased the cumulative score of skin response to a battery of antigens, the proliferative response of blood lymphocytes to PHA, and the production of IL-2. The helper T cell number, immunoglobulin levels, and IL-1 production were not affected (85).

In rats, vitamin E deficiency reduces spleen cell proliferation in response to ConA (86) but increases natural killer (NK) cell activity (87). The mechanisms by which vitamin E deficiency increases NK activity is probably related to an *in vivo* activation by free radicals generated in the absence of the antioxidant. High doses of vitamin E in mice increase antibody responses to sheep red blood cells, tetanus toxoid, and resistance to infectious challenge (88).

Vitamin B_6 (Pyridoxine)

Pyridoxal-5-phosphate, the active form of vitamin B_6, is a coenzyme required for the metabolism of amino acids involving decarboxylation, transamination, and desulfuration, and for the metabolism of lipids and nucleic acids. Pyridoxine deficiency in humans, although fairly common, is usually found in combination with deficiencies of other B-complex vitamins such as riboflavin and/or PEM. In guinea pigs, the number of blood lymphocytes is decreased, whereas the number of neutrophils is increased (88). In rats, vitamin B_6 deficiency induces thymus and spleen atrophy, decreased spleen lymphocyte proliferation in response to PHA, and decreased antibody responses to sheep red blood cells (89).

Vitamin C (Ascorbic Acid)

Severe vitamin C deficiency, or scurvy, manifested by bleeding gums, is rare. Subclinical deficiency, however, is not uncommon, even in industrialized, wealthy countries (90). Severe vitamin C deficiency in humans has no significant detrimental effects on lymphocyte numbers and proliferative responses (91). Ingestion of large doses of ascorbic acid (1 to 3 g/day) does, however, significantly enhances PHA-induced lymphocyte proliferation by two- to threefold above pretreatment levels (92).

In guinea pigs, vitamin C deficiency is known to prolong skin allograft survival (93) and to impair cell-mediated cytotoxicity (94), DTH to tuberculin, and the bactericidal capacity of neutrophils against *Actinomyces viscosus* (95). Antibody-mediated immunity is not altered by vitamin C deficiency.

Folic Acid Deficiency

Folic acid is required for the biosynthesis of nucleic acids by serving as a methyl group carrier. Folic acid deficiency is very common in humans, especially children and pregnant women. It is second only to iron deficiency as a cause of nutritional anemia. Folic acid deficiency, as well as the rare vitamin B_{12} deficiency, impair iron metabolism or iron incorporation into heme. In pregnant women, folic acid deficiency impairs skin response to DNCB and lymphocyte proliferation, both of which return to normal after folate therapy (96). Folic acid deficiency in humans does not affect phagocytosis and bactericidal capacity of neutrophils for *Staphylococcus aureus,* whereas vitamin B_{12} reduces these functions (88). In rats, folic acid deficiency reduces spleen weight, T cell numbers in the thymus and blood, splenic lymphocyte response to PHA, and cytotoxic T cell activity (88).

Iron Deficiency

Iron deficiency is one of the most common nutritional disorders in humans, affecting 10% to 20% of the world population. The deficiency predominantly affects children and women of the childbearing age. In nutritional surveys, iron deficiency is usually identified by anemia. However, serum ferritin levels, transferrin saturation and erythrocyte protoporphyrin identify increasing degrees of iron deficiency that precede the onset of iron deficiency anemia (97).

Iron is essential for the activity of enzymes required for DNA synthesis and for intracellular killing mechanisms of phagocytes.

Iron-deficient children have been found to have reduced absolute blood lymphocyte counts, decreased absolute and relative T lymphocytes counts, and decreased lymphocyte proliferative responses to T cell mitogens and several antigens (98–101). Most studies have found a defect in cell-mediated immunity in iron-deficient patients (102). Although phagocytosis is generally unimpaired, bactericidal capacity of neutrophils is severely reduced (103). Following iron replacement without modification of other nutrient intake, the impaired functions are usually corrected within 3 months (100,103).

Circulating B lymphocytes, immunoglobulin levels, antibody responses to tetanus and diphtheria toxoids, and complement C3 levels are generally unaltered (104). Elevated immunoglobulin levels have been occasionally reported in infected iron-deficient children.

In humans, especially children from developing countries, the role of iron deficiency in immunologic abnormalities may be difficult to evaluate, since it is often associated with other nutritional deficiencies. This may explain the sometimes contradictory results reached in various studies. Interestingly, in the case of iron deficiency alone and iron deficiency combined with zinc deficiency, the absolute lymphocyte counts are more decreased in iron deficiency alone, whereas skin response to DNCB is more depressed in the combined deficiencies (101).

Results from animal studies in which pure iron deficiency has been induced provide evidence for the impaired cell-mediated immunity caused by or associated with iron deficiency. These studies have confirmed the following to be impaired by iron deficiency: skin response to DNCB (105), proliferative response of spleen cells to PHA, ConA, and bacterial LPS (106), proliferative responses of thymocytes to T-cell mitogens (107), natural killer cells and killer cell activity (108), cytotoxicity of T cells against allogeneic tumor cells (109), production of IL-1 (110) and IL-2 (111), antibody responses to tetanus toxoid (112), production of antibodies to sheep red blood cells *in vitro* (113,114), macrophage function (115), and neutrophil myeloperoxidase and bactericidal capacity (116).

Although the impairment of these immune responses have been attributed to reduced activity of iron-dependent and iron-containing enzymes, there is also the possibility that part of the decreased cell-mediated immunity may be due to differences in the number of immunocompetent T cells. Iron deficiency decreases the percentage of immunocompetent T cells, helper T cells, and suppressor T cells by approximately 50%. Iron repletion *in vivo* corrects the relative numbers of immunocompetent T cells, skin responses to DNCB, and lymphocyte proliferative responses. *In vitro* repletion of iron, however, does not correct impaired lymphocyte functions (106,107,117).

The iron available to immune cells may be further decreased locally during infections with bacteria-secreting siderophores. For example, the presence of certain outer-membrane proteins in cystic fibrosis isolates suggests that *Pseudomonas aeruginosa* grows under iron-restricted conditions in the lung of cystic fibrosis patients (118). Iron deprivation in turn favors selection and maintenance of mucoid *P. aeruginosa* (119) and may also lead to the secretion of specific *P. pyoverdins*, i.e., siderophores (120).

Zinc Deficiency

Zinc is a component of over 200 metalloenzymes including thymidine kinase, ribonucleic acid (RNA) polymerase, deoxyribonucleic acid (DNA) polymerase, and ribonuclease, which are required for cell division (121,122). Zinc has also been shown to be an essential cofactor for thymulin, one of the thymic hormones and a potent B-cell mitogen (123).

Zinc deficiency was first recognized in humans in 1961 (124). Today, zinc deficiency is commonly found in many diseases (122,123) including AIDS (125-128), malabsorption syndrome, chronic renal disease, cirrhosis of the liver, sickle-cell disease, acrodermatitis enteropathica (AE), and other chronically debilitating diseases. Old age, pregnancy, lactation, and alcoholism are also associated with zinc deficiency. Manifestations of chronic zinc deficiency include: growth retardation, male hypogonadism, skin changes, poor appetite, mental lethargy, and delayed wound healing, all of which are reversible with zinc supplementation. A more severe deficiency produces dermatological manifestations, diarrhea, loss of hair, mental disturbances, and intercurrent infections with opportunistic organisms (121,122).

The effect of zinc deficiency on immunity is best studied in AE, an inherited disorder of zinc absorption characterized by symmetrical mucocutaneous lesions, diarrhea, growth failure, and frequent severe infections with fungi, viruses, and bacteria. The immune system in AE is affected by lymphoid atrophy and depletion of lymphocytes.

Thymic atrophy in children with PEM and zinc deficiency has been documented by radiologic examination. Zinc supplementation increased plasma zinc levels as well as the size of the thymus. Several mechanisms for lymphoid atrophy have been postulated (129): (a) a decrease in the number of T and B cells due to reduced *in vivo* antigen-induced cellular proliferation (121,122), (b) a reduction of serum thymulin levels and the consequent impairment of T lymphocyte maturation (130,131), (c) an elevation of free-cortisol levels that may be toxic for lymphocytes (132), and (d) a possibility that zinc deficiency causes shifts in lymphocyte populations in various tissue compartments (122).

Immunological studies of AE patients have demonstrated a reduction in lymphocyte counts and in the proportion of helper T cells. Helper cell activity for both B-cell and suppressor T-cell function is also decreased (122,133). In addition, zinc deficiency impairs the ability of lymphocytes to produce antigen- and mitogen-stimulated lymphokines (134). All these immunological changes could be corrected by zinc supplementation (121,129,135-137).

There is strong evidence that the elderly are more susceptible to some infectious diseases and that this enhanced susceptibility is associated with immunologic dysfunction (138) and a high incidence of mild zinc deficiency (139-141). Immunologic dysfunction in zinc deficiency has been associated with decreased erythrocyte nucleoside phosphorylase activity (142).

Studies have demonstrated that zinc deficiency in rodents results in rapid atrophy of the thymus with preferential involution of the cortex, decreased DTH reactions, decreased cytotoxic T-killer activity and natural killer cell activity, greatly depressed antibody responses to both T-cell-dependent (TD) and T-cell-independent antigens, and reduced expression of Fc and C3b receptors on macrophages (123,129). These immunological effects of zinc deficiency have been associated with the enhanced susceptibility of deprived mice and rats to challenge with various pathogens (129).

Copper Deficiency

Copper deficiency, although rare in humans, is occasionally found in premature infants, in patients receiving total parenteral nutrition, and in patients diagnosed with Menkes's disease, a congenital X-linked copper deficiency syndrome (143). Very little information exists on cell-mediated immunity in patients with copper deficiency. The relative and absolute blood T- and B-cell numbers are either normal or in the low-normal range (144,145). The proliferative responses of lymphocytes to mitogens are either normal (145) or decreased (144). The secondary antibody response to bacteriophage oX-174 was severely decreased in one patient with copper deficiency (145). Immunoglobulins levels, antibody responses to *Salmonella typhi*, and C3 and C4 levels have been reported to be normal (144).

Animal studies have demonstrated strong evidence of the role of copper deficiency on the immune response. In mice, copper deficiency induces thymus atrophy and splenomegaly. Serum levels of thymulin hormone required for the differentiation of T lymphocytes are decreased (146). The percentages of total T cells, helper T cells, and, to a lesser extent, suppressor T cells are decreased (147,148). The proliferative responses of spleen cells to ConA, PHA and, to a lesser extent, to LPS are decreased (147). Natural killer cell cytotoxicity (149), T-dependent antibody response to keyhole-limpet hemocyanin (149), and microbicidal activity of phagocytic cells are also abnormally low in copper-deficient mice or rats. Copper deficiency increases delayed inflammatory responses (150) but does not affect prostaglandin E_2 biosynthesis. *In vitro*, copper-deficient culture medium does not alter the production of IL-1 and IL-2 by murine spleen cells (151). However, the addition of copper to the culture medium enhances murine splenic T-lymphocyte proliferation in response to ConA and PHA (152). The absolute and/or relative number of B cells in the spleen of copper-deficient animals is increased.

The mechanisms by which copper deficiency alters cell-mediated immunity are not known. A defect in iron mobilization from liver cells or to changes in composition of membrane proteins and lipids have been suggested (153). Copper is found in superoxide dismutase and may thus contribute to the detoxification of oxygen radicals.

Selenium Deficiency

Selenium (Se) is an integral part of the red blood enzyme, glutathione peroxidase, which reduces hydroperoxides and protects membrane lipids against oxidant damage. Se deficiency has been described in residents of low-soil-Se areas (154) and in patients receiving total parenteral nutrition (155,156). In animals, abnormalities have been described in all host defense components, including neutrophil function, and antibody and cell-mediated immunity (157). Further information in humans is needed to understand the possible clinical implications of these abnormalities.

NUTRITIONAL ASPECTS OF SPECIFIC INFECTIONS

Human Immunodeficiency Virus (HIV) Infection

The interactions among HIV infection, nutrition, and immunity are complex and difficult to define. Immunological abnormalities caused by the HIV infection and by malnutrition clearly overlap (Table 4).

Immunologic Changes in HIV Infection

The major pathogenic process of HIV infection includes binding of the HIV envelope glycoprotein gp 120 on the HIV to the CD4 molecule on both T cells and

TABLE 4. *Immunological abnormalities caused by HIV infection and by nutritional abnormalities which have been described in HIV infected patients*

Host defense	HIV infection	Malnutrition	
		PEM	Zinc
Cell-mediated immunity			
Thymus	?	D	D
CD4 cells	SD	D	D
CD8 cells. Suppressor cells	N	?	?
Cytotoxic cells	I	D	?
CD4/CD8 ratio	SD	D	D
Blastogenesis. Mitogens	N/D	D	D
Antigens	D	D	D
LK secretion	D	D	D
NK cells and function	D	D	D
Antibody-mediated immunity			
B lymphocytes	I	N/I	N
Serum Igs	I	N/I	N
Secretory IgA	?	D	?
Specific antibodies	D	N/D	N
Complement			
CH_{50}	?	D	?
Components C3	D	D	?
C4	D	N	?
PMN numbers	N/I/D	N/I	?
Chemotaxis	?	D	?
Killing	D	D	
Monocytes			
Activation markers (HLA II)	D	?	?
Killing	D	D	?
Tumor necrosis factor	I	N/I	?
Neopterin	I	?	?

N, normal; D, decreased; SD, severely decreased; I, increased.

monocyte/macrophages with subsequent functional impairment and ultimate destruction of the CD4+ helper T cell (158). Helper T cells play a pivotal role in the control of the immune response (158–160). Cells of the macrophage lineage are generally not destroyed but serve as a reservoir of virus. It was first believed that the elimination of CD4+ T cells *in vivo* was due to a direct cytopathic effect of the virus. However, the natural history of HIV infection suggests now that other mechanisms are also involved, and that the progression of the infection is intimately associated with the normal functioning of the immune system (161). Infection with HIV causes a gradual suppression of immunological function that leads to a diverse spectrum of opportunistic diseases.

In order to understand the possible role of nutrition in this process it is important to understand the immunological changes caused by the HIV. The hallmark of the immune defect in AIDS is a marked reduction in absolute numbers of the helper/inducer (CD4+) subset, and a relatively stable or raised number of the cytotoxic (CD8+) subset, resulting in an inverted CD4/CD8 ratio (158–160). Although reports on *in vitro* mitogen-induced lymphocyte blastogenic responses in AIDS are contradictory, responses to antigens are clearly depressed. Decreased IL-2, IL-2 receptors, and IFN-γ production have also been observed in these patients (158–160,162). Decreased antibody-dependent cellular cytotoxicity (163) and cytolytic function of NK cells are associated with disease progression. This latter abnormality can be reversed with exogenous IL-2 *in vitro* (164).

With respect to antibody-mediated immunity, polyclonal activation of B cells and elevated levels of serum immunoglobulin (particularly IgA) are common in the early stages of infection. In spite of the hypergammaglobulinemia observed in AIDS, there is a deficient antibody response to new antigens (158,160,165).

Macrophages and monocytes are generally not destroyed as a result of HIV infection. They do show a defect at the level of HLA class II expression that can impair antigen-presenting cell function. Functional abnormalities in these cells have been demonstrated by reduced chemotaxis, Fc-dependent phagocytosis, low levels of intracellular killing, and nonspecific cytotoxic and hydrogen peroxide release. Elevated levels of TNF-α have been found in the sera of AIDS patients; elevated levels of this cytokine are produced *in vitro* by monocytes from HIV-1 infected individuals. The autocrine/paracrine induction of HIV expression by TNF-α on HIV infected cells may result in the spread of HIV to uninfected cells (161). Neopterin, a metabolite of guanosine triphosphate, produced by activated macrophages, is a useful indicator of the progression of HIV infection (166–168). Neutrophils from HIV-infected patients have high levels of peroxidase activity (169). Neutrophil bactericidal activity, however, is impaired in these patients (170).

Nutritional Status of Patients with AIDS

Many patients with AIDS are wasted; the occurrence of opportunistic infections and tumors are often preceded by weight loss and asthenia. Malnutrition, which can cause a variety of immunological abnormalities similar to AIDS, may, therefore, predispose to opportunistic infections, which, in turn, cause or exacerbate AIDS (171). The clinical syndrome in AIDS usually includes anorexia, weight loss, and significant malnutrition (172–174). In children, symptomatic HIV infections are an important cause of failure to thrive (175,176). An evaluation of hemophiliac children with asymptomatic HIV infection showed that 40% were malnourished compared to 4.5% of the noninfected children with hemophilia (177). Weight loss in adults with AIDS and failure to thrive in children are probably due to the combined effects of the catabolic response to HIV infection, anorexia, fever, opportunistic infections, diarrhea, and malabsorption (178–180).

Specific nutrient deficits have also been observed in AIDS patients. Some patients have vitamin E deficiency, manifested clinically as the yellow nail syndrome, which improves with vitamin E supplementation (181,182). Zinc deficiency and acrodermatitis enteropathica have been observed in children and adults (125–128). Severely diminished plasma and red cell levels of selenium have been observed independently of malabsorption or disease duration (183). Serum iron concentrations have been found to be significantly reduced and ferritin levels to be significantly higher in AIDS patients compared to patients with persistent generalized lymphadenopathy (184). This suggests that infectious agents draw on body iron stores and that phagocytic cells, while ingesting those agents, incorporate the iron when synthesizing and releasing ferritin. Hence, the malnutrition commonly seen in HIV-infected patients may further impair their immune response. Nutritional support of the HIV-infected patient may slow the progression of the disease process stemming the usual development of AIDS and death.

Mycobacterial Infections

Nutritional factors may also play a role in the wide variability in susceptibility to tuberculosis. Vitamin D_3 deficiency has been postulated as a factor in predisposing certain ethnic groups to tuberculosis. Dark-skinned immigrants from the Indian subcontinent to the United Kingdom have serum vitamin D_3 concentrations well below, and rates of tuberculosis 20 to 30 times higher, than lighter-skinned Britons (185). *In vitro* studies have shown that the addition of 1,25(OH)$_2$-vitamin D_3 inhibits the multiplication of virulent *Mycobacterium tuberculosis* in cultured human macrophages, suggesting a connection of vitamin D_3, sunlight, and immunity to tuberculosis (186). American blacks have a higher incidence of *M. tuberculosis* infections measured by tuberculin conversion (187). However, the contribution of vitamin D_3 to this increased risk is difficult to evaluate since only 25-(OH)-vitamin D_3 is decreased in this population, and not the active metabolite, $1,25(OH)_2$-vitamin D_3 (188). Vitamin D_3 may also have a deleterious effect in tuberculosis. It has been shown to increase the release of TNF by macrophages suggesting that, at least in some individuals, vitamin D_3 may be indirectly responsible for the fever and weight loss that characterize tuberculosis (189). The particular relationship between vitamin D_3 and tuberculosis needs to be understood within population subsets to avoid enhancing the risk of increased TNF release and increased malnutrition because of inappropriate therapy.

BCG immunization is important in preventing tuberculosis in many developing nations. Two important questions are (a) How does malnutrition affect the measurement of tuberculin reactivity after BCG immunization?, and (b) Should BCG be given to children who are malnourished? Ganapathy and Chakraborty (190) found no difference in tuberculin reactivity between 1- and 9-year-old normal and malnourished Indian children. However, Colombian infants with grade I and II malnutrition immunized with BCG at birth (when they were presumably well nourished) had significantly reduced DTH to tuberculin at 8 weeks of age (191). These differences may be due to age and nutritional status differences at the time of initial exposure to mycobacterial antigens, and also to differences in selective nutrient deficiencies in different study populations.

Conflicting results have been reported from studies in which malnourished children have been immunized with BCG. Harland (192) found lower tuberculin responses in these children 4 to 6 weeks after BCG immunization when testing with a low tuberculin dose (2 TU). No differences were observed, however, with an increased dosage of 20 TU. Renutrition repaired tuberculin reactivity without the need for BCG revaccination, suggesting that antigen recognition was not defective. Ziegler and Ziegler (193) observed that immunization of children with PEM and preexisting tuberculin reactivity did not result in decreased tuberculin reactivity 9 to 11 weeks later. However, tuberculin reactivity was clearly decreased in those children with PEM who were not presensitized to tuberculin, suggesting an antigen recognition defect in children with PEM. Satyanarayana et al. (194) immunized 1- to 5-year-old Indian children with moderate to severe PEM and kwashiorkor. Only kwashiorkor patients had decreased DTH to tuberculin 6 months postimmunization. Leukocyte migration inhibition *in vitro* was normal in all groups tested. Seth et al. (195) immunized 1- to 6-year-old children and observed a lower percentage of positive tuberculin reactions in those with PEM. However, she also observed hyperergic reactions in some children with severe PEM. Normal and malnourished children had normal *in vitro* leukocyte migration inhibition (195). Kielmann et al. (46) observed a lower percentage of tuberculin positivity 235 days after BCG vaccination in PEM, but there was no difference, after 735 days, between those whose nutritional status improved and those whose weight-for-age had decreased. Patients with kwashiorkor had a greater degree of unresponsiveness than those with marasmus. Rivera et al. (196) found that tuberculin reactivity in Mexican children with PEM was determined by the degree of wasting, but not chronic undernutrition, as reflected by stunting. This implies that in chronically malnourished children who do not develop marasmus or marasmus-kwashiorkor, there is a certain degree of adaptation. In dietary protein–deficient guinea pigs, BCG immunization failed to protect against a respiratory challenge with virulent *M. tuberculosis* (197).

These results suggest that both antigen recognition and the measurement of tuberculin sensitivity *in vivo* (DTH) can be affected by malnutrition, particularly kwashiorkor. However, there is no contraindication for immunizing malnourished children with BCG. Even children with severe PEM can develop strong tuberculin reactivity *in vivo* after BCG immunization, and reactivity *in vitro* does not seem to be affected. Furthermore, renutrition improves tuberculin reactivity without need for revaccination. The critical issue of differentiating tuberculin hypersensitivity from protective immunity against mycobacterial disease has not been resolved and clearly needs further investigation.

Tuberculosis has become the leading cause for morbidity and mortality in HIV-infected individuals (198). BCG immunization is a defense against the resurgence of tuberculosis. The nutritional aspects of these two pandemics need to be considered as an integral part of any prevention and treatment strategy.

EVALUATION OF PATIENTS WITH INFECTION AND MALNUTRITION

A complete evaluation of a patient with infections should include appropriate indicators of both the nutritional status and the status of the various host defense mechanisms (Table 5). Although such evaluations are likely to be performed on obviously malnourished patients with chronic infections, they are rarely done in patients with acute infections whose nutritional status is apparently normal. The immunological and nutritional assessment of patients with acute infections is hampered by the fact that the more commonly performed tests reflect chronic rather than acute changes. For instance, a patient with a severe acute infection who is not being adequately nourished may develop selective nutrient de-

TABLE 5. *Immunologic and nutritional evaluation of patients with suspected immunodeficiency and malnutrition*

Initial evaluation	Advanced evaluation
Immunological evaluation	
Cell-mediated immunity	
CBC, lymphocyte count	Lymphocyte subpopulations
PA and lateral chest X-ray to evaluate the thymus	Blastogenic responses to antigens and mitogens
Delayed hypersensitivity	Cytokines and lymphokines
Antibody-mediated immunity	
Serum protein electrophoresis	B lymphocyte numbers
Serum immunoglobulin levels including IgG subclasses	Specific antibody responses to proteins and polysaccharides
In vitro immunoglobulin production	
Phagocytosis	
Neutrophil count and smear	Chemotaxis
	Superoxide generation
	Opsonophagocytosis
Complement	
Serum hemolytic complement	Individual components
Quantitation of C3 and C4	
Acute-phase reactants (chronic inflammation)	
C-reactive protein	Inflammatory mediators, TNF
Ceruloplasmin	
Alpha$_1$-acid-glycoprotein	
Nutritional evaluation	
Height and weight	Prealbumin
Total protein and albumin	Retinol-binding protein
Hemoglobin	Vitamin levels
Fe and ferritin	
Zn and trace elements	

ficiencies that in turn may decrease the capability of mounting a specific immune response against the offending pathogen. This relevant acute deficiency is unlikely to be reflected in the levels of circulating lymphocytes or immunoglobulins. As the techniques of molecular biology become more accessible to clinicians, our ability to understand the specific relationships among the offending infectious agent, the nutritional status, and the capability to enhance the specific host defense mechanisms required to best fight the identified pathogen will increase. Understanding the potentially noxious inflammatory response will, in addition, help us to tailor case-specific therapeutic approaches that lead to the clearance of infection without an undue increase in the detrimental aspects of the host response. This expertise is dependent on much needed basic and clinical research.

DIFFERENTIAL DIAGNOSIS

The differential diagnosis of immunological abnormalities that result from correctable nutritional deficiencies includes all primary immunodeficiency syndromes (1), immunodeficiencies caused by immunosuppressive and cytoreductive drugs, and immunodeficiencies caused by neoplasias and infectious agents, e.g., HIV (Table 6). Most tumors and infectious agents will cause immunodeficiency syndromes through changes in the nutritional status, and not through a direct immunosuppressive effect of the primary disease.

The differential diagnosis of the immunological abnormalities of severe protein-energy malnutrition and either severe combined immunodeficiency (SCID) or pediatric AIDS is complicated by the fact that both immunodeficiency syndromes may have secondary malnutrition. Some SCIDs have characteristic genetic or biochemical markers, e.g., X-linked inheritance, and adenosine deaminase or nucleoside phosphorylase deficiency, which are not seen in any form of malnutrition. In general, when there is very profound lymphopenia and absent lymphocyte blastogenic responses to mitogens, a primary immu-

TABLE 6. *Differential diagnosis of immunological abnormalities caused by nutritional deficiencies*

Cutaneous anergy with normal lymphocyte numbers
    Moderate protein energy malnutrition
    Viral infections (and some immunizations)
    Corticosteroids and immunosuppressive drugs
    Suppressor mechanisms for specific antigens
Lymphopenia, deficient lymphocyte function *in vitro*
    Severe protein energy malnutrition
    Vitamin A deficiency
    Zinc deficiency
    Severe combined immunodeficiencies
    AIDS
Secretory IgA deficiency
    Protein energy malnutrition
Specific antibody deficiency
    Protein-energy malnutrition
    Age related unresponsiveness to bacterial polysaccharides (<2 years of age)
    Primary specific antibody deficiencies?
Complement deficiencies (several components)
    Protein-energy malnutrition
    Complement deficiencies of newborns and young infants
    Complement consumption in infections, autoimmune disorders
Mild neutrophil and macrophage killing defects
    Iron deficiency
    Zinc deficiency
    Copper deficiency
    Vitamin C deficiency
    Vitamin B$_{12}$ deficiency
    Protein-energy malnutrition

nodeficiency syndrome is likely to be present. HIV infections and PEM rarely cause the profound lymphocyte unresponsiveness to mitogens seen in patients with SCID. Nutritional treatment of SCID patients does not restore lymphocyte function.

It is now possible to measure IL-2 secretion and the effect of exogenous IL-2 on lymphocyte proliferative responses. Some forms of SCID have been found to respond *in vitro* and *in vivo* to exogenous administration of IL-2 (199,200). IL-2 deficiencies seen in HIV-infected patients (201,202) and in patients with chronic infections such as leprosy and tuberculosis do not improve with exposure to *in vitro* IL-2 (203,204). It is important to establish similar data for IL-2 and other lymphokines in other forms of malnutrition and immunodeficiency syndromes in order to be able to differentiate the various forms of immunodeficiency, each of which requires a very different therapeutic approach.

NUTRITIONAL TREATMENT OF THE INFECTED AND MALNOURISHED PATIENT

Prevention of Secondary Immunodeficiencies Due to Malnutrition

Prevention of immunodeficiencies due to malnutrition is the most important goal of nutritional care. In newborns, breast-feeding significantly reduces the incidence and severity of infections (205). The decrease of gastrointestinal infections in particular has been attributed to secretory IgA and other antimicrobial components present in breast milk, which may act locally in the gastrointestinal tract of the newborn infant (206). Human milk leukocytes are also capable of producing factors that participate in cell-mediated immunity, e.g., interferon (207,208). Breast milk was found to significantly enhance spontaneous proliferation and T-cell blastogenic responses at 6 days and 6 weeks of age, suggesting a systemic effect (209). Transmission by breast milk factors of cell-mediated immunity to specific microbial antigens, e.g., tuberculin, remains controversial (210,211). However, a recent study has suggested a more vigorous cellular response to BCG in infants breast-fed at the time of immunization (212).

In healthy children, a well-balanced diet is probably adequate for the development and maintenance of host defenses after infancy. There is no evidence that amounts of any dietary component beyond daily requirements would offer additional protection to a normal individual.

Special nutritional support of patients with debilitating diseases, e.g., cystic fibrosis, cancer, or HIV infection, is essential in preventing a vicious cycle of secondary immunodeficiencies, infection, and further malnutrition.

Realimentation and Nutritional Support of Malnourished Children

Realimentation and nutritional support of malnourished children is essential. If chronic infections, e.g., giardiasis and diarrhea, are present, a vigorous effort to eliminate the infection needs to be made even if the infection is not overly symptomatic or life-threatening. Further research will help define strategies for the enhancement of specific immune responses with immunoregulatory nutrients and vitamins.

Nutritional Intervention in Patients with Ongoing Infections

This is an area where much more information is needed before clear recommendations can be made. If there is no evidence for preexisting malnutrition, the risk for exaggerating hypersensitivity and inflammation rather than protective immunity needs to be considered.

Downregulation of Undesirable Inflammatory Responses

Dietary immunoregulation promises to become an important way of regulating immune responses and decreasing exaggerated inflammatory responses. Long-chain polyunsaturated fatty acids present in fish oil have been reported to have an anti-inflammatory effect reducing leukotriene generation by neutrophils and monocytes (213), and suppressing the synthesis of IL-1 and of tumor necrosis factor (214).

Scavenging of Damaging Oxygen Radicals

Bacterial infections are potent stimulators of superoxide and hydrogen peroxide by PMN. When these radicals are not effectively detoxified by superoxide dismutase and the Se-glutathione system, they can cause damage to host cells. Vitamin E, riboflavin, vitamin B_6, zinc, copper, and selenium play a crucial role in the removal of oxygen radicals. A deficiency in these nutrients may contribute to inflammatory damage during infections in malnourished children. As our capability to diagnose selective nutrient deficiency improves, it should be possible to increase the therapeutic use of some nutrients as a way of decreasing tissue damage.

REFERENCES

1. Berger M, Sorensen RU. Immune defects associated with recurrent infections. *Adv Pediatr Infect Dis* 1989;4:111–138.
2. Tonegawa S. Somatic generation of antibody diversity. *Nature* 1983;302:575–581.

3. Marrack P, Kappler J. The T cell receptor. *Science* 1987;238:1073–1079.
4. Lafaille JJ, Haas W, Coutinho A, Tonegawa S. Positive selection of gamma-delta-T cells. *Immunol Today* 1990;11:75–78.
5. Vogler LB, Lawton AR. Ontogeny of B cells and humoral immune functions. *Clin Immunol Allergy* 1985;5:235–252.
6. Weiss A, Imboden J, Hardy K, Manger B, Terhorst C, Stobo J. The role of the T3/antigen receptor complex in T-cell activation. *Annu Rev Immunol* 1986;4:593–619.
7. Gajewski TF, Schell SR, Fitch FW. Evidence implicating utilization of different T cell receptor-associated signaling pathways by TH1 and TH2 clones. *J Immunol* 1990;144:4110–4120.
8. Gilman AG. G proteins: transducers of receptor-generated signals. *Annu Rev Biochem* 1987;56:615–645.
9. Diamantstein T, Osawa H. The interleukin-2 receptor, its physiology and a new approach to a selective immunosuppressive therapy by anti-interleukin-2 receptor monoclonal antibodies. *Immunol Rev* 1986;92:5–27.
10. Robb RJ. Interleukin 2: the molecule and its function. *Immunol Today* 1984;5:203–209.
11. Mossman TR, Coffman RL. Two types of mouse helper T-cell clone. Implications for immune regulation. *Immunol Today* 1987;8:10–14.
12. Gajewski TF, Schell SR, Nau G, Fitch FW. Regulation of T-cell activation: differences among T-cell subsets. *Immunol Rev* 1989;111:79–109.
13. Livingston DH, Appel SH, Sonnenfeld G, Malangoni MA. The effect of tumor necrosis factor-alpha and interferon-gamma on neutrophil function. *J Surg Res* 1989;46:322–326.
14. Sawyer DW, Donowitz GR, Mandell GL. Polymorphonuclear neutrophils: an effective antimicrobial force. *Rev Infect Dis* 1989;11:S1532–S1544.
15. Brain SD, Williams TJ. Leukotrienes and inflammation. *Pharmacol Ther* 1990;46:57–66.
16. Minghetti PP, Norman AW. 1,25(OH)2-Vitamin D3 receptors: gene regulation and genetic circuitry. *FASEB J* 1988;2:3043–3053.
17. Rigby WFC, Denone S, Fanger MW. Regulation of lymphokine production and human T lymphocyte activation by 1,25 dihydroxyvitamin D3. *J Clin Invest* 1987;79:1659–1664.
18. Abe J, Moriya Y, Saito M, Sugawara Y, Suda T, Nishi Y. Modulation of cell growth, differentiation, and production of interleukin-3 by 1,25 dihydroxyvitamin D3 in the murine myelo-monocytic leukemia cell line WEHI-3. *Cancer Res* 1986;46:6316–6321.
19. Old LJ. Polypeptide mediator network. *Nature* 1987;326:330–331.
20. Sherry B, Cerami A. Cachectin/tumor necrosis factor exerts endocrine, paracrine, and autocrine control of inflammatory responses. *J Cell Biol* 1988;107:1269–1277.
21. Klasing KC. Nutritional aspects of leukocytic cytokines. *J Nutr* 1988;118:1436–1446.
22. Jayaraman S, Martin C, Dorf ME. Enhancement of in vivo cell-mediated immune responses by three distinct cytokines. *J Immunol* 1990;144:942–951.
23. Maury CPJ. Tumour necrosis factor—an overview. *Acta Med Scand* 1986;220:387–394.
24. Gamble JR, Harlan SJ, Klebanoff SJ, Vadas MA. Stimulation of the adherence of neutrophils to umbilical vein endothelium by recombinant tumor necrosis factor. *Proc Natl Acad Sci USA* 1985;82:8667–8671.
25. Nathan CF. Neutrophil activation on biological surfaces. *J Clin Invest* 1987;80:1550–1560.
26. Shalaby MR, Palladino MA Jr, Hirabayashi SE, Eessalu TE, Lewis GD, Shepard HM, Aggarwal BB. Receptor binding and activation of polymorphonuclear neutrophils by tumor necrosis factor-alpha. *J Leukoc Biol* 1987;41:196–204.
27. Shalaby MR, Agarwall BB, Rinderknecht E, Svedersky LP, Finkle BS, Paladine MA. Activation of human polymorphonuclear neutrophil function by interferon-gamma and tumor necrosis factor. *J Immunol* 1985;135:2069–2073.
28. Ghiara P, Boraschi D, Nencioni L, Ghezzi P, Tagliabue A. Enhancement of in vivo immune response by tumor necrosis factor. *J Immunol* 1987;139:3676–3679.
29. Scheurich P, Thoma B, Ucer U, Pfizenmaier K. Immunoregulatory activity of recombinant human tumor necrosis factor (TNF)-alpha: induction of TNF receptors on human T cells and TNF-alpha mediated enhancement of T cell responses. *J Immunol* 1987;138:1786–1790.
30. Philip R, Epstein LB. Tumor necrosis factor as immunomodulator and mediator of monocyte cytotoxicity induced by itself, gamma-interferon and interleukin-1. *Nature* 1986;326:86–89.
31. Fleck A. Clinical and nutritional aspects of changes in acute-phase proteins during inflammation. *Proc Nutr Soc* 1989;48:347–354.
32. Beutler B, Cerami A. Cachectin and tumour necrosis factor as two sides of the same biological coin. *Nature* 1986;320:584–588.
33. Vaisman N, Schattner A, Hahn T. Tumor necrosis factor production during starvation. *Am J Med* 1989;87:115.
34. Schattner A, Steinbock M, Tepper R, Schonfeld A, Vaisman N, Hahm T. Tumour necrosis factor production and cell-mediated immunity in anorexia nervosa. *Clin Exp Immunol* 1990;79:62–66.
35. Gordon JE, Scrimshaw NS. Infectious disease in the malnourished child. *Med Clin North Am* 1970;54:1495–1508.
36. Chandra RK. Nutritional deficiency and susceptibility to infection. *Bull WHO* 1979;57:167–177.
37. Whittle HC, Mee J, Weberlinska J, Yalsubu A, Onuora C, Gomwalk N. Immunity to measles in malnourished children. *Clin Exp Immunol* 1980;42:144–151.
38. Bhaskaram P, Madhusudham J, Radhakrishna KV, Reddy V. Immune response in malnourished children with measles. *J Trop Pediatr* 1986;32:123–126.
39. Suskind RM, Thanangkul O, Damongsak D, Leitzmann C, Suskind L, Olson E. The malnourished child: clinical, biochemical, and hematological changes. In: Suskind RM, ed. *Malnutrition and the immune response.* New York: Raven Press, 1977;1–8.
40. Gomez F, Galvan RR, Craviato J, Frank S. Malnutrition in infancy and childhood with special reference to Kwashiorkor. *Adv Pediatr* 1955;7:131–139.
41. Waterlow JC. Classification and deficiency of protein-calorie malnutrition. *Br Med J* 1972;2:566–569.
42. Chandra RK, Selli V, Bhujavala, Ghai OP. Polymorphonuclear leukocyte function in malnourished Indian children. In: Suskind RM, ed. *Malnutrition and the immune response.* New York: Raven Press, 1977;259–264.
43. Edelman R, Kulapongs P, Suskind RM, Olson RE. Leukocyte mobilization in Thai children with kwashiorkor. In: Suskind RM, ed. *Malnutrition and the immune response.* New York: Raven Press, 1977;265–269.
44. Rich KC, Neumann CG, Stiehm ER. Neutrophil chemotaxis in malnourished Ghanaian children. In: Suskind RM, ed. *Malnutrition and the immune response.* New York: Raven Press, 1977;271–275.
45. Douglas SD, Schopfer K. The phagocyte in protein-calorie malnutrition. In: Suskind RM, ed. *Malnutrition and the immune response.* New York: Raven Press, 1977;231–243.
46. Kielmann AA, Uberoi IS, Chandra RK, Mehra VL. The effect of nutritional status on immune capacity and immune responses in preschool children in a rural community in India. *Bull WHO* 1976;54:477–483.
47. Chandra RK. Serum complement components in malnourished Indian children. In: Suskind RM, ed. *Malnutrition and the immune response.* New York: Raven Press, 1977;329–332.
48. McMurray DN, Watson RR, Reyes MA. Effect of renutrition on humoral and cell-mediated immunity in severely malnourished children. *Am J Clin Nutr* 1981;34:2117–2126.
49. Jackson CM. *The effects of inanition and malnutrition upon growth and structure.* Philadelphia: Blakiston, 1925;285.
50. Mugewa JW. The lymphoreticular system in kwashiorkor. *J Pathol* 1971;105:105–109.
51. Jambon B, Ziegler O, Maire B, et al. Thymulin (facteur thymique serique) and zinc contents of the thymus glands of malnourished children. *Am J Clin Nutr* 1988;48:335–342.
52. Neumann CG, Stiehm ER, Swenseid A, Ferguson AC, Lawlor G. Cell-mediated immune response in Ghanian children with protein-calorie malnutrition. In: Suskind RM, ed. *Malnutrition and the immune response.* New York: Raven Press, 1977;77–89.

53. Chandra RK. Serum thymic hormone activity in protein-energy malnutrition. *Clin Exp Immunol* 1979;38:228–230.
54. Chandra RK. Immunocompetence in undernutrition. *J Pediatr* 1972;81:1184–1200.
55. Kulapongs P, Suskind RM, Vithayasai V, Olson ED. In vitro cell-mediated immune response in Thai children with protein-calorie malnutrition. In: Suskind RM, ed. *Malnutrition and the immune response.* New York: Raven Press, 1977;99–104.
56. Chandra RK, Gupta S, Singh H. Inducer and suppressor T cell subsets in protein-energy malnutrition: analysis by monoclonal antibodies. *Nutr Res* 1982;2:21–26.
57. Salimonu LS, Johnson AOK, Williams AIO, Iyabo-Adeleye G, Osunkoya BO. Lymphocyte populations and antibody levels in immunized malnourished children. *Br J Nutr* 1982;48:7–14.
58. Neumann CG, Lawlor GI, Stiehm ER, et al. Immunologic responses in malnourished children. *Am J Clin Nutr* 1975;28:89–104.
59. Sellmeyer E, Bhettay E, Truswell AS, Meyers OL, Hansen JDL. Lymphocyte transformation in malnourished children. *Arch Dis Child* 1972;47:429–435.
60. Bhaskaram P, Sivakumar B. Interleukin-1 in malnutrition. *Arch Dis Child* 1986;61:182–185.
61. Kauffman CA, Jones PG, Kluger MJ. Fever and malnutrition: endogenous pyrogen/interleukin-1 in malnourished patients. *Am J Clin Nutr* 1986;44:449–452.
62. Schlesinger L, Ohlbaum A, Greg L, Stekel A. Cell-mediated immune studies in marasmic children from Chile: delayed hypersensitivity, lymphocyte transformation and interferon production. In: Suskind RM ed. *Malnutrition and the immune response.* New York: Raven Press, 1977;91–98.
63. Suskind RM, Sirisinha S, Edelman R, et al. Immunoglobulins and antibody response in Thai children with protein-energy malnutrition. In: Suskind RM, ed. *Malnutrition and the immune response.* New York: Raven Press, 1977;185–190.
64. Stiehm R. Humoral immunity in malnutrition. *Fed Proc* 1980;39:3093–3097.
65. Chandra RK. Reduced secretory antibody response to live attenuated measles and poliovirus vaccines in malnourished children. *Br Med J* 1975;2:583–585.
66. Sirisinha S, Suskind RM, Edelman A, Asvapaka C, Olson RE. Secretory IgA in Thai children with protein-calorie malnutrition. In: Suskind RM, ed. *Malnutrition and the immune response.* New York: Raven Press, 1977;195–199.
67. McMurray DN, Rey H, Casazza LJ, Watson RR. Effect of moderate malnutrition on concentrations of immunoglobulins and enzymes in tears and saliva of young Colombian children. *Am J Clin Nutr* 1977;30:1944–1948.
68. McMurray DN, Yetley EA, Burch T. Effects of malnutrition and BCG vaccination on macrophage activation in guinea pigs. *Nutr Res* 1981;1:373–384.
69. Majunder MSI, Ali A. Immune response of Peyer's patch cells in rabbit on low protein. *Nutr Res* 1987;7:671–675.
70. Mengheri E, Bises G, Gaetani S. Differentiated cell-mediated immune response in zinc deficiency and in protein malnutrition. *Nutr Res* 1988;8:801–812.
71. Ahmed F, Jones DB, Jackson AA. Effect of undernutrition on the immune response to rotavirus infection in mice. *Ann Nutr Metab* 1990;34:21–31.
72. Petro TM. Effect of reduced dietary protein intake on regulation of murine in vitro polyclonal T lymphocyte mitogenesis. *Nutr Res* 1985;5:263–276.
73. Zile MH, Cullum ME. The functions of vitamin A: current concepts. *Proc Soc Exp Biol Med* 1983;172:139–152.
74. Milton RC, Reddy V, Naider AN. Mild vitamin A deficiency and childhood morbidity. *Am J Clin Nut* 1987;46:827–829.
75. Thurnham DI. Vitamin A deficiency and its role in infection. *Trans R Soc Trop Med Hyg* 1989;83:721–723.
76. Bhaskaram P, Reddy C. Cell-mediated immunity in iron and vitamin A deficient children. *Br Med J* 1975;3:522.
77. Bhaskaram P. Immune response and infection in relation to vitamin A and iron deficiency in children. In: Taylor TC, Jenkins NK, eds. *Proceedings of the XIIIth International Congress of Nutrition.* New York: Libbey, 1985;132–135.
78. Krishman S, Bhyan UN, Talwar GP, Ramalingaswani V. Effect of vitamin A and protein-calorie undernutrition on immune response. *Immunology* 1974;27:383–392.
79. Chandra RK, Au B. Single nutrient deficiency and cell-mediated immune responses. III: Vitamin A. *Nutr Res* 1981;1:181–185.
80. Mark DA, Nauss KM, Baliga BS, Suskind RM. Depressed transformation response by splenic lymphocytes from vitamin A deficient rats. *Nutr Res* 1981;1:489–497.
81. Nauss KM, Phua CC, Ambrogi L, Newberne PM. Immunological changes during progressive stages of vitamin A deficiency in rat. *J Nutr* 1985;115:909–918.
82. Murthy KK, Suskind SAL, Venkatash V, Edwardo BJ, Suskind RM. Decreased T lymphocyte function and interleukin-2 production associated with vitamin A deficiency. *6th International Congress of Immunology* 1986;86.
83. Pasantiempo AM, Taylor CE, Ross CA. Effects of early stages of vitamin A deficiency on the immune response to streptococcus pneumoniae SSS-III. *FASEB J* 1989;3:A663,Abstr 2537.
84. Mark DA, Baliga BS, Suskind RM. Vitamin A deficiency and cellular immune responses: Relocation of competent cells? *XIIIth International Congress of Nutrition, Brighton,* 1985;146.
85. Meydani SN, Barklund MP, Liu S, et al. Effect of vitamin E supplementation on immune responsiveness of healthy elderly subjects. *FASEB J* 1989;3:A1057,Abstr 4828.
86. Bendich A, Gabriel E, Machlin LJ. Dietary vitamin E requirement for optimum immune responses in the rat. *J Nutr* 1986;116:675–681.
87. Bendich A, Gabriel E, Machlin LJ. Role of dietary vitamin E on natural killer cell lysis. *XIIIth International Congress of Nutrition,* Brighton, 1985;77.
88. Gershwin ME, Beach RS, Hurley LS, eds. *Nutrition and immunity.* New York: Academic Press, 1985;228–258.
89. Chandra RK, Au B, Heresi G. Single nutrient deficiency and cell-mediated immune responses. II: Pyridoxine. *Nutr Res* 1981;1:101–106.
90. Bowering J, Lowenberg RL, Morrison MA. Nutritional studies of pregnant women in East Harlem. *Am J Clin Nutr* 1980;33:1987–1996.
91. Kay NE, Holloway DE, Hutton SW, Bones ND, Duane WC. Human T-cell functions in experimental ascorbic acid deficiency and spontaneous scurvey. *Am J Clin Nutr* 1982;36:127–130.
92. Anderson R, Oosthuizen R, Maritz R, Theron A, Van Rensberg AJ. The effects of increasing weekly doses of ascorbate on certain cellular and humoral immune functions in normal volunteers. *Am J Clin Nutr* 1980;33:71–76.
93. Kalden JR, Guthy EA. Prolonged skin allograft survival in vitamin C deficient guinea pigs. *Eur Surg Res* 1972;4:114–119.
94. Anthony LE, Kurahara CG, Taylor KB. Cell-mediated cytotoxicity and humoral immune response in ascorbic acid deficient guinea pigs. *Am J Clin Nutr* 1979;32:1691–1698.
95. Goldschmidt MC, Masin WJ, Brown LR, Wyde PR. The effect of ascorbic acid deficiency on leukocyte phagocytosis and killing of *Actinomyces viscosus. Int J Vitam Nutr Res* 1988;58:326–334.
96. Gross RL, Reid JVO, Newberne PM, Burgess B, Marston R, Hift MW. Depressed cell-mediated immunity in megaloblastic anemia due to folic acid deficiency. *Am J Clin Nutr* 1975;28:225–232.
97. Cook JD, Finch CA. Assessment of iron status of a population. *Am J Clin Nutr* 1979;32:2115–2119.
98. Chandra RK, Saraya AK. Impaired immunocompetence associated with iron deficiency. *J Pediatr* 1975;86:899–902.
99. McDougall LG, Anderson R, McNab GM, Katz J. The immune response in iron deficient children: impaired cellular defense mechanisms with altered humoral components. *J Pediatr* 1975;86:833–843.
100. Krantman HJ, Young SR, Ank BJ, et al. Immune function in pure iron deficiency. *Am J Dis Child* 1982;136:840–844.
101. Kemahli AS, Babacan E, Cavdar AO. Cell-mediated immune responses in children with iron deficiency and combined zinc deficiency. *Nutr Res* 1988;8:129–36.
102. Grosh-Worner I, Grosse-Wilde H, Bender G, Shafer KH. Lymphocyte function in children with iron deficiency. *Klin Wochenschr* 1984;62:1091–1093.
103. Walter T, Arrendoch S, Avenato M, Stekel A. Effects of iron

therapy on phagocytosis and bactericidal activity in neutrophils or iron deficient infants. *Am J Clin Nutr* 1986;44:877–882.
104. Bagchi K, Mohanram M, Reddy V. Humoral immune response in children with iron deficiency anemia. *Br Med J* 1980;1:1249–1251.
105. Kuvibidila S, Baliga BS, Suskind RM. Effects of iron deficiency anemia on delayed cutaneous hypersensitivity in mice. *Am J Clin Nutr* 1981;34:2635–2640.
106. Kuvibidila S, Nauss KM, Baliga BS, Suskind RM. Impairment of blastogenic response of splenic lymphocytes from iron deficient mice: in vivo repletion. *Am J Clin Nutr* 1983;37:15–25.
107. Kuvibidila S, Dardenne M, Savino W, Lepol F. Influence of iron deficiency on selected thymus functions in mice: thymulin biological activity, T cell subsets and thymocyte transformation. *Am J Clin Nutr* 1990;51:228–232.
108. Sherman AR, Lockwood JF. Impaired natural killer cell activity in iron-deficient rat pups. *J Nutr* 1987;117:567–571.
109. Kuvibidila S, Baliga BS, Suskind RM. The effects of iron deficiency on cytolytic activity of mice spleen and peritoneal cells against allogenic tumor cells. *Am J Clin Nutr* 1983;38:238–244.
110. Helyar L, Sherman AR. Iron deficiency and interleukin-1 production by rat leucocytes. *Am J Clin Nutr* 1987;46:346–352.
111. Kuvibidila S, Murthy KK, Suskind RM. Iron deficiency and interleukin-2 (IL-2) production by murine spleen cells. *FASEB J* 1989;3:A664(abstr 2545).
112. Nalder BM, Mahoney AW, Ramakrishnen R, Hendricks DG. Sensitivity of the immunological response to nutritional status of rats. *J Nutr* 1972;102:535–542.
113. Kochanowski BA, Sherman AR. Decreased antibody formation in iron-deficient rat pups—effect of iron repletion. *Am J Clin Nutr* 1985;41:271–284.
114. Kuvibidila S, Baliga BS, Suskind RM. Generation of plaque forming cells in iron deficient anemic mice. *Nutr Rep Int* 1982;26:861–871.
115. Kuvibidila S, Wade S. Macrophage function as studied by the clearance of 125I-labeled polyvinyl pyrrolidone in iron-deficient and iron-repleted mice. *J Nutr* 1987;117:170–176.
116. Mackler B, Pearson R, Ochs H, Finch CA. Iron deficiency in the rat: effects on neutrophil activation and metabolism. *Pediatr Res* 1984;18:549–551.
117. Kuvibidila S, Baliga BS, Nauss KM, Suskind RM. Impairment of blastogenic response of splenic lymphocytes from iron deficient mice: in vitro repletion. *Am J Clin Nutr* 1983;37:557–565.
118. Brown MRW, Anwar H, Lambert PA. Evidence that mucoid *Pseudomonas aeruginosa* in the cystic fibrosis lung grows under restricted conditions. *FEMS Microb Lett* 1984;21:113–117.
119. Boyce JR, Miller RV. Selection of nonmucoid derivatives of mucoid *Pseudomonas aeruginosa* is strongly influenced by the level of iron in the culture medium. *Infect Immun* 1982;37:695–701.
120. Cox CD, Adams P. Siderophore activity of pyoverdin for *P. aeruginosa*. *Infect Immun* 1985;48:130–138.
121. Prasad A. Essential trace elements in human health and disease. *J Am Coll Nutr* 1985;4:1–2.
122. Chandra RK. Trace elements and immune response. *Clin Nutr* 1987;6:118–125.
123. Fraker PJ, Gershwin ME, Good RA, Prasad A. Interrelationships between zinc and immune function. *Fed Proc* 1986;45:1474–1479.
124. Prasad AS, Halsted JA, Nadimi M. Syndrome of iron deficiency anemia hepatosplenomegaly, hypogonadism, dwarfism, and geophagia. *Am J Med* 1961;31:532–546.
125. Weiner RG. AIDS and zinc deficiency. *JAMA* 1984;252:1409–1410.
126. Tong TK, Andrew LR, Albert A, Mickell JJ. Childhood acquired immune deficiency syndrome manifesting as acrodermatitis enteropathica. *J Pediatr* 1986;108:426–428.
127. Fabris N, Mocchegiani E, Galli M, et al. AIDS, zinc deficiency, and thymic hormone failure. *JAMA* 1988;259:839–840.
128. Falutz J, Tsoukas C, Gold P. Zinc as a cofactor in human immunodeficiency virus-induced immunosuppression. *JAMA* 1988;259:2850–2851.
129. Chandra RK. Trace element regulation of immunity and infection. *J Am Coll Nutr* 1985;4:5–16.
130. Chandra RK, Herresi G, Au B. Serum thymic factor activity in deficiencies of calories, zinc, vitamin and pyridoxine. *Clin Exp Immunol* 1980;42:322–335.
131. Chandra RK. Serum thymic hormone activity and cell-mediated immunity in healthy neonates, preterm infants, and small-for-gestational age infants. *Pediatrics* 1981;67:407–411.
132. DePasquale-Jardieu P, Fraker PJ. Further characterization of the role of corticosterone in the loss of humoral immunity in zinc-deficient A/J mice as determined by adrenalectomy. *J Immunol* 1980;124:2650–2655.
133. Alford RM. Metal cation requirements for phytohemagglutinin-induced transformation of human peripheral blood leukocytes. *J Immunol* 1970;104:698–703.
134. Bendtzen K. Differential role of Zn^{2+} in antigen and mitogen-induced lymphokine production. *Scand J Immunol* 1980;12:489–492.
135. Barnes PM, Moynahan EJ. Zinc deficiency in acrodermatitis enteropathica: multiple dietary intolerance treated with synthetic diet. *Proc R Soc Med* 1973;66:327–329.
136. Oleske JM, Wesphal ML, Shore S, Gorden D, Bogden JD, Nahamias A. Zinc therapy of depressed cellular immunity in acrodermatitis enteropathica: its correction. *Am J Dis Child* 1979;133:915–918.
137. Allen JL, Kay NE, McClain CJ. Severe zinc deficiency in humans: association with a reversible T-lymphocyte dysfunction. *Ann Intern Med* 1981;95:154–157.
138. Walford PL. Immunology and aging. *Am J Clin Pathol* 1980;74:247–253.
139. Beisel WR. Single nutrients and immunity. *Am J Clin Nutr* 1982;35:417–468.
140. Standstead HH, Hendrikesen LK, Greger JL, Prasad AS, Good RA. Zinc nutriture in the elderly in relation to taste acuity, immune response, and wound healing. *Am J Clin Nutr* 1982;36:1046–1059.
141. Bogden JD, Oleske JM, Munves EM, Lavenhar MA, et al. Zinc and immunocompetence in the elderly: baseline data on zinc nutriture and immunity in unsupplemented subjects. *Am J Clin Nutr* 1987;47:101–109.
142. Cossack ZT. T-lymphocyte dysfunction in the elderly associated with zinc deficiency and subnormal nucleoside phosphorylase activity: effect of zinc supplementation. *Eur J Cancer Clin Oncol* 1989;25:973–976.
143. Underwood EJ. Copper. In: Underwood, EJ, ed. *Trace elements in humans and animal nutrition*, 3rd ed. London: Academic Press, 1971;57.
144. Pedroni E, Bianchi E, Ugazio AG, Burgio GR. Immunodeficiency and steely hair. *Lancet* 1975;1:1303–1304.
145. Sullivan JL, Ochs HD. Copper deficiency and the immune system. *Lancet* 1978;2:686.
146. Vyas D, Chandra RK. Thymic factor activity, lymphocyte stimulation response and antibody producing cells in copper deficiency. *Nutr Res* 1983;3:343–349.
147. Lukacewycz OA, Prohaska JR, Meyer SG, Schmidtke JR, Hatfield SM, Marder P. Alterations in lymphocyte subpopulations in copper-deficient mice. *Infect Immun* 1985;48:644–647.
148. Mulhern SA, Koller LD. Severe or marginal copper deficiency results in a graded reduction in immune status in mice. *J Nutr* 1988;118:1041–1047.
149. Koller LD, Mulhern SA, Frankel PC. Immune dysfunction in rats fed a diet deficient in copper. *Am J Clin Nutr* 1987;45:997–1006.
150. Jones JD. Effects of dietary copper depletion on acute and delayed inflammatory responses in mice. *Res Vet Sci* 1984;37:205–210.
151. Flynn A, Loftus MA, Finke JH. Production of interleukin-1 and interleukin-2 in allogeneic mixed lymphocyte cultures under copper, magnesium and zinc deficient conditions. *Nutr Res* 1984;4:673–679.
152. Flynn A. In vitro levels of copper, magnesium and zinc required for mitogen stimulated T lymphocyte proliferation. *Nutr Res* 1985;5:487–495.
153. Korte JJ, Prohaska JR. Dietary copper deficiency alters protein and lipid composition of murine lymphocyte plasma membranes. *J Nutr* 1987;117:1076–1084.
154. Rea HM, Thomson CD, Campbell DR, Robinson MF. Relation

between erythrocyte selenium concentrations and glutathione peroxidase (EC 1.11.1.9) activities of New Zealand residents and visitors to New Zealand. *Br J Nutr* 1979;42:201–208.
155. Baker SS, Lerman RH, Krey SH, Crocker KS, Hirsh EF, Cohen H. Selenium deficiency with total parenteral nutrition: reversal of biochemical and functional abnormalities by selenium supplementation: a case report. *Am J Clin Nutr* 1983;38:769–774.
156. Cohen HJ, Chovaniec ME, Mistretta D, Baker SS. Selenium repletion and glutathione peroxidase-differential effects on plasma and red blood cell enzyme activity. *Am J Clin Nutr* 1985;41:735–747.
157. Kiremidjian-Schumacher L, Stotzky G. Selenium and immune responses. *Environ Res* 1987;42:277–303.
158. Seligmann M. Immunological features of human immunodeficiency virus disease. *Baillieres Clin Haematol* 1990;3:37–63.
159. Spickett GP, Dalgleish AG. Cellular immunology of HIV-infection. *Clin Exp Immunol* 1988;71:1–7.
160. Sattentau QJ. HIV infection and the immune system. *Biochem Biophys Acta* 1989;989:255–268.
161. Rosenberg ZF, Fauci AS. Immunopathogenic mechanisms of HIV infection: cytokine induction of HIV expression. *Immunol Today* 1990;11:176–180.
162. Murray HW, Rubin BY, Masur H, Roberts RB. Impaired production of lymphokines and immune (gamma) interferon in the acquired immunodeficiency syndrome. *N Engl J Med* 1984;310:883–889.
163. Tyler DS, Stanley SD, Nastala CA, Austin AA, et al. Alterations in antibody-dependent cellular cytotoxicity during the course of HIV-1 infection. *J Immunol* 1990;144:3375–3384.
164. Brenner BG, Dascal A, Margolese RG, Wainberg MA. Natural killer cell function in patients with acquired immunodeficiency syndrome and related diseases. *J Leukoc Biol* 1989;46:75–83.
165. Lane HC, Masur H, Edgar LC, et al. Abnormalities of B-cell activation and immunoregulation in patients with the acquired immunodeficiency syndrome. *N Engl J Med* 1983;309:453–458.
166. Melmed RN, Taylor JMG, Detels R, Bozorgmehri M, Fahey JL. Serum neopterin changes in HIV-infected subjects: indicator of significant pathology, CD4 T cell changes, and the development of AIDS. *J Acquir Immune Defic Synd* 1989;2:70–76.
167. Kramer A, Wiktor SZ, Fuchs D, Milstien S, Gail MH, et al. Neopterin: a predictive marker of acquired immune deficiency syndrome in human immunodeficiency virus infection. *J Acquir Immune Defic Synd* 1989;2:291–296.
168. Fahey JL, Taylor JMG, Detels R, Hofmann B, et al. The prognostic value of cellular and serologic markers in infection with human immunodeficiency virus type 1. *N Engl J Med* 1990;322:166–172.
169. D'Onofrio G, Mancine S, Tanburrini E, Margo G, Ortora L. Giant neutrophils with increased peroxidase activity. Another evidence of dysgranulopoiesis in AIDS. *Am J Clin Pathol* 1987;87:584–587.
170. Murphy PM, Lane HC, Fauci AS, Gallin JI. Impairment of neutrophil bactericidal capacity in patients with AIDS. *J Infect Dis* 1988;158:627–630.
171. Jain VK, Chandra RK. Does nutritional deficiency predispose to acquired immune deficiency syndrome? *Nutr Res* 1984;4:537–543.
172. Kotler DP, Wang J, Pierson RN Jr. Body composition studies in patients with the acquired immunodeficiency syndrome. *Am J Clin Nutr* 1985;42:1255–1265.
173. Moseson M, Zeleniuch-Jacquotte A, Belsito DV, Shore RE, Marmor M, Pasternack B. The potential role of nutritional factors in the induction of immunologic abnormalities in HIV-positive homosexual men. *J Acquir Immune Defic Synd* 1989;2:235–247.
174. Chelluri L, Jastremski MS. Incidence of malnutrition in patients with acquired immunodeficiency syndrome. *Nutr Clin Pract* 1989;4:16–18.
175. Rubinstein A, Sicklick M, Gupta A, et al. Acquired immunodeficiency with reversed T4/T8 ratios in infants born to promiscuous and drug-addicted mothers. *JAMA* 1983;249:2350–2356.
176. Lesbordes JL, Chassignol S, Ray E, et al. Malnutrition and HIV infection in children in the Central African Republic. *Lancet* 1986;2:337–338.
177. Kuvibidila S, Warrier R, Suskind D, Sarpong D, Deselle B, Suskind RM, Andes W. Nutritional status of hemophiliacs with and without infection with the human immunodeficiency virus (HIV). *Nutr Res* 1989;9:1197–1206.
178. Malebranche R, Guerin JM, Larouche AC, et al. Acquired immunodeficiency syndrome with severe gastrointestinal manifestations in Haiti. *Lancet* 1983;2:873–878.
179. Dworkin B, Wormser GP, Rosenthal WS, et al. Gastrointestinal manifestations of the acquired immunodeficiency syndrome: a review of 22 cases. *Am J Gastroenterol* 1985;80:774–778.
180. Modigliani R, Bories C, Le Charpentier Y, et al. Diarrhea and malabsorption in acquired immune deficiency syndrome: a study of four cases with special emphasis on opportunistic protozoan infestations. *Gut* 1985;26:179–187.
181. Chernosky ME, Finley VK. Yellow nail syndrome in patients with acquired immunodeficiency disease. *J Am Acad Dermatol* 1985;13:731–736.
182. Ayres S Jr. Yellow nail syndrome controlled by vitamin E therapy. *J Am Acad Dermatol* 1986;15:714–715.
183. Dworkin BM, Rosenthal SW, Wormser GP, Weiss L. Selenium deficiency in the acquired immunodeficiency syndrome. *JPEN J Parenter Enteral Nutr* 1986;10:405–407.
184. Blumberg BS, Hann HWL, Mildvan D, Mathur U, Lustbader E, London WT. Iron and iron binding proteins in persistent generalized lymphadenopathy and AIDS (letter). *Lancet* 1984;2:347.
185. Davies PDO. A possible link between vitamin D deficiency and impaired host defence to mycobacterium tuberculosis. *Tubercle* 1985;66:301–306.
186. Crowle AJ, Ross EJ, May MH. Inhibition by 1,25(OH)$_2$-vitamin D$_3$ of the multiplication of virulent tubercle bacilli in cultured human macrophages. *Infect Immun* 1987;55:2945–2950.
187. Stead WW, Senner JW, Reddick WT, Lofgren JP. Racial differences in susceptibility to infection by mycobacterium tuberculosis. *N Engl J Med* 1990;322:422–427.
188. Bell NH, Greene A, Epstein S, Oexmann MJ, Shaw S, Shary J. Evidence for alteration of the vitamin D–endocrine system in blacks. *J Clin Invest* 1985;76:470–473.
189. Rook GAW, Taverne J, Leveton C, Steele J. The role of gamma-interferon, vitamin D3 metabolites and tumour necrosis factor in the pathogenesis of tuberculosis. *Immunology* 1987;62:229–234.
190. Ganapathy KT, Chakraborty AK. Does malnutrition affect tuberculin hypersensitivity reaction in the community. *Indian J Pediatr* 1982;49:377–382.
191. McMurray DN, Loomis SA, Casazza LJ, Rey H, Miranda R. Development of impaired cell-mediated immunity in mild and moderate malnutrition. *Am J Clin Nutr* 1981;34:68–77.
192. Harland PSEB. Tuberculin reactions in malnourished children. *Lancet* 1965;2:719–721.
193. Ziegler HD, Ziegler PB. Depression of tuberculin reaction in mild and moderate-protein-calorie malnourished children following BCG vaccination. *Johns Hopkins Med J* 1975;137:59–64.
194. Satyanarayana K, Bhaskaram P, Seshu VC, Reddy V. Influence of nutrition on postvaccinal tuberculin sensitivity. *Am J Clin Nutr* 1980;33:2334–2337.
195. Seth V, Kukreja N, Sundaram KR, Malaviya AN, Seth SD. In vivo and in vitro correlation of cell mediated immune response in preschool children after BCG in relation to their nutritional status. *Indian J Med Res* 1982;75:360–365.
196. Rivera J, Habicht JP, Torres N, et al. Decreased cellular immune response in wasted but not in stunted children. *Nutr Res* 1986;6:1161–1170.
197. McMurray DN, Mintzer CL, Bartow RA, Parr RL. Dietary protein deficiency and mycobacterium bovis BCG affect interleukin-2 activity in experimental pulmonary tuberculosis. *Infect Immun* 1989;57:2606–2611.
198. Selwyn PA, Hartel D, Lewis VA, et al. A prospective study of the risk of tuberculosis among intravenous drug users with human immunodeficiency virus infection. *N Engl J Med* 1989;320:545–550.
199. Pahwa R, Chatila T, Pahwa S, et al. Recombinant interleukin-2 therapy in severe combined immunodeficiency disease. *Proc Natl Acad Sci USA* 1989;86:5069–5073.
200. Chatila T, Wong R, Young M, Miller R, Terhorst C, Geha RS. An immunodeficiency characterized by defective signal transduction in T lymphocytes. *N Engl J Med* 1989;320:696–702.

201. Rook AH, Masur H, Lane HC, et al. Interleukin-2 enhanced the depressed natural killer and CMV specific cytotoxic activities of lymphocytes from patients with acquired immune deficiency syndrome. *J Clin Invest* 1983;72:398–403.
202. Gluckman JC, Klatzmann D, Cavaille-Coll M, et al. Is there correlation of T-cell proliferative functions and surface marker phenotypes in patients with acquired immune deficiency syndrome of lymphadenopathy syndrome? *Clin Exp Immunol* 1985;60:8–16.
203. Haregewoin A, Godal AT, Mustafa AS, Belehu A, Yemaneberhan T. T-cell conditioned media reverse T-cell unresponsiveness in lepromatous leprosy. *Nature* 1983;303:342–344.
204. Toossi Z, Kleinhenz ME, Ellner J. Defective interleukin-2 production and responsiveness in human pulmonary tuberculosis. *J Exp Med* 1986;163:1162–1172.
205. Cunningham AS. Morbidity in breast-fed and artificial-fed infants. II. *J Pediatr* 1979;95:685–689.
206. Welsh JK, May JT. Anti-infective properties of breast milk. *J Pediatr* 1979;94:1–9.
207. Emodi G, Just M. Interferon production by lymphocytes in human milk. *Scand J Immunol* 1974;3:157–160.
208. Lawton JWM, Shortridge KF, Wong RLC, Ng MH. Interferon synthesis by human colostral leukocytes. *Arch Dis Child* 1979;54:127–130.
209. Stephens S, Brenner MK, Duffy SW, Lakhani PK, Kennedy CR, Farrant J. The effect of breast-feeding on proliferation by infant lymphocytes. *Pediatr Res* 1986;20:227–231.
210. Schlesinger JJ, Covelli HD. Evidence for transmission of lymphocyte responses to tuberculin by breast feeding. *Lancet* 1977;2:529–532.
211. Keller MA, Rodriguez AL, Alvarez S, Wheeler NC, Reisinger D. Transfer of tuberculin immunity from mother to infant. *Pediatr Res* 1987;22:277–281.
212. Pabst HF, Godel J, Grace M, Cho H, Spady DW. Effect of breast feeding on immune response to BCG vaccination. *Lancet* 1989;1:295–297.
213. Lee TH, Hoover RL, Williams JD, et al. Effect of dietary enrichment with eicosanoic and docosahexaenoic acids on in vitro neutrophil and monocyte leukotriene generation and neutrophil function. *N Engl J Med* 1985;312:99–108.
214. Endres S, Ghorbani R, Kelley VE, et al. The effect of dietary supplementation with n-3 polyunsaturated fatty acids on the synthesis of interleukin-1 and tumor necrosis factor by mononuclear cells. *N Engl J Med* 1989;320:265–271.

CHAPTER 13

Endocrine Changes in Malnutrition

Alfred Tenore and Alfonso Vargas

Malnutrition is a problem not limited to underdeveloped countries. The high incidence of undernutrition in hospitalized patients makes malnutrition, and its ramifications, clinically relevant in advanced societies, as well.

Protein-energy malnutrition (PEM), the term currently used to designate malnutrition, encompasses a number of nutritional deficiency syndromes. It must be understood, however, that PEM is a multifactorial disease and as such it is not possible, nor appropriate, to isolate dietary factors from other factors, including infections. In this review, the term *malnourished child* will refer to a child suffering from protein-energy malnutrition, i.e., kwashiorkor and/or marasmus.

CLINICAL CHANGES IN MALNUTRITION

The physiological and biochemical changes that occur in chronic malnutrition are directed toward survival, which takes precedence over all other nonessential, non–life sustaining "luxury" types of functions. One such luxury is growth; hence, growth failure is one of the most consistent clinical signs of chronic malnutrition.

Anthropometric evidence of growth failure is determined by the analysis of height-for-age, corrected for genetic potential, weight-for-height, and weight-for-age (Table 1). Weight-for-height is most appropriate for diagnosing acute malnutrition, which, in its severest form, is characterized as "wasting." Height-for-age, on the other hand, is a determinant of chronic, ongoing malnutrition, which ultimately leads to the status known as "stunting." Weight-for-age is, however, a poor criterion for differentiating acute from chronic malnutrition.

The ultimate consequence of starvation is, of course, death. Death results from the critical loss of body protein, a loss that affects muscle and immune function and occurs long before the body depletes its primary energy stores (fat). In order to spare protein and maintain a constant energy supply to the brain, the body responds to insufficient food intake by reducing urea excretion. The energy supply, which is also the primary fuel of the brain, is glucose. During the first hours of fasting (depending on the size of the child), glucose comes from glycogen stores. Once glycogen is depleted, glucose is derived from amino acids via gluconeogenesis. In order to spare protein, however, the brain progressively shifts from a glucose fuel system to a ketone fuel system. The ketone bodies (β-hydroxybutyrate and acetoacetate) are produced in the liver from free fatty acids (FFA), which come from adipose tissue lipolysis of triglyceride fat stores. In terms of cellular fuel production, there are three chronologically progressive mechanisms activated when food intake is deficient (Table 2).

A. Tenore: Department of Pediatrics, University of Udine, Udine, Italy 33100.
A. Vargas: Department of Pediatrics, Louisiana State University School of Medicine, New Orleans, Louisiana 70112.

TABLE 1. *Growth failure in malnutrition*

Type of malnutrition	Height-for-age	Weight-for-age	Weight-for-height
Ongoing			
Acute (short duration)	Normal	Low	Low
Chronic (long duration)	Low	Low	Low
Past	Low	Low	Normal

Modified from ref. 1.

TABLE 2. *Mechanisms activated to maintain adequate supply of fuel during the three phases of fasting*

Phase	Substrate	Intermediary	Fuel
Postprandial	Glycogen breakdown		Glucose
Early fast	Protein breakdown	Amino acids	Glucose
Late fast	Fat breakdown	Triglycerides, FFA	Glucose, ketones

NUTRIENT-HORMONE INTERACTIONS

A very tight, synergistic interaction exists between hormones and nutrients. Strong evidence confirms that many hormones directly influence the transport of nutrients across membranes and that adequate supplies of nutrients are required to produce the effects signaled by hormones. Hormones not only influence the nutritional requirements of individual cells but also affect the nutrient environment upon which different types of tissues depend. Thus, a particular hormone may exert a catabolic effect in one tissue and in so doing may be increasing the substrates necessary to provoke an anabolic effect in another (Table 3). However, it is just as important to remember that the nutritional environment will also be instrumental in controlling the preferential secretion of one hormone over another. This differential type of hormone secretion and action becomes vitally important during malnutrition for maintaining life-sustaining functions.

Homeostasis and homeorrhesis are, therefore, important concepts relative to this mechanism. Homeostasis is described as a mechanism of rapid adjustment of the internal environment with the purpose of maintaining physiologic equilibrium in states such as fasting or acute starvation. Homeorrhesis, which occurs in malnutrition, has been used by Bauman and Currie (2) to describe the mechanism by which an organism partitions nutrients to tissues in order to support growth or other physiologic processes. From these mechanisms, the concepts of anabolic and catabolic hormones have emerged. For instance, if the so-called anabolic hormones exert their effects in a "fed state," an increased protein content of both viscera and muscle will occur; in the "fasted state," however, these hormones will continue to support muscle protein synthesis preferentially at the expense of visceral proteins. It becomes clear that the presence of "anabolic" hormones in a malnourished child would be counterproductive; conversely, the presence of "catabolic" hormones, which function to protect the viscera when nutrients are in short supply, would be ideal.

ADAPTATION AND MALNUTRITION

"The salient feature of life, the secret of its resistance, is adaptability to change." Selye (3) is implying, of course, that the essential factor of survival is the ability of "stressed" organisms to undergo physical or physiological changes. In this context, he has also proposed that the most important function of hormones is in differentiation and adaptation, with the adrenal cortex being central to the adaptive response (4). Adaptation is not the ultimate goal, however, but, rather, a means of survival, with each disturbing influence inducing a compensatory mechanism aimed at neutralizing or repairing the disturbance.

Gopalan (5) proposed that the individual child's ability to adapt to restricted food intake determined the type of PEM that would result. Castellanos and Arroyave (6) indicated that although the majority of children would adapt sufficiently to develop only a mild degree of malnutrition, the adaptation mechanisms of others would result in marasmus, and, to a lesser extent, kwashiorkor.

TABLE 3. *Effects of hormones on carbohydrates, proteins, and fats*

| Hormone | Proteins | | Carbohydrates | Fats |
	Synthesis	Breakdown		
Growth hormone	Muscle		Insulin-like (acute)	Lipolysis
			Insulin-antagonist	Inhibits lipogenesis
Thyroid	Liver	Muscle	Glycogenolysis	Lipolysis
			Gluconeogenesis	
Insulin	Muscle		Glycogen synthesis (liver)	Lipogenesis
	Liver		Inhibits glycolysis	Inhibits lipolysis
Androgens	Muscle			
Glucocorticoids	Viscera	Muscle	Glycogen synthesis	Redistribution
			Gluconeogenesis (permissive)	

Modifications of the endocrine system represent adaptation of the organism to an altered nutritional state. Changes, therefore, are more relevant not so much in terms of what the change is, but rather why it occurs and what it means.

HORMONES AND MALNUTRITION

Current data describing the endocrine status in malnourished children would appear to be contradictory if one were looking at single effects from single causes. Malnutrition is not, however, a single, delineated entity but rather a combination of entities in a continuum of degrees. These entities have varying etiologies, including a deficiency in nutrient intake, malabsorption, and excessive nutrient losses. Apparently contradictory endocrine data can be explained by the following:

1. Malnutrition is a heterogeneous state encompassing a spectrum of components and conditions from mild to severe and from simple to complex.
2. It is highly improbable that any study can identify two children, let alone an entire population, malnourished to the same degree.
3. Adaptive responses function in response to the degree of malnutrition, barring any complicating factors such as infection.

All of the apparently contradictory data are probably correct, each study describing a particular segment of the continuum of endocrine changes that occur on the basis of the duration and severity of the malnutrition and on the composition of the diet. The individual responses limit our ability to describe a particular hormone as high, normal, or low in malnutrition. We can, however, attempt to explain the pathogenesis of observed endocrine changes, such as the endocrine and metabolic changes in marasmus and kwashiorkor (Table 4).

TABLE 4. *Metabolic and hormone changes in marasmus and kwashiorkor*

	Marasmus	Kwashiorkor
Metabolic		
Albumin, total proteins	Low-normal	Low
Amino acids	Normal	Low
Cholesterol and triglycerides	Normal	Low
Nonesterified fatty acids	Elevated	Elevated
Glucose	Normal	Normal/low
Glucose tolerance	Normal	Impaired
Binding proteins	Normal	Low
Endocrine		
Adrenal-functional unit cortisol	Very high	High
Cortisol response to ACTH	Exaggerated	Normal to poor
Aldosterone[a]	Normal	Elevated
Catecholamines[a]	Low	Low
Thyroid-functional unit		
Thyroxine	Normal/low	Low
Triiodothyronine	Low	Low
Reverse T_3	Elevated	Elevated
TSH[a]	(Low—normal—high)	
TSH response to THR[a]	(Normal to abnormal)	
Gonad-functional unit		
LH and FSH[a]	(Low—normal—high)	
Testosterone[a]	Low	Low
Testoterone response to HCG[a]	(subnormal)	
Pancreas-functional unit		
Insulin	Low/normal	Normal/low
Insulin response to stimuli	Normal	Poor
Glucagon[a]		
Growth-promoting functional unit		
Growth hormone	Low/normal/high	High
GH response to stimuli	Poor	Normal
Somatomedin-C	Low	Low
Miscellaneous		
Prolactin[a]	Low	Normal/high
Prolactin response to TRH[a]	(low—normal—high)	

The responses cited above are by no means unanimous but represent tendency reported by most of the published data.

[a] Denotes that there is little agreement concerning the status of secretory response.

ADRENAL GLAND

Cortisol, ACTH, Aldosterone, and Catecholamines

Anatomic-histopathologic evidence of the adrenals in malnutrition indicates a state of hypocortisolemia. Although, in most reports, the adrenals have been found to be anatomically small, adrenal enlargement has also been reported in some cases of kwashiorkor (7,8). However, since these anatomic findings reflect the consequence of extreme malnutrition and since elevated cortisol levels have been found in malnourished individuals, the data may imply that initial hyperactivity may be followed by adrenal exhaustion and atrophy.

It has been suggested that the rise in plasma cortisol may not be a feature of malnutrition, per se, but a response to various associated stress factors, particularly infection. However, Lunn et al. (9) reported not only a significant correlation between severity of infection and plasma cortisol levels but also a progressive increase in plasma cortisol levels with increasing deficits in body weight.

Current data indicate that the elevated plasma levels of cortisol may be due to the varying influence of the following three factors:

1. decreased metabolic clearance rate (10)
2. prolonged half-life (11)
3. stress
   (a) metabolic stress of malnutrition (11)
   (b) stress of infection (9,12).

Insufficient and contradictory data exist in the literature on the functional status of the pituitary corticotrophs. Some evidence indicates hyposecretion, whereas other evidence implies a state of hypersecretion. Support of the former is based on findings that (a) the adrenals of malnourished rats respond to adrenocorticotropic hormone (ACTH) with an increase in protein and RNA concentration and in weight (13), and (b) in some patients, exogenous ACTH showed a normal adrenal reserve (10,11,14). Evidence favoring a state of hypersecretion comes from the finding (a) that dexamethasone has been shown to cause incomplete suppression of plasma cortisol levels (10,11), and (b) there is absence of diurnal variation in cortisol secretion (11,15).

Cortisol levels in marasmus have been found to be significantly higher than in kwashiorkor; synthetic ACTH had an exaggerated response in increasing cortisol secretion in marasmic children, in contrast to a quasi-normal or less than normal response in kwashiorkor (14). Normal levels of aldosterone, but an elevated secretion rate, were found in marasmus; increased levels but with a normal secretion rate were found in kwashiorkor (16).

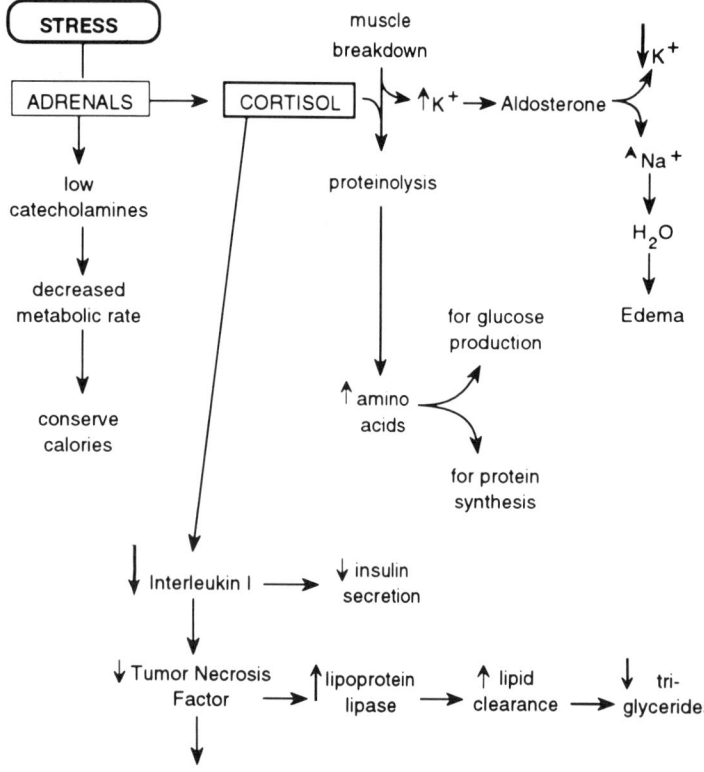

FIG. 1. Rationale for the adrenal response to malnutrition.

Functional Significance (Fig. 1)

According to Selye (4), cortisol is at the center of the adaptive response to a particular stimulus. The catabolic action of cortisol provides the required amino acids, from muscle, for organs with a high protein turnover. Furthermore, the action of the increased cortisol level spills into immunologically related alterations that can affect metabolism, as well as host-defense mechanisms, setting the stage for possible infections. Steroids have been shown to inhibit transcriptional and post-transcriptional expression of both cachectin/tumor necrosis factor (CTNF) and interleukin-1 (IL-1), which are directly related to carbohydrate, protein, and lipid metabolism (17,18).

The increase in aldosterone may be involved, at least in part, in two important adaptive mechanisms: (a) increased sodium reabsorption to combat the decreased plasma volume in PEM, and (b) increased potassium excretion, to combat the tendency of potassium to accumulate from catabolic breakdown of muscle proteins.

Existing data on catecholamine secretion are conflicting. Certainly alterations in catecholamine levels may play a part in maintaining homeorrhesis during malnutrition. It has been shown that during experimental fasting there is suppression of the sympathetic nervous system leading to a decrease in the metabolic rate and the conservation of calories (19).

PANCREAS

Insulin, Glucagon, and Glucose

The histologic changes in the pancreas of animals generally point to reduced beta-cell function. In children dying from PEM, however, the histology of the islets of Langerhans generally appears to be normal (20).

Basal insulin levels in children with PEM appear to be low. Fasting levels of plasma insulin, however, appear normal, depending on whether fasting blood glucose levels were normal or low. In some cases, insulin secretion after glucose administration can be augmented by the addition of IV glucagon, suggesting impaired release mechanisms rather than deficient synthesis (21). Insulin resistance has been described (22). However, resistance is not due to an abnormal molecule as assessed by chromatography but may be due to an increase in circulatory factors known to be associated with insulin resistance, such as growth hormone (GH), cortisol, or free fatty acids (23). In fact, impaired tolerance to a glucose or amino acid load has also been described in malnutrition (24).

Insulin secretion has also been found to directly correlate with body potassium content in kwashiorkor (25). Potassium depletion, possibly a consequence of aldosterone secretion (Fig. 1), and/or diarrhea would be further stimuli to inhibiting insulin secretion.

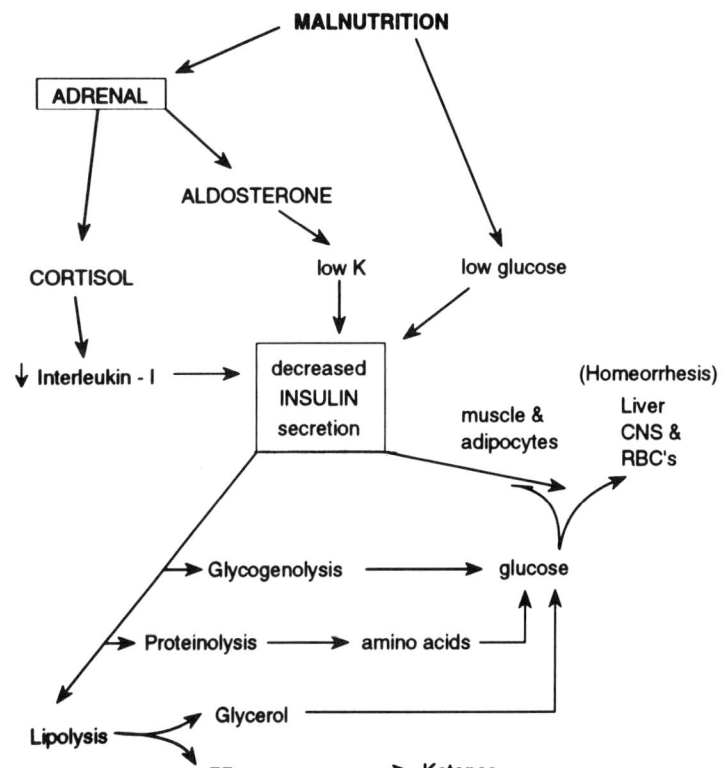

FIG. 2. Rationale for the insulin response to malnutrition.

Information regarding insulin degradation and clearance rates in humans is not available. The available animal data indicate that these metabolic parameters are normal.

There are also few studies of glucagon secretion. Poor glucagon response to arginine has been reported. Lower glucagon levels in blood samples of hypoglycemic children compared to those from normoglycemic children with malnutrition have also been reported (26).

One cannot speak of insulin without considering glucose homeostasis, which is of paramount importance in the successful adaptation to PEM. The response of blood glucose to epinephrine and glucagon has been found to be defective in kwashiorkor (27,28). This might imply a defect in hepatic glycogenolysis. Conversely, the response of blood glucose to epinephrine and glucagon has been found to be exaggerated in marasmus (27). This may be secondary to hyperactivity of the adrenal cortex.

Functional Significance (Fig. 2)

A situation that favors low insulin levels will cause glycogen breakdown (to produce glucose), protein breakdown (to furnish amino acids for glucose production), and fat breakdown (to furnish ketones as an alternate fuel source). The low insulin levels will diminish glucose uptake by insulin-dependent tissues, thus allowing more glucose to be available to the brain and other obligate glucose users.

GROWTH HORMONE AND SOMATOMEDIN-C

Although data from animal studies indicate that pituitary size is reduced with histologic evidence of marked depletion and degranulation of acidophils, suggesting hypofunction, serum growth hormone levels in marasmus have been found to be low, normal, or elevated (29). In diseases associated with severe wasting or caloric deprivation, GH levels, both basally and after stimulation, have been found to be markedly elevated (30,31). These levels seem predicated on the degree and the associated consequences of malnutrition.

The elevated GH levels do not correlate with fasting blood glucose, as they would in normal individuals, but appear to be related to at least three factors: plasma albumin, amino acids, and somatomedin-C.

A correlation ($r = .7$) has been found between GH levels and a reduction in plasma albumin (32). Growth hormone increases and somatomedin-C decreases when albumin falls to levels less than 2.5 g/dl (33–35). However, correction of the hypoalbuminemia with intravenous albumin infusion does not result in a decrease in the GH levels (36). Interestingly, milk feeding for 1 day has been shown to bring about a fall in GH levels without altering the serum concentration of albumin (36).

In addition to serum albumin, an inverse relationship has also been observed between serum amino acid levels and GH; this has been considered more likely to be the stimulus for GH secretion (33,37). However, again no correlation exists after administering amino acids, except if the amino acid is alanine. An inverse correlation between basal serum GH and alanine levels has been reported that persists during therapy with alanine (38). Since alanine is the amino acid precursor to gluconeogenesis, its inverse correlation with GH levels may imply a possible feedback relationship between GH and carbohydrate metabolism (39).

The feedback relationship between GH and somatomedin-C is probably the most plausible explanation for the elevated GH secretion in malnutrition (40,41). Low somatomedin-C levels have been demonstrated in PEM, although the actual mechanism is still not clear.

Functional Significance (Fig. 3)

The low insulin and elevated cortisol levels, which are known to inhibit somatomedin-C, together with the general failure of the liver to synthesize protein, may all contribute to the low somatomedin-C levels. The primary factor appears to be the low somatomedin-C level, which, depending on the degree of PEM, leads to a secondary increase in GH. The lack of alanine, which is a

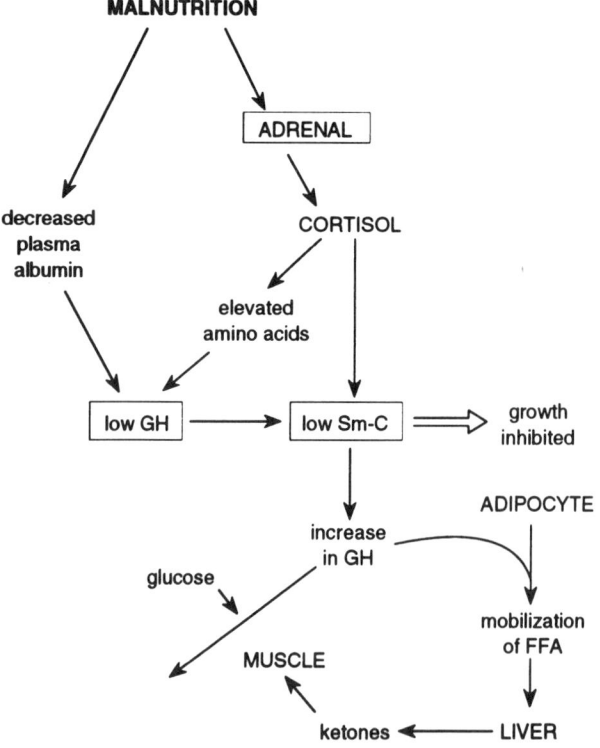

FIG. 3. Rationale for the growth hormone (GH) and somatomedin-C (Sm-C) response to malnutrition.

reflection of inadequate gluconeogenesis, may be an alternative stimulus for GH secretion. The increased GH and low somatomedin-C levels would deviate substrates away from growth toward metabolic homeostasis, such as mobilization of free fatty acids from adipose tissue stores and inhibition of glucose uptake by muscle cells, making more of it available to the brain and obligate glucose users.

THYROID GLAND

Thyroxine (T_4), Triiodothyronine (T_3), Reverse-T_3, Thyroid-Stimulating Hormone (TSH), and Thyroxine-Binding Globulins

Anatomic studies of the thyroid from malnourished infants revealed the gland to be atrophied with collapsed follicles of irregular shape, washed-out colloid, and extensive fibrosis, strongly reminiscent of hypofunctional or resting states (42,43). The histologic picture of pituitary thyrotrophs from protein-depleted rats is not, however, indicative of a decreased TSH secretory state (44).

There is a relatively unified scientific opinion regarding thyroid function. It is generally agreed that PEM is characterized by thyroid hypofunction. Total T_4 (TT_4) tends to be low (45), whereas free T_4 (FT_4) tends to be normal (46). In addition, both TT_3 and FT_3 have been found to be low (47). Other thyroid-related factors, such as reverse-T_3 (rT_3), have been found to be elevated (48); basal TSH may be low (49), normal (47), or high (45); and the thyroxine-binding globulins (TBG and TBPA) are reduced (49,50).

It has been suggested that reduction of both TT_4 and TT_3 may be due to impaired thyroidal secretion rate, low levels of binding proteins, and iodine deficiency from fecal loss.

Large quantities of inorganic or nonhormonal iodine leak from the altered gland throughout the course of malnutrition (51). This phenomenon, which is reported in several other disease conditions, is confirmed by unusually high mono- and diiodinated compounds in the bloodstream of children with PEM (52). In addition, the discharge of significant amounts of radioactive material following the perchlorate test provides indirect evidence for an intrathyroidal organification defect (53).

The low levels of binding proteins are probably the direct result of inadequate protein intake and the subsequent failure of hepatic biosynthesis of these proteins.

With regard to iodide deficiency from high fecal loss and malabsorption, it has been shown that the biological half-life of intestinal ^{131}I given orally to fasting children with PEM is greatly increased (5 hr 44 min) when compared to healthy children (45 min), demonstrating some degree of intestinal malabsorption involving dietary iodine (54). The residual radioactivity found in the stools of children with PEM indicates that fecal loss of dietary

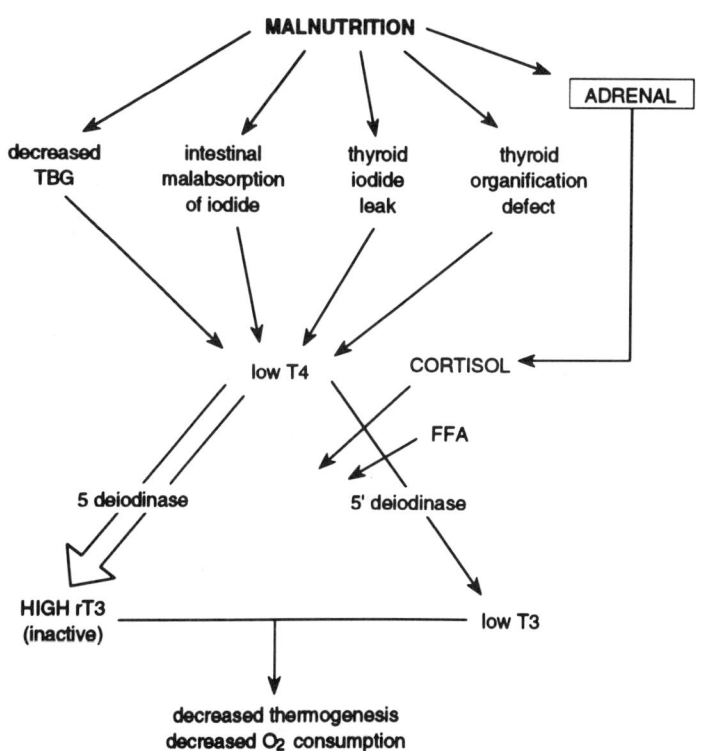

FIG. 4. Rationale for the thyroid hormones' response to malnutrition.

iodine due to malabsorption represents about 10% of intake.

Reverse-T_3 levels are elevated in malnutrition because of suppression of the normally active 5'-deiodinase enzyme and activation of the normally suppressed 5-deiodinase enzyme. Control of the 5- and 5'-deiodinase enzyme activity is dependent on three important factors: (a) free fatty acids and (b) corticosteroids, both of which are elevated in PEM, inhibit the 5'-deiodinase enzyme; (c) carbohydrates, which are relatively scarce in PEM, stimulate 5'-deiodinase. In fact, the depressed T_3 levels of starvation are rapidly corrected by refeeding as little as 100 kilocalories (Cal) of pure carbohydrate; neither protein nor fat, however, significantly influences recovery of T_3 (55).

Restoration of T_3 levels to normal in malnourished subjects is associated with a prompt and significant increase in urinary nitrogen excretion. This increase is primarily in the form of urea, implying increased availability to the liver of glucogenic substrates (56). The increase in urinary excretion of 3-methylhistidine, which is not parallel to the increased excretion of ammonia and urea nitrogen, indicates that muscle breakdown probably does not provide the glucogenic substrate to the liver, but that the substrate supporting the increased urinary ammonia and urea excretion is probably derived from hepatic proteolysis.

The thyroid-related abnormalities encountered in PEM are related to severity and duration. In short-term and mild malnutrition, the observed abnormalities are confined to the thyroid hormonal transport system; the normal feedback mechanism maintains euthyroidism. In long-term and severe malnutrition, the peripheral adaptive measures are overwhelmed and the thyroid gland may undergo various involuted processes, which, in children, invariably lead to hypothyroidism.

Functional Significance (Fig. 4)

The reduction of active thyroid hormones and the shifting to the formation of inactive metabolites (rT_3) will decrease thermogenesis and oxygen consumption leading to conservation of energy and protein.

GONADS

Sex Hormones: Luteinizing Hormone (LH) and Follicle-Stimulating Hormone (FSH)

The variability in pituitary and gonadal function has been thought to be related to the degree of malnutrition. Information from animal (57) and human (7) studies concerning the anatomical and histopathologic changes of the gonads suggests the presence of diminished gonadal activity. Insufficient data exist on the activity state of the pituitary gonadotrophs.

The secretory profile of sex-related hormones indicates a difference between the adult and child. In the adult, testosterone levels (58), as well as estradiol levels, tend to be low in both sexes. However, LH and FSH tend to be high in some and low in others regardless of the level of testosterone. Human chorionic gonadotropin (HCG) stimulation produced a subnormal testosterone response in malnourished as well as renourished patients. Therefore, there is ample evidence of primary gonadal damage in adults during malnutrition irrespective of changes in the pituitary. In the child, basal LH and FSH levels have been reported to be normal (59) or decreased (60), and to exhibit a poor response of LH to luteinizing hormone releasing hormone (LH-RH) stimulation (61). Therefore, whereas the adult appears to have primarily gonadal failure, the major abnormality found in children is gonadotropin deficiency.

Functional Significance

In the male, the absence of androgens shuts off muscle protein synthesis so that amino acids can be diverted to more important life-sustaining organs. In both sexes, the absence of androgens prevents dispersion of protein synthesis to occur in such pubertal-related events as development of secondary sex characteristics and bone and linear growth. In females, absence of sex hormones delays reproductive capacity until pregnancy can be supported with adequate nutritional intake.

PROLACTIN

Prolactin studies are primarily related to adults and results are not uniform. Some investigators have found high prolactin levels in PEM that are attributed to suppression of pubertal development by directly inhibiting gonadotropin releasing hormone (GnRH) secretion (59). Others have found low basal prolactin levels in children and adults with either decreased or increased responses after thyrotropin releasing hormone (TRH) stimulation (62,63).

Higher prolactin levels have been reported in children with kwashiorkor than in children with marasmus (60). The functional significance of the altered prolactin levels in PEM is unknown, largely because the normal metabolic role of prolactin is unknown except for its involvement in lactation.

SUMMARY AND CONCLUSIONS

Based on current information presented, the following conclusions may be drawn:

A. Observed changes in hormone secretions appear to reflect an adaptive response to the lack of adequate body fuel.
B. The role played by hormones in such an adaptive response is to
   1. increase the amount of usable fuel from endogenous sources (i.e., increase in cortisol and, if necessary, growth hormone)
   2. assure that the produced fuel is utilized by those body structures that are involved with life-sustaining functions (i.e., low insulin)
   3. inhibit all unnecessary expenditure of fuel (energy) for

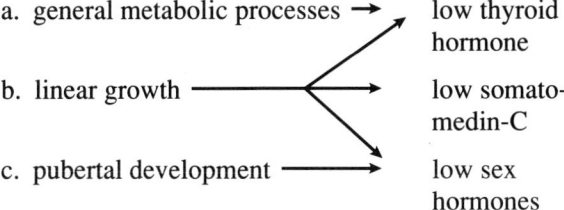

a. general metabolic processes → low thyroid hormone
b. linear growth → low somatomedin-C
c. pubertal development → low sex hormones

The extent to which the hormones will be increased or decreased depends upon the degree of malnutrition and the degree of adaptation. These factors may be the basis of contradictory data describing the endocrine status in malnourished children. The word *degree* implies a myriad of situations that may potentially exist within the status of malnutrition and adaptation.

Malnutrition, itself, encompasses a spectrum of situations, from the mildest to the most severe and from simple to highly complex. It is highly improbable that, within any study, two children, let alone a whole cohort, will be malnourished to the same degree.

The adaptive process responds to the existing degree of malnutrition, and may be altered by any complicating factors, for example, infection. This may explain the apparently contradictory data that are the results of studies describing a particular segment of the continuum of adaptive endocrine changes occurring in individual cases of malnutrition. The data, as they pertain to each study, are most likely all correct. It is important, therefore, to be acutely aware of what the behavior of a particular hormone implies is happening in the malnourished patient rather than what the behavior of a particular hormone is in malnutrition.

Marasmus

When energy intake is deficient, the body begins to furnish energy from endogenous sources (Fig. 5). Cortisol, crucial to this adaptive process, breaks down muscle protein to furnish amino acids. The existing endocrine milieu favors the uptake of amino acids by the liver, maintaining normal liver function (despite muscle wasting). Synthesis of apolipoproteins proceeds normally and triglycerides are not trapped in the liver. This adaptive process continues, as long as energy is not replaced from exogenous sources, until other factors upset the delicate homeorrhetic balance. The ultimate cessation of the adaptive process may be related to the adaptive process itself, which, in an attempt to maintain equilibrium, begins a process of decompensation. One example is the chronically elevated cortisol secretion that invariably affects immune processes, setting the stage for infection.

Kwashiorkor

Infection, with its increased demands on an already depleted body, leads to decompensation (Fig. 5). Cortisol can no longer adequately furnish amino acids from muscle protein catabolism. The decrease in amino acids becomes the major constraint on protein synthesis in the liver and at the same time stimulates growth hormone secretion, which mobilizes FFA from adipose tissue stores in an attempt to maintain adequate amounts of fuel. The liver, being unable to maintain adequate protein synthesis, affects, among other processes, the levels of apolipoproteins, binding proteins and enzymes. Because of decreased apolipoprotein synthesis, triglycerides are not released, resulting in fatty infiltration of the liver. With no intervention, including combating infection and replacing energy, the cycle repeats itself with continued decompensation until death supervenes.

One does not have to travel to the most remote parts of underdeveloped countries to find malnutrition. Second-

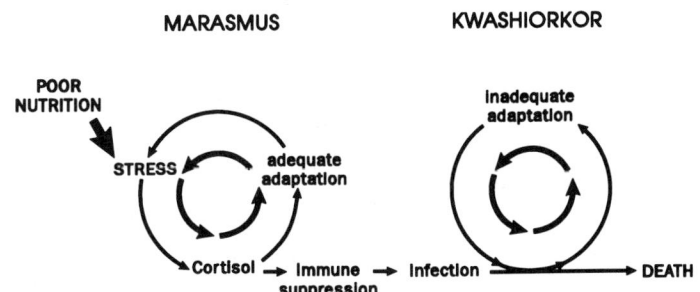

FIG. 5. Adequate and inadequate adaptation to malnutrition resulting in marasmus and kwashiorkor.

ary malnutrition, the result of many commonly encountered chronic diseases, must be appreciated as a problem to be dealt with vigorously as a specific disease entity, not simply another feature of the basic disease.

Although the endocrine changes observed in PEM tend to be adaptive, that is, are mechanisms to conserve energy and direct essential substrates to life-sustaining functions, concomitant complications or the deleterious ramifications of prolonged adaptive measures may, in the long run, defeat this purpose.

REFERENCES

1. Seoane N, Latham M. Nutritional anthropometry in the identification of protein calorie malnutrition in childhood. *J Trop Ped Envir Child Hlth* 1971;17:98–104.
2. Bauman DE, Currie WB. Partitioning of nutrients during pregnancy and lactation: a review of mechanisms involving homeostasis and homeorrhesis. *J Dairy Sci* 1980;63:1514–1528.
3. Selye H. Hormones and resistance. *J Pharm Sci* 1971;60:1–28.
4. Selye H. The story of the adaptation syndrome. *Acta* Montreal, 1952.
5. Gopalan C. Kwashiorkor and marasmus. Evolution and distinguishing features. In: McCance RA, Widdowson EM, eds. *Calorie deficiencies and protein deficiencies.* London: Churchill, 1968;49–58.
6. Castellanos H, Arroyave G. Role of the adrenal cortical system in the response of children to severe protein malnutrition. *Am J Clin Nutr* 1961;9:186–195.
7. Zubiran S, Gomez-Mont F. Endocrine disturbances in chronic human malnutrition. *Vitam Horm* 1953;11:97–132.
8. Trowell HC, Davies JNP, Dean RFA. *Kwashiorkor.* London: Arnold, 1954.
9. Lunn PG, Whitehead RG, Baker BA. Progressive changes in serum cortisol, insulin and growth hormone concentrations and their relationship to the distorted aminoacid pattern during the development of kwashiorkor. *Br J Nutr* 1973;29:399–422.
10. Smith SR, Bledsoe T, Chhetri MK. Cortisol metabolism and the pituitary-adrenal axis in adults with protein-calorie malnutrition. *J Clin Endocrinol Metab* 1975;40:43–52.
11. Alleyne GAO, Young VH. Adrenocortical function in children with severe protein-calorie malnutrition. *Clin Sci* 1967;33:189–200.
12. Samuel AM, Kadival GV, Patel BD, Desai AG. Adrenocorticosteroids and corticosteroid binding globulins in protein-calorie malnutrition. *Am J Clin Nutr* 1976;29:889–894.
13. Munro HN, Hutchinson WC, Ramaiah TR, Neilson FJ. The influence of diet on the weight and chemical constituents of the rat adrenal gland. *Br J Nutr* 1962;16:387–395.
14. Jaya Rao KS, Srikontia SG, Gopalan C. Plasma cortisol levels in protein-calorie malnutrition. *Arch Dis Child* 1968;43:365–367.
15. Beitens IZ, Kowarski A, Migeon CJ, Graham G. Adrenal function in normal infants and in marasmus and kwashiorkor: cortisol secretion, diurnal variation of plasma cortisol and urinary excretion of 17-hydroxycorticoids, free corticoids and cortisol. *J Pediatr* 1975;86:302–308.
16. Beitens IZ, Graham GG, Kowarski A, Migeon CJ. Adrenal function in normal infants and in marasmus and kwashiorkor: plasma aldosterone concentration and aldosterone secretion rate. *J Pediatr* 1974;84:444–451.
17. Beutler B, Krochin N, Milsark IW, Luedke C, Cerami A. Control of cachectin (tumor necrosis factor) synthesis—mechanism of endotoxin resistance. *Science* 1986;232:977–980.
18. Knudson PJ, Dinarello CA, Strom TB. Glucocorticoids inhibit transcriptional and post-transcriptional expression of interleukin-1 in U937 cells. *J Immunol* 1987;139:4129–4134.
19. Landsberg L, Young JB. Fasting, feeding and regulation of sympathetic nervous system. *N Engl J Med* 1978;298:1295–1301.
20. Viteri F, Behar M, Arroyave G. Clinical aspects of protein malnutrition. In: Munro HN, Allison JB, eds. *Mammalian protein metabolism.* vol 2. New York: Academic Press, 1964;523–528.
21. Becker DJ, Pimstone BL, Hansen JDL, Hendricks S. Insulin secretion in protein-calorie malnutrition: I. Quantitative abnormalities and the response to treatment. *Diabetes* 1971;20:542–551.
22. Becker DJ, Pimstone BL, Hansen JDL, MacHutchon B, Drysdale A. Patterns of insulin response to glucose in protein-calorie malnutrition. *Am J Clin Nutr* 1972;25:499–505.
23. Becker DJ, Murray PJ, Hansen JDL, Pimstone BL. Circulating "big" insulin in PCM. *Br J Nutr* 1973;30:345–350.
24. Cahill GF, Herrera MG, Morgan AP, Soeloner TS, Steinke J, Levy PL, Reichard GA, Kipnis DM. Hormone-fuel interrelationships during fasting. *J Clin Invest* 1966;45:1751–1769.
25. Becker DJ, Mann MD, Weinkwe E, Pimstone BL. Early insulin release and its response to potassium supplementation in protein calorie malnutrition. *Diabetologia* 1975;11:237–239.
26. Buchanan N, Moddley G, Eyberg C, Bloom SR, Hansen JDL. Hypoglycemia associated with severe kwashiorkor. *S Afr Med J* 1976;50:1442–1446.
27. Jaya Rao KS. Kwashiorkor and marasmus. Blood sugar levels and response to epinephrine. *Am J Dis Child* 1965;110:519–522.
28. Milner RDG. Metabolic and hormonal responses to glucose and glucagon in patients with infantile malnutrition. *Ped Res* 1971;5:33–39.
29. Srebnik HH, Nelson MM, Simpson ME. Reduced growth hormone content in anterior pituitaries of rats on protein-free diets. *Proc Soc Exp Biol Med* 1959;101:97–99.
30. Tenore A, Berman WF, Parks JS, Bongiovanni AM. Basal and stimulated serum growth hormone concentration in inflammatory bowel disease. *J Clin Endocrinol Metab* 1977;44:622–628.
31. Merimee TJ. Endocrine manifestations of systemic disease. *Clin Endocrinol Metab* 1979;8:453–466.
32. Pimstone BL, Barbezat G, Hansen JDL, Murray P. Studies on growth hormone secretion in protein calorie malnutrition. *Am J Clin Nutr* 1968;21:482–487.
33. Samuel AM, Deshpand UR. Growth hormone levels in protein-calorie malnutrition. *J Clin Endocrinol Metab* 1972;35:863–867.
34. Raghuramulu N, Rao KSJ. Growth hormone secretion in protein-calorie malnutrition. *J Clin Endocrinol Metab* 1974;38:176–180.
35. Mohan PS, Rao KSJ. Plasma somatomedin activity in protein calorie malnutrition. *Arch Dis Child* 1979;54:62–64.
36. Becker DJ, Pimstone BL, Hansen JDL, Hendricks S. Serum albumin and growth hormone in kwashiorkor and the nephrotic syndrome. *J Lab Clin Med* 1971;78:865–871.
37. Suskind R, Amayatakul R, Leitzmann C, Olson RE. Interrelationships between growth hormone and aminoacid metabolism in protein-calorie malnutrition. In: Gardner LI, Amacher P, eds. *Endocrine aspects of malnutrition.* Santa Ynez, CA: The Kroc Foundation, 1973;99–113.
38. Pimstone BL, Becker DJ, Hansen JDL. Human growth hormone in protein-calorie malnutrition. In: Pecile A, Muller EE, eds. *Growth and growth hormone.* Proc 2nd Int Symp on Growth Hormone, Milan-Italy. Amsterdam: Excerpta Medica Foundation, 1972;389–401.
39. Felig P, Pozefsky T, Marliss E, Cahill GF Jr. Alanine: key role in gluconeogenesis. *Science* 1970;167:1003–1004.
40. Grant DB, Hambley J, Becker DJ, Pimstone BL. Reduced sulphation factor in undernourished children. *Arch Dis Child* 1973;48:596–600.
41. Hintz RL, Suskind R, Amatayakui K, Thanangkul O, Olson R. Plasma somatomedin and growth hormone values in children with protein-calorie malnutrition. *J Pediatr* 1978;92:153–159.
42. Stirling GA. The thyroid in malnutrition. *Arch Dis Child* 1962;37:99–102.
43. Ejeckham GC, Attah EB. The thyroid gland in kwashiorkor. A pathologic study. *J Trop Pedit Envir Child Hlth* 1975;21:298–300.
44. Florsheim WH, Suhr BZ, Mirise RT, Williams AD. Thyroid function in protein-depleted rats. *J Endocrinol* 1970;46:93–99.
45. Pimstone BL, Becker DJ, Hendricks S. TSH response to synthetic thyrotropin-releasing hormone in human protein-calorie malnutrition. *J Clin Endocrinol Metab* 1973;36:779–783.
46. Parra A, Klish W, Cuellar A, Serrano PA, Garcia G, Argote RM, Conseco L, Nichols BL. Energy metabolism and hormonal profile

47. Ingenbleek Y, Beckers C. Triiodothyronine and thyroid stimulating hormone in protein-calorie malnutrition in infants. *Lancet* 1975;2:845–847.
48. Chopra IJ, Smith SR. Circulating thyroid hormones and thyrotropin in adult patients with protein-calorie malnutrition. *J Clin Endocrinol Metab* 1975;40:221–227.
49. Graham GG, Baerth JM, Claeyssen G, Suskind R, Greenberg AH, Thompson RG, Blizzard RM. Thyroid hormonal studies in normal and severely malnourished infants and small children. *J Pediatr* 1973;83:321–331.
50. Ingenbleek Y, DeVisscher M, DeNayer P. Measurement of prealbumin as index of protein-calorie malnutrition. *Lancet* 1972;2:106–108.
51. Ingenbleek Y. In: Delange F, Fisher DA, Malvaux P, eds. *Pediatric and adolescent endocrinology*, vol 14. Basel: Karger, 1985; 345–368.
52. Godard C, Lemarchand-Beraud T. Plasma thyrotropin levels in severe infantile malnutrition. *Horm Res* 1973;4:43–52.
53. Jaya Rao KS, Raghuramula N, Srikantia SG. Thyroid function in kwashiorkor. *Indian J Med Res* 1971;59:1300–1304.
54. Ingenbeek Y, Beckers C. Evidence for intestinal malabsorption of iodine in protein-calorie malnutrition. *Am J Clin Nutr* 1973;26:1323–1330.
55. Azizi F. Effect of dietary composition on fasting induced changes in serum thyroid hormones and thyrotropin. *Metabolism* 1978;27:935–942.
56. Vignati L, Finley RJ, Haag S, Aoki TT. Protein conservation during prolonged fast: a function of triiodothyronine levels. *Trans Assoc Am Physicians* 1978;91:169–179.
57. Gopalan C. Endocrines in malnutrition. *Indian J Med Sci* 1956;10:370–374.
58. Smith SR, Chhetri MK, Johanson AJ, Radfar N, Migeon C. The pituitary-gonadal axis in men with protein-calorie malnutrition. *J Clin Endocrinol Metab* 1975;41:60–69.
59. Olusi SO, Orrell DH, Morris P, McFarlane H. A study of endocrine function in protein energy malnutrition. *Clin Chim Acta* 1977;74:261–269.
60. Chakravarty I, Sreedhar R, Ghosh K, Bulusi S. Circulating gonadotropin profile in severe cases of protein malnutrition. *Fertil Steril* 1982;37:650–654.
61. Pimstone BL, Becker DJ, Kronheim S. LH and FSH response to gonadotropin-releasing hormone in normal and malnourished infants. In: Radioimmunoassay, methodology and application in physiology and in clinical studies. *Horm Metab Res* Suppl 1974;5:179–183.
62. Becker DJ, Vinik AI, Pimstone BL, Paul M. Prolactin responses to thyrotropin-releasing-hormone in protein-calorie malnutrition. *J Clin Endocrinol Metab* 1975;41:782–783.
63. Di Maio S, Capano G, Sandomenico ML, Zaccaria S, Guarino A, Ecuba P, Mariano A. Prolactin and thyroid hormones in malnourished children. *Riv Ital Pediatr* (IJP) 1989;15:1–9.

CHAPTER 14

Malnutrition and Mental Development

Janina R. Galler and Robert N. Ross

Understanding the tangled relationship of early malnutrition, brain development, and mental function has become an urgent problem in the last two or three decades. Widespread implementation of public health measures has permitted increasing numbers of children to survive episodes of severe malnutrition; many of these children are now of reproductive age and, indeed, are having children of their own. Assessing the quality of life they experienced in their earliest years and its etiological role in malnutrition, and evaluating the enduring impact of early childhood malnutrition are thus of utmost importance.

Throughout the world, as many as half the children in pediatric wards, particularly in poor communities, suffer from either primary or secondary malnutrition. This problem exists not only in developing countries, where it affects 40% to 60% of the population, but also in wealthier nations, including the United States. As we learn to deal with the acute effects of malnutrition and their sequelae, which are, for the most part, physical, we are confronted by a growing awareness that long-term psychological effects remain to be addressed.

EFFECT OF MALNUTRITION ON MENTAL DEVELOPMENT

The effect of malnutrition on mental and physical development depends on a number of factors. Both the *type* and *severity* of malnutrition are very important, regardless of whether the condition is severe, overwhelming protein-energy malnutrition, simple protein deficiency, or, more commonly, vitamin, iron, or essential mineral deficiencies. The *timing of malnutrition* in the child's brain development is also important. The critical period occurs from the second trimester prenatally through the second year of life (1,2). This is the stage of most rapid brain growth and development. If nutritional deficits of any degree occur during this time, the likelihood of long-lasting effects is much greater than if such deficits were to occur later in the life of the child. Effects occurring during this "critical period" are generally thought to be irreversible.

Another factor is the *duration* of malnutrition. Clearly, a long period of malnutrition can be expected to produce more severe deficits than a shorter period. The problem during early malnutrition is the continued, uninterrupted privation during critical growth periods. Compounding the effects of duration is the extent to which positive and negative *environmental factors* are superimposed on the episode of malnutrition. Research on the effects of early childhood malnutrition has been complicated, however, by the fact that environmental factors can either exacerbate or ameliorate outcome. Poverty, ignorance, and poor medical attention, for example, can increase the risk of malnutrition and will almost certainly adversely affect the result. On the other hand, education, rapid medical response, and positive parental influence can minimize the long-term effects. Finally, there are the baffling *intrinsic factors* that predispose some children to suffer adverse effects of malnutrition, whereas other, apparently similar, children in apparently similar circumstances seem to escape.

Animal Models

Animal models have been particularly useful in providing information on how malnutrition can affect brain and mental development (3,4). We should be aware, however, that animal models are not a completely faithful reproduction of the clinical phenomena under study; behavior is not directly comparable from one species to another. Well-designed studies, however, can provide in-

J. R. Galler, R. N. Ross: Center for Behavioral Development and Mental Retardation, Boston University School of Medicine, Boston, Massachusetts 02118.

valuable information about the human condition because, although the specific repertoire of human and animal behaviors may differ, the biochemical and cellular bases of those behaviors—the structure and function of the nervous system—are sufficiently common to permit many valid comparisons. Moreover, animal studies that encompass a range of behavioral outcomes are most likely to be relevant to the human condition. The research advantages in animal studies include the ability to exercise rigorous experimental controls and to manipulate conditions, and, because of the shortened life span and reproductive period of laboratory animals, to study the effects of malnutrition over an animal's full life and through subsequent generations.

Animal studies have found that malnutrition early in life disrupts normal brain development at the cellular and biochemical levels (5). Moreover, functional disturbances persist throughout life (6,7). Our own laboratory studies have demonstrated that many of the mental or behavioral effects of malnutrition may continue for up to three to four generations (8,9).

Human Studies

Immediate Effects

The findings of our animal studies corroborate our clinical observations. When small children are *concurrently malnourished,* neurological and behavioral manifestations are the direct outcome of metabolic disturbances associated with nutritional privation; profound effects on brain and behavior can be observed. Autopsy data show reduced brain weight in malnourished children (10,11). Children with malnutrition have grossly pathological EEGs (12) and abnormal responses to auditory evoked potentials (13).

The effect on behavior is also negative (Table 1). Children with primary or secondary malnutrition associated with one of a number of medical conditions are apathetic and less active (14–16). They show delays on all developmental scales (17). Most marked is the delay in language development (18,19). Abnormal crying patterns are similar to those seen in children with CNS dysfunction (20). Cardiac habituation, or the decline in heart rate as an infant becomes accustomed to an unfamiliar stimulus, does not occur as rapidly as in the normal infant (21).

TABLE 1. *Behavioral effects of current malnutrition*

Apathy
Developmental delays
Delays in language development
Abnormal crying patterns and habituation
Altered mother–infant interaction

Significantly, the behavioral abnormalities are likely to have an adverse effect on the mother-infant relationship (22). When a baby is ill, there is generally increased suckling, clinging, and dependence on the mother. In many instances, particularly when malnutrition is associated with disadvantage and poverty, aberrant mothering and reduced stimulation of the baby may also contribute to the occurrence of malnutrition (19,23).

For 3 years we have been following 87 mother-infant pairs in a population of Mayan Indians in the southern Yucatán. Chronic malnutrition is extremely common in this region. Our aim is to identify factors in early childhood that influence the patterns of a child's subsequent growth and development. In two of the four communities in our study, a community-based intervention program taught each mother simple information about the nutrition, health, and mental development of her child. In a preliminary study of this population, 26 babies, between 6 and 12 months of age, were classified into two groups: mildly to moderately malnourished and well nourished. We documented the differences between the babies as well as interaction between caretakers and babies (24).

This population is unusual in that there are multiple caretakers, not simply the parents. The significant differences between the malnourished and well-nourished infants included increased fussing in the undernourished babies. Responses of caretakers were also altered. Caretakers looked at the well-nourished babies more often than at undernourished babies. They also brought toys to the attention of well-nourished babies more frequently. Undernourished babies, however, were held more often than were well-nourished babies.

These findings are important, not only because they reflect the differences in nutritional status of the children, but also because they indicate an interference in the normal pattern of caretaker-infant interaction that may prevent the malnourished baby from acquiring essential learning experiences from its environment. Thus, developmental delays resulting from malnutrition may be compounded by experiences that fundamentally differ from those of healthy babies. This is an important consideration regardless of whether the malnourished child is in the Yucatán or in a more prosperous clinical setting.

Babies in this sample were also evaluated for temperament, using behavioral profiles compiled from maternal reports (25). These profiles were based on temperament scales assumed to measure stable behavioral characteristics as early as *in utero* (26–27). Based on a classification system of nine behavioral categories, we found that 79% of the well-nourished Mayan babies were classified as "easy" babies and only 21% as "difficult" babies. These frequencies compared favorably with American, Canadian, and English populations, where 75% to 85% babies are described as being easy. However, in our malnourished group, the proportion of easy babies was 45% and difficult babies, 55%. The shift toward a greater incidence of difficult babies may have adverse effects on the caretaker-infant interaction. Conversely, a "difficult" temperament may be adaptive in an underprivileged setting, resulting in more attention by caretakers (28).

Recovery

Rapid physiologic and metabolic changes take place during *recovery* from malnutrition, as the organism attempts to restore adequate levels of growth and maturation (29). These efforts are not totally successful, however, as shown by continuing brain and behavioral deficits during this period. Children who were malnourished during the critical periods of brain development were found to have reduced head circumference at later ages (30). Many studies of malnourished children have used this as a marker of the damage that the child has experienced, although there are often difficulties in making accurate measurements. Gross changes in the EEG are no longer observed. However, auditory evoked potentials continue to be abnormal (13).

The period during recovery from malnutrition is especially important because interventions at this time may be particularly beneficial. Unfortunately, because the child is medically cleared, there is a strong probability that the more subtle behavioral deficits will go unnoticed (Table 2). For example, once adequate nutritional support is provided, apathy disappears; concomitantly there is a dramatic increase in motor and exploratory skills. In contrast to these changes, however, are continued delays in language and mental development. Numerous studies report that these deficits in developmental quotients continue even when a child has "recovered" from malnutrition (31–33). Indeed, rehabilitation programs often seem to consider recovery complete without regard to the long-term cognitive-behavioral problems that may still exist. Therefore, although the physical signs of recovery are the most obvious and the easiest to measure, physicians must be acutely conscious of the more subtle cognitive and emotional signs. These may be most significant precisely because they are so slow to manifest themselves.

Long-Term Sequelae

Most evidence for permanent behavioral deficits from an episode of malnutrition comes from several studies that have followed previously malnourished children up to adolescence or early adulthood (34–40). Head circumference is reduced, especially following a history of marasmus in the first 2 years of life (41). Although alpha rhythm may be reduced, gross changes in EEG are no longer present once a child has been adequately provided with nutritional support (37). Recent reports using computed tomography (CT) scans show underdevelopment of the temporoparietal region (42). The functional implication of this structural change remains to be elucidated. One sees soft neurologic signs in children at least through 18 years of age (43). These children are clumsy and their fine motor skills are impaired. However, at these later ages, they do not demonstrate any type of gross neurological deficits.

The most striking effects of early malnutrition are behavioral and mental (Table 3). IQ tests, the most commonly applied measure in long-term studies of malnutrition, indicate deficits in cognitive development (34,43–46). This is especially true in children with marasmus who may have been more severely affected than those with kwashiorkor as a result of the earlier onset and more chronic course. Our own studies, however, comparing the two disorders with a similar age of onset, failed to show any consistent differences in IQ (43).

The usefulness of IQ tests, especially in cross-cultural studies, may be limited (47). Consequently, other kinds of cognitive measures have also been applied, including tests of intersensory integration, Piagetian tasks, and assessments of school performance. These have generally been thought to be more appropriate because they are less culture-bound than standard IQ tests.

Intersensory integration, or the ability to transfer information from one sensory modality to another, may be impaired long after the episode of malnutrition (48,49). This has been associated with learning disabilities (50). Reduced performance on Piagetian tests has also been documented (43,51). In addition, previously malnourished children demonstrate impaired school performance (49,52–54). This is characterized by lower marks, reduced scores on achievement tests, and attentional deficits. In fact, the impaired school child is largely determined by attentional deficits rather than by IQ (55). Finally, children with previous malnutrition may also demonstrate low self-esteem.

TABLE 2. *Behavioral effects during recovery from malnutrition*

Reversal of apathy
Improved motor and exploratory skills
Continued delays in language and mental development
Reduced developmental quotient

TABLE 3. *Behavioral function: long-term effects of early malnutrition through adolescence*

Decreased IQ scores
Delayed cognitive development (Piaget)
Impaired intersensory integration
Impaired school performance
Attention-deficit disorder (60% vs 15%)
Low self-esteem

The Barbados Study

The long-term effects of early malnutrition are illustrated by our longitudinal study, conducted in Barbados over a 23-year period. We followed approximately 320 children, half of whom had experienced severe infantile malnutrition.

Barbados, a small island with a population of 250,000, was ideal as a study site. The National Nutrition Centre, under the aegis of the Ministry of Health, was established in the mid-1960s. Since its inception, over 2,100 cases of malnutrition, from mild to severe, were referred there, in part the result of malnutrition being considered a reportable disease.

In addition, socioeconomic conditions are stable in Barbados. The population is relatively homogeneous and accessible. With a literacy rate of 99%, living standards are higher than in most other developing countries. Education and health records are carefully maintained and readily available. Because of these factors, it is easier to generalize findings in malnourished children to more developed parts of the world and to control for the role of environmental disadvantage.

We studied nearly every child born on the island between 1967 and 1972 who had a single episode of severe malnutrition in the first year of life. These children had been hospitalized with either marasmus or kwashiorkor. We compared these children to a group of healthy children, on whom we also had prenatal, perinatal, and postnatal information, who had no history of malnutrition. Comparison children were drawn from the same socioeconomic group and were mostly classmates of the index children. Both groups had documented prenatal care, no prenatal or postnatal complications, and birth weights greater than 2,268 g. The children were matched by a number of factors, including socioeconomic level, age, and sex. Because we looked at the neurologic and brain function of these children, the groups were also matched for handedness.

The children were comprehensively evaluated at three points in their lives: during early school age, during early adolescence, and during late adolescence. Examinations were made of cognitive function, behavior, neurologic function, and physical growth and development. We also documented the home-environmental conditions in which the children were being reared. The children now range in age from 18 to 23 years; a number have their own offspring, whom we are also planning to study.

Children with previous marasmus or kwashiorkor show a marked and significant shift to the left in IQ, having roughly 12.5 points less than the nonmalnourished controls (43). This difference persisted even after controlling for socioeconomic factors and conditions in the home environment. The statistically significant 12.5 point difference in IQ may not, in fact, be of major functional significance in the social and environmental setting in which these children were to live as adults.

Probably the most dramatic and persistent outcome of our study was the increased frequency of attention-deficit disorder among previously malnourished children (53). We first investigated this problem by asking teachers who had both index and comparison children in one classroom to describe the behavior of the children. The teachers had no way of knowing the differences in the children's nutritional histories. Yet it was evident that teachers could predict that history based on the child's present behavioral pattern. Children with poor nutritional histories had short attention spans, poor memory, were easily distracted, were not as cooperative as other children, were restless, and had the constellation of symptoms generally associated with the diagnosis of attention-deficit disorder. We found that 60% of our previously malnourished children suffered from attention-deficit disorder as opposed to 15% of the controls; 15% compares favorably with American statistics of school-age children. Further evaluations by teachers and parents (56) confirmed these findings. Thus, several different sources of data emphasized both the high frequency of attention-deficit disorder and the finding that such deficits persist through 18 years of age.

All children in Barbados take an academic qualifying examination at age 11 that determines the local high schools to which they will be assigned. Children who do not pass are assigned to trade schools. Responding to the concern of the Ministry of Education in Barbados as to why some children perform poorly, we compared the scores of previously malnourished children with those of controls. We found that the controls had significantly higher scores than those who had been malnourished (57). Children who had survived either marasmus or kwashiorkor performed similarly, showing a significant shift to the left in the scores. The control group, on the other hand, had the same distribution of scores found in the general population of Barbadian children.

Closer analysis showed that the single most important factor determining the difference on the 11-plus examination was whether or not the child had an attention-deficit disorder. There was a significant correlation ($r = .85$) between the presence of attention deficit as reported by teachers when children were as young as 5 to 8 years of age and low scores subsequently on the 11-plus examination. IQ performance at the earlier ages was also correlated, though less strongly, with later 11-plus scores. Because appropriate interventions at an early age may improve prognosis, the ability to predict these problems early is important.

In contrast to permanent impairment of the behavior and mental development, physical growth of children with histories of malnutrition ultimately "caught up." This was true although, initially, we documented small stature throughout childhood in our population, especially in girls (58). We also reported a delayed onset of puberty especially in girls with histories of marasmus. However, by the time the children completed puberty, we reported complete catch-up with respect to physical size (59). In our estimation, these findings support the theory that previously malnourished children can achieve a genetic growth potential given adequate nutritional and environmental support.

One of the most perplexing topics concerning nutrition and mental development is the role of environment and social background in the prognosis after an episode of malnutrition (60). Environment includes not only socioeconomic indices but also measures of the specific experiences available to the child in the home. Although some studies have indicated a strong environmental influence, our well-controlled study indicated that environmental factors, including microenvironmental and socioeconomic factors, did not play a major role in the outcome of the Barbadian children. The independent effects of malnutrition may be more striking when there is a greater variation in existing degrees of poverty.

Because studies have demonstrated that adequate nutrition alone is not sufficient to reverse long-term deficits in brain and behavioral development after recovery from malnutrition, knowledge of the child's environmental background is essential in designing suitable interventions (61). Children provided with cognitive stimulation in addition to improved nutrition have been shown to perform at control or near-normal levels. The series of studies of Jamaican children by Grantham-McGregor et al. (62,63) are especially convincing in supporting this conclusion. These investigators have shown that relatively simple interventions were effective in 6-year-olds who experienced severe malnutrition in the first 2 years of life.

CONCLUSIONS

There are several conclusions to be drawn from the review of the literature. First, later behavioral deficits arising from early moderate to severe malnutrition are much more permanent than physical deficits. Not surprisingly, medical practitioners and policymakers have only monitored physical growth when measuring the impact of interventions. Second, of the range of behavioral and cognitive effects, the most striking is the increase in occurrence of attention-deficit disorder in children who had early malnutrition. Third, these effects are independent of the social background of the child. However, a disadvantaged home environment augments the effects of early malnutrition. This is especially important in considering malnutrition in severely underprivileged settings and also in many cases of environmentally caused failure-to-thrive in Western countries. Finally, generational effects may be present as a partial explanation of why "poverty breeds poverty."

Considering the adverse outcome of infantile malnutrition, pediatricians and other health providers should be prepared to identify and treat this disorder. Clinicians should recognize that malnutrition may be an etiologic factor in behavior deficits. Children with low birth weight, failure-to-thrive, and other evidence of early nutritional deficits should be monitored on a regular basis. Follow-up beyond the period of illness and throughout the school years is indicated.

Mental functions are more sensitive than physical growth as measures of recovery from early malnutrition. It is therefore unfortunate that many national nutrition programs have been evaluated only on the basis of documenting physical growth patterns of participants. For example, the lack of clear effects on physical growth was a reason cited in the termination of national school breakfast and lunch programs for underprivileged children. Because factors in the home environment may contribute to or exacerbate the effects of malnutrition, these also should be monitored. Obviously, this would necessitate the involvement of experts in mental health or social work.

We conclude that public policy must change to include early comprehensive interventions for groups at risk for malnutrition. We have much to learn in our own country (as well as in other industrialized nations) of the worldwide experience with early childhood malnutrition.

SUMMARY

There is no quick fix for the long-term effects of malnutrition; merely saving a child's life is only the beginning. Public policy in the United States must change to include early comprehensive interventions for children at risk. Studies such as ours have shown that final success depends on a long-term rehabilitation program that monitors and treats growth and development along several physical, cognitive, and emotional dimensions.

REFERENCES

1. Dobbing J. The later development of the brain and its vulnerability. In: Davis JA, Dobbing J, eds. *Scientific foundations of pediatrics.* Philadelphia: W.B. Saunders, 1974;565–577.
2. Dobbing J, Smart JL. Early undernutrition, brain development and behavior. In: Barnett SA, ed. *Ethology & development,* vol 47. London: Heinemann, Clinics in Developmental Medicine, 1973;16–36.
3. Galler JR, Kanis K. Animal models of malnutrition applied to brain research. In: Rassin D, Haber B, Drujan B. eds. *Basic and clinical aspects of nutrition and brain development.* New York: Alan R. Liss, 1987;57–73.

4. Fleischer SF, Turkewitz G. The use of animals for understanding the effects of malnutrition on human behavior: models vs a comparative approach. In: Galler JR, ed. *Nutrition and behavior.* New York: Plenum Press, 1984;37–57.
5. Diaz-Cintra S, Cintra L, Galvan A, Aguilar A, Kemper T, Morgane PJ. Effects of prenatal protein deprivation on the postnatal development of granule cells in the fascia dentata. *J Comp Neurol* (in press).
6. Bronzino JD, Austin LaFrance RJ, Morgane PJ. Effects of prenatal protein malnutrition on perforant path kindling in the rat. *Brain Res* 1990;515:45–50.
7. Tonkiss J, Galler JR, Formica RN, Shukitt-Hale B, Timm RR. Fetal protein malnutrition impairs acquisition of a DRL task in adult rats. *Physiol Behav* 1990;48:73–77.
8. Galler JR, Seelig C. Home-orienting behavior in rat pups: the effects of two and three generations of rehabilitation following intergenerational malnutrition. *Dev Psychobiol* 1981;14:541–548.
9. Galler JR, Propert K. Maternal behavior following rehabilitation of rats with intergenerational malnutrition. II. Contribution of mothers and pups to deficits in lactation-related behaviors. *J Nutr* 1981;111:1337–1342.
10. Winick M, Rosso P. Head circumference and cellular growth of the brain in normal and marasmic children. *J Pediatr* 1969;74:774–778.
11. Chase HP, Canosa CA, Dabiere CS, Welch NN, O'Brien D. Postnatal undernutrition and human brain development. *J Ment Defic Res* 1974;18:355–366.
12. Nelson GK. The electroencephalogram in kwashiorkor. *Electroencephalogr Clin Neurophysiol* 1959;8:459.
13. Barnet AB, Weiss JP, Sotillo MV, Ohrlich ES, Sakurovich ZM, Cravioto J. Abnormal auditory evoked potentials in early infancy malnutrition. *Science* 1978;201:450–452.
14. Bowlby J. Separation anxiety. *Int J Psychoanal* 1960;41:89.
15. Meneghello J. *Desnutricion en el lactante mayor (Distrofia poliurencial).* Santiago, Chile: Central de Publicaciones, 1979.
16. Grantham-McGregor SM. Studies in behavior and malnutrition in Jamaica. *Royal Soc Trop Med* 1988;82:7–9.
17. Grantham-McGregor SM, Stewart ME. The relationship between hospitalization, social background, severe protein energy malnutrition and mental development in young Jamaican children. *Ecol Food Malnutr* 1980;98:151–156.
18. Cravioto J, Robles B. Evolution of adaptive and motor behavior during rehabilitation from kwashiorkor. *Am J Orthopsychiatry* 1965;35:449–464.
19. Cravioto J, DeLicardie ER. Environmental correlates of severe clinical malnutrition and language development in survivors from kwashiorkor or marasmus. In: *Nutrition, the nervous system and behavior.* PAHO Publication No. 251, 1972;73–94.
20. Lester BM. Spectrum analysis of the cry sounds of well-nourished and malnourished infants. *Child Dev* 1976;47:237–241.
21. Lester BM. Cardiac habituation of the orienting response to an auditory signal in infants of varying nutritional status. *Dev Psychol* 1975;11(4):432–442.
22. Galler JR, Ricciuti HN, Crawford MA, Kucharski LT. The role of mother-infant interaction in nutritional disorders. In: Galler JR, ed. *Nutrition and behavior.* New York: Pelnum Press, 1984;269–300.
23. Cravioto J, DeLicardie ER. Microenvironmental factors in severe protein-energy malnutrition. In: Scrimshaw NS, Behar M, eds. *Nutrition and agricultural development: significance and potential for the tropics.* New York: Plenum Press, 1976;25–35.
24. Cervera MD, Galler JR. Caretaker-infant interaction and malnutrition among the Mayans. (*Submitted for publication*).
25. Galler JR, Cervera MD. Infantile malnutrition and temperament among the Mayans. (*Submitted for publication*).
26. Chess TA, Birch S, Hertzig NG, Korn ME. *Behavioral individuality in early childhood.* New York: New York University Press, 1963.
27. Carey WB, McDevitt SC. Revision of the infant temperament questionnaire. *Pediatrics* 1978;61(5):735–739.
28. deVries MW. Temperament and infant mortality among the Masai of East Africa. *Am J Psychiatry* 1984;141:1189–1194.
29. Ramos-Galvan RR, Mariscal AC, Viniegra CA, Perez DB. Denutricion en el nino. *Impresiones Modernas,* Mexico City, Mexico, 1969;535–551.
30. Graham G. Growth during recovery from infantile malnutrition. *J Am Med Wom Assoc* 1966;21:737–742.
31. Stoch MB, Smythe PM. Does undernutrition during infancy inhibit brain growth and subsequent intellectual development? *Arch Dis Child* 1963;38:546–552.
32. Chase HP, Martin HP. Undernutrition and child development. *N Engl J Med* 1970;282:933–939.
33. Grantham-McGregor SM, Powell C, Stewart ME, Schofield WN. Longitudinal study of growth and development of young Jamaican children recovering from severe malnutrition. *Dev Med Child Neurol* 1982;24:321–331.
34. Richardson SA, Koller H, Katz M, Albert K. The contributions of differing degrees of acute and chronic malnutrition to the intellectual development of Jamaican boys. *Early Hum Dev* 1978;2(2):163–170.
35. Evans DE, Moodie AD, Hansen JDL. Kwashiorkor and intellectual development. *S Afr Med J* 1971;45:1414–1426.
36. Stoch MB, Smythe TM, Moodie AD, Bradshaw D. Psychosocial outcome and CT findings after growth undernourishment during infancy: a twenty-year developmental study. *Dev Med Child Neurol* 1982;24:419–436.
37. Bartel PR, Griesel RD, Freiman I, Rosen EU, Geefhuysen J. Long-term effects of kwashiorkor on the electroencephalogram. *Am J Clin Nutr* 1979;32:753–757.
38. Fisher MM, Killeross MC, Simonsson M, Elgie KA. Malnutrition and reasoning ability in Zambian school children. *Trans R Soc Trop Med Hyg* 1972;66:471–478.
39. Hoorweg J, Stanfield JP. The effects of protein energy malnutrition in early childhood on intellectual and motor abilities in later childhood and adolescence. *Dev Med Child Neurol* 1976;18:330–350.
40. Galler JR, Ramsey F, Morley DS, Archer E. The long term effects of early kwashiorkor compared with marasmus. IV. Performance on the national high school entrance examination. *Pediatr Res* 1990;28:235–239.
41. Hoorweg J, Stanfield JP. The effects of protein energy malnutrition in early childhood on intellectual and motor abilities in later childhood and adolescence. *Dev Med Child Neurol* 1976;18:330–350.
42. Stoch MB, Smythe TM, Moodie AD, Bradshaw D. Psychosocial outcome and CT findings after growth undernourishment during infancy: a twenty-year developmental study. *Dev Med Child Neurol* 1982;24:419–436.
43. Galler JR, Ramsey F, Salt P, Forde V. The long term effects of early kwashiorkor compared with marasmus. II. Intellectual performance. *J Pediatr Gastroenterol Nutr* 1987;6:847–854.
44. Winick M, Meger KK, Harris RC. Malnutrition and environmental enrichment by early adoption. *Science* 1975;190:1173–1175.
45. Birch HG, Pineiro C, Alcalde E, Toca T, Cravioto J. Relation of kwashiorkor in early childhood and intelligence at school age. *Pediatr Res* 1971;5:579–585.
46. Stoch MB, Smythe PM. 15-year developmental study on effects of severe undernutrition during infancy on subsequent physical growth and intellectual functioning. *Arch Dis Child* 1976;51:327–336.
47. Pollitt E, Thomson C. Protein-calorie malnutrition and behavior: a view from psychology. In: Wurtman RJ, Wurtman JJ, eds. *Nutrition and the brain,* vol 2, New York: Raven Press, 1977;261–306.
48. Cravioto J, DeLicardie ER, Birch HG. Nutrition, growth and neurointegrative development: an experimental and ecologic study. *Pediatrics* 1966;38(2)(Pt.I):319–372.
49. Pereira SM, Sundararaj R, Begum A. Physical growth and neurointegrative performance of survivors of protein-energy malnutrition. *Br J Nutr* 1979;42:165–171.
50. Birch HG, Lefford A. Two strategies for studying perception in "brain damaged" children. In: Birch HG, ed. *Brain damage in children.* Baltimore: Williams and Wilkins, 1964;46.
51. Agarwal DK, Upadhyay SK, Agarwal KN. Influence of malnutrition on cognitive development assessed by Piagetian tasks. *Acta Paediatr Scand* 1989;78:115–122.
52. Lien NM, Meyer KK, Winich M. Early malnutrition and "late" adoption: a study of their effects on the development of Korean orphans adopted into American families. *Am J Clin Nutr* 1977;30:1734–1739.
53. Galler JR, Ramsey F, Solimano G, Lowell WE. The influence of

early malnutrition on subsequent behavioral development. II. Classroom behavior. *J Child Psychiatry* 1983a;22:16–22.
54. Richardson SA, Birch HG, Hertzig ME. School performance of children who were severely malnourished in infancy. *Am J Ment Defic* 1973;77(5):623–637.
55. Galler JR, Ramsey F, Solimano G. The influence of early malnutrition on subsequent behavioral development. III. Learning disabilities as a sequel to malnutrition. *Pediatr Res* 1984;18:309–313.
56. Galler JR, Ramsey FE. A follow-up study of the influence of early malnutrition on development. Behavior at home and at school. *J Am Acad Child Adolesc Psychiatry* 1989;28(2):254–261.
57. Galler JR, Ramsey F, Morley DS, Archer E. The long term effects of early kwashiorkor compared with marasmus. IV. Performance on the national high school entrance examination. *Pediatr Res* 1990;28:235–239.
58. Galler JR, Ramsey F, Solimano G, Propert K. Sex differences in the growth of Barbadian school children with early malnutrition. *Nutr Rep Int* 1983;27:503–517.
59. Galler JR, Ramsey F, Salt P, Archer E. The long term effects of early kwashiorkor compared with marasmus. I. Physical growth and sexual maturation. *J Pediatr Gastroenterol Nutr* 1987;6: 841–846.
60. Galler JR. The interaction of nutrition and environment in behavioral development. In: Dobbing J, ed. *Early nutrition and later achievement.* New York: Academic Press, 1987;175–207.
61. Rush D. The behavioral consequences of protein-energy deprivation and supplementation in early life: an epidemiological perspective. In: Galler JR, ed. *Nutrition and behavior.* New York: Pelnum Press, 1984;5:119–154.
62. Grantham-McGregor SM, Schofield W, Powell C. Development of severely malnourished children who received psychosocial stimulation: six-year follow-up. *Pediatrics* 1987;79:247–254.
63. Grantham-McGregor SM, Schofield W, Haggard D. Maternal-child interaction in survivors of severe malnutrition who received psychosocial stimulation. *Eur J Clin Nutr* 1989;43:45–52.

CHAPTER 15

Nutritional Implications of Vegetarianism for Children

Johanna T. Dwyer

This chapter explores nutritional implications of the various types of vegetarian diets fed to children. These diets cannot be categorized as completely positive or negative. Rather, they differ, in important ways, from usual nonvegetarian diets. Understanding these differences is essential when one is involved in the health supervision and nutritional counseling of vegetarian children and their parents.

The implications of vegetarianism begin in fetal life; vegetarian diets consumed during pregnancy may influence the nutritional status of the infant at birth. Vegetarian diets during lactation may alter milk composition and influence later child growth. Vegetarianism in the first two decades of life, before growth has ceased, presents special reasons for concern because the increased nutrient needs of that period must be met to support optimal growth. Child growth and development, either positive or negative, is, therefore, contingent on how the vegetarian diet is planned.

Vegetarian diets for children, if properly planned are, however, compatible with excellent growth and development. The onus of appropriate planning falls on parents and health care providers who must, therefore, be well informed about nutrition.

BACKGROUND

Vegetarian diets fed to children in the United States vary from healthful to dangerous. Vegetarian parents, like some omnivorous parents, may fail to understand the nutritional steps necessary to promote optimal child growth and development. Concerns about vegetarianism before full growth is reached are physiologically based. Health service providers may not always be alert to some of these problems.

Vegetarian diets that sustain adults in good health are not necessarily appropriate for infants, young children, and adolescents. The nutrient density, e.g., the protein, vitamins, or minerals per kilocalorie (Cal), of pediatric diets must be higher because nutrient needs prior to maturity are elevated when they are expressed on a per kilocalorie basis. Also, in early infancy, as breast-feeding declines, vegan diets, consisting of plant foods that are low in caloric density and high in bulk, may be difficult to consume in sufficient quantity to meet the weanling's energy needs. Stomach capacity is limited and on usual feeding schedules it is difficult for infants to consume enough food to meet energy needs if the caloric density of the diet is less than 0.5 Cal/g.

The problem of inadequate feeding among vegetarian parents is not always due to a lack of knowledge. Some parents hold rigid views about health and child rearing that are at variance with conventional pediatric recommendations. They may plan their children's diets, but the basis of that plan fails to incorporate present knowledge of nutritional science. In addition, a minority of vegetarian parents reject immunization, the use of vitamin and mineral supplements, and other health safeguards, increasing the health-risks for their children (1).

There are, however, vegetarian diets for children that are not only adequate but beneficial. They depend on a sound knowledge of nutritional science, preventive medicine, and careful design (2).

An optimal vegetarian diet for children would include sufficient energy, protein, vitamins, and minerals; a balance in energy-yielding nutrients; moderation in constituents posing health problems, such as saturated fats and

J. T. Dwyer: Frances Stern Nutrition Center, Boston, Massachusetts 02111.

cholesterol; avoidance of excessive bulk; appropriateness with respect to the child's age and developmental level; and hygiene in food preparation (3). Optimum design would also take into account the specific nutrition-related needs and problems for each age. Pregnant and lactating women, infants, and children differ at each stage of growth, as do the diet-related problems that may arise.

CLASSIFICATION OF VEGETARIAN DIETS

There is a wide variety of vegetarian diets, ranging from healthful to risky. Classification is usually determined by the extent of animal food use. Semivegetarians eat no red meat but do eat some chicken and fish. Lacto-ovovegetarians add only milk products and eggs to their diets. Lactovegetarians add milk and dairy products, but no eggs. Vegans, i.e., total vegetarians, consume no animal foods at all. Near-vegans, such as macrobiotic vegetarians, eat so little animal food that deficiencies similar to those common in unplanned vegan diets are likely to arise.

The foods eaten, and avoided, by these different types of vegetarians result in differing nutrient intakes, with correspondingly different risks and benefits (1). Other characteristics of vegetarians also influence the health risks and benefits they experience. These include use or non-use of vitamin and mineral supplements; use or non-use of enriched, refined, and processed foods; use or non-use of alcohol, tobacco, and various drugs, either over-the-counter, prescription, or illicit (4). Vegetarian groups in the United States differ considerably (Table 1). They vary from the highly health conscious and aware, such as Seventh Day Adventists, who consume well-planned and nutritionally well-balanced diets, to those whose attitudes and practices pose potential health problems.

VEGETARIAN DIETS DURING PREGNANCY

Diet is one of the important factors setting the stage for the nutritional status of the infant at birth. Pregnancy increases the needs for energy, calcium, vitamins A, C, and D, iron, folic acid, vitamin B_{12}, and protein, and increases the importance of nutritional counseling for the pregnant vegetarian (Table 2) (4).

Protein needs during pregnancy increase by 30 g/day and by 20 g/day during lactation. If the biological value of the protein is low, as it is likely to be on monodiets consisting of only one or a few plant protein sources, protein intakes must increase even more (5).

In counseling, patients must learn to use complemen-

TABLE 1. Types of vegetarianism common in children

Type of vegetarianism and group	Supplements common	Close medical supervision	Other comments
Vegan-like			
Macrobiotics	No	No	Avoid sugar; smoking permitted
Rastafarians	No	No	Avoid salt, preserved foods, additives, and alcohol; marijuana is used in a religious ritual
Vegans	No but varies	No but varies	
Black Hebrews	No	No	
Fruitarians	Probably no	Probably no	
Vegetarian			
Lactovegetarian			
The Farm	Yes	Yes	
Yogic groups (some)	Unknown	Unknown, varies	Restrictions vary
Hare Krishnas	No	Probably no	Avoid alcohol, tobacco; use natural and organic foods
Hindu immigrants	Varies	Yes	
Lacto-ovovegetarians			
Seventh Day Adventists	Yes	Yes	Avoid tobacco, alcohol, highly processed foods
Anthroposophics	Yes	Unknown	Avoid tobacco, alcohol
Transcendental meditators	Yes	Yes	
Yogic	Varies	Varies	Restrictions vary by group and sect
Semivegetarians			
Non–red meat eaters	Yes	Yes	

Adapted with permission from ref. 3.

tary plant proteins, such as a combination of grains and legumes, to produce an amino acid mix that meets the body's needs for protein (Table 2) (6,7).

During pregnancy, iron needs rise greatly to, at least, 3.5 mg/day absorbed, versus nonpregnant needs of 1.5 mg/day. On vegan diets, only nonheme iron, which tends to be very poorly absorbed, is present. Even when ascorbic acid intake is high, and nonheme iron absorption is increased, absorption remains lower than it is on high animal-protein diets (8).

Calcium intakes during pregnancy must also increase. The 1989 *Recommended Dietary Allowances* (RDA) suggests increases of 200 mg calcium and phosphorus per day, from 800 to 1,000 mg. Calcium absorption is influenced by vitamin D nutritional status. During pregnancy, vitamin D needs rise from 5 to 10 μg (i.e., from 200 to 400 IU) per day. Even many nonpregnant women in northerly latitudes of the United States and Canada probably do not obtain enough vitamin D during winter.

The increased nutrient needs of the pregnant lacto-ovovegetarian are easily met by simple dietary adjustments, and recommendations differ little from those given to omnivores (7,9). In fact, the common practice among many vegetarians, especially lacto-ovovegetarians, to increase and liberalize the variety of foods in their diets during pregnancy helps to assure good nutrition (10).

It is more difficult to meet the greatly increased nutrient needs per kilocalorie when the woman is a vegan vegetarian. Vegan diets exclude the usual sources of necessary nutrients, and lack of information about alternative sources, or additional dietary restrictions, continue their exclusion. It is important, therefore, that the pregnant vegan receive adequate counseling and support, particularly if her vegetarianism is relatively recent. Information on rich sources of nutrients that are often low in vegan diets is now available (11).

Vegan vegetarians who are willing to liberalize their dietary intakes during pregnancy improve the probabilities that their diets will be satisfactory. For example, the outcomes of pregnancy among the vegan-like vegetarians at the "Farm," a vegetarian commune in Tennessee, were good when diets were coupled with prenatal care, iron, calcium and vitamin supplements, and mixed protein diets (12). Other pregnant and nonpregnant women, on less restrictive vegetarian regimens, appeared to have satisfactory intakes of vitamin B_6 (13), zinc (14), and taurine, although urinary taurine excretion was low in other studies (15).

Vegan diet planning becomes more complicated if the pregnant woman eats a purely vegan diet, refuses mineral and vitamin supplements, and/or if personal beliefs keep her from using prenatal care. This has been noted in some Native Americans and also among Indian and Asian women living in Western countries. In one such immigrant group, although birth weights were satisfactory and calcium biochemical indices were normal, zinc intakes and biochemical indices were low (16). In another group of pregnant Asian immigrants on nearly vegan diets, nutritional osteomalacia was reported. Bone mineral content was less than that of controls, with serum calciums also low. In part, this may be because the women resided in England, where milk is not fortified with vitamin D, as it is in the United States (17).

Common problems of pregnant vegans include inadequate weight gain, as well as low intakes of protein, calcium, zinc, vitamin B_{12}, iron (with resulting anemias), and, in some instances, deficiencies of iodide and vitamin D (9).

Vegan women tend to weigh less when they become pregnant; their pregnancy weight gain may also be less than that of nonvegetarians. Some may even be in negative energy balance. When their energy needs are not met, body or dietary protein will be catabolized, further increasing protein needs from dietary sources. Thus, vegan patients should be urged, from the inception of pregnancy, to increase total energy intake by increasing the number of meals they eat per day (7).

Vegan life-styles often contribute to increased risk of iron deficiency anemia. First, there are the risks imposed by inadequately bioavailable iron sources. In addition, vegan women often are anemic at the onset of pregnancy. Some of these women also refuse to take the usual prophylactic iron supplements of 30 to 60 mg of elemental iron per day, or the larger therapeutic doses of iron, which may be needed if iron deficiency anemia is already present. Without such supplements, even among nonvegetarian women, depletion of iron stores is likely to develop in pregnancy.

In addition, some vegans refuse prenatal care. Others present for prenatal care very late or refuse medical assistance during labor and delivery, including blood transfusions. If hemorrhage or other complications that deplete iron stores occur, iron deficiency anemia may become severe.

For vegan women who do not drink vitamin D-fortified milk, vitamin D supplements in quantities approximating the recommended dietary allowances are recom-

TABLE 2. *Counseling the pregnant vegetarian*

Establish rapport and trust in medical and health care
Reinforce positive nutrition and other life-style practices, e.g., no smoking, avoidance of alcohol and illicit drugs
Ascertain dietary practices and proscribed foods
Assure both quality and quantity of nutrient sources
Prioritize nutritional concerns
Investigate attitudes and life-style practices
Help patient choose appropriate dietary change
Individualize counseling and guidance
Simplify the information given
Follow up nutrition practices and status

Adapted from ref. 7.

mended. If these are not acceptable, adequate exposure to the sun or use of cod liver oil may be helpful, although neither of these is as reliable and standardized a source as are supplements. Calcium requirements rise during pregnancy by 200 mg/day. If calcium supplements are acceptable, these should be suggested. Most vegan foods are low in calcium; soy milk, for example, unless it is fortified with calcium, provides only 20% of the calcium of cow's milk. If diets are high in phosphorus and protein, calcium excretion may also rise. If vitamin D nutriture is also low, secondary hyperparathyroidism may develop, even in nonvegetarians. This phenomenon has been observed in nonpregnant nonvegetarians during the winter months in the northeastern part of the United States, and is probably widespread in similar latitudes elsewhere (18). Counseling should stress the need for alternative food sources of calcium and vitamin D that deliver adequate intake in vegans. If supplements are not acceptable, a liberalization of the diet to a lacto-ovovegetarian pattern that includes vitamin D–fortified milk products can be helpful.

Thanks to public health efforts during the past century, vitamin D–deficiency rickets has been rare in this country since World War II (19). Vitamin D–deficiency rickets in vegan infants and children, which has been reported recently, is easily avoidable. Counseling is of increased importance to help vegan mothers understand the ramifications of poor vitamin D intake so they can tend to their own vitamin D needs as well as protect their infants and young children from this easily preventable deficiency disorder.

The recommended dietary allowance for vitamin B_{12} rises from 3 to 4 μg/day during pregnancy. Although pregnancy increases the absorption of vitamin B_{12} from the gastrointestinal tract, the amounts provided in vegan diets are so low, and stores are often already so depleted, that these physiological adjustments do not insure against deficiency. In one recent study, a prenatal deficiency of vitamin B_{12} in a vegan mother was continued in the infant after birth by the inadequate content of vitamin B_{12} in the mother's breast milk (20).

Vitamin B_{12} is lacking in virtually all plant foods. Many vegan foods, such as tempeh, miso, dulse, kelp, soy sauce, and bean sprouts have vitamin B_{12} activity if microbiological assays are used, but the forms of vitamin B_{12} produced are not bioavailable to humans. Also, some forms of seaweed have enough plankton attached to them to provide some vitamin B_{12}. However, seaweed varies in the amount of plankton it contains, and it, too, is an unreliable source of vitamin B_{12} in the vegan diet (20).

VEGETARIAN DIETS DURING LACTATION

Vegetarians are more likely to breast-feed their infants, and to do so for a longer period of time than omnivores. The effects of vegetarian diets during lactation are, therefore, of prime importance.

In general, the quantity of human milk produced by vegetarians is comparable to that of omnivores. The quality varies, however, depending on the type of vegetarian diet consumed, particularly in vitamin D, calcium, vitamin B_{12}, and protein levels (21).

Vitamin D in human milk is always relatively low in comparison to the infant's needs, 4 to 9 IU per liter, even in omnivores. Since the infant needs at least 400 IU of vitamin D per day, and few young infants consume as much as a liter of milk per day, vitamin D from breast milk alone is grossly insufficient to meet the infant's needs for vitamin D after a few months postpartum. Even among women who supplement their dietary intakes with vitamin D, the milk still is lower in vitamin D than is probably sufficient for infants who suckle for much of the first year of life. The highly publicized contention that there exists a previously undiscovered water-soluble form of vitamin D in breast milk was disproven several years ago, but many vegetarians continue to believe that this is true (22,23). Vegan women, especially those who are rarely exposed to the sun and who fail to consume vitamin D–fortified foods or vitamin supplements, are especially likely to have low vitamin D levels in their milk. Indeed, some chronically vitamin D–deficient vegan mothers may be in a state of secondary hyperparathyroidism during lactation. Neither supplementation of the maternal diet nor sunlight exposure alone may be sufficient to make human milk high enough in vitamin D to assure optimal mineralization and to prevent rickets in later infancy among infants with no other source of vitamin D in their diets (24,25). The current RDA for vitamin D is 300 IU (7.5 μg) from birth to 6 months of age, and 400 IU until 24 years of age. Cases of rickets among breast-fed infants of both vegetarian and nonvegetarian mothers, when lactation is extended for several months or years, continue to be reported.

Nutritional counseling should, therefore, stress that all infants receive 300 IU of vitamin D per day. Since exposure to sunlight may be insufficient in northerly latitudes during winter months, recommended alternative sources would include vitamin D–fortified cow's milk or soy formula, a water-miscible vitamin D supplement, or cod liver oil, if it is more acceptable. Use of a water-miscible form averts the problem of lipid pneumonia, which may result from lipid-soluble forms.

The RDA for calcium are 800 mg/day for nonpregnant women over 25 years of age, 1,200 mg/day for younger women, and 1,200 mg/day during pregnancy and lactation. The calcium in human milk is fixed in amount, approximately 320 mg/l. Milk production is usually 750 ml/day. Such intakes result in 240 mg calcium being available to the infant. High-calcium diets or calcium supplements do not increase the calcium in breast milk, but they may minimize demineralization in mothers.

During lactation, adaptive changes occur in calcium

metabolism to spare maternal calcium losses. But losses of calcium may still be considerable, probably 50 mg of bone calcium per day, even when calcium intakes are adequate. No clear relationship has been detected, however, between bone health and number of pregnancies or lactation histories among omnivorous women who consume recommended amounts of calcium (26,27).

Women on lactovegetarian and lacto-ovovegetarian diets get plenty of calcium and vitamin D from the milk they drink, at least in the United States, where milk is fortified with vitamin D. However, vegan diets are often low in calcium and vitamin D and secondary hyperparathyroidism is common. Although their serum calciums are normal, and even after vitamin supplementation of individuals whose 25 hydroxyvitamin D levels were low, high parathyroid hormone levels persist.

One interpretation suggests that a secondary hyperparathyroidism helps vegetarians maintain normal serum calcium levels (28). Supporting this is a recent study of lactating women on vegan-like diets. Their 1,25-dihydroxyvitamin D levels were over a third higher than controls who were also lactating, although all had highly increased serum parathyrin levels (29). This indicates that supplementation of at least 1,200 mg elemental calcium and 400 IU vitamin D are appropriate to minimize maternal losses during lactation. Vegans may require supplemental sources to reach these intake levels.

The requirement for vitamin B_{12} during lactation rises from 2 to 2.6 μg/day. Outputs in human milk vary from 0.2 to 0.8 μg/l, so it is important to assure that vitamin B_{12} intakes are adequate. Human milk levels generally reflect serum B_{12} levels, and serum levels tend to reflect long-term stores. Vegans are at particular risk of having low levels of vitamin B_{12} in their breast milk.

Occasionally, vitamin B_{12} deficiencies have been reported among breast-fed infants of vegans or other very strict vegetarian women that cannot be explained by undiagnosed inborn errors of metabolism (30). With vitamin B_{12} treatment, consisting of pharmacologic doses of the nutrient, hematological and neurological problems of such infants reverse (31). Lactating vegan Indian women, immigrants to Western countries, were found to have such frank vitamin B_{12} deficiency that they developed very low vitamin B_{12} levels in their milk and a megaloblastic anemia (32). Anemia in macrobiotic American mothers and their infants is also occasionally a biochemical sign of vitamin B_{12} deficiency (33).

The mothers' urinary methylmalonic acid levels, which are indicative of vitamin B_{12} deficiency, are increased; their serum vitamin B_{12} levels are low. Their infants also have very high levels of urinary methylmalonic acid. Among those infants with the highest levels, vitamin B_{12}, either orally or by injection, reversed this biochemical indicator.

Nutritional counseling should stress the importance of both mother and infant receiving supplements of 100 to 300 μg/day of vitamin B_{12}.

Protein is rarely a problem in vegetarian or vegan diets during pregnancy and lactation. Most vegetarian women increase their food choices during lactation, and protein intake rises. In fact, their prepregnancy intake is rarely insufficient. The protein content of their milk tends to remain constant during lactation. With extended lactations, that is, over 7 months, the protein content of human milk may decrease very slightly, but this is not of practical significance (10). Levels of amino acids are altered, however. For example, among women on vegan diets whose taurine intakes are virtually zero, plasma and breast milk taurine levels are only slightly lower than nonvegetarians, although urinary excretion of taurine is only half that of omnivores (34). L-carnitine is also lower in vegans than in omnivores, since the main source of carnitine is meat. Breast milk carnitine, especially in the free and short- or medium-chain acyl carnitine esters is low among vegetarians. This is not thought to be due to a lysine or methionine deficiency (35).

The amount of fat in the breast milk of vegetarian women is relatively constant. Human milk reflects both the fatty acid composition of the diet and also that of adipose tissue stores (36). Adipose tissue fatty acids reflect diet over the longer term, that is, weeks or months (36a). Up to a certain upper limit, the longer vegetarians stay on vegan diets, the more certain fatty acids, such as arachidonic acid, increase (29,37). The milk of vegetarian women, and especially that of vegans, has a lower proportion of fatty acids from animal fat and a higher percent of polyunsaturates from vegetable fats than milk from omnivores (10). Thus, vegetarian milk has more C 12:0, C 14:0, more linoleic and other polyunsaturated fatty acids, and less saturated and monounsaturated C:16 and C:18 fatty acids than that of omnivores. But, eventually, an upper level of alteration is achieved, after which, even in omnivores, the C:16 and C:18 fatty acid content does not rise (38).

VEGETARIAN INFANTS FROM BIRTH TO SIX MONTHS OF AGE

Infants have been fed successfully on the human milk of lactovegetarian mothers for millennia. The many advantages of extended breast-feeding have recently been rediscovered in Western countries. Breast milk production and infant growth are excellent if the mother eats an adequate vegetarian or vegan diet, and if the infant is fed frequently on demand. Breast milk production in Western countries is generally 750 ml until 6 months of age. This provides roughly 525 Cal/day. Assuming an energy need of 108 Cal/kg for infants under 6 months, the energy provided by usual breast milk outputs should suffice until the infant reaches a weight of 5 kg. If, of course, breast milk yields are lower, starvation at the breast may occur unless energy needs are supplemented.

There are other risks when very small infants or in-

TABLE 3. *Milk substitutes used by vegetarians and their suitability of feeding for infants under 1 year of age*

Nutritionally complete and suitable	Nutritionally incomplete and unsuitable
Breast milk	Cow's milk (undiluted)
Soy formulas (Isomil, Prosobee)	Goat's milk
	Ewe's milk
Liquid soy milk formulas	Nondairy creamer
	Honey water and crushed sesame seeds
	Kokkoh (cereal pap of rice, barley, and beans)

fants suffering from a congenital or acquired illnesses are fed less-than-optimal vegetarian diets. These include problems resulting from the marginal levels of vitamins D and B_{12} in the milk of vegan mothers. Supplementation can ameliorate these potential problems.

It is essential to know the appropriate versus inappropriate food for infants in early infancy if breast-feeding is not possible (Table 3). Mixtures other than fortified infant formula or human milk are usually inadequate for young infants in energy as well as in other nutrients. Parents should be discouraged from their use. Unfortunately, vegan mothers who adhere to philosophical groups with special food beliefs, such as macrobiotics, Black Hebrews, and Rastafarians, are especially likely to use inadequate mixtures during weaning. The mixtures that have been found to cause problems include Kokkoh, a cereal pap of rice, barley, and beans, which is frequently fed to macrobiotic infants; honey water with ground-up sesame seeds; and diluted nondairy creamer (39).

VEGETARIANISM IN LATER INFANCY: 6 TO 18 MONTHS

Recent studies demonstrate that the difficulties resulting from unplanned and inadequate vegetarian diets in infancy generally arise after 6 months of age (Table 4). The growth velocity of infants in industrialized societies slows after 4 to 6 months because not enough calories are provided from the usual suckling patterns. Breast milk output provides approximately 750 ml of milk (yielding 525 Cal) until 6 months of age, and 600 ml (yielding 420 Cal) thereafter, not enough to support growth and the infant's increased body size. Current energy recommendations for infants are 108 Cal/kg/day until 6 months, 98 Cal/kg/day from 6 to 12 months, and 102 Cal/kg/day thereafter. Since a normal 1-year-old infant weighs at least 9 kg, it is apparent that a supplementary source of calories is necessary for energy needs.

Vegan families pose particular problems because vegan diets used at weaning often have a very low caloric density per unit volume, especially if infant diets are based on cereal gruels. Weaning is also a period of high vulnerability for infants being weaned to vegetarian diets, which are likely to be high in dietary fiber and bulk, low in caloric density, and low in certain essential vitamins and minerals, such as vitamins D and B_{12}, calcium, and iron (40–49).

Energy is a particular problem at weaning among vegans. Dry cereals and legumes provide 3 to 4 Cal/g, but during preparation they absorb varying amounts of water. Rice and wheat absorb 2.5 to 3 times their weight; usual feeds provide about 1 Cal/g cooked weight. Corn (maize)–based feeds absorb 6 times their weight in water and, often, only provide a caloric density of 0.5 Cal/g. If gruels are further diluted during feeding, the caloric density may be even lower. Since a meal for an infant may be 300 ml or less, unless the infant is fed many times a day, or other energy sources are provided, energy intakes are likely to be inadequate. The use of nut butters, oils, and concentrated mixtures of cereals and legumes to supplement dilute feeds can be helpful.

Protein may also become a problem among some vegan infants. On usual American mixed diets the digestibility of protein is 96%. Vegetable proteins are often lower in protein quality, however (50–52). Protein digestibility may be important to take into account when proposing diets for infants and very small children fed vegan diets.

Because the animal-protein intake of lacto-ovovegetarians is often similar to the 66% consumed by most omnivores in the United States, adjustments for protein quality in amino acids or for digestibility are seldom necessary. Vegan and near-vegan diets, which consist of little or no animal protein, may require such adjustments. The practical effects are relatively small in most cases, however, since most American vegetarians eat ample amounts of protein.

An example of required adjustments is outlined in the 1989 RDA (5). On mixed diets containing 67% animal and 33% vegetable protein, the RDA for a 1- to 3-year-old preschool child is 1.2 g/kg. On a diet of 33% animal

TABLE 4. *Recommended protein intakes on three different diets for a 3-year-old preschool child*

Dietary pattern	Protein digestibility relative to reference protein	Limiting adjusted amino acid recommended dietary allowance
Usual omnivorous (67% animal protein)	100%	Not applicable 1.1 g/kg
Semivegetarian (33% animal protein)	92%	Lysine 1.4 g/kg
Vegan (100% vegetable protein)	88.5%	Tryptophan 1.7 g/kg

and 67% vegetable protein, with a digestibility of 92%, the RDA is 1.4 g/kg. For vegans, it would be 1.7 g/kg, using only the vegetable protein sources specified, and digestibility would fall to only 88%. The limiting amino acid would be tryptophan.

Deficiencies of carnitine among infants and children on vegan diets have been reported (53,54). It is unclear, however, if these are of functional significance. If carnitine is essential in human beings, it is most likely to be so in prematures. Studies of carnitine deficiency in premature vegan infants would seem to warrant special consideration.

Among the risks of micronutrient deficiency in later infancy are rickets and iron deficiency anemia.

Rickets is especially common among vegans, such as macrobiotics, Rastafarians, Black Hebrews, and non–milk drinking Pakistani or Indian infants, and in children suffering from malabsorption syndromes. Risks increase without vitamin D supplementation and for infants in the northern parts of the country.

Iron deficiency anemia is most common in vegans; it is also more common in vegetarians than in omnivores. The prevalence in vegan infants is due to the lower bioavailability of iron in the plant foods generally used for weaning. Most of these foods, like Kokkoh, which are naturally low in iron to begin with, are not fortified or enriched with iron. When parents refuse other sources of iron supplementation, iron deficiency is likely in the weanling.

Problems of undernutrition may also arise in later infancy, especially among vegans. Although vitamin B_{12} deficiency is rare, when it does occur it is usually in unsupplemented vegan infants breast-fed exclusively by a mother with very low vitamin B_{12} stores (55,60a). Failure to thrive, also common in vegan infants, results from insufficient supplementation of energy (3,41,44,45,55,56). Other nutrient deficiencies, such as of protein, calcium, zinc, and phosphorus, are also found, but more rarely, among vegans.

On vegan diets, protein needs are considerably increased by the decreased digestibility and altered biological value of the proteins consumed (Table 4), (80a). When vegan diets are very high in fiber, growth failure may result from the decreased bioavailability of amino acids and nitrogen as well as malabsorption (50).

In contrast, failure to thrive is rare among lacto-ovo- and lactovegetarian children, such as Seventh Day Adventists (56–59).

Vegetarian parents should be made aware of the potential nutritional deficits in infants 6 to 18 months old and of ways to avoid them. Energy intake can be increased by adding oils or sugars. Vitamin and mineral supplements may prevent deficiencies or correct them if they already exist. Concern is most warranted for the infants on vegan diets. No risks are likely on lacto-ovovegetarian diets when iron and vitamin D supplements are given (2,60,61).

VEGETARIAN PRESCHOOL CHILDREN 18 MONTHS TO 5 YEARS OLD

Well-planned vegetarian diets have many health advantages for children over the age of 2. These diets tend to be low in saturated fat, total fat, and cholesterol, high in fiber and complex carbohydrates, and high in fruits and vegetables. Such a dietary pattern is appropriate for children over age 2 and adults (62,63). The danger of inadequate diet decreases in children as growth velocity decreases and as children are able to eat enough food, independently, so that catch-up growth occurs.

Preschool-age vegetarian children on lacto-ovo, lacto-vegetarian, and semivegetarian diets rarely have problems. The children more likely to have problems are vegans. They often experience lags in height, weight, and fatness, although, in Western countries, these are small and often fall within normal limits (3,33,44,45,55,59). Iron-deficiency anemia, in this age group, is especially common among vegans, and is also occasionally reported among vegetarians. Among vegans, there is also the rare report of other deficiencies such as of zinc, vitamin B_{12}, and calcium.

VEGETARIAN DIETS IN PRIMARY SCHOOL CHILDREN

Most school-age vegetarian children in Western countries appear to be in good nutritional status. Generally, from ages 5 to 11 years they exhibit gradual, steady growth. Nutritional risks due to increased nutrient requirements seem to be few; there are few reports of adverse health findings.

VEGETARIAN DIETS AMONG ADOLESCENTS

Adolescence produces another sharp divergence between the relatively good nutritional status of vegetarians and that of vegans living in this, and other, affluent countries.

In general, well-planned semivegetarian, lacto-ovo- and lactovegetarian diets for adolescents are nutritionally satisfactory and, in fact, positive in many respects. They conform with the latest recommendations of the Diet and Health Report of the National Academy of Sciences and of the American Heart Association. Vegetarian life-styles, which often include refraining from smoking and drinking, are also beneficial to health. Vegetarian adolescents who drink milk and/or eat eggs have few nutritional problems. Vegetarian diets also seem to have little effect on age of menarche (64). There may be some effect on the menstrual cycle of vegans, although these findings have not been substantiated (65–69). Amenorrhea has been reported among vegetarian athletes, but hypocaloric, rather than vegetarian, diets per se may have been the cause (70). In anorectic adolescents who have adopted vegetarian diets, low-energy intakes, again, rather than vegetarianism may be responsible for the observed amenorrhea (59). However, the issue is by no means closed and some aspects of vegetarian diets, such as low fat intakes, may, in fact, be associated with alterations in sex hormone metabolism (20a,71,72).

Although iron status may be a problem for all teenagers during puberty, it may be exacerbated in vegetarians because of the lower bioavailability of plant sources of iron and the lack of heme iron in their diet (73). In addition, there are several reports of vegetarian athletes who have developed iron deficiency anemia due to occult blood loss in addition to possibly low intakes (74,75). Zinc may also fall short of the RDA levels.

The risks of vegan diets during adolescence are increased because of a lack of planning. During the pubertal growth spurt, growth is very rapid. The intake of the vegan adolescent may be insufficient to prevent rickets, iron deficiency anemia, declines in zinc status, and to maintain growth velocity at normal levels. In extreme cases, the pubertal growth spurt may even be delayed a few months by very restrictive vegetarian diets (64).

When weights are very low, menstrual cycling may also be abnormal or absent. This should not be confused with anorexia nervosa, which sometimes masquerades as veganism (59). The effects of vegan diets on reproductive hormones is an area of active investigation that warrants further study.

Poor mineralization of bone is an added concern in the vegan adolescent's diet. Calcium needs during adolescence are very high (e.g., 1,200 mg), and they are very difficult to meet on vegan diets, even when green leafy vegetables, nuts, seeds, and calcium-fortified soy milk are available. It is also very difficult to plan vegan diets that meet the RDA for zinc. The bioavailability of zinc is especially low in plant foods as a result of the presence of fiber and phytates. Zinc molar ratios of phytate to zinc are very high, often ten times higher than on omnivorous diets, a sign of very low zinc bioavailability.

Vegan adolescents should be counseled regarding the importance of sufficient energy intake to assure good growth. They should be aware of the necessity for supplementation of calcium, iron, possibly zinc, and vitamins B_{12} and D (76,77). Vegetarian adolescents may also benefit from iron and, possibly, zinc supplements. All adolescents should keep their ascorbic acid and iron intakes high, via whole-grain and fortified cereals, to prevent iron deficiency anemia.

SUMMARY

If they are well planned, vegan and vegetarians diets promote excellent health, even before full growth has been achieved. After growth has ceased, they can also promote excellent health (4,78–81). Dietary recommendations, issued by the Institute of Medicine of the National Academy of Sciences (62), stress moderation in the intake of high fat animal foods for everyone and suggest that semivegetarian eating patterns may be beneficial.

For vegetarians, dietary advice is usually sufficient for correcting intake problems. Vegan parents, who eat no animal foods at all, require more detailed dietetic counseling because food sources of several key nutrients are low in their diets, and other constraints may further limit what is considered acceptable fare (82–89). The expertise and detailed knowledge of dietitians is important.

Medical supervision of vegetarians, especially vegans, is also important since life-style, as well as diet restrictions, may have negative health ramifications.

In conclusion, the nutritional implications of vegetarianism in childhood may be positive or negative. Parental attitudes, practices, and the availability of sound nutritional advice make the difference.

ACKNOWLEDGMENT

Partial support for preparation of this chapter was provided from training grant MCJ 9120 to Dr. Dwyer from the U.S. Department of Health and Human Services.

REFERENCES

1. Position of the American Dietetic Association: vegetarian diets. *J Am Diet Assoc* 1988;88(3):351.
2. Vyhmeister IB, Register UD, Sonnenberg IM. Safe vegetarian diets for children. *Pediatr Clin North Am* 1977;24:203–210.
3. Jacobs C, Dwyer JT. Vegetarian children: appropriate and inappropriate diets. *Am J Clin Nutr* 1988;48:811–818.
4. Dwyer JT. Health aspects of vegetarian diets. *Am J Clin Nutr* 1988;48:712–738.
5. Johnston PK. Getting enough to grow on. *Am J Nurs* 1984;84(3):336–339.
6. Mutch PB. Food guides for the vegetarian. *Am J Clin Nutr* 1988;48(suppl 3):913–919.
7. Johnston PK. Counseling the pregnant vegetarian. *Am J Clin Nutr* 1988;48:901–905.
8. Worthington Roberts BS, Breskin MW, Monsen ER. Iron status of premenopausal women in a university community and its relationship to habitual dietary sources of protein. *Am J Clin Nutr* 1988;47:275–279.
9. Dwyer JT. Vegetarian diets in pregnancy and lactation: recent studies of North Americans. *J Canad Dietetic Assoc* 1983;44:27–34.
10. Finley A, Lonnerdal B, Dewey KG, Grivetti LE. Breast milk composition: fat content and fatty acid composition in vegetarians and nonvegetarians. *Am J Clin Nutr* 1985;41:787–800.
11. Truesdell DD, Whitney EN, Acosta PB. Nutrients in vegetarian foods. *J Am Diet Assoc* 1984;84(1):28–35.
12. Carter JP, Furman T, Hutchenson HR. Preeclampsia and reproductive performance in a community of vegans. *South Med J* 1987;80:692–697.
13. Shultz TD, Leklem JE. Nutrient intake and hormonal status of premenopausal vegetarian Seventh Day Adventists and premenopausal nonvegetarians. *Nutr Cancer* 1983;4(4):247–259.
14. Abu Assal MJ, Craig WJ. The zinc status of pregnant vegetarian women. *Nutr Rep Int* 1984;29(2):485–494.
15. Naismith DJ, Rana SK, Emery PW. Metabolism of taurine during reproduction in women. *Hum Nutr Clin Nutr* 1987;41C(1):37–45.

16. Ward RJ, Araham R, McFadyen IR, Haines AD, North WR, Patel M, Bhatt RV. Assessment of trace metal intake and status in a Gujerati pregnant Asian population and their influence on the outcome of pregnancy. *Br J Obstet Gynaecol* 1988;95(7):676–682.
17. Fonseca V, Agnew J, Dandona P. Secondary hyperparathyroidism and bone density. *Br Med J* 1985;290:555–556.
18. Krall EA, Sahyoun N, Tannenbaum S, Dallal GE, Dawson Hughs B. Effect of vitamin D on seasonal variations in PTH secretion in postmenopausal women. *N Engl J Med* 1989;321:1777–1783.
19. Eisenberg L. From circumstances to mechanism in pediatrics during the Hopkins century. *Pediatrics* 1990;85:42–49.
20. Herbert V. Vitamin B12 plant sources, requirements, assay. *Am Clin Nutr* 1988;48:852–858.
20a. Hill PB, Garbaczewski L, Daynes G, Gaire KS. Gonadotrophin release and meat consumption in vegetarian women. *Am J Clin Nutr* 1986;43:37–41.
21. Finley DA, Lonnerdal B, Dewey KG, Grivetti LE. Inorganic constituents of breast milk from vegetarian and nonvegetarian women: relationships with each other and with organic constituents. *J Nutr* 1985;115(6):772–781.
22. Tsang RC. The quandary of vitamin D in the newborn infant. *Lancet* 1983;1:1370–1372.
23. Greer FR, Tsang RC. Vitamin D in human milk: is there enough? *J Pediatr Gastroenterol Nutr* 1983;2:5227–5281.
24. Roberts CC, Chan GM, Folland D, Rayburn C, Jackson R. Adequate bone mineralization in breastfed infants. *J Pediatr* 1989;99:192–196.
25. Greer FR, Searey JE, Lem RS, Steichen JJ, Steichen Asche PS, Tsang RC. Bone mineral content and serum 25-hydroxyvitamin D concentrations in breast fed infants with or without supplemental vitamin D: 1 year follow up. *J Pediatr* 1982;100:919–922.
26. Koetting CA, Wardlow GM. Wrist, spine and hipbone density in women with variable histories of lactation. *Am J Clin Nutr* 1988;48:1479–1481.
27. Lambke B, Bruhdin B, Moberg P. Changes of bone mineral content during pregnancy and lactation. *Acta Obstet Gynecol* 1977;56:217–219.
28. Dandona P, Mohiuddin J, Weerakoon JW, Freedman DB, Fonseca V, Healy T. Persistence of parathyroid hypersecretion after vitamin D treatment in Asian vegetarians. *J Clin Endocrinol Metab* 1984;59:535–537.
29. Specker BL, Tsang RC, Ho M, Miller D. Effect of vegetarian diet on serum 1,25 dihydroxyvitamin D concentrations during lactation. *Obstet Gynecol USA* 1987;70(6):870–874.
30. Gambon RC, Lentze MJ, Rossi E. Megaloblastic anemia in one of monozygous twins breast fed by their vegetarian mother. *Eur J Pediatr* 1986;145:570–571.
31. Sklar R. Nutritional vitamin B12 deficiency in a breast fed infant of a vegan diet mother. *Clin Pediatr* 1986;25(4):219–221.
32. Bijur AM, Desai AG. Composition of breast milk with reference to vitamin B12 and focic acid of Indian mothers. *Indian J Pediatr* 1985;52:147–150.
33. Specker BL, Miller D, Norman EJ, Greene H, Hayes KC. Increased urinary methylmalonic acid excretion in breast-fed infants of vegetarian mothers and identification of an acceptable dietary source of vitamin B12. *Am J Clin Nutr* 1988;47(1):89–92.
34. Rana SK, Sanders TAB. Taurine concentration in the diet, plasma, urine and breast milk of vegans compared with omnivores. *Br J Nutr* 1986;56(1):17–27.
35. Barth CA, Roos N, Nottbohm B, Erbersdobler HF. L carnitine concentrations in milk from mothers on different diets. In: Schaub J, ed. *Composition and physiological properties of human milk.* Amsterdam: Elsevier, 1985;229–239.
36. Plakke T, Berkel J, Beynen AC, Hermus RJ, Katan MB. Relationship between the fatty acid composition of the diet and that of the subcutaneious adipose tissue in individual human subjects. *Hum Nutr Appl Nutr* 1983;37(5):365–372.
36a. Specker BL, Wey HE, Miller D. Differences in fatty acid composition of human milk in vegetarian and nonvegetarian women: long term effect of diet. *J Pediatr Gastroenterol Nutr* 1987;6:764–768.
37. Stammers JP, Hull D, Abraham R, McFadyen IR. High arachidonic acid levels in the cord blood of infants of mothers on vegetarian diets. *Br J Nutr* 1989;61(1):89–97.
38. Finley DAC, Lonnerdal B. Fatty acid composition of breast milk from vegetarian and nonvegetarian lactating women. In: Schaub J, ed. *Composition and physiological properties of human milk.* Amsterdam: Elsevier, 1985;203–212.
39. Robson JRK. Food faddism. *Pediatr Clin Nutr* 1977;24:189–201.
40. James JA, Clark C, Ward PS. Screening Rastafarian children for nutritional rickets. *Br Med J* 1985;290(6472):899–900.
41. Close GC. Rastafarianism and the vegans syndrome. *Br Med J* 1983;286:(6363):473.
42. Shinwell ED, Gorodischer R. Totally vegetarian diets and infant nutrition. *Pediatrics* 1982;70(4):582–586.
43. Curtis JA, Kooh SW, Fraser D, Greenberg ML. Nutritional rickets in vegetarian children. *Can Med Assoc J* 1983;128(2):150–152.
44. Dagnelie PC, Van Staveren WA, Verschuren SAJM, Hautvast JGAJ. Nutritional status of infants aged 4–18 months on macrobiotic diets and matched omnivorous control infants: a population based mixed longitudinal study. I. Weaning pattern, energy, and nutrient intake. *Eur J Clin Nutr* 1989;43:311–324.
45. Dagnelie PC, Van Staveren WA, Vergote FJVRA, Burema J, Van t'Hof MA, Van Klaveren JD, Hautvast JGAJ. Nutritional status in infants aged 4–18 months on macrobiotic diets and matched omnivorous control infants: a population based mixed longitudinal study. II. Growth and psychomotor development. *Eur J Clin Nutr* 1989;43:325–338.
46. Rona RJ, Chinn S, Duggal S, Driver AP. Vegetarianism and growth in Urdu, Gujarati, and Punjabi children in Britain. *J Epidemiol Community Health* 1987;41(3):233–236.
47. Henderson JB, Dunnigan MG, McIntosh WB, Abdul Motalaal AA, Gettinby G, Glekin BM. The importance of limited exposure to ultraviolet radiation and dietary factors in the etiology of Asian rickets: a risk factor model. *Q J Med* 1987;63(241):413–425.
48. Stenhammer L. Coeliac disease presenting as vitamin D deficiency rickets in a vegetarian child. *Acta Paediatr Scand* 1985;74(6):972–973.
49. Hellebostad M, Markestad T, Seger Halvorsen K. Vitamin D deficiency rickets and vitamin B12 deficiency in vegetarian children. *Acta Paediatr Scand* 1985;74(2):191–195.
50. Acosta PB. Availability of essential amino acids and nitrogen in vegan diets. *Am J Clin Nutr* 1988;48(suppl 3):868–874.
51. Position of the American Dietetic Association: Vegetarian diets: technical support paper. *J Am Diet Assoc* 1988;88(3):352–355.
52. Hopkins DT. Effects of variation in protein digestibility. In: Bodwell CE, Adkus JS, Hopkins DT, eds: *Protein quality in humans: assessment and in vitro estimation,* Westport, CT; AVI Publishing, 1981;169–193.
53. Lombard KA, Olson AL, Nelson SE, Rebouche CJ. Carnitine status of lactoovovegetarians and strict vegetarian adults and children. *Am J Clin Nutr* 1989;50:301–306.
54. Etzioni A, Levy J, Nitzan M, Erde P, Benderly A. Systemic carnitine deficiency exacerbated by a strict vegetarian diet. *Arch Dis Child* 1984;59(2):177–179.
55. Sanders TA. Growth and development of British vegan children. *Am J Clin Nutr* 1988;48(suppl 3):822–825.
56. Dwyer JT, Andrew EM, Berkey C, Valadian I, Reed RB. Growth in new vegetarian preschool children using the Jenss Bayley curve fitting techniques. *Am J Clin Nutr* 1983;37:(5):815–827.
57. Dwyer JT, Dietz WH, Andrews EM, Suskind RM. Nutritional status of vegetarian children. *Am J Clin Nutr* 1982;135:204–216.
58. Van Staveren WA, Dhuyvetter JH, Bons A, Zeelen M, Hautvast JG. Food consumption and height weight status of Dutch preschool children on alternative diets. *J Am Diet Assoc* 1985;85(12):1579–1584.
59. O'Connor MA, Touyz SW, Dunn SM, Beaumont PJ. Vegetarianism in anorexia nervosa? A review of 116 consecutive cases. *Med J Aust* 1987;147(11–12):540–542.
60. Findley DA. Effects of vegetarian diets on composition of human milk. In: Hamosh M, Golman AS, eds. *Human lactation 2. Maternal and environmental factors.* New York: Plenum Press, 1986;83–92.
60a. Stollhoff K, Schulte FJ. Vitamin B12 and brain development. *Eur J Pediatr* 1987;146(2):201–205.
61. Truesdell DD, Acosta PB. Feeding the vegan infant and child. *J Am Diet Assoc* 1985;85(7):837–840.
62. Committee on Diet and Health. *Diet and health: implications for chronic disease risk.* Washington: National Academy Press, 1989.

63. Weidmen W, Kwiterovich P, Jesse MJ, Nugent E. Diet in the healthy child. *Circulation* 1983;67:1411A–1414.
64. Kissinger DG, Sanchez A. The association of dietary factors with the age of menarche. *Nutr Res* 1989;7(5):471–479.
65. Pirke KM, Schwiger U, Laessle R, Dichout B, Schweiger M, Waechtler M. Dieting influences the menstrual cycle: vegetarian vs nonvegetarian diet. *Fertil Steril* 1986;46(6):1083–1088.
66. Fentiman IS, Caleffi M, Wang DY, Hampson SJ, Hoare SA, Dwa HG. Diurnal variations in prolactin and growth hormone levels in normal premenopausal vegetarian and omnivorous women. *Nutr Cancer* 1986;8(4):239–245.
67. Adlercreutz H, Fotsis T, Bannwart C, Hamalainen E, Bloigu S, Ollus A. Urinary estrogen profile determination in young Finnish vegetarian and omnivorous women. *J Steroid Biochem* 1986;24(1):289–296.
68. Hill P, Garbaczewski L, Haley N, Wynder EL. Diet and follicular development. *Am J Clin Nutr* 1984;39:771–777.
69. Shultz TD, Leklem JE. Vitamin B6 status and bioavailability in vegetarian women. *Am J Clin Nutr* 1987;46(4):647–651.
70. Slavin J, Lutter J, Cushman S. Amenorrhea in vegetarian athletes. *Lancet* 1984;1(8392):1474–1475.
71. Shultz TD, Wilcox RB, Spuehler JM, Howie BJ. Dietary and hormonal interrelationships in premenopausal women: evidence for a relationship between dietary nutrients and plasma prolactin levels. *Am J Clin Nutr* 1987;46:905–911.
72. Frisch RE. Amenorrhea, vegetarianism, and/or low fat. *Lancet* 1984;1(8384):1024.
73. Helman AD, Darnton Hill I. Vitamin and iron status in new vegetarians. *Am J Clin Nutr* 1987;45:785–789.
74. Jacobs MB, Wilson W. Iron deficiency anemia in a vegetarian runner. *JAMA* 1984;252(4):481–482.
75. Liebman M, Landis WH, Trollinger HR, Sykes J, Irvin BC. Effects of exercise training and a vegetarian diet on mineral status and plasma lipids in female runners. *Nutr Rep Int* 1987;35(5):1059–1071.
76. Ashkenazi S, Weitz R, Varsano I, Mimounit M. Vitamin B12 deficiency due to a strictly vegetarian diet in adolescence. *Clin Pediatr* 1987;26(12):662–663.
77. Lewis NM, Kies C, Fox HM. Vitamin B12 status of lacto ovo vegetarian and omnivore subjects fed controlled lactovegetarian, vegan and omnivore diets. *Nutr Rep Int* 1986;34(2):197–206.
78. Yanez E, Uauy R, Acarias I, Barrera G. Longterm validation of 1 gm of protein per kilogram body weight from a predominantly vegetable mixed diet to meet the requirements of young adult males. *J Nutr* 1986;116(5):865–872.
79. Agarwal DK, Agarwal KN, Shankar R, Bhatia BD, Mishra KP, Tripathi BN. Determination of protein requirements on vegetarian diet in healthy female volunteers. *Ind J Med Res* 1984;79:60–67.
80. Rudy CA. Vegetarian diets for children. *Pediatr Nurs* 1984;10(5):329–333.
80a. Sanders TA. Vegetarian and macrobiotic diets. *Midwife Health Visit Community Nurse* 1988;24(5):154–155.
81. Hebert JR. Relationship of vegetarianism to child growth in south India. *Am J Clin Nutr* 1985;42(6):1246–1254.
82. Bindra GS, Gibson RS. Iron status of East Indian predominantly lactoovo vegetarian immigrants to Canada: a model approach. *Am J Clin Nutr* 1986;44(5):643–652.
83. Akesson B, Ockerman PA. Selenium status in vegans and lactovegetarians. *Br J Nutr* 1985;53:199–205.
84. Davies CJ, Crowder M, Reid B, Dickerson JWT. Bowel function measurements of individuals with different eating patterns. *Gut* 1986;27(2):164–169.
85. Debski B, Finley DA, Picciano MF, Lonnerdal B, Milner J. Selenium content and glutathione peroxidase activity of milk from vegetarian and nonvegetarian women. *J Nutr* 1989;119(2):215–220.
86. Finley DA, Dewey KG, Lonnerdal B, Grivetti LE. Food choices of vegetarians and nonvegetarians during pregnancy and lactation. *J Am Diet Assoc* 1985;85(6):678–685.
87. Matthews JH, Wood JK. Megaloblastic anemia in vegetarian Asians. *Clin Lab Hematol* 1984;6(1):1–7.
88. McNeill DA, Ali PS, Song YS. Mineral analyses of vegetarian, health, and conventional food: magnesium, zinc, copper and manganese content. *J Am Diet Assoc* 1985;85(5):569–572.
89. Mills PK, Annegers JF, Phillips RL. Animal product consumption and subsequent fatal breast cancer risk among Seventh Day Adventists. *Am J Epidemiol* 1988;127(3):440–453.

CHAPTER 16

Clinical and Laboratory Assessment of the Malnourished Child

Reinaldo Figueroa-Colon

Accurate assessment of a child's nutritional status is an important element of pediatric care. Its goals are to determine if a child is, or may imminently become, malnourished; to ascertain the risks of nutrition-related complications; and to provide guidelines for short- and long-term therapy (1). Successful nutritional assessment is predicated on an awareness of nutritional deficiencies secondary to other processes: disease states that precipitate specific nutrient depletion; drug, radiation, or surgical therapies with detrimental nutritional effects; inborn errors of metabolism involving nutrient utilization; the varied results of intervention with oral/enteral or parenteral nutritional support regimens (2). In addition, sensitivity to nutritional needs may mitigate the problem of increased morbidity, as well as possible mortality, in hospital patients subsisting on marginal levels of nutrition (3,4).

While easily recognizable clinical signs and symptoms appear only in the advanced stages of nutritional depletion, nutritional status can be satisfactorily assessed earlier by dietary history combined with a physical and psychosocial examination (Table 1). When a child is determined to be at risk of becoming nutritionally depleted, precipitating factors such as inadequate intake, reduced absorption, excessive losses, impaired utilization, or increased requirements must be established (5).

Although monitoring intake is important in the nutritional management of a child at risk of becoming malnourished, other elements play a key role in successful therapy (6). As a child's nutrient supply decreases and/or demand increases, the organism undergoes a series of adaptive changes, designed mainly to protect more vital functions (7). Tissue stores and available pools are first utilized and depleted before significant alterations in other systems arise. As these adaptive changes begin failing, however, physiologic and metabolic abnormalities follow and clinical manifestations become evident. The terminal stage is reached when growth and development are impaired and vital functions become compromised. At this stage, the diagnosis is clinically evident, and the laboratory has little role in diagnosis. Laboratory assessment may, however, be very useful in assessing prognosis and effective monitoring.

CLINICAL AND DIETARY HISTORY

Nutritional evaluation should include a complete psychosocial, medical, and food intake history. Primary malnutrition, essentially the result of inadequate intake, may result from aberrations in the maternal-child relationship, lack of parental education, poverty, restricted allergy diets, and extremes of food faddism. Secondary malnutrition may be a consequence of congenital malformations, infectious disease, trauma, malignancy and its treatment, or any chronic disorder involving a major organ system such as the liver, kidney, lung, heart, or gastrointestinal tract. Secondary malnutrition may also result from anorexia nervosa, nutrient loss, e.g., from malabsorption or nephrosis, an increased metabolic rate, e.g., from congestive heart failure or burns, a decreased efficiency in the utilization of nutrients, as in infection, and alteration in the metabolism of nutrients resulting from drugs or nutrient interactions or antagonisms.

R. Figueroa-Colon: Departments of Pediatrics and Nutrition Sciences, Division of Pediatric Gastroenterology and Nutrition, University of Alabama at Birmingham, Children's Hospital of Alabama, Birmingham, Alabama 35233.

TABLE 1. Levels of nutritional assessment in relationship to the natural history of disease

Stage	Condition	Assessment Method
Predisposing factors	Inadequate intake	Psychosocial evaluation
	Reduced absorption / Impaired utilization / Excessive losses / Increased requirements	Clinical and dietary history
Adaptive changes	Depletion of reserves	Biochemical analysis
	Physiologic and metabolic abnormalities	
Clinical manifestations	Wasting or delayed growth	Anthropometric measurements
	Specific anatomic findings	Physical examination

The Psychosocial History

When growth is significantly delayed, and/or medical examination has indicated a child at risk, the psychosocial history is an important element in assessing or eliminating the possibility of environmental influences on intake. Factors to discern are inadequate income to purchase food, inadequate facilities for preparing or storing food, religious/cultural beliefs related to food intake, such as extreme vegetarianism or periodic fasting, and a parental lack of knowledge about nutritional needs. Other contributory factors may be the number of people living with the child, alcohol or drug use in the home, child abuse in which food is withheld as punishment, or psychological problems that may result in under- or overeating.

Dietary Intake History

Methods for collecting dietary intake data include 24-hr recall, food diary, food frequency (8), and observed intake. A 24-hr recall involves having the subject, or caretaker, recall everything consumed during the preceding 24-hr period. The food diary requires the subject, or caretaker, to weigh or measure and record everything consumed during a 3- to 7-day period. In the food frequency method, the subject or caretaker is asked how often and in what quantities specific foods are consumed (9). In this method, it is important to request information about consumption of fats, oils, sugar, and other sweets since, although they are calorically dense and nutritionally poor, they are often overlooked. It is also valuable to ask specifically if any foods are being restricted or promoted.

Although the methods described are considered valid for determining mean nutrient intakes in population groups, their accuracy in determining individual dietary intake is vulnerable to such factors as the respondent's memory and cooperativeness, as well as the skill of the interviewer (8,10). These variables are presumed to cancel each other out in large surveys, in which only the mean values of a population are considered.

There are specific problems with each of the methods. Although the 24-hr recall may be accurate for estimating the intake of infants or young children whose diet contains a small number of items, it may provide less accurate information when intake is more diversified (11). In addition, more reliable data may be produced when the recall is administered at successive visits; there seems to be a greater awareness of food intake when subjects know they will be queried (12). A 24-hr recall, without warning, is no more than a test of memory and should be conducted only as a practice run and the data discarded (12). Another problem with the 24-hr recall is that diet on the recalled day may not be representative (12). In addition, subjects or caretakers may tell the physician what they think the physician wants to hear (13), or they may actually change their eating habits when they are being monitored. Generally, the "flat-slope" syndrome is a problem intrinsic to 24-hr recalls, in which small intakes tend to be over- and large intakes underreported.

There is controversy concerning the number of days necessary for food diaries to give an accurate assessment, ranging from 3 to 7 days. It is generally acknowledged, however, that because food intake is significantly different on weekends (14), no matter what the length of the record, at least 1 weekend day should be included. In addition to this problem, subjects keeping a food diary may change their eating patterns (15), or alter what they actually record, in order to ease the burden of record-keeping or "please" the physician (13).

Intake Observation

The goal of intake observation is to accurately calculate caloric intake by careful weighing and measuring the food served against that left uneaten. Subjects must be monitored to assure that no other foods have been consumed and that all food noted as eaten was consumed by the subject, not given or thrown away. In the hospitalized patient, intravenous feedings must also be included. Tallies are then translated into estimations of protein, fat, carbohydrate, vitamin, mineral, as well as total calorie (energy) content.

The Recommended Dietary Allowances (RDA) are the nutritional standards against which diets being studied are usually compared (16). They comprise a list of levels of nutrient intake adequate to meet the known nutritional needs of practically all healthy persons (16), as defined by the Committee on Dietary Allowances of the Food and Nutrition Board. These are recommendations for average daily amounts within population groups and should not be confused with requirements for an individual with specific needs (16). In addition, intake below an RDA level does not necessarily indicate deficiency nor malnutrition since, with the exception of calories, which are estimated in the 50th percentile for each age group, the RDAs for each nutrient are purposely calculated at the 98th percentile for each age group (Fig. 1).

ENERGY EXPENDITURE

Energy expenditure can be precisely measured in the laboratory with either direct or indirect calorimetry. With direct calorimetry, the subject is placed in a thermally insulated water-cooled suit or chamber and body heat production is used to determine energy expenditure. This technique is laborious and expensive. Indirect calorimetry determines energy expenditure by measuring the rate of exchange of respiratory gases, i.e., oxygen consumption and carbon dioxide production. Both processes must be assessed for whether the energy expenditure measured actually reflects the physiologic situation under nonmeasurement conditions. Unfortunately, neither method lends itself to field studies.

Energy expenditure is traditionally calculated from indirect reporting methods that compare food intake diaries to activity diaries and information from automatic monitors of physical activity and heart rate (10,17). The inaccuracy of these methods is largely attributable to a reliance on memory and subject honesty. In addition, these methods tend to interfere with the subject's life-style.

The most accurate method of measuring energy expenditure in free-living humans is the doubly labeled water method. It is noninvasive, convenient, and not impaired by the need for active subject participation. In this indirect method, two isotopes of water, (^2H_2O and $H_2^{18}O$), are administered and their disappearance rates from a body fluid, e.g., saliva or urine, monitored. The disappearance rate of ^2H_2O reflects water output, whereas that of $H_2^{18}O$ reflects water output plus carbon dioxide production. The difference between these two disappearance rates is a measure of carbon dioxide production. Energy expenditure is calculated from the carbon dioxide production rate and the energy equivalent per mole of carbon dioxide, adjusted for the respiratory quotient as measured, or estimated, from the diet. The doubly labeled water method has been validated against the traditional indirect method in adults (18–25), preterm infants (26), and postsurgical infants (27). Investigators have successfully used it for assessing the energy requirements necessary for catch-up growth in malnour-

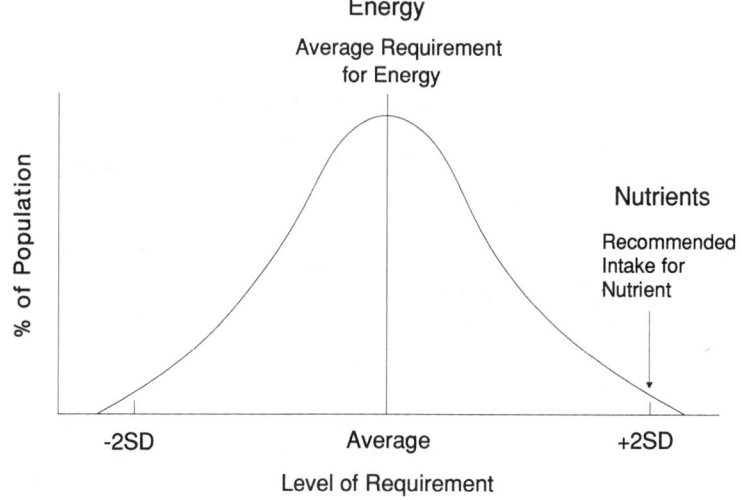

FIG. 1. Estimated requirements for energy and nutrients for each age group population.

ished infants by demonstrating that the unusually large energy expenditures per kilogram of body weight in these children are due to their large proportion of fat-free body (FFB) mass that results from fat store depletion. They also were able to identify energy use as either maintenance or growth (28). The method is noninvasive and nonrestrictive, and provides accurate measurements of energy expenditure in free-living subjects, regardless of nutritional status or age. The disadvantages of the doubly labeled water method are that the $H_2^{18}O$ is expensive and its analysis is not universally available.

PHYSICAL EXAMINATION

Once the patient's clinical and dietary history is known, the next step in nutritional assessment is a complete physical examination with a careful evaluation for signs of nutritional depletion. Symptoms such as apathy, irritability, pallor, edema, obesity, or emaciation are easy to detect. However, clinical signs often attributable to nutritional deficiency may be nonspecific for a given nutrient, the result of several nutrient deficiencies, or caused by trauma, environmental and climatic exposure, infection, or allergy (Table 2). These signs should be regarded essentially as clues and interpreted in the context of dietary and biochemical findings.

When clinical and dietary history and physical examination indicate a state of malnutrition, anthropometric and biochemical assessments may be used for confirmation and quantification.

ANTHROPOMETRIC MEASUREMENTS

The National Center for Health Statistics' growth charts have become an important tool for pediatricians interested in assessing a patient's growth against an expected norm. They provide age-related standards for weight, height, and/or growth velocity, the most useful anthropometric measurements to assess nutritional status of children (29,30). The norms were derived from a larger cross section of the United States population than previous standards.

Anthropometric indices have been used extensively to assess the nutritional status of children in developing countries. An early classification, by Gomez et al. (31), is based on weight-for-age criteria. Children weighing between 90% and 75% of the norm for a particular age are designated as having first-degree (mild) malnutrition; those weighing between 75% and 60% are second-degree (moderate); less than 60% is classified as third-degree (severe) malnutrition. Jelliffe (32) designated four levels of malnutrition: weights between 90% and 80%, 80% and 70%, 70% and 60%, and less than 60% of the age-related norm.

Weight-for-age, however, fails to consider the effect of differences in height. Two children of the same weight and age may have entirely different nutritional states depending on their height. In addition, an age-independent system for predicting nutritional status is necessary since exact age is frequently unknown in developing countries (29).

A classification system based on the concepts of height-for-age and weight-for-height was developed by Waterlow (33,34). Height-for-age, which is age-dependent, serves as an indicator of the chronicity of undernutrition. Weight-for-height, on the other hand, is age-independent and is an indicator of the state of acute undernutrition.

Waterlow's concepts are appropriate because a child with energy deficiency resulting from inadequate intake, reduced absorption, excessive losses, impaired utilization, or increased requirements presents first with failure to gain weight. During the adaptive process, the child begins to use fat and muscle mass as an energy source. The term for this state of short-term, or early, malnutrition, in which there is weight loss but during which linear growth is not yet affected, is *wasting*. The result of a prolonged deficiency state that causes obvious retardation in linear growth is *stunting*. The short stature associated with many chronic pediatric diseases is a manifestation of chronic undernutrition.

Based on Waterlow's classification, children are either normal; stunted, i.e., height deficit for age; wasted, i.e., weight deficit for height; or both stunted and wasted (Fig. 2). Stunting is graded by comparing actual heights to the 50th percentile for a given age: heights greater than 95% of the norm—grade 0; 95% to 90%—grade 1; 90% to 85%—grade 2; less than 85%—grade 3. Wasting is defined similarly against the 50th percentile for weight/height: weights greater than 90% of the standard—grade 0; 90% to 80%—grade 1; 80% to 70%—grade 2; less than 70%—grade 3.

There are several other important parameters used for screening and preliminary assessment. Included among these is the midarm circumference. Although not age-independent, midarm circumference varies very little between 1 and 4 years of age (29). Its classification system uses 80%, 70%, and 60% of the standard to distinguish mild, moderate, and severe malnutrition (35). Variations of this technique include midarm circumference in relation to arm length (36) and midarm circumference in relation to head circumference (37). All standards for midarm circumference appear to correlate closely with both weight-for-age and weight-for-height (38,39).

The frequent use of skin-fold measurements to estimate body fatness is the result of the assumption that the subcutaneous fat mantle reflects the total amount of body fat and that the selected measurement sites represent the average thickness of the entire mantle. In fact, separate studies have shown that only 42% of the total body fat of a full-term neonate and 32% in a female adult

TABLE 2. *Selected clinical findings associated with nutritional deficiencies*

Organ	Finding	Nutritional deficiency to be considered
General	Underweight, short stature	Calories
	Overweight	[Excess calories]
	Edematous, decreased activity level	Protein
Subcutaneous tissue	Decreased fat fold	Calories
	Increased fat fold	[Excess calories]
	Edema	Protein, thiamin, vitamin E in preemies
Skin (face)	Moon face, diffuse depigmentation	Protein
	Nasolabial seborrheic dermatitis	Riboflavin, niacin, pyridoxine
Mucous membranes	Pale	Anemia
Hair	Lack of curl, dull, altered texture, thin or sparse, depigmented, easily plucked	Protein
	Hair loss	Zinc, biotin, essential fatty acids
	Coiled, corkscrew-like	Vitamin A, ascorbic acid
Lips	Angular stomatitis	Riboflavin
	Cheilosis	B-complex vitamins
Gums	Swollen, bleeding	Ascorbic acid
	Reddened gingiva	[Excess vitamin A]
Teeth	Caries	Fluoride
	Mottled, pitted enamel	[Excess fluoride]
Tongue	Smooth, pale, atrophic	Anemia
	Red, painful, denuded, edema	Niacin, riboflavin, vitamin B_{12}
Nails	Spoon-shaped, koilonychia	Iron
Muscles	Decreased muscle mass (wasting)	Protein, calories
	Tender calves	Thiamin
Neurologic	Ophthalmoplegia, foot drop	Thiamin, vitamin E
	Ataxia, sensory loss, motor weakness	Vitamin B_{12}, vitamin E
	Psychomotor change, mental confusion and irritability	Protein
	Loss of vibratory sense, deep tendon reflexes	Thiamin, vitamin B_{12}
	Sensory loss, motor weakness	Thiamin
	Peripheral neuropathy	Pyridoxine
Skin (general)	Generalized dermatitis	Zinc, biotin, essential fatty acids
	Symmetrical dermatitis of skin exposed to sunlight, thickened pressure points, trauma	Niacin
	Follicular hyperkeratosis	Vitamin A
	Petechiae, purpura, ecchymosis perifollicular hemorrhage	Ascorbic acid, vitamin K
	Scrotal, vulval dermatitis	Riboflavin
Eyes	Dry (xerosis) conjunctiva, keratomalacia, Bitot's spots	Vitamin A
	Circumcorneal injection	Riboflavin
	Photophobia	Zinc
	Conjunctival pallor	Anemia
Skeletal	Costochondral beading (rachitic rosary), pigeon chest, Harrison's groove, knock-kneed or bowed legs, craniotabes, frontal and parietal bossing, persistently open anterior fontanel	Vitamin D
	Epiphyseal enlargement	Vitamin D, ascorbic acid
	Bone tenderness, hemorrhages, frog-leg position	Ascorbic acid
Gastrointestinal	Hepatomegaly (fatty infiltration)	Protein
Cardiovascular	Tachycardia, cardiomegaly, congestive heart failure	Thiamin
	Cardiomyopathy	Selenium
Endocrine	Hypothyroidism, goiter	Iodine
	Glucose intolerance	Chromium
	Hypogonadism, delayed puberty	Zinc
Other	Altered taste	Zinc
	Delayed wound healing	Zinc, ascorbic acid
	Parotid enlargement	Protein

Compiled from several sources.

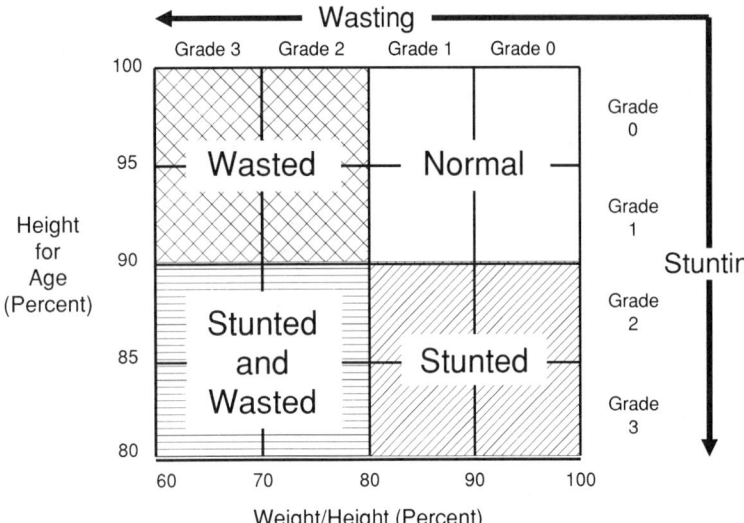

FIG. 2. Classification of protein-energy malnutrition. (Adapted from ref. 33.)

reside in the subcutaneous compartment (40,41). The potential inaccuracy of assuming that skin fold will represent the body as a whole is easily demonstrated by observing the wide differences in body fat distribution among individuals. In addition, accurate, reproducible measurement of the skin fold is difficult in a normal individual and perhaps impossible in an edematous or obese one. Skin-fold measurements at various sites could minimize some of the limitations of this method. Measurement of skin fold is useful and recommended, however, for the longitudinal assessment of a patient's response to nutritional therapy.

When weight-for-height indices were applied to hospitalized pediatric patients in the United States, almost one-third of the patients were classified as "malnourished" (42–44). This is significant since decreased weight-for-height has been associated with increased morbidity as well as prolonged hospital stay (42,45). A similar relationship was not found with decreased height-for-age, suggesting a more deleterious effect on morbidity by wasting than stunting (42).

The demonstration of the effect of nutritional deficiency on morbidity heightens the need for routine assessment of hospitalized patients to identify those who require nutritional support. This will most likely be achieved by a combination of anthropometric and biochemical measurements. Once nutritional support has been instituted, its efficacy can be monitored by changes in the anthropometric variables including weight, arm circumference, skin-fold thickness and, after a period of time, length. Once valid standards are developed, even better monitoring will occur by the use of biochemical indices of nutritional status or biochemical indicators of body composition. Until such indices are developed, however, weight and height are the most useful and simplest measures to assess nutritional status.

INDIRECT METHODS OF BODY COMPOSITION DETERMINATION IN CHILDREN

Measurements of body composition are important components of nutritional assessment; body weight is the most common measure for all ages. In adults, changes in weight are commonly equated with a change in adiposity, although, particularly in young adults, a vigorous exercise program could increase weight as a result of increased muscle mass. Changes in weight in the pediatric patient are more difficult to interpret. If weight gain is assumed to simply be a product of growth, with an appropriate mixture of fat and FFB mass, the possibility that it may be due to increased composition of salt and water may be overlooked. The composition of the weight gain is, therefore, essential to understanding the nutritional status of the child. Reference models for measuring the body composition of children include a fetus (46), a male infant during the first year of life (47), children from birth to 10 years (48), a 9-year-old boy (49), and a male adolescent (50).

One model of body composition is the two-component system in which the body is considered a composition of fat and FFB mass. This system provides the basis for most body composition studies with children and adults. A simple model of body composition is as follows:

Body weight = fat + fat free body mass (FFB)

Body weight = fat + total body water + protein + carbohydrate + mineral

Body weight = fat + intracellular fluid + extracellular fluid + protein + carbohydrate + mineral.

Fat is the most variable body component, ranging from about 5% to over 50% of body weight; the normal range is narrower, between approximately 10% and 30%. The infant *in utero* increases its fat content from about 2.2% at 1 kg to about 12% at term, presumably in preparation for extrauterine life (46). From birth to 6 months of age, body fat rises from 12% to about 25% (47). This striking change in body fat content may be due to the infant's need for energy homeostasis and thermoregulation as well as its high energy intake combined with little activity. With increasing age and mobility, fat content drops and muscle mass increases. This continues until preadolescence, at which time, in both sexes, there is an increase in fat content, which persists and increases in females but wanes in males (50).

Protein content increases from about 11.4% at birth (47) to about 17.5% in boys and 15% in girls at age 10 years (48). About 0.5% of body weight (0.6% of FFB) is carbohydrate. The remaining component is principally mineral, about 80% of which is osseous. Mineral content gradually rises from 2.5% at birth (47) to about 4.8% at 10 years of age, altering the density of the FFB mass (48).

Water content, greatest during fetal life, is about 88% of body weight at 24 weeks' gestation (46) and about 75% at term (47). After birth, it drops rapidly to about 60% at 4 months of age (47). From then until adolescence, it ranges between 55% and 64% (50). The drop in water content is caused by a rise in body-fat content and a drop in the relative water content of the FFB mass.

Growth alters the proportions of intracellular fluid (ICF) and extracellular fluid (ECF). The ICF initially is about 25% to 30% of body weight but by adolescence constitutes 35% to 40%, principally because the child's muscle mass increases with growth. At the same time, ECF slowly drops from about 40% to about 20% to 25% of body weight. ECF and total body water are often used to estimate ICF; thus, errors of ECF estimation compound errors in ICF estimation.

In each major component, there are differences between the sexes, which are obvious from early life and become pronounced in preadolescence and adolescence.

The development of constants for estimation of body composition has come from a 4.5-year-old boy (51), a few adult human cadaver dissections (40), and from the results of indirect estimates of FFB composition in human subjects. All of these pose specific problems. The five adult cadavers, who had died from various illnesses, are not likely to be representative of living humans; preferable subjects would be individuals who had experienced sudden accidental death. Further, in several instances the analyses were incomplete with respect to minerals, including potassium. The 4.5-year-old boy, who died of tuberculosis meningitis, appeared to be seriously depleted of water and potassium. The indirect methods of measurement are limited by the inaccurate assumption that the components of the body maintain a relatively constant composition, which is not true in childhood.

These methods, once their limitations have been understood, have been used successfully by several investigators (47,48,52). The basic problem is to adjust for the chemical immaturity of the growing child compared to the chemical maturity of the adult when estimating FFB mass or percent fat in children. Using age- and sex-specific estimates of the water, potassium, and density of FFB mass provides more accurate estimates of body composition in children and adolescents (Table 3). The estimated relative composition of FFB mass in Fomon's study (48) does not add up to 100 because the small, "constant" percentage of carbohydrate (0.6%) is not included (Table 3). The protein content of the FFB mass in Lohman's (52) estimates is derived by subtraction:

$$100 - \text{water} - \text{mineral} = \text{protein}.$$

Stable Isotope Techniques

Neutral fat does not bind water, so the measurement of total body water provides an estimate of the FFB compartment of the body. This can be accomplished, noninvasively, by the oral administration of water labeled with a known amount of the stable isotopes deuterium (^{2}H) or oxygen 18 (^{18}O) (53). Because the water content of FFB mass is constant in healthy subjects, total body water can be estimated, after a suitable period of equilibration, by determining the dilution of the isotope within a body fluid such as serum, saliva, or urine. Although this method is simple, its clinical application is limited because the assays for ^{2}H isotopes of hydrogen might exchange with nonaqueous hydrogen of protein and carbohydrate, resulting in an overestimation of body water content (54). Although expensive, ^{18}O does not appear not to have this problem (55).

Bioelectrical Impedance Analysis

Bioelectrical impedance analysis (BIA), recently developed, is based on the principle that a weak electric current passes through the body via the FFB mass, rather than through fat (56). The impedance to electrical flow, therefore, will vary in proportion to the amount of fat free tissue present. This method has been validated in adults with densitometry and total body water by isotope dilution (57,58). However, it does not appear to be precise. Small, normal, changes in body water appear to make significant differences in the estimate of FFB mass. Because of its attributes of ease and convenience, it is hoped that further honing of this method will improve both its validity and its precision. Presently, however, because impedance is proportional to the geometry of

TABLE 3. *Estimated composition of the fat-free mass (FFM) during growth*

Age (yr)	Compartments of the FFM (%)			Potassium (g/kg)	Density (g/ml)
	Water	Protein	Mineral		
Males					
Birth	80.6	15.0	3.7	1.92	1.063
1	70.0	16.6	3.7	2.21	1.068
3	77.5	17.8	4.0	2.39	1.074
5	76.6	18.5	4.3	2.49	1.078
7–9	76.8	18.1	5.1	2.40	1.081
9–11	76.2	18.4	5.4	2.45	1.084
11–13	75.4	18.9	5.7	2.52	1.087
13–15	74.7	19.1	6.2	2.56	1.094
15–17	74.2	19.3	6.5	2.61	1.096
17–20	74.0	19.4	6.6	2.63	1.099
Females					
Birth	80.6	15.0	3.7	1.92	1.064
1	78.8	16.9	3.7	2.24	1.069
3	77.9	17.7	3.7	2.38	1.071
5	77.6	18.0	3.7	2.42	1.073
7–9	77.6	17.5	4.9	2.32	1.079
9–11	77.0	17.8	5.2	2.34	1.082
11–13	76.6	17.9	5.5	2.36	1.086
13–15	75.5	18.6	5.9	2.38	1.092
15–17	75.0	18.9	6.1	2.40	1.094
17–20	74.8	19.2	6.0	2.41	1.095

Data from birth to 5 years adapted from ref. 48; data for other ages adapted from ref. 52.

the conductor, e.g., its length and configuration, and because the geometry of the conductor is constantly altered during growth, causing the electrical impedance of FFB mass to change progressively with age, this method is difficult to use in children (59).

Total Body Electrical Conductivity

Total body electrical conductivity (TOBEC) also measures FFB mass by electrical means. This method is based on the principle that individuals placed in an electromagnetic field perturb the field (60). The degree of perturbation depends on the amount and the volume of distribution of the electrolytes present. Because electrolytes reside exclusively in FFB mass, this compartment can be estimated. Using phantoms of infants composed of electrolyte solutions and corn oil, researchers (61) validated a TOBEC system developed for use with human infants. The TOBEC system was sensitive to changes in total electrolyte content and fluid volume of the phantoms. TOBEC is a rapid, safe, and noninvasive method for precisely determining body composition. Its major limitations are lack of portability and expense (55).

Ideal Method of Body Composition Determination

The ideal method of body composition measurement in children should be accurate to within the limits that make it clinically relevant. It should be sensitive enough to detect changes in fatness and leanness over a short period of time. Any assumptions should be well defined; it should be easy to use with both normal and sick children. Finally, it should be safe, simple, noninvasive, and cost-effective.

Indirect Methods of Body Composition Determination in Adults

Methods for measuring body composition in adults, including densitometry, total body potassium, and neutron activation are impractical for use with children. Densitometry determines the density of an individual by dividing actual weight by the amount of weight lost when the person is completely submerged in water. Since the densities of fat and FFB compartments are assumed to be constant, it is possible to calculate the proportion of each compartment when the density of the whole body is known. Its use in young children and/or severely ill patients is limited by the fact that they cannot be submerged in water. In older children, the method may be also be limited because during maturation, the density of the FFB mass changes, thus invalidating one of the basic assumptions of the method.

Because naturally occurring potassium (^{39}K) contains a fixed proportion (0.0118%) of the radioactive isotope ^{40}K, the total body potassium is calculated by measuring the amount of ^{40}K present in the body. Counting time is long and requires isolation in a special chamber, which may not be possible with a child or an ill person. An even more severe limitation results from the lack of uniform potassium content of the FFB mass. The potassium content of visceral organs such as the liver tends to differ from that of skeletal muscle and, since the relative weight of viscera to skeletal muscle varies with age, the potassium content of the FFB mass will vary, making this method more inaccurate in children.

Finally, the radiation exposure involved in the neutron activation method makes it unacceptable for use with children.

BIOCHEMICAL ASSESSMENT

Biochemical Indices of Nutritional Status

Accurate assessment of nutritional status is dependent on appropriate biochemical testing combined with thorough clinical and dietary histories, physical findings, and anthropometric measurements. Tests should be chosen with regard to availability, cost, predictive value, sensitivity, specificity, reliability, and validity (Table 4) (62).

Serum Protein Measurements

Nutritionists (63) have stated that the "ideal" protein for measurement would have a short biologic half-life, would respond to a protein-deficient diet, reflecting deficiency by decreased blood concentration, would have small reserves, a rapid rate of synthesis, a fairly constant catabolic rate, and be responsive only to protein and energy restriction (Fig. 3). Unfortunately, we are far from having found the ideal protein marker.

The serum protein concentration in the blood is dependent not only on protein deficiency but also on a large number of physiologic and pathologic variables. For instance, liver and renal disease, as well as hydration state, will affect serum protein values. The presence of an acute response to trauma, infection, inflammation, neoplasia, or any other tissue damage, may also influence protein measurements. Table 5 compares the major characteristics of the more commonly measured proteins.

Albumin

Serum albumin concentration is the most common indicator of protein nutritional status. The body pool of albumin is large (4 to 5 g/K) and almost 60% is extravascular; the biologic half-life is 18 to 20 days. The serum concentration is a balance between hepatic synthesis and degradation.

The control of hepatic synthesis is not completely understood, although it may be inhibited by infection and inflammation (7). Synthesis may be increased following injury, which may result in low serum values due to peripheral redistribution or increased catabolism (64). In the early stages of malnutrition, the albumin, first mobilized from the extravascular pool, will maintain serum concentration for some time. Decreased serum albumin concentrations only develop later as undernutrition continues. In other words, the child in an early stage of protein-energy deficiency who presents simply with a failure to gain weight is using fat and muscle mass stores as an energy source but maintaining visceral protein synthesis. As malnutrition progresses, and fat and muscle stores are depleted, serum albumin depletion becomes evident. Albumin depletion rapidly occurs with the introduction of superimposed infection and cessation of visceral protein synthesis.

Serum albumin is useful in the assessment of the severity and prognosis of acute or chronic malnutrition complicated by infection and/or trauma. Patients with marasmus or simple starvation often have a normal serum albumin concentration, whereas those with superimposed infection generally have a gradually decreasing serum albumin (65,66).

Studies have indicated that low albumin concentrations are associated with increased morbidity and mortality (7). Thus, within the context of weight-for-height response, measurement of serum albumin may be useful for the longitudinal assessment of the patient's response to nutritional therapy. As in all biochemical tests, however, results must be interpreted in an individualized clinical context.

The relationship of hypoalbuminemia to the edema associated with such malnourished states as kwashiorkor is not clear (7). Edema is not only a result of a decreased albumin and colloid osmotic pressure, but has more complex mechanisms (67,68). Serum albumin is affected by the hydration state of the patient, the acute phase response to sepsis or trauma, and hepatic disease. Hypoalbuminemia is seen in children being treated for malignant tumors; it is unrelated to dietary intake, but dependent upon the inflammatory response (69). Renal and gastrointestinal protein loss can result in profound depression in serum values.

Transferrin

Transferrin, the major transport protein for iron, is synthesized in the liver. Most of its body pool is intravascular and it has a half-life of 8 to 9 days. About one-third of the available transferrin is bound to the serum iron.

Many factors other than protein-energy deficiency affect transferrin. Iron deficiency results in increased hepatic synthesis and very high levels. In contrast, decreases are seen in many inflammatory states, liver and renal disease, as well as in hemolytic anemias. Infection will turn off visceral protein synthesis including that of transferrin.

TABLE 4. *Biochemical tests for nutritional assessment of minerals and vitamins*

Nutrient	Initial screening	Nutrient evaluation	Special tests
Calcium		Serum calcium, bone x-rays	Bone densitometry, calcium balance, serum parathyroid hormone
Phosphorus		Serum phosphorus	
Magnesium		Serum magnesium	
Iron	Hemoglobin, hematocrit, RBC indices, RBC morphology	Serum iron, ferritin, iron-binding capacity, transferrin saturation	Bone marrow iron, free RBC protoporphyrin, iron isotope studies
Zinc		Serum zinc	RBC zinc, WBC zinc, salivary zinc, hair zinc, zinc isotope turnover
Copper		Serum copper, serum ceruloplasmin	RBC copper, 24-hr urine copper, hair copper, RBC superoxide dismutase, radiocopper turnover
Iodine		Serum thyroxine, serum thyroid stimulation hormone	
Selenium		RBC selenium, RBC glutathione peroxidase	
Vitamins			
A		Serum retinol, serum carotene	Serum retinol-binding protein, dark adaptation test
D		Serum 25-hydroxy-D, serum calcium, serum phosphorus, serum alkaline phosphatase, bone x-rays	Serum 1,25-dihydroxy-D, serum vitamin D_2, serum parathyroid hormone
E		Serum tocopherol	RBC hemolysis test, tocopherol transport capacity
K		Prothrombin time	Clotting time, serum vitamin K
Thiamin (B_1)		RBC transketolase activity	24-hr urine thiamin, thiamin pyrophosphate stimulation test
Riboflavin (B_2)		RBC glutathione reductase activity	24-hr urine riboflavin, blood pyruvate
Niacin (B_3)		Whole blood NAD	24-hr urine methylnicotinamide, urine 2-pyridone
Pyridoxine (B_6)		Serum pyridoxine, serum pyridoxal phosphate	RBC glutamate-oxaloacetate transaminase or RBC glutamate-pyruvate transaminase index, urine pyridoxine, urine 4-pyridoxic acid, tryptophan load test
C		Serum ascorbate	WBC ascorbate, blood ascorbate, tyrosine load test
B_{12}	Hemoglobin, RBC indices, RBC morphology	Serum vitamin B_{12}	Urine methylmalonic acid, RBC vitamin B_{12} Schilling test
Folate	Hemoglobin	Serum folate	RBC folate, urine formiminoglutamic acid
Pantothenic acid			Serum pantothenate, 24-hr urine pantothenate
Biotin			Plasma or RBC biotin, 24-hr urine biotin

Adapted from ref. 62.
NAD, nicotinamide-adenine dinucleotide.

Prealbumin

Prealbumin, i.e., thyroxine-binding prealbumin and transthyretin, carries thyroxine and, together with retinol-binding protein, transports vitamin A. Prealbumin, which is synthesized in the liver, has a half-life of 2 days.

Prealbumin is sensitive to acute changes in nutritional status, and it decreases rapidly in the face of infection or when calories and/or protein intake is suddenly decreased (7). Even when protein intake is adequate, severe calorie restriction will result in a decrease in 3 to 4 days (70,71). Concentrations usually return rapidly to normal with adequate nutritional therapy (72–74). Failure to re-

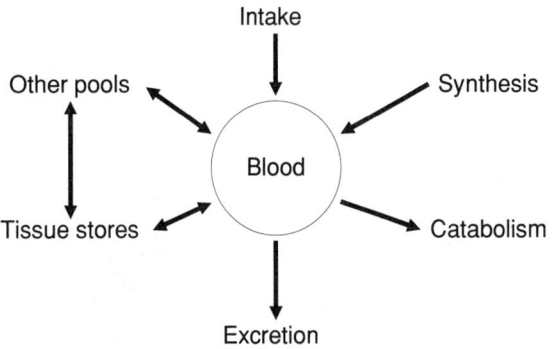

FIG. 3. Factors influencing blood concentration of nutrients. (Adapted from ref. 7.)

verse decreased concentrations with adequate intake is indicative of a poor prognosis (75).

The use of prealbumin is limited because it is very sensitive to infection and the inflammatory response, and because of the incidence of infection and inflammation in hospitalized patients (7). In addition, decreased values may be indicative of liver or iron metabolic disorders, whereas increased levels have been observed in renal disease (7,76). Prealbumin is also not useful as an indicator for stopping nutritional support because its values often return to normal as soon as adequate intake begins.

Retinol-Binding Protein

Retinol-binding protein, which is responsible for the transport of vitamin A, is produced by the liver and has a half-life of 12 hr. Most clinical studies have demonstrated a direct correlation between retinol-binding protein and prealbumin in response to protein-energy deprivation and nutritional therapy (77). Like prealbumin, retinol-binding protein in blood will increase when the diet is sufficient in calories but still deficient in protein (78). It may be a better indicator of recent dietary intake than protein status. Low values are seen in vitamin A deficiency, zinc deficiency, hyperthyroidism, liver disease, and as part of the acute-phase response (7).

Fibronectin

Fibronectin, a cold-insoluble globulin, and a nonspecific, nonimmune serum opsonin is a relatively new biochemical indicator used for the assessment of visceral protein status. Fibronectin, a large glycoprotein with a half-life between 4 and 24 hr, is synthesized by several cell types, including endothelial cells, fibroblasts, and hepatocytes (7). Studies have demonstrated decreased levels in states of acute nutritional deprivation with a return to normal levels when sufficient caloric intake has been instituted, even with a continued protein deficiency (79–81). The mechanism underlying the decrease in plasma fibronectin is unknown. Further clinical studies are necessary to validate its use.

Amino-Acid Profiles

No convincing evidence exists that the measurement of plasma amino acid concentrations, or their profiles in blood, has any specific role in the diagnosis or management of protein-energy malnutrition. However, monitoring plasma amino acids has been helpful in patients on total parenteral nutrition (7).

Evaluating Tests of Nutritional Status

Successful nutritional monitoring is dependent on a clinician's understanding of the limitations of each test. This knowledge must be combined with a thorough

TABLE 5. Serum protein measurements in the evaluation of nutritional status

Protein	Half-life	Clinical use	Limitations
Albumin	18–20 days	For prognosis and duration of hospitalization	Liver and renal disease, hydration, inflammation
Transferrin	8–9 days	None	Disorders of iron metabolism, liver and renal disease, inflammation
Prealbumin	2 days	Monitoring acute depletion and maybe prognosis	Responds more to calories than protein, liver and renal disease, disorders of iron metabolism, inflammation
Retinol-binding protein	12 hr	Similar to prealbumin	Vitamin A and zinc deficiency, liver disease, inflammation
Fibonectin	4–24 hr	Acute depletion and prognosis	Reference ranges not well studied, inflammation
Amino-acid profiles	Many	? Monitoring parenteral nutrition	Many

Adapted from ref. 7.

knowledge of nutrition, metabolism, and pathophysiology. A precise definition of the clinical and laboratory questions that need to be answered will lead to better use of the laboratory for nutritional assessment.

Biochemical Indices of Body Composition

Urinary Creatinine Excretion and Creatinine Height Index

Creatinine, the breakdown product of creatine, is derived mainly from muscle. Muscle creatine phosphate transfers high-energy phosphate bonds to adenosine diphosphate (ADP) to form adenosine triphosphate (ATP). The rate of conversion of creatine to creatinine is relatively constant. Creatinine is excreted by the kidney. The daily (24-hr) urinary excretion is relatively stable, reflecting muscle mass and, therefore, lean body mass. Unfortunately, several factors influence the levels of urinary creatinine excreted: renal function, hydration state, normal urinary output, duration of bed rest, recent high protein intake, age limits, and catabolic states such as infection, trauma, stress, or surgery (7). The measurement of creatinine excretion has been combined with the individual's height to obtain an index that is an estimate of body protein reserve (82). The creatinine/height index (CHI) is calculated as follows:

$$\text{CHI} = \frac{\text{24-hr urine creatinine excretion (mg)}}{\text{24-hr urine creatinine excretion for a well-nourished child of the same height (mg)}} \times 100.$$

This index is dependent on the accuracy of the 24-hr urine collection, the creatinine measurement in the patient, and the reliability of reference tables. A CHI under 40% is regarded as evidence of severe protein depletion; 40% to 60%, moderate depletion; and 60% to 80%, mild depletion. Normal values for 24-hr creatinine excretion for height have been reported (83,84).

Nitrogen Balance

Nitrogen balance or nitrogen retention studies give no information about protein stores or nutritional status. They reflect very short-term protein metabolism and dietary intake. Nitrogen balance studies should involve a 24-hr measurement of nitrogen intake and a 24-hr measurement of urinary nitrogen excretion. The constant 4 (g/24 hr) is used to account for other losses of nitrogen in the stool, through the skin, or elsewhere. Nitrogen intake is estimated by dietary protein (g/24 hr) divided by 6.25, which is the average amount of nitrogen in most dietary protein. Liver and renal disease, disturbances in hydration, and some drugs may affect the results.

$$\text{Nitrogen balance} = \frac{\text{Protein intake (g/24 hr)}}{6.25} - [\text{Urine Urea Nitrogen (g/24 hr)} + 4].$$

$$\text{Nitrogen intake} = \frac{\text{Protein intake (g/24 hr)}}{6.25}.$$

Amino Acid Infusions Using Stable Isotopes

The preceding equations are indirect, somewhat crude estimates of protein metabolism. Several investigators have measured the incorporation of an amino acid directly into protein (85). Such studies can provide information about intake, excretion, synthesis, and catabolism. Stable isotopic techniques may be more routinely employed in future clinical studies.

APPLICATION OF NUTRITIONAL ASSESSMENT

An effective program of nutritional support includes evaluation of the patient's nutritional status, determination of the etiology of nutritional depletion, and the development and implementation of a treatment and monitoring plan. Initial screening can be performed using a history of weight loss, the current weight-for-height, a listing of medical diagnoses, and the serum albumin value (86). Patients with recent weight loss of greater than 5% of body weight, a decreased weight-for-height, diagnoses associated with the development of malnutrition, or a decreased serum albumin, merit further evaluation. Patients are then divided into three categories: those for whom nutritional therapy is imperative, those for whom it is advisable, and those who should do well without nutritional intervention (86).

Patients who need immediate therapy include those with moderate to severe malnutrition. In addition, patients with marginal serum albumins who are markedly stressed should receive nutritional therapy prior to procedures such as surgery, radiation, or chemotherapy, as should those with extensive burn injury, major trauma, or surgical sepsis, regardless of initial nutritional status.

Patients with milder nutritional deficits require continued surveillance for evidence of further depletion and at least maintenance nutritional support if full repletion is not feasible.

Those patients who are initially normal, do not have chronic disease, and do not encounter markedly stressful situations in the hospital, should do well without nutritional support. However, normal patients who develop infection, are starved, or undergo major surgery require reevaluations in 1 to 2 weeks.

SUMMARY

In healthy children, normal growth is predicated on adequate nutritional intake. Malnutrition is also the most important cause of growth retardation in children with disease. For that reason, routine nutritional assessment should be considered an integral part of optimal pediatric care.

Comprehensive nutritional assessment involves evaluation by clinical, dietary, anthropometric, and biochemical methods. Each method has strengths and limitations, and no single measure provides a comprehensive assessment of nutritional status.

Clinical evaluation remains the simplest, most widely available and most reproducible method. It may reveal specific signs of malnutrition including wasting, stunting, pallor, apathy, and obesity. The family and medical history may indicate present health status as well as environmental and psychosocial factors that impinge on that status. Dietary evaluation helps explain observed clinical or biochemical abnormalities and may suggest appropriate intervention. Its usefulness is limited by difficulty in accurate assessment and extrapolating short-term histories to long-term practices.

Anthropometric assessment is helpful in detecting deficiencies or excesses as compared to recognized standards. Most useful are indices for weight and height. Skin-fold measurement may be used for the longitudinal assessment of a patient's response to nutritional therapy.

Although anthropometric measures provide an easy, quantitative means of nutritional assessment, they can only identify nutritional problems that have resulted in measurable change. More subtle subclinical changes may need biochemical evaluation.

Biochemical assessment is used to identify specific nutritional abnormalities including anemia, iron deficiency, or hypoproteinemia before these conditions are clinically apparent. However, because biochemical tests are specific for a particular nutrient, a deficiency must be suspected on the basis of clinical assessment. In hospitalized patients, many biochemical tests are ineffectual because they are profoundly affected by the underlying disease, inflammation, or therapy. As a result, nutritional status often has more impact on the interpretation of commonly performed biochemical tests than biochemical tests affect the assessment of nutrition.

Current research promises to produce major advances in the area of clinical nutritional assessment. Investigators are exploring techniques for evaluating body composition with the use of stable isotopes, impedance, and total body electrical conductivity. Presently, however, these assessment procedures are not easily accessible, are time-consuming, and expensive.

Recognizing the relationship between health status and body fat distribution, advances are also occurring in the technology for measuring energy expenditure in free-living subjects, regardless of nutritional status or age.

In the end, however, the value of any test is dependent on the sophistication and understanding of the clinician who is using it.

REFERENCES

1. Zerfas AJ, Shorr IJ, Neumann CG. Office assessment of nutritional status. *Pediatr Clin North Am* 1977;24:253–272.
2. Solomons NW. Assessment of nutritional status: functional indicators of pediatric nutriture. *Pediatr Clin North Am* 1985;32:319–334.
3. Apelgren KN, Rombeau JL, Twomey PL, Miller RA. Comparison of nutritional indices and outcome in critically ill patients. *Crit Care Med* 1982;10:305–307.
4. Harvey KB, Moldawer LL, Bistrian BR, Blackburn GL. Biological measures for the formulation of a hospital prognostic index. *Am J Clin Nutr* 1981;34:2013–2022.
5. Herbert V. The five possible causes of all nutrient deficiency: illustrated by deficiency of vitamin B_{12} and folic acid. *Am J Clin Nutr* 1973;26:77–86.
6. Kerr GR, Lee ES, Lam MKM, et al. Relationships between dietary and biochemical measures of nutritional status in HANES I data. *Am J Clin Nutr* 1982;35:294–308.
7. Benjamin DR. Laboratory tests and nutritional assessment, protein-energy status. *Pediatr Clin North Am* 1989;36:139–161.
8. Graham AM. Assessment of nutritional intake. *Proc Nutr Soc* 1982;41:343–348.
9. American Diabetes Association. *A guide for the professional: the effective application of exchange lists for meal planning.* New York: American Diabetes Association, 1986.
10. Acheson KJ, Campbell IT, Edholm OG, Miller DS, Stock MJ. The measurement of food and energy intake in man—an evaluation of some techniques. *Am J Clin Nutr* 1980;33:1147–1154.
11. Queen PM, Boatright SL, McNamara MM, et al. Nutritional assessment of pediatric patients. *Nutr Support Serv* 1983;3:23–29.
12. Beal VA. The nutritional history in longitudinal research. *J Am Diet Assoc* 1967;51:426–432.
13. MacLean WC, Graham G. *Pediatric nutrition in clinical practice.* Menlo Park, CA: Addison-Wesley, 1982.
14. Beaton GH, Milner J, Corey P, et al. Sources of variance in 24-hour dietary recall data: implications for nutrition study design and interpretation. *Am J Clin Nutr* 1979;32:2546–2559.
15. Stunkard AJ, Waxman M. Accuracy of self-reports of food intake. *J Am Diet Assoc* 1981;79:547–551.
16. National Research Council, Commission on Life Sciences, Food and Nutrition Board. *Recommended Dietary Allowances,* 10th ed. Washington, DC: National Academy Press, 1989.
17. Acheson KJ, Campbell IT, Edholm OG, Miller DS, Stock MJ. The measurement of daily energy expenditure—an evaluation of some techniques. *Am J Clin Nutr* 1980;33:1155–1164.
18. Schoeller DA, van Santen E. Measurement of energy expenditure in humans by doubly-labeled water method. *J Appl Physiol* 1982;53:955–959.
19. Klein PD, James WPT, Wong WW, et al. Calorimetric validation of the doubly-labeled water method for determination of energy expenditure in man. *Hum Nutr Clin Nutr* 1987;38C:95–106.
20. Coward WA, Prentice AM, Murgatroyd PR, et al. Measurement of CO_2 and water production rates in man using ^2H, ^{18}O-labeled H_2O: comparisons between calorimeter and isotope values. In: van ES AJH, ed. *Human energy metabolism: physical activity and energy expenditure measurements in epidemiological research based upon direct and indirect calorimetry.* Wageningen, The Netherlands: Euro-Nutr, 1987(Series no 5);126–128.
21. Schoeller DA, Webb P. Five-day comparison of the doubly labeled water method with respiratory gas exchange. *Am J Clin Nutr* 1984;40:153–158.
22. Westerterp KR, Schoffelen PFM, Saris WHM, van Hoor F. Measurement of energy expenditure using doubly-labeled water: a validation study. In: van ES AJH, ed. *Human energy metabolism:*

physical activity and energy expenditure measurements in epidemiological research based upon direct and indirect calorimetry. Wageningen, The Netherlands: Euro-Nutr, 1984(Series no 5); 129–131.
23. Coward WA, Prentice AM. Isotope method for the measurement of carbon dioxide production rate in man. *Am J Clin Nutr* 1985;41:659–663.
24. Schoeller DA, Ravussin E, Schutz Y, Acheson KJ, Baertschi P, Jequier EL. Energy expenditure by double labeled water: validation in humans and proposed calculation. *Am J Physiol* 1986;250:R823–R830.
25. Schoeller DA. Measurement of energy expenditure in free-living humans using doubly labeled water. *J Nutr* 1988;118:1278–1289.
26. Roberts SB, Coward WA, Schlingenseipen K-H, Nohria V, Lucas A. Comparison of the doubly labeled water ($^2H_2{^{18}O}$) method with indirect calorimetry and a nutrient-balance study for simultaneous determination of energy expenditure, water intake, and metabolizable energy intake in preterm infants. *Am J Clin Nutr* 1986;44:315–322.
27. Jones PJH, Winthrop AL, Schoeller DA, Swyer PR, Smith J, Filler RM, Heim J. Validation of doubly labeled water for assessing energy expenditure in infants. *Pediatr Res* 1987;21:242–246.
28. Fjeld CR, Schoeller DA, Brown KH. A new model for predicting energy requirements of children during catch-up growth developed using doubly labeled water. *Pediatr Res* 1989;25:503–508.
29. Cooper A, Heird WC. Nutritional assessment of the pediatric patient including the low birth weight infant. *Am J Clin Nutr* 1982;35:1132–1141.
30. Hamil PVV, Drizd TA, Johnson CL, Reed RB, Roche AF, Moore WM. Physical growth: National Center for Health Statistics Percentiles. *Am J Clin Nutr* 1979;32:607–629.
31. Gomez F, Ramos-Galvan R, Frenk S, Cravioto-Munoz J, Chavez R, Vasquez J. Mortality in second and third degree malnutrition. *J Trop Pediatr* 1956;2:77–83.
32. Jelliffe DB. *Assessment of the nutritional status of the community.* Geneva: World Health Organization, WHO Monograph Series no 53, 1966.
33. Waterlow JC. Classification and definition of protein-calorie malnutrition. *Br Med J* 1972;3:566–569.
34. Waterlow JC. Note on the assessment and classification of protein-energy malnutrition in children. *Lancet* 1973;2:87–89.
35. Jelliffe DB, Jelliffe EFP. The arm circumference as a public health index of protein calorie malnutrition of early childhood. XX. Current conclusions. *J Trop Pediatr* 1969;15:253–260.
36. Arnhold R. The arm circumference as a public health index of protein calorie malnutrition of early childhood. XVII. The QUAC stick: a field measure used by the Quaker Service Team in Nigeria. *J Trop Pediatr* 1969;15:243–247.
37. Kanawati AA, McLaren DS. Assessment of marginal malnutrition. *Nature* 1970;228:573–575.
38. Rutishauser IHE. The arm circumference as a public health index of protein calorie malnutrition of early childhood. V. Correlations of the circumference of the mid upper arm with weight and weight for height in three groups in Uganda. *J Trop Pediatr* 1967;15:196–197.
39. Trowbridge FL, Staehling N. Sensitivity and specificity of arm circumference indicators in identifying malnourished children. *Am J Clin Nutr* 1980;33:687–696.
40. Forbes GB. Methods for determining composition of the human body. *Pediatrics* 1962;29:477–494.
41. Moore FD, Lister J, Boyden CM, Ball MR, Sullivan N, Dagher FJ. The skeleton as a feature of body composition: values predicted by isotope dilution and observed by cadaver dissection in an adult human female. *Hum Biol* 1968;40:135–188.
42. Merritt RJ, Suskind RM. Nutritional survey of hospitalized pediatric patients. *Am J Clin Nutr* 1979;32:1320–1325.
43. Parsons HG, Francoeur TE, Howland P, Spengler RF, Pencharz PB. The nutritional status of hospitalized children. *Am J Clin Nutr* 1980;33:1140–1146.
44. Cooper A, Jakobowski D, Spiker J, Floyd T, Ziegler MM, Koop CE. Nutritional assessment: an integral part of the preoperative pediatric surgical evaluation. *J Pediatr Surg* 1981;16:554–561.
45. Long CL, Schiller WR, Blackmore WS, Geiger JW, O'Dell M, Henerson K. Muscle protein catabolism in the septic patient as measured by 3-methylhistidine excretion. *Am J Clin Nutr* 1977;30:1349–1352.
46. Ziegler EE, O'Donnell AM, Nelson SE, Fomon SJ. Body composition of the reference fetus. *Growth* 1976;40:329–341.
47. Fomon SJ. Body composition of the male reference infant during the first year of life. *Pediatrics* 1967;40:863–870.
48. Fomon SJ, Haschke F, Ziegler EE, Nelson SE. Body composition of reference children from birth to age 10 years. *Am J Clin Nutr* 1982;35:1169–1175.
49. Haschke F, Fomon SJ, Ziegler EE. Body composition of a nine-year-old reference boy. *Pediatr Res* 1981;15:847–849.
50. Haschke F. Body composition of the male reference adolescent. *Acta Paediatr Scand (Suppl)* 1983;307:11–23.
51. Widdowson EM, McCance RA, Spray CM. The chemical composition of the human body. *Clin Sci* 1951;10:113–125.
52. Lohman TG. Applicability of body composition techniques and constants for children and youths. *Exerc Sport Sci Rev* 1986;14:325–357.
53. Schoeller DA, van Santen E, Petersen DW, Dietz W, Jaspan J, Klein PD. Total body water measurements in humans with ^{18}O and ^2H labeled water. *Am J Clin Nutr* 1980;33:2686–2693.
54. Schloerb PR, Friis-Hansen BJ, Edelman IS, Solomon AK, Moore FD. The measurement of total body water in the human subject by deuterium oxide dilution. *J Clin Invest* 1950;29:1296–1310.
55. Lukaski HC. Methods for the assessment of human body composition: traditional and new. *Am J Clin Nutr* 1987;46:537–556.
56. Nyboer J. *Electrical impedance plethysmography,* 2nd ed. Springfield, IL: Charles C Thomas, 1970.
57. Lukaski HC, Bolonchuk WW, Hall CA, Siders WA. Estimation of fat free mass in humans using the bioelectrical impedance method: a validation study. *J Appl Physiol* 1986;60:1327–1332.
58. Kushner RF, Shoeller DA. Estimation of total body water by bioelectrical impedance analysis. *Am J Clin Nutr* 1986;44:417–424.
59. Hansman C. Anthropometry and related data: anthropometry, skinfold thickness measurements. In: McCammon RW, ed. *Human growth and development.* Springfield, IL: Charles C Thomas, 1970.
60. Harrison GGA, Van Itallie TB. Estimation of body composition: a new approach based on electromagnetic principles. *Am J Clin Nutr* 1982;35:1176–1179.
61. Klish WJ, Forbes BG, Gordon A, Cochran WJ. New method for the estimation of lean body mass in infants (EMME instrument): validation in non-human models. *J Pediatr Gastroenterol Nutr* 1984;3:199–204.
62. Lo CW. Laboratory assessment of nutritional status. In: Walker WA, Watkins JB, eds. *Nutrition in pediatrics basic science and clinical application.* Boston/Toronto: Little, Brown, 1985.
63. Haiden M, Haiden SQ. Assessment of protein-calorie malnutrition. *Clin Chem* 1984;30:1286–1299.
64. Dahn MS, Jacobs LA, Smith S, Lange P, Mitchell RA, Kirkpatrick JR. The significance of hypoalbuminemia following injury and infection. *Am Surg* 1985;51:340–343.
65. Forse RA, Shizgal HM. Serum albumin and nutritional status. *J Parenter Enteral Nutr* 1980;4:450–454.
66. Anonymous. Laboratory tests in protein-calorie malnutrition. *Lancet* 1973;1:1041–1042.
67. Golden MHN. Protein deficiency, energy deficiency and the oedema of malnutrition. *Lancet* 1982;1:1261–1265.
68. Golden MHN, Golden BE, Jackson AA. Albumin and nutritional oedema. *Lancet* 1980;1:114–116.
69. Merritt RJ, Kalsch M, Roux LD, Ashley-Mills J, Siegel SS. Significance of hypoalbuminemia in pediatric oncology patients: malnutrition or infection? *J Parenter Enteral Nutr* 1985;9:303–306.
70. Fischer JE. Plasma proteins as indicators of nutritional status. In: Lewenson SM, ed. *Nutritional assessment, present status, future directions and prospects.* Report on the Second Ross Conference on Medical Research, Ross Laboratories, Columbus, Ohio, 1982.
71. Tuten MB, Wogt S, Dasse F, Leider Z. Utilization of prealbumin as a nutritional parameter. *J Parenter Enteral Nutr* 1985;9:709–711.
72. Carpentier YA, Barthel J, Bruyns J. Plasma protein concentration in nutritional assessment. *Proc Nutr Soc* 1982;41:405–417.

73. Ingebleek Y, Van Den Schneck HG, De Nayer P, De Visschen M. Albumin, transferrin and the thyroxine binding prealbumin/retinol binding protein (TBPA-RBP) complex in assessment of malnutrition. *Clin Chim Acta* 1975;63:61–67.
74. Large S, Neal G, Glover J, Thanangkul O, Olson RE. The early changes in retinol-binding proteins and prealbumin concentrations in plasma of protein-energy malnourished children after treatment with retinol and an improved diet. *Br J Nutr* 1980;43:393–402.
75. Bourry J, Milano G, Caldani C. Assessment of nutritional proteins during the parenteral nutrition of cancer patients. *Ann Clin Lab Sci* 1982;12:158–162.
76. Delpeuch F, Cornu A, Chevalier P. The effect of iron deficiency anemia on two indices of nutritional status, pre-albumin and transferrin. *Br J Nutr* 1980;43:375–379.
77. Shetty PS, Watrasiewicz KE, Jung PT, James WPT. Rapid-turnover transport proteins: an index of subclinical protein-energy malnutrition. *Lancet* 1979;2:230–232.
78. Golden MHN. Transport proteins as indices of protein status. *Am J Clin Nutr* 1982;35:1159–1165.
79. McKone TK, Davis AT, Dean RE. Fibronectin: a new nutritional parameter. *Am Surg* 1985;51:336–339.
80. Scott RL, Sohmer PR, MacDonald MG. The effect of starvation and repletion on plasma fibronectin in man. *JAMA* 1982;248:2025–2027.
81. Yoder MC, Anderson DC, Gopalakrishna GS, Douglas SD, Polin RA. Comparison of serum fibronectin, prealbumin, and albumin concentrations during nutritional repletion in protein-calorie malnourished infants. *J Pediatr Gastroenterol Nutr* 1987;6:84–88.
82. Forbes GB, Bruining GJ. Urinary creatinine excretion and lean body mass. *Am J Clin Nutr* 1976;29:1359–1366.
83. Viteri FE, Alvarado J. The creatinine height index: its use and the estimation of protein depletion and repletion in protein-calorie malnourished children. *Pediatrics* 1970;46:696–706.
84. Cheek DB. *Human growth: body composition, cell growth, energy and intelligence.* Philadelphia: Lea & Febiger, 1968.
85. Matthews DE, Bier DM. Stable isotope methods for nutritional investigation. *Annu Rev Nutr* 1983;3:309–339.
86. Merritt RJ, Blackburn GL. Nutritional assessment and metabolic response to illness of the hospitalized child. In: Suskind RM, ed. *Textbook of pediatric nutrition.* New York: Raven Press, 1981.

CHAPTER 17

Nutritional Support of Children in the Intensive Care Unit

Murray M. Pollack

In 1930, Sir David Cuthbertson, a clinical chemist at the Royal Infirmary in Glasgow, observed that patients with injuries as minor as long bone fractures had substantially increased nitrogen losses with a concomitant depletion of protein stores (1). Subsequently, he realized that injuries and other critical illnesses cause unique metabolic consequences (2). This pioneering work led to a significant, clinically relevant, understanding of the metabolic and nutritional impact of critical illness.

The nutritional failure of critical illness, unlike that of simple starvation, rapidly results in malnutrition, contributing to the dysfunction of the most important organ systems (Fig. 1). In many critically ill patients, nutritional failure is an important determinant of outcome. Emphasis on prevention and treatment of nutritional depletion is one of the most significant, recent critical care advances.

M. M. Pollack: Departments of Anesthesiology and Pediatrics, Critical Care Medicine, George Washington University and Children's Neonatal Medical Center, Washington, D.C. 20010.

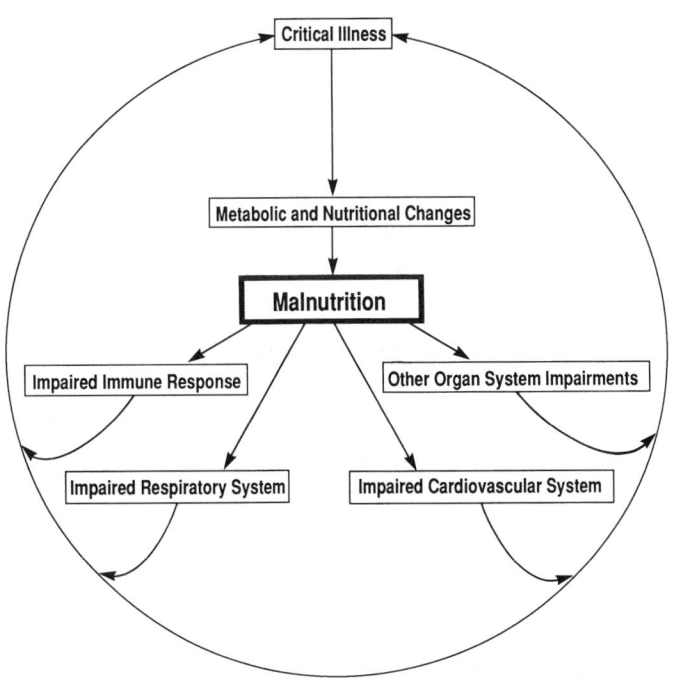

FIG. 1. The relationship of critical illness to malnutrition.

THE METABOLIC RESPONSE TO CRITICAL ILLNESS

Nutritional support for critically ill children depends on understanding the basic metabolic profiles of life-threatening disease. For patients with minor stress, the physiology is equivalent to simple starvation. For more critically ill children, however, important consequences include hypermetabolism with autocanabalism, hyperglycemia, insulin resistance, increased fat mobilization, increased fat utilization, nitrogen depletion, fat depletion, and acute and chronic protein-energy malnutrition. The hypermetabolic response to critical illness is proportionate to the severity of the insult, returning to baseline as the injury abates. Long bone fractures generally increase basal metabolic rate by 20%, sepsis increases the rate by 50%, and severe burns increase the rate by 80% to 100%.

Neuroendocrine changes mediate the nutritional response to critical illness and consist of basic, important elements. The global response, especially to critical illnesses such as sepsis and trauma, includes serum elevations of catecholamines, cortisol, glucagon, and growth hormone. Infusion of cortisol, glucagon, and epinephrine in normal volunteers duplicates the metabolic stress response and demonstrates that multiple hormones, acting synergistically, are required for the "normal" response to critical illness (3). The severity of the neuroendocrine response is proportionate to the clinical severity of illness. Although characteristic neuroendocrine *temporal* changes have been proposed, they have not been confirmed for pediatric patients nor for the vast majority of diagnoses in the pediatric ICU.

The neuroendocrine changes appear to be mediated by peptides produced, primarily, by macrophages and polymorphonuclear leukocytes. Recent research indi-

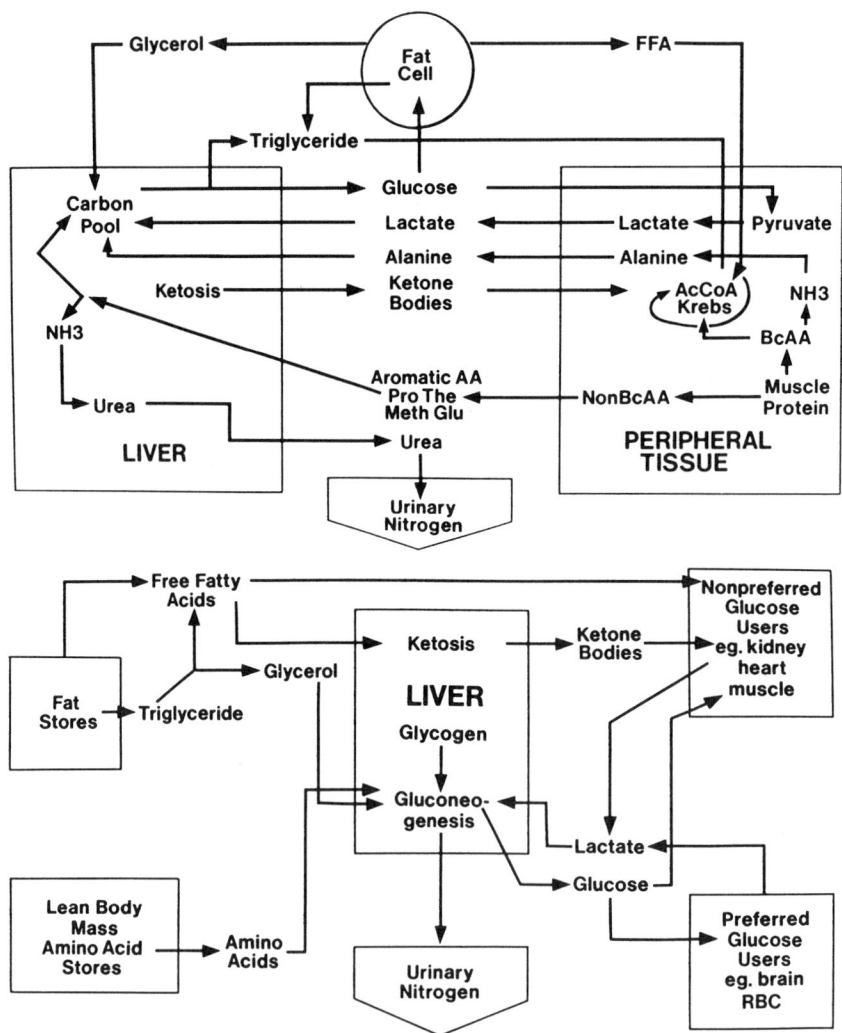

FIG. 2. Acute nonstress fasting (*top*) and stress (*bottom*) metabolic flow diagrams. In the acute nonstress fasting state, the initial fuel is glucose, which, over time, shifts to fat. Protein sparing is accomplished as lactate and alanine recycle from glucose. During acute stress, there is simultaneous utilization of carbohydrates, fats, and amino acids. Peripheral tissues utilize endogenous branch-chain amino acids (autocanabalism), increasing protein breakdown, and urinary nitrogen excretion. (Reproduced from ref. 83, with permission.)

cates that these mediators are central to the neuroendocrine and nutritional response to injury as well as the cardiopulmonary and systemic responses to critical illness. The major mediators currently considered controllers of the stress response are tumor necrosis factor and interleukin-1. Interleukin-1, especially, may be a central mediator of the nutritional consequences of critical illness because it induces fever, leukocytosis, increased gluconeogenesis, and acts directly on muscle to increase proteolysis resulting in the net breakdown of protein. A small peptide isolated from the serum of septic patients, which may be a degradation product of interleukin-1, has similar effects (4,5). Changes in tumor necrosis factor are temporally correlated with temperature, adrenocorticotropic hormone (ACTH), and white blood cell counts after endotoxin injection. Tumor necrosis factor is acknowledged to induce cachexia (6,7). The control of the metabolic and nutritional response by mediators indicates that efforts to alter the response, either with nutritional support or hormonal infusions, will be relatively difficult.

There are clinically important patterns of substrate utilization during critical illness (Fig. 2). The most important pattern is muscle proteolysis and nitrogen loss (autocanabalism). Although protein loss is minimized in starvation, it is accelerated during critical illness, presumably due to the anti-insulin hormones (catecholamines, glucagon, cortisol) and peptides such as tumor necrosis factor and interleukin-1. Branch-chain amino acids from proteolysis, which normally supply only 6% to 7% of energy requirements, may supply up to 25% of the total energy supply (8). The branch-chain amino acids from proteolysis are used directly by the muscle, brain, heart, and other tissues as energy substrates and for hepatic gluconeogenesis.

The second clinically important general pattern of substrate utilization is the alteration of fat and glucose metabolism. Normally, hyperglycemia with hyperinsulinemia inhibits fat mobilization and oxidation. However, in most critical illnesses, fat mobilization increases in spite of the occurrence of hyperglycemia (Fig. 2). Fat becomes the preferable energy source for most tissues, providing up to 75% to 90% of energy. Gluconeogenesis is, at least in part, responsible for the hyperglycemia classically seen in the stress response. These global changes appear to be largely due to increases in glucagon, cortisol, and catecholamines, occurring despite the elevated glucose and insulin concentrations (3,9).

The final result of critical illness is a metabolic response that is very different from simple starvation (Table 1; Fig. 2). Starvation physiology minimizes energy expenditure and conserves nutrients, especially nitrogen. Starvation without critical illness reduces metabolic requirements, and converts to a fat-based energy system. The result is a low respiratory quotient (0.7). Critical illness, on the other hand, causes increased energy usage and requires endogenous nutrients, especially protein.

TABLE 1. *Metabolic response to critical illness versus starvation*

Variable	Critical illness	Starvation
Energy requirements	+ to +++	−
Primary fuels	Mixed	Fat
Protein breakdown	+++	+
Amino acid oxidation	+++	+
Ureagenesis	+++	+
Hepatic protein synthesis	+++	+
Total body protein synthesis	−	−
Gluconeogenesis	+++	+
Ketone production	+	++++
Rate of malnutrition development	+++	+

Modified from ref. 10.
+, increased; −, decreased.

The fuels for critical illness are mixed, resulting in a higher respiratory quotient (0.85).

MALNUTRITION IN CRITICALLY ILL CHILDREN

Protein-energy malnutrition (PEM) is a common and important consequence of pediatric critical illness. PEM occurs very early in the course of critical illness. A survey of 50 consecutive patients with nonsurgical disease, conducted within 48 hr of admission to a pediatric ICU, revealed that 16% had acute protein-energy malnutrition, 20% had deficiencies in their somatic protein stores, and 18% had deficiencies in their fat stores. Visceral protein stores, as evaluated by albumin levels, were decreased in over 60%. These data are even more impressive since all children with chronic organ failure and malignancies were excluded. Children under 2 years of age were more likely to develop PEM than older children (11). Significantly, children with acute PEM early in their ICU course had more physiologic instability and a greater chance of dying than those without PEM (12).

In a 6-month prevalence study, the nutritional status of all medical and surgical patients in a pediatric ICU was assessed anthropometrically. The prevalence of acute PEM was found to be 19% and chronic PEM was 18%. Somatic protein store depletions and fat store depletions were 21% and 14%, respectively. The children at highest risk for nutritional depletion were those less than 2 years of age and surgical patients of any age (13). Children remaining in the ICU for prolonged time periods who were treated with aggressive enteral and parenteral support generally showed consistent improvement in their nutritional parameters.

The most important factor in the development of PEM is increased energy expenditure. The resting energy expenditure of children with critical illness varies with the extent of the stress. In noncritically ill patients, resting energy expenditure is about 10% above basal because it includes the specific dynamic action of food. Degrees of stress, as typified by long bone fractures, sepsis, and severe burns, increase metabolic rates of adult patients by approximately 20%, 50%, and 80% to 100%, respectively. Several pediatric studies have confirmed that critically ill children, as well as adults, have resting energy expenditures substantially above basal metabolic rates. Tilden et al. (14) studied 18 children with traumatic injuries and found that resting energy expenditure was 48% greater than that estimated from the Harris-Benedict equation. The respiratory quotient was 0.82, similar to most adult studies, indicating a mixed substrate utilization, with the primary fuel being fat. The relative energy contribution of fat, carbohydrate, and protein was 53%, 33%, and 14%, respectively, corroborating studies in adults. Finally, Tilden et al. found that the energy response was in proportion to the severity of injury. Winthrop et al. (15) measured energy expenditure in 19 children after blunt trauma but found only a 14% increase in measured energy expenditure compared to basal metabolic rate. However, their patients were less ill than those of Tilden et al. A study of patients with a greater variety of diseases showed much greater variability, with energy expenditures varying from basal to approximately 50% greater than basal (16).

Protein loss leading to protein depletion in children also appears to be comparable to adults. Urinary nitrogen losses in two pediatric critical care studies were much greater than that expected from simple starvation and similar to studies of traumatically injured adult patients (14,17).

Not only is the metabolic rate increased in proportion to the stress, other activities in the critical care unit consume energy, as well. Breathing, itself, for patients with respiratory disease may consume large amounts of energy. Normal respiration consumes 1% to 3% of total oxygen consumption. In respiratory failure, the oxygen cost of breathing averages 30% of the respiratory oxygen consumption; in individual patients, the oxygen cost of breathing may be equivalent to the oxygen consumption of the rest of the body (18). For children with bronchiolitis, the work of breathing, which is an indirect measure of the caloric requirements for respiration, averages 6 times normal and may reach 40 times the expected energy expenditure (19). In addition, chest physical therapy increases oxygen consumption by approximately 40%, doing a chest radiograph increases oxygen consumption by approximately 30%, dressing changes by approximately 25%, visitation by approximately 20%, and passive range of motion by approximately 20% (20). Therefore, the daily routines of ICU patients increase energy requirement over the measured resting energy expenditure in proportion to the amount of activity and effort devoted to the activity. Even a patient's state of agitation may substantially add to energy expenditures. Providing routine sedation and pain relief will decrease resting energy expenditure by 5% to 10% (21). In the more severely agitated patient, paralysis decreases oxygen consumption by up to 58% (22).

The striking tendency of children to develop PEM with critical illness is attributable to several factors. First, children have greater caloric requirements per weight than adults. This relatively greater energy requirement exists because the major metabolic organs (brain, kidneys, liver, heart) make up 16% to 17% of body weight in children versus 5% to 6% in adults. In particular, the brain of a child consumes about 60% of the basal energy requirement compared to only 20% in adults (23).

In addition, children have lower caloric reserves than adults, especially infants less than 1 year old. Fat represents only about 1% of a premature infant's weight, 16% of a full-term infant's weight, and 20% of the weight of a 1-year-old child. Protein stores change similarly (24). These lower nutritional reserves cause children to withstand nutritional stress less well than adults and help to account for the increased risk of young children to PEM.

Many children also have decreased caloric intake prior to a critical illness leading to depletion of their nutritional reserves. Moreover, weight loss is exaggerated by conversion to an energy system that utilizes protein from muscle breakdown as a fuel. Muscle is 80% water and 20% solid matter; caloric content of 1 kg of muscle is only about 800 kilocalories (Cal), in contrast to 7,000 Cal contained in a kilogram of fat. If 1,000 Cal of energy were supplied by muscle, 1.25 kg of weight loss would occur; if the same energy were supplied by fat, only 0.14 kg of weight loss would result. This muscle catabolism may result in dramatic wasting, even when caloric requirements are not excessive.

A significant reason why many children in pediatric ICUs develop PEM is that the severe chronic disease for which they are hospitalized may be associated with decreased nutritional reserves. A multi-institutional study of pediatric ICUs found that 22% to 48% of admissions had chronic disease severe enough to limit life expectancy to less than adult age or to prevent independent functioning (25). An in-depth analysis of a single ICU indicated that 24% of patients had nonlimiting chronic disease and 31% had chronic, life-limiting disease. Nine percent of these children were admitted because of an exacerbation of their chronic disease, and 10% were mentally retarded (4% with chromosomal disorders) (26). Finally, chronically ill children consume a much larger percentage of the days of ICU care than their numeric percentage. Seven percent of the patients in a pediatric ICU stayed 2 weeks or more, consuming approximately 50% of all bed days (27). There is a very high likelihood, therefore, that patients in an ICU will be chronically ill, either from illness present prior to admission or from illness necessitating their current admission.

ORGAN SYSTEM DYSFUNCTIONS AND NUTRITIONAL DEPLETIONS

The physiologic consequences of nutritional depletion are critically important to outcome in severely ill children. Depletion of protein and energy body stores results in a characteristic pattern of physiologic dysfunctions that may severely affect the critically ill child. This progression of events starts with decreased muscle mass, and continues to decreased visceral proteins, impaired immune response, impaired wound healing, impaired organ function, and death (28). For children such as those with bronchopulmonary dysplasia, whose major hope is the growth of new lung tissue, nutritional depletion may severely decrease chances of achieving a normal life.

The Immune System

Critically ill children have increased susceptibility to infection. The nosocomial infection rate in pediatric intensive care units is substantially higher than in routine hospital areas and may be a determining factor in outcome (29). Although the increased incidence of infection is undoubtedly multifactorial, macronutrient depletion has a significant detrimental effect on all aspects of the immune response including the cell-mediated system, the phagocytic system, and, to a lesser extent, the B-cell system (30–32). Other nutrient deficiencies, such as of zinc, iron, magnesium, pyridoxine, folic acid, and vitamins A and E, may also result in impaired immune function (33,34). Malnutrition severe enough to depress immune status may be an important indicator of mortality risk. Patients with malnutrition severe enough to depress cell-mediated immunity have increased mortality rates (35).

The Respiratory System

The clinically important effects of starvation on the respiratory system may be the most amenable to nutritional therapy. In the respiratory system, the muscles act as a pump, the lungs as an exchange mechanism, and the brain and chemoreceptors as "controller" of respiratory function. Each component may become dysfunctional secondary to nutritional depletion.

The most important respiratory muscles are the diaphragm and intercostal/accessory muscles. Respiratory muscle wasting occurs as a result of nutritional depletion. Arora and Rochester (36,37) demonstrated that diaphragmatic muscle mass is reduced in proportion to the total body weight loss. Malnutrition may produce reductions in muscle strength substantial enough to effect the need for mechanical ventilation in patients with acute or chronic respiratory disease. Muscle dysfunction includes inspiratory and expiratory muscle weakness as well as decreased endurance. Important for clinical assessment, the respiratory muscle weakness is out of proportion to the amount of muscle wasting, implying that undernourishment might affect the fuel availability and/or the biochemical functioning of the muscle as well as gross loss of tissue (38). Micronutrient depletion, especially hypophosphatemia and hypomagnesemia, may also cause muscle weakness severe enough to result in respiratory failure (39,40). Repletion of malnourished patients results in a return of respiratory strength within several weeks in proportion to the gain in body weight (41–43). The patterns of functional return indicate that strength may return prior to a return of the actual respiratory muscle mass, indicating that the initial restoration of strength is on a biochemical basis followed by actual repletion of muscle mass (44).

The effects of starvation on the lung parenchyma are less directly relevant to most patients' care. Emphysematous changes are seen in humans with severe starvation. More pertinent to critical care, however, is the observation that acute nutritional deprivation results in decreased surfactant and other pulmonary proteins, and decreased lung growth (44–46). These effects may be important contributors to the development of atelectasis and parenchymal dysfunction in ICU patients. Since decreased compliance and increased intrapulmonary shunting are major components of respiratory disease in the ICU, their potential exacerbation by atelectasis, which occurs as a result of nutritional depletion, is significant. Observations in nutritionally depleted animals that may have clinical significance in humans include changes in the mechanical properties of the lung and changes in pulmonary connective tissue (44).

The effect of nutritional status on the control of respiration may be one of the most critical effects of nutritional deprivation. First, nutritional depletion results in rapid, shallow respirations and a decreased number of sighs, both of which might contribute to the development of atelectasis and pneumonia (47,48). Second, nutritional deprivation for as short as 12 hr may reduce hypoxic and hypercarbic ventilatory drive (49,50). The loss of hypoxic ventilatory response may be dramatic with a blunting of the hypoxic response until dangerously low PaO_2 levels are reached. Therapy with amino acid infusions or enteral protein may restore normal respiratory control within hours (50,51). This lack of hypoxic and hypercarbic drive may be a contributor to the respiratory acidosis of bronchopulmonary dysplasia patients and may also account for the rapid respiratory improvement seen in some patients soon after restarting nutritional support.

The Cardiovascular System

Cardiac dysfunction resulting from various causes is extremely common in critically ill children. Because cardiac performance may be the determining factor for survival, prevention of cardiac dysfunction from nutritional depletion is very important. Malnourished patients with cardiac disease have increased operative mortality and longer hospital stays (52).

The long-held belief that cardiac muscle and, therefore, performance was spared by starvation was refuted by Keyes and his associates (53) in the 1940s. They demonstrated that 25% loss of body weight resulted in bradycardia, hypotension, decreased stroke volume, and decreased cardiac output. Electrocardiographic changes of undernutrition include sinus bradycardia, increased Q-T interval, and decreased voltage. In the 1970s, Viart (54) reported that catheterized malnourished children demonstrated hemodynamic profiles of prolonged circulation times, bradycardia, hypotension, decreased cardiac index, decreased stroke volume, and decreased cardiac work. The most severely malnourished children had hemodynamic profiles of severe, hypovolemic shock. Both cardiac index and stroke volume, the most important clinical indices, were significantly correlated with the degree of weight loss. The cardiac index was also significantly correlated with serum albumin concentration.

Animal studies corroborate that nutritional depletion depresses cardiac performance, most importantly, contractility. Abel et al. (55) found nutritionally depleted dogs had both abnormal ventricular compliance and contractility. Alden et al. (56) found decreased contractility as well as findings consistent with decreased numbers of beta receptors.

Cardiac performance is also affected by deficiencies in trace elements, vitamins, and inorganic ions. Thiamine is involved as a cofactor in energy production; selenium deficiency is associated with cardiomyopathy; calcium, phosphorus, magnesium, and potassium are important in electrical excitation and mechanical coupling of myocardial cells.

The acute effect of nutritional repletion on cardiac performance is not established. Abel et al. (57) were unable to show that, in severely malnourished dogs, nutritional repletion for 2 months was effective in normalizing cardiac performance. However, cardiac muscle mass clearly increases in anorexia nervosa patients during nutritional repletion (58).

Other Physiologic Consequences of PEM

Other physiologic consequences of malnutrition are less important to the general pediatric ICU population. Malnourished patients are hypovolemic, a physiologic state that interferes with their ability to respond to life-threatening physiologic dysfunction (59). Gastrointestinal changes include mucosal atrophy, decreased intestinal motility and malabsorption, and decreased pancreatic function, all of which interfere with the delivery of enteral nutrition (60). The bacterial overgrowth associated with these conditions could also be an important source of sepsis. Malnutrition may depress important serum proteins. For example, fibronectin, a circulating opsin important in phagocytosis, is depressed after starvation (61). Renal effects are controversial: some studies do not find the kidney critically affected by nutritional depletion, others report reduced glomerular filtration rate, reduced ability to handle solute loads, and polyuria (62,63). The hematologic effects of nutritional depletion include anemia, with depressed stem cell function and depressed erythropoietin synthesis. Finally, hepatic effects of malnutrition include decreased visceral protein synthesis, depressed microsomal activity, and eventual hepatic insufficiency (63).

THE NUTRITIONAL EVALUATION OF CRITICALLY ILL PATIENTS

Accurate nutritional assessment of critically ill patients is difficult. Classical nutritional evaluation includes, for acute nutritional status, weight-for-length; for chronic nutritional status, length-for-age; for fat stores, triceps skin-fold thickness; for somatic protein stores, midarm muscle circumference; and for anergy and visceral protein assessment, total lymphocyte counts and skin testing. Although these assessments may be used for critically ill children, in the acute phase of illness they may simply yield confusing or misleading information (64). First, many critically ill patients have a capillary leak syndrome that causes edema formation and requires fluid boluses for cardiovascular support. Therefore, total body water may be substantially changed, resulting in nonnutritional changes in body weight, midarm circumferences, and triceps skin-fold thickness. Length is always difficult to accurately assess, especially when ICU equipment interferes with measuring instruments. Lymphopenia, commonly associated with nutritionally caused impaired immune function, may be influenced by the primary disease process. Anergy, also associated with nutritionally caused impaired immune function, is affected by many factors other than nutrition in ICU patients including viral and bacterial sepsis, uremia, hepatitis, trauma, burns, hemorrhage, malignancy, drugs, including steroids, immunosuppressants, cimetidine, and even surgery and anesthesia (34).

Visceral protein assessment is also difficult. Albumin, the most commonly assessed visceral protein, is frequently given exogenously during volume resuscitation and, with a half-life of approximately 20 days, does not adequately reflect the rapid nutritional changes occurring with critical illness. Transferrin, prealbumin, and retinol-binding protein, with half-lives of 8 days, 2 days, and 10 hr, respectively, are much better candidates for visceral protein assessment because of their shorter half-lives. However, they are dependent on hepatic synthesis. Since hepatic function is affected by many ICU factors (e.g., hypoxic/ischemic injury, sepsis, congestive heart failure), accurate nutritional assessment of visceral protein status is frequently difficult.

The lack of an accurate nutritional assessment should not be used as an excuse for withholding nutritional support since the concept of nutritional support in the ICU now encompasses metabolic support for organ function for all critically ill patients. Many of the nutritional evaluation difficulties will resolve after the first few days of intensive care, especially after the acute phase of therapy is over.

NUTRITIONAL SUPPORT IN PEDIATRIC CRITICAL CARE

Conceptually, nutrient delivery to critically ill children, especially during the early phase of illness, has become metabolic support. The goal at this stage of illness is to support organ function and prevent, if possible, impaired immune, cardiovascular and respiratory system dysfunctions. Therefore, nutritional evaluation is not important in determining the need for nutritional support since the amount of support will be primarily determined by the severity of illness and the ability to provide parenteral and enteral therapy to an unstable patient. During the early phase of illness, the nutritional goal is the maintenance of lean body mass. During this hypermetabolic phase of critical illness, growth or repletion of body mass is exceptionally difficult. After the hypermetabolic phase of illness passes, the patient will revert to more normal metabolic physiology. Major goals of parenteral nutrition at that time are repletion of lost body stores of nitrogen and energy, and maintenance of growth. Table 2 indicates the most important organ system dysfunctions and when each responds to nutritional therapy. Generally, resolution of the organ system dysfunctions associated with malnutrition takes days to weeks.

Parenteral nutrition aimed at providing metabolic support or minimizing the loss of lean body mass should begin soon after the resuscitation phase of the illness. In practice, this usually is within the first 3 days and often within the first 24 hr. During this phase of therapy, limitations on fluid delivery may restrict the amount of parenteral nutrition delivered. Close cooperation with the pharmacy to provide individualized, concentrated solutions will ameliorate this limitation.

Metabolic support starts with an estimation of energy requirements. This is best accomplished by the direct measurement of metabolic rate because clinical estimates or those from formulas are frequently inaccurate (65). Commercially available metabolic carts make this practical in ICUs. Caloric estimates from metabolic carts should be derived from multiple measurements taken throughout the day and night. There is, however, no indication that outcome is improved by their use. In addition, increases of up to 20% of measured caloric needs may result from the activities of critical care, such as state of agitation, chest physical therapy, etc. Metabolic carts will not necessarily assess these.

Basal metabolic rate can be determined from standard formulas, such as the Harris-Benedict or Aub-Dubois formulas, or computed and adjusted for the degree of stress based on adult data. Basal metabolic rates for children, with adjustment factors for degree of stress, have been determined (Tables 3 and 4). With the exception of severe burns, most stress factor adjustments should not exceed 160% of basal energy expenditure. Maintenance energy requirements are approximately 150% of basal requirements; therefore, substantially greater-than-normal intakes will not be necessary to provide the necessary calories. This is consistent with recent data demonstrating that septic and respiratory failure patients had metabolic requirements only 15% greater than expected (66–68).

How caloric intake should be divided among fat, carbohydrate, and protein is a source of substantial disagreement. In general, at least 4% of calories should be linoleic acid in order to prevent fatty acid deficiency. When possible, this should be given daily, since infusions of the large amounts of glucose characteristic of parenteral nutrition can suppress the release of linoleic acid from adipose tissue, causing the development of linoleic acid deficiency within 1 week (69). Although no absolute amount of carbohydrate is required, in nonstressed, fasted individuals, provision of 25% of energy requirements as carbohydrate will minimize nitrogen loss (34). In patients following hip replacement, maintenance of intracellular, high-energy phosphate bonds is improved when glucose is part of the parenteral nutrition protocol, strongly indicating that glucose is important for the maintenance of cellular energy levels (70). In practice, division of the nonprotein calories equally between fat and carbohydrate is a reasonable approach. Fat and carbohydrate

TABLE 2. *Clinically significant organ system dysfunctions and their times to respond to nutritional therapies*

Organ system dysfunction	Response to therapy
Respiratory	
Decreased muscle strength	Weeks
Depressed central respiratory drive	Hours
Cardiovascular	
Decreased cardiac output	Weeks
Decreased contractility	Weeks
Immune	
Increased susceptibility to infection	?

TABLE 3. *Energy requirements of critically ill children (66)[a]*

Age	Basal energy requirements (Cal/kg/day)
<3 months	55
1 year	55
5 years	45
10 years	38
16 years	27
Adult	26

[a] Data are shown for males. Requirements of females are slightly less.

TABLE 4. Approximate stress factors[a]

Representative stress state	Stress factor
Simple starvation	1.0
Postoperative recovery: uncomplicated surgery	1.0
Sepsis (moderate)	1.3
Sepsis (severe)	1.6
Trauma: mild (e.g., long bone fracture)	1.2
Trauma: central nervous system (sedated)	1.3
Trauma: moderate to severe	1.5
Burns (proportionate to burn size)	up to 2.0

[a] Multiply basal metabolic weight by stress factor for approximate energy requirements.

seem to have equivalent effects on energy use and nitrogen sparing (71,72).

Nitrogen excretion is directly related to energy requirements (73). As energy consumption increases, alanine is used in increasing amounts for gluconeogenesis and branch-chain amino acids are used in greater amounts as a direct energy source, especially for skeletal muscles. Concomitant with the increased nitrogen excretion, protein turnover is increased by up to 100% (74). Nitrogen balance may also be influenced by the type of protein delivered. Multiple studies demonstrate that branch-chain–enriched protein solutions increase the efficient utilization of protein (75–77). Daly et al. (77) demonstrated that forearm amino acid flux was significantly improved by the administration of solutions with 45% branch-chain amino acids compared to the more frequently used 25% branch-chain amino acids formulations (77). However, no improved outcomes have been demonstrated by administering branch-chain–enriched solutions and the nitrogen sparing effects can be duplicated by simply giving more of the standard, non–branch-chain–enriched protein solutions.

Nitrogen balance can be maximized by delivering nitrogen in proportion to the estimated energy requirements. In general, the more protein delivered, the less the effect of the amount of energy delivered. Nitrogen intake can be maximized by providing calorie/nitrogen ratios of approximately 100:1 for severely stressed patients and about 150:1 for noncritically stressed patients. In practice, this is usually equivalent to 2 to 3 g/kg/day of protein for most infants, 1.5 to 2 g/kg/day for most children, and 1 to 2 g/kg/day for adults. Repletion of protein stores in children following severe stress is generally similar to the provision of protein for growth.

Micronutrients are frequently abnormal in critically ill children. Electrolytes, especially sodium, potassium, magnesium, calcium, and phosphorus must be measured frequently and provided in individualized amounts. Disorders of these nutrients are common. Therefore, although routine amounts of these nutrients are delivered in parenteral nutrition, frequent monitoring and correction of demonstrated disorders may be necessary. Trace minerals have not been specifically studied in critically ill children. We deliver routine amounts of trace minerals in our parenteral nutrition solutions with frequent monitoring of their status.

COMPLICATIONS OF PARENTERAL NUTRITION IN CRITICALLY ILL CHILDREN

Adverse effects of parenteral nutrition in the critically ill child primarily involve the cardiorespiratory system. High glucose loads will increase carbon dioxide production, even when the respiratory quotient does not exceed 1.0 (66,78). Administration of parenteral nutrition to patients with major sepsis and trauma increased carbon dioxide production by 57%, oxygen consumption by 30%, and minute ventilation by 71%. Patients with mild to moderate injury had 121% increase in minute ventilation along with a 21% increase in oxygen consumption and a 53% increase in carbon dioxide production. These increased ventilatory requirements could result in respiratory failure, or difficulty in weaning from mechanical ventilation in patients with compromised respiratory function (79,80). Fat solutions used for about half of the calories will both ameliorate these effects, because of the lower respiratory quotient, and minimize the respiratory complications of high glucose loads for patients with compromised respiratory status (80–82).

SUMMARY

Although the techniques of nutritional delivery for critically ill patients are similar to those for routine care patients, the goals and objectives are different. Critically ill patients do not have a simple starvation physiology. Rather, they have metabolic profiles of hypermetabolism and proteolysis that exacerbate the loss of lean body mass. The controllers of this response are believed to be the same mediators responsible for the critical illness. Therefore, nutritional support can only be expected to ameliorate the effects of critical illness.

During the early phases of critical illness, the purpose of nutritional support is to minimize the negative nitrogen balance and attempt, as much as possible, to provide metabolic support for organ function. After the critical phase of illness, patients revert to more normal physiologies and can be managed along more traditional avenues of nutritional support.

REFERENCES

1. Cuthbertson DP. The disturbance of metabolism produced by long bony and non-bony injury, with notes on certain abnormal conditions of bone. *Biochem J* 1930;24:1244–1263.

2. Cuthbertson DP. Post-shock metabolic response. *Lancet* 1942;1:433–436.
3. Bessey PQ, Watters JM, Aoki TT, Wilmore DW. Combined hormonal infusion simulates the metabolic response to injury. *Ann Surg* 1984;200:264–280.
4. Baracos V, Rodemann HP, Dinarelli CA, et al. Stimulation of muscle degradation and prostaglandin E_2 release by leukocytic pyrogen (interleukin-1). *N Engl J Med* 1983;308:553–558.
5. Clowes GH, George BC, Villee CA Jr, et al. Muscle proteolysis induced by a circulating peptide in patients with sepsis or trauma. *N Engl J Med* 1983;308:545–552.
6. Mitchie HR, Manogue KR, Spriggs DR, et al. Detection of circulating tumor necrosis factor after endotoxin administration. *N Engl J Med* 1988;318:1481–1486.
7. Tracey KJ, Wei H, Manogue KR, et al. Cachectin/tumor necrosis factor induces cachexia, anemia, and inflammation. *J Exp Med* 1988;167:1211–1227.
8. Elwyn DE. Nutritional requirements of stressed patients. In: Shoemaker WC, Ayres S, Grenvik A, et al., eds. *Textbook of critical care,* 2nd ed. Philadelphia: WB Saunders, 1989;1085–1092.
9. Shamoon HR, Hendler R, Sherwin RS. Synergistic interaction among antiinsulin hormones in the pathogenesis of stress hyperglycemia in humans. *J Clin Endocrinol Metab* 1981;52:1235–1241.
10. Cerra FB. Nutrition in trauma, stress, and sepsis. In: Shoemaker WC, Ayres S, Grenvik A, et al., eds. *Textbook of critical care,* 2nd ed. Philadelphia: WB Saunders, 1989;1118–1125.
11. Pollack MM, Wiley JS, Holbrook PR. Early nutritional depletion in critically ill children. *Crit Care Med* 1981;9:580–583.
12. Pollack MM, Ruttimann UE, Wiley JS. Nutritional depletion in critically ill children: association with physiologic instability and increased quantity of care. *JPEN J Parenter Enteral Nutr* 1985;9:309–313.
13. Pollack MM, Wiley JS, Kanter R, et al. Malnutrition in critically ill infants and children. *JPEN J Parenter Enteral Nutr* 1982;6:20–24.
14. Tilden SJ, Watkins S, Tong TK, et al. Measured energy expenditure in pediatric intensive care patients. *Am J Dis Child* 1989;143:490–492.
15. Winthrop AL, Wesson DE, Pencharz PB, et al. Injury severity, whole body protein turnover, and energy expenditure in pediatric trauma. *J Pediatr Surg* 1987;22:534–537.
16. Chwals WJ, Lally KP, Woolley MM, et al. Measured energy expenditure in critically ill infants and young children. *J Surg Res* 1988;44:467–472.
17. Mickell JJ. Urea nitrogen excretion in critically ill children. *Pediatrics* 1982;70:949–955.
18. Field S, Kelly SM, Macklem PT. The oxygen cost of breathing in patients with cardiorespiratory disease. *Am Rev Respir Dis* 1982;126:9–13.
19. Stokes GM, Milner AD, Groggins RC. Work of breathing, intrathoracic pressure and clinical findings in a group of babies with bronchiolitis. *Acta Paediatr Scand* 1981;70:689–694.
20. Weissman C, Kemper M, Damask MC, et al. The effect of routine intensive care interactions on metabolic rate. *Chest* 1984;86:815–818.
21. Swinamer DL, Phang PT, Jones RJ, et al. Effect of routine administration of analgesia on energy expenditure in critically ill patients. *Chest* 1988;93:4–10.
22. Clifton GL, Robertson CS, Choi SC. Assessment of nutritional status of head-injured patients. *J Neurosurg* 1986;64:895–901.
23. Holiday MA. Metabolic rate and organ size during growth from infancy to maturity and during late gestation and early infancy. *Pediatrics* 1971;47:169–179.
24. Heird WC, Driscoll JM, Schullinger JN, et al. Intravenous alimentation in pediatric patients. *J Pediatr* 1972;80:351–372.
25. Pollack MM, Ruttimann UE, Getson PR, et al. Accurate prediction of pediatric intensive care outcome: a new quantitative method. *N Engl J Med* 1987;316:134–139.
26. Glass NL, Pollack MM, Ruttimann UE. Pediatric intensive care: who, why, and how much. *Crit Care Med* 1986;14:222–226.
27. Pollack MM, Wilkinson JD, Glass NL. Long-stay pediatric intensive care patients: outcome and resource utilization. *Pediatrics* 1987;80:855–860.
28. Steffee WP. Malnutrition in hospitalized patients. *JAMA* 1980;244:2630–2635.
29. Donowitz LG. High risk of nosocomial infection in the pediatric critical care patient. *Crit Care Med* 1986;14:26–28.
30. Ackerman AD. Conditions that predispose the critically ill child to infection. In: Rogers MC, ed. *Textbook of pediatric intensive care.* Baltimore: Williams and Wilkins, 1987;789–842.
31. Dionigi R, Gnes F, Bonera A, et al. Nutrition and infection. *JPEN J Parenter Enteral Nutr* 1979;3:62–68.
32. Suskind RM. *Malnutrition and the immune response.* New York: Raven Press, 1977.
33. Beisel WR, Edelman R, Nauss K, et al. Single-nutrient effects on immunologic functions. Report of a workshop sponsored by the Department of Food and Nutrition and its nutrition advisory group of the American Medical Association. *JAMA* 1981;245:53–58.
34. Jeejeebhoy KN. Nutrition in critical illness. In: Shoemaker WC, Ayres S, Grenvik A, et al., eds. *Textbook of critical care,* 2nd ed. Philadelphia: WB Saunders, 1989;1093–1118.
35. Meakins JL, Pietsch JB, Bubenick O, et al. Delayed hypersensitivity: indicator of acquired failure of host defenses in sepsis and trauma. *Ann Surg* 1977;186:241–250.
36. Arora NS, Rochester DF. Effects of general nutritional and muscular status on the human diaphragm. *Am Rev Respir Dis* 1977;115:84s.
37. Arora NS, Rochester DF. Effects of body weight and muscularity on human diaphragm muscle mass, thickness, and area. *J Appl Physiol* 1982;52:64–70.
38. Arora NS, Rochester DF. Respiratory muscle strength and maximal voluntary ventilation in undernourished patients. *Am Rev Respir Dis* 1982;126:5–8.
39. Dhingra S, Solven F, Wilson A, et al. Hypomagnesemia and respiratory muscle power. *Am Rev Respir Dis* 1984;129:497–498.
40. Agusti AGN, Torres A, Estopa R, et al. Hypophosphatemia as a cause of failed weaning: the importance of metabolic factors. *Crit Care Med* 1984;12:142–143.
41. Kelly SM, Rosa A, Field S, et al. Inspiratory muscle strength and body composition in patients receiving total parenteral nutrition therapy. *Am Rev Respir Dis* 1984;130:33–37.
42. Mansell AL, Andersen JC, Muttart CR, et al. Short-term pulmonary effects of total parenteral nutrition in children with cystic fibrosis. *J Pediatr* 1984;104:700–705.
43. Russell DM, Walker PM, Leiter LA, et al. Metabolic and structural changes in skeletal muscle during hypocaloric dieting. *Am J Clin Nutr* 1984;39:503–513.
44. Weissman C, Hyman AI. Nutritional care of the critically ill patient with respiratory failure. *Crit Care Clin* 1987;3:185–203.
45. D'Amours R, Clerh L, Massaro D. Food deprivation and surfactant in adult rats. *J Appl Physiol* 1983;55:1413–1417.
46. Gail DB, Massaro GD, Massaro D. Influence of fasting on the lung. *J Appl Physiol* 1977;42:88–92.
47. Askanazi J, Elwyn DH, Silverberg PA, et al. Patterns of ventilation in postoperative and acutely ill patients. *Crit Care Med* 1979;7:41–46.
48. Rosenbaum SH, Askanazi J, Hyman AI, et al. Respiratory patterns in profound nutritional depletion. *Anesthesiology* 1979;50(suppl):366 (abstract).
49. Doeckel RC Jr, Zwillich CW, Scopggin CH, et al. Clinical semistarvation: depression of hypoxic ventilatory response. *N Engl J Med* 1979;295:358–361.
50. Zwillich CW, Sahn SA, Weil JV. Effect of hypermetabolism upon respiratory gas exchange in normal man. *J Clin Invest* 1977;60:900–906.
51. Weissman C, Askanazi J, Rosenbaum S, et al. Amino acids and respiration. *Ann Intern Med* 1983;98:41–44.
52. Walesby RK, Goode AW, Spinks TJ, et al. Nutritional status of patients requiring cardiac surgery. *J Thorac Cardiovasc Surg* 1979;77:570–576.
53. Keyes A, Henschel A, Taylor HL. Size and function of the human heart at rest in semistarvation and in subsequent rehabilitation. *Am J Physiol* 1947;50:153–169.
54. Viart P. Hemodynamic findings in severe protein-calorie malnutrition. *Am J Clin Nutr* 1977;30:334–348.
55. Abel RM, Grimes JB, Alonso D, et al. Adverse hemodynamic and

ultrasonic changes in dog hearts subjected to protein-calorie malnutrition. *Am Heart J* 1979;97:733–744.
56. Alden PB, Madoff RD, Stahl TJ, et al. Ventricular dysfunction from malnutrition: a controlled prospective study in a canine model. *Crit Care Med* 1986;14:338 (abstract).
57. Abel RM, Paul J. Failure of short-term nutritional convalescence to reverse the adverse hemodynamic effects of protein-calorie malnutrition in dogs. *JPEN J Parenter Enteral Nutr* 1979;3:211–214.
58. Gottidiener JS, Gross HA, Henry WL, et al. Effects of self-induced starvation on cardiac size and function in anorexia nervosa. *Circulation* 1978;58:425–433.
59. Viart P. Blood volume (^{51}Cr) in severe protein-calorie malnutrition. *Am J Clin Nutr* 1976;29:25–37.
60. Suskind RM. Gastrointestinal changes in the malnourished child. *Pediatr Clin North Am* 1975;22:873–883.
61. Scott RL, Sohmer PR, MacDonald MG. The effect of starvation and repletion on plasma fibronectin in man. *JAMA* 1982;248:2025–2027.
62. Paniagua R, Santos D, Munoz R, et al. Renal function in protein-energy malnutrition. *Pediatr Res* 1980;14:1260–1262.
63. Cerra FB. Nutrition in the critically ill: modern metabolic support in the intensive care unit. In: Chernow B, Shoemaker WC, eds. *Critical care. State of the art.* Fullerton, CA: The Society of Critical Care Medicine, 1986;1–17.
64. Pollack MM. Nutritional failure and support in pediatric intensive care. In: Shoemaker WC, Ayres S, Grenvik A, et al., eds. *Textbook of critical care,* 2nd ed. Philadelphia: WB Saunders, 1989;1125–1128.
65. Weissman C, Kemper M, Askanazi J, et al. Resting metabolic rate of the critically ill patient: measured versus predicted. *Anesthesiology* 1986;64:673–679.
66. Askanazi J, Carpenter YA, Elwyn DH, et al. Influence of total parenteral nutrition on fuel utilization in injury and sepsis. *Ann Surg* 1980;191:40–46.
67. Roulet M, Detsky AS, Marliss EB, et al. A controlled trial of the effect of parenteral nutritional support on patients with respiratory failure. *Clin Nutr* 1983;2:97–101.
68. Baker JP, Detsky AS, Stewart S, et al. Randomized trial of total parenteral nutrition in critically ill patients: metabolic effects of varying glucose-lipid ratios as the energy source. *Gastroenterology* 1984;87:53–59.
69. Wene JD, Connor WE, DenBesten L. The development of essential fatty acid deficiency in healthy men fed fat free diets intravenously and orally. *J Clin Invest* 1975;56:127–134.
70. Liaw KY, Askanazi J, Michelsen CB, et al. Effect of postoperative nutrition on muscle high energy phosphates. *Ann Surg* 1988;200:340–344.
71. Nordenstrom J, Askanazi J, Elwyn DH, et al. Nitrogen balance during total parenteral nutrition, glucose versus fat. *Ann Surg* 1983;197:27–33.
72. Rubecz I, Mestyan J, Varga P, et al. Energy metabolism, substrate utilization, and nitrogen balance in parenterally fed postoperative neonates and infants. *J Pediatr* 1981;98:42–46.
73. Kinney JM, Elwyn DH. Protein metabolism and injury. *Am Rev Nutr* 1983;3:433–440.
74. Kien CL, Young VR, Rohrbaugh DK, et al. Increased rates of whole body protein synthesis and breakdown in children recovering from burns. *Ann Surg* 1978;187:383–391.
75. Bower RH, Kern KA, Fischer JE, et al. Use of branch-chain amino acid–enriched solutions in patients under metabolic stress. *Am J Surg* 1985;149:266–270.
76. Cerra FB, Mazuki JE, Chute E, et al. Branched chain metabolic support: a prospective, randomized, double-blind trial in surgical stress. *Ann Surg* 1984;199:286–291.
77. Daly JM, Mihranian MH, Kehoe JE, et al. Effects of postoperative infusion of branched chain amino acids on nitrogen balance and forearm muscle substrate flux. *Surgery* 1983;94:151–158.
78. Askanazi J, Rosenbaum SH, Hyman AI, et al. Respiratory distress secondary to high carbohydrate loads of total parenteral nutrition. *JAMA* 1980;243:1444–1447.
79. Askanazi J, Elwyn DH, Silverberg PA, et al. Respiratory distress secondary to a high carbohydrate load: a case report. *Surgery* 1980;87:596–598.
80. Covelli HD, Black JW, Olsen MW, et al. Respiratory failure precipitated by high carbohydrate loads. *Ann Intern Med* 1981;95:579–581.
81. Askanazi J, Nordenstrom J, Rosenbaum SH, et al. Nutrition for the patient with respiratory failure: glucose versus fat. *Anesthesiology* 1981;54:373–377.
82. Heymsfield SB, Head A, McManus CB, et al. Respiratory, cardiovascular, and metabolic effects of enteral hyperalimentation: Influence of formula, dose and composition. *Am J Clin Nutr* 1984;40:116–130.
83. Cerra FB. Metabolic support of the systemic septic response. In: Sibbald WJ, Sprung CL, eds. *Perspectives on sepsis and septic shock.* Fullerton, CA: Society of Critical Care Medicine, 1986;235–256.

CHAPTER 18

Energy and Protein Metabolism in the Pediatric Burn Patient

Hugo F. Carvajal

The morbidity and mortality associated with thermal injuries have significantly decreased in the past two decades. Aggressive nutritional support, by the enteral route, stands out as one of the most important contributing factors to this development (1). In addition to improving the nutritional status of patients, enteral nutrition restores cell-mediated immunity, promotes protein retention, and facilitates wound healing (2).

By maintaining the normal gastrointestinal barrier and thus preventing endotoxin and bacterial translocation from the GI tract, enteral feedings have also been associated with a decrease in the metabolic response to injury (3,4). Since the parenteral administration of nutrients in equivalent quantities has failed to prevent bacterial translocation, direct stimulation of the enterocyte appears to be a key factor in this response (5,6).

METABOLIC RESPONSE TO THERMAL INJURY

Burn injuries are among the most catastrophic of injuries. They are associated with the most severe alterations in body metabolism and neuroendocrine responses ever described for an illness or injury (Fig. 1). Without adequate nutritional support, the burn patient cannot avoid protein-energy malnutrition and significant immunologic deficits which, almost certainly, influence the prognosis.

Maximal physiologic responses have been demonstrated in humans and animals with 50% burn (7). Heat losses by convection, conduction, or radiation, and water losses by evaporation, however, are not limited to the 50% burn ceiling. Instead, these losses remain proportional to burn size and depth (from 0% to 100%) and contribute to increased nutritional demands.

The time course for these posttraumatic responses was first described by Cuthbertson (8) in 1932. Two distinct time periods were identified: an early "ebb" phase and a subsequent "flow" phase.

The Ebb Phase

The ebb phase is short; it lasts hours, or, at most, a couple of days. First, the brain receives a sensory signal that tissue injury has occurred. This effects a release of corticotropin (ACTH) and antidiuretic hormone (ADH) by the hypothalamus, in response to pain, fear, hypoxia, or hypovolemia. This phase is dominated by α-adrenergic receptor stimulation and catecholamine secretion, and is characterized by redistribution of blood from the skin to vital organs (9). Plasma cortisol, aldosterone, and growth hormone levels become markedly elevated and insulin secretion is curtailed. Hyperglycemia results from (a) increased sympathetic activity; (b) secretion of epinephrine, with a consequent inhibition of insulin release; (c) insulin resistance; and (d) increased gluconeogenesis and glycogenolysis secondary to cortisol and glucagon secretion (10,11).

In contrast to adults, pediatric patients, particularly infants, have difficulty maintaining glucose homeostasis. During the immediate postburn period, children are predisposed to hypoglycemia, rather than hyperglycemia, because of higher basal energy expenditure, increased heat loss from high surface area to weight ratios, and limited glycogen stores (11,12).

Soon after the burn, ADH is secreted, and a state of antidiuresis develops. This may persist beyond restoration of plasma volume (13). Aldosterone secretion pro-

---

H. F. Carvajal: Division of Pediatric Critical Care Unit, Humana Women's and Children's Hospital, San Antonio, Texas 78229.

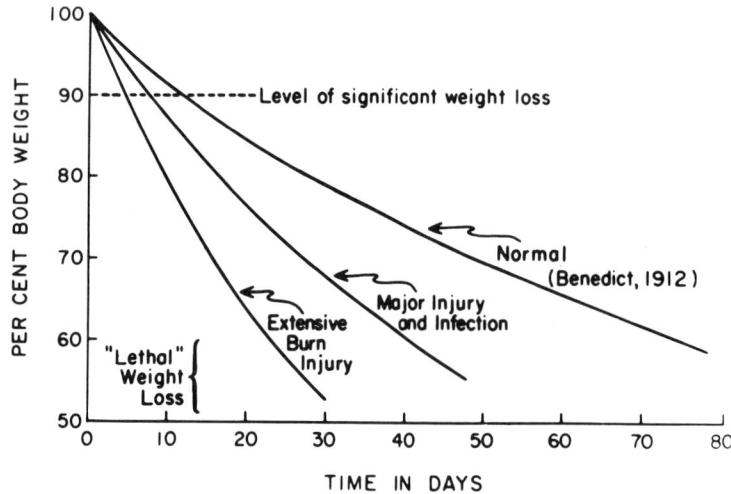

FIG. 1. Extensive burn injury accelerates weight loss and requires vigorous nutritional support. Reproduced from ref. 45, with permission.

motes sodium retention and potassium excretion. The cumulative effect of these two hormones leads to significant oliguria (even after intravascular volume is restored) and edema formation, secondary to salt and water retention (9).

An increase in vascular permeability, which becomes evident during the first 15 to 30 min after the injury, persists for 8 to 12 hr (14), and leads to extravasation of fluid into the interstitial compartment. A dramatic decrease in intravascular volume ensues and edema and hypoperfusion of peripheral tissues takes place.

Soon after the burn, cardiac output falls (15) and, despite adequate volume replacement, remains at levels below normal (16). Increased sympathetic discharges are thought to mediate this response (17), but the exact mechanism remains to be elucidated.

Thus, during the immediate postburn period, the endocrine system orchestrates several physiologic and biochemical changes designed to benefit the host. Salt and water conservation takes place in order to support the circulation and improve tissue perfusion. Hepatic glucose production is enhanced to provide the fuel necessary for vital organ function, white and red cell metabolism, and wound healing. Skeletal muscle proteolysis provides the amino acid precursors for gluconeogenesis and hepatic protein synthesis. Finally, epinephrine, glucagon, and growth hormone promote lipolysis and make abundant quantities of free fatty acids available for utilization as the principal sources of energy.

The Flow Phase

The flow phase usually begins at 24 hr postinjury; it lasts several days and is characterized by hypermetabolism, increased cardiac output, and increased oxygen consumption. Accelerated tissue catabolism, increased urinary nitrogen losses, and altered glucose metabolism are also invariably present. The degrees of hypermetabolism correlates with the extent of the injury (7).

Burn patients also develop a 1°C to 2°C elevation in body temperature. This resetting of the body's internal "thermostat" is not associated with any symptomatology (7,18).

After the first 24 hr, and assuming adequate volume replacement, the cardiac index increases to levels as high as 6 to 8 l/m^2 of body surface. This is a compensatory response to increased oxygen demands that may also be associated with increased O_2 extraction by the tissues. However, in some cases, the utilization of oxygen by injured tissues is impaired and a dissociation between flow and O_2 extraction may occur (7). The increased blood flow is directed to the surface rather than to deep underlying tissues (18). Either a metabolic block for O_2 utilization occurs or the increased flow is directed to supporting regenerative processes in the wound that do not require oxygen (7). Splanchnic blow flow is also increased, but in proportion to O_2 utilization.

The heat produced in the burn patient is derived from fat oxidation and the major portion of heat produced is the result of biochemical inefficiency (11). Heat production, however, appears to be distributed in a normal fashion, i.e., two-thirds produced in visceral tissues and one-third in the extremities.

Although energy demands may be augmented by the increased work of breathing and tachycardia, most of the energy is utilized for synthetic and reparative processes. These include gluconeogenesis, erythropoiesis, leukocyte production, and synthesis of acute-phase reactants and other proteins, particularly albumin (12).

To facilitate wound healing, the skin temperature is raised. This increased heat production imposes a metabolic cost on the patient, further contributing to tissue catabolism and disruption of body mass.

The increased metabolic rate that follows trauma can be aggravated by cold exposure, pain, anxiety, and other treatment-related factors, as well as various complications, including associated infections.

Insulin concentrations may return to normal during

the flow phase but hyperglycemia usually persists. This is, in part, related to increased gluconeogenesis promoted by cortisol secretion (12). The liver does not appear to be the only, or even the central, organ for gluconeogenesis to take place. Instead, the gut (enterocyte) is transformed from an organ of glucose utilization to one of primary glucose release (19) and it interacts with the liver in the synthesis of new glucose. Glutamine (instead of glucose) becomes the alternate fuel for the enterocyte (20,21) and the three carbon compounds produced are reused by the liver to form new glucose. The release of alanine by the gut is enhanced, and it also becomes a key gluconeogenic precursor.

Although fat represents the primary fuel for resting skeletal muscle, the injured tissues and certain specialized cells of the wound (fibroblasts, macrophages, and leukocytes) continue to metabolize glucose anaerobically and develop a large capacity for lactate production. The latter is then recycled in the Cori cycle. Most of the available glucose is utilized by the wound. Glucose utilization by the CNS does not appear to be increased, and the resting muscle and nonburned skin use only a minimum of this fuel during injury (18).

It is interesting that, during injury, gluconeogenesis, glycogenolysis, and lipolysis are relatively resistant to suppression by glucose infusions (22). This is probably related to glucocorticoid and epinephrine secretion, the key hormones during the flow phase. Through stimulation of mitochondrial glutaminase activity (23,24), glucocorticoids promote the use of glutamate as a source of energy by the enterocyte.

In addition to the various alterations in protein and amino acid metabolism discussed above, a generalized breakdown of muscle protein is also present. This occurs in both the burned and unburned extremities and leads to progressive wasting of skeletal muscle mass.

Amino acids (AA) are released from muscle in high quantities, but the composition of AA efflux does not reflect the composition of muscle protein. Alanine and glutamine constitute 50% to 60% of the amino acids released but neither one makes up more than 6% of muscle protein. Likewise, the branch-chain AA, which represent 15% of the muscle protein, comprise only 6% of the released amino acids. Alanine and glutamine are believed to function as amino donors for α-ketoglutarate, yielding the corresponding branch-chain ketoacid and glutamate. α-Ketoglutarate can be converted in muscle to Krebs cycle intermediates, and glutamate can be used in the synthesis of glutamine or alanine. These two compounds appear to be the most important, if not most essential, means of nitrogen transfer from muscle to viscera.

During stress, fat is the primary nutrient. When fat stores are depleted, protein becomes the secondary fuel. Although fat supplementation is essential in order to curtail visceral protein metabolism, the best way to accomplish this remains a source of controversy. Alterations in triglyceride, cholesterol, carnitine, fatty acids, lipoprotein, and prostaglandin have been reported in burn patients (25). Because polyunsaturated fatty acids (PUFA) of the ω-6 variety (linoleic acid) in high concentrations have been shown to be immunosuppressants and, since glucose is a more effective energy source than fat, the current trend is to use high carbohydrate loads with low levels of fat, particularly ω-6 PUFA (3,26,27).

NUTRITIONAL REQUIREMENTS

Burn injury patients in the United States are often well nourished before the insult. Despite this, the increased energy demands of a severe burn are such that unless an aggressive nutritional program can be promptly implemented, protein-energy malnutrition is bound to occur.

The total energy requirement of the burn patient represents the sum of several contributing factors, including the basal metabolic rate (BMR), the specific dynamic action (SDA) of ingested food substances, the energy necessary for a specific level of activity, and the requirements of the burn injury itself (11).

ESTIMATION OF CALORIC REQUIREMENTS

Several methods have been recommended to estimate caloric requirements in burn patients (2,3,24–29). Extrapolation from adults to children has also been attempted, but for the most part these formulas result in considerable error (27).

Measurement of actual needs by direct or indirect calorimetry is fraught with considerable difficulties (30–32). Despite monumental efforts, currently available equipment and methodology do not permit accurate measurement of calorie expenditure in the unintubated patient (33–39).

Maintenance caloric needs can be calculated from recommended dietary allowance (RDA) tables from the Food and Nutrition Board of the National Research Council (40) or they can be approximated by using the body surface area formula as follows:

Maintenance caloric requirements =

1,800 kilocalories(Cal)/m_2/day.

Hildreth and Carvajal (31) used total body surface area and burned surface to estimate optimal caloric intake.

Burn caloric requirements =

2,200 Cal/m^2 of body surface burned/24 hr.

Body surface burned is calculated by multiplying the patient's body surface area (BSA) in square meters by the percent burned divided by 100. For example, for a 2-year-old child of 0.5 m^2 BSA with a 40% burn:

$$\text{Body surface burned} = \frac{0.5 \text{ m}^2 \times 40}{100} = 0.2 \text{ m}^2.$$

The use of the above formula in 53 acutely burned children resulted in weight gain, decreased morbidity and mortality, and a shortened hospital stay. Patients who gained weight ($N = 40$), had an average burn of $35\% \pm 2\%$, and a mean age of 6 ± 1 years. These patients were presumed to have received adequate nutrition with a daily caloric intake exceeding that recommended by the surface area formula. The average weight gain varied from 1% to 6% depending on the time of discharge. The longer the patients remained in the hospital, the more weight they gained.

Patients who lost weight ($N = 12$) were older (mean age 9 ± 1 year), had larger burns (mean burn $47\% \pm 5\%$), and their daily caloric intake was less than recommended by the formula. These patients were also subjected to an increased number of surgical procedures.

It is still uncertain whether "optimal" caloric intake, as recommended by the formula, would have induced weight gain in the latter group of patients. Because of their larger body surface and body surface burned, these patients presumably required a higher caloric intake. The authors assume that failure to gain weight was probably due to an inability to meet the daily caloric needs, which, in most cases, was due to

1. fluid intake limitations (fluid restriction)
2. decreased enteral intake resulting from frequent surgical procedures
3. complications such as diarrhea, vomiting, or septicemia, which temporarily precluded the use of the enteral route and limited caloric intake.

DETERMINATION OF PROTEIN REQUIREMENTS

In 1980, Alexander et al. (2) reported that, in burned children, a high-protein diet was associated with improved survival and fewer episodes of sepsis. Higher serum levels of total protein, transferrin, C-3, and immunoglobulin G (IgG) were also observed. Although this study and others favor the use of high-protein diets, an animal study done by Dominioni et al. (41) suggests that certain limits should not be surpassed. In this study, protein concentrations of greater than 40% of the calories resulted in increased liver fat deposition, diarrhea, and decreased survival.

Our current recommendation is that 18% of the calories be derived from protein, although values as high as 25% may generally be considered safe. In fact, Alexander et al. (2) recently proposed the use of a high-protein, low-fat, high-carbohydrate formula for pediatric burn patients. This formulation, the Shriners' burn diet, provides 20% of the calories as whey protein, 2% as arginine, 0.5% as histidine, and 0.5% as cysteine. The diet also provides 15% of the nonprotein calories as fat (half from fish oil and half by a linoleic acid–rich source) and 85% as carbohydrate (3). Prospective studies are underway to determine its effectiveness in pediatric burn cases.

VITAMIN AND MINERAL REQUIREMENTS

Dietary allowances for vitamins and minerals have been established for healthy people in the United States (Table 1) (40). Thiamine, riboflavin, niacin, and vitamin B_6, components of essential enzymes and coenzymes, are needed to metabolize carbohydrate, fat, and protein. As energy requirements increase, requirements for these vitamins also increase. Deficiencies in vitamins A and D, ascorbic acid, thiamine, riboflavin, pyridoxine, niacin, pantothenic acid, and folic acid are associated with reduced host resistance to infection. Vitamin A is important for wound healing (18,27), and ascorbic acid is needed for collagen synthesis.

While specific vitamin deficiencies have been demonstrated in burned patients, adverse effects have also been reported when excessive amounts of fat or water soluble vitamins have been added to the diet. It is, therefore, important to exercise caution when contemplating vitamin supplementation.

Minerals essential to human nutrition may be classified as: a) those present in large quantities (sodium, potassium, calcium, magnesium, and phosphorous) b) those present in trace amounts (iron, zinc, copper, iodine, selenium, fluoride, manganese, and chromium).

In burn patients, sodium and potassium requirements are proportional to the extent and depth of the burn, the metabolic response, water requirements, and heart and kidney function. Concentrations of sodium and potassium of 50 and 30 mEq/l of parenteral and enteral fluids, respectively, are optimal in patients with normal cardiovascular and kidney function. Sodium and potassium requirements increase as the losses of these ions are enhanced in the form of burn exudate, excessive diuresis, or even the inappropriate secretion of antidiuretic hormone.

We currently recommend that sodium be supplemented so that all fluids the patient receives contain a total of 50mEq/l (13). Potassium supplementation must also be undertaken to prevent the development of hypokalemia, paralytic ileus, and feeding intolerance.

Hypophosphatemia is a common and serious complication of major trauma, burns, and other conditions that are associated with massive diuresis (diabetes mellitus, diabetes insipidus), total parenteral nutrition (TPN), increased metabolic requirements, acid base imbalance, etc. The consequences of severe hypophosphatemia include red blood cell dysfunction, leukocyte dysfunction, CNS dysfunction, and rhabdomyolysis (39,40). If the

TABLE 1. *Recommended dietary allowances: designed for the maintenance of good nutrition of practically all healthy people in the United States*

	Age, yr	Minerals					
		Calcium, mg	Phosphorus, mg	Magnesium, mg	Iron, mg	Zinc, mg	Iodine, μg
Infants	0.0–≤0.5	360	240	50	10	3	40
	0.5–1.0	540	360	70	15	5	50
Children	1–3	800	800	150	15	10	70
	4–6	800	800	200	10	10	90
	7–10	800	800	250	10	10	120
Males	11–14	1,200	1,200	350	18	15	150
	15–18	1,200	1,200	400	18	15	150
Females	11–14	1,200	1,200	300	18	15	150
	15–18	1,200	1,200	300	18	15	150

	Age, yr	Fat-soluble vitamins			Water-soluble vitamins						
		Vitamin A, μg RE[a]	Vitamin D, μg[b]	Vitamin E, mg α-TE[c]	Vitamin C, mg	Thiamine, mg	Riboflavin, mg	Niacin, mg NE[d]	Vitamin B_6, mg	Folacin, μg[e]	Vitamin B_{12}, μg[f]
Infants	0.0–≤0.5	420	10	3	35	0.3	0.4	6	0.3	30	0.5
	0.5–1.0	400	10	4	35	0.5	0.6	8	0.6	45	1.5
Children	1–3	400	10	5	45	0.7	0.8	9	0.9	100	2.0
	4–6	500	10	6	45	0.9	1.0	11	1.3	200	2.5
	7–10	700	10	7	45	1.2	1.4	16	1.6	300	3.0
Males	11–14	1,000	10	8	50	1.4	1.6	18	1.8	400	3.0
	15–18	1,000	10	10	60	1.4	1.7	18	2.0	400	3.0
Females	11–14	800	10	8	50	1.1	1.3	15	1.8	400	3.0
	15–18	800	10	8	60	1.1	1.3	14	2.0	400	3.0

Adapted from ref. 40.
[a] RE indicates retinol equivalents. 1 retinol equivalent = 1 μg retinol or 6 μg β-carotene.
[b] Vitamin D as cholecalciferol. 10 μg cholecalciferol = 400 International Units (IU) of vitamin D.
[c] α-TE indicates α-tocopherol equivalents. 1 mg/day of α-tocopherol = 1 α-TE.
[d] NE indicates 1 NE (niacin equivalent) is equal to 1 mg of niacin or 60 mg of dietary tryptophan.
[e] Folacin indicates allowances for dietary sources as determined by *Lactobacillus casei* assay after treatment with enzymes (conjugates) to make polyglutamyl forms of the vitamin available to the test organism.
[f] The recommended dietary allowances for vitamin B_{12} in infants are based on average concentration of the vitamin in human milk. The allowances after weaning are based on energy intake (as recommended by the American Academy of Pediatrics) and consideration of other factors, such as intestinal absorption.

condition is recognized early, oral supplementation with one of the commercially available phosphorous preparations usually suffices to restore sodium homeostasis. Otherwise parenteral therapy may be needed.

Zinc deficiencies have been associated with impaired cellular immunity, poor wound healing, impaired protein synthesis, anorexia, and altered taste and smell. Increased zinc requirements have been reported in burn patients, but no controlled studies to date have documented direct benefits from zinc supplementation (11).

Without more evidence, vitamin and mineral supplements for burned children should not exceed established guidelines for healthy individuals, unless a deficiency is documented.

DELIVERY TECHNIQUES AND AVAILABLE DIETS

Optimal resuscitation of pediatric burn patients almost always can be accomplished with colloid-containing solutions, a surface area formula, and a program that imposes limits on fluid intake, minimizing edema formation and organ failure (13). By following such a procedure, total serum protein and albumin levels are maintained within narrow ranges and enteral feedings can be tolerated earlier (13). Patients who are breathing spontaneously, with no evidence of smoke inhalation or organ failure, may generally be offered enteral feedings 24 hr postinjury. Milk, or an appropriate infant formula, may be offered by mouth or nasogastric tube, its quantity progressively increased as parenteral fluids are proportionally decreased. The second day is a transitional period, during which tolerance to feedings, and the capacity of the GI tract to absorb nutrients, is determined. From the third day, the enteral route is used almost exclusively to provide fluids, minerals, and nutrients; sodium and potassium supplementation is begun, and maintained at fixed levels thereafter.

Although caloric intake is a primary consideration, every effort is made to provide isotonic formulas that are lactose-free and have a caloric density less than 27 Cal/oz. In general, 75% of the calories needed can be provided by means of liquid diets and 25% by solid food.

To minimize the risk of vomiting, aspiration, and/or diarrhea, fluids are given by continuous intragastric infusion. For patients who are intubated, comatose, or septic, nasoduodenal feedings, via a Dubhoff catheter, are used instead. A standard high-calorie, high-protein diet is first offered on day 3. By day 5 or 6 the patients are consuming adequate calories via solid foods.

An important consideration is the weekly "mapping" of the wounds in order to recalculate actual fluid and caloric requirements and minimize the problems of overfeeding and excessive sodium and potassium supplementation.

ALBUMIN REPLACEMENT

Despite adequate caloric intake, hypoalbuminemia, secondary to protein losses in burn exudate, continues to recur. This usually persists until the burn wound is less than 20% of the body surface and hepatic protein synthesis is restored. Until then, albumin supplementation is necessary to prevent hypoalbuminemia and its consequences. In most cases, 100 to 150 g of albumin per square meter burned per week is needed to maintain the serum albumin levels above 2.5 g/dl, the colloidosmotic pressure above 15 mm Hg, and to prevent the development of secondary hyperaldosteronism. Albumin may be administered intravenously as a 5% solution in 0.33 normal saline solution over 4–6 hr. In most cases repeat doses must be given every other day.

Although other visceral proteins, such as transferrin, retinol-binding protein, and thyroxin-binding prealbumin, have a shorter half-life than albumin and, thus, are preferred for monitoring nutritional status, a patient who is able to tolerate enteral feedings well and maintain weight, adequate electrolyte, protein, and acid base balance is, in most cases, adequately nourished.

Every effort should be made to minimize energy demands by reducing external stresses (pain, anxiety, fear, and reduced body temperature) that stimulate the release of catecholamines and raise energy requirements. Use of narcotics and sedatives should be balanced to ensure the comfort of the patient, while avoiding undue sedation. Hypothermia should be prevented through heating devices as well as regulation of the environmental temperature. This is particularly important during procedures such as hydrotherapy, debridement and grafting, and dressing changes.

REFERENCES

1. Carvajal HF, Parks DH. Survival statistics in burned children. *J Trauma* 1981;21:221–227.
2. Alexander JW, MacMillan BG, Stinnett JC, et al. Beneficial effects of aggressive protein feeding in severely burned children. *Ann Surg* 1980;192:505.
3. Alexander JW, Gottschlich RD. Nutritional immunomodulations in burned patients. *Crit Care Med* 1990;18:S149–S153.
4. Alverdy JC. The GI tract as an immunologic organ. *Contemp Surg* 1990;35:14–19.
5. Alverdy JC, Aoys E, Moss GS. Total parenteral nutrition promotes bacterial translocation from the gut. *Surgery* 1988;104:185–190.
6. Alverdy JC, Chi HS, Sheldon GF. The effects of parenteral nutrition on gastrointestinal immunity. The importance of enteral stimulation. *Ann Surg* 1985;202:681–684.
7. Aulick LH, Wilmore DW. Hypermetabolism in trauma. In: Girardies L, Stock MJ, eds. *Mammalian thermogenesis.* London: Chapman and Hall, 1983;259–304.
8. Cuthbertson DP. Observations on the disturbance of metabolism produced by injury to the limbs. *Q J Med* 1932;25:233–246.
9. Arturson G. Metabolic changes and nutrition in children with severe burns. *Prog Pediatr Surg* 1981;14:81–109.
10. Wilmore DW, Mason AD Jr, Pruitt BA Jr. Insulin response to glucose in hypermetabolic burn patients. *Ann Surg* 1976;183:314.
11. Souba WW, Schindler BA, Carvajal HF. Nutrition and metabolism. In: Carvajal HF, Parks DH, eds. *Burns in children.* Chicago: Yearbook Medical Publishers, 1988;119–144.
12. Weise K, Saritsky A. Endocrine manifestations of critical illness in the child. *Pediatr Clin North Am* 1987;34:119–127.
13. Carvajal HF. A physiologic approach to fluid therapy in severely burned children. *Surg Gynecol Obstet* 1980;150:379–384.
14. Carvajal HF, Linares HA, Brouhard BH. Relationship of burn size to vascular permeability changes in rats. *Surg Gynecol Obstet* 1979;149:193–202.
15. Carvajal HF, Reinhard JA, Traber DL. Renal and cardiovascular functional response to thermal injury in dogs subjected to sympathetic blockade. *Circ Shock* 1976;3:287–298.
16. Carvajal HF, Parks DH. The optimal composition of burn resuscitation fluids. *Crit Care Med* 1988;16:695–699.
17. Turner R, Carvajal HF, Traber DL. Effects of ganglionic blockade upon renal and cardiovascular dysfunction induced by thermal injury. *Circ Shock* 1977;4:103–113.
18. Wilmore DW, Aulick LH, Mason AD Jr, et al. The influence of the burn wound on local and systemic responses to injury. *Ann Surg* 1977;186:444.
19. Souba WW, Wilmore DW. Gut-liver interaction during accelerated gluconeogenesis. *Arch Surg* 1985;120:66–70.
20. Souba WW, Smith RJ, Wilmore DW. Glutamine metabolism by the intestinal tract. *JPEN J Parenter Enteral Nutr* 1985;9:608–617.
21. Windwelles HG. Glutamine utilization by the small intestine. *Adv Enzymol* 1982;53:201–237.
22. Wolfe RR, Goodenough RD, Burke JF, et al. Response of protein and urea kinetics in burned patients to different levels of protein intake. *Ann Surg* 1983;197:163–171.
23. Souba WW, Smith RJ, Wilmore DW. Effects of glucocorticoids on glutamine metabolism in visceral organs. *Metabolism* 1985;34:450–456.
24. Fox AD, Kripke SA, Berman JM, et al. Dexamethasone administration induces increased glutaminase specific activity in the jejunum and colon. *J Surg Res* 1988;44:391–396.
25. Gottschlick MM, Alexander JW. Fat kinetics and recommended dietary intake in burns. *JPEN J Parenter Enteral Nutr* 1987;11:80–85.
26. Alexander JW. Nutrition and infection. New perspectives for an old problem. *Arch Surg* 1986;121:966–972.
27. Andrassy RJ. Practical rewards of enteral feeding for the surgical patient. *Contemp Surg* 1989;35:20–24.
28. Curreri PW. Nutritional replacement modalities. *J Trauma* 1979;19(suppl 11):906–908.
29. Pleban WE. Nutritional support of burned patients: Bridgeport Hospital Burn Unit. *Conn Med* 1979;43:767–768.
30. Sutherland AB, Batchelor ADR. Nitrogen balance in burned children. *Ann NY Acad Sci* 1969;150:700–710.
31. Hildreth M, Carvajal HF. Caloric requirements in burned children. A simple formula to estimate daily requirements. *J Burn Care Rehabil* 1980;3:78–80.
32. Bartlett RH, Allyn PA, Medley T, et al. Nutritional therapy based on positive caloric balance in burned patients. *Arch Surg* 1977;112:974–980.

33. Ireton CS, Turner WW, Hunts JL, et al. Evaluation of energy expenditures in burn patients. *JADA* 1986;86:331–333.
34. Weissman C, Damas MC, Askanazi J, et al. Evaluation of a noninvasive method for the measurement of metabolic rate in human. *Clin Sci* 1985;69:135–141.
35. Daly JM, Heymsfield SB, Head A, et al. Human energy requirements: overstimulation by widely used prediction equation. *Am J Nutr* 1985;42:1170–1174.
36. Westenskow DR, Cutler C, Wallace WD. Instrumentation for monitoring gas exchange and metabolic rate in critically ill patients. *Crit Care Med* 1984;12:183–187.
37. Mann S, Westenskow DR, Houtchens BA. Measured and predicted caloric expenditure in the acutely ill. *Crit Care Med* 1985;13:173–177.
38. Chwals WH, Lally KP, Woolley MM, et al. Measured energy expenditure in critically ill infants and young children. *J Surg Res* 1988;44:467–472.
39. Elia M, Livesey C. Theory and validity of indirect colorimetry during net lipid synthesis. *Am J Clin Nutr* 1988;47:591–607.
40. Committee on Dietary Allowances. *Recommended dietary allowances,* 9th ed. Washington, DC: National Academy of Science, 1980.
41. Dominioni L, Orrawin T, Cheng-Hui F, et al. Enteral feeding in burn hypermetabolism: nutritional and metabolic effects of different levels of caloric and protein intake. *JPEN J Parenter Enteral Nutr* 1985;9:269–279.
42. Stratford F, Seiffer E, Rettina G, et al. Impaired wound healing due to cyclophosphamide alleviated by supplemental vitamin A. *Surg Forum* 1980;31:224–225.
43. Prockop DJ, Guzman NA. Collagen diseases and biosynthesis of collagen. *Hosp Pract* 1977;12:61–68.
44. Knochel JP. The pathophysiology and clinical characteristics of severe hypophosphatemia. *Arch Intern Med* 1977;137:203–220.
45. Souba WW, Bessey PQ. Nutritional support of the trauma patient. *Infect Surg* 1984;3:727–736.

CHAPTER 19

Parenteral Support of the Hospitalized Child

William C. Heird

The first successful clinical use of modern parenteral nutrition was reported by Wilmore and Dudrick (1) in 1968. The patient, an infant with virtually no remaining small intestine, grew and developed normally for several months while receiving only parenterally delivered nutrients. Since this dramatic demonstration, parenteral nutrition has been used widely in a variety of pediatric patients. Initially, it was used almost exclusively in treatment of infants requiring multiple operative procedures for correction of congenital or acquired lesions of the gastrointestinal tract (2) and in infants and children with intractable diarrhea (3). In these patients, who usually cannot be fed for weeks to months, the ability to maintain or improve nutritional status has played a major role in reversing previously low survival rates to the high survival rates characteristic of these conditions today (4). The efficacy of parenteral nutrition in these groups of patients, in fact, led to its use in any patient with obvious intolerance of enterally delivered nutrient regimens.

Today, low birth weight (LBW) infants (i.e., infants weighing less than 2,500 g at birth) account for the largest percentage of pediatric patients receiving parenteral nutrition. Approximately 7% of all infants born in the United States are in this category. Of these, approximately 15%, or about 1% of all infants, weigh less than 1,500 g at birth. Many of the total population and virtually all of the latter group cannot tolerate more than very small amounts of enterally delivered nutrients during the early days or weeks of life. Moreover, because of their limited endogenous nutrient stores and a relatively high rate of ongoing energy expenditure (5), these infants are at great risk for developing malnutrition or actual starvation during the early neonatal period. For example, the endogenous stores of the 1,000-g infant are probably sufficient to support survival without exogenous nutrients for only about 5 days (6). For these reasons, virtually all infants who weigh less than 1,500 g at birth and many larger LBW infants receive some or all of their total nutrient intake during the early days to weeks of life by the parenteral route.

Despite the widespread use of parenterally delivered nutrients in pediatric patients, the expectations of the therapy often are either over- or underrated. This is particularly true if the many problems associated with this therapy are ignored, resulting in inappropriate use of parenteral nutrition in patients who can tolerate enterally delivered nutrients or, if these problems are exaggerated, resulting in failure to provide parenteral nutrition to patients for whom it is indicated. These misinterpretations may well result from the many aspects of the technique that remain poorly understood.

In this chapter, many of the intricacies and expectations of parenteral nutrition, as viewed by the author, are discussed and the techniques of parenteral nutrition developed and followed reasonably successfully for the past 20 years at the Babies Hospital in New York are described. In addition, some of the unsolved and potential problems related to parenteral nutrition are reviewed. An understanding of these problems is an important first step toward enhancing the efficacy of what is undoubtedly one of the most important medical advances of recent years.

TECHNIQUES OF PARENTERAL NUTRITION

Parenteral nutrition therapy (1,7) entails infusion of a hypertonic nutrient solution at a constant rate into a vessel with rapid flow. This usually is accomplished by placing an indwelling catheter in the superior vena cava with the tip of the catheter just above the right atrium. The catheter frequently is inserted through a surgical cutdown into either the internal or external jugular vein. This route is preferable in the young infant, but in older

---

W. C. Heird: Department of Pediatrics, Baylor College of Medicine, Children's Nutrition Research Center USDA/ARS, Houston, Texas 77030.

children and adolescents the catheter may be placed percutaneously through the subclavian vein. Regardless of the route of placement, the proximal portion of the catheter usually is tunneled subcutaneously to exit some distance from the site of insertion, usually at the anterior chest. The channeling of the catheter to an exit site distant from the phlebotomy site and the application of an occlusive dressing over the exit site help protect the catheter from both inadvertent dislodgment and contamination by microorganisms.

The inferior vena cava also is a large vessel with rapid flow; hence, catheters placed in this vessel with the tip just below the right atrium should be equally effective. However, since introduction of a catheter through a cutdown in the groin area may increase the risk of infection, inferior vena cava catheters are less popular than superior vena cava catheters. Although some argue that such catheters, if tunneled subcutaneously to an exit site on the abdominal wall or the thigh, represent no greater risk with respect to infection than the usual superior vena cava catheters (8), firm data substantiating this argument are not available.

Silastic rather than polyvinyl catheters are preferred. This is because the latter, once in place, have a tendency to become very rigid. Currently, silastic catheters with a polyvinyl cuff on the portion that is tunneled subcutaneously are quite popular. The cuff promotes fibroblast proliferation which, in turn, helps secure the catheter. Such catheters are mandatory for successful home parenteral nutrition and, in many centers, they are used almost exclusively for in-hospital parenteral nutrition. Their major disadvantage is that they must be removed surgically.

Since reducing the complications of central vein delivery of concentrated nutrient mixtures requires considerable effort and expense, many advocate infusion of parenteral nutrition regimens by peripheral vein. However, unless fluid intake is excessive, the amount of nutrients that can be delivered by peripheral vein is limited. More liberal use of parenteral lipid emulsions helps compensate for the limited energy intake. Nonetheless, if fluid intake is limited to a total volume of 150 ml/kg/day, glucose concentration of the infusate is limited to 10% and intravenous lipid intake is limited to 3 g/kg/day, the maximum energy intake that can be delivered by peripheral vein is approximately 80 kilocalories (Cal)/kg/day (6). Although the growth achievable with such an intake and the duration that such intakes can be maintained are less than with conventional central vein parenteral nutrition regimens, there are a number of patients for whom such regimens may be preferable.

COMPOSITION OF NUTRIENT INFUSATE

The parenteral nutrition infusate, whether delivered by central or peripheral vein, must include a nitrogen source as well as adequate energy, electrolytes, minerals, and vitamins (Table 1).

Nitrogen Source

Several crystalline amino acid mixtures are available for use as the nitrogen source of parenteral nutrition regimens (Table 2). The amount of amino acids provided usually ranges from 2 to 4 g/kg/day. According to Zlotkin et al. (9), the parenteral amino acid intake required to assure a rate of nitrogen accretion equal to the intrauterine rate (i.e., ~300 mg/kg/day) is approximately 3 g/kg/day. This amino acid intake with an energy intake of 80 Cal/kg/day results in a rate of weight gain approximating the intrauterine rate (i.e., approximately 15 g/kg/day). Greater amino acid and energy intakes, of course, will support even higher rates of nitrogen retention and weight gain.

Anderson et al. (10) found that LBW infants receiving

TABLE 1. *Composition of nutrient infusates suitable for central vein and peripheral vein infusion*

Component	Central vein (amount/kg/day)	Peripheral vein (amount/kg/day)
Crystalline amino acids (g)	3–4	2.5–3.0
Glucose (g)	20–30	15
Lipid emulsion (g)	0.5–3.0	0.5–3.0
Sodium (mEq)	3–4	3–4
Potassium[a] (mEq)	2–4	2–4
Calcium (mg)	40–60	40–60
Magnesium (mEq)	0.25	0.25
Chloride (mEq)	3–4	3–4
Phosphorus[a] (mmol)	~1.5	1.5
Zinc (μg)	200	200–400
Copper (μg)	20	
Iron[b]		
Other trace minerals[c]		
Vitamins (MVI-Pediatric)[d]		
Total volume	120–130	150

[a] Hyperphosphatemia may occur if the phosphorus intake exceeds the amount accompanying a daily potassium intake of 2 mEq/kg as a mixture of KH_2PO_4 and K_2HPO_4; thus, if a potassium intake of more than 2 mEq/kg/day is required, the additional potassium should be given as KCl.

[b] Iron dextran (Imferon, Fisons Corp., Bedford, MA) often is added to the infusate of patients requiring prolonged parenteral nutrition therapy. At Babies Hospital, the dose is limited arbitrarily to 0.1 mg/kg/day. Alternatively, the indicated intramuscular dose can be used intermittently, either as the sole source of iron or as an additional dose.

[c] See text and Table 5.

[d] 5 ml of MVI-Pediatric (Armour Pharmaceutical Co., Chicago, IL) reconstituted as directed, provides 80 mg vitamin C, 700 μg vitamin A, 10 μg vitamin D, 1.3 mg thiamine, 1.4 mg riboflavin, 1.0 mg pyridoxine, 17 mg niacin, 5 mg pantothenic acid, 7 mg vitamin E, 20 μg biotin, 140 μg folic acid, 1 μg vitamin B_{12}, and 200 μg vitamin K_1 (cf. most recent suggested intakes, Table 4).

TABLE 2. Composition of available parenteral amino acid mixtures (mg/g) and that of human milk

Amino acid	Aminosyn (Abbott)	Aminosyn-PF (Abbott)	Travasol (B) (Travenol)	FreAmine III (McGaw)	Trophamine (McGaw)	Neopham (Cutter)	Human milk[a]
Isoleucine	72	76	48	70	82	49	57
Leucine	94	119	62	91	140	110	95
Lysine	40	68	58	73	82	83	70
Methionine	44	18	58	53	33	20	21
Phenylalanine	52	43	62	56	48	42	44
Threonine	16	52	42	40	42	56	47
Tryptophan	80	18	18	15	20	22	17
Valine	30	65	46	66	78	56	61
Histidine	30	32	44	30	48	33	24
Cyst(e)ine	0	0	0	0	<3	0	19
Tyrosine	9	6	4	0	23[b]	8	47
Taurine	0	7	0	0	2	5	0
Alanine	128	70	207	70	53	99	37
Aspartate	0	53	0	0	32	64	92
Glutamate	0	82	0	0	50	111	180
Glycine	128	38	207	140	37	33	26
Proline	86	82	42	112	68	88	79
Serine	42	50	0	59	38	59	50
Arginine	98	123	103	95	122	64	42

[a] Data provided by Ross Laboratories, Columbus, OH.
[b] Mixture of L-tyrosine and N-acetyl-L-tyrosine.

an amino acid intake of 2.5 g/kg/day and an energy intake of 60 Cal/kg/day during the first week of life retained nitrogen at a mean rate of ~175 mg/kg/day, whereas similar infants receiving the same energy intake with no amino acids experienced nitrogen losses of ~130 mg/kg/day. Although neither group gained weight, it is well known that changes in weight during the first week of life are difficult to interpret. Older LBW infants receiving similar intakes usually do not lose weight or exhibit slow rates of weight gain (9,11). It is likely, therefore, that these intakes are close to maintenance requirements.

The quality of the parenteral amino acid intake also appears to be important in determining the parenteral requirement for amino acids. Duffy et al. (12) found that nitrogen retention was greater in infants receiving a crystalline amino acid mixture than in infants receiving an isonitrogenous and isocaloric regimen containing casein hydrolysate. In addition, protein synthesis accounted for a greater percentage of total nitrogen flux in those who received the crystalline amino acid regimen. Helms et al. (13) observed that nitrogen retention was more efficient (i.e., 78% of intake) in infants who received a regimen containing a parenteral amino acid mixture designed for infants than in those who received a regimen containing a "general-purpose" parenteral amino acid mixture (i.e., 66% of intake).

Explaining why one regimen is better utilized than another is not easy. In the Helms study (13), the regimen resulting in better utilization provided more cyst(e)ine and tyrosine, both considered indispensable for the infant but rarely present in parenteral amino acid mixtures (Table 2). This is an unlikely explanation, however, since, in the Duffy study (12), the less efficiently utilized nitrogen source contained more tyrosine and cyst(e)ine (12).

Energy Intake

Theoretically, an energy intake approximating the resting energy expenditure (i.e., 50 to 65 Cal/kg/day) is sufficient for maintenance (i.e., prevention of weight loss, provided amino acid intake is adequate), whereas an energy intake in excess of resting energy expenditure is necessary to produce weight gain. Since energy expenditure is dependent upon a variety of factors, the resting energy requirement varies considerably among infants. The total energy intake necessary to produce a specific rate of weight gain also varies, although not as much as the resting energy requirement. For example, the resting energy expenditure of infants with bronchopulmonary dysplasia is ~10% greater than that of infants without bronchopulmonary dysplasia (14). Hence, the resting energy requirements of such infants is ~10% greater than that of infants without bronchopulmonary dysplasia. However, the additional energy intake required to produce a specific rate of weight gain is not likely to be any greater than that required to produce the same rate of weight gain in infants without bronchopulmonary dysplasia. Thus, the total energy requirement of infants with bronchopulmonary dysplasia is less than 10% greater than the requirement of infants without this condition. This reasoning is probably also true for infants with other conditions (e.g., infection).

According to Zlotkin et al. (9), LBW infants who receive an energy intake of 80 Cal/kg/day with a concomitant amino acid intake of 3 g/kg/day gain weight at approximately the intrauterine rate. Theoretically, each additional 10 Cal of energy intake will result in an additional gram of weight gain. This additional weight gain, however, represents primarily deposition of adipose tissue. Hence, a greater energy intake is not particularly desirable unless it is accompanied by a greater amino acid intake thereby supporting greater rates of both protein and fat deposition.

The effect of energy intake on nitrogen utilization also must be considered. The usual concept, developed primarily in animals and adults, is that utilization of protein intake improves as energy intake increases. There is, however, an upper level of energy intake beyond which additional increases will not further improve utilization of a specific protein intake (15,16). Zlotkin et al. (9) observed that low birth weight infants had greater retention of nitrogen at amino acid intakes of either 3 or 4 g/kg/day when energy intake was 80 versus 50 Cal/kg/day. Pineault et al. (11) observed a statistically significant effect of an energy intake of 80 versus 60 Cal/kg/day on retention of nitrogen at an amino acid intake of 2.7 g/kg/day. These data suggest that an amino acid intake of 2.7 g/kg/day is reasonably well utilized, although perhaps not maximally so, at an energy intake of 60 Cal/kg/day.

The effect of distribution of energy intake on amino acid utilization also may be important. Certainly, the nitrogen-sparing effect of carbohydrates in the absence of nitrogen intake is not shared by fat (17). Whether or not parenterally administered glucose versus lipid differentially affects utilization of concomitantly administered amino acids is less well understood. Studies in adults suggest both that the two energy substrates are equal in this regard (18) and that lipid exerts no such effect unless glucose provides the bulk of the resting energy requirement (19). This apparent discrepancy may reflect differences in the patient populations of the two studies (i.e., stable, depleted adults in the former and stressed, burned patients in the latter). Pineault et al. (11) studying the effects of parenteral lipid intakes of 3 and 1 g/kg/day at total energy intakes of both 60 and 80 Cal/kg/day, found that the plasma concentration of most amino acids was lower in infants who received the higher carbohydrate regimens at both total energy intakes. Although this finding suggests better amino acid utilization with the higher carbohydrate regimens, the rates of nitrogen retention did not differ significantly.

Glucose, the only energy source of early parenteral nutrition regimens, is still the major energy source of most regimens. Since a glucose intake greater than 15 g/kg/day rarely is tolerated by any infant on the first day of therapy and since the amount tolerated by LBW infants frequently is less, glucose intake must be increased gradually over the first few days of therapy. Daily increases of 2 to 5 g/kg are well tolerated by all but the most immature infants.

Parenteral Lipid Intake

Any infant who receives a fat-free parenteral nutrition regimen is likely to develop essential fatty acid deficiency within a relatively short period of time. Preterm and nutritionally depleted infants do so within days, particularly if growth is rapid (20). Thus, sufficient amounts of a parenteral lipid emulsion to prevent this deficiency (i.e., 0.5 to 1.0 g/kg/day) are indicated. The maximum intakes recommended are 2 g/kg/day for the LBW infant and 3 g/kg/day for the older infant (21).

Currently, parenteral lipid emulsions containing soybean oil (e.g., Intralipid and Liposyn III) and a mixture of safflower and soybean oils (e.g., Liposyn II) are available (Table 3). Egg yolk phospholipid is the emulsifying agent of all emulsions and the emulsion particles of all are roughly the size of chylomicrons or very low-density lipoprotein (VLDL). After infusion, the triglyceride portion of these particles is hydrolyzed by endothelial lipoprotein lipase; the free fatty acids and glycerol released are metabolized by the usual mechanisms (22).

The ability of infants to hydrolyze the infused emulsion particles increases with increasing gestational age but, at any gestational age, the small-for-gestational-age (SGA) infant has a lower capacity for hydrolysis than one of appropriate size (23). This probably is true for the malnourished versus the well-nourished older infant, as well. A number of clinical conditions, e.g., infection, surgical stress, and malnutrition, also adversely affect hydrolysis (22).

Theoretically, if the rate of lipid infusion does not exceed the rate of hydrolysis, dramatic changes in plasma triglyceride concentration are unlikely. However, if the rate of lipid infusion exceeds the rate of hydrolysis, plasma triglyceride concentration rises and may affect

TABLE 3. *Composition of representative parenteral lipid emulsions*

Component	Soybean oil emulsion[a]	Soybean/safflower oil emulsion[b]
Soybean oil (g/l)	100[c]	50[c]
Safflower oil (g/l)	—	50[c]
Egg yolk phospholipid (g/l)	12	up to 12
Glycerol (g/l)	22.5	25
Fatty acids (% of total)		
16:0	10	8.8
18:0	3.5	3.4
18:1	26	17.7
18:2	50	65.8
18:3	9	4.2
Particle size (μm)	0.5	0.4

[a] Intralipid, Kabi-Vitrum, Sweden.
[b] Liposyn II, Abbott Laboratories, N. Chicago, IL.
[c] 20% emulsions also are available; these contain twice as much of the oils but roughly the same amounts of all other ingredients.

adversely both pulmonary diffusion (24,25) and polymorphonuclear leukocyte function (26,27). In either situation, if the rate of hydrolysis exceeds the rate at which the released free fatty acids are oxidized, the plasma concentration of free fatty acids will rise. Since free fatty acids displace bound bilirubin from albumin (28), this possibility is of some concern in infants with hyperbilirubinemia. Unfortunately, the concentration of free fatty acids likely to displace albumin-bound bilirubin *in vivo* is not known.

A low plasma carnitine concentration, common in infants and adults receiving carnitine-free parenteral nutrition regimens (29,30) may inhibit fatty acid oxidation. Although most clinical trials of carnitine supplementation show no effect on fatty acid oxidation (31,32), one study in which carnitine was added following a prolonged period of carnitine-free parenteral nutrition shows that carnitine, under these circumstances, improves fatty acid oxidation (33).

The amount of the soybean oil emulsions necessary to prevent essential fatty acid deficiency (i.e., 2% to 4% of total energy intake or approximately 0.5 g/kg/day) is likely to be tolerated by almost all infants. Since the linoleic acid content of safflower oil (~75%) is higher than that of soybean oil (~50%), an even smaller dose of the safflower plus soybean oil emulsion should provide the linoleic acid requirement. Linolenic acid, a component of soybean but not safflower oil, also is an essential fatty acid (34) and, since the requirement for linolenic acid is unknown, it is not clear that a dose of 0.5 g/kg/day of the mixed emulsion is sufficient.

The most prudent approach for use of the currently available lipid emulsions, particularly in those infants who are likely to experience difficulties in hydrolyzing parenteral lipid emulsions or infants with hyperbilirubinemia, is to limit intake initially to 0.5 g/kg/day. Subsequently, as tolerance of the emulsion is demonstrated and/or hyperbilirubinemia resolves, intake can be increased. This approach is common in clinical practice and appears to be based on the assumption that slow introduction of the lipid emulsion increases the ability to utilize it. The data of Brans et al. (35) suggest otherwise. These data suggest that the plasma triglyceride and free fatty acid concentrations of LBW infants receiving parenteral lipid emulsions, regardless of the method or duration of infusion, is a function of the amount of emulsion administered over a specific period of time. Plasma triglyceride and free fatty acid concentrations remained within an acceptable range as long as the dose of emulsion was less than 2 to 3 g/kg/day. Thus, in infants who are likely to tolerate the recommended dose, this dosage can be introduced almost immediately. On the other hand, gradual introduction is advisable in the smaller infant, the SGA infant, and the infant who is infected or is experiencing other complications associated with delayed triglyceride hydrolysis. In such infants, the graded introduction permits monitoring lipid tolerance before intake is increased.

A recent study (36) suggests that LBW infants hydrolyze the 20% soybean oil emulsion better than the 10% emulsion. In fact, the total amount of triglyceride tolerated appears to be at least 100% greater when the 20% rather than the 10% emulsion is used (37). The proposed mechanism is the lower phospholipid/triglyceride ratio of the 20% versus the 10% emulsion. Since phospholipid is known to inhibit lipoprotein lipase (22), this is a logical explanation. If these findings are confirmed by others, it is likely that current recommendations for use of parenteral lipid emulsions will change.

Intakes of Electrolytes, Minerals, and Vitamins

The requirements for electrolytes, minerals, and vitamins, particularly those for electrolytes and minerals, vary considerably from patient to patient. For this reason, Table 1 reflects the amounts provided by early parenteral nutrition regimens, i.e., the same intakes provided in maintenance parenteral fluid therapy, and subsequently found to be appropriate for the majority of infants requiring parenteral nutrition (38).

The amounts of sodium and potassium required are particularly tenuous. Because of immature renal function, very small LBW infants often require greater intakes of sodium to maintain a normal plasma sodium concentration. In addition, nutritionally depleted infants often require quite high potassium intakes to maintain a normal plasma potassium concentration. Thus, frequent monitoring of plasma electrolyte concentrations and appropriate reformulation of the nutrient infusate to maintain normal plasma electrolyte concentrations is recommended for all infants, particularly during the first few days of parenteral nutrition.

The suggested parenteral intakes of phosphorus and magnesium were established in the same manner as the recommended electrolyte intakes. These intakes, too, appear to be adequate for most infants and children but frequent monitoring of the plasma concentration with appropriate reformulations of the infusate are recommended. This is particularly important for the nutritionally depleted patient.

Because of the insolubility of calcium phosphate, most commonly used parenteral nutrition regimens do not provide an adequate calcium intake. For example, the fetus deposits calcium at a rate of ~100 mg/kg/day during the last trimester of gestation (5), but parenteral nutrition regimens rarely provide more than 40 to 60 mg/kg/day (1 to 1.5 mmol/kg/day). More calcium can be provided if phosphorus intake is decreased, but a phosphorus intake of <1.5 mmol/kg/day is likely to result in hypophosphatemia.

The lower pH of some of the newer amino acid mixtures allows provision of more calcium without sacrificing phosphorus intake. Using this approach to maximize calcium phosphate solubility, Koo et al. (39) studied the effects of regimens providing calcium and phosphorus intakes of either 0.5 or 1.5 to 2.0 mmol/dl of both. Although the vitamin D content of both regimens was the same (i.e., 25 IU/dl), serum 1,25-dihydroxy-D concentrations of the high calcium/phosphorus group remained stable and within the normal range, whereas serum 1,25-dihydroxy-D concentrations of the low calcium/phosphorus group were high. Tubular reabsorption of phosphorus also was stable and consistently less than 90% in the high calcium/phosphorus group but was consistently greater than 90% in the low calcium/phosphorus group. It appears, therefore, that delivery of higher calcium and phosphorus intakes produces minimal stress to calcium and phosphorus homeostatic mechanisms, whereas delivery of lower intakes stresses these mechanisms. Whether the higher intakes result in more optimal skeletal mineralization is less clear; serum alkaline phosphatase activity of the two groups did not differ.

The greater solubility of calcium phosphate at low temperatures raises serious concerns about the safety of the three-in-one or complete parenteral nutrient infusates, i.e., glucose, amino acids, and the lipid emulsion combined, in one bottle, with required electrolytes, minerals, and vitamins. Since these infusates must be administered without an in-line filter and since the presence of the lipid in the infusate obscures any precipitate of calcium phosphate that may occur either upon removal from refrigeration and warming or during infusion, their use seems unwise. This is particularly true if efforts are being made to maximize calcium and phosphorus intakes.

TABLE 4. *Suggested parenteral intakes of vitamins (43)*

Vitamin	Preterm infants (amount/kg/day)[a]	Term infants and children (amount/day)[b]
Vitamin A (μg)	280	700
Vitamin E (mg)	2.8	7
Vitamin K (μg)	80	200
Vitamin D (μg)	4	10
(IU)	160	400
Ascorbic acid (mg)	25	80
Thiamin (mg)	0.48	1.2
Riboflavin (mg)	0.56	1.4
Pyridoxine (mg)	0.4	1.0
Niacin (mg)	6.8	17
Pantothenic acid (mg)	2.0	5
Biotin (μg)	8.0	20
Folate (μg)	56	140
Vitamin B_{12} (μg)	0.4	1.0

[a] Total daily dose should not exceed that recommended for term infants and children. A dose of 2 ml of reconstituted MVI-Pediatric provides the recommended amount/kg/day of all vitamins except ascorbic acid.
[b] These amounts are provided by 5 ml of reconstituted MVI-Pediatric (Armour Pharmaceutical Co.).

TABLE 5. *Suggested parenteral intakes of trace minerals (43)[a]*

Trace mineral	Preterm infants (μg/kg/day)	Term infants (μg/kg/day)
Zinc	400	250[b]
Copper	20	20
Selenium	2.0	2.0
Chromium	0.20	0.20
Manganese	1.0	1.0
Molybdenum	0.25	0.25
Iodide	1.0	1.0

[a] If parenteral nutrients are used as a supplement for tolerated enteral feedings or as the sole source of nutrients for <4 weeks, only zinc is needed.
[b] 100 mg/kg/day for infants > 3 months of age.

Mixtures of vitamins for parenteral use have been available since the early days of parenteral nutrition and these mixtures have been used to formulate parenteral nutrition infusates. Dosages administered, in fact, were (and are) determined by the multivitamin preparations available. Prior to the recent availability of trace mineral preparations suitable for parenteral use, frequent plasma and/or blood transfusions were used to provide the needed trace minerals. Reports of zinc and copper deficiencies demonstrated the inadequacy of this approach and led to zinc and copper additives. Currently, other trace minerals for which a deficiency has been demonstrated in patients receiving parenteral nutrition, e.g., selenium (40), chromium (41), and molybdenum (42), also are available.

Little definitive information is available concerning the parenteral requirements of either vitamins or trace minerals. Research concerning the parenteral requirements of these nutrients is hindered by the difficulties of performing accurate retention studies as well as the difficulties both of measuring plasma concentrations using small volumes and of interpreting the data obtained. Recent recommendations for parenteral vitamin and trace mineral intakes are based on the most reliable information available but very little of this information reflects data from randomized trials of various intakes (Tables 4 and 5) (43).

DELIVERY OF NUTRIENT INFUSATES

The nutrient infusate, whether delivered by central or peripheral vein, should be infused at a constant rate using one of several available constant infusion pumps. The use of a 0.22-μm filter between the catheter and the administration tubing is advocated by some, including the author; others feel that this precaution is not necessary.

Radiographic confirmation of correct catheter position is mandatory before infusion by central vein is begun. Otherwise, the hypertonic nutrient mixture may be infused into an undesired site. Regular and meticulous care of the central vein catheter also is essential for prolonged, safe, complication-free use. Attention to this detail seems to be the most important factor in preventing infection. It is recommended that the occlusive dressing at the catheter exit site be changed at least three times a week. Each time, the skin area should be cleaned thoroughly with both a defatting and an antiseptic agent and an antiseptic ointment as well as a fresh occlusive dressing should be applied. Unnecessary use of the catheter for purposes other than delivery of the nutrient infusate, particularly for blood transfusions and blood sampling, is discouraged. With meticulous care, a single catheter, particularly one with a polyvinyl cuff, can be used safely for months to years.

Many patients tolerate the same infusate for the total duration of parenteral nutrition. Others, however, require frequent adjustment of one or more components of the infusate. It is important, therefore, to be able to change the concentration of one or more components in response to clinical and chemical monitoring or to increase the volume in response to diarrheal and other ongoing losses.

INDICATIONS FOR PARENTERAL NUTRITION

Most agree that any patient who is unable to tolerate adequate enteral feedings for a significant period of time will benefit from parenterally administered nutrients. There is less agreement, however, concerning the definition of "significant period of time" and the specific indications for central versus peripheral vein delivery.

A reasonable guideline for defining a "significant period of time" is the extent to which endogenous nutrient stores are likely to be eroded if nutrient intake is inadequate for the total duration of enteral feeding intolerance. For example, a large infant who must forego enteral feedings for only a few days is unlikely to experience serious erosion of endogenous nutrient stores, whereas a small infant or a large infant with preexisting nutritional depletion is likely to experience further depletion of already limited endogenous stores with even a short period of starvation.

Peripheral vein delivery of nutrient infusates is often chosen over central vein because of the perception that it is easier and less time-consuming. This perception, however, is not supported by fact. The supervision required for successful peripheral vein delivery is at least equal to that required for successful central vein delivery. In addition, since a single infusion site rarely lasts for more than 24 hr, considerable time and effort are required to maintain peripheral vein infusions. Furthermore, the complications associated with the two routes of delivery are similar when expressed per day of therapy, albeit different in nature and seriousness (44). Delivery routes should be chosen, therefore, by the appropriateness for a patient's clinical condition and nutritional needs rather than by the perceived ease of a particular technique.

Since regimens that can be delivered by peripheral vein tend to maintain existing body composition, this route is a logical one for a normally nourished infant who is likely to tolerate an adequate enteral regimen within 1 to 2 weeks. Central vein delivery, on the other hand, is more appropriate for infants likely to be intolerant of enteral feedings for longer than 2 weeks. This differentiation is based both on the likely difficulty of maintaining peripheral vein infusions for more than 2 weeks and the fact that a more concentrated nutrient mixture can be delivered by central vein.

Factors such as nutritional status, duration of illness, and prior clinical course also must be considered when choosing between peripheral and central vein delivery. In this regard, infants with a reasonably good nutritional status who become intolerant of enteral feedings within the first few days of life (e.g., the term infant with a surgically correctable lesion of the intestine) are appropriate candidates for a peripheral vein regimen. Smaller neonates with the same condition (e.g., an SGA infant with the same surgically correctable lesion), however, are candidates for central vein delivery. Infants who require parenteral nutrition after the first few weeks of life following a complicated clinical course characterized by inadequate nutritional intake (e.g., the infant with intractable diarrhea or some infants with necrotizing enterocolitis) also are likely to require central vein delivery. Not only are such infants likely to be nutritionally depleted, they are unlikely to tolerate peripheral infusions for an additional 2 weeks.

EXPECTATIONS OF PARENTERAL NUTRITION

Growth

There is little doubt that parenteral nutrition regimens delivered by central vein produce normal growth of infants and children and regrowth of depleted adults. In infants, a regimen delivering 2.5 to 3.0 g/kg/day of amino acids and 100 Cal/kg/day reliably produces rates of weight gain and nitrogen retention, respectively, of 10 to 15 g/kg/day and 200 to 300 mg/kg/day. Increases in length also occur in infants receiving such regimens but, in the author's experience, the increase in length often lags behind the increase in weight and weight-for-length soon exceeds the 50th percentile value. Since adjusting energy intake in response to the rates of increase in weight and length produces proportionate growth, i.e., maintenance of weight for length at or around the 50th percentile, it is likely that the disproportionate growth is a result of excessive energy intake and, hence, excessive fat deposition. Disproportionate growth, of course, is only a problem in patients who are dependent upon parenteral nutrients for months rather than weeks. In the usual patient, weight-for-length is frequently low when parenteral nutrition is started; thus, a disproportionate increase in weight during the early period of parenteral nutrition is not necessarily undesirable.

Composition of Weight Gain

Although commonly assumed, there is no definitive evidence that infants and adults receiving parenteral nutrients retain more water than those receiving enteral nutrients. Nonetheless, the disproportionate weight loss following sudden cessation of parenteral nutrients suggests that this may be at least partially true. The fact that edema is uncommon, however, suggests that the excess water is in part intracellular or that it does not exceed 10% of extracellular volume.

Applying the principle of energy balance to the data of Zlotkin et al. (9) provides some insight into the probable composition of weight gain of infants receiving only parenteral nutrients. The retained protein of infants receiving amino acid and energy intakes of 3 g/kg/day and 80 Cal/kg/day, i.e., ~300 mg/kg/day of nitrogen, or 1.9 g of protein, accounts for only a small portion of the total weight gain of 15 g/kg. Further, assuming that the coefficient of hydration of lean body mass is 0.8, deposition of lean body mass accounts for only 9.5 g of the total daily weight gain of 15 g/kg. To account for the remaining 5.5 g/kg as fat, metabolizable energy intake would have to exceed resting energy expenditure by at least 50 Cal/kg/day; since total energy intake was 80 Cal/kg/day, resting energy expenditure, in turn, would have to be only 30 Cal/kg/day.

Although no energy expenditure data are available, this rate of resting expenditure is considerably lower than the rate of 45 to 50 Cal/kg/day reported by other investigators in infants receiving only parenteral nutrients (45). Thus, the calculations fall short by at least 1 g/kg/day. Although some of this could be fat derived from the roughly 1 g/kg/day of amino acids not stored as new protein, some also could be water. Alternatively, these calculations simply may not be sufficiently precise to permit complete agreement between intake and storage calculations. More precise data concerning the composition of weight gain is hindered by a lack of available methods.

Gastrointestinal Function During Parenteral Nutrition

The one unquestioned clinical indication for parenteral nutrition is to maintain or restore the nutritional status of patients with deranged gastrointestinal function. Thus, there is considerable interest in the consequences of this therapy with respect to gastrointestinal function. In normal animals, parenteral nutrition, like starvation, results in an appreciable decrease in enteric mucosal mass (46–48). On the other hand, parenteral nutrition following a period of starvation in rats prevents a further decrease in mucosal mass but does not support regrowth of the enteric mucosa as does refeeding with chow (49).

The effect of parenteral nutrition on mucosal enzyme activities is unclear. Some studies suggest that the specific activity of several disaccharidases decreases relative to that of control animals (46), whereas others suggest that the specific activity of these enzymes do not differ between control animals and animals treated with parenteral nutrition (49). Since the type of dietary sugar intake affects the specific activity of most disaccharidases, these discrepancies may be related to the nature of the diet consumed by the control animals of the various studies.

The few available clinical studies of the effects of parenteral nutrition on intestinal tract structure and function do not demonstrate morphological involution (50,51). On the other hand, disaccharidase activities, which are usually low when parenteral nutrition begins, are not fully restored until enteral intake is reinstituted (51).

Two recent studies in LBW infants suggest that infants who receive seemingly negligible amounts of enterally delivered nutrients during the period of parenteral nutrition are more easily weaned from parenteral to enteral nutrients (52,53). The mechanism of this apparent effect is not known but it is tempting to speculate that it is related to the different pattern of release of various enteric hormones between fed and unfed (i.e., parenterally fed) infants (54).

COMPLICATIONS OF PARENTERAL NUTRITION

There are two general categories of complications associated with parenteral nutrition—those related to the technique, particularly the presence of an indwelling catheter, and those related to the infusate. The former category usually is referred to as catheter-related complications and the latter as metabolic complications.

The major catheter-related complication is infection. Although many of the infusate components support growth of various microorganisms (55,56), a contaminated infusate rarely is the underlying cause of infection. Rather, most infections appear to result from improper care of the catheter, particularly failure to follow meticulously the requirement for frequent changes of the dressing covering the catheter exit site.

Other catheter-related complications include malposition, dislodgment, and thrombosis, including superior (or inferior) vena cava thrombosis. Malposition can be avoided by radiographic confirmation of the location of the catheter tip prior to initial infusion of the hypertonic nutrient infusate and reconfirmation as indicated thereafter. The other catheter-related complications cannot be avoided completely but their incidence can be kept to an acceptable level if careful attention is paid to all procedures involving use and care of the catheter.

The major complications associated with infusion of nutrients by peripheral vein are thrombophlebitis and either skin or subcutaneous sloughs secondary to infiltration of the hypertonic infusate. Infection is much less common with peripheral vein than with central vein delivery; if it occurs, it is more likely to be due to a contaminated infusate.

The causes of the metabolic complications of parenteral nutrition include two general categories—those related to the concentration of various components of the infusate, and those related to the infusate components, per se (Table 6). Since the infusates delivered by central vein and peripheral vein are qualitatively similar, the latter group of complications are independent of the route of delivery. There are, however, likely to be fewer complications related to the composition of the infusate with the less-concentrated peripheral vein regimens.

TABLE 6. *Metabolic complications of parenteral nutrition and their most common cause*

Disorder	Most common cause
Disorders related to metabolic capacity of patient relative to intakes of various nutrients	
Hyperglycemia	Excessive intake secondary either to excessive concentration or excessive infusion rate, e.g., pump dysfunction; change in metabolic state, e.g., infection
Hypoglycemia	Sudden cessation of infusion
Azotemia	Excessive amino acid intake, either absolute or in relation to concurrent energy intake
Electrolyte, mineral (major and trace) and vitamin disorders	Excessive or inadequate intake
Disorders related to infusate components	
Abnormal plasma aminograms	Amino acid pattern of nitrogen source
Hypercholesterolemia/ phospholipidemia	Characteristics of lipid emulsion
Abnormal fatty acid pattern	Characteristics of lipid emulsion or its route of metabolism
Hepatic disorders	Unknown

Since a glucose concentration of more than 10% is impractical for peripheral vein regimens, glucose intolerance, except perhaps in very immature infants, is much less frequent with this route of delivery. Electrolyte and mineral disorders associated with both routes of delivery usually result from an inaccurate assessment of ongoing needs and, hence, inadequate or excessive provision. Theoretically, electrolyte disorders also can result from hyperglycemia if sufficiently severe to cause osmotic diuresis and excessive loss of electrolytes.

Some of the complications associated with early amino acid mixtures, e.g., metabolic acidosis related to the use of hydrochloride salts of the cationic amino acids (57) and hyperammonemia related either to the preformed ammonia content of hydrolysates (58) or to inadequate arginine intake [i.e., <0.5 mmol/kg/day (59)], are no longer problems. The major concern with respect to the metabolic consequences of currently available amino acid mixtures is that few result in a completely normal plasma amino acid pattern (60). This concern is based, in part, on the long-recognized coexistence of mental retardation and elevated plasma concentrations of specific amino acids in patients with various inborn errors of metabolism. In addition, the fact that the plasma concentration of many amino acids is low rather than high in patients receiving parenteral nutrition suggests that the intake of these amino acids may be inadequate. Also, plasma concentrations of the indispensable or conditionally indispensable amino acids, cyst(e)ine and tyrosine, are quite low, possibly because these amino acids, which are either unstable or insoluble in aqueous solution, are not present in appreciable amounts in any available parenteral amino acid mixture.

Animal studies demonstrate that the abnormal plasma amino acid pattern associated with administration of parenteral nutrition regimens is accompanied by an abnormal tissue amino acid pattern (61). Although this relationship is not necessarily a direct one, the abnormal plasma and tissue amino acid patterns are of concern with respect to possible adverse effects on ongoing whole-body protein synthesis as well as synthesis of various neurotransmitters within the central nervous system and synthesis of other derivatives of specific amino acids, e.g., glutathione and carnitine. Unfortunately, these areas have not been studied sufficiently to warrant major concern or to allay fears.

MONITORING

Successful parenteral nutrition is predicated on careful monitoring. This includes clinical and chemical monitoring to detect metabolic and/or catheter-related complications as well as monitoring the intake of each nutrient and the results of that intake. Clinical monitoring requires considerable nursing time. Frequent observations are necessary to prevent infiltration of the nutrient infusate delivered by peripheral vein and to assure long-term function of the central vein catheter. This requires personnel familiar with the intricacies of all aspects of the intravenous infusion apparatus, including the various constant infusion pumps essential for both central and peripheral vein delivery.

An established schedule for chemical monitoring allows detection of most metabolic complications in sufficient time to permit prompt correction (Table 7). The schedule suggested differs somewhat from other monitoring schemes. For example, instead of routinely monitoring blood glucose, it suggests checking the urine regularly for the presence of glucose (at least three times daily and perhaps even more frequently during the first few days of the technique) and determining blood glucose concentrations only when glucosuria is present. This is because the blood glucose concentration is not likely to be high enough to cause problems if the urine is free of glucose.

Direct measurement of plasma osmolality also is unnecessary. In the absence of hyperglycemia, plasma osmolality can be estimated with sufficient accuracy as twice the plasma sodium concentration; with hyperglycemia, plasma osmolality can be estimated as twice the sodium concentration plus the plasma glucose concentration divided by 18. In addition, the derangements of the plasma amino acid pattern incident to use of available parenteral amino acid mixtures are predictable from the pattern of the mixture of amino acids used (60); thus, this expensive and difficult-to-obtain determination is unnecessary.

The cause of the hepatic dysfunction that develops during the course of parenteral nutrition in many patients (62) is not known. Nonetheless, the fact that such dysfunction occurs and occasionally progresses to cirrhosis and death mandates careful assessment and monitoring of hepatic function. The indices listed in Table 7 are adequate for this purpose.

Periodic visual or nephelometric inspection of the plasma for presence of lipemia is the usual method of monitoring to ensure safe and efficacious use of intravenous fat emulsions. However, neither method accurately detects elevated plasma triglyceride and free fatty acid concentrations (63). Actual chemical determinations of both triglyceride and free fatty acid concentrations are required. Since microtechniques for these assays are not routinely available or, if available, are performed only two or three times per week, such monitoring is not practical. A reasonable compromise is to inspect the plasma frequently, either visually or by nephelometry, and to determine actual triglyceride and free fatty acid concentrations once or twice weekly. This is particularly important during the initial period of parenteral nutrition and/or when the patient develops a clinical condition likely to interfere with triglyceride hydrolysis. Other serum lipid abnormalities associated with use of parenteral lipid emulsions (hypercholesterolemia, hyperphospholipidemia, deranged fatty acid patterns of serum and tissue lipids) are predictable, perhaps unavoidable, and/or of questionable clinical relevance; thus, monitoring to detect them is not necessary.

UNANSWERED QUESTIONS

Perhaps the major unanswered question concerning parenteral nutrition is the extent to which this route of delivery affects the requirements for various nutrients. For example, the parenteral energy intake required to produce a specific rate of weight gain appears to be less than that required when nutrients are delivered by the enteral route. Conversely, the parenteral amino acid (or nitrogen) requirement appears to be greater than that required by the fed infant. In addition, some usually dispensable amino acids appear to be indispensable for the patient receiving only parenterally delivered nutrients. It also appears that the amount of lipid that can be utilized when it is administered intravenously is less than when it is ingested by mouth.

TABLE 7. *Suggested monitoring schedule during parenteral nutrition*

Variables to be monitored	Suggested frequency (per week)[a]	
	Initial period	Later period
Growth variables		
Weight	7	7
Length	1	1
Head circumference	1	1
Metabolic variables		
Blood or plasma		
Electrolytes	2–4	1
Ca, Mg, P	2	1
Acid base status	2	1
Urea nitrogen	2	1
Albumin	1	1
Liver function studies	1	1
Lipids[b]		
Hemoglobin	2	1
Urine glucose	2–6/day	2/day
Prevention and detection of infection		
Clinical observations (activity, temperature)	Daily	Daily
WBC and differential	As indicated	As indicated
Cultures	As indicated	As indicated

[a] "Initial period" refers to the time before full intake is achieved as well as any period during which metabolic instability is present or suspected (i.e., postoperative period, presence of infection). "Later period" refers to the time during which the patient is in a metabolic steady state.

[b] See text.

Energy Requirements

LBW infants receiving a parenteral energy intake of 80 Cal/kg/day with a protein intake of 3 g/kg/day gain weight at a rate of ~15 g/kg/day (9). In contrast, LBW infants receiving an enteral intake of 120 Cal/kg/day and a protein intake of 2.8 g/kg/day gain weight at only a slightly greater rate (64). Some of this apparent difference in requirement, of course, is related to the greater fecal energy losses of enterally fed infants. However, the metabolizable energy intake of infants who ingest 120 Cal/kg/day usually is at least 100 Cal/kg/day—substantially greater than the total parenteral energy intake of 80 Cal/kg/day.

Another possible reason for the apparent greater rate of weight gain of infants receiving parenterally versus enterally delivered regimens is the possibility that parenterally delivered regimens result in deposition of more water. However, evidence to confirm or refute this possibility is lacking. Lower resting energy expenditure, secondary, presumably, to the fact that the gastrointestinal tract is bypassed, also may contribute to the apparently lower energy requirement of infants receiving only parenteral nutrients. Rather than a single explanation, it is likely that all of the discussed differences contribute to the apparently lower parenteral versus enteral energy requirement.

Amino Acid Requirements

Despite fecal losses of up to 15% of intake, most infants retain 70% or more of ingested protein (65). In contrast, infants receiving only parenteral nutrients have minimal fecal losses of nitrogen but retain only 60% to 65% of intake (66). Thus, the nitrogen intake that must be provided by the parenteral route to result in a specific rate of nitrogen retention is greater than the amount that must be provided enterally. The reason for this is not clear but may be related to the difference in the amino acid pattern of most available parenteral amino acid mixtures versus the pattern of a high-quality dietary protein such as human milk (Table 2).

Because cystine and tyrosine are only sparingly soluble and cysteine is unstable in aqueous solution, they are not present in appreciable amounts in any currently available parenteral amino acid mixture. Moreover, presumably because of inadequate intakes, plasma cyst(e)ine and tyrosine concentrations of infants receiving these mixtures are quite low. Further, these low plasma concentrations are not altered by greater intakes, respectively, of methionine and phenylalanine (60).

Hepatic activity of cystathionase, one of the enzymes required for endogenous conversion of methionine to cysteine, is known to be low at birth and for some time postnatally (67,68). This developmental deficit is an acceptable explanation for the low plasma cyst(e)ine concentrations of infants receiving cyst(e)ine-free parenteral nutrition regimens. However, since there appears to be no developmental delay in hepatic phenylalanine hydroxylase activity (69), the low plasma tyrosine concentrations of infants receiving tyrosine-free parenteral nutrition regimens is not as easily explicable on this basis.

According to Chawla et al. (30), adults receiving cyst(e)ine- and tyrosine-free parenteral nutrition regimens also have much lower plasma concentrations of cyst(e)ine and tyrosine than patients receiving a cyst(e)ine- and tyrosine-free elemental enteral diet. Moreover, plasma concentrations of taurine, which is synthesized endogenously from cysteine, as well as carnitine, creatine, and choline, all of which require a methyl group from S-adenosylmethionine for endogenous synthesis, also are lower in those receiving the parenteral regimen. These differences in plasma concentrations between patients receiving similar enterally versus parenterally administered regimens suggest that parenterally delivered methionine is metabolized by a pathway other than the transsulfuration pathway, the first intermediate of which is S-adenosylmethionine. The specific reason for the apparent parenteral requirement for tyrosine is less clear but a similar mechanism seems reasonable.

In both adults and infants, then, it appears that parenterally administered methionine and phenylalanine are not metabolized by the usual pathways and, therefore, are not effectively converted, respectively, to cyst(e)ine and tyrosine. Although evidence is lacking, it seems reasonable to suspect that metabolism of other amino acids also may differ as a function of route of delivery.

Cysteine hydrochloride is soluble and also is reasonably stable for short periods of time; thus, it can be used to supplement parenteral nutrition infusates. However, cysteine supplementation (70,71) appears to have no beneficial effect on nitrogen retention, perhaps because the tyrosine content of the control regimens of these studies also was low and any beneficial effect of cysteine intake on nitrogen retention was masked by concurrent tyrosine deficiency. One of the newer parenteral amino acid mixtures contains a soluble tyrosine derivative, N-acetyl-L-tyrosine (Table 2). Although the absolute efficacy of this derivative has not been determined, infants receiving this mixture have higher plasma tyrosine concentrations than infants receiving other mixtures (66,72). Indeed, Helms et al. (13) attributed the greater nitrogen retention of infants receiving a parenteral regimen containing this amino acid mixture (i.e., 78% of intake) versus a regimen containing another parenteral amino acid mixture (i.e., 66% of intake) to the mixture's content of N-acetyl-L-tyrosine plus cysteine supplementation.

A more thorough knowledge of the differences in metabolism of parenterally versus enterally administered amino acids will help clarify the reasons for the apparent differences in amino acid requirements when nutrients are delivered by the parenteral versus the enteral route. This information is crucial for the design of more efficacious parenteral amino acid mixtures.

Lipid Requirements

Many of the metabolic abnormalities related to the composition and/or metabolism of available parenteral lipid emulsions are better understood than those related to available parenteral amino acid mixtures (22). The most pressing concern, perhaps, is the fatty acid pattern of serum and tissue lipids associated with use of available parenteral lipid emulsions. All available emulsions contain linoleic and linolenic acids, the parent fatty acids, respectively, of the n-6 and n-3 fatty acid families; however, none contains the longer-chain, more unsaturated fatty acids of either family (Table 3). The potential inability of the infant to elongate and desaturate the parent fatty acids (73) gives rise to at least the following two concerns.

First, arachidonic acid, an elongated and desaturated derivative of linoleic acid, is a precursor of many prostaglandin series. Thus, if it cannot be formed from linoleic acid, infants receiving available lipid emulsions, theoretically, may develop arachidonic acid deficiency and, in turn, derangements in prostaglandin production. Indeed, the arachidonic content of serum and erythrocyte phospholipid decreases in infants receiving available emulsions and, in these infants, urinary excretion of a stable metabolite of prostaglandin E is very low (74). Although not associated with recognized clinical abnormalities, this association is disturbing. Unfortunately, it has received very little attention.

Second, since appreciable amounts of the longer-chain, more unsaturated members of both the n-3 and n-6 fatty acid families accumulate during development, particularly in the developing central nervous system (75,76), the possibility that the infant cannot convert the parent fatty acids of either family to these longer-chain, more unsaturated derivatives raises concerns regarding the fatty acid pattern of tissue lipids (Table 8). Currently, this concern is largely theoretical. Whether the fatty acid pattern of lipids deposited by infants receiving only parenteral nutrients is abnormal as well as whether such an abnormal pattern, if it occurs, is associated with functional abnormalities remains unknown.

SUMMARY AND CONCLUSIONS

After a quarter-century of use, it is clear that the technique of parenteral nutrition is an established component of medical practice. It also is clear that the technique has contributed to the decrease in mortality and morbidity associated with many of the conditions for which it has been used. On the other hand, the technique has been associated with a variety of problems. Some of these have resulted from failure to appreciate the importance of many of the intricacies of the technique. Others are related to lack of knowledge, particularly concerning the effects of bypassing the gastrointestinal tract. This lack of knowledge, in turn, has inhibited the pace at which improved devices and products for formulating "optimal" nutrient infusates have been introduced.

These problems notwithstanding, the benefits of the technique outweigh its risks in those patients for whom it is indicated. With further research and, hence, better insight into a variety of physiological concerns raised by the technique, better products are likely to be developed. These, in turn, undoubtedly will further enhance the efficacy of this deceptively simple technique.

TABLE 8. *Accretion of n-6 and n-3 fatty acids in the developing human brain*

Fatty acid	Fetal (mg/wk)	Postnatal (mg/wk)
Total n-6	31	78
18:2	<1	2
20:4	19	45
Total n-3	15	4
18:3	<1	<1
Total	181	149

From refs. 75 and 76, with permission.

REFERENCES

1. Wilmore DM, Dudrick SJ. Growth and development of an infant receiving all nutrients by vein. *JAMA* 1968;203:860–864.
2. Filler RM, Eraklis AJ, Rubin VG, Das JB. Long term parenteral nutrition in infants. *N Engl J Med* 1969;281:589–594.
3. Keating JP, Ternberg JL. Amino acid-hypertonic glucose treatment for intractable diarrhea in infants. *Am J Dis Child* 1971;122:226–228.
4. Heird WC. Nutritional support of the pediatric patient. In: Winters RW, Greene HL, eds. *Nutritional support of the seriously ill patient.* New York: Academic Press, 1983;157–179.
5. Ziegler EE, O'Donnell AM, Nelson SE, et al. Body composition of the reference fetus. *Growth* 1986;40:329–341.
6. Heird WC. Parenteral nutrition. In: Grand RJ, Sutphen JL, Dietz WH Jr, eds. *Pediatric nutrition: theory and practice.* Boston: Butterworths, 1987;747–761.
7. Dudrick SJ, Wilmore DW, Vars HM, et al. Long term parenteral nutrition with growth, development, and positive nitrogen balance. *Surgery* 1968;64:134–142.
8. Mulvihill SJ, Fonkalsrud EW. Complication of superior versus inferior vena cava occlusion in infants receiving central total parenteral nutrition. *J Pediatr Surg* 1984;19:752–757.
9. Zlotkin SH, Bryan MH, Anderson GH. Intravenous nitrogen and energy intakes required to duplicate in utero nitrogen accretion in prematurely born human infants. *J Pediatr* 1981;99:115–120.
10. Anderson TL, Muttart C, Bieber MA, et al. A controlled trial of glucose vs. glucose and amino acids in premature infants. *J Pediatr* 1979;94:947–951.
11. Pineault M, Chessex P, Bisaillon S, et al. Total parenteral nutrition

in the newborn: impact of the quality of infused energy on nitrogen metabolism. *Am J Clin Nutr* 1988;47:298–304.
12. Duffy B, Gunn T, Collinge J, et al. The effect of varying protein quality and energy intake on the nitrogen metabolism of parenterally fed very low birth weight (1600 G) infants. *Pediatr Res* 1981;15:1040–1044.
13. Helms RA, Christensen ML, Mauer EC, et al. Comparison of a pediatric versus standard amino acid formulation in preterm neonates requiring parenteral nutrition. *J Pediatr* 1987;110:466–472.
14. Weinstein MR, Oh W. Oxygen consumption in infants with bronchopulmonary dysplasia. *J Pediatr* 1981;99:958–961.
15. Munro HN. General aspects of the regulation of protein metabolism by diet and hormone. In: Munro HN, ed. *Mammalian protein metabolism, vol I. Biochemical aspects of protein metabolism.* New York: Academic Press, 1964;381–481.
16. Calloway DH, Spector H. Nitrogen balance as related to caloric and protein intake in active young men. *Am J Clin Nutr* 1954;2:405–412.
17. Brennan MF, Moore FD. An intravenous fat emulsion as a nitrogen sparer: comparison with glucose. *J Surg Res* 1973;14:501–504.
18. Jeejeebhoy KN, Anderson GK, Nakhooda AF, et al. Metabolic studies in total parenteral nutrition with lipid in man: comparison with glucose. *J Clin Invest* 1976;57:125–136.
19. Long JM III, Wilmore DW, Mason AD Jr, et al. Effect of carbohydrate and fat intake on nitrogen excretion during total intravenous feeding. *Ann Surg* 1977;185:417–422.
20. Friedman Z, Danon A, Stahlman MT, et al. Rapid onset of essential acid deficiency in the newborn. *Pediatrics* 1976;58:640–649.
21. Committee on Nutrition, American Academy of Pediatrics. Use of intravenous fat emulsions in pediatric patients. *Pediatrics* 1981;68:738–743.
22. Heird WC. Lipid metabolism in parenteral nutrition. In: Fomon SJ, Heird WC, eds. *Energy and protein needs during infancy.* New York: Academic Press, 1986;215–229.
23. Andrew G, Chan G, Schiff D. Lipid metabolism in the neonate. I. The effect of intralipid infusion on plasma triglyceride and free fatty acid concentrations in the neonate. *J Pediatr* 1976;88:273–278.
24. Greene HL, Hazlett D, Demaree R. Relationship between intralipid-induced hyperlipidemia and pulmonary function. *Am J Clin Nutr* 1976;29:127–135.
25. Perreira GR, Fox WW, Stanley CA, et al. Decreased oxygenation and hyperlipidemia during intravenous fat infusions in premature infants. *Pediatrics* 1980;66:26–30.
26. Loo LS, Tang JP, Kohl S. The inhibition of leukocyte cellular cytotoxicity to herpes simplex virus in vitro and in vivo by intralipid. *J Infect Dis* 1982;146:64–70.
27. Cleary TC, Pickering LK. Mechanisms of intralipid effect on polymorpho-nuclear leukocytes. *J Clin Lab Immunol* 1983;11:21–26.
28. Odell GB, Cukier JO, Ostrea EM Jr, et al. The influence of fatty acids on the binding of bilirubin to albumin. *J Clin Med* 1977;89:295–307.
29. Penn D, Schmidt-Sommerfeld E, Pascu F. Decreased carnitine concentration in newborn infants receiving total parenteral nutrition. *Early Hum Dev* 1979;4:23–28.
30. Chawla RK, Berry CJ, Kutner MH, et al. Plasma concentrations of transsulfuration pathway products during nasoenteral and intravenous hyperalimentation of malnourished patients. *Am J Clin Nutr* 1985;42:577–584.
31. Schmidt-Sommerfeld E, Penn D, Wolf H. Carnitine deficiency in premature infants receiving total parenteral nutrition: effect of L-carnitine supplementation. *J Pediatr* 1983;102:931–935.
32. Orzali A, Donzelli F, Enzi G, et al. Effect of carnitine on lipid metabolism in the newborn. I. Carnitine supplementation during total parenteral nutrition in the first 48 hours of life. *Biol Neonate* 1983;43:186–190.
33. Helms RA, Whitington PF, Mauer EC, et al. Enhanced lipid utilization in infants receiving oral L-carnitine during long-term parenteral nutrition. *J Pediatr* 1986;109:984–988.
34. Holman RT, Johnson SB, Hatch TF. A case of human linolenic acid deficiency involving neurological abnormalities. *Am J Clin Nutr* 1982;35:617–623.
35. Brans YW, Andrew DS, Carrillo DW, et al. Tolerance of fat emulsions in very-low-birth-weight neonates. *Am J Dis Child* 1988;142:145–152.
36. Haumont D, Deckelbaum RJ, Richelle M, et al. Plasma lipid and plasma lipoprotein concentrations in low birth weight infants given parenteral nutrition with twenty or ten percent lipid emulsion. *J Pediatr* 1989;115:787–793.
37. Haumont D, Richelle M, Deckelbaum RJ, Dahlan W, Carpentier YA. Excess liposomal phospholipid content of IV fat emulsions impairs lipid clearance and alters lipoprotein patterns in LBW infants. *Pediatr Res* 1989;25:291A(abstract).
38. Heird WC, Winters RW. Total parenteral nutrition: the state of the art. *J Pediatr* 1975;86:2–16.
39. Koo WWK, Tsang RC, Steichen JJ, et al. Parenteral nutrition for infants: effect of high versus low calcium and phosphorus content. *J Pediatr Gastroenterol Nutr* 1987;6:96–104.
40. Kien CL, Ganther HE. Manifestations of chronic selenium deficiency in a child receiving total parenteral nutrition. *Am J Clin Nutr* 1983;37:319–328.
41. Jeejeebhoy KN, Chu RC, Marliss EB, et al. Chromium deficiency, glucose intolerance, and neuropathy reversed by chromium supplementation, in a patient receiving long-term total parenteral nutrition. *Am J Clin Nutr* 1977;30:531–538.
42. Abumrad NN, Schneider AJ, Steel D, et al. Amino acid intolerance during prolonged total parenteral nutrition reversed by molybdate therapy. *Am J Clin Nutr* 1981;34:2551–2559.
43. Greene HL, Hambidge KM, Schanler R, et al. Guidelines for the use of vitamins, trace elements, calcium, magnesium, and phosphorus in infants and children receiving total parenteral nutrition: report of the subcommittee on pediatric parenteral nutrient requirements from the committee on clinical practice issues of the American Society for Clinical Nutrition. *Am J Clin Nutr* 1988;48:1324–1342.
44. Jacobowski D, Ziegler MD, Perreira G. Complications of pediatric parenteral nutrition: central versus peripheral administration. *JPEN J Parenter Enteral Nutr* 1979;3:29(Abstract).
45. Rubecz I, Mestyan J, Varga P, Klujber L. Energy metabolism, substrate utilization, and nitrogen balance in parenterally fed postoperative neonates and infants. *J Pediatr* 1981;98:42–46.
46. Levine GM, Deren JJ, Steiger E, et al. Role of oral intake in maintenance of gut mass and disaccharidase activity. *Gastroenterol* 1974;67:975–982.
47. Johnson LR, Copeland EM, Dudrick SJ, et al. Structural and hormonal alterations in the gastrointestinal tract of parenterally fed rats. *Gastroenterol* 1975;68:1177–1183.
48. Feldman EJ, Dowling RH, McNaughton J, et al. Effects of oral versus intravenous nutrition on intestinal adaptation after small bowel resection in the dog. *Gastroenterol* 1976;70:712–719.
49. Mones RL, Heird WC, Rosensweig SN. Unpublished data.
50. Shwachman H, Lloyd-Still JD, Khaw KT, et al. Protracted diarrhea of infancy treated with intravenous alimentation. II. Studies of small intestinal biopsy results. *Am J Dis Child* 1973;125:365–368.
51. Greene HL, McCabe DR, Merenstein GB. Intractable diarrhea and malnutrition in infancy: changes in intestinal morphology and disaccharidase activities during treatment with total intravenous nutrition or oral elemental diets. *J Pediatr* 1975;87:695–704.
52. Dunn L, Hulman S, Weiner J, et al. Beneficial effects of early hypocaloric enteral feeding on neonatal gastrointestinal function: preliminary report of a randomized trial. *J Pediatr* 1988;112:622–629.
53. Slagle TA, Gross SJ. Effect of early enteral substrate on subsequent feeding tolerance. *J Pediatr* 1988;113:526–531.
54. Lucas A, Bloom SR, Aynsley-Green A. Metabolic and endocrine effects of depriving preterm infants of enteral nutrition. *Acta Paediatr Scand* 1983;72:245–249.
55. Goldman DA, Martin WT, Worthington JW. Growth of bacteria and fungi in total parenteral nutrition solutions. *Am J Surg* 1973;126:314–318.
56. McKee KT, Melly MA, Greene HL, et al. Gram-negative bacillary sepsis associated with use of lipid emulsion in parenteral nutrition. *Am J Dis Child* 1979;133:649–650.
57. Heird WC, Dell RB, Driscoll JM Jr, et al. Metabolic acidosis resulting from intravenous alimentation mixtures containing synthetic amino acids. *N Engl J Med* 1972;827:943–948.

58. Johnson JD, Albritton WL, Sunshine P. Hyperammonemia accompanying parenteral nutrition in newborn infants. *J Pediatr* 1972;81:154–161.
59. Heird WC, Nicholson JF, Driscoll JM Jr, et al. Hyperammonemia resulting from intravenous alimentation using a mixture of synthetic L-amino acids: a preliminary report. *J Pediatr* 1972;81:162–167.
60. Winters RW, Heird WC, Dell RB, et al. Plasma amino acids in infants receiving parenteral nutrition. In: Greene HL, Holliday MA, Munro HN, eds. *Clinical nutrition update: amino acids.* Chicago: American Medical Association, 1977;147–154.
61. Malloy MH, Rassin DK, Heird WC, Gaull GE. Plasma-cerebrum amino acid relationships during total parenteral nutrition (TPN). *Pediatr Res* 1979;13:404(abstract).
62. Merritt RJ. Cholestasis associated with total parenteral nutrition. *J Pediatr Gastroenterol Nutr* 1980;5:9–22.
63. Schreiner RL, Glick MR, Nordschow CD, et al. An evaluation of methods to monitor infants receiving intravenous lipids. *J Pediatr* 1979;94:197–200.
64. Kashyap S, Schulze KF, Forsyth M, et al. Growth, nutrient retention, and metabolic response in low birth weight infants fed varying intakes of protein and energy. *J Pediatr* 1988;113:713–721.
65. Heird WC, Kashyap S, Schulze KF, et al. Nutrient utilization and growth. In: Goldman A, Atkinson SA, Hanson LA, eds. *Human lactation 3: the effects of human milk on the recipient infant.* New York: Plenum Press, 1987;9–21.
66. Heird WC, Dell RB, Helms RA, et al. Amino acid mixture designed to maintain normal plasma amino acid patterns in infants and children requiring parenteral nutrition. *Pediatrics* 1987;80:401–408.
67. Sturman JA, Gaull GA, Räihä NCR. Absence of cystathionase in human liver: is cystine essential? *Science* 1970;169:74–76.
68. Zlotkin SH, Anderson GH. The development of cystathionase activity during the first year of life. *Pediatr Res* 1982;16:65–68.
69. Räihä NCR. Phenylalanine hydroxylase in human liver during development. *Pediatr Res* 1973;7:1–4.
70. Zlotkin SH, Bryan MH, Anderson GH. Cysteine supplementation to cysteine-free intravenous feeding regimens in newborn infants. *Am J Clin Nutr* 1981;34:914–923.
71. Malloy MH, Rassin DK, Richardson CJ. Total parenteral nutrition in sick preterm infants: effects of cysteine supplementation with nitrogen intakes of 240 & 400 mg/kg/d. *J Pediatr Gastroenterol Nutr* 1984;3:239–244.
72. Heird WC, Hay W, Helms RA, et al. Pediatric parenteral amino acid mixture in low birth weight infants. *Pediatrics* 1988;81:41–50.
73. Clandinin MT, Chappell JE, Heim PR, et al. Fatty acid utilization in perinatal de novo synthesis of tissues. *Early Hum Devel* 1981;5:355–366.
74. Friedman Z, Frolich JC. Essential fatty acids and the major urinary metabolites of the E prostaglandins in thriving neonates and in infants receiving parenteral fat emulsions. *Pediatr Res* 1979;13:926–932.
75. Clandinin MT, Chappell JE, Leong S, et al. Intrauterine fatty acid accretion rates in human brain: implications for fatty acid requirements. *Early Hum Devel* 1980;4:121–129.
76. Clandinin MT, Chappell JE, Leong S, et al. Extrauterine fatty acid accretion in infant brain: implications for fatty acid requirements. *Early Hum Devel* 1980;4:131–138.

CHAPTER 20

Enteral Support of the Hospitalized Child

George J. Fuchs III

The intestinal tract is the preferred route of nutritional support because it is considered to be more "physiologic," and because it obviates potential complications associated with parenterally delivered nutrition including infection, cholestasis, thrombosis, and significantly higher cost. In addition, unlike parenterally delivered nutrients, intraluminal nutrition results in the morphologic and functional recovery of the gastrointestinal tract (1–4). Pancreatic enzymes, intestinal mass, and disaccharidase activity are greater in animals receiving enteral, as opposed to parenteral, nutrition (5–8). Optimal maintenance and restoration of intestinal function results from the direct interface between nutrients and the intestinal lumen as well as from the effect of enteric hormones induced by enteral feedings (5,9). Many of the advantages of enteral alimentation may be due to nutrients and growth factors not present in parenteral solutions. The role of glutamine and short-chain fatty acids derived from dietary fiber are of particular current interest (10,11).

G. J. Fuchs III: Department of Pediatrics, Louisiana State University School of Medicine, New Orleans, Louisiana 70112.

INDICATIONS

The prevalence of secondary undernutrition in hospitalized children has highlighted the need for vigorous nutritional support. Merritt and Suskind (12) found that one-half of the children in a large children's hospital had evidence of acute or chronic protein-energy malnutrition. Several similar surveys in other urban hospitals have confirmed the extent of this as a major problem in children hospitalized for a variety of illnesses (Table 1). The great majority of these children are secondarily undernourished as a result of a specific underlying disorder (Table 2) (13). Although malnutrition is commonly the result of reduced food intake, abnormal nutrient losses, or increased requirements, inadequate intake sufficient to meet requirements is clearly the most frequent cause. Anorexia may accompany any severe medical or surgical illness. Iatrogenic reasons for inadequate nutrient intake such as prolonged nil per os (NPO) status for diagnostic testing or even the lack of recognition of nutritional needs unfortunately is often involved in the genesis of malnutrition during hospitalization.

The inability to tolerate oral feedings often results in a state of malnutrition. Problems that affect intake include esophageal strictures, esophagitis, and invasive carci-

TABLE 1. *Protein-energy malnutrition in hospitalized children*

Authors, year	% with acute protein-energy malnutrition	Weight or height criteria	Comments
Merritt and Suskind, 1979 (12)	36	<90% std	Patients > 3 months old
Parsons et al., 1980 (33)	12	<5th percentile	Upon admission
Cooper et al., 1981 (34)	54	<90% std	Neonate rate higher
Cooper and Heird, 1982 (35)	46	<90% std	Neonate rate higher
Pollack et al., 1982 (36)	39	<90% std	Intensive-care patients
Leleiko et al., 1986 (37)	12	<5th percentile	Upon admission

Adapted from ref. 30.
Std, standard.

TABLE 2. *Disease states often associated with protein-energy malnutrition in children*

> Low birth weight
> Short bowel syndrome
> Cystic fibrosis
> Mucosal disease
>   Celiac disease
>   Milk protein enteropathy
>   Infectious enteritis
>   Soy protein enteropathy
>   Tropical sprue
>   Allergic gastroenteritis
>   Intractable diarrhea
>   Immune deficiency disorders
> Chronic liver disease
> Inflammatory bowel disease
> Chronic renal disease
> Congenital heart disease
> Burns and trauma
> Anorexia nervosa
> Cancer

nomas, as well as an altered sensorium due to trauma, central nervous system tumors, or infections. Malnutrition may also result from the chronic, intermittent nausea and intractable vomiting associated with several disorders. A damaged intestinal mucosa that precipitates severe diarrhea and malabsorption, or the pancreatic insufficiency accompanying cystic fibrosis or Shwachman's disease may also lead to a malnourished state.

SELECTION OF CHILDREN TO RECEIVE ENTERAL NUTRITION

Most hospitalized children have a sufficiently intact and functional gastrointestinal tract that enables them to be fed enterally rather than requiring the parenteral route (Fig. 1). Proper nutritional assessment and monitoring of the pediatric patient will identify children presently undernourished or at risk of becoming malnourished and for whom nutritional support should be considered. It is essential that a system is institutionalized so that every child admitted to the hospital is evaluated and monitored. Simple anthropometric measurements are frequently overlooked allowing the malnourished child to go unrecognized. Specific nutrient deficiencies and requirements should be quantitated, an appropriate program instituted, and the response to the nutritional therapy serially monitored.

ROUTE OF ADMINISTRATION OF ENTERAL NUTRITION

If a child is able, oral feedings with a hypercaloric diet or a complex nutritional supplement such as Carnation Instant Breakfast, Ensure, Ensure Plus, or Sustecal is the obvious first choice. When this is not viable, "tube-feedings" may be indicated (Table 3). Nasoenteral feedings, in order of preference, are nasogastric, nasoduodenal, and nasojejunal placement of an enteral tube. Nasogastric feedings have the advantages of ease of placement and fewer complications as compared to transpyloric administration. Nasogastric feedings are considered to be more "physiologic," i.e., the antimicrobial and digestive properties of the stomach remain involved in the feeding process. Gastric acid is an essential component of the gastric barrier that prevents infection and overgrowth of the small bowel with enteropathogens and nonpathogens, respectively. The digestive properties of

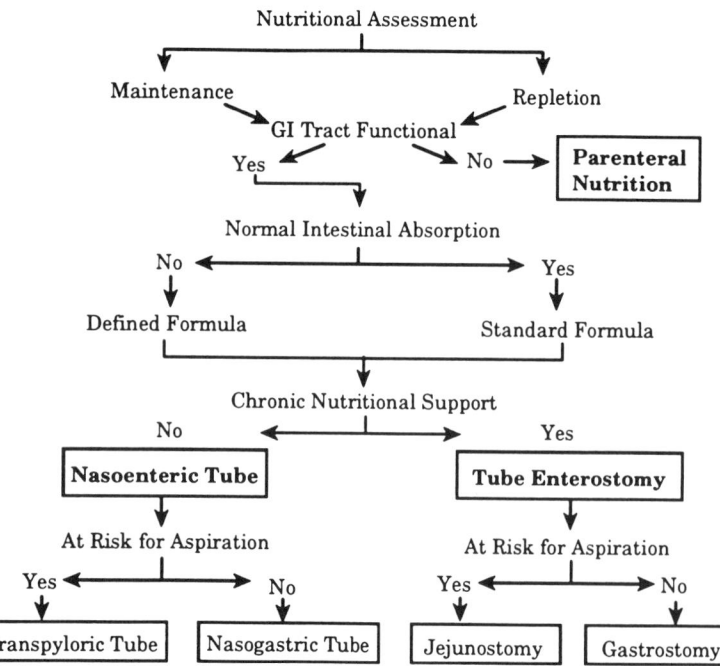

FIG. 1. Enteral nutrition algorithm.

TABLE 3. *Route of administration of enteral nutrition*

Nasoenteral
  Nasogastric
  Nasoduodenal
  Nasojejunal
Tube enterostomy
  Cervical pharyngostomy/esophagostomy
  Gastrostomy
  Jejunostomy

gastric acid and the grinding and mixing action of the stomach are also retained with nasogastric feedings (14). Similarly, the direct and indirect induction of pancreaticobiliary secretions and certain enteric hormones remain largely intact (5,6).

Transpyloric feedings are necessary in patients at unacceptable risk of aspiration (Table 4). Such patients, many of whom are institutionalized, include those with primary neuromuscular disorders or abnormalities secondary to psychomotor retardation involving mechanisms of normal glutination and swallowing. Normal gastric emptying is disrupted in several disease states resulting in intermittent vomiting and possible aspiration. Abnormal lower esophageal motility can be of sufficient severity as to cause reflux and aspiration of gastric contents. Unless there is structural gastric outlet obstruction, or functional or structural intestinal obstruction, a prokinetic agent such as metoclopramide or cisapride can be given and the tube allowed to be carried into the small bowel with peristaltic activity. Patients should be carefully selected to receive transpyloric rather than nasogastric feedings since nasoduodenal and nasojejunal feedings have specific disadvantages. A transpyloric feeding tube is frequently more difficult to establish, particularly in those children with functional or structural gastric outlet obstruction. When this occurs, placement with simultaneous fluoroscopic monitoring is attempted, resulting in additional cost and radiation exposure. Inadvertent removal of the feeding tube or expulsion by forceful regurgitation is not infrequent and requires tube replacement. Nasojejunal, and to a lesser extent nasoduodenal, tube feedings may need to be administered continuously or a therapeutic formula utilized depending on the absorptive capacity of the intestine. This significantly increases the cost because of the need for an infusion pump and/or specialized formulas.

TABLE 4. *Indications for transpyloric feedings*

Abnormal swallowing mechanism
Comatose patient
Delayed gastric emptying
Incompetent lower esophageal sphincter
Intractable vomiting

ENTEROSTOMY FEEDINGS

Enterostomy tube feedings are indicated when chronic use of the nasoenteral route precipitates pharyngeal irritation and discomfort, and an increased risk for aspiration. The various types of enterostomy feedings include cervical pharyngostomy/esophagostomy, gastric, or jejunal placement. In practice, it is rare that cervical pharyngostomy/esophagostomy is desirable or necessary. Many of the advantages and disadvantages of nasogastric versus transpyloric feedings are relevant when considering the need for gastrostomy versus enterostomy (Table 5). The delivery of nutrients to the stomach via gastrostomy simulates normal feeding in much the same manner as the nasogastric route. An intermittent bolus feeding regimen is usually more successful with gastric feedings than jejunal feedings, obviating the need for costly infusion pumps and specialized formulas. If necessary, it is possible to convert a gastrostomy tube to a transpyloric enterostomy without the use of anesthesia. The advent of percutaneous endoscopic gastrostomy (PEG) tube placement reduces the cost and postoperative morbidity of the procedure when compared to surgical placement (15,16). A PEG can be placed at the bedside or endoscopy suite with intravenous sedation, or in the surgical suite with general anesthesia in the case of younger, uncooperative children. Compared to surgical placement, recovery from the PEG procedure is much faster, and feedings are introduced sooner. With the more commonly used techniques, surgical placement of gastrostomy tubes causes gastroesophageal reflux in as many as 60% of children, resulting in the usual practice of performing a concomitant antireflux procedure with its attendant perioperative risk and potential for postoperative complications (17,18). It is encouraging that the PEG does not appear to cause gastroesophageal reflux, although further study is needed to confirm this impres-

TABLE 5. *Enterostomy feedings*

Type	Possible advantages	Possible disadvantages
Gastrostomy	Simulates normal feeding	Aspiration
	Intermittent bolus regimen	Gastroesophageal reflux
	Percutaneous endoscopic placement	Dumping syndrome
	Conversion to transpyloric route	
Jejunostomy	Decreased risk of aspiration	General anesthesia
		Continuous infusion
		Tube occlusion
		Specialized formula

sion. Disadvantages of a gastrostomy tube include the risk of aspiration if gastroesophageal reflux is coexistent and unrecognized or develops postoperatively. This concern is particularly relevant when a simultaneous antireflux procedure is not routine. The dumping syndrome rarely occurs as the result of gastrostomy tube placement alone, but generally occurs within the context of a concomitant antireflux procedure. Jejunostomy tube placement has the advantage of minimizing the risk of aspiration, but usually requires the use of general anesthesia for placement and the use of costly therapeutic formulas. As previously discussed, jejunal feeds are provided by continuous rather than bolus administration to prevent inducing diarrhea and malabsorption. The internal diameter of jejunostomy tubes is significantly narrower than gastrostomy tubes and the tubes are therefore prone to occlusion by the formula or medicine infusate. When this occurs, reoperation is necessary.

SELECTION OF FORMULA FOR ENTERAL FEEDINGS

With the vast array of commercially available formulas, selection of the most appropriate formula is based on a child's individual requirements and underlying physiology or pathophysiology. Diet formulations are often designated as "infant" or "adult" (Appendix 1 and 2). Infant formulas are generally reserved for children less than 1 year of age. Specialized infant and adult formulas exist in a variety of formulations including those for children with unique requirements resulting from specific illnesses. Polymeric formulas that contain whole protein and complex carbohydrates are recommended for children with intact intestinal, biliary, and pancreatic function (Table 6). The fat of polymeric formulas is partly or entirely long-chain triglycerides (LCT). Home-prepared blenderized diets, although less expensive, are less preferable because of longer preparation time, greater risk of tube occlusion due to greater viscosity, and a higher incidence of diarrhea that may result from contamination (19–21).

The term *elemental diet* signifies a "predigested" formula containing amino acids, glucose, and a low fat content in the form of medium-chain triglycerides (MCT). Elemental formulas contain protein, carbohydrates, fats, additives, vitamins, and minerals in their most elemental and easily absorbable form. Most contain protein hydrolyzed to amino acids or peptides, minimally complex carbohydrates in the form of short-chain polymers of glucose or disaccharides other than lactose, and MCT alone or combined with essential fatty acids or a small quantity of LCT. On occasion, commercial formulas fail to meet the special needs of certain infants and, less often, certain older children. Modular components are available in such cases to construct "designer" formulas (Appendix 3).

TABLE 6. *Categorization of enteral diets*

Polymeric diets	Whole protein nitrogen source and complex carbohydrate for use in children with normal or near-normal gastrointestinal function
Chemically defined elemental diets	Predigested nutrients: most diets have lower fat content often with partial MCT fat source for use in children with impaired gastrointestinal function
Specially formulated predigested diets	
Cirrhosis	Amino acid nitrogen source
Portosystemic encephalopathy	High concentration branched-chain amino acids, low concentrations aromatic amino acids; indication still disputed
Stress	Amino acid nitrogen source High concentration branched-chain amino acids may contain more than 1 Cal/ml energy; indications still disputed

Adapted from ref. 31.
MCT, medium-chain triglycerides.

ADMINISTRATION OF ENTERAL NUTRITION

A polyurethane tube is preferable because it is pliable, relatively long-lasting, and has the greatest internal to external diameter (Table 7). There are several approaches to initiate feedings, many of which are based on strong feelings rather than rationale. In children who are closely monitored and who are not nutritionally unstable, it is reasonable to select an appropriate formula and to administer 100% of the therapeutic goal via continuous or intermittent feedings. This method is generally well tolerated and is preferable to the "graded" feeding approach of gradually increasing the concentration and/

TABLE 7. *Feeding tubes for delivery of enteral nutrition*

Tube	Advantages	Disadvantages
Polyvinylchloride (PVC)	Rigidity makes PVC easier to place, less likely to collapse with vigorous aspiration	Rigidity increases risk of perforation; should be changed every 3 days
Silicone (Sialastic)	Remains pliable, less patient discomfort	For equivalent external diameter, silicone has a smaller internal diameter than polyurethane
Polyurethane	Remains pliable, less patient discomfort	

or volume of the formula over several hours or days. It is the fastest and most direct way to determine the need for supplemental parenteral nutrition and often shortens the hospital stay by days. Further, graded feedings may unnecessarily delay the provision of adequate nutrition. There is little physiologic basis for the notion that graded feedings induce tolerance to a formula over the relatively brief time commonly employed by advocates of this method. However, when children are intolerant to a formula, graded feeding or a combination of enteral and parenteral nutrition may be required until tolerance to total enteral nutrition is achieved. Keohane et al. (22) compared graded feeding (concentration increased over a 4-day period) to "full-strength" (430 mmol/kg) feeding. No difference was noted in frequency of nausea, bloating, or abdominal cramps. However, individuals receiving the graded feeding regimen had more diarrhea. Nitrogen intake and absorption were greater in the individuals receiving full-strength feedings.

Intermittent feedings are generally preferred as they are considered to simulate normal feeding better than continuous feeding, are considerably less expensive as they avoid the need for feeding pump, and allow the patient more mobility since the child is not tethered to a pump. Continuous feedings are required and offer definite advantages in instances of severe intestinal disease or when the feedings are directly delivered to the small intestine to avoid "dumping." Parker et al. (23) demonstrated improved absorption of fat, nitrogen, calcium, zinc, and copper with continuous compared to intermittent feedings in children with severe intestinal disease. Further, body weight was significantly greater during the period of continuous feedings as compared to the period of intermittent bolus feedings.

ASSESSMENT OF ENTERAL FEEDINGS

Regular monitoring of anthropometric measurements, biochemical indices, and specific nutrients are important for children on therapeutic enteral nutrition. Serial weights help assess progress toward the goal weight, and provide information on fluid intake and hydration status.

Tolerance to an enteral feeding regimen is determined by the presence or absence of nausea, vomiting, abdominal cramping, or diarrhea. The routine practice of determination of gastric aspirate volumes to guide the rate and volume of the administration of the formula has many advocates but is not based on objective proof of efficacy. This practice often results in insufficient delivery or premature cessation of feedings. The assumption that a specific gastric volume at a specific time after a feeding is normal or abnormal disregards the multiple variables that determine effective gastric emptying including lower esophageal sphincter pressure, inherent gastric motility, and intragastric pressure. Examining the gastric "residual" is useful if a patient experiences abdominal distention, respiratory difficulties, or retching in order to determine the possible relationship to delayed gastric emptying. Close observation of the patient for these signs and a subsequent appropriate response generally avoids problematic regurgitation. Stool characteristics often relate to the type of formula being utilized, so it is worthwhile to carefully define diarrhea. A stool volume less than 15 to 20 cc/kg/day and the absence of stool-reducing sugars or fat on microscopic examination are indicative of normal stool and the absence of carbohydrate or fat malabsorption, respectively, regardless of the frequency, consistency, or color of the stool output.

COMPLICATIONS OF ENTERAL NUTRITION

Cataldi-Betcher et al. (24) examined the frequency and nature of complications associated with various enteral feedings delivered by a variety of routes in 253 hospitalized patients. Although complications were rare, diarrhea, vomiting, and occlusion of the feeding tube were the most frequent (Table 8). Diarrhea in such patients is usually not directly related to the feeding but rather associated with specific medications taken concurrently (25,35). Medications with a known laxative effect such as magnesium hydroxide antacids and those that contain sorbitol are often the cause of diarrheal stool. Many patients are often also receiving antibiotics in which case the diarrheal stool must be examined for evidence of *Clostridium difficile* as well as other enteric pathogens

TABLE 8. *Complications of enteral nutrition*

Complication	% of patients	% of total complications
Enteral		
Vomiting	1.5	13.3
Diarrhea	2.3	20.0
GI bleed	0.8	6.6
Mechanical		
Aspiration	0.8	6.6
Occlusion	1.6	13.3
Metabolic		
Hypokalemia	0.4	3.3
Hyperkalemia	0.8	6.6

Modified from ref. 24.

TABLE 10. *Vomiting*

Cause	Response
Intraesophageal placement of nasogastric tube	Avoid by documenting proper tube placement radiographically
Mechanical obstruction (prolapse of G-tube, gastritis/ulcer, etc.)	Evaluate radiographically, retract and secure tube, medical therapy
Functionally delayed gastric emptying	Continuous infusion, metoclopramide, reduce fat content of formula, reduce caloric density of formula, transpyloric EN

(Table 9). A recent investigation demonstrated an association of antibiotic-associated diarrhea with a high concentration of *Candida* in the stool (26). The diarrhea resolved with clearance of *Candida* from the stool upon withdrawal of the antibiotic or with the oral administration of an antifungal agent. The susceptibility of blenderized feedings to bacterial contamination simulating the diarrhea of small bowel bacterial overgrowth highlights the advantage of the well-designed commercial formulas.

MCT or LCT, often added to a formula to increase its energy concentration, has a tendency to separate and to be unintentionally administered as a bolus. A large bolus of lipid may overwhelm the absorptive capacity of the intestine, resulting in diarrhea in much the same fashion as a dose of mineral oil. Utilizing small volumes of the formula/lipid mixture during continuous feedings, decreasing the concentration of lipid, or adding an emulsifier usually remedies this problem. Unrecognized disorders of the small bowel, liver, or pancreas may result in carbohydrate or fat malabsorption. Once identified, continuous rather than intermittent infusion of the original formula may be helpful or, alternatively, a more appropriate formula should be selected depending upon the specific malabsorptive disorder and offending nutrient. When diarrhea is not attributable to any of the factors outlined above, addition of dietary fiber to the feeding may be useful (11).

Vomiting often occurs as the result of misplacement of the nasogastric feeding tube into the esophagus (27). Alternatively, vomiting may have its origin in mechanical obstruction of the gastric outlet due to edema and spasm of a stress-related or peptic ulcer or gastritis (Table 10). The possibility of intra-abdominal adhesions needs to be considered in those patients with previous abdominal surgery. The use of contemporary gastrostomy tubes avoids the complication of prolapse and gastric outlet obstruction known to occur with the balloon Foley-type catheter/tube. Vomiting due to gastric dysmotility may respond to the use of continuous rather than bolus feedings. Reducing nutrients that contribute to delayed gas-

TABLE 9. *Diarrhea*

Cause	Comments	Response
Concomitant antibiotics	Commonly associated with diarrhea in patients receiving EN, mechanism unknown (*Candida*?)	Modify antibiotic regimen (*Lactobacillus*?)
Bacterial contamination of formula	Associated with blenderized feedings or large volumes of formula hanging at room temperature	Use commercial formulas, hang smaller volumes, change or clean infusion set regularly
Enteric infection	Stool C + S, WBC, occult blood, O + P, *C. difficile* toxin	Depends on etiology
Bolus administration of supplemental lipid	Observe formula for separation of lipid fraction	Add emulsifier (Tween 80)
	Diarrhea stools occur at completion of EN container	Reduce volume of supplemental lipid
Malabsorption		
Carbohydrate	Stool RS ± hydrolysis	Continuous infusion of formula, substitute or restrict causitive nutrient, TPN in refractory cases
Fat	Stool pH, breath hydrogen test Stool microscopy, balance study	

C + S, culture and sensitivity; EN, enteral nutrition; O + P, ova and parasites; RS, reducing substances; TPN, total parenteral nutrition.

TABLE 11. *Complications of enterostomy tubes*

Wound infection or dehiscence
Intestinal obstruction
Leakage of gastric contents
Inadvertent tube removal
Occlusion of jejunal tube

---

tric emptying such as hypercaloric or hyperosmolar formulas and formulas high in fat concentration is often helpful. In the absence of mechanical obstruction, a prokinetic agent such as metoclopramide to enhance gastric emptying should be administered or, alternatively, in children not responsive to conservative measures, transpyloric feedings should be used. The potentially life-threatening complication of aspiration of regurgitated gastric contents is an absolute indication for transpyloric feeding or, if necessary, parenteral nutrition.

Feeding tubes, particularly smaller-bore jejunal tubes, should be routinely irrigated and highly viscous medications should be avoided to prevent tube occlusion. Nasogastric feeding is commonplace because of the ease of placement and improved patient acceptability of the pliable and durable polyurethane enteric feeding tubes. However, children who are uncooperative or have anatomic abnormalities, impaired consciousness or paralysis, endotracheal intubation or tracheostomy are at a defined risk for tube misplacement capable of disastrous consequences (28). Complications including pneumothorax, intrapulmonary feeding, abscess, or empyema, and death from intrapulmonary placement of nasoenteric feeding tubes have been estimated to occur in approximately 0.3% of adult patients (29). Direct visualization using laryngoscopy, endoscopy, or fluoroscopic guidance will ensure proper placement. However, pre- and postplacement anteroposterior chest radiographs following the usual "blind" placement are equally reliable, safer, and easily obtained at the bedside. Insufflation of air and auscultation over the midepigastrium is commonly employed to confirm tube position, but can be misleading.

Children with enterostomy tubes are at risk for additional complications (Table 11). Wound infection or dehiscence may complicate the immediate postoperative period, whereas leakage of gastric contents around a gastrostomy tube or intestinal obstruction from adhesions or as the result of prolapse of the Foley-type tube occurs later. Inadvertent tube removal is particularly problematic with nasojejunal tubes or jejunostomies because of the additional effort and exposure to radiation or surgical replacement, respectively. The smaller-bore jejunostomy tubes often become occluded.

Severe constipation and fecal impaction from inactivity or depression, decreased colonic motility, a deficiency of dietary fiber, or specific medications are common complaints with chronic enteral tube nutrition. They may be avoided by eliminating medications known to predispose to constipation and by the use of formulas containing fiber. A stool softener such as lactulose titrated to induce the desired stool volume and frequency may be required in refractory children. The chronic use of laxatives is rarely necessary and is best avoided.

CONCLUSION

Enterally provided nutrition is unquestionably the preferred method of nutrition support. With the accumulation of shared experience and the introduction of advanced formulas, equipment, and techniques, enteral nutrition is now indicated in most children who previously required total intravenous nutrition. Careful consideration, application of the knowledge and available tools, and recognition of potential complications enable most children to be nutritionally supported with the exclusive or partial use of enteral nutrition.

REFERENCES

1. Feldman EJ, Dowling RH, McNaughton J, Peters TJ. Effects of oral vs intravenous nutrition on intestinal adaptation after small bowel resection in the dog. *Gastroenterology* 1976;70:712–719.
2. Levine GM, Deren JJ, Yezdimir E. Small bowel resection: oral intake is the stimulus for hyperplasia. *Am J Digest Dis* 1976;21:542–546.
3. Eastwood GL. Small bowel morphology and epithelial proliferation in intravenously alimented rabbits. *Surgery* 1977;82:613–620.
4. Weser E, Vandeventer A, Tawil T. Stimulation of small bowel mucosal growth by midgut infusion of different sugars in rats maintained by total parenteral nutrition. *J Pediatr Gastroenterol Nutr* 1982;1:411–416.
5. Johnson LR. Regulation of gastrointestinal growth. In: Johnson LR, ed. *Physiology of the gastrointestinal tract,* 2nd ed. New York: Raven Press, 1987;301–334.
6. Johnson LR, Schanbacher LM, Dudrick SJ, Copeland EM. Effect of long-term parenteral feeding on pancreatic secretion and serum secretin. *Am J Physiol* 1977;233:E524–E529.
7. Levine GM, Deren JJ, Steiger E, Zinno R. Role of oral intake in maintenance of gut mass and disaccharidase activity. *Gastroenterology* 1974;67:975–982.
8. Morin CL, Ling V, Van Caillie M. Role of oral intake on intestinal adaptation after small bowel resection in growing rats. *Pediatr Res* 1978;12:268–271.
9. Johnson LR, Copeland EM, Dudrick SJ, Lighten Berger, LM, Castro GA, et al. Structural and hormonal alterations in the gastrointestinal tract of parenterally fed rats. *Gastroenterology* 1975;68:1177–1183.
10. Proceedings of an international glutamine symposium. Glutamine metabolism in health and disease-basic science and clinical aspects. *JPEN J Parenter Enteral Nutr* 1990;14(suppl):39S–146S.
11. Palacio JC, Rombeau JL. Dietary fiber. A brief review and potential application to enteral nutrition. *Nutr Clin Pract* 1990;5:99–106.
12. Merritt RJ, Suskind RM. Nutritional survey of hospitalized pediatric patients. *Am J Clin Nutr* 1979;32:1320–1325.
13. Fuchs GJ. Secondary malnutrition in children. In: Suskind R, Suskind L, eds. *The malnourished child.* New York: Raven Press, 1990;23–36.
14. Thor PJ, Copeland EM, Dudrick SJ, Johnson, LR, et al. Effect of long-term parenteral feeding on gastric secretion in dogs. *Am J Physiol* 1977;232:E39–E43.

15. Gauderer MW, Stellato TA. Percutaneous endoscopic gastrostomy in children: the technique in detail. *Pediatr Surg Int* 1991;6:82–87.
16. Benkov KJ, Kazlow PG, Waye JD, Leleiko NS. Percutaneous endoscopic gastrostomies in children. *Pediatrics* 1986;77:248–250.
17. Flake AW, Shopene C, Ziegler MM. Anti-reflux gastrointestinal surgery in the neurologically handicapped child. *Pediatr Surg Int* 1991;6:92–94.
18. Jolley JG, Tunell WP, Hoelzer DJ, Thomas S, Smith EI. Lower esophageal pressure changes with tube gastrostomy: a causative factor of gastroesophageal reflux in children? *J Pediatr Surg* 1986;21:624–627.
19. Casewell MW. Nasogastric feeds as a source of Klebsiella infection for intensive care patients. *Research and Clinical Forums* 1979;1:101–105.
20. Keighley MRB, Mogg B, Beatley S, Allan C. "Home brew" compared with commercial preparations for enteral feeding. *Br Med J* 1982;284:163.
21. Moore MC, Greene HL. Tube feeding of infants and children. *Pediatr Clin North Am* 1985;32:401–417.
22. Keohane PP, Attrill H, Love M, Frost P, Silk DBA. Relation between osmolality of diet and gastrointestinal side effects in enteral nutrition. *Br Med J* 1984;288:678–680.
23. Parker P, Stroop S, Greene H. A controlled comparison of continuous versus intermittent feeding in the treatment of infants with intestinal disease. *J Pediatr* 1981;99:360–364.
24. Cataldi-Betcher EL, Seltzer MH, Slocum BA, Jones KW, et al. Complications occurring during external nutrition support: A prospective study. *JPEN J Parenter Enteral Nutr* 1983 Nov-Dec; 7(6):546–552.
25. Edes TE, Walk BE, Austin JL. Diarrhea in tube-fed patients: feeding formula not necessarily the cause. *Am J Med* 1990;88:91–93.
26. Danna PL, Urban C, Bellin E, Rahal JJ. Role of candida in pathogenesis of antibiotic-associated diarrhoea in elderly inpatients. *Lancet* 1991;337:511–514.
27. Benya R, Langer S, Mobarhan S. Flexible nasogastric feeding tube tip malposition immediately after placement. *JPEN J Parenter Enteral Nutr* 1990;14:108–109.
28. Broughton WA, Green AE, Hall MW, Bass JB. The technique of placing a nasoenteric tube. *J Crit Illness* 1990;5:1101–1105.
29. Roubenoff R, Ravich WJ. The technique of avoiding feeding tube misplacement. *J Crit Illness* 1989;4:75–79.
30. Merritt RJ. Enteral feeding: who needs support? In: Balistreri WF, Farrell MR, eds. *Enteral feeding: scientific basis and clinical applications*. Report of the 94th Ross Conference on Pediatric Research. Columbus, OH: Ross Laboratories, 1988.
31. Silk DBA. Diet formulation and choice of enteral diet. *Gut* 1986;27:40–46.
32. Greene MG, ed. The Harriet Lane handbook, 12th ed. St. Louis: Mosby, 1991.
33. Parsons HG, Francoeur TE, Howland P, Spengler RF, et al. The nutritional status of hospitalized children. *Am J Clin Nutr* 1980;33:1140–1146.
34. Cooper A, Jakobowski D, Spiker J, Floyd T, et al. Nutritional assessment: an integral part of the preoperative pediatric surgical evaluation. *J Pediatr Surg* 1981;16:554–560.
35. Cooper A, Heird WC. Nutritional assessment of the pediatric patient including the low-birthweight infant. *Am J Clin Nutr* 1982;35:1132–1141.
36. Pollack MM, Wiley JS, Kauter R, Holbrook PR, Malnutrition in critically ill infants and children. *JPEN* 1982;6:20–24.
37. LeLeiko NS, Luder E, Friedman M, Fersel J, Benkov K. Nutritional assessment of pediatric patients admitted to an acute-care pediatric service utilizing anthropometric measurements. *JPEN* 1986;10:166–168.

CHAPTER 21

Nutrient-Drug Interactions in Children

Mark J. S. Miller

GENERAL DESCRIPTION OF DRUG-INDUCED ALTERATIONS IN NUTRITIONAL STATUS

Diagnosis of Drug-Induced Malnutrition

It is common to experience great difficulty in determining if a specific drug therapy is the cause of malnutrition. As a general guideline the following approach is useful. There should be an immediately antecedent or current history of drug intake. However, it should be recognized that nutritional deficiencies are slow in onset as tissue stores can often match unmet dietary intake. Thus, it is common for drug therapy to be chronic in nature (1). Single or multiple hypovitaminoses are the most common problems, particularly deficiencies in B vitamins, in part because of their lower tissue stores. To avoid merely inferring that a nutritional deficiency is associated with drug administration it is advisable, where possible, to demonstrate causality, e.g., to determine if drug withdrawal reverses the clinical findings (2).

Effects on Nutrient Synthesis

In addition to dietary intake, nutrients can be synthesized within the distal alimentary canal by enteric bacteria, e.g., vitamin K. Modification of gut flora number and/or function by broad spectrum antibiotics may impair systemic vitamin K levels by reducing vitamin K production by enteric flora (3). Another example is small-chain fatty acids, which are produced by colonic flora from dietary substrates that have not been metabolized by the small intestine. These organic acids are utilized as a source of energy by the colonic mucosa. Broad-spectrum antibiotics would also limit this source of nutrition, although there is little evidence that the colonic mucosa is subsequently compromised.

Nutrient Absorption

Drugs may impair nutrient absorption by directly binding the nutrient within the alimentary canal (Table 1). The subsequent prevention of the nutrient absorption will lead to enhanced fecal excretion and reduced bioavailability. Through solubility characteristics, drugs or their vehicles/solvents may modify nutrient absorption by modifying their intraluminal disposition. Carotene, for example, is highly soluble in mineral oil. Co-consumption of carotene with mineral oil may limit carotene bioavailability.

This effect on nutrient solubility may be evident if a drug alters the function of the exocrine pancreas or bile secretion in response to food ingestion. As a result of impaired pancreatic or bile acid coordination fat, carbohydrate and protein digestion and absorption may be compromised (4). Drugs may also impair intestinal transport processes for specific nutrients, which may lead to inadequate nutrient absorption.

Effects on Nutrient Distribution and Excretion

Once a nutrient is absorbed, it is still susceptible to altered disposition and utilization in the presence of drugs. Nutrients that are highly bound to plasma proteins or tissue binding sites are susceptible to direct competition for these binding sites by drugs, which can lead to nutrient displacement and increased nutrient metabolism/excretion. Examples of this are the interactions between salicylates and folate for plasma proteins (3).

Drugs may also form direct complexes with circulating nutrients, e.g., the formation of Schiff bases between vitamin antagonists and vitamin B_6 and folate. The re-

---

M. J. S. Miller: Department of Pediatrics, Louisiana State University School of Medicine, New Orleans, Louisiana 70112.

TABLE 1. Primary intestinal absorptive defects induced by drugs

Drug	Usage	Malabsorption of fecal nutrient loss	Mechanism
Mineral oil	Laxative	Carotene, Vitamins A, D, K	Physical barrier
			Nutrients dissolve in mineral oil and are lost
			Micelle formation ↓
Phenolphthalein	Laxative	Vitamin D, Ca	Intestinal hurry
			K depletion
			Loss of structural integrity
Neomycin	Antibiotic to "sterilize" gut	Fat, nitrogen, Na, K, Ca, Fe, lactose, sucrose, vitamin B_{12}	Structural defect
			Pancreatic lipase ↓
			Binding of bile acids (salts)
Cholestyramine	Hypocholesterolemic agent Bile acid sequestrant	Fat, vitamins A, K, B_{12}, D, Fe	Binding of bile acids (salts) and nutrients, e.g. Fe
Potassium chloride	Potassium repletion	Vitamin B_{12}	Ileal pH ↓
Colchicine	Anti-inflammatory agent in gout	Fat, carotene, Na, K, Vitamin B_{12}, lactose	Mitotic arrest
			Structural defect
			Enzyme damage
Biguanides Metformin, phenformin	Hypoglycemic agents (in diabetes)	Vitamin B_{12}	Competitive inhibition of B_{12} absorption
p-Aminosalicylic acid	Antituberculosis agent	Fat, folate, vitamin B_{12}	Mucosal block in B_{12} uptake
Sulfasalazine (Azulfidine)	Anti-inflammatory agent in ulcerative colitis, and regional enteritis	Folate	Mucosal block in folate uptake
			Folate antagonist
Sodium bicarbonate	Antacid	Folate	Inhibition gastric acid secretion
Cimetidine	H_2 receptor antagonist	Vitamin B_{12} (protein-bound)	

sulting complexes lead to a hyperexcretion of these nutrients in the urine and with prolonged administration, nutrient depletion. Increased nutrient excretion may occur via the feces, particularly with drug-induced intestinal damage, e.g., iron loss with neomycin or nonsteroidal and steroidal anti-inflammatory drugs. Deleterious effects of drugs on intestinal mucosal integrity may also impair the nutrient absorptive properties of the intestine.

Effects on Nutrient Metabolism

Drugs that act as vitamin antagonists (Table 2) may result in marked effects in children, resembling vitamin deficiency. These drugs have a marked diversity of therapeutic applications, and deleterious side effects can be largely negated by vitamin supplementation. Enzymes that regulate the levels of active forms of nutrients are target sites for drug interactions. Hepatic cytochrome P-450 mixed-function oxidase systems are of particular importance.

Effects on Appetite

Nutrient delivery may be influenced by drugs that modify appetite (5). These drug-induced effects on appetite may reflect central and peripheral actions and, in some cases, may affect taste acuity (Table 3).

Drugs that decrease appetite may have central actions leading to nausea and vomiting. These effects may reflect toxic effects of the therapeutic agents.

Drugs that cause sedation (alcohol, central-acting antihypertensives) may also attenuate appetite. Drugs that suppress appetite through peripheral effects predominantly influence gastrointestinal function, e.g., bulking agents that cause gastric distention, laxatives that may

TABLE 2. Drugs that are vitamin antagonists

Folate (folacin) antagonists	Methotrexate
	Pyrimethamine
	Triamterene
	Trimethoprim
	Pentamidine isethionate
	Sulfasalazine
	Triazinate
Vitamin B_6 antagonists	Isoniazid
	Hydralazine
	Cycloserine
	Levodopa
	Penicillamine
Riboflavin antagonist	Boric acid
Vitamin B_{12} antagonist	Nitrous oxide
Vitamin K antagonists	Coumarin anticoagulants
	Cephalosporin antibiotics
Vitamin D antagonists	Isoniazid
	Phenytoin
	Phenobarbital

TABLE 3. *Drugs affecting appetite and food intake*

Drugs that may decrease appetite	Drugs that may increase appetite	Drugs that may impair taste or taste acuity
Alcohol	Anabolic steroids	Antineoplastic agents
Aluminum hydroxide (antacid)	Benzodiazepines	Captopril
Amphetamines and various sympathomimetics	Cyproheptadine	Clofibrate
Antihypertensive agents	Glucocorticoids	Griseofulvin
Clonidine	Insulin	Lincomycin
Guanabenz	Oral contraceptives	Lithium
Methyldopa	Phenothiazines (psychotic patients)	Metronidazole
Antineoplastic agents	Sulfonylureas	Penicillamine
Bulk-forming agents (methylcellulose)	Tricyclic antidepressants (especially in newly treated depressed patients)	Phenytoin
Colchicine		Potassium iodide and bromide-containing medications
Digitalis glycosides		
Penicillamine		
Estrogens		
Furosemide and other loop diuretics		
Hydralazine		
Isoniazid		
Methotrexate		
Mineral oil (laxative)		
Pyrimethamine		
Spironolactone		
Sulfasalazine		
Thiazide diuretics		

cause intestinal hurry, or other agents that may cause gastrointestinal injury, cramping, and discomfort. Some drugs may enhance appetite, with insulin and corticosteroids being common examples. Appetite may also be influenced by drugs that modify taste sensation or acuity (Table 3).

DRUG-VITAMIN INTERACTIONS

Water-Soluble Vitamins

Intestinal absorption of folate is subject to drug inhibition at several levels. Drugs may inhibit the activity of

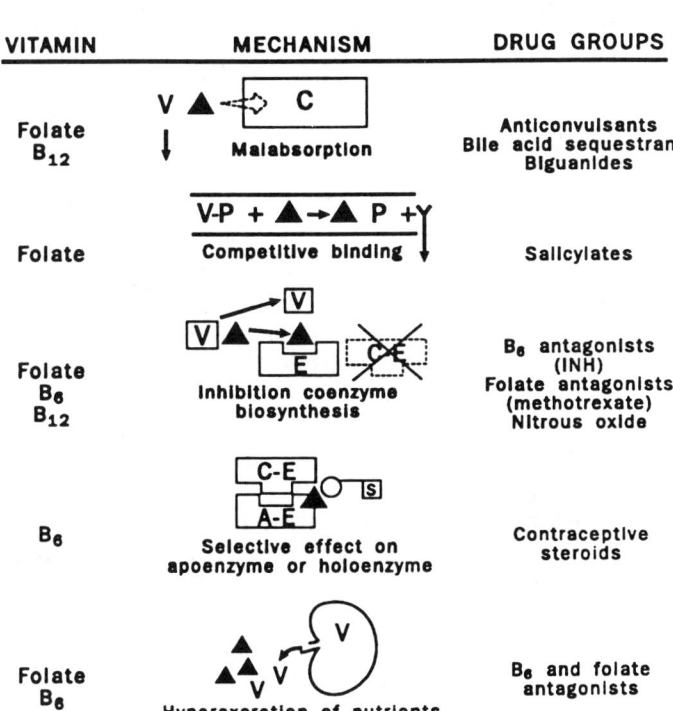

FIG. 1. Mechanisms for drug-induced depletion of vitamin B_6, folate, and vitamin B_{12}. V, vitamin; P, plasma protein; C-E, co-enzyme; ▲, drug; C, cell; E, activating enzyme; A-E, apoenzyme; S, substrate. (Adapted from ref. 3.)

folate conjugase, which is responsible for converting pteroylheptaglutamate and other pteroylpolyglutamates to pteroylmonoglutamate, which is the form of folate that is readily absorbed. Drugs that alter luminal pH may affect folate solubility, as well as direct interactions with intestinal binding and transport processes (3). Drugs that modify reduction and methylation pathways in the intestine can affect folate redistribution to systemic sites. In children, the drugs of greatest concern to folate absorption are sulfasalazine and diphenylhydantoin.

Acute folate deficiency with severe reactions accompany the administration of folate antagonists, e.g., methotrexate, triamterene, pyrimethamine, pentamidine, and sulfasalazine. Folate supplementation can minimize these reactions for the course of the drug therapy.

Vitamin B_{12} absorption can be impaired by drugs that bind to intrinsic factor and by agents that limit gastric acid output (H_2 antagonists, proton pump inhibitors). Agents like cholestyramine and neomycin may precipitate the vitamin B_{12}–intrinsic factor complex within the intestinal lumen, leading to excessive excretion in the feces. Neomycin as well as a number of other drugs (Fig. 1) may impair the intestinal absorption of vitamin B_{12} as a result of epithelial damage. Vitamin B_6 levels are most commonly influenced by hydrazide drugs, as they form Schiff bases with pyridoxal phosphate and the complex is excreted in the urine (Fig. 2).

Flavin absorption can be impaired by agents that increase intestinal propulsion (thyroxine, cathartics) in the proximal small intestine, the major site of riboflavin and

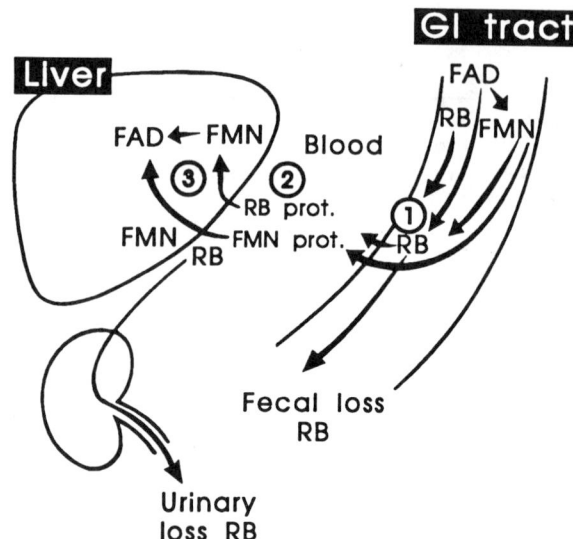

FIG. 3. Flavin absorption, transport, biotransformation, and excretion. Sites of drug interaction: (1) absorption: thyroxine, cathartics; (2) dissociation from plasma proteins: boric acid; (3) coenzyme biosynthesis: alcohol. (Adapted from ref. 3.)

flavin mononucleotide (FMN) absorption. In this situation, "intestinal hurry" through this specific region of absorption will promote riboflavin excretion in the feces (Fig. 3).

Riboflavin and FMN are transported in the portal venous system bound to plasma proteins. This binding may be inhibited by boric acid ingestion, which will then lead to excessive urinary loss of riboflavin; the nonbound form is readily cleared from the circulation by the kidneys. Alcoholic cirrhosis of the liver is associated with impaired hepatic coenzyme synthesis and flavin adenine dinucleotide (FAD) formation.

Fat-Soluble Vitamins

To obtain sufficient amounts of the fat-soluble vitamins (A, D, and K) from dietary sources, the function of the pancreaticobiliary system and small intestine must be intact and coordinated (Figs. 3 and 4). The most common site of drug-induced complications involves interactions with bile acids (3). Bile acid sequestrants (cholestyramine, colestipol) can cause deficiencies in vitamin A, D, and K by limiting their solubility and, hence, absorption. These complications are readily overcome with vitamin supplements (Fig. 4).

Neomycin has significant effects on vitamin K levels by impairing epithelial absorption as well as vitamin K production by intestinal flora. Vitamin A and carotene deficiency along with vitamin K may be affected by neomycin-induced fatty acid precipitation and impairment of micellular solubilization (Fig. 5).

Mineral oil may promote the excretion of fat-soluble

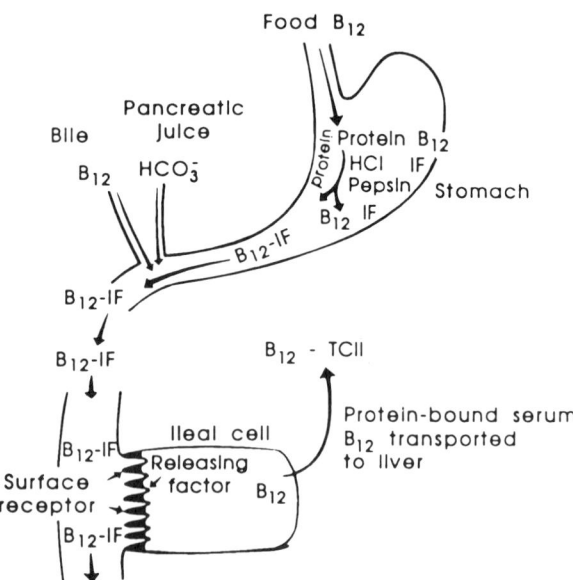

FIG. 2. Absorption of vitamin B_{12}. Sites of drug interaction: stomach: cimetidine; gut lumen: cholestyramine, neomycin; ileal surface receptor: para-aminosalicylic acid (PAS), colchicine, neomycin, ethanol, KCl, biguanides. IF, intrinsic factor. (Adapted from ref. 3.)

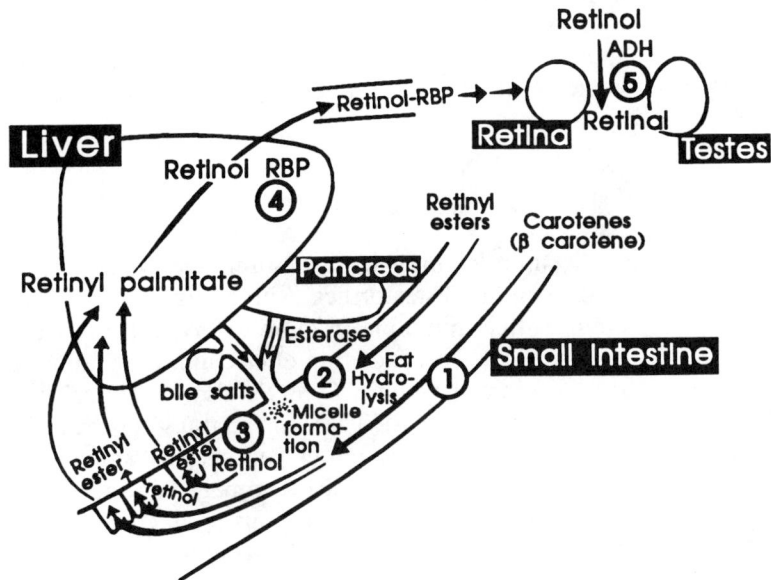

FIG. 4. Vitamin A absorption, transport, storage, and utilization. Sites of drug interaction: (1) mineral oil, (2) neomycin, (3) cholestyramine, (4) and (5) ethanol. (Adapted from ref. 3.)

vitamins by virtue of their solubility in mineral oil (3). However, this problem can be greatly lessened if the mineral oil is not administered with meals. The absorption of fat-soluble vitamins may be affected by drugs that cause steatorrhea, e.g., phenolphthalein, calcium carbonate, phenidone.

DRUG-INDUCED MINERAL DEPLETION

Generally, drug-induced mineral depletion arises from three types of interactions: (a) malabsorption, (b) gastrointestinal damage, and (c) excessive urinary losses.

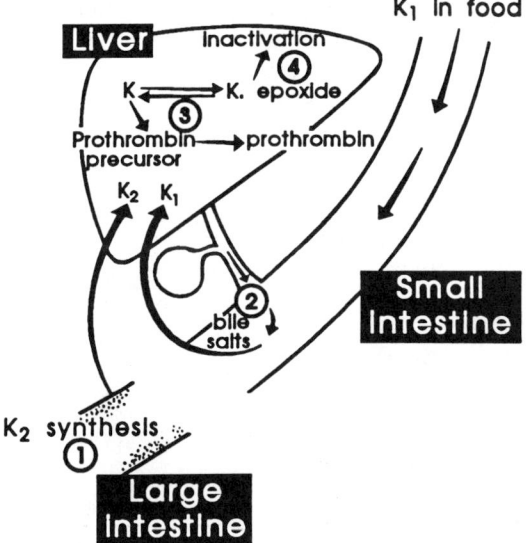

FIG. 5. Vitamin K: sources, absorption, and metabolism. Sites of drug interaction: (1) broad spectrum antibiotics, (2) cholestyramine, (3) coumarin anticoagulants, (4) anticonvulsants. (Adapted from ref. 3.)

Sodium

Hyponatremia, not unexpectedly, may accompany diuretic therapy or agents that interfere with the renin-angiotensin-aldosterone axis (Table 4). In addition, agents that modify the secretion of antidiuretic hormone (chlorpropamide, tolbutamide) may promote sodium excretion. Hypernatremia can be caused by glucocorticoid therapy due to enhanced renal and intestinal absorption, unless the glucocorticoid used is devoid of mineralocorticoid properties.

Potassium

Hypokalemia is commonly associated with loop and thiazide diuretics, laxative abuse, and glucocorticoid and mineralcorticoid therapy (Table 5). Drugs that cause ele-

TABLE 4. *Drugs that induce changes in serum sodium levels*

Drugs that increase sodium level (hypernatremia)	Drugs that decrease sodium level (hyponatremia)
Diazoxide	Chlorpropamide
Carbenicillin	Vincristine
Sodium sulfate	Cyclophosphamide
	Carbamazepine
	Amitriptyline
	Thioridazine
	Clofibrate
	Hydrochlorothiazide
	Polythiazide and other thiazides
	Metalazone
	Mannitol
	Spironolactone
	Captopril
	Licorice

TABLE 5. *Drugs that induce changes in serum potassium levels*

Drugs that increase potassium level (hyperkalemia)	Drugs that decrease potassium level (hypokalemia)
Hypertonic mannitol	Amphotericin B
Aminocaproic acid	p-Aminosalicylic acid
Isoniazid	Carbenoxolone
Phenformin	Gentamicin
Spironolactone	Lithium carbonate
Succinylcholine	Chlorthalidone
Triamterene	Furosemide
Indomethacin	Ethacrynic acid
Amiloride	Hydrochlorothiazide and other thiazides
	Albuterol (salbutamol)
	Corticosteroids
	Salicylates (aspirin)
	Tetracycline (degraded)

TABLE 6. *Drugs that induce changes in serum magnesium levels*

Drugs that increase magnesium level (hypermagnesemia)	Drugs that decrease magnesium level (hypomagnesemia)
Magnesium sulfate	Thiazides
Magnesium antacids	Furosemide
Lithium carbonate	Ethacrynic acid
	Ammonium chloride
	Mercurial diuretics
	Neomycin
	Gentamicin
	Cephalothin
	Methoxyflurane
	Ethanol
	CIS-platinum

vated serum potassium levels primarily act by limiting sodium-potassium exchange (aldosterone antagonists).

Magnesium

Hypomagnesemia may be caused by excessive renal excretion induced by diuretics that act on the proximal convoluted tubule (thiazides and mercurial diuretics). Drug-induced steatorrhea may be associated with enhanced fecal loss of magnesium through the formation of magnesium soaps (Table 6).

Excessive serum magnesium levels, although uncommon, are associated with drugs that have a high magnesium component, e.g., magnesium sulfate or magnesium antacids.

Calcium

Dietary calcium, like magnesium, may be influenced by drug-induced steatorrhea, with undigested fats combining with intraluminal calcium to form calcium soaps and excessive fecal excretion of calcium. Drug-induced modification of vitamin D levels also dictate calcium homeostasis (Table 7). These interactions may be registered at multiple levels but glucocorticoids, anticonvulsants, and mineral oil are of primary concern. Light barriers may limit the endogenous production of vitamin D_3 from ultraviolet (UV) light effects on the dermis, but it is unlikely that UV screens are used in the excessive amounts required to bear influence on vitamin D_3 homeostasis (Fig. 6).

Bile acid sequestrants may impair the intestinal absorption of dietary vitamin D_2 and D_3. Similarly, mineral oil and anticonvulsants directly impair calcium absorption from the intestine. Drugs that affect liver function, specifically bile acid formation and cytochrome P-450 (formation of the 25-OH forms of D_3 and D_2) may also indirectly affect calcium homeostasis (6) (Tables 7 and 8) (6).

Chelating agents may promote excessive urinary excretion of calcium. Some antacids may impair intestinal phosphate absorption, which may secondarily influence calcium absorption, although there is a growing trend to use calcium-based antacids, as opposed to sodium, which under some circumstances may elevate calcium levels. Excessive calcium loads do not promote a prolonged hypercalcemia due to the marked capacity of the kidneys to clear calcium from the circulation.

Iron

Drug-induced iron depletion may result from agents that bind to inorganic iron or heme in the intestinal lumen, e.g., cholestyramine, which then promote fecal iron loss. Nonsteroidal anti-inflammatory drug-induced gastrointestinal damage and occult blood loss are major causes of drug-induced iron depletion in children. Simi-

TABLE 7. *Drugs affecting vitamin D and calcium transport*

Drugs	Usage	Malabsorption	Mechanism
Prednisone (other glucocorticoids)	Allergic and collagen diseases	Calcium	Calcium transport ↓
Phenobarbital	Anticonvulsants	Calcium	Accelerated catabolism of vitamin D and active metabolites
Phenytoin	Anticonvulsants	Calcium	
Primidone	Anticonvulsants	Calcium	
Glutethimide	Sedative	Calcium	

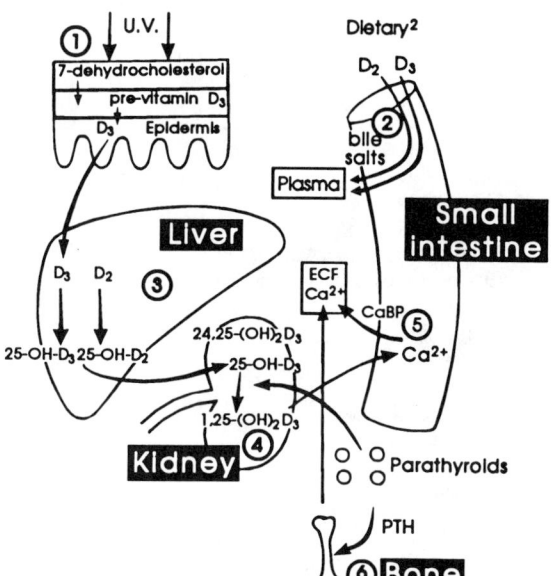

FIG. 6. Vitamin D and the calcium homeostatic mechanism showing sites of drug interaction: (*1*) light barriers, (*2*) bile acid sequestrants, (*3*) anticonvulsants—isoniazid (INH), (*4*) INH, (*5*) and (*6*) mineral oil and anticonvulsants. (Adapted from ref. 3.)

lar effects may also be apparent with high-dose glucocorticoids.

Zinc

Zinc depletion may result from D-penicillamine or diuretic therapy; both promote urinary excretion of zinc by chelation of plasma zinc and impaired tubular reabsorption, respectively. Zinc is primarily stored in skeletal muscles; these stores are subject to depletion by agents that promote skeletal muscle catabolism, e.g., glucocorticoids.

TABLE 8. *Drugs that induce changes in serum calcium level*

Drugs that increase calcium level (hypercalcemia)	Drugs that decrease calcium level (hypocalcemia)
Thiazides	Phosphate laxatives
Vitamin D and metabolites	Sodium phytate
Isotretinoin	Sodium cellulose phosphate
Etretinate	EDTA
Calcium carbonate	Furosemide
	Ethacrynic acid
	Phenobarbital
	Phenytoin
	Phenolphthalein
	Bisacodyl
	Primidone
	Glutethimide
	Corticosteroids

INFLUENCE OF DIET ON DRUG METABOLISM AND DISPOSITION

Timing of Meals

Drug absorption is greatly influenced by the presence of food in the stomach; depending on the drug and the ingested food, drug absorption may be decreased, delayed, or enhanced (Table 9). These effects may be due to the formation of a physical barrier that limits drug absorption and/or the formation of drug-food complexes that may either promote or hinder drug absorption (7,8). For example, a fatty meal may promote the absorption of lipid-soluble drugs, whereas antibiotics that are susceptible to degradation by gastric acid have a decreased absorption when food is in the stomach. In particular, foodstuffs that delay gastric emptying (fats, casein) may further promote this diminution of antibiotic absorption (9). The casein and calcium components of milk may form insoluble chelates with some drugs, e.g., tetracyclines and phenytoin, limiting their absorption (10).

Binding sites linked to absorption of some drugs may be influenced by high-protein meals, e.g., high intraluminal levels of amino acids following a protein-rich meal may compete with binding sites for levodopa and methyldopa, thereby decreasing their absorption.

Drug absorption may be merely delayed rather than decreased when consumed with food. This means that the amount of drug that is absorbed is not reduced but the time-course of its absorption is prolonged. This may influence efficacy by potentially reducing the peak plasma levels of the drug. Table 9 also displays a list of drugs that have enhanced absorption when taken with meals, usually the result of alterations in solubility or pancreatobiliary cooperation (11).

Drug Disposition

As drug disposition is greatly influenced by body composition, total body water, and plasma proteins, nutrition has long-term implications on drug actions and bioavailability as well as the acute interactions outlined above. In general, acidic drugs (phenytoin, barbiturates, nonsteroidal anti-inflammatory drugs) bind avidly to albumin; malnourished states that lead to decreased albumin synthesis and levels may cause a marked increase in the free drug concentration, and subsequently potentiate drug effects or toxicity. Basic drugs (propranolol, lidocaine, quinidine) primarily bind to globulins and may be similarly influenced by malnourished states that affect hepatic synthesis of globulins.

Free fatty acids can bind to some drugs and as a result drug disposition may be modified by the types of meals or fasting states where there is increased triglyceride breakdown to fatty acids (12).

TABLE 9. *Effects of food in the stomach on drug absorption*

Drugs with absorption *decreased* by food in the stomach	Drugs with absorption *delayed* by food in the stomach	Drugs with absorption *enhanced* by food in the stomach
Ampicillin	Acetaminophen	Carbamazepine
Aspirin	Aspirin	Chlorothiazide
Atenolol	Cefaclor capsules	Diazepam
Captopril	Cephalexin capsules	Dicumarol
Cephalexin suspension	Cimetidine	Erythromycin estolate
Doxycycline	Digoxin	Erythromycin ethylsuccinate suspension
Erythromycin stearate	Furosemide	Griseofulvin
Hydrochlorothiazide	Metronidazole	Hetacillin
Isoniazid	Quinidine	Hydralazine
Levodopa	Sulfonamides	Lithium
Methyldopa		Metoprolol
Nafcillin		Nitrofurantoin
Oxytetracycline		Propoxyphene
Penicillin G or V		Propranolol
Phenobarbital		Spironolactone
Propantheline		
Rifampin		
Tetracycline		

Drug Metabolism

Cytochrome P-450–related enzymes of the mixed-function oxidase system of the liver and gut mucosa are primary regulators of drug levels, particularly because of a high rate of exposure as a result of the first-pass effect. The activity of this mixed function oxidase system and other detoxifying enzyme systems can be attenuated by diets deficient in essential amino acids (particularly sulfur-containing amino acids) ascorbic acid, α-tocopherol, retinol, essential fatty acids and minerals (magnesium, calcium, zinc, selenium, and potassium) (13). Conversely, a high protein–low carbohydrate diet may enhance metabolism of drugs that are eliminated by sulfation-dependent reactions, due to the high intake of sulfur-containing amino acids with this diet (Table 10) (14).

Drug Excretion

Both the biliary and renal excretory routes of drug elimination can be influenced by diet. High-fiber diets can promote the fecal elimination of drugs particularly those with an extensive enterohepatic recirculation. Conversely, high-protein and high-fat diets will promote bile formation and thereby reduce the elimination of drugs with a marked enterohepatic recirculation.

Food components that influence urinary pH can readily modify renal drug absorption and excretion (Table 11). Low protein diets can elevate urinary pH from approximately 5.9 to 7.5. Specific food groups that lower urinary pH will increase the elimination of weak bases (and decrease the elimination of weak acids), and the converse is true for food groups that alkalinize the urine.

WHEN IS A NUTRIENT A DRUG?

There is a growing body of evidence that digestive fragments of dietary proteins exert drug-like actions on the gastrointestinal tract and systemic sites. The best characterized are opioid peptides derived from gluten

TABLE 10. *Dietary factors that increase drug metabolism*

High-protein, low-carbohydrate diet
Sulfur-containing amino acids
Charcoal broiling
Vegetables (cabbage, brussels sprouts)
Coffee, tea, cocoa (methylxanthine-containing beverages)
Dietary fiber (and other factors influencing intestinal microflora)

TABLE 11. *Foods that influence urinary pH and drug excretion*

Foods that acidify the urine (may increase elimination of weak bases or decrease elimination of weak acids)	Foods that alkalinize the urine (may increase elimination of weak acids or decrease elimination of weak bases)
Bread	Milk
Bacon	Vegetables: all types except corn and lentils
Vegetables: corn, lentils	Almonds
Fish	Chestnuts
Fowl	Coconuts
Shellfish	Fruits: all types except cranberries, plums, and prunes
Eggs	
Cheese	
Peanut butter	
Fruit: cranberries, plums, prunes	

and casein. Many other active ingredients have not been fully isolated but exert a range of drug-like effects on enteric flora (β-lactamase induction, carbohydrate fermentation), intestinal propulsion, hormone secretion, inflammatory and immune responses, platelet aggregability, ventilation, and appetite. For more complete reviews of this field, readers are referred to the recent reviews of Hamosh et al. (15) and Miller et al. (16). The implication of this growing field is that nutrient-drug interactions may extend to drug-drug interactions with the generation of biologically active compounds during nutrient digestion.

SUMMARY

Drug-nutrient interactions represent an often overlooked source of nutritional deficiencies. This chapter is meant to serve as a brief outline of the types of interactions that may occur and how they may be overcome or negated. Drug-nutrient interactions may occur at many levels: nutrient intake, synthesis, absorption, transport, metabolism, disposition, and excretion. However, interactions can be predicted with a basic understanding of the mechanism of absorption, action, utilization, and fate of individual nutrients and drugs. Children may be particularly sensitive to these interactions, based on the nutritional demands of growth and maturation. In addition, for certain drugs, altered pharmacokinetics in children, compared to adults, may enhance the likelihood of drug-nutrient interactions. Finally, as it is now well recognized that certain foods contain and/or are metabolized to biologically active components, these interactions may take on drug-drug qualities.

REFERENCES

1. Roe DA. Therapeutic significance of drug-nutrient interactions in the elderly. *Pharmacol Rev* 1984;36(Suppl):109S–122S.
2. Roe DA. *Diet and drug interactions.* New York: AVI Publishing, 1989.
3. Roe DA. *Drug-induced nutritional deficiencies,* 2nd ed. Westport, CT: AVI Publishing, 1985.
4. Roe DA. Drugs, diet, and nutrition. *Am Pharm* 1978;18:62–66.
5. Garabedian-Ruffalo SM, Ruffalo RL. Drug and nutrient interactions. *Am Fam Physician* 1986;33:165–174.
6. Olness K. Nutritional consequences of drugs used in pediatrics. *Clin Pediatr* 1985;24:417–420.
7. Vassell ES. Complex effects of diet on drug disposition. *Clin Pharmacol Ther* 1984;36:285–296.
8. Welling PG. Interactions affecting drug absorption. *Clin Pharmacokinet* 1984;9:404–434.
9. Osman MA, Pontel RB, Schuna A, Sandstrom WR, Welling PG. Reduction in oral penicillamine absorption by food, antacid and ferrous sulfate. *Clin Pharmacol Ther* 1983;33:465–470.
10. George CF. Food, drugs and bioavailability. *Br Med J* 1984;289:1093–1094.
11. Melander A. Influence of food and different nutrients on drug bioavailability. *World Rev Nutr Diet* 1984;43:34–44.
12. Royer RJ, Debry G, Ulmer M, Bannworth B. Food and drug interactions. *World Rev Nutr Diet* 1984;43:117–128.
13. Sonawane BR, Coates PM, Yaffe SJ, Koldovsky O. Influence of perinatal nutrition on hepatic drug metabolism in the adult rat. *Dev Pharmacol Ther* 1983;6:323–332.
14. Bidlack WR, Hamilton Smith C. The effect of nutritional factors on hepatic drug and toxicant metabolism. *J Am Diet Assoc* 1984;84:892–898.
15. Hamosh M, Hong MH, Hamosh P. Beta-casomorphin: mild β-casein derived opioid peptides. In: Lebenthal E, ed. *Textbook of gastroenterology and nutrition in infancy.* New York: Raven Press, 1989.
16. Miller MJS, Witherly SA, Clark DA. Casein: a milk protein with diverse biologic consequences. *Proc Soc Exp Biol Med* 1990;195:143–159.

CHAPTER 22

Nutrition and the Adolescent

Johanna T. Dwyer

Within an historical perspective, adolescents in the United States are now blessed with excellent health and, although problems remain, there is good reason to believe that this trend will continue. This chapter reviews the nutritional needs of adolescents contrasted with what they actually eat and why. Emphasis is placed on adolescents at especially high risk for nutritional problems including dieters, athletes, and those with disabilities. Nutritional goals for the year 2000, as well as steps to enhance fitness during adolescence, are reviewed.

Compared to their counterparts one century ago, adolescents in the United States today are physically healthier, better nourished and, although they are less physically active, probably better off as a group. They also compare favorably to adolescents in other countries.

But problems remain: malnutrition still afflicts subgroups of adolescents, especially those in disadvantaged minorities and those with chronic diseases and handicapping conditions. Iron deficiency anemia, as well, remains a problem.

There are, in addition to the traditional problems of adolescent nutrition, the new morbidities. Anorexia nervosa, other eating disorders, and alcohol and drug abuse have become far more frequent as precursors to undernutrition. Excessive participation in very competitive sports is another potential etiological factor as are diet-related risks of chronic degenerative diseases. The most widespread problem of adolescent nutrition in the United States is, however, overnutrition, the imbalances and excesses of which affect all adolescents, rich and poor. Finally, there are adolescents with special food and nutrition problems due to long-term developmental and health needs associated with handicapping conditions.

J. T. Dwyer: Frances Stern Nutrition Center, Boston, Massachusetts 02111.

NUTRITIONAL NEEDS OF ADOLESCENTS

Adolescents need highly nutritious diets. The pubertal growth spurt of the second decade of life relies on energy and nutrients to build body tissue, necessitating a higher intake of nutrients per kilocalorie (Cal). Thereafter, the larger size and altered body composition achieved during the growth spurt, and consolidated with further physiological changes in later adolescence, must be maintained by dietary intakes. The onset of menses, for example, increases iron needs in females; increased lean body mass of males and females increases needs for protein on an absolute basis. Energy intake must parallel the changes in physical activity and life-style common during adolescence. In addition, therapeutic modification of intake may be required as a result of disease processes that alter absorption, metabolism, or excretion of nutrients.

The recommended dietary allowances (RDA) are considerably higher for adolescents than they are for younger children or adults, especially if they are expressed on a nutrients-per-calorie basis (Table 1).

Nutrient needs differ by sex and change as biological maturation proceeds during adolescence, correlating

TABLE 1. *Percent changes in selected recommended allowances per 1,000 kilocalories for adolescents of various ages*

Nutrient	11- to 14-year-olds		15- to 18-year-olds	
	Males	Females	Males	Females
Protein	17%	8%	9%	12%
Calcium	74	40	45	50
Iron	41	0	18	0
Vitamin A	16	0	3	0
Ascorbic acid	−3	−17	−3	0
Magnesium	−17	0	10	7
Zinc	16	0	−4	0

Source: 1990 Recommended Dietary Allowances.

TABLE 2. Reference adolescents, Recommended Dietary Allowances, revised 1989

Age group (years)	Males		Females	
	Weight (pounds)	Height (inches)	Weight (pounds)	Height (inches)
7–10	62	52	62	52
11–14	99	62	101	62
15–18	145	69	120	64

TABLE 4. Selected recommended dietary allowances (RDA) for pregnant versus nonpregnant adolescents percent increase per 1,000 kilocalories

Nutrient needs compared to RDA for nonpregnant, nonlactating adolescent	% increase in RDA by age group pregnant	
	Age: 11–14	15–18
Protein	15%	15%
Calcium	12	12
Iron	77	77
Vitamin A	12	12
Vitamin C	23	3
Magnesium	1	6
Zinc	9	9
Folic Acid	98	98
Vitamin B_{12}	0	0
Vitamin D	−3	−3
Iodide	9	9

more closely with biological maturity than with chronological age. These differences are obscured in the *Recommended Dietary Allowances* (1), which presents needs by chronological, rather than biological, age. Biological maturity assessments are appropriate in dietary planning for adolescents, especially for those who have special diet-related problems. This is best accomplished using sexual maturity ratings (SMR).

Sex differences in nutrient needs become especially pronounced during adolescence. These differences are due, largely, to sex-specific changes in body size, and are reflected in the summary of RDA reference individuals (Table 2). Differences are also apparent in the RDA recommended energy intakes, revised in 1989, which are based on estimates of resting energy expenditures plus light to moderate activity levels (Table 3).

The female's growth spurt is, generally, about 2 years earlier than the male's. Most females are pubertal before they reach 10 years of age, peripubertal between 10 and 14 years, and reach later adolescence by 15 years of age. In contrast, males are, most usually, pubertal under 12 years of age, peripubertal from 12 to 17, and reach later adolescence by 18 years or older. As a result, at the inception of adolescence, early-maturing girls may be larger than boys of the same age, and have equal or greater needs for some nutrients, since they are experiencing the rapid changes in height and weight that occur during the peripubertal period. Males, however, as adolescence proceeds, tend to gain more height, weight, and lean body mass than do girls. These are important factors in understanding the difference in nutritional needs of males and females during various periods of adolescence.

The inception of the pubertal growth spurt differs, not only between males and females, but also within each sex. It varies from 9.7 to 13.3 years in females, and from 11.7 to 15.3 years in males. Although its duration is usually the same, about 3 to 4 years, the variability of its timing contributes to the diversity of nutrient needs of teenagers of similar chronological ages.

Age at onset of the pubertal growth spurt may, also, be associated with later health. Recent studies suggest, for example, that females who experience puberty early, end up more obese as adults than do peers who begin puberty later.

In addition to the normal needs of adolescence, events such as pregnancy, lactation, or illness have an impact on nutritional requirements. The needs of pregnant and lactating teenagers are greatly elevated, not only over those of their nonpregnant peers, but over those of older pregnant women as well (Tables 4 and 5).

YEAR 2000 GOALS FOR NUTRITION

The 10-year plan, published in 1989 by the United States Department of Health and Human Services to promote good health and disease prevention would, if accomplished, lessen preventable diet-related problems and decrease morbidity and mortality from a variety of

TABLE 3. Recommended Energy Intakes, 10th edition, 1989

Age	Males			Females		
	Calories per pound	Total calories	Range	Calories per pound	Total calories	Range
7–10	32	2,000	1,600–2,400	32	2,000	1,600–2,400
11–14	25	2,500	2,000–3,000	21	2,200	1,760–2,640
15–18	19	3,000	2,600–3,600	18	2,200	1,760–2,640
19–24	18	2,900	2,320–3,480	17	2,200	1,760–2,640

TABLE 5. *Selected recommended dietary allowances for lactating versus nonlactating adolescents: percent increase per 1,000 calories*

Nutrient needs compared to RDA for nonlactating adolescents	Age:	% Increase in RDA by age group	
		Lactating first 6 months 11–14 & 15–18 years	Lactating second 6 months 11–14 & 15–18 years
Protein		15%	15%
Calcium		−19	−19
Iron		−18	−18
Vitamin A		32	22
Vitamin C		55	22
Magnesium		3	7
Zinc		27	7
Folic Acid		27	26
Vitamin B_{12}		10	9
Vitamin D		−18	−18
Iodide		9	9

causes by the year 2000 (2). Many of these goals are targeted toward problems prevalent today in the American adolescent population.

Overweight

Goal: To reduce the overall prevalence of overweight adolescents to less than 15% of the population, and assure that at least 75% of all teenagers with weight problems learn, and employ, sound practices relating to dieting and physical activity.

Minorities, especially low-income African-Americans and Hispanics, may need special attention, since they are especially likely to be overweight today. All teenagers need to improve their knowledge of factors involved in weight loss. Those who have a weight problem need to adopt sensible dieting practices and increased physical activity.

Anemia

Goal: To reduce the prevalence of iron deficiency anemia in low-income teenage pregnant women, in whom it is especially prevalent.

Increased iron intake is important for all teenagers, especially girls, who often have very low iron intakes. Currently, the RDA for iron remains static at 15 mg per day for females, throughout adolescence, to compensate for menstrual losses. RDA for males, on the other hand, decrease from only 12 mg at 11 to 14 years of age to 10 mg, thereafter. Although 15 mg represents a reduction from the previously published RDA of 18 mg, it remains a higher recommendation than for males.

Low Calcium Intakes

Goal: To increase calcium intakes, by assuring that teenagers consume at least three servings of calcium-rich foods daily.

It is now recognized that peak bone mass is probably not attained until age 25. The latest edition of the RDA extended the calcium and phosphorus allowances, of 1,200 mg, to 24 years of age for both men and women. Many adolescent girls and young women fail to meet this recommendation in their daily diets. This may slow or prevent the achievement of peak bone mass and increase later risks of osteoporosis.

Diet-Related Risks of Hyperlipidemias and Other Risk Factors for Chronic Degenerative Diseases

Goal: At least 75% of teenagers should be able to identify the major food sources of fat; dietary fat intakes will not exceed 30% of total calories; saturated fat intakes will not exceed 10% of calories.

Teenagers must be able to recognize diet-related risk factors for heart disease, hypertension, cancer, and osteoporosis and to understand the methods for minimizing them. Of special importance is altering the type and amount of fat in the diet. This may be accomplished by the use of the Dietary Guidelines for Americans published by the United States Department of Health and Human Services and the Department of Agriculture, and school nutrition-education programs which would be part of a required health curriculum from preschool to grade 12 (3).

Improving the health and nutritional status of adolescents involves, in addition to specific nutrition changes, many other objectives.

Fitness, as a long- and short-term goal, should be a primary objective of all adolescents. Programs are needed that help adolescents understand the importance of fitness as well as how to attain it by planning more physically active lives for themselves. Adolescents must be taught the added benefits of greatly increased physical activity and exercise, sports training, and/or competitive athletics. This may entail encouragement from professionals and family who must help some adolescents overcome problems or fears that inhibit participation in such activities, as well as help the teenagers develop more positive attitudes about themselves and their bodies (4,5).

It is important for adolescents to understand the reason for fitness. Cosmetic aspects should not be emphasized; rather, the importance, to outcome, of long-term adherence to a well-designed plan should be stressed. An example of this might be lifelong aerobic exercise in order to help ensure cardiovascular fitness, maintenance of weight at appropriate levels, and suppleness.

Encouraging physical activity in children and adolescents helps to establish exercise as a lifelong habit, teaches relevant skills, and develops endurance, muscle strength, and flexibility. A physically active life also reduces the prevalence of obesity, injuries associated with disuse, the potential for osteoporosis and coronary artery disease, helps with rehabilitation from illness and injury, and increases self-esteem.

The appropriate program varies according to age group. All children and adolescents, however, should have daily physical activity designed to improve endurance, fitness, and strength in various muscle groups. The program should develop skills that will allow a variety of exercise choices in later life. Special programs should be designed for those students especially poor in fitness and those who have a disability, including obesity. For optimal results, these school programs should be coordinated with health and nutrition education programs, and should be fun, in order to assure continued participation.

It is especially important for parents to encourage family-based physical activities, both by involvement and by providing appropriate facilities for such fun and games.

In addition to physical activity, adolescents must understand the necessity of good nutrition as an absolute component of optimal fitness. Toward this end, all adolescents must be taught to assess their own nutritional status, to monitor their own growth, and to understand their nutrient needs and how these needs change with growth (6,7).

It is essential that adolescents learn what differentiates "good" from "poor" eating habits and how to alter the latter. They must know what nutrient needs must be met, especially iron and calcium, which often tend to be low. At the same time, dietary fat, saturated fat, cholesterol, sodium, and sugar should be identified as foods to be eaten in moderation. Alcohol, if used at all in later adolescence, should be recognized as a substance to be strictly limited. Behaviors that increase the likelihood of choking accidents, such as "wolfing" food, should also be avoided.

Adolescents suffering from conditions or diseases that pose special risks to nutrition and fitness need more specific, individualized attention. Those who are obese need to learn to reduce body fatness by sensible diet and exercise, and to maintain their weights at appropriate levels by healthful means. Those who are overly lean must be helped to achieve more appropriate levels, also through sensible diet. Adolescents afflicted with chronic degenerative diseases need to be taught dietary and life-style alterations that act in concert with any prescribed medical treatment. This includes the diet-related aspects of chronic diseases as well as the dietary aspects of handicapping conditions. And, of course, in the pregnant teenager, nutritional needs of both the mother and infant must be considered.

ADOLESCENTS AT HIGH RISK FOR NUTRITIONAL PROBLEMS

Adolescents at high risk for nutritional problems are not randomly distributed within the population. Rather, they fall into specific groups defined by demography, socioeconomic status, physical characteristics, and other factors. They are largely poor, rural, and/or minority groups, especially African-Americans, Hispanics, and Native Americans. Adolescents with several of these characteristics are at especially high risk.

Adolescents at high risk because of physical characteristics include the obese, those with congenital defects, inborn errors of metabolism or other potentially handicapping conditions, as well as those with risk factors for chronic degenerative diseases, such as hypertension or hypercholesterolemia, and those who are already ill with diseases such as diabetes mellitus or renal disease that require special dietary measures for their control. Pregnancy and lactation in the teenager are also important risk factors.

Other conditions that present risk factors and are also associated with poor nutritional status include emotional problems that precipitate eating disorders, mental retardation, mental illness, and alcohol or drug abuse. When social disabilities such as these are present with physical disabilities, the risks to nutritional status are greatly increased.

EXAMPLES OF DISEASES AND CONDITIONS POSING SPECIAL RISKS TO NUTRITION AND FITNESS OF ADOLESCENTS

Teenage Dieters

The American food supply is inexpensive, abundant, tasty, and readily available, maximizing the likelihood of overindulgence. Concomitantly, and ironically, modern fashion emphasizes leanness, pressuring adolescents to limit intake in order to conform to "standards of beauty." Dieting to lose weight is more common among adolescent girls than among any other age group in the

TABLE 6. *Self-evaluation of weight status by American primary and secondary school students: response to question "Are you the right weight?"*

	Elementary (N = 2,061)	Junior high (N = 1,529)	Senior high (N = 1,399)
Overweight	12%	20%	21%
Underweight	14	12	12
About right	67	63	65
Don't know	8	4	2

Source: Louis Harris Associates, 1989, Kellogg's Child Nutrition Survey.

United States. A recent national survey of schoolchildren in the United States illustrates the high prevalence of dieting (Table 7) (8). It revealed that a third of all elementary students, over two-fifths of all junior high school students, and nearly half of all senior high school students reported that they had been on weight-losing diets at some time in their lives. The question of health benefits was definitely secondary in most cases, appearance and weight loss being the main reason for diet alterations. The survey also indicated that many adolescents are discontented about their own weight status, seeing themselves as less attractive than their close friends. Two-thirds of junior and senior high school students described themselves as being at the right weight (Table 6). However, although a fifth of the students interviewed believed they were overweight and one-tenth thought they were underweight, over four-fifths of these students considered their close friends to be at the appropriate weight and less than 5% believed these friends to be overweight (8).

There are many reasons to be concerned about excessive emphasis on dieting. First, there is a major difference between short-term weight loss and lifetime weight control. Long-term weight control is achieved by a realistic assessment of one's body and appropriate changes in life-style that include physical activity as well as moderation in dietary intake. Strict dieting during the pubertal growth spurt, in addition to its lack of long-term effect, can adversely affect linear growth and may lead to menstrual abnormalities. Later in adolescence chronic dieting may be associated with decreased intakes of iron, calcium, and other nutrients that are already low in the diets of adolescent girls.

In addition, although dieting, per se, does not cause eating disorders, one must be concerned with the occasional association. For example, although dieting behavior does not precipitate anorexia nervosa unless other psychiatric problems are also present, dieting episodes often precede the onset of binges in bulimic individuals (9). In other words, the combination of dieting and occasional binging is not necessarily predictive of eating disorders. It is only when dieting disintegrates into chronic, pathologically disorganized eating behavior that is associated with psychological disturbance, or other signs, including amenorrhea, extreme weight loss, frequent vomiting, laxative abuse, regular diet pill use, or fasting, that an eating disorder may be present (10,11).

In spite of the considerable trend toward adolescent dieting, adolescent obesity is not decreasing and, in fact, is probably becoming more prevalent (12). There is good evidence of an increasing trend toward obesity in young African-American and adult Caucasian females over the past several decades (13). It appears concomitantly with a related problem: physical inactivity. Fitness is low among youth (14). Less than half of all adolescents, and probably even fewer of those with weight problems, engage in physical activity of the sort that is likely to continue into the adult years (5).

The multiple precursors of obesity reinforce the need for a multifaceted program of prevention. Obesity prevention programs must include education in fitness through physical activity, nutrition, body assessment, and healthful weight control rather than weight loss. Family-based interventions, which incorporate these programs for the entire family, may have a greater impact. Several excellent guides are available, including Shapedown (15) and the publication of the Interdisciplinary Committee on Children and Weight (16). These books emphasize an integrated program for long-term change similar to what has been described. School-based obesity prevention programs should be encouraged to supplement and support these other efforts.

TABLE 7. *Self-reported dieting behavior in American primary and secondary school students: response to question "Have you ever been on a diet?"*

	Elementary (N = 2,061)	Junior high (N = 1,529)	Senior high (N = 1,399)
Yes, have dieted	32%	42%	48%
Lose weight to look better	(12%)	(23%)	(29%)
Health reasons	(6%)	(4%)	(5%)
Both	(9%)	(12%)	(12%)
Don't know, other	(5%)	(3%)	(2%)
No	65	55	50
Don't know	3	2	2

Source: Louis Harris Associates, 1989, Kellogg's Child Nutrition Survey.

Adolescent Athletes

In spite of their concerns about fitness, body composition, and health, adolescent athletes may also run into trouble (17). Nutritional deficiencies among athletes may occur either as a result of excessive energy output during training or due to a purposely low energy intake for activities requiring a slim body.

Adolescents who are involved in activities in which a lean physique is advantageous, such as runners, gymnasts, figure skaters, and ballet dancers, may fall victim to undernutrition, amenorrhea, and eating disorders. Those engaged in training and competition since childhood may be at particular risk. In ballet dancers, for example, although energy output is not greatly elevated, food intake tends to be very low and signs of eating disorders are common (18). Similarly, gymnasts attain low weights by limiting food intakes as well as by increased energy outputs (19). In females, the delays in menarche and amenorrhea that may result have negative effects, not only on physical growth, but upon bone health, resulting in stress fractures and low mineral density of bone, among other problems. The lower bone density also increases the potential of osteoporosis.

All adolescent athletes should understand the long-term ramifications of their diet. They should be given a dietary regime that will meet their energy needs, improve their athletic performance, and maintain an appropriate body fatness. Those who are involved in heavy training and competitive sports have especially great need for expert advice.

Adolescent athletes often indulge in fasting and thirsting themselves to lose weight, especially immediately before competition when they wish to compete in a lower weight category. The main danger of short-term fasting is dehydration. Fasting for several days during training may reduce muscle glycogen stores, which may also reduce endurance and performance in activities requiring anaerobic power, especially during a final sprint.

Anabolic steroids are used by many adolescent athletes to build strength and muscle mass (20). Aside from the fact that they are illegal and barred from use in most competitive sports, they also have toxic effects. Growth failure may occur as a result of use during puberty since anabolic steroids lead to premature closing of the epiphyses. They also have profound effects on reproductive hormones. In females, there is masculinization; in males, breast growth, reduced libido, and acne. Lipid metabolism is altered, with increases in atherogenic low-density lipoprotein (LDL) cholesterol and decreases in high-density lipoprotein (HDL) cholesterol to dangerous levels, and, in some cases, liver damage. In a third or more of chronic users, moderate to severe psychiatric symptoms may be present, including "roid rage" (21,22). There is, therefore, no question of the danger of steroids, which is even more severe in the adolescent than the adult.

"Doping," or the use of prescription drugs to improve performance, is not limited to anabolic steroids use. Narcotics, depressants, diuretics, beta blockers, and pharmacologic doses of caffeine and alcohol, although banned by the United States and the International Olympic committees, have also been used.

Adolescent athletes often spend large sums of money on unproven nutrient supplements as ergogenic aids to increase athletic performance. These include a wide variety of "magic" substances such as amino acids, special vitamin mixtures, gelatin, carnitine, wheat germ oil, bee pollen, honey, calcium pangamate, phosphorus, lecithin, aspartate, ginseng, inosine, and lipotrophic factors that have little or no benefit to performance. In addition to being unnecessary, some substances, such as the fat-soluble vitamins A and D and vitamin B_6, may be toxic in large quantities.

Dehydration is an added risk to adolescents engaged in competitive sports. Adequate hydration during athletic events is important to compensate for sweat losses and to maintain normal body temperature in order to avoid heat illness. Special fluids are not necessary; water will suffice. But, during competition, thirst alone is not an adequate indicator of hydration, and mandatory fluid consumption schedules may be needed. After exercise, drinking past the point of thirst, to rehydrate the body, is important.

Diets for fitness should be well balanced, varied, low in fat, and appropriate in energy and fluids. Recommended intakes of carbohydrate are high, 55% of total calories or more. Protein needs are slightly elevated but easily met in the usual American diet. Needs for vitamins and minerals are in the normal range.

Carbohydrate needs are best supplied by starches rather than sugar. High-carbohydrate, low-fat diets are good for general health and especially appropriate for fitness reasons. A large intake of carbohydrates loads glycogen into muscles. Previously, it was believed that muscles had to be glycogen-depleted by exhaustive exercise before beginning the high-carbohydrate diet. This has now been disproven. Carbohydrate loading can be practiced daily by simply consuming a carbohydrate-rich diet, exercising regularly, and taking enough rest. There are no hazards associated with this type of regimen. It is effective in improving performance in endurance events, and may also be helpful in activities requiring power.

In summary, diets that promote general and nutritional health also promote good physical performance. Special diets for athletes are not necessary. Good nutrition for optimal fitness matches energy intakes and outputs. Periods of fasting are not encouraged. Steps to avoid dehydration are taken. Diets are planned to be balanced, moderate, and varied. Prescription drugs for "doping," including steroids, and unproven ergonomic aids of all sorts, are to be avoided.

ADOLESCENTS WITH SPECIAL DEVELOPMENTAL AND HEALTH NEEDS

Nutrition is also an important component in the care of adolescents with special developmental and health needs: those who have inborn errors of metabolism and congenital defects that began at birth as well as those whose disabilities begin in childhood and adolescence. Adolescents whose health problems involve dietary adjustments run higher risks of nutritional problems and psychological distress related to food than do healthy adolescents. In addition, when a child or adolescent has a chronic disease, growth may be affected by the disease as well as by malnutrition secondary to the condition.

Nutrition counseling and intervention can help mitigate, or even eliminate, preventable causes of poor growth. Unfortunately, financial constraints, disorganized health services, as well as other perceived priorities often hamper incorporation and use of nutritional assistance.

Nutritional problems among handicapped adolescents vary, ranging from the need for help with managing food and feeding to the need for therapeutic diets that control the disease, prevent secondary malnutrition, and improve the quality of life. These problems in the adolescent who is handicapped further complicate the difficult weaning from dependence on parents for feeding and care, to the independence coveted by all children of this age.

With an ultimate goal of preventing problems resulting from inadequate intake, including poor growth and development, the optimum nutritional program will help the adolescent manage food choices independently while taking into account the constraints imposed by disease. Some conditions, such as diabetes mellitus, renal disease, phenylketonuria, and severe allergies require special diets to control the disease. Although occasional lapses are to be expected, it is important to keep noncompliance low so that it does not become a medical issue or a source of family conflict (23,24). Therapeutic modifications can be adapted to teen life-styles and teenagers can be taught to assume control of their intakes (25). Individualization can help to reduce noncompliance with therapeutic diets. Psychosocial and physiological adaptations also improve when appropriate care is provided (26).

Many conditions have a prevalence of less than 1 per 1,000. These include hemophilia, leukemia, muscular dystrophy, sickle-cell anemia, blindness, phenylketonuria, chronic renal failure, and cystic fibrosis. Nutritional counseling can often bring dramatic improvements in the quality of life, and the growth and health of those afflicted. Phenylketonuria and cystic fibrosis are two examples.

Phenylketonuria

The prevalence of phenylketonuria is approximately 0.01 per 1,000. It is a rare but striking example of how nutritional attention can preserve normal function and maximize development. It is now clear that mental retardation due to phenylketonuria can be reduced by the continuation of therapeutic diets throughout adolescence (27,28). It is a challenge to the adolescents, to the parents, to the school authorities, as well as to the skills of the nutritionist to plan and adhere to diets that permit normal growth and a socially normal life while restricting phenylalanine-containing foods. The reward is greater mental capacity (29–31).

Cystic Fibrosis

Cystic fibrosis afflicts approximately 0.2 per 1,000 adolescents. Dietary and respiratory therapy are essential to promote good growth and help to minimize crises in this heredity disease affecting the gastrointestinal tract and lungs.

Other Conditions

Other, slightly more common conditions, with prevalences that vary from 1 to 38 per 1,000 are arthritis, asthma, central nervous system injury, cerebral palsy, cleft lip and palate, congenital heart disease, diabetes mellitus, Down syndrome, mental retardation of varying degrees, and seizure disorders. Although not all children who suffer from these conditions have nutritional problems, they run higher risks of such difficulties and deserve screening. Two examples are given below.

Diabetes Mellitus

Diabetes mellitus has a prevalence of 1.8 per 1,000. Better adherence to prescribed diet, drug therapy, and exercise decreases risks of complications such as hypoglycemia and ketoacidosis. There is also the exciting possibility that dietary alterations can yield long-term health benefits by decreasing the complications arising from atherosclerosis, vascular, and kidney disease (32–34).

Obesity, Hypertension, Cholesterol, and Glucose

Obesity, hypertension, high serum cholesterol, and high blood glucose are among the most common conditions. They form a lethal cobweb of interactive risks, increasing risks for each other, as well as for other health problems. This heightens their need for control. Environmental changes can be helpful (35,36).

CONCLUSION

American adolescents can be healthy. They have the potential to develop into mature, productive adults. Even those who are at special risk of nutritionally related health problems can be helped to mitigate, or eliminate, those problems through nutritional counseling and therapeutic diets (37). As a nation we must devote the attention and resources necessary to this end (38).

ACKNOWLEDGMENT

Partial support from training grant MCJ 9120 to Dr. Dwyer from the Maternal and Child Health Service, U.S. Department of Health and Human Services, permitted the preparation of this manuscript.

REFERENCES

1. Subcommittee for the Tenth Edition of the RDA. *Recommended Dietary Allowances*, 10th ed. Washington, DC: National Academy Press, 1989.
2. U.S. Department of Health and Human Services. *Year 2000 goals: promoting health, preventing disease: objectives for the nation* (draft). Washington, DC: Office of the Assistant Secretary, U.S. Department of Health and Human Services, 1989.
3. *U.S. Department of Health and Human Services and USDA dietary guidelines for Americans*. Washington, DC: U.S. Government Printing Office, 1990.
4. American Academy of Pediatrics. *Sports medicine: health care for young athletes*. Elk Grove Village, IL: American Academy of Pediatrics, 1983.
5. Pate R, Ross J. Fitness of children and adolescents. *Annu Rev Public Health*. New York: Academic Press, 1988.
6. Dwyer J. Promoting good nutrition for today and the year 2000. *Pediatr Clin North Am* 1986;33:799–822.
7. Gong EJ, Spear BA. Adolescent growth and development: implications for nutritional needs. *J Nutr Ed.* 1988;20:273–279.
8. Louis Harris Associates. *The Kellogg's child nutrition survey*. New York: Louis Harris Associates, 1989.
9. Johnson C. Anorexia nervosa and bulimia. In: Coates TA, Petersen A, Perry C, eds. *Promoting adolescent health: a dialogue on research and practice*. New York: Academic Press, 1988.
10. Adams L, Shafer M. Early manifestations of eating disorders in adolescents: defining those at risk. *J Nutr Ed* 1988;20:307–313.
11. Mallick M, Whipple T, Huerta E. Behavioral and psychological traits of weight conscious teenagers. *Adolescence* 1987;22:157–168.
12. Gortmaker S, Dietz WH, Sobol AN, Wehler C. Increasing pediatric obesity in the U.S. *Am J Dis Child* 1987;14:535–540.
13. Harlan WR, Landis J, Flegal K, et al. Secular trends in body mass in the United States 1950–1980. *Am J Epidemiol* 1988;128:1065–1074.
14. President's Council on Physical Fitness and Sports. *Youth physical fitness in 1985*. Ann Arbor, MI: Institute for Social Research, 1986.
15. Shapedown. *Weight management program for adolescents*. Larkspur, CA: Balboa, 1987.
16. Interdisciplinary Committee on Children and Weight. *Children and weight: what health professionals can do about it*. Berkeley, CA: Cooperative Extension and Beef Council, 1988.
17. Dwyer JT. *Adolescent nutrition and fitness*. Washington, DC: Office of Technology Assessment, U.S. Government Printing Office, 1989.
18. Benson J, Gillien DM, Bourdt K, Loosli AR. Inadequate nutrition and chronic calorie restriction in adolescent ballerinas. *Physician Sports Med* 1985;13:79–90.
19. Van Erp-Baart LW, Fredrix TC, Lavaleye PC, et al. Energy intake and energy expenditure of top female gymnasts. *Children and Exercise* 1985;9:194–202.
20. Buckley WE, Yesalis CE, Friedl KE, et al. Estimated prevalence of anabolic steroid use among male high school seniors. *JAMA* 1988;260:3441–3445.
21. Pope HG, Katz DL. Affective and psychotic symptoms associated with anabolic steroid use. *Am J Psychiatry* 1988;145:487–490.
22. Wright JE, Stone MH. NSCA statement on anabolic drug use. *NSCA J* 1985;7:45–59.
23. Siegel D. Adolescents and chronic illness. *JAMA* 1987;257(24):3396–3399.
24. Crumette B. Assessing the impact of illness upon an adolescent and family. *Matern Child Nurs J* 1983;12:155–167.
25. Perrin E, Ramsey B, Sandler H. Competent kids: children and adolescents with a chronic illness. *Child Care Health Dev* 1987;13(1):13–32.
26. McAnarney E. Social maturation: a challenge for handicapped and chronically ill adolescents. *J Adolesc Health Care* 1985;6:90–101.
27. Clarke W, Gates R, Hogan S, et al. Neuropsychological studies on adolescents with phenylketonuria returned to phenylalanine restricted diets. *Am J Ment Retard* 1987;92(3):255–262.
28. Lou H, Guttler F, Lykkelund C, et al. Decreased vigilance and neurotransmitter synthesis after discontinuation of dietary treatment for PKU in adolescents. *Eur J Pediatr* 1985;144(1):17–20.
29. Hunt M, Bery H, White P. Phenylketonuria, adolescence, and diet. *J Am Diet Assoc* 1985;85(10):1328–1334.
30. Schmidt H, Mahle M, Michel U, Pietz J. Continuation vs. discontinuation of low phenylalanine diet in PKU adolescents. *Eur J Pediatr* 1987;146(suppl 1):A17–19.
31. Naughten E, Kiely B, Saul I, Murphy D. Phenylketonuria: outcome and problems in a "Diet For Life" clinic. *Eur J Pediatr* 1987;146(suppl 1):A23–24.
32. Powers M. *Handbook of diabetes nutritional management*. Rockville, MD: Aspen, 1987.
33. Tamborlane W, Sherwin R. Diabetes control and complications: new strategies and insights. *J Pediatr* 1985;102:805–813.
34. Gabbay K. Treatment of diabetes mellitus. In: Grand R, Sutphen J, Dietz WD, eds. *Pediatric nutrition: theory and practice*. Boston: Butterworth, 1987.
35. Massachusetts Medical Society Committee on Nutrition. Fast food fare: consumer guidelines. *N Engl J Med* 1989;321:752–755.
36. Auld GW, Smiciklas-Wright H, Shannon BM. School health interventions for adolescents at nutritional risk: a survey of health teachers, nurses and coaches. *J Nutr Ed* 1988;20:319–325.
37. Tebbi C, Cummings K, Zevon M, et al. Compliance of pediatric and adolescent cancer patients. *Cancer* 1986;58(5):1179–1184.
38. Forbes GB, Woodruff CW, eds. Committee on Nutrition, American Academy of Pediatrics. *Pediatric nutrition handbook*, 2nd ed. Elk Grove Village, IL: American Academy of Pediatrics, 1985.

CHAPTER 23

Nutritional Considerations in the Treatment of Anorexia Nervosa and Bulimia

Michael J. Pertschuk

Eating disorders were "discovered" about 10 years ago by the media, and about 100 to 300 years ago by medicine, but have existed for millennia. *Anorexia nervosa* was a term coined in the 1870s by Sir William Gull (1) to label weight loss brought about by self-imposed starvation. Gull went on to become Queen Victoria's personal physician, the Queen obviously not being one of his anorectic patients.

The first case report of anorexia nervosa, describing a patient with "nervous consumption," was written almost 200 years before by Richard Morton (2), a prominent English physician. Retrospective analyses of histories of the saints have suggested the existence of the disorder in medieval times. One author has traced a possible description back to 660 AD (3–5).

Although bulimia, as a formal diagnosis, only dates to 1980, its origins may be more ancient than anorexia. Xenophon, around 400 BC, wrote of "fames canina" or "dog hunger," characterized by uncontrolled eating without apparent satiation (6,7).

Despite their historical credentials, eating disorders have a uniquely contemporary nature that may be reflected in their apparently recent increase in incidence. In this chapter, anorexia nervosa and bulimia nervosa, disorders characterized by abnormal food consumption, will be reviewed from a nutritional perspective. Although it is obvious that these diagnoses have more extensive components, they can be neither understood nor treated without knowledge of their nutritional aspects.

DEFINITIONS

Anorexia nervosa is defined in the current psychiatric diagnostic manual, the *Diagnostic and Statistical Manual of Disorders* (DSM IIIR) (8), by self-induced weight loss, intense fear of gaining weight, distorted body image, and for women, amenorrhea. Anorexia officially begins with weight loss to a level at or below 85% of ideal body weight (%IBW). Previously, the official weight was under 75% IBW (6,9). The change from a 75% IBW to an 85% IBW standard reflects a meaningful difference in the level of malnutrition and the type and extent of physical findings likely to be observed. With the weight criterion being entirely arbitrary, someone with all the other clinical stigma of anorexia, but at 86% IBW, may still require treatment, especially if that patient has had a >10% reduction in %IBW.

Distorted body image refers specifically to an inability to correctly judge body size. Many, although not all, anorectic patients see themselves as either normal weight or overweight despite the emaciation that is apparent to everyone else. The presence of other signs of anorexia, including amenorrhea, hypotension, hypothermia, bradycardia, loss of scalp hair, and development of lanugo hair are, individually, dependent on the degree and duration of malnutrition.

Anorectics can be categorized by their means of weight loss, a distinction that is not part of the formal diagnosis. "Restrictors" lose weight purely through severe dieting or dieting combined with overexercise. Those who eat more, but purge, have been variously labeled as "bulimic anorectics," "purgers," or "bulimarexic." Purging anorectics, in addition to self-inducing vomiting, may also abuse laxatives or diuretics.

M. Pertschuk: Department of Psychiatry, University of Pennsylvania, Graduate Hospital, Philadelphia, Pennsylvania 19146.

Both weight loss strategies can achieve equally low weights. There are differences, however, that go beyond behavioral distinctions. Physical findings can differ, and it has been argued that purgers may more closely resemble bulimics in their personality profiles than restricting anorectics.

Bulimia nervosa is characterized by binge eating, a subjective sense of lack of control over eating, a preoccupation with weight and thinness, and a pattern of compensatory behavior to counter the weight gain potential of binging. The DSM IIIR sets as a minimum binge frequency for diagnosis two episodes a week for a period of 3 months (8). Unfortunately, binges by their nature are hard to quantify. Where does overeating end and binging begin? If a patient eats large quantities of food more or less continuously throughout a day, is that counted as one long binge or many? This is not just academic hair splitting. Epidemiological studies, outcome research, and clinical decisions are all affected by such distinctions.

Purging is not a prerequisite for the diagnosis of bulimia by DSM IIIR criteria; it is the combination of binging and some compensatory behavior. The latter may be vomiting or laxative abuse, but can also be fasting or exercise.

Although anorexia and bulimia are two distinct diagnoses, as many as half of bulimic patients may have had a previous anorexic episode. Often this episode went undiagnosed and untreated, and is only identified in retrospect. Treated anorexia can also evolve into bulimia. In one study, almost a third of the patients treated in a behaviorally oriented weight gain program went on to develop a pattern of binge eating during a 2-year follow-up period (10). Although less common, bulimics have also been known to become anorexic.

EPIDEMIOLOGY

Eating disorders are primarily seen in societal strata where there is an abundance of food, where binging is possible because of food availability, and where limiting consumption is a conspicuous statement rather than a necessity. Women with anorexia outnumber men approximately 10 or 15 to 1. The female to male ratio for bulimia appears to be approximately the same. Anorexia has its peak incidence in the mid- to late teens. Bulimia peaks somewhat later, in the early 20s. The age range for both disorders is broad, extending from preteen years passed middle age.

Incidence for anorexia has been reported in the range of 1 to 8 cases per 100,000 person years (11). For the specific population at greatest risk, namely middle and upper middle class adolescent girls, the prevalence of anorexia has been estimated as high as 1% (12). The wide variance in reported prevalence for bulimia, from a high of 19% to a low of under 1% for female college undergraduates, reflects the stringency of diagnostic criteria applied (13,14). In a recent study utilizing the DSM IIIR criteria, a prevalence rate of 1% was reported for college women (15). Behavioral self-reports in this study would have supported a rate closer to 2% had the data been interpreted in a slightly different fashion.

Most investigators looking at trends in case findings have observed severalfold increases in the diagnosis of anorexia (16,17) from the 1960s, 1970s, and 1980s versus the 1930s, 1940s, and 1950s. In one of the most careful retrospective studies, however, the author failed to find a significant change in incidence from 1930 to 1980 (11).

There are no data for bulimia since it was not an officially recognized diagnosis until 1980.

PREMORBID NUTRITIONAL STATUS

For disorders capable of wreaking such nutritional havoc, the premorbid state is strikingly unremarkable. Most anorectics are at or near normal weight prior to weight loss; the same is usually true of bulimics. There are exceptions. A small but noticeable minority has a prior history of obesity. Another small subset of anorectics, but not bulimics, has a history of chronic low weight.

Most often, anorexia and bulimia start from the same, innocent point. A teenage girl or young adult woman decides she needs to lose a few pounds. She begins a diet, often without a definite goal weight or diet plan beyond just "cutting back." The diet becomes increasingly stringent as lower weights are achieved. The bulimics part company from the anorectics when overwhelming hunger leads to an episode of binge eating which, after being repeated, becomes an established pattern. Purging follows as a means to compensate for the calories consumed. Although the weight that was originally lost may be regained, most bulimics remain at a weight below their original baseline.

Bulimics usually have two components of abnormal eating: a pattern of moderate to severe dietary restriction and dramatic episodes of binging during which they eat large quantities of foods they would otherwise deny themselves. A typical "in-control" diet reported by patients is little or no breakfast, and for lunch and dinner a salad, with or without diet dressing, and possibly a small quantity of cottage cheese or plain yogurt. When more is consumed, which, for most patients, is either in the late afternoon or evening, a binge ensues. Binges tend to be mixtures of candy, starches like french fries or chips, cookies, ice cream, doughnuts, and sometimes one or more fast food meals (hamburger, fries, and a milk shake). Total caloric intake during a binge can exceed 10,000 kilocalories (Cal). A minority of bulimics binge on "health foods," that is, foods such as vegetables, rice cakes, etc.

Anorectics are more "successful" at controlling their eating. Restricting anorectics tend to follow diets very similar to those of the bulimics on their "good" days, i.e., small meals with most of their limited calorie intake from vegetables. More than half of anorectic patients may be described as "pseudovegetarians" (18). Red meat is avoided, not out of humanitarian concerns, but because of fear of fats and caloric density. Protein sources are usually limited to cottage cheese, yogurt, and occasionally, broiled fish or poultry. Total caloric intake for most restricting anorectics is under 800 Cal per day.

Purging anorectics typically restrict for all but one meal a day, often a meal where they are forced by circumstance to eat with others. Small to average portions are consumed but are purged shortly thereafter. Patients with this pattern follow it either because they find more severe restriction too uncomfortable, or because friends or family members insist on the patient's eating.

NUTRITIONAL ASSESSMENT

Anorexia Nervosa

Physical findings, in anorexia nervosa, are dependent on the purging/restricting status and the extent and duration of the illness. Most of the research data are based on moderate to severe anorexia with patients generally below 80% IBW. The 80% to 85% range for restricting anorexics is something of a "twilight zone," with relatively little data. Clinical experience suggests that, for this group, routine chemistries, trace metals, and blood count are generally normal. For restricting anorexics, however, with weight under 80% IBW, a number of abnormalities have been reported.

In anorexia, serum electrolytes tend to be normal in the absence of purging. Serum protein and albumin are usually within normal limits unless the patient is severely malnourished; most patients appear to maintain a normal serum protein until their weight reaches approximately 60% IBW. Total iron binding capacity is a more sensitive measure of protein status, however, and can be below normal values at weights between 70% to 80% IBW.

Anorexics differ significantly in plasma and erythrocyte amino acid concentrations from well-nourished control populations and from third-world starving populations (19). Plasma threonine, valine, isoleucine, and leucine were lower in anorectics than normal controls, whereas plasma glycine was significantly higher. Plasma threonine, valine, leucine, lysine, and cystine were lower for third-world starving populations than in the anorectics. In the context of protein-energy malnutrition, anorectics appear to be midway between normal controls and third-world patients. This is most likely the result of the anorectic diet, which, while severely restricted, is probably higher in protein than that of the third-world group.

The white blood cell count, in anorectics, is usually mildly depressed in the 3.0 to 4.0 $\times 10^3$ range with a relative lymphocytosis. Red blood cell count, hemoglobin, and hematocrit tend to be either at the low end of normal or in the mildly anemic range. Trace minerals have been variously reported as normal or low (20,21). Vitamin levels are usually within normal limits, although hypovitaminosis A and hypercarotenemia have been reported (22). Liver enzymes are usually mildly elevated. Cholesterol is often in the low normal range, but can be elevated. The elevation does not reflect dietary indiscretion, but rather an apparent abnormality of fat metabolism. Triglycerides are usually in the low normal range.

Thyroxine (T_4) is normal, whereas triiodothyronine (T_3) is mildly depressed, reflecting reduced conversion of T_4 to T_3 (23). Serum cortisol levels are elevated (24), and do not suppress with dexamethasone. Luteinizing hormone levels drop with consequent reduced ovarian stimulation and a decrease in estradiol levels. For males, there is evidence of a decrease in testosterone (25).

Anorectics lose their glycogen stores, and periodic hypoglycemia can be a problem. Associated with severe weight loss, blood sugar values as low as 25 mg% have been observed.

Transient marked elevations in creatine phosphokinase (CPK) have been documented. This reflects muscle breakdown from overly vigorous exercise coupled with inadequate fluid intake.

Bone density is often decreased in anorectics who have been ill for a year or more (26). Because most patients are at an age when bone density would normally be increasing, it is not clear whether the low values reflect absolute mineral loss or a failure to increase bone mineral content. Elevated serum cortisol levels can promote calcium loss. Inadequate calcium intake can lead to failure in bone calcification or, if intake is too low, to loss of bone calcium. Decreased estrogen levels can also lead to reduction in the deposition of calcium in bone.

Blood urea nitrogen (BUN) and serum creatinine values are usually normal. Glomerular filtration rates are reduced (27). Skeletal and cardiac muscle mass is reduced. Decreased cardiac volumes have been demonstrated along with decreases in maximal heart rate and maximal oxygen uptake in response to exercise (27). The reduction in lean body mass of the GI tract and abdominal muscles causes the stomach to ride lower in the abdomen and to be less well constrained. The resulting tendency for the stomach to bulge more noticeably after meals is usually interpreted by the anorectic patient as a sign of fat, producing even more psychological distress.

Reduced brain mass has been demonstrated by computerized tomography studies. There is an increase in the external and less frequently internal CSF (5). Because of a correlation between elevated serum cortisol levels and increase in CSF space, it has been speculated that elevated cortisol, and not simply malnutrition, is responsible for the decrease in brain mass.

Metabolic rates as demonstrated by indirect calorimetry are usually low, with observed rates in the range of 70% to 80% of values predicted by the Harris-Benedict equation. Immune function usually remains intact until weight loss is far advanced. Anorectics will often remark that they feel fine and seem to have fewer colds than their normal weight peers or family members. When weight approaches 60% IBW, immune function is compromised and patients become demonstrably anergic (28).

Almost all of the above changes are reversible with improved nutrition. Blood counts normalize. The alterations in plasma and erythrocyte amino acids are, for the most part, reversed (19). Liver enzymes normalize as does serum cortisol. Serum cholesterol, if elevated acutely, returns to normal. These are changes that can be seen within weeks of the initiation of successful nutritional treatment. Normalized estrogen levels usually require several months of sustained normal or near-normal weight. Ninety percent ideal body weight is an approximate level cited for return of menses, an occurrence that may be related to percent body fat (29).

There are limited data on changes in bone, brain, and muscle mass with nutritional rehabilitation. One small unpublished study reported improvement in bone density with weight recovery, although values remained below normal. There was a decrease in CSF levels for almost half the anorectics in a study that followed a group of patients through nutritional recovery (5). It was also noted that, for some patients, decreased brain mass persisted a year after weight recovery. Fluid and fat can be replaced more rapidly than protein, and lean body mass may require months to normalize, although longitudinal data on body composition in anorexia are lacking.

Metabolic rate quickly rises with nutritional repletion, and may nearly double (30). Metabolic needs for anorectics may remain high for a period of months after weight recovery (31), possibly because of the continued need for extra calories to rebuild lean body mass. One study demonstrated that anorectics with a previous history of overweight needed fewer calories for weight gain than anorectics who were normal weight premorbidly, suggesting an overall lower metabolic rate (32).

A change that may not be reversible is loss of growth. Although most anorexia begins after most or all linear growth has been achieved, patients who develop chronic anorexia in their preteen or early teenage years may miss out on their adolescent growth spurt (33). This may inhibit the incentive for recovery. As one patient told us, overcoming her anorexia would just mean facing life as a "normal midget." The effectiveness of growth hormone treatments for such patients is not yet known.

There are only a few differences in findings for purging anorectics, as compared with "restrictors." Dehydration, hypochloremia, hypokalemia, and metabolic alkalosis can result from frequent vomiting and/or laxative and diuretic abuse. Dehydration may artifactually increase both white and red blood cell counts. Serum amylase may be elevated as a result of chronic parotid irritation secondary to vomiting. BUN may be elevated through dehydration. There are also data to suggest that purging anorectics may have somewhat lower metabolic needs than restrictors (34).

Prolonged Q-T intervals may be present on the EKG as a consequence of hypokalemia. Marked orthostasis may be superimposed on the usual hypotension of anorectics because of dehydration.

The mortality rate for anorexia nervosa has been reported in the range of 1% to 5% (35). One long-term study, which followed patients for 30 years, found a mortality rate of 18% (36). The majority of deaths in this study were suicides, reflecting the associated psychopathology. Medical complications responsible for death in anorexia include sepsis, renal failure, heart failure, and hypoglycemia. Sometimes the immediate cause is iatrogenic, as when the severely depleted and precariously functioning anorectic is mismanaged with regard to fluid and electrolytes.

Bulimia Nervosa

Patients with bulimia nervosa generally show far less disturbance on laboratory assessment. Electrolytes may be abnormal from frequent vomiting, laxative, and/or diuretic abuse. Hypokalemia, hypochloremia, and metabolic alkalosis as well as dehydration can all be observed. Amylase, often elevated in association with frequent vomiting, may be a useful marker for severity of the disorder (37). Red and white blood cell counts may be artifactually elevated because of dehydration. BUN may be elevated for the same reason. Moderate increases may occur in cholesterol and triglycerides secondary to foods consumed during binges. Metabolic rate, measured by indirect calorimetry, may be under predicted values, perhaps by as much as 10% to 15%. Whether this lower rate is primary to the disorder or secondary to eating pattern is unclear.

Morbidity with bulimia nervosa can be significant. Dental problems are the most frequent complication, the result of the erosion of enamel after prolonged periods of frequent vomiting. Painful swelling of the parotids, chronic esophagitis, and hiatal hernia are also possible consequences of continued vomiting. With extended use of laxatives, usually in large quantities for 5 years or more, the colon can become atonic. We have seen two patients who have required either partial or total colon resection.

The mortality rate for bulimia nervosa is not known. Although rupture of the stomach from binging has been reported, such events appear to be rare. Theoretically, cardiac arrhythmia from electrolyte imbalance would be the most common cause of death. However, after having treated well over 500 bulimic patients during the past 10 years, we have yet to see a fatality.

NUTRITIONAL REHABILITATION

Anorexia Nervosa

The strategy for nutritional rehabilitation will depend on the degree of patient cooperation and extent of medical jeopardy. A modicum of patient cooperation is always necessary. The less restrictive the treatment setting, the more cooperation is required. Even intravenous hyperalimentation, at a minimum, requires that the patient does not pull out the line or dump the hyperalimentation solution in the sink.

Most patients are ambivalent about treatment. Except in rare instances of extreme denial, patients are partially aware of the disruption they have caused in their lives and the medical risks they run. How accepting they are of treatment will depend on the balance between the fears and pain they experience as a result of their illness versus the anticipatory pain and fears they have of treatment and recovery. For almost all patients, there comes a point at which the balance shifts in favor of attempting recovery; some, however, reach this point only when they are in grave danger of physical collapse.

There are three routes of nutritional rehabilitation and four possible settings. Nutrition can be provided by mouth, tube, or IV. This can be accomplished in a home, partial hospital, residential, or hospital setting. Obviously, not all routes work with all settings. Except under unusual circumstances, tube feedings [total enteral nutrition (TEN)] or intravenous hyperalimentation [total parenteral nutrition (TPN)] will be performed only in a hospital. Table 1 shows the various permutations of level of cooperation, medical risk, treatment setting, and route of feeding.

Nutritional rehabilitation should almost always be done in the context of a comprehensive treatment plan. The "almost" refers to the exception of a "grave" medical situation in which the patient's life is in acute danger and immediate medical intervention is essential with or without the niceties of an entire program.

At a minimum, outpatient treatment should involve regularly scheduled psychotherapy. More intensive inpatient treatment usually includes a combination of individual, group, and family therapy. Free time is structured through planned activities in occupational, recreational, or limited physical therapy. Considerable and competent nursing is essential for patient support whether the designated route of nutritional rehabilitation takes place within a hospital, day treatment program, or in a residential setting.

Comprehensive treatment of anorexia will also include nutritional education either through counseling or formal classes. Many patients are pseudoknowledgeable about nutrition. Although they may know the caloric content of foods, they have major misconceptions of

TABLE 1. *Treatment and treatment settings*

Patient cooperation	Medical risk	Setting	Route
Good	Minimal (patient stable at weight over 80% IBW)	Home	Oral
Good	Mild (patient stable at weight between 75% and 80% IBW)	Home or partial hospital	Oral
Fair (patient will cooperate with a structured program but will do little on her own)	Mild	Partial hospital, residential, or hospital	Oral
Fair	Significant (patient's weight between 62% and 75% IBW, with clinical findings consistent with malnutrition, but without acute medical jeopardy)	Residential or hospital	Oral
Poor (patient consents to treatment but refuses to eat)	Significant	Hospital	TEN or TPN followed by oral when more cooperative
Fair	Grave (patient's weight under 62% IBW and/or presence of acute medical compromise)	Hospital	Oral (brief trial) if unsuccessful, TEN or TPN
Poor	Grave	Hospital	TEN or TPN
None	Grave	Hospital commitment	TEN or TPN

IBW, ideal body weight; TEN, total enteral nutrition; TPN, total parenteral nutrition.

their own needs. What is true for others, they feel, is not true for them. They need far less food than anyone else; weight dangerously low for others is normal for them. Nutritional instruction, and evidence such as abnormal laboratory tests, may correct some misconceptions. Changing such beliefs is, however, slow and difficult. Some emotional progress toward recovery is necessary before patients become open to accepting any nutritional information.

When patients are to eat their way out of anorexia, i.e., use the oral route, two basic strategies have been utilized. For outpatient and partial hospital settings with good patient cooperation, a diet of regular food is prescribed. This usually starts at a level of intake greater than the patient has been consuming, but well under what is needed for sustained weight gain. A frequently prescribed range is between 1,000 and 1,200 Cal.

At home, some means of meal monitoring is generally recommended, often by family and friends when available. A behavioral contract may be drawn up in which expectations regarding meals and weight are written out in detail. Most contracts include agreed upon consequences for meeting or falling short of expectations. In inpatient settings, meals are usually monitored by nursing or other staff, often with contracted consequences for meeting or not meeting calorie or food exchange quotas.

The diet is gradually advanced until an amount of food is consumed consistent with sustained weight gain, frequently between 2,500 and 3,200 Cal. The rate of advance depends on patient tolerance, medical danger, and the amount of weight that must be gained. Even though there may be no medical reason to push for rapid weight gain, realities of limited insurance reimbursement in partial hospital, residential, or hospital settings may necessitate encouraging patients to gain weight within a circumscribed time period.

Generally, it has not proved necessary to place patients on esoteric diets to achieve nutritional rehabilitation. A normally balanced regimen incorporating fats, proteins, and carbohydrates is adequate. Vitamin and mineral supplements are frequently prescribed early in the process when caloric intake may be insufficient to cover all needs. The absolute number of calories necessary for 1 kg of weight gain varies significantly. In one study, a range of 4,500 to almost 13,000 Cal was reported (34). The variance was thought to reflect differing levels of patient activity.

In our own treatment program, we respect nutritionally adequate dietary patterns that predate the onset of anorexia, e.g., a kosher diet and/or vegetarian diet that includes dairy products. Dietary quirks adopted after the onset of anorexia, e.g., "pseudo-vegetarianism," are not permitted.

When patients on the oral route are unwilling to meet caloric requirements, dietary supplements are often utilized. This can be done for a single meal or routinely to replace missing calories until the patient will take all nutrition as normal food.

An alternate oral strategy is initiating treatment with liquid supplements only. The rationale is that patients' fears of eating may be mitigated since the supplement may appear more like medicine than food. These fears relate to the concern both of becoming fat and of being unable, once eating has begun, to stop. Typically, initial intake is about 1,000 to 1,200 Cal, which is advanced by increasing the concentration and volume of the supplement until a predetermined percentage of normal weight or a fully normal weight is reached.

Liquid supplements have the additional advantage of being sufficiently monotonous to act as an incentive for patients to eat real food. The disadvantage is that supplements do nothing to educate the patient about eating normally. This is of particular concern when inpatient treatment time is restricted.

Total enteral nutrition (TEN) is an alternative for patients refusing to eat. The procedure still requires some patient cooperation: consent is required for tube placement; patients must be willing to leave tubes in place. TEN has the advantage, over TPN, of better caloric absorption via the patient's gastrointestinal tract. There are few complications, either with tube insertion or feedings. With continuous feedings, the patient can be cycled so that TEN is done overnight, keeping interference with daytime therapeutic activities to a minimum. Success is predicated on the patient refraining from surreptitiously disposing of the TEN solution.

Concomitantly with TEN, the patient can be encouraged to eat. This is especially easy if TEN is being given overnight so the patient is not especially full during the day. The quantity of supplement provided can be titrated against the amount the patient has taken by mouth. When the patient begins taking most calories orally, TEN is discontinued. This can serve as a potent reinforcer of eating.

The major limitation of the procedure is psychological. Patients sometimes perceive tube placement as the equivalent of oral rape. This is especially true if TEN is presented as a punitive measure. In such cases, patients are less likely to give consent. Even under optimal conditions, in an entirely supportive environment, tube feedings seem prone to heighten patient resentment.

Total parenteral nutrition (TPN) is the other alternative when patients refuse to eat. It is the converse of TEN, psychologically more acceptable, but fraught with medical complications. The approach is so clearly medical and so removed from eating that many patients find it the least threatening approach to nutritional rehabilitation. Some will explicitly state that it allows them to gain weight without working at it, or taking any responsibility. They do not have to worry about losing control over eating because, in fact, they are not eating. If they gain weight it is the "fault" of the doctors. Implicit in this is the expectation that once the plug is pulled on the IV pump, they can resume starvation.

The medical risks with TPN are not specific to anorexia, but may be greater because of the depleted condition of these patients. Placement of a subclavian line can be more difficult because of extreme emaciation. Pneumothorax and hemopneumothorax occur with some frequency. Line-related sepsis is a concern in the severely anorectic patient with compromised immune function. In one series, virtually all the anorectics on TPN developed liver enzyme elevations (37). Electrolyte disturbances brought about by errors in fluid replacement can be lethal. At one university hospital, before all the nuances of the technique were understood, TPN led to hypophosphatemia with progressive paralysis and death in a severely anorectic patient (38). Even as knowledge has increased, imbalances remain possible. Recently, hypophosphatemia, which developed in one patient immediately after a course of TPN, resulted in transient paralysis.

As with TEN, TPN can be cycled and titrated against the amount of food consumed. Depending on how uncomfortable the patient is with the procedure, this may or may not be an incentive to increase oral intake.

TEN and TPN are definitely second choices to oral feeding. The patient learns nothing about normal eating when these are the exclusive means of nutritional repletion. They may allow the patient to avoid taking responsibility for recovery. Further, the medical risks can be significant, especially with TPN.

There are two primary rationales for the use of these two approaches. First, they can be lifesaving. If the patient is in immediate medical jeopardy and refuses to take oral nourishment adequate to quickly resolve the danger, TEN and TPN are the only alternatives. Second, when depression, brought about by malnutrition, reduces motivation toward recovery or when impaired judgment, resulting from severe malnutrition, impairs efforts toward recovery, TEN or TPN may be initiated with the hope that once the patient's nutritional state is improved, there will be enhanced participation in treatment (39,40).

In fact, TEN or TPN are the only options with the totally noncompliant patient; conversely, they are neither necessary nor legal when such patients are medically stable. For the patient at immediate risk, TEN or TPN must be done under strict supervision to prevent the patient's removing the line or tube or disposing of nutritional solutions. In such situations, the courts will respond to an appropriate petition for provision of treatment.

Results, with improved nutrition, vary. Some patients improve psychologically to the extent of becoming willing participants in treatment; some, at least, learn how to avoid such situations in the future; others resume starvation as soon as TEN or TPN is withdrawn. For the last group, rehospitalization every few months for TEN or TPN can become a way of life.

Bulimia Nervosa

By comparison, nutritional repletion in bulimia is an easy, straightforward matter, invariably a brief procedure requiring 2 or 3 days at most. The heroics of TEN or TPN are unnecessary. IV fluids may sometimes be needed for rehydration and restoration of electrolyte balance. Some patients with frequent vomiting, laxative, and/or diuretic abuse run chronically low potassium levels, which can be rectified with oral potassium supplements until better control is achieved.

The major thrust of nutritional rehabilitation of bulimic patients is to alter the dysfunctional pattern of eating, which includes restrictive dieting, binge eating, and, often, purging. The therapeutic strategy usually includes some behavioral intervention.

In its simplest form, such intervention involves individual outpatient therapy utilizing self-monitoring and direct behavioral counseling for managing meals and free time. The patient tracks intake using a diet log. When possible, meals are taken with friends or family either at restaurants or using preportioned foods. Activities are planned to occupy time that might otherwise be used for binging and purging. This treatment requires a high level of patient motivation and a substantial degree of patient control.

For adolescents living at home, family members can be enlisted to help with structuring meals and free time. As with family interventions for anorexia, a behavioral contract may be written with clear expectations and assignments for everyone involved. All meals may be taken with a family member with specific plans for the patient to remain with the family after meals. Bathroom access may be limited. This approach is dependent on both patient and family cooperation.

When the patient is unable to make changes within the home, a partial hospital, residential facility, or hospital may be used. These more-structured programs usually include supervised meals with designated postprandial observation periods and/or activities scheduled to preclude purging. Bathroom access may be limited and possibly supervised. Free access to food is either limited or nonexistent. As with anorexia, these behavioral interventions are made within the context of an appropriate, intensive program of psychotherapy.

As the patient is able to approximate a more normal pattern of eating, the structure is gradually eliminated. Supervision and prohibitions are discontinued with the patient assuming more responsibility. The ultimate goal is to have the patient eat with a semblance of normality, if not spontaneity, and to continue to do so with only outpatient support.

An alternative strategy, which has frequently been combined with a behavioral approach, is the use of antidepressant medication. It was fortuitously observed in the early 1980s that some depressed bulimic patients given antidepressant medication experienced a reduction or elimination of binge impulses. The effect appeared to be independent of improvement in mood and was confirmed in several controlled trials (41,42). Although the exact mechanism by which antidepressants achieve a reduction in binging is unknown, the effect may be due to the resultant increase in serotonin and/or norepinephrine levels. The former neurochemical has been implicated in appetite regulation. No one antidepressant has been reliably demonstrated to be more effective in bulimia than another, although some clinicians claim to have found monamine oxidase inhibitors and serotonin uptake blockers superior to the tricyclic antidepressants.

The initial enthusiasm for antidepressants has diminished because it has become apparent that often their effectiveness diminishes with time. Some patients use the temporary control over binging to lose more weight by further restriction of intake. When the drug effectiveness lessens, binge impulses return and patients are back where they started. Alternatively, when the period of relative control that antidepressants provide is successfully used to alter behavioral patterns, including restrictive eating, the end of drug effectiveness may find the patient in better control of the disorder.

A significant number of bulimics have sought assistance through self-help groups such as Overeaters Anonymous (OA). OA offers considerable support and definite guidelines. Foods with refined flour and sugar are prohibited and treated as substances of abuse. The line of demarcation drawn around certain foods is somewhat artificial; virtually any food can be consumed during a binge. Nonetheless, although there have been no formal studies, there are unquestionably individuals who have been helped by this approach.

BEYOND NUTRITION

Nutrition constitutes an important element in the highly complex problem of eating disorders. Concomitant psychological problems are, of course, also profound; the fear of attempting to live a normal life for many of these patients can be overwhelming. For some bulimic patients, binging may be just one of several impulse control problems that can include alcoholism, drug abuse, shoplifting, and sexual promiscuity. Depression, personality disorder, as well as childhood physical and sexual abuse, are frequently part of the history for both anorexics and bulemics.

As awareness of the complexity of eating disorders has increased, it has been questioned whether recovery is a realistic possibility. From experience, it is evident that recovery is possible, but may be a long-term process rather than a discrete event. Especially when the problem has been chronic over years, treatment becomes a matter of helping the patient put together his or her life piece by piece. Treatment should incorporate long-term support for the patient until the ultimate goal is reached: the reestablishment or, in some cases, the beginning, of an independent life.

REFERENCES

1. Gull W. Anorexia nervosa (apepsia hysterica). *Br Med J* 1873;2:527.
2. Morton R. *Phthisiologia: or, a treatise of consumptions.* London: Smith and Walford, 1694.
3. Bell RM. *Holy anorexia.* Chicago: University of Chicago Press, 1985.
4. Rampling D. Ascetic ideals and anorexia nervosa. In: Szmukler GI, Slade PD, Harris P, Benton D, Russel GFM, eds. *Anorexia nervosa and bulimic disorders.* Oxford: Pergamon Press, 1986;89–94.
5. Ploog DW, Pirke KM. Psychobiology of anorexia nervosa. *Psychol Med* 1987;17:843–859.
6. American Psychiatric Association. *Diagnostic and statistical manual of disorders,* 3rd ed. Washington, DC: American Psychiatric Association, 1980.
7. Casper R. The pathophysiology of anorexia nervosa and bulimia nervosa. *Annu Rev Nutr* 1986;6:299–316.
8. American Psychiatric Association. *Diagnostic and statistical manual of disorders,* 3rd ed, revised. Washington, DC: American Psychiatric Association, 1987.
9. Feighner JP, Robins E, Guze SB, Woodruff RA, Winokur G, Munoz R. Diagnostic criteria for use in psychiatric research. *Arch Gen Psychiatry* 1972;26:57–63.
10. Pertschuk MJ, Edwards N, Pomerleau OF. A multiple baseline approach to behavioral intervention in anorexia. *Behav Ther* 1978;9:368–376.
11. Lucas AR, Beard CM, O'Fallon WM, Kurland LT. Anorexia nervosa in Rochester, Minnesota: a 45-year study. *Mayo Clin Proc* 1988;63:433–442.
12. Crisp AH, Palmer RL, Kalucy RS. How common is anorexia nervosa? A prevalence study. *Br J Psychiatry* 1976;128:549–554.
13. Halmi KA, Falk JR, Schwartz E. Binge-eating and vomiting, a survey of a college population. *Psychol Med* 1981;11:697–706.
14. Stunkard AJ, Schotte DE. Bulimia versus bulimic behaviors on the college campus. *JAMA* 1987;258:1213–1215.
15. Drewnowski A, Hopkins SA, Kessler RC. The prevalence of bulimia nervosa in the US college student population. *Am J Pub Hlth* 1988;78:1322–1325.
16. Szmukler G, McCance C, McCrone L, Hunter D. Anorexia nervosa: a psychiatric case register study from Aberdeen. *Psychol Med* 1986;16:49–58.
17. Jones DJ, Fox MM, Babigian HM, Hutton HE. Epidemiology of anorexia nervosa in Monroe County, New York: 1960–1976. *Psychosom Med* 1980;42:551–558.
18. O'Connor MA, Touyz SW, Dunn SM, Beumont PJV. Vegetarianism in anorexia nervosa? A review of 116 consecutive cases. *Med J Aust* 1987;147:540–542.
19. Halmi KA, Struss AL, Owen WP, Stegink LD. Plasma and erythrocyte amino acid concentrations in anorexia nervosa. *JPEN J Parenter Enteral Nutr* 1987;11:458–464.
20. Casper RC, Kirschner B, Sandstead JJ, Jacob RA, Davis JM. An evaluation of trace metals, vitamins, and taste function in anorexia nervosa. *Am J Clin Nutr* 1980;33:1801–1808.
21. Hall RCW, Hoffman RS, Beresford TP, Wooley B, Tice L, Klassen Hall A. Hypomagnesemia in patients with eating disorders. *Psychosomatics* 1988;29:264–272.
22. Silverman JA. Medical consequences of starvation. In: Darby PL,

Garfinkel DM, Garner DM, Coscina DV, eds. *Anorexia nervosa: recent developments in research.* New York: Liss, 1983;293–299.
23. Moshang T, Parks JS, Baker L, et al. Low serum triiodothyronine in patients with anorexia nervosa. *J Clin Endocrinol Metab* 1975;40:470–473.
24. Doerr P, Fichter M, Pirke KM, Lund R. Relationship between weight gain and hypothalamic pituitary adrenal function in patients with anorexia nervosa. *J Steroid Biochem* 1980;13:529–537.
25. Hall A, Delahunt JW, Ellis PM. Anorexia nervosa in the male: clinical features and follow-up of nine patients. In: Szmukler GI, Slade PD, Harris P, Benton D, Russell GFM, eds. *Anorexia nervosa and bulimic disorders.* Oxford: Pergamon Press, 1985;315–321.
26. Crosby LO, Kaplan FS, Pertschuk MJ, Mullen JL. The effect of anorexia nervosa on bone morphometry in young women. *Clin Orthop* 1985;201:271–277.
27. Fohlin L. Body composition, cardiovascular and renal function in adolescent patients with anorexia nervosa. *Acta Paediatr Scand* 1977;(Suppl)268:7–20.
28. Pertschuk MJ, Barot L, Crosby L, Mullen JL. Immunocompetency in anorexia nervosa. *Am J Clin Nutr* 1982;35:968–972.
29. Frisch RE. Food intake, fatness and reproductive ability. In: Vigersky RA, ed. *Anorexia nervosa.* New York: Raven Press, 1977;149–162.
30. Dempsey DT, Crosby LO, Pertschuk MJ, Feurer ID, Buzby GP, Mullen JL. Weight gain and nutritional efficacy in anorexia nervosa. *Am J Clin Nutr* 1984;39:236–242.
31. Kaye WH, Gwirtsman T, Ebert MH, Peterson R. Caloric consumption and activity levels after weight recovery in anorexia nervosa: a prolonged delay in normalization. *Int J Eat Dis* 1986;5:489–502.
32. Walker J, Roberts SL, Halmi KA, Goldberg SC. Caloric requirements for weight gain in anorexia nervosa. *Am J Clin Nutr* 1979;32:1396–1400.
33. Pugliese MT, Lifshitz F, Grad G, Fort P, Marks-Katz M. Fear of obesity: a cause of short stature and delayed puberty. *N Engl J Med* 1983;309:513–518.
34. Kaye WH, Gwirtsman HE, Obarzanek E, George T, Jimerson DC, Ebert MH. Caloric intake for weight maintenance in anorexia nervosa: nonbulimics require greater caloric intake than bulimics. *Am J Clin Nutr* 1986;44:435–443.
35. Seidensticker JF, Tzagournis M. Anorexia nervosa—clinical features and long term follow-up. *J Chronic Dis* 1968;21:361–367.
36. Theander S. Research on outcome and prognosis of anorexia nervosa and some results from a Swedish long-term study. *Int J Eat Dis* 1983;2:167–174.
37. Gwirtsman HE, Kay WH, George DT, Carosella NW, Greene RC, Jimerson DC. Hyperamylasemia and its relationship to binge-purge episodes: development of a clinical, relevant laboratory test. *J Clin Psychiatry* 1989;50:196–204.
38. Pertschuk MJ, Forster J, Buzby G, Mullen JL. The treatment of anorexia nervosa with total parenteral nutrition. *Bio Psychiatry* 1981;16:539–550.
39. Keys A, Brozek J, Heuschel A, Mickelson O, Taylor HL. *The biology of human starvation.* Minneapolis: University of Minnesota Press, 1950.
40. Laessle RG, Schweiger U, Pirke KM. Depression as a correlate of starvation in patients with eating disorders. *Biol Psychiatry* 1988;23:719–725.
41. Hughes PL, Wells SA, Cunningham CJ, et al. Treating bulimia with desipramine. *Arch Gen Psychiatry* 1986;43:182–186.
42. Walsh BT, Stewart JW, Roose SP, Gladis M, et al. Treatment of bulimia with phenelzine. *Arch Gen Psychiatry* 1984;41:1105–1109.

CHAPTER 24

Nutritional Considerations in the Development and Treatment of Psychosocial-Deprivation Dwarfism

Alfonso Vargas and Alfred Tenore

Psychosocial-deprivation dwarfism remains, as it has been for over 20 years, somewhat a mystery. Psychosocial-deprivation dwarfism is defined clinically by the presence of severe growth retardation, emotional disturbance, bizarre behavior, and atypical eating and drinking patterns. A key factor in almost all cases of psychosocial-deprivation dwarfism is, however, child neglect and/or abuse (1–5). In fact, most, if not all, of the problems of this syndrome resolve by improving the patient's environment.

Diagnosis of psychosocial-deprivation dwarfism as a defined entity is difficult. This is, first of all, because of the endocrine and nutritional disturbances that overlap the psychosocial aspects of this disease. In addition, histories, which form the basis of the diagnosis, may often be of questionable accuracy since they are taken from caretakers considered to be psychopathological themselves. Mothers of patients may, for example, state that their children eat excessively and, therefore, have to be restricted, without seeing the conflict in this (1).

The mystery of psychosocial-deprivation dwarfism will be resolved when adequate studies determine its etiology. Controversy often is polarized. The basic scientific question in this condition is whether it is possible with adequate, and even excessive, nutritional intake, to have severe growth retardation secondary to pathological, psychosocial, and environmental stresses, or whether this syndrome is the direct result of inadequate nutrient intake secondary to child neglect and abuse (1,4). If, in fact, growth failure can occur in the face of adequate nutritional intake, studies are needed to verify the system by which "caloric wastage" ensues from chronic stress and aberrational behavior. In addition, studies are needed to determine the role of nutritional intake in these children, both its contribution to the syndrome and its significance to the prognosis.

The term *psychosocial-deprivation dwarfism*, rather than the more commonly used *psychosocial dwarfism*, is used in this chapter because of the confirmed role of deprivation in the pathophysiology (Table 1).

ETIOLOGY

Most children who are diagnosed with psychosocial-deprivation dwarfism are brought in for evaluation after they have had the syndrome for some time. As a result, neither the origin of the disease nor the sequence of its development are clearly understood. One theory is

TABLE 1. *Psychosocial-deprivation dwarfism: equivalent terminology*

Psychosocial-deprivation dwarfism
Psychosocial dwarfism
Abuse dwarfism
Reversible hyposomatotropism
Reversible somatotropin deficiency
Deprivation dwarfism
Maternal-deprivation dwarfism
Emotional-deprivation dwarfism
Psychogenic growth retardation
Psychosocial growth retardation
Psychosomal dwarfism

A. Vargas: Department of Pediatrics/Endocrinology, Louisiana State University School of Medicine, New Orleans, Louisiana 70112.
A. Tenore: Department of Pediatrics, University of Udine, Udine, Italy 33100.

that psychosocial stress mediates, in some way, central nervous system neurotransmitter responses (5) involving one or several pathways including the dopaminergic, catecholaminergic, cholinergic, serotoninergic, γ-aminobutyric acidergic, histaminergic, and enkephalinergic pathways. This neurotransmitter change leads to hypothalamic-pituitary changes that result, it is hypothesized, in the inhibition of growth hormone releasing hormone (GHRH) and increased growth hormone inhibiting hormone (somatostatin) (6). This is clearly shown by the growth hormone deficiency found in many patients who demonstrate depressed growth hormone response to standard stimulation tests (i.e., intravenous arginine infusion, insulin-induced hypoglycemia, L-dopa, or clonidine administration) (1–4,7–12). A decreased 24-hr growth hormone secretory pattern, similar to that found in the syndrome of growth hormone neurosecretory dysfunction, which returns to normal with therapeutic intervention, has been reported (9). Insulin-like growth factor–1 (IGF-1 or somatomedin-C) serum concentrations are also lower than the normal range for chronological age, contributing to the decrease, or cessation, of linear growth (1,8–10).

Further studies are needed to demonstrate the contribution of nutritional deprivation to the neurological changes found in these children. Although there are significant social and physiological differences, the child with psychosocial dwarfism can be compared, somewhat, with the child who is chronically undernourished, stunted, and who has a decreased growth hormone response to standard stimulation tests (13) and depressed IGF-1 levels (see chapter 13, *Endocrine Changes in Malnutrition*). It has been observed that although children with primary protein-energy malnutrition have elevated circulating growth hormone, the growth hormone response to standard stimulation tests is depressed. In the primarily malnourished child these neuroendocrine changes are reversed by improved nutrient intake. Studies are needed to determine how much of the improvement seen in psychosocial-deprivation dwarfism is related to increased nutritional intake.

Other endocrine changes include decreased adrenocorticotropic hormone (ACTH) secretion and diminished cortisol production. However, no true state of adrenal insufficiency has been documented (1–4,8). Although thyroid hormone studies have reflected normal or low-normal serum concentrations of thyroxine (T_4) and triiodothyronine (T_3), thyroid-stimulating hormone (TSH) serum levels are not elevated and no evidence of transient or true reversible hypothyroidism has been found (4,8). In a few teenage patients, significant pubertal developmental delay has been observed, suggesting that gonadotropin releasing hormone (Gn-RH) and the gonadotropins luteinizing hormone (LH) and follicle-stimulating hormone (FSH) production and/or secretion are also affected by the proposed regulatory changes in the neurotransmitters, similar to that observed in anorexia nervosa (10–12).

None of the features of psychosocial deprivation is pathognomonic. The etiology almost always includes a dysfunctional parent or family within the framework of an abnormal social environment. In one study, personality disorders were common in mothers of children treated for deprivation (14). In an investigation of 14 cases of "garbage eaters," 10 cases had mothers who restricted food (4).

The characteristic clinical findings in children with psychosocial-deprivation dwarfism include:

1. emotional disturbances including temper tantrums, apathy, depression, and withdrawal
2. sleep disorders such as insomnia and sleep wandering
3. bizarre behavior, pain agnosia, self-inflicted injuries
4. bizarre eating behavior including polyphagia, gorging and vomiting, stealing food, and eating from garbage and animal dishes
5. bizarre drinking behavior including polydypsia and drinking stagnant water, toilet bowl water, fish tank water, or dishwater
6. developmental lags and decreased performance in cognitive testing (1,4,5,11,15).

Because nutritional intake prior to the diagnosis is usually obtained from the history, it is hard to ascertain what the intake actually had been. Several authors have reported excessive caloric intake with no sign of malabsorption or significant diarrhea associated with poor weight gain and lack of growth. No satisfactory explanation has resolved the intriguing question of the "missing calories," if, indeed, there are missing calories. Krieger (4), in studies involving home-feeding, describes a case in which a child gained 70 g/day with measured intake. In two endocrine studies, Krieger found both nutritional and sensory deprivation in patients with the deprivation syndrome. Nutritional intake needs to be investigated more extensively to determine its role as an etiological factor and as a factor in improved status.

It is essential, in the case of a child suspected of having psychosocial-deprivation dwarfism, that a very careful history complement a thorough clinical and laboratory investigation to determine diagnosis.

DIAGNOSIS

Although the incidence of psychosocial-deprivation syndrome is not clear, the Stanford University Pediatric Endocrinology Clinic found that 8 (3%) out of 263 children with true growth retardation were diagnosed with this syndrome (16). In a review of several studies, twice as many boys have been diagnosed as girls (boys, 56% to 77% vs girls, 33% to 54%) (17).

Children with psychosocial-deprivation dwarfism are severely growth retarded, often ≤ -2.5 SD from the mean height-for-age, with a bone maturation index or bone age ≤ -2 SD from the mean. In the initial stages, when these deviations are not present, the diagnosis is more difficult. In that case, a height-velocity standard curve (cm/year), using determinations that span several months, is valuable. When growth stunting is severe, growth velocity may become negligible (0 to 2 cm/year), as in severe hypothyroidism, severe renal failure, or, less commonly, severe growth hormone deficiency (1,4,8–10,12).

Characteristics usually revealed in the psychosocial history include emotional disturbances ranging from severe temper tantrums to apathy, withdrawal, and depression. Abnormal eating behavior includes polyphagia, gorging and vomiting, and inappropriate food sources such as animal dishes and garbage cans. Abnormal drinking patterns include polydipsia and inappropriate sources such as toilet bowls and fish tanks. Sleep disorders are characterized by insomnia or sleep wandering. Self-destructive behavior and pain agnosia also coexist. Developmental lags are increasingly apparent as the disease progresses. Enuresis and encopresis are common. Poor performance in cognitive testing has also been reported (5,8,12).

The functional endocrine changes in psychosocial-deprivation dwarfism are similar to those of other chronic disorders in which secondary metabolic and nutritional changes occur. Several characteristics are, however, unique to this syndrome:

1. normal or decreased growth hormone response to stimulus with low serum IGF-1 values (1,4,8,9)
2. decreased amplitude in growth hormone spontaneous pulses; the preserved frequency of pulses suggests a pattern similar to that observed in growth hormone neurosecretory dysfunction (6,9)
3. decreased ACTH response to stimulus by metyrapone testing (although there are no data on corticotropin releasing hormone (CRH) stimulation, available data demonstrate a preserved serum cortisol rise in response to exogenous administration of ACTH, indicating adequate adrenal cortex activity) (1,5,8).

Because most patients are not underweight for height, at clinical presentation they do not appear to be malnourished. Chapter 13 describes in detail the parameters necessary for evaluation of a malnourished child including biochemical and hormonal profiles, radiological studies, and urine and stool examinations. These help determine whether organic causes may be present to explain the child's growth failure.

Although growth deficits are usually attributable to inadequate intake, children with psychosocial-deprivation dwarfism are often reported to have had a caloric intake at or above a reasonable range for the weight of the child. Scientific documentation of adequate nutrient intake associated with such growth failure needs further documentation. It has been suggested, however, that if growth deficits can be attributed to "caloric wastage" secondary to chronic stress, the resulting neutral or modestly negative caloric balance may slow linear growth while allowing the child to maintain an adequate weight-for-height (5,8,12).

TREATMENT

The neglect/abuse factor in psychosocial-deprivation syndrome makes it essential that there is an integrated approach to the care of the child including the services of a pediatrician, nutritionist, social worker, psychologist, and child psychiatrist, all of whom participate in the early evaluation and treatment of the child (5).

The diagnosis of psychosocial-deprivation dwarfism is confirmed when improvement follows environmental change. This may occur when the patient is either moved to a more nurturing environment or when intervention has resolved the family's psychopathology (5,8,18). This "treatment" almost invariably leads to rather dramatic changes, including weight gain with catch-up growth, and behavioral-developmental improvement. As has been stated, controlled studies are needed to confirm the role of nutrition intervention in these demonstrated improvements. In cases where the environment has not, in fact, really changed or where the original psychosocial stress factors return, deceleration and stunting of growth will recur despite appropriate nutrient intake (1,4,5,8).

Response to human pituitary growth hormone and recombinant human growth hormone in children with psychosocial-deprivation dwarfism has been poor, although when combined with a positive environmental change, growth velocity increases and "catch-up" growth occurs (19). It is well documented, however, that there is no need for such therapy since behavioral and endocrine changes are rapid once patients are placed under the care of a loving staff, relatives, or foster parents (1,7–9,18).

Psychotherapy for the child and the family are almost always needed for reasonable recovery. Some children may be allowed to return to their original homes with ongoing counseling and supervision. Sadly, many children must be removed from their families for prolonged periods of time, often permanently (1,4,5,11,12,15).

When patients remain in a supportive environment the prognosis is good for continued growth, weight gain, and adolescent development. Intellectual recovery is also significant (5). Serious psychological scarring has, however, been reported. If patients do return to their original homes, frequent monitoring is essential to assure that the environment does not revert to its original, destructive pattern (5).

CONCLUSION

Psychosocial-deprivation dwarfism is a unique syndrome in which a child demonstrates growth retardation associated with bizarre behavior including very abnormal eating and drinking patterns. It is almost always associated with a pathological, abusive home environment. Its dramatic therapeutic response to a supportive environment causes it to be somewhat analogous to the environmentally stressed, nutritionally deprived, growth-retarded child from the third world. The pathophysiology of this syndrome suggests that chronic stress-induced central nervous system neurotransmitter regulatory changes may be part of its etiology (6,9). Because problems often recur when recovered patients return to their original environments, it is likely that etiologic agents are capable of a recurrent effect on the child. Identification of the neuroendocrine changes that precede the growth failure may be dependent on an accurate description of the patient's early psychosocial milieu as well as of the documented nutritional intake.

Psychosocial-deprivation dwarfism differs from protein-energy malnutrition in that baseline serum growth hormone concentrations are detectable or elevated in protein-energy malnutrition and undetectable or low in psychosocial-deprivation dwarfism. The elevated growth hormone levels in children with primary protein-energy malnutrition dramatically decrease within 24 hr of the first protein meal (20). The lack of response to growth hormone administration in children with psychosocial dwarfism indicates that the child needs appropriate environmental and nutritional support to effect optimal growth.

The characteristically abnormal environment from which patients with psychosocial-deprivation dwarfism emerge highlights the psychogenic factor in the etiology of this syndrome (11,15,18). Further studies are necessary, however, to better understand the pathophysiology of this disorder, including the role of nutrient intake in its cause and its treatment.

No matter what the physiology is, however, the basis of this syndrome is deprivation. Charles Dickens, himself, was a victim of deprivation. It is not surprising that his literature is replete with mishandled and abused, but extraordinarily "good," children who, in the end, defeat their abusers (18), after surviving the horrors of this abuse. As Oliver Twist pleaded with dramatic elegance, "Don't turn me out of doors to wander in the streets again."

REFERENCES

1. Brasel JA. Review of findings in patients with emotional deprivation. In: Gardner LI, Amacher P, eds. *Endocrine aspects of malnutrition—marasmus, kwashiorkor and psychosocial deprivation.* Santa Ynez, CA: Kroc Foundation, 1973;115–127.
2. Frasier SD. Abnormalities of growth. In: Collu R, Ducharme JR, Guyda H, eds. *Comprehensive endocrinology series—pediatric endocrinology.* New York: Raven Press, 1981;167–204.
3. Kaplan SA. Growth and growth hormone: disorders of the anterior pituitary. In: Kaplan SA, ed. *Clinical and pediatric endocrinology.* Philadelphia: WB Saunders, 1990;1–60.
4. Krieger I. Endocrines and nutrition in psychosocial deprivation in the U.S.A.: comparison with growth failure due to malnutrition on an organic basis. In: Gardner LI, Amacher P, eds. *Endocrine aspects of malnutrition—marasmus, kwashiorkor and psychosocial deprivation.* Santa Ynez, CA: Kroc Foundation, 1973; 129–162.
5. Green WH, Campbell M, David R. Psychosocial dwarfism: a critical review of the evidence. *J Am Acad Child Psychiatry* 1984;23:39–48.
6. Bercu BB. Growth hormone neurosecretory dysfunction: Update. In: Bercu BB, ed. *Basic and clinical aspects of growth hormone.* New York: Plenum Press, 1988;119–141.
7. Ruch W, Bubl R, Eggli E. Psychosocial dwarfism in three siblings. *Helv Paediatr Acta* 1988;43:233–239.
8. Sarr M, Job JC, Chaussain JL, Golse B. Psychogenic growth retardation. Critical study of diagnostic data. *Arch Fr Pediatr* 1987;44:331–338.
9. Stanhope R, Adlard P, Hamill G, Jones J, Skuse D, Preece MA. Physiological growth hormone secretion during recovery from psychosocial dwarfism: a case report. *Clin Endocrinol (Oxf)* 1988;28:335–339.
10. Blunk W, Morrot M, Borner S. Zur Differentialdiagnose des psychosozialen Minderwuchses. *Pediatr Grenzgeb* 1990;29:K4–6.
11. Money J. The syndrome of abuse dwarfism (psychosocial dwarfism or reversible hyposomatropism)—behavioral data and a case report. *Am J Dis Child* 1977;131:508–513.
12. Mouridsen SE, Nielsen S. Reversible somatotropin deficiency (psychosocial dwarfism) presenting as a conduct disorder and growth hormone deficiency. *Dev Med Child Neurol* 1990;32:1087–1104.
13. Brown PI, Brasel JA. Endocrine changes in the malnourished child. In: Suskind RM, Lewinter-Suskind L, eds. *The malnourished child.* Nestlé Nutrition Workshop Series, vol 19. New York; Raven Press, 1990;213–228.
14. Fischhoff J, Whitten CG, Pettit MG. A psychiatric study of mothers of infants with growth failure secondary to maternal deprivation. *J Pediatr* 1971;79:209–215.
15. Sonis WA, Spiliotis B, Maymi-Gascue M, Schuman E, Bercu BB. Maturational arrest: an experiment in nature. *J Am Acad Child Adolesc Psychiatry* 1987;26:277–280.
16. Werther GA. Causas no endocrinas del retardo de crecimiento. In: Hintz RL, Rosenfeld RG, eds. *Trastornos del crecimiento.* Barcelona: Ancora S.A., 1987;87–115.
17. Rudolf MCJ, Hochberg Z. Are boys more vulnerable to psychosocial growth retardation? *Dev Med Child Neurol* 1990;32:1022–1025.
18. Gardner LI. The endocrinology of abuse dwarfism—with a note on Charles Dickens as child advocate. *Am J Dis Child* 1977;131:505–507.
19. Root AW, Diamond F. Effects of human growth hormone in normal short children and in patients with intrauterine growth retardation, glucocorticoid-induced stunting of growth, osteochondrodystrophies and other disorders. In: Bercu BB, ed. *Basic and clinical aspects of growth hormone.* New York: Plenum Press, 1988;311–325.
20. Suskind RM, Amatayakul K, Leitzmann C, Olson RE. Interrelationships between growth hormone and amino acid metabolism in protein-calorie malnutrition. In: Gardner LI, Amacher P, eds. *Endocrine aspects of malnutrition—marasmus, kwashiorkor and psychosocial deprivation.* Santa Ynez, CA: Kroc Foundation, 1973;99–114.

CHAPTER 25A

Childhood Obesity

William H. Dietz

Obesity is the most prevalent nutritional disease of children and adolescents in the United States. This chapter focuses on the most important aspects of the identification, clinical approach, and therapy of childhood obesity.

IDENTIFICATION

The reliability of various anthropometric measures of fatness depends on each measure's correlation with total body fat, determined either by underwater weighing, isotope dilution, or ^{40}K counting. Although this problem has not been studied extensively in pediatric patients, both triceps skin-fold thickness (TSF) and body mass index (BMI: weight in kilograms divided by height in meters^2) appear to have similar correlation coefficients with total body fat (1). A TSF greater than the 85th percentile for children of the same age and sex has been used in the past to determine obesity. The appropriate cutoff point for the body mass index has not yet been established.

Clinically, plots of weight and height on the National Center for Health Statistics growth charts are the easiest first approximation of the degree of overweight. For preadolescent children, the height/weight chart on the back of the form is sufficient. A weight-for-height in excess of the 95th percentile indicates that the child is overweight; ideal body weight is defined as the 50th percentile of weight for children of the same height age and sex. In adolescents, calculation of ideal body weight depends on the assumption that weight should fall within 120% of the same percentile for height. Therefore, obesity is considered a weight-for-height that is in excess of 120%, i.e.,

$$\frac{\text{actual weight}}{\text{weight-for-height}} > 120\%.$$

In most children overfatness will be readily apparent, so that the standard growth charts can be used. Triceps skin-fold measurements are essential to determine whether children who are mildly overweight have an excess of body fat or fat free mass. For example, children who are muscular, or who have a large frame will be overweight, but not overfat. Such children may have a weight-for-height that is greater than the 95th percentile, but their TSF will be within the normal range.

When discussing excessive fatness with families, we rarely use the term *obesity,* even though the term is more commonly used by the general public to describe morbid fatness. Most families appear to prefer the word *overweight* regardless of how obese their child is. Therefore we describe our patients as overweight rather than obese, although the dichotomous definition is more commonly used in medical settings. However, for the purpose of this chapter, we will use the term *obesity* to describe the child or adolescent with a triceps skin fold in excess of the 85th percentile.

Within populations, considerable debate still exists regarding the most appropriate measure of obesity. We have used baseline measures of TSF obtained during the National Health Examination Survey to demonstrate increases in the prevalence of childhood obesity between 1965 and 1980 (2). However, over the same time period, no changes were observed in body mass index (3). Although our results have been criticized because of the difficulties inherent in the standardization of TSF measures between surveys (4), the BMI is not a direct measure of fatness. Therefore, if a population is becoming less fit and fatter simultaneously, the BMI could remain constant, whereas the TSF would increase (5).

CLINICAL APPROACH

First Encounter

Patients with chronic obesity in our clinic require an hour for the first visit. We require both parents in an

---

W. H. Dietz: Department of Pediatrics, Tufts University School of Medicine, Boston, Massachusetts 02111.

intact family, and where possible the significant other (friend, grandparent, etc.) in a single parent family to attend the first visit. This approach has several important advantages. First, a family visit enlarges the scope and the focus of the problem. From the outset the problem is redefined as a family rather than an individual difficulty. Second, a family visit allows us to determine in a relatively unbiased setting how important the problem is to each of the family members, to establish whether they agree on its causes, and to assess whether they think weight loss is possible. We also seek information from the parents regarding their own history of obesity, and the types of difficulties that they encountered when they were overweight. Such information often initiates an alliance with the parents at the outset of treatment, particularly if the health professional's attitude is nonjudgmental and sympathetic. This approach may also help establish parental ambivalence regarding food restrictions. For example, obese parents who link a child's success at weight reduction to their own ability to adhere to a diet may be less consistent regarding food restriction than parents who have never been obese.

Because the psychosocial consequences of obesity are so prevalent, and because peer group discrimination is often the factor that prompts a family to seek therapy and may act as a powerful catalyst for change, we often ask early in the course of the interview if obesity has had any significant social consequences. Children as young as 5 or 6 years of age have already learned to distinguish children who are overweight, and consistently rank overweight children as less desirable playmates (6). Teasing on the playground and exclusion from games is commonplace. As a result, overweight children and adolescents often prefer the company of younger children who are less likely to discriminate against them.

With advancing age, discrimination becomes more subtle and institutionalized. For example, acceptance rates to prestigious colleges were significantly lower for obese girls matched for performance with nonobese girls (7). Among the most time-consuming and painful experiences for obese children and adolescents is shopping for clothes. Very few clothes of any quality are designed and manufactured for the obese child or adolescent, despite the high prevalence of the disorder. The recent trend in baggy clothing has been a boon to the obese pediatric population, and it seems reasonable to assume that the demand for such clothes by an increasingly overweight pediatric population may have produced or sustained the trend.

Dietary History

Recent studies indicate that both normal and overweight adolescents underreport food intake and that underreporting was greater among the obese cohort (8). Because the obese cohort underreported energy intake by almost 30%, we no longer rely on a dietary history to determine caloric requirements. Currently, we combine a history of usual dietary intake with a history of frequency of intake of high–caloric-density foods. These methods in combination allow us to identify foods that can be eliminated for calorie reduction without a drastic alteration in the dietary pattern. Although objective data are lacking, this approach may enhance long-term dietary adherence.

Family History

The family history should focus on other members of the extended family who have been overweight, in an effort both to determine the prevalence of obesity within the family and to begin to approach the potential myths that underlie the disease. For example, if the prevailing notion within the family is that the child is overweight, just as the rest of the family is overweight, and that everyone is destined to be overweight, obesity may be viewed as an index of family membership that will be particularly resistant to therapy. However, if the family believes that the child can lose weight, we frequently prescribe a dietary modification at the time of the first visit.

Other aspects of the family history may also be used to estimate and heighten concern about the potential morbidity of obesity. A strong family history of non–insulin-dependent diabetes mellitus (type II diabetes mellitus) increases the risk that diabetes may occur in the obese patient later in life. Type II diabetes is rare in the pediatric patient, although it does occasionally occur in obese adolescents with a strongly positive family history (9). Likewise, strong family histories of hypertension, hypercholesterolemia, or evidence of early atherosclerotic cardiovascular disease all heighten the risk of future disease if obesity is allowed to persist. Emphasis that weight reduction will reduce the risk of these complications may also increase the potential for adherence.

REVIEW OF SYSTEMS

The review of systems should stress potential causes or consequences of obesity. Although social discrimination against obese children is widespread, self-esteem may remain unaffected (10). Mild mental retardation, learning disabilities, or congenital syndromes, such as myelodysplasia or Down syndrome, identify children at risk for the disease, as well as a family constellation associated with a potentially vulnerable child. Recurrent headaches that have recently increased in frequency or severity identify children or adolescents in whom a hypothalamic tumor must be sought and excluded.

The patient's involvement in, and capacity for, exercise should be determined. Obese adolescents are observably less active than their nonobese counterparts (11). However, the energy costs of activity are greater, because of the increased mass to be moved. These observations explain why the energy spent on activity by obese adolescents does not differ from that of the nonobese (12).

Time spent viewing television is directly related to the prevalence of obesity, probably because television viewing promotes both inactivity and increased food consumption (13). The reduced fitness observed among children who watch more television (14) suggests that the effects of television on activity may be more important than the effects of television on food intake. Strategies to decrease television viewing may significantly reduce the prevalence of childhood obesity in the United States.

Additional areas to be considered include daytime somnolence, nocturia, and abdominal or extremity pain. Daytime somnolence may be the most important indication of sleep apnea or primary alveolar hypoventilation. The majority of affected patients have a history of snoring, and a history of frank apneic episodes is present in approximately 30% (15). Despite the anxiety about this problem, families rarely discuss it spontaneously. Based on published data, the potential mortality of sleep apnea or primary alveolar hypoventilation is 30% (16).

Nocturia may be the only symptom of type II diabetes mellitus. In contrast to adults, where truncal fat distribution appears to be a major risk factor for abnormal glucose tolerance and other cardiovascular sequelae of obesity, no convincing evidence suggests that fat distribution plays a major role in the occurrence of cardiovascular risk factors in children and adolescents. In part, the lack of such data is attributable to the lack of control for body fatness in such studies. The problem is also complicated by the centrifugal distribution of fatness that occurs normally during puberty (17).

In our clinic, the prevalence of encopresis appears increased, although our analysis of data from the National Health Examination Survey suggests that neither enuresis nor encopresis occur with increased frequency in an unselected obese population of either children or adolescents (W. H. Dietz and S. L. Gortmaker, unpublished observations). Steatohepatitis (18) and cholecystitis (19) must also be considered in the differential diagnosis of abdominal pain in the obese pediatric patient, particularly if recent weight reduction has occurred (20).

Hip pain may suggest imminent slipped capital femoral epiphysis. Although this disorder is rare, the majority of patients in whom it occurs are obese (21). Chronic ankle strain or pain may reflect the effect of increased weight bearing. In addition, obesity may delay the recovery time from minor injuries.

PHYSICAL EXAMINATION

Obesity has a variety of effects on growth, psychosocial development, and disease. Among the most benign of these are the effects of excessive fatness on growth. Obese children are generally taller at all ages than other children of the same age and sex, as well as taller than expected for their genetic potential. Ultimate height, however, remains unaffected.

The effects of obesity on growth may affect how the pediatrician discusses the problem with the family. Because an obese 5-year-old may be the size of an 8-year-old, or an obese 10-year-old may be the size of a 14-year-old, the expectations and interactions of those who meet them for the first time may be inappropriate for the child's age. One potential consequence for health professionals is that the child's ability to comprehend dietary instructions may be overestimated.

One of the most important clues that a problem other than energy imbalance may be contributing to obesity is a height less than the 50th percentile, or a height less than expected for genetic potential. Many of the congenital or acquired syndromes associated with obesity, such as Prader-Willi syndrome or Cushing's syndrome, are associated with short stature.

Growth charts can also be used to demonstrate to families the duration of weight maintenance required for their children to achieve ideal weight by "growing into their weight." The demonstration is accomplished by assuming that the height percentile will remain constant, and by drawing a line horizontally across the growth chart from the present weight until it intersects the same percentile on the weight chart. The current age is then subtracted from the age at which the intersection occurs to estimate the length of time required to achieve ideal body weight.

Obesity is also associated with advanced bone age, early menarche (22), and increased fat free mass (23). Early menarche associated with obesity may be difficult to distinguish from early menarche due to other causes, and may occasionally require the assistance of an endocrinologist. Fat free mass accounts for approximately 20% of the increased weight in obesity (24) and is associated with an increase in metabolic rate (12). Whether the increase in fat free mass represents muscular hypertrophy or the increase in the nuclear mass of adipocytes remains unclear.

Blood pressure, taken with an appropriate-size cuff, will exclude hypertension. Approximately half of all hypertensive children or adolescents are obese. Hypertension in obese patients with Bardet-Biedl syndrome, formerly called Laurence-Moon-Biedl, (25) is most likely of renal origin. In obese adolescents, however, hypertension may be attributable to chronic sodium retention that results from hyperinsulinism (26). As in adults, modest weight reduction may have a marked impact on blood pressure and sensitivity to sodium (27).

In patients with a history of headache, a fundoscopic examination and careful neurologic examination are essential to exclude the possibility of a hypothalamic tumor. We have never seen a child in whom this diagnosis has been the presenting cause of obesity, although obesity frequently occurs following resection of a craniopharyngioma.

Enlarged tonsils in patients with sleep apnea suggest the usefulness of a tonsillectomy, which may be lifesaving. Such children should be monitored in an intensive care unit following surgery because retropharyngeal swelling may produce respiratory obstruction.

Increased fatty breast tissue may embarrass boys, who may refuse to go swimming or remove their shirts because of the fear that they will be called girls. These patients should be reassured that their breast enlargement is due to excess fat that will diminish as they lose weight, and that they are not becoming girls.

Hirsutism and amenorrhea in adolescent girls should suggest the possibility of polycystic ovary disease (28). Obesity appears to play a major role in the genesis of this disease because of the role of adipose tissue in the aromatization of estrogens (29). Weight reduction in adults may reverse many of the abnormalities associated with polycystic disease, suggesting that obesity may play a causal role (30).

In young children, severe obesity may produce abnormalities of the lower extremities, such as bowing of the femur or tibia (Blount disease) (31). Affected children commonly exhibit a waddling gait. The bowing is readily apparent on physical examination, but the bony abnormality should be confirmed radiologically. This abnormality is directly related to the severity of obesity (31). Surgical correction is usually required. The disease will recur following surgery if obesity persists.

INTERVENTION

Despite the mystique that surrounds obesity, weight loss cannot be achieved without a negative energy balance. Therefore, the cornerstones of therapy are an increase in activity and/or a reduction in energy intake. Neither can be achieved without substantial and sustained adherence by the family.

Obesity is not a problem that easily fits traditional models of therapy, because substantial behavioral change on the part of the child and the family is required. Obesity is not often viewed as a disease in the same category as an infection. Medications are ineffective, and simplistic recommendations rarely work. The family context of obesity, and the information necessary to effective therapy cannot be adequately elicited in a short visit. Furthermore, although the mother is the parent who usually accompanies the child to the pediatrician's office, she, too, is a member of a larger system. Fathers also determine what food is purchased, prepared, served, and consumed. A focus on the family at the outset not only has the advantage of permitting a detailed observation of the family's interaction around the child's obesity, but gives the family the implicit message that the focus of change is broader than the child.

Dietary Modification

Weight reduction programs require a design for the whole family rather than patient-specific changes. Family food selection patterns are easier to adjust than those of isolated individuals within the family. Although no clinical method exists to establish the level of caloric intake necessary to achieve a negative caloric balance, dietary histories and a modified food frequency questionnaire may be used to identify high caloric density foods usually consumed. Because a significant portion of patients overdrink, rather than overeat, consideration of milk, soft drinks, and juice intake is essential. This approach results in a broad plan of recommended and excluded foods rather than specific diets. A more formal approach that categorizes foods as limited, acceptable, or free has also been used successfully (32).

The goals of weight reduction for children and adolescents must be appropriate to the age of the patient and the severity of disease. Mildly overweight children whose growth is incomplete may achieve ideal body weight by weight maintenance. For more severely overweight children, loss of one to two pounds per month is entirely reasonable.

More restrictive diets in a routine clinic setting should be used cautiously in children and adolescents. Twenty per cent of adolescents studied on these diets in the past have had nitrogen losses that have occurred without plateau for the duration of the hypocaloric dietary study period (33). In addition, one of the adolescents we studied using a 24-hr Holter monitor developed repeated asymptomatic episodes of bi-, tri-, and quadrigeminy while consuming hypocaloric diets with and without carbohydrate. Although the clinical implications of her arrhythmias are unclear, these findings emphasize the caution with which such diets must be used. Additional information regarding the content and application of hypocaloric diets is presented elsewhere including the following chapter (34).

Activity

The second major intervention consists of increases in activity. Although we believe that television viewing constitutes a major source of inactivity, and that reduction in television time will increase the amount of time spent in more energy-expensive activities, no data yet support this assumption. Rates of weight reduction do not appear significantly different in programs that have included an exercise component. Nonetheless, in both school and clinic programs that have incorporated exercise, long-term success rates appear improved (35,36).

Exercise should be structured on an individual basis. Massively overweight children may achieve maximal energy expenditure during a brisk walk. For such children, prescriptions for jogging are likely to fail. Exercise that becomes part of daily routine, such as walking to or from school, the use of stairs, or outside play after school may stand the greatest likelihood of long-term adherence. As with dietary alterations, the goal is long-term adherence to the modifications proposed.

Commercial Programs

Although many commercial programs exist to treat obese adults, few similar resources are available for adolescents, and none for children. Adolescent participation in programs aimed at adults is often inappropriate. Adult programs are generally directed at women. The concerns of adults and the problems that limit their weight reduction are not commonly shared by adolescents. As a result, adolescents often feel out of place. In addition, many adult programs rely on highly restrictive diets that should not be used routinely to treat adolescent obesity.

Adherence

Adherence usually requires changes in family behavior. Identification of those families that are unlikely to change, or the specific focus for change in those families that are capable of change, is the first task for the pediatrician.

Obesity in an infant may reflect overfeeding that resulted from a misinterpretation of the infant's cues by inexperienced or anxious parents. Such parents will respond to an infant's restlessness or fretting by feeding, rather than comforting. This pattern may be apparent in cases of maternal depression, where the focus on the infant provides a distraction from the mother's preoccupation with her own problems. Excessive feeding also occurs in single children, or the first grandchild in extended families. In such families, food is just one of the many attentions lavished on the infant.

In preschool children, excessive fatness may reflect difficulties with limit-setting. This pattern may appear in parents who are overwhelmed by grief, stress, or depression, in families in which parents cannot tolerate a child's anger or withdrawal, or in families where parents are preoccupied with their own obesity. The latter type of family commonly reports that its child is preoccupied with food, which, in fact, is often substantiated by observation. In such families, either no limits exist with respect to food intake, or the limits are inconsistent. Children rapidly learn that parents will eventually accede to persistent demands for food. Food may also gain them attention from an otherwise preoccupied parent. The preoccupation with food may persist long after the original stimulus for its development has passed.

Work in our clinic has defined several family prototypes common to severe obesity (37). The first of these is known as the triple-decker family. These are extended families that occupy successive floors in the three-story, three-family homes common in Boston. Triple-decker families typically consist of grandparents who live on the first floor, a single mother and her child or children who live on the second floor, and a sibling of the mother on the third floor. In such families there are two sets of parents (the mother and her parents), and two sets of children (the mother and her children). The lines of authority within such families are often confused. Frequently the grandparents exert as much authority over the child as the mother, and a cross-generational alliance exists between the grandparents and the child. Under such circumstances, it is difficult for the parent to set effective limits on the child's food intake, because her authority may be bypassed by sympathetic grandparents, who may not share the mother's perception of the child's weight as a problem. Effective therapy requires access to all those involved.

Another pattern is seen in families in which one parent is also obese. In such families, an overt conflict about the child's weight may mask a covert conflict between the parents about the obese parent's weight; the conflict between the parents about the child's weight is a surrogate for the struggle between the parents. Often the overweight parent is overinvolved with the overweight child. In the clinic, overinvolvement is indicated by statements by the obese parent that the parent and child share the same problem, that their obesity has the same antecedents, or that it is inevitable that the child will grow up to be like the parent. Weight loss is unlikely as long as conflict between the parents persists.

Finally, in some families, both parents may be united in their insistence that the child lose weight. These families are characterized by a more overt conflict than exists in those in which one parent is obese. Such parents frequently report that their child "doesn't care" about his or her weight, and that they, the parents, have "given up." The problems within such a family, where the adolescent is given the responsibility for his or her weight, present as serious a dilemma for the professional as those families in which the parents overidentify with the problem. Weight reduction in such cases often requires that the struggle for independence shift to other behaviors.

Because of the time required, the extensive information necessary for an adequate assessment, the sense of ineffectiveness that obesity provokes, and the lack of training in family therapy and behavior modification, the pediatrician may not be the health professional best suited for the long-term treatment of childhood obesity. Nonetheless, no one is better suited to initiate therapy, to provide the family with an assessment of the child's health, and to convey to them the psychosocial and medical consequences of persistent disease.

Above all, the treatment of obesity requires humility. Families may not be concerned, ready, or able to change at the time that we think they should. Under such circumstances, we must be patient, despite the urgency and concern that we feel. The families and patients who deserve our greatest efforts, however, are those who are ready to achieve and maintain weight reduction.

REFERENCES

1. Roche AF, Siervogel RM, Chumlea WC, et al. Grading fatness from limited anthropometric data. *Am J Clin Nutr* 1981;34:2831–2838.
2. Gortmaker SL, Dietz WH, Sobol AM, et al. Increasing pediatric obesity in the United States. *Am J Dis Child* 1987;141:535–540.
3. Harlan WR, Landis JR, Flegal KM, et al. Secular trends in body mass in the United States. *Am J Epidemiol* 1988;128:1065–1074.
4. Flegal KM, Harlan WR, Landis JR. Secular trends in body mass in the United States, 1960–1980. *Am J Epidemiol,* 1988;128:1065–1074.
5. Gortmaker SL, Dietz WH. Measures of fatness in epidemiologic investigations. *Am J Epidemiol,* 1990;132:194–195.
6. Staffieri JR. A study of social stereotype of body image in children. *J Pers Soc Psychol* 1967;7:101–104.
7. Canning H, Mayer J. Obesity—its possible effect on college acceptance. *N Engl J Med* 1966;275:1172.
8. Bandini LG, Schoeller DA, Dietz WH. Validity of reported energy intake in obese and nonobese adolescents. *Am J Clin Nutr* 1990;52:421–425.
9. Chiumello G, del Guercio MJ, Camelutti M, et al. Relationship between obesity, chemical diabetes and beta pancreatic function in children. *Diabetes* 1969;18:238–243.
10. Kaplan KM, Wadden TA. Childhood obesity and self esteem. *J Pediatr* 1986;109:367–370.
11. Bullen BA, Reed RB, Mayer J. Physical activity of obese and nonobese adolescent girls appraised by motion picture sampling. *Am J Clin Nutr* 1964;14:211.
12. Bandini LG, Schoeller DA, Dietz WH. Energy expenditure in obese and nonobese adolescents. *Pediatr Res* 1990;27:198–203.
13. Dietz WH, Gortmaker SL. Do we fatten our children at the TV set? Television viewing and obesity in children and adolescents. *Pediatrics* 1985;75:807–812.
14. Tucker LA. The relationship of television viewing to physical fitness and obesity. *Adolescence* 1986;21:797–806.
15. Malloy GB Jr, Fiser DH, Jackson R. Sleep-associated breathing disorders in morbidly obese children and adolescents. *J Pediatr* 1989;115:892–897.
16. Riley DJ, Santiago TV, Edelman NH. Complications of obesity—hypoventilation syndrome in childhood. *Am J Dis Child* 1976;130:671–674.
17. Mueller WH. Changes with age of the anatomical distribution of fat. *Soc Sci Med* 1982;16:191–196.
18. Moran JR, Ghishan FK, Halter SA, Greene HL. Steatohepatitis in obese children: a cause of chronic liver dysfunction. *Am J Gastroenterol* 1983;78:374–377.
19. Bennion LJ, Knowler WC, Mott DM, Spagnola AM, Bennett PH. Development of lithogenic bile during puberty in Pima Indians. *N Engl J Med* 1979;300:873–876.
20. Liddle RA, Goldstein RB, Saxton J. Gallstone formation during weight-reduction dieting. *Arch Intern Med* 1989;149:1750–1753.
21. Chung S. Diseases of the developing hip joint. *Pediatr Clin North Am* 1977;24:857–870.
22. Dietz WH Jr. Obesity in infants, children and adolescents in the United States. I. Identification, natural history and aftereffects. *Nutr Res* 1981;1:117–137.
23. Forbes GB. Lean body mass and fat in obese children. *Pediatrics* 1964;34:308–314.
24. Dietz WH, Bandini LG, Schoeller DA, Gortmaker S. Diagnosis of obesity in adolescents and young adults. In: Berry EM, Blondheim SH, Eliahou HE, Shafrin E, eds. *Recent advances in obesity research,* vol 5. London: John Libbey, 1987;9–15.
25. Green JS, Palfrey JS, Hamett JD, et al. The cardinal manifestations of Bardet-Biedl syndrome, a form of the Laurence-Moon-Biedl syndrome. *N Engl J Med* 1989;321:1002–1009.
26. Rocchini AP, Katch V, Kveselis D, et al. Insulin and renal sodium retention in obese adolescents. *Hypertension* 1989;14:367–374.
27. Rocchini AP, Key J, Bondie D, et al. The effect of weight loss on the sensitivity of blood pressure to sodium in obese adolescents. *N Engl J Med* 1989;321:580–585.
28. McKenna TJ. Pathogenesis and treatment of polycystic ovary syndrome. *N Engl J Med* 1988;318:558–562.
29. McDonald PC, Edman CD, Hemsell DL, et al. Effect of obesity on conversion of plasma androstenedione to estrone in postmenopausal women with and without endometrial cancer. *Am J Obstet Gynecol* 1978;130:448–455.
30. Kopelman PG, White N, Pilkinton TE, et al. The effect of weight loss on sex steroid secretion and binding in massively obese women. *Clin Endocrinol* 1981;14:113–116.
31. Dietz WH Jr, Gross WL, Kirkpatrick JA Jr. Blount disease (tibia vara): another skeletal disorder associated with childhood obesity. *J Pediatr* 1982;101:735–737.
32. Epstein LH, Squires S. *The stop-light diet for children.* Boston: Little, Brown, 1988.
33. Dietz WH. Metabolic aspects of dieting in childhood obesity. In: Krasnegor NA, Grave GD, Kutchmer, eds. *A biobehavioral perspective.* Caldwell, NJ: Telford Press, 1988;173–182.
34. Dietz WH Jr. Childhood obesity: susceptibility, cause and management. *J Pediatr* 1983;103:676–686.
35. Epstein LH, Wing RR, Valoski A. Childhood obesity. *Pediatr Clin North Am* 1985;32:363–379.
36. Brownell KD, Kaye FS. A school-based behavior modification, nutrition education, and physical activity program for obese children. *Am J Clin Nutr* 1982;35:277–283.
37. Harkaway JE. Family intervention in the treatment of childhood and adolescent obesity. In: Harkaway JE, ed. *Eating disorders.* Rockville, MD: Aspen, 1987.

CHAPTER 25B

Treatment of Childhood Obesity

Reinaldo Figueroa-Colon, T. Kristian von Almen, and Robert M. Suskind

Studies in the United States confirm the growing prevalence of obesity in children and adolescents (1). Early detection and treatment of obesity are essential. The percentage of obese children who become obese adults is 14% at age 6 months (2), 41% at age 7 years (3), and about 70% at 10 to 13 years of age (4,5). Nonobese children who become obese with advancing age are far less common. Conversely, if an obese child does not lose weight by the end of adolescence, the odds against his/her doing so as an adult are 28 to 1 (6).

T. K. von Almen: Children's Hospital of New Orleans, New Orleans, Louisiana 70118.

R. Figueroa-Colon: Departments of Pediatrics and Nutrition Sciences, Division of Pediatric Gastroenterology and Nutrition, University of Alabama at Birmingham, Childrens Hospital of Alabama, Birmingham, Alabama 35233.

R. M. Suskind: Department of Pediatrics, Louisiana State University School of Medicine, New Orleans, Louisiana 70112.

Childhood obesity occurs as a result of a complex interaction between genetic and environmental factors. Studies implicating genetic influences include those showing differences in energy expenditure between offspring of obese and nonobese parents (7–9), adoption studies demonstrating a significant relationship between adoptees and their biological parents (10–12), overfeeding studies of identical twins (13), and, at the cellular level, lipoprotein lipase activity studies in obese individuals (14,15). Environmental factors that have affected the prevalence of obesity include season, geographic region, population density (16), socioeconomic factors (17–19) including education, income, family size (20), and activity levels (21). The combination of genetic and environmental influences justifies efforts toward successful treatment of childhood obesity. Successful treatment of obesity is predicated on a decreased caloric intake and increased energy expenditures. Success can be enhanced

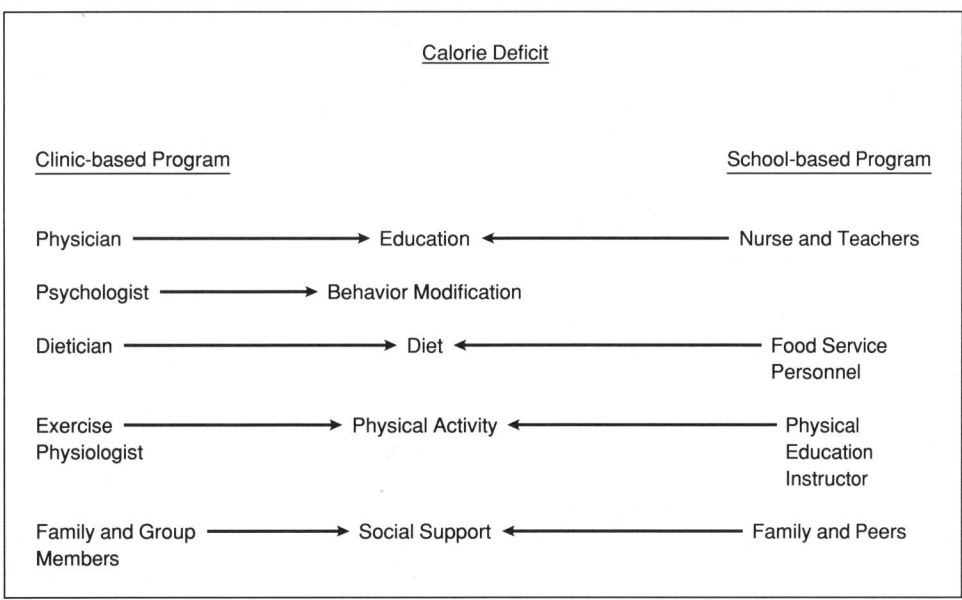

FIG. 1. Conceptual model in the treatment of childhood obesity.

by nutrition education, behavior modification, physical activity, social support, and the patient's willingness to make changes (Fig. 1).

The goals of a treatment program for childhood obesity should (a) be appropriate for the child's age and developmental status, (b) result in significant weight reduction to within 20% of the ideal weight-for-height, and (c) inculcate long-term appropriate eating and physical activity habits that result in weight maintenance but do not hinder growth and development. The treatment includes caloric intake reduced to below energy expenditure, increased physical activity, and modification of eating behavior. The type of diet depends on the age of the child and the severity of the obesity. Because growth is a factor in childhood obesity, diets must provide adequate protein, minerals, and vitamins to support lean body mass and linear growth (22).

TREATMENT

Diet

Protein-Sparing Modified Fast (PSMF) Diet

Very low calorie diets are effective in the medical management of childhood obesity. These diets are typically less than 800 kilocalories (Cal) per day, and contain high biological value protein, with added vitamins, minerals, and small amounts of carbohydrate (23). One such diet developed by Blackburn and Bistrian for adults, and modified by Merritt and Suskind for children (24), is the high-protein/low-calorie protein-sparing modified fast (PSMF) diet (25–30).

Hospitalized adolescents have been studied metabolically while on the PSMF diet (24,31–39). The diet was found to be safe and effective for children who lost weight while preserving lean body mass. In the weight reduction program at Children's Hospital of New Orleans, we have compared PSMF with the traditional hypocaloric balanced diet (40). The PSMF diet (Table 1) consists of 1.5 to 2.0 g of biologically high-quality protein per kilogram ideal body weight per day and provides 600 to 800 Cal daily. Total dietary fat intake is low, ranging from 27 to 36 g per day. The protein sources of the PSMF diet include lean beef (fat trimmed and unmarbled) such as round steak, chicken and turkey (skin removed), fish (if canned, water-packed), and other seafood such as shrimp, crab, oysters, and clams. Four cups of raw or two cups of cooked nonstarchy vegetables are recommended daily. Free food (e.g., pickles, spices, lemon, lime, unsweetened gelatin, and artificial sweetener) are allowed *ad libitum*. Daily supplements include one multivitamin with minerals and iron, 25 mEq of potassium in the form of Morton Lite Salt (Morton Thiokol) or K-lyte (Mead Johnson Laboratories) and 800 mg elemental calcium as four tablets of Tums (Lewis-Howe). A 5-mg tablet of vitamin K, Mephyton (Merck, Sharp and Dohme) is taken weekly. Additionally, children drink a minimum of 2 liters/day of water or calorie-free fluids.

After 10 weeks of being on PSMF or after having reached 120% of ideal weight/height, the child is started on a balanced deficit diet of 1,000 to 1,200 cal. The child's intake is gradually increased during the next 2 to 3 months to provide for maintenance of weight loss and adequate growth.

Hypocaloric Balanced (HCB) Diet

The American Diabetes Association HCB diet reduces caloric intake to 30% to 40% of usual intake. It divides foods into six groups (milk, vegetable, fruit, bread and starch, meat, and fat) and is designed to contain 20% protein, 30% fat, and 50% carbohydrate (41). The deficit is achieved by eliminating foods of high caloric density such as butter, gravy, cheese, mayonnaise, salad dressing, fried foods, and whole milk. The HCB diet poses no recognized hazard for continued growth during weight reduction (42).

The "traffic-light" diet (43) divides foods into five groups (fruits and vegetables, grains, milk and dairy, high protein, and other foods). Foods are then divided into the three "traffic-light" colors: green (go), yellow (caution), and red (stop). Green foods are vegetables that contain less than 20 cal per serving. Yellow foods, taken from each group, have 20 cal per average serving. Red foods, also from each group, are foods that exceed the caloric value of a yellow food. Reduced-calorie foods designed to resemble red foods (e.g., low-calorie lasagna) are considered red foods because, theoretically, dieters will not break the habit of eating regular lasagna by substituting low- for high-calorie lasagna. A food also becomes "red" when combined with other red foods (as in a casserole) or when eaten in excess of over 300 cal per serving. This helps teach that it is not simply the food but the portion that is important. The "traffic-light" diet incorporates nutritional balance within a design for weight loss.

Hypocaloric Liquid Diets

Liquid diets have become popular; many adults find it easier to drink a premade or easily mixed drink than to "count calories" (44–46). One study (39) with eight adolescents, however, revealed poor compliance and a high attrition rate. Further studies are needed to determine the role of hypocaloric liquid diets in the treatment of childhood obesity.

TABLE 1. *Protein-sparing modified fast*

DIET

600 to 800 Cal/day
1.5 to 2.0 g protein/kg ideal body weight/day
25 g/day carbohydrates, low starch vegetables
Water or calorie-free fluids: at least 2 liters/day
Daily supplements: Ca 800 mg/day (4 Tums/day), KCl 25 mEq/day, multivitamins with minerals
Vitamin K (Mephyton): 5 mg/week

Foods allowed

Protein

Lean beef (fat trimmed and unmarbled) such as roast, steak, ground round (hamburger)
Chicken, turkey (remove skin)
Fish (if canned, water-packed)
Seafood such as shrimp, lobster, oyster, clams

Vegetables (4 servings/day)
Serving size: 1/2 cup cooked or juice, 1 cup uncooked

Okra	Broccoli	Artichokes	Cabbage
Beets	Radishes	Sauerkraut	Brussels sprouts
Onion	Eggplant	Cauliflower	Spinach
Squash	Chicory	Tomato juice	Mushroom
Tomato	Asparagus	Bamboo shoots	Beans, green
Rhubarb	Watercress	Vegetable juice	Pepper, green or red
Carrots			

Serving size: 2 cups uncooked

Lettuce	Endive	Greens
Cabbage	Spinach	Chard
Cucumber	Romaine	Collard
Zucchini	Mushrooms	Dandelion
Celery	Chinese cabbage	Mustard
	Green onion	Turnip
		Kohlrabi

Free food

Tea	Rennet	Clear broth
Lime	Spices	Dill or sour pickle
Salt	Mustard	Artificial sweetener
Lemon	Bouillon	Gelatin (unsweetened)
Coffee	Vinegar	Low calorie salad dressing
Pepper	Diet sodas	[Catsup (limit to 1 tbsp/day)] [BBQ sauce (limit to 1 tbsp/day)]

Foods to avoid

Oil	Liver	Cereals	Hamburger	Fried foods
Nuts	Sugar	Sausage	Cold cuts	Peanut butter
Eggs	Cream	Cheese	Avocados	Flour, cornmeal
Pork	Fruits	Breads	Mayonnaise	Starchy vegetables
Milk	Butter	Wieners	Margarine	Regular chewing gum
Bacon	Olives			

Safety Measures During Dietary Restriction

One advantage of the PSMF diet is that ketonuria, which occurs within 2 days, can be monitored daily to assess compliance. However, some subjects, under carefully controlled conditions, have had losses of nitrogen, lymphopenia, and decreases in transferrin and C_3 (24,33,38). Nitrogen losses are mitigated when carbohydrate is added to the diets (38). These metabolic changes appear to have no clinical significance.

Hypocaloric diets may result in a temporary reduction in growth velocity (47–49). Two studies using PSMF diet

(34,39) have reported contradictory findings regarding its impact on linear growth. In one study, most of the children had growth velocities below the 50th percentile (34); the other (39) reported that linear growth was maintained in all five children. Linear growth was not, however, compared to growth velocity standards for age and sex. No current data suggest that a temporary delay in linear growth velocity in obese children is associated with permanent stunting. Close monitoring of a child's growth during weight reduction is recommended.

Exercise

Treatment programs are structured with either aerobic activities and/or a change in life-style activity. Aerobic activities are running, walking, cycling, or swimming, and they are done several times per week at a specific duration and intensity (Table 2). The goal is to increase caloric expenditure and improve fitness. Activity intensity is also important.

Life-style activity is less structured and does not require intensity. Although this program can be made isocaloric to an aerobic program, the intensity of the physical activity is likely to be lower and fitness effects may not be as pronounced. If the goal of the activity is to produce weight loss, then the energy expenditure, and not the physical activity intensity, is the important factor.

Many people do not sustain participation in physical activity programs (50). The most important factor in predicting nonadherence is intensity; subjects adhere less to higher-intensity programs (51). Thus, activity programs must be evaluated both in terms of weight change goals and potential adherence.

Fitness may be measured to assess comparative effects of programs, but fitness should not be considered an end point (52). In addition, weight change itself has been shown to improve fitness when fitness is measured via treadmill or step tests (52).

Physical activity programs (53) should incorporate (a) frequency—3 to 5 times per week; (b) intensity—50% to 60% maximal ability (50% to 60% maximal heart rate); (c) duration—15 min initially, building to 30 to 40 min; (d) mode—use of large muscles, such as walking, jogging, swimming, or cycling; (e) interest—patient-dependent, such as tennis, dancing, skating; (f) enjoyment—an important factor in adherence; (g) incorporation into functional activities, such as walking to school, taking stairs versus elevators, bicycles versus cars; and (h) reducing passive "activities" such as frequent TV watching, lying down after school or meals, spending time with friends who do not like active play.

Behavior Modification

Obesity is a result of more than just the satisfaction of hunger. Habit and interpersonal relationships are also contributory factors. Understanding and treating childhood obesity must take these into consideration (54–56).

Approaches that attempt to ameliorate obesity by modifying behavior must first analyze the discrete behaviors centered around eating, e.g., the type and frequency of food consumed as well as the behaviors antecedent and consequent to food consumption. When these behaviors are understood, programs to modify them can be designed.

Family-based approaches analyze the structure and function of impinging relationships, exploring behaviors that, explicitly or implicitly, influence fatness, activity and food consumption. These two approaches, incorporated into a multidisciplinary childhood obesity program, increase long-term treatment effectiveness.

Successful behavior modification is often dependent on the available support systems. In order to provide the appropriate support, parents, as well as children, must understand the types of programs as well as the techniques.

The two overall methods of behavior modification are the "gradual shift" (shaping) and "all or none" (replacement/omission) approaches. Techniques supporting these methods include diet and activity self-monitoring,

TABLE 2. *Calories expended in various physical activities*

Exercises	Calories per min	Time (min)
Archery	3.5–5	45–60
Backpacking	6–13.5	30–45
Badminton	5–11	20–30
Basketball (nongame)	3.5–11	20–30
Baseball	4.7	45–60
Bicycling	3.5–10	20–30
Bowling	2.5–5	45–60
Calisthenics (aerobic dancing)	5	20–30
Canoeing (2.5–4.0 mph)	3.5–10	30–45
Dancing (social, square)	3.5–8	20–30
Fencing	7.5–12	30–40
Fishing (stream, wading)	6–8	30–45
Football (touch)	7–12	20–35
Golf (walking)	5–9	45–60
Handball	10–15	15–30
Hiking	3.5–8	30–45
Horseback riding	3.5–10	20–45
Horseshoes	2.5–3.5	60–90
Judo and karate	13	15–25
Paddleball (racket) and squash	10–15	30–60
Rowing	5–15	30–45
Running		
12-min mile (5 mph)	10	20–60
8-min mile (7.5 mph)	15	15–30
6-min mile (10 mph)	20	15–30
5-min mile (12 mph)	25	15–30
Sailing	3–6	30–60
Scuba diving	6–10	30–60

goal setting, stimulus control, cue elimination, behavior substitution, exploration of alternatives to overeating, and parental support (Table 3).

1. *Diet and activity self-monitoring* requires the child to keep a daily diary of all foods eaten and activities undertaken. The goal is to help children and parents become aware of energy requirements and expenditures.
2. Children are also encouraged to *set weekly goals* for weight loss. Appropriate praise and material rewards are given for goal attainment.

TABLE 3. *Behavioral modification of weight-reduction programs*

Self-monitoring
  Diary of dietary record
    Each time that patients eat they write down precisely what they eat, how much, at what time of day, where they were, whom they were with, and how they felt
  Diary of activity log
    Each time that patients exercise they write down the mode of activity, the duration, and the intensity
Control of the stimuli that precede eating
  Shopping
    Shop for food after eating
    Shop from a list
    Avoid ready-to-eat foods
    Do not carry more cash than needed for shopping
  Plans
    Plan to limit food intake
    Substitute exercise for snacking
    Eat meals and snacks at scheduled times
    Do not accept food offered by others
  Actions
    Store all food out of sight
    Remove food from inappropriate places in the house
    Do not put serving dishes on the table
    Use smaller plates
    Avoid being the food server
    Leave the table immediately after eating
    Do not save leftovers
  Holidays and parties
    Plan intake before each party
    Eat a low-calorie snack before parties
    Practice polite ways to decline food
    Do not get discouraged by an occasional setback
Development of techniques to control the act of eating
  Drink a glass of water before starting to eat
  Prepare foods one portion at a time
  Put fork down while chewing
  Chew thoroughly before swallowing
  Leave some food on the plate
  Pause in the middle of the meal
  Do nothing else while eating (i.e., reading, watching television)
Reinforcement of the prescribed behaviors: in treatment sessions, patients learn how to obtain rewards for their changed behavior by learning to:
  Solicit help from family and friends
  Teach family and friends to provide help in the form of praise and inexpensive material rewards
  Utilize self-monitoring records as basis for rewards
  Plan specific rewards for specific behaviors

3. *Stimulus control,* or the avoidance of situations that encourage overeating, is taught. An example is understanding the ways in which to cope with parties and ordering in restaurants.
4. *Cue elimination,* i.e., elimination of those foods that both tempt and induce obesity, is encouraged. An example is banning purchase of high-fat and high-calorie foods.
5. *Behavior substitution* is the technique of initiating a noneating activity at a time when food would normally be consumed, e.g., going for a walk after school rather than heading for the kitchen to "snack." It also means becoming aware when overeating occurs as a result of boredom and learning to substitute other activities.
6. *Parental support:* Parents become part of the "team." They are instructed in weight-losing techniques, on setting up consistent enforceable limits, on how to provide positive reinforcement for weight-losing behaviors and how to ignore behaviors incompatible with weight loss.

CLINIC- AND SCHOOL-BASED PROGRAMS

Multidisciplinary interventions have replaced one-on-one dietary instruction by a physician. These medically supervised programs usually use groups to teach dietary restriction, nutrition, exercise, behavior modification and family life-style change (Fig. 1). Such programs have demonstrated short-term success (57,58), although some long-term studies indicate recidivism rates similar to those reported in adults. In two studies, 80% to 100% of children returned to preclinic levels of obesity 7 to 9 years after treatment (59,60). Other studies, however, reported more favorable results 5 (61) and 10 (62) years after treatment.

Intervention is usually clinic/hospital- or school-based (Fig. 1). In either setting, the treatment team usually consists of a physician, dietitian, psychologist, and exercise physiologist. Therapy may be group or individual. Group intervention has the decided advantage of providing a support system beyond that of the therapeutic team. A school-based program provides an additional support group, i.e., peers who may provide moral support to a child who needs to lose weight. In addition, school resources and the environment are conducive to successful management of childhood obesity (63–67); schools allow easy access to children providing both continuity, concentrated contact, and cost-effectiveness. Intervention also takes place within the context of the child's natural environment removing the stigma of hospital-based programs. In addition, schools provide the possibility of intervention before the obesity becomes severe; they are a unique place for the dissemination of information to children and their families.

The presence of both peer groups and significant adults in schools offers backup support for the obesity team. The physical layout of the school, including classrooms, gymnasium, and outdoor fields are excellent for the educational as well for as the physical activity components of the obesity programs (66). Finally, because maintenance of weight loss requires long-term, sustained effort, the continuum of time provided through schools is invaluable, especially when weight control programs are started early and incorporated into the total school system (64).

The four elements that are common among several school-based obesity programs (53) include (a) integration of behavior modification, nutrition education, physical activity, and familial support; (b) structured physical activities, four or five times per week, with encouragement and incentives to participate during nonschool hours; (c) team approach, including teachers, physical education instructors, school nurses, counselors, and/or lunchroom supervisors; (d) parent involvement for ensuring home support for the development of new behaviors.

Nutrition and Physical Education Program

Despite their preoccupation with food, obese individuals generally know little about nutrition and are particularly vulnerable to popular myths (68). The most important factor the obese child must learn is that any diet that reduces caloric intake below caloric expenditure will produce weight loss. The most important thing the professional must learn is the patient's eating preferences. In that way, dietary design can incorporate foods that the patient can eat indefinitely.

The following components are essential to an effective nutrition education program (53): (a) teaching the critical aspects of quality nutrition, i.e., food groups, serving requirements, and variety; (b) developing an understanding of intake-expenditure balance; (c) teaching the impact of high-calorie–low-nutrition snacks on weight; (d) teaching selectivity in fast-food intake; (e) teaching selectivity in "snack" intake; (f) alerting children to the myths incorporated into media advertising; (g) teaching the way to read food labels.

Acquisition of the skills as well as the positive attitude necessary for lifetime participation in physical activities are important components of weight maintenance. Although physical education programs may foster this, obese children often lack the motivation, self-confidence, stamina, and motor skills necessary to successfully join with their peers. Their frustration often leads to complete withdrawal from participation. This may be obviated by providing a separate physical education class designed exclusively for overweight children.

Optimally, schools could be used to support an integrated environment designed to promote a healthier lifestyle. Health education could teach students how to monitor diet and exercise behavior, how to recognize when changes are needed, how to initiate those changes, and how to monitor and maintain their success. Nutrition courses could emphasize the long-term problems resulting from high-fat, high-calorie "snacking." School cafeterias could serve low-calorie, low-fat meals, and vending machines could offer snacks that have reduced fat, sugar, and sodium (69,70). Further research is needed to determine the most effective way schools could be used to have a significant impact on children's eating and physical activity behavior.

Behavior Modification

Psychosocial morbidity associated with childhood obesity is of concern. Negative, early stereotyping frequently sets up aberrant behavior and emotional responses in these children. Five- and six-year-old children characterize children with the endomorphic or obese body type as "lazy," "ugly," and "stupid" (71). Obese children have demonstrated significantly lower body self-esteem than normal-weight children (72,73). Further research will broaden understanding of the psychological impact of obesity during childhood and enhance treatment efforts.

Standardized, self-reporting, psychosocial questionnaires for parents, teachers, and children allow health professionals to document participants' perspectives on a variety of parameters. This is essential for understanding both the obese children as well as the adults with whom they have contact. Questionnaire completion time is approximately 30 min.

Questionnaires

For Parents

The Achenbach Child Behavior Checklist (74) measures common child behavior problems from the perspective of the parent. Parameters include aggression, cruelty, hyperactivity, and withdrawal. Normative and clinic-referred norms are available.

The Family Environment Scale–Form R (75) measures family interactional patterns from the parent's perspective. It is composed of ten subscales each divided into three categories: relationship, personal growth, and system maintenance.

For Teachers

The Achenbach Teacher Behavior Checklist (74) measures common child behavior problems from the perspective of the teacher.

For Children

The Culture-Free Self-Esteem Inventory (76) is a child-reported self-esteem measure. Parameters include perception of general, social, academic, and parent assessments. Normative data and data from special populations are available.

The Child Depression Inventory (77) is a child self-report measuring depression. Score is comparable to normative values.

The State-Trait Anxiety Inventory in Children (78) reliably assesses fear and anxiety in children. Normative data are available.

The Piers-Harris Self-Concept Scale (79) is a child self-report measuring self-esteem. The test score is positively correlated with the degree of self-esteem.

Social Support

Success in treating childhood obesity is dependent on a complex support network that includes the family, the peer group, and health professionals.

Parents exert a powerful influence on the eating, activity, and attitude patterns of their children. They determine what food enters the house, and they establish the emotional environment that may impinge on eating behavior. It is generally felt that the parental role in the treatment of a child's obesity needs to be most structured for younger children; adolescents may require more independence.

Family-based behavioral treatment for obese 6- to 12-year-old children was examined for its effect on weight and growth over 10 years (62). Obese children and their parents were randomized to three groups, each of which was provided similar diet, exercise, and behavior modification training but differed in reinforcement for weight loss and behavioral change (62). In one group, parents and children were reinforced for behavioral change and weight loss; in the second group, only children were reinforced for behavioral change and weight loss; in the control group, families were reinforced only for attendance (62). Children in the group in which both parent and child were reinforced showed significantly greater decreases in percent overweight after 5 and 10 years (-11.2% and -7.5%, respectively) than children in the control group ($+7.9\%$ and $+14.3\%$, respectively). Children in the group that only reinforced children showed an increase in percent overweight after 5 and 10 years ($+2.7\%$ and $+4.5\%$, respectively) (62). Height, on the other hand, showed no difference among the three groups. At 10 years, a child's height was correlated with the height of the parents of the same sex ($r = .78$); children were 1.8 cm taller than their parents (62).

This study provides evidence of the importance of family reinforcement in the long-term treatment of childhood obesity. It also satisfies concerns regarding the effect of weight regulation on linear growth (62).

Involvement of peers appears to be helpful in successful treatment of obese children. It is especially helpful when nonobese children learn not to tease a child for being overweight and to be openly supportive of changes in weight and eating patterns. Support of health professionals including the pediatrician, nutritionist, and psychologist is also an important factor in a child's success in losing weight.

SUMMARY

The multidisciplinary approach to weight loss in children combines nutrition education, behavioral modification, psychosocial support, dietary restriction, and increased physical activity designed to gradually mobilize fat stores while preserving lean body mass. Hypocaloric diets promote rapid weight loss and a reduction in risk factors. They are not appropriate for weight maintenance programs. A more long-term approach stresses maintenance of weight loss, and includes exercise, behavior modification, and family and social involvement. Success is enhanced by family, peer group, and health professional support. Although schools have the potential of contributing to both treatment and prevention of childhood obesity, more research is needed to define and clarify their potential role.

The results of a 10-year follow-up of behavioral, family-based treatment program for obese children (62) provide the first evidence that treatment of obesity in childhood can produce effects that persist into young adulthood. Although still overweight, the children in the treatment group showed significantly greater decreases in percent overweight than control children. Treatment, which was relatively conservative, involved a nutritious, low-fat diet with regular exercise.

Childhood obesity is an intellectual challenge but it is not an intractable problem. Successful management of obesity can improve the quality of life and reduce the morbidity and mortality associated with childhood obesity. Obesity-prone people who wish to control their weight must learn to eat defensively and to maintain a relatively high level of physical activity (80).

REFERENCES

1. Gortmaker SL, Dietz WH JR, Sobol AM, Wehler CA. Increasing pediatric obesity in the United States. *Am J Dis Child* 1987;141:535–540.
2. Charney M, Goodman HC, MacBride M, Lyon B, Pratt B. Childhood antecedents of adult obesity: do chubby infants become obese adults? *N Engl J Med* 1976;295:6–9.
3. Stark D, Atkins E, Wolff DH, Douglas JWB. Longitudinal study of obesity in the National Survey of Health and Development. *Br Med J* 1981;283:12–17.

4. Abraham S, Collins C, Nordsieck M. Relationship of child weight status to morbidity in adults. *Public Health Rep* 1970;86:273–284.
5. Birch LL. Effects of peers models' food choices and eating behaviors on preschoolers' food preferences. *Child J Dev* 1980;51: 489–496.
6. Stunkard AJ, Burt V. Obesity and the body image. II. Age at onset of disturbances in the body image. *Am J Psychiatry* 1967;123: 1443–1447.
7. Roberts SB, Savage J, Coward WA, Chew B, Lucas A. Energy expenditure and intake in infants born to lean and overweight mothers. *N Engl J Med* 1988;318:461–466.
8. Bogardus C, Lillioja S, Ravussin E, et al. Familial dependence of the resting metabolic rate. *N Engl J Med* 1986;315:96–100.
9. Ravussin E, Lillioja S, Knowler WC, et al. Reduced rate of energy expenditure as a risk factor for body-weight gain. *N Engl J Med* 1988;318:467–472.
10. Stunkard AJ, Sorensen TIA, Hanis C, et al. An adoption study of human obesity. *N Engl J Med* 1986;314:193–198.
11. Stunkard AJ, Harris JR, Pedersen NL, McClearn GE. The body-mass index of twins who have been reared apart. *N Engl J Med* 1990;322:1483–1487.
12. Macdonald A, Stunkard AJ. Body-mass indexes of British separated twins. *N Engl J Med* 1990;322:1530.
13. Bouchard C, Tremblay A, Despres JP, et al. The response to long-term overfeeding in identical twins. *N Engl J Med* 1990;322: 1477–1482.
14. Kern PA, Ong JM, Saffari B, Cary J. The effects of weight loss on the activity and expression of adipose-tissue lipoprotein lipase in very obese humans. *N Engl J Med* 1990;322:1053–1059.
15. Reitman JS, Losmakos FC, Howard BV, Taskinen MR, Kuusi T, Nikkila EA. Characterization of lipase activities in obese Pima Indians, decreases with weight reduction. *J Clin Invest* 1982;70:791–797.
16. Dietz WH Jr, Gortmaker SL. Factors within the physical environment associated with childhood obesity. *Am J Clin Nutr* 1984;39:619–624.
17. Garn SM, Clark DC. Trends in fatness and the origins of obesity. *Pediatrics* 1976;57:443–456.
18. Goldblatt PB, Moore ME, Stunkard AJ. Social factors in obesity. *JAMA* 1965;192:1039–1044.
19. Garn SM, Bailey SM, Cole PE, Higgins ITT. Level of education, level of income, and level of fatness in adults. *Am J Clin Nutr* 1977;30:721–725.
20. Ravelli GP, Belmont L. Obesity in nineteen-year old men: Family size and birth order associations. *Am J Epidemiol* 1979;109:66–70.
21. Dietz WH Jr, Gortmaker SL. Do we fatten our children at the television set? Obesity and television viewing in children and adolescents. *Pediatrics* 1985;75:807–812.
22. Committee on Nutrition American Academy of Pediatrics. Nutritional aspects of obesity in infancy and childhood. *Pediatrics* 1981;68:880–883.
23. Wadden TA, Stunkard AJ, Brownell KD. Very low calorie diets: their efficacy, safety, and future. *Ann Intern Med* 1983;99: 675–684.
24. Merritt RJ, Bistrian BR, Blackburn GL, Suskind RM. Consequences of modified fasting in obese pediatric and adolescent patients. I. Protein-sparing modified fast. *J Pediatr* 1980;96:13–19.
25. Bistrian BR, Blackburn GL, Stanbury JB. Metabolic aspects of a protein-sparing modified fast in the dietary management of Prader-Willi obesity. *N Engl J Med* 1977;296:774–779.
26. Bistrian BR, Blackburn GL, Stanbury JB. Metabolic aspects of a protein-sparing diet and brief fast on nitrogen metabolism in mildly obese subjects. *J Lab Clin Med* 1977;89:1030–1035.
27. Blackburn GL, Bistrian BR, Flatt TP. Role of a protein-sparing modified fast in a comprehensive weight reduction program. In: Howard A, ed. *Recent advances in obesity research. I.* London: Newman, 1975;279–283.
28. Lindner PG, Blackburn GL. Multidisciplinary approach to obesity utilizing fasting modified by protein-sparing therapy. *Obesity Bariat Med* 1976;5:198–216.
29. Bistrian BR, Blackburn GL, Flatt TP, Sizer J, Scrimshaw NS, Sherman M. Nitrogen metabolism and insulin requirements in obese diabetic adults on a protein-sparing modified fast. *Diabetes* 1976;25:494–504.
30. Bistrian BR. Clinical use of a protein-sparing modified fast. *JAMA* 1978;240:2299–2302.
31. Merritt RJ. Treatment of pediatric and adolescent obesity. *Int J Obes* 1978;2:207–214.
32. Merritt RJ, Bistrian BR. The natural history and treatment of obesity in childhood. In: Blackburn GL, ed. *Obesity.* Boston: Center for Nutritional Research, 1977;1–48.
33. Pencharz PB, Motil KJ, Parsons HG, Duffy BJ. The effect of an energy-restricted diet on the protein metabolism of obese adolescents: nitrogen-balance and whole body nitrogen turnover. *Clin Sci* 1980;59:13–18.
34. Archibald EH, Harrison JE, Pencharz PB. Effect of a weight-reducing high-protein diet on the body composition of obese adolescents. *Am J Dis Child* 1983;137:658–662.
35. Pencharz PB, Clarke R, Archibald EH, Vaisman N. The effect of a weight-reducing diet on the nitrogen metabolism of obese adolescents. *Can J Physiol Pharmacol* 1988;6:1469–1474.
36. Stallings VA, Archibald ED, Pencharz PB. Potassium, magnesium, and calcium balance in obese adolescents on a protein-sparing modified fast. *Am J Clin Nutr* 1988;47:220–224.
37. Stallings VA, Archibald EH, Pencharz PB, Harrison JE, Bell LE. One-year follow up of weight, total body potassium, and total body nitrogen in obese adolescents treated with the protein-sparing modified fast. *Am J Clin Nutr* 1988;48:91–94.
38. Dietz WH Jr, Schoeller DA. Optimal dietary therapy for obese adolescents: comparison of protein plus glucose and protein plus fat. *J Pediatr* 1982;100:638–644.
39. Brown MR, Klish WJ, Hollander J, Campbell MA, Forbes GB. A high protein, low calorie liquid diet in the treatment of very obese adolescents: long-term effect on lean body mass. *Am J Clin Nutr* 1983;38:20–31.
40. Figueroa-Colon R, von Almen TK, Franklin FA, Schuftan C, Suskind RM. Clinical and biochemical responses to a comprehensive outpatient weight reduction program for children and adolescents, comparison of two hypocaloric diets. (submitted)
41. American Diabetes Association. *A guide for the professional: the effective application of exchange lists for meal planning.* New York: American Diabetes Association, 1986.
42. Dietz WH Jr. Childhood obesity: susceptibility, cause and management. *J Pediatr* 1983;103:676–686.
43. Epstein LH, Wing RR, Valoski A. Childhood obesity. *Pediatr Clin North Am* 1985;32:363–379.
44. Genuth SM, Castro JH, Vertes V. Weight reduction in obesity by outpatient semistarvation. *JAMA* 1974;230:987–991.
45. Vertes V, Genuth SM, Hazelton IM. Supplemented fasting as a large-scale outpatient program. *JAMA* 1977;238:2151–2153.
46. Vertes V, Genuth SM, Hazelton IM. Precautions with supplemented fasting. *JAMA* 1977;238:2142–2150.
47. Wolff OH. Obesity in childhood. *Q J Med* 1955;24:109–114.
48. Brook CDG, Lloyd JK, Wolff OH. Rapid weight loss in children. *Br Med J* 1974;3:44–45.
49. Dietz WH Jr, Hartug R. Changes in height velocity of obese preadolescents during weight reduction. *Am J Dis Child* 1985;139: 705–707.
50. Oldridge NB. Compliance and exercise in primary and secondary prevention of coronary heart disease: a review. *Prev Med* 1982;11:56–70.
51. Epstein LH. Adherence to exercise in obese children. *J Cardiol Rehabil* 1984;4:185–195.
52. Epstein LH, Wing RR, Kolske R, Ossip DJ, Beck S. A comparison of lifestyle change and programmed aerobic exercise on weight and fitness changes in obese children. *Behav Res Ther* 1982;13: 651–655.
53. Ward DS, Bar-Or O. Role of the physician and physical education teacher in the treatment of obesity at school. *Pediatrician* 1986;13:44–51.
54. Dietz WH. Childhood obesity. *Ann NY Acad Sci* 1987;499:47–54.
55. Epstein LH, Valoski A, Koeske R, Wing RR. Family-based behavioral weight control in obese young children. *J Am Diet Assoc* 1986;86:481–484.
56. Ganley RM. Epistemology, family patterns and psychosomatics: the case of obesity. *Fam Process* 1986;25:437–451.
57. Epstein LH, Wing RR, Koeske R, Andrasik F, Ossip DJ. Child and parent weight in a family-based behavior modification program. *J Consult Clin Psychol* 1981;49:674–685.

58. Epstein LH, Wing RR, Koeske R, Valoski A. The effects of diet plus exercise on weight change in parents and children. *J Consult Clin Psychol* 1984;52:429.
59. Lloyd JK, Wolf OH, Whelan WS. Childhood obesity: a long-term study of height and weight. *Br Med J* 1981;2:145–148.
60. Ginsberg-Fellner F, Knittle J. Weight reduction in young obese children: effects on adipose tissue and cellularity and metabolism. *Pediatr Res* 1981;15:1381–1389.
61. Epstein LH, Wing RR, Koeske R, Valoski A. Long-term effects of family-based treatment of childhood obesity. *J Consult Clin Psychol* 1987;55:91–95.
62. Epstein LH, Valoski A, Wing RR, McCurley J. Ten-year follow-up of behavioral, family-based treatment for obese children. *JAMA* 1990;264:2519–2523.
63. Seltzer CC, Mayer J. An Effective weight control program in a public school system. *Am J Public Health* 1970;60:679–689.
64. Collip PJ. An obesity program in public schools. *Pediatr Ann* 1975;4:276–282.
65. Botvin GJ, Cantlon A, Carter BJ, Williams CL. Reducing adolescent obesity through a school health program. *J Pediatr* 1979;95:1060–1062.
66. Brownell KD, Kaye FS. A school-based behavior modification nutrition education, and physical activity program for obese children. *Am J Clin Nutr* 1982;35:277–283.
67. Wolf MC, Cohen KR, Rosefeld JC. School-based interventions for obesity: current approaches and future prospects. *Psychol Sch* 1985;22:187–200.
68. Stunkard AJ. Conservative treatments for obesity. *Am J Clin Nutr* 1987;45:1142–1154.
69. Frank GC, Webber LS, Berenson GS. Dietary studies of infant and children: The Bogalusa Heart Study. In: Coates TJ, Petersen AC, Perry C, eds. *Promoting adolescent health.* New York: Academic Press, 1982.
70. Parcel GS, Simons-Morton B, O'Hara N, Baranowski T, Kolbe L, Bee D. School promotion of healthful diet and exercise behavior: an integration of organizational change and social learning theory intervention. *J Sch Health* 1987;57:150–157.
71. Staffieri JR. A study of social stereotype of body image in children. *J Pers Soc Psychol* 1967;7:101–104.
72. Mendelson BK, White DR. Relation between body-esteem and self-esteem of obese and normal children. *Percep Mot Skill* 1982;54:899–905.
73. Mendelson BK, White DR. Development of self-body-esteem in overweight youngsters. *Dev Psychol* 1985;21:90–96.
74. Achenbach TM, Edelbrock CS. *Manual for the Child Behavior Checklist and Revised Child Behavior Profile.* Burlington, VT: Department of Psychiatry, University of Vermont, 1983.
75. Moos RH, Moos BS. *Family Environment Scale (Form R) Manual.* Palo Alto, CA: Consulting Psychologists Press, 1984.
76. Battle J. *Culture-Free SEI Self-Esteem Inventories for Children and Adults.* Seattle, WA: Special Child Publications, 1981.
77. Kovacs M. Ratings scales to assess depression in school-aged children. *Acta Paedopsychiatricia* 1981;45:305–315.
78. Spielberger CD, Gorsuch RI, Lushene RE. *Manual for the State-Trait Anxiety Inventory.* Palo Alto, CA: Consulting Psychologists Press, 1970.
79. Piers EV. *Piers-Harris Children's Self-Concept Scale revised manual.* Los Angeles: Western Psychological Services, 1984.
80. Van Itallie TB. Bad news and good news about obesity. *N Engl J Med* 1986;314:239–240.

CHAPTER 26

Dyslipidemia in Childhood

Raynorda F. Brown, Cynthia Cole Franklin, Binh Dac Ho, and Frank A. Franklin, Jr.

In adults, there is a correlation between coronary heart disease (CHD) and dyslipoproteinemia (DLP). Dietary saturated fat and cholesterol are considered the major environmental causes of hypercholesterolemia. There is strong evidence that the risk of CHD may be reduced by lowering the levels of total and low-density lipoprotein (LDL) cholesterol (C).

This chapter summarizes the rationale and approach to the screening, diagnosis, and management of DLP in children.

RATIONALE FOR INITIATING CONTROL OF CHILDHOOD DYSLIPOPROTEINEMIA

Atherosclerotic Lesions During Childhood

The atherosclerotic process begins in childhood, but only becomes clinically manifest later in life (1). The earliest lesion, the fatty streak, is a lipid-containing intimal lesion. On gross appearance, the lesions are yellow in color and flat or only slightly elevated. Histologically, the earliest phase is an accumulation of small groups of foam cells, i.e., macrophages filled with cholesterol ester. With advancing age, the lesions progressively accumulate smooth muscle cells in the extracellular matrix of the intima. In contrast, the fibrous plaque is a firm, gray-white, glistening and translucent, elevated, lumen-occupying, intimal lesion. It is composed of a thick, fibrous connective tissue cap with varying amounts of lipid overlaying a more concentrated lipid core. The histologic hallmark is a greatly increased extracellular collagen component accompanied by numerous adjoining smooth muscle cells with or without lipid droplet inclusions.

Fatty streaks can be seen by 5 years of age. Initially appearing in the aorta, they do not appear in the coronary arteries until the second decade of life. Fibrous plaques usually begin developing after 20 years of age.

In children and young adults followed in the Bogalusa Heart Study (BHS), the extent of the aortic fatty streaks was significantly correlated with both serum total cholesterol (TC) and LDL-C ($r = .67$ for each correlation) (2). An inverse correlation between the fatty streaks and the ratio of high-density lipoprotein (HDL)-cholesterol (HDL-C) to LDL-cholesterol (LDL-C) plus very low-density lipoprotein (VLDL) cholesterol (VLDL-C) ($r = -.35$) was also observed.

Adverse Lipoprotein Patterns from Childhood into Adulthood: Tracking

Adverse lipoprotein (LP) patterns (elevated TC and LDL-C, and decreased HDL-C) in childhood appear to persist into adulthood. This permits the identification of children at high risk for future cardiovascular disease (CVD). The maintenance of rank order over time among individuals of the same age is called "tracking." Tracking of TC in children is strong but not as strong as in adults (3–12). Smoking, truncal obesity, and physical inactivity produce and promote persistent adverse LP during childhood (9,13).

Association of TC and LP Levels in Children with CHD in Adults

Children in countries with the highest rate of CHD have higher TC levels than children in those countries with a lower rate of CHD.

R. F. Brown: Department of Pediatrics, Louisiana State University School of Medicine, New Orleans, Louisiana 70112.

C. C. Franklin, F. A. Franklin: Departments of Pediatrics and Nutritional Services, Division of Pediatric Gastroenterology and Nutrition, University of Alabama at Birmingham School of Medicine, Children's Hospital of Alabama, Birmingham, Alabama 35233.

B. D. Ho: Department of Biomedical Engineering, Tulane University School of Medicine, New Orleans, Louisiana 70118.

There is a strong correlation between the TC of children and adults within the same country. In the United States, the CHD mortality under age 60 was 2.9 times higher among the first- and second-degree relatives of the high-TC children (TC > 95th percentile) (14). The combined morbidity and mortality from CHD was 1.8 times higher in grandfathers of the high-TC children (15). Fathers of children with LDL-C or VLDL-C above the 75th percentile had a rate of CHD that was 2.2 times higher when there were two consecutive determinations than when there was only a single determination (5). Thus, children with consistently increased TC have two to three times more CHD in their families.

The major CV risk factors that are found in offspring of parents with premature CHD include elevated TC, lower HDL-C levels, higher apolipoprotein B (Apo B) and Apo B/Apo A-I levels (16). In offspring of positive CHD white families, an increase in LDL-C is associated with an increase in premature CHD (17). In contrast, offspring of positive CHD black families have an increased prevalence of lower HDL-C (17).

High CV Risk Life-Styles from Childhood into Adulthood

CV risk in adulthood is increased as a result of lifestyle characteristics developed during childhood, including smoking, obesity, patterns of eating, and exercise. Smoking experimentation occurs early among white boys, 17% by age 8. Although augmented smoking may progress gradually, the habit is usually established by age 14 (18). The frequency of remission of obesity by age 14 is related inversely to age and to the severity of the obesity (19,20). A significantly obese 7-year-old who exceeds 160% ideal body weight has a 60% chance of becoming an obese adult (19,20).

FACTORS INFLUENCING LIPID LEVELS

In order to provide the appropriate intervention, it is important to understand the factors that affect childhood/adolescent LP levels. Interindividual variability in LP levels is the result of the interaction of environmental/cultural factors, both dietary and nondietary, with an individual's genotype.

NONMODIFIABLE FACTORS

Age

Regardless of the culture, serum lipid levels are similar at birth. The mean for TC, triglycerides (TG) and HDL-C are 69.4, 41.6, and 31 mg/dl, respectively (21–37).

Major shifts in the lipoprotein profile are observed during two important developmental phases: 0 to 2 years of age and adolescence (26,32,36,38–42). By age 14 days, the TC levels of Apo B–containing LP have doubled. By age 2 years, the mean serum TC levels approach the young adult level. The changes observed are primarily due to the exogenous fat consumed, starting in the newborn period (43).

In contrast, the dynamic changes observed during adolescence are primarily race and gender determined. By 9 years of age, race-related differences in lipoproteins are clearly established. Characteristically, black children show lower VLDL-C, higher HDL-C, and a higher ratio of cholesterol to Apo B in LDL than whites (44–46). The characteristic gender-related difference is a progressive increase of the ratio of LDL-C to HDL-C and marked decrease of HDL-C/Apo A-I ratio, especially among white males (47,48). These LP shifts establish the adult patterns and have important clinical implications for future development of CHD.

Familial Aggregation

Familial aggregation of lipids and LP is mediated both by heredity and the shared environment. The parent-child correlation (0.2 to 0.4) is a composite of both genetic and cultural (environmental) heritability (49–51). There is a very significant contribution of genetic heritability to population variation in TC and LP (45% to 68%) compared to the marginal environmental contribution (5% to 22%) (52–58). This genetic contribution to LP is largely polygenic with little evidence of major monogenic effects.

Race

Race-related differences in lipoproteins are observed during infancy and persist into adulthood (42,47). Black children have higher TC (+4%) and HDL-C (+12%) than do whites. They also have higher levels of HDL_2 (+5% to 12%) (46,48). In contrast, white children have higher TG (+11%) and VLDL-C (+34%) levels. Also, they have a lower ratio of cholesterol to Apo B in LDL than do blacks. These racial differences become more pronounced in older adolescents and young adult males.

Gender/Pubertal Development and Sex Hormones

Endogenous sex steroid hormones during puberty may account for the sexual divergence of the LP profile observed between males and females, especially among whites (45,59). Estradiol increases HDL-C and decreases VLDL-C. Testosterone decreases HDL-C and increases VLDL-C. Similar effects occur when exogenous sex hormones are administered clinically (60). Upon withdrawal of the sex hormone, the LP profile returns to baseline.

MODIFIABLE DIETARY AND ACTIVITY FACTORS

Fat and Carbohydrates

Dietary factors represent the most important environmental influence on serum lipoproteins. Decreased cholesterol intake is associated positively with changes in serum TC and LDL-C levels in infants and preschoolers (61). Serum TC levels tend to be lower among formula-fed babies than those receiving cow's or human milk (43). The cholesterol intake of preschoolers influences the serum TC and LDL-C levels. The association is not, however, as readily apparent among adolescents and adults. In cross-cultural studies of children, the concentration of TC was shown to be related to the percentage of energy from saturated fatty acids (SFA) (62). For each 1% change in the percentage of dietary energy from SFA, TC increases 1.74 mg/dl. For HDL-C, there is a negative relationship to the percentage of dietary energy from carbohydrate. For an increase of 10% in the percentage of dietary energy from carbohydrate, HDL-C decreases 2.9 mg/dl. Both inter- and intracountry studies suggest that increased levels of TC, and LDL-C in children are associated with higher intakes of protein, SFA, and cholesterol, whereas increased HDL levels are associated with lower intakes of carbohydrate (13,62).

Alcohol

In several populations of children, HDL-C, LDL-C, and TG were positively related to alcohol intake. In the LRC Prevalence Study, for every increment of 1 oz of alcohol per week, HDL-C was higher by 0.55 mg/dl in males and by 1.04 mg/dl in females; LDL-C was higher by 0.70 mg/dl in males and by 2.07 mg/dl in females; TG was 1.07 mg/dl higher in males and 2.14 mg/dl higher in females (54). In the Bogalusa Heart Study, young males who consumed alcohol had increased Apo A-I levels of 5 mg/dl; females increased by 7 mg/dl (63). There was no alcohol-related change in HDL-C/Apo A-I. These studies suggested that alcohol consumption changes the HDL particle composition in a uniform manner and does not alter TC/HDL-C.

Physical Activity and Adiposity

Decreased physical activity and adiposity are causally related in children (64,65). Both produce adverse LP patterns. The degree of physical activity is related directly to HDL-C and inversely to TC/HDL-C ratio (66). It has been suggested that physical activity may lower TG and raise HDL-C independent of its effects on body fatness.

Adiposity, whether expressed by weight-for-height or by subcutaneous fat, is associated with adverse LP patterns in children, i.e., increased TC, LDL-C, and TG, and decreased HDL-C. Longitudinal data suggest an amplification of the adverse impact of adiposity on LP. Those with adiposity in the 85th percentile had a higher adverse LP ratio (LDL-C/HDL-C) at baseline and a greater increase (57%) over a 5-year period than those with triceps skin fold in the lower 15th percentile (5). Sexual maturation with increased adiposity results in a synergistic effect to lower HDL-C. Persistent truncal obesity is associated with long-term tracking of elevated blood pressure and TC from childhood into adulthood (67). Thus, the degree of adiposity in children is associated with the emergence of an adverse LP pattern that increases in magnitude with pubertal development and persists into young adulthood.

MODIFIABLE NONDIETARY FACTORS

Cigarette Smoking

Smoking has a similar adverse effect on lipoprotein profiles in children as in adults. It increases plasma free fatty acids and decreases plasma HDL_2-C (antiatherogenic portion) (54,68). Higher VLDL-C and lower HDL-C levels occur among cigarette smokers, especially girls (69). Compared to nonsmokers, smoking an average of eight cigarettes per day resulted in a decrease in HDL-C of 6.1 mg/dl, an increase LDL-C of 4.1 mg/dl, and an increased TG of 9.4 mg/dl (54,68). Cigarette smoking during adolescence and early adulthood contributed to an adverse LP pattern including lowering both Apo A-I and HDL-C, particularly in white males (63). It also appears to lower HDL-C independent of the association with TG, body composition, age, and alcohol intake (63,69).

Anticonvulsants

Anticonvulsants, which are medications commonly prescribed for children, affect LP levels (70,71). Phenobarbital, carbamazepine, phenytoin, and primidone are associated with an increased TC and HDL-C. Valproic acid appears to have no effect, a discrepancy that has yet to be explained. Among the HDL subfractions, almost all of the increase attributable to anticonvulsant treatment is in the HDL_2 fraction (71). Anticonvulsant therapy produces significantly higher Apo-A levels although there is no effect on Apo-B (71). Several anticonvulsants increase, predominantly, the Apo A-I–rich HDL_2, which may be related to the induction of the hepatic smooth endoplasmic reticulum (72,73).

Oral Contraceptives

Exogenous steroid hormones influence the concentrations of lipids and lipoproteins. Oral contraceptives contain both synthetic estrogens and progestins, which have an androgenic effect. The estrogen used in oral contraceptives are almost exclusively ethinyl estradiol and mestranol. The progestins commonly used in these formulations are the testosterone-derived 19-nor- agents, for instance, norethisterone or norgestrel (74).

Estrogens are potent lipid-altering agents, causing an increase in HDL-C and a decrease in LDL-C. The impact of progesterone on lipids and LP is less clear. The 19-nor- progestins appear to cause adverse LP patterns similar to testosterone. Thus, the specific lipid and LP effects are influenced by the oral contraceptive dose and composite of estrogen and progestin (74).

SCREENING TO IDENTIFY DYSLIPIDEMIC CHILDREN

Controversy over the most effective strategy to identify DLP children exists among the major policy-making groups. Some advocate the selective screening approach: children chosen based on a specific family history of CVD determinants. Others propose screening all children.

Universal Screening

Universal screening is justified by the difficulty in identifying high-risk children. Only 48% of high-risk children are identified through a family history of DLP or premature CVD, in combination or alone. In single-parent households, where the family history may be less complete, the likelihood of identification is even less.

Universal screening for TC in capillary blood, as part of a school-based program, is recommended for all 5- to 8-year-old children (Fig. 1). Alternatively, screening may be done in the physician's office. Reliable TC measurements are easily and inexpensively obtained. The development of the desktop analyzer to accurately and inexpensively analyze fingerstick TC provides an easy, accessible screening tool. Between 5 and 8 years of age, distributions of lipid and LP are well established and stable, and they track well. Rescreening should take place between 15 and 18 years of age since adverse patterns can emerge during adolescence. Those with levels ≥ 200 mg/dl should be retested. The second TC level obtained may be lower due to regression to the mean. In

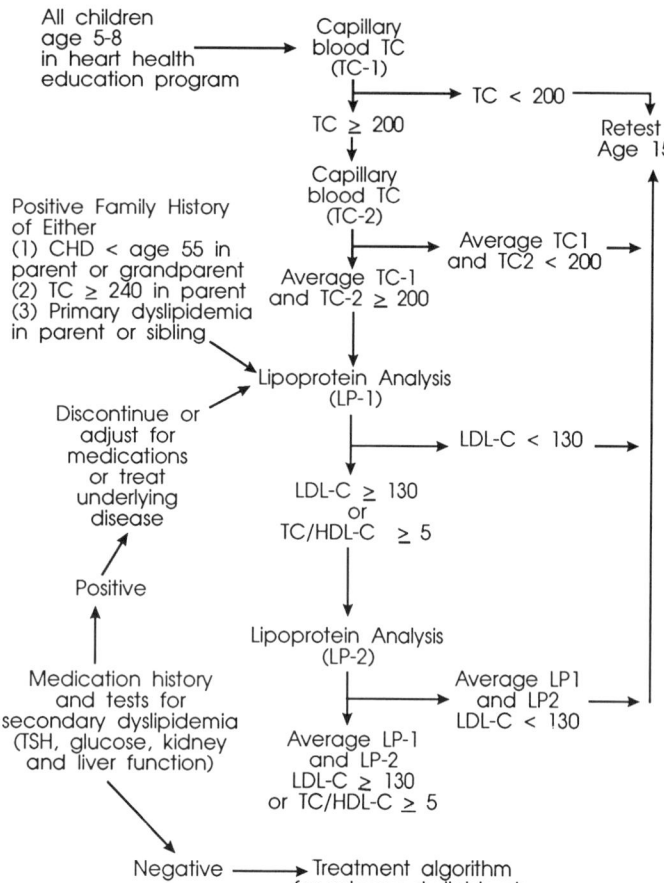

FIG. 1. Algorithm for screening of children to diagnose primary dyslipoproteinemia. (From ref. 139, with permission.)

the Lipid Research Clinics (LRC), the mean TC of children with an initial TC ≥ 95th percentile was 6% lower 6 weeks later (75,76). Children with an average TC > 200 on two measurements should have an LP profile performed (75,77,78). Children with a positive family history should have LP measurements in addition to a TC measurement. Follow-up of children with TC ≥ 90th percentile to identify those with LDL-C > 95th percentile has a sensitivity of 0.8 and a positive predictive value of 0.4. Thus, these cutoff points are efficient, cost-effective, and have a good benefit-risk ratio. They form the basis of a strong, well-accepted screening program.

The Elements of Selective Screening

1. Multiple measurements to confirm the abnormality and to establish baseline levels: repeated measurements of lipids and LPs improve the accuracy in establishing individual risk as well as establishing a baseline prior to diet or drug therapy (79,80). Variations can be minimized by standardizing procedures, including the position during blood drawing; the length of time the tourniquet is in place; sampling only during times of "normal" health, weight, and dietary intake; and using laboratories that meet the National Cholesterol Education Program (NCEP) standards (80–82).

2. Ruling out secondary dyslipoproteinemia: Many conditions, including hypothyroidism, chronic renal failure, nephrotic syndrome, cholestatic liver disease, hepatitis, hepatoblastoma, diabetes mellitus, systemic lupus erythematosus, dysgammaglobulinemia, glycogen storage disease, and growth hormone deficiency can cause elevated TC and/or TG (21,37,83–87). In addition, medications including glucocorticoids, androgenic steroids, estrogens, anticonvulsants, and retinoic acid can cause DLP. Thyroid-stimulating hormone (TSH), albumin, globulins, fasting glucose, tests of liver function (bilirubin, AST, ALT, and GGT) and kidney function [blood urea nitrogen (BUN), creatinine] should be performed on DLP children.

The likelihood of secondary DLP is very small if the child has been identified in school screening, is in the appropriate grade for age, has normal growth parameters, has not been hospitalized with a significant illness, has a negative review of systems and medication history, has been screened as a newborn for congenital hypothyroidism, and/or has a positive family history of premature CHD. If a potential DLP-producing medication is identified, the medication should be discontinued if clinically indicated, and the child retested. If discontinuation is not possible clinically, the potential effect of the medication should be taken into account in evaluating the extent of the abnormal LP pattern. In some children, DLP results from an underlying primary DLP that is aggravated by a disease or medication. If no underlying disease or medication is identified, the child should be considered to have primary DLP.

3. Assessing familial aggregation and the genetic basis of DLP: First-degree relatives of children with primary DLP should have LP determinations and follow-up if adverse patterns are demonstrated. A three-generation family pedigree should be drawn that includes ages, lipid and LP levels, clinical manifestations, age of onset of CVD and xanthomas, and presence of other CV risk factors including smoking, high blood pressure, obesity, and diabetes mellitus. The lipid and LP measurements in first-degree, and selectively, second-degree, relatives, combined with a family history, suggest the transmission of a dominant monogenic disorder such as familial hypercholesterolemia (FH), familial combined hyperlipidemia, or familial hypertriglyceridemia. The appearance of other CV risk factors such as obesity, diabetes, high blood pressure, and cigarette smoking may indicate a familial proclivity. In addition, a positive family history for CVD may be an independent CV risk factor beyond the classic CV risk factors (88,89). In families where the family history is significantly positive beyond the extent of the abnormalities in routine LP testing, it may be valuable to assess the levels of Apo B, Apo A-I, and LP (a) (90,91).

4. Assessing general health, nutritional status, and extent of lipid deposition: Routine pediatric physical examination should include carefully performed standardized blood pressure (BP) monitoring. Children with primary DLP should be examined for soft tissue and tendon xanthomas, and aortic, femoral, dorsalis pedis, and posterior tibial pulses. Height and weight, body fat distribution, and pubertal development are also essential measurements. Previous growth records, as well as parental heights and weights, may be useful in predicting growth potential. They may also be useful in the prediction of future LP levels and in the appropriateness of prescribed therapy.

INFORMING THE FAMILY OF THE DIAGNOSIS AND INITIATING COUNSELING

Providing Information

Families must understand that primary DLP is related to genetics as well as environment, both of which influence diet, body composition, and physical activity. They must have a basic appreciation of lipids and LP as well as know what are considered "normal" LP, BP, and growth in children. Percentile grids should be used for height, weight, and weight-for-height as well as for lipids, LP, skin folds, and BP. The range of variation in a child's lipid and LP measurement and the need for multiple measurements in order to reduce this variation should be explained to parents. This will help them to understand the continuous nature of risk rather than the artificial dichotomy of normal versus abnormal.

This positive approach, that is, emphasizing a child's ability to control both genetic and environmental components of the lipid and LP levels is essential to the success of the program. The diet's expected efficacy, i.e., TC and LDL-C lowered by 10%, should be emphasized. In general, since most children present with an initial LDL-C < 200 mg/dl, the family can be advised that medications are unlikely to be necessary. If a prolonged period of diet therapy does not lower LDC-C adequately, however, recommendations can include the use of a safe, effective, and well-tolerated medication.

Obtaining Commitment to Behavioral Change While Relieving Guilt and Anxiety

Family involvement is an important element in the ultimate success of the program. Although the child is expected to accept responsibility for the diet, it is valuable to explore collectively and individually the worries, goals, and expectations of each family member. Parents should understand the importance of their support, especially in facilitating behavioral changes. This includes purchasing and preparing appropriate foods as well as going exclusively to restaurants in which these foods can be ordered. Each family member must also understand the importance of being a positive role model, which means following the same fat-modified diet, exercising, and not smoking. The health care team functions both to help families understand these responsibilities as well as to give families support, expertise, and answers to the never-ending questions regarding cholesterol.

The question of risk should be discussed with the family to allay the normal anxiety concerning the potential for death during childhood. With the exception of homozygous familial hypercholesterolemia, the likelihood of a child developing symptomatic CVD in the next 30 years is extremely low, a risk almost eliminated by DLP control and avoidance of cigarette smoking (92,93). Parents must understand that the child is not "sick" and there is no "heart disease." This helps to avoid the problems of cardiac nondisease, that is, inappropriate restriction of physical activity and assumption of the role of a sick child (94). Anxieties about the risks of the therapy, particularly of medications, can be relieved by discussing the risks and benefits of alternative treatments, and by involving the family in decision-making.

EFFECTIVE AND SAFE THERAPY FOR DYSLIPOPROTEINEMIC CHILDREN

Diet

1. Nutrient composition: Dietary goals for DLP children are the achievement of ideal body weight with normal linear growth velocities; total fat at 30% of dietary energy (calories), with ≤7% of dietary energy from SFA, 14% from monounsaturated fatty acids (MUFA), and 9% from polyunsaturated fatty acids (PUFA); cholesterol limited to <75 mg/1,000 kilocalories (Cal) (Fig. 2). This diet must maintain sufficient energy, protein, vitamins, and minerals to meet the recommended dietary allowances (RDA) which, in turn, should sustain normal growth, development, and health.

Results from recent studies indicate that mean dietary energy intakes for United States children are 13% to 16% from protein, 34% to 39% from fat, 13% to 14% from SFA, 5% to 7% from PUFA, with cholesterol intakes of 126 to 176 mg per 1,000 Cal (95–97). The major objective of the cholesterol lowering diet is a 50% reduction in SFA. As SFA are reduced, fat decreases to 30% of dietary energy and dietary cholesterol decreases proportionately.

2. Efficacy of a fat-modified diet: Dietary modification has an effect on lipids and LP in normal and familial hypercholesterolemic (FH) children (Table 1). A low-cholesterol (<300 mg/day), low–total fat and PUFA-rich [ratio of PUFA to SFA (P/S > 1] diet can achieve a 10% to 20% decrease in the TC in normal children and children with FH (98–105). Lowering occurs primarily in LDL-C (106,107). No added benefit results from increasing the P/S to >2.0 (102). Stein et al. (107) observed an 8% decrease in TC and 11% decrease in LDL-C on a low cholesterol (151 mg), high P/S (1.5) diet. A diet with similar P/S but with higher dietary cholesterol (528 mg) was associated with only a 4% decrease in TC. Decreasing the P/S to 1.0 was associated with 6% lowering in TC. The typical American diet was associated with a 2% lowering. None of these fat modifications had a significant effect on HDL-C. This suggests that lowering dietary cholesterol and increasing P/S within these ranges can be achieved on an outpatient basis. These modifications have equal and additive effects on lowering TC and LDL-C without reducing HDL-C.

Fernandes et al. (108), using a cholesterol-free vegetarian diet that was modestly higher in P/S, lowered TC 10% below the levels of the fat-modified diet. Because the decrease is greater than expected solely from the restriction in cholesterol and increase in P/S, it suggests an additional effect from the shift to largely vegetable protein. Incorporating soy protein into a high-P/S (1.5) low-cholesterol (180 mg) diet lowered TC an additional 10% and LDL-C an additional 8% below the levels of the fat-modified diet (109). HDL-C, however, also decreased an additional 11%. A textured vegetable protein lowered TC and LDL-C an additional 19% with only a small increase in HDL-C (110). These studies suggest that decreasing SFA and cholesterol, increasing PUFA, and incorporating vegetable protein in the diets of United

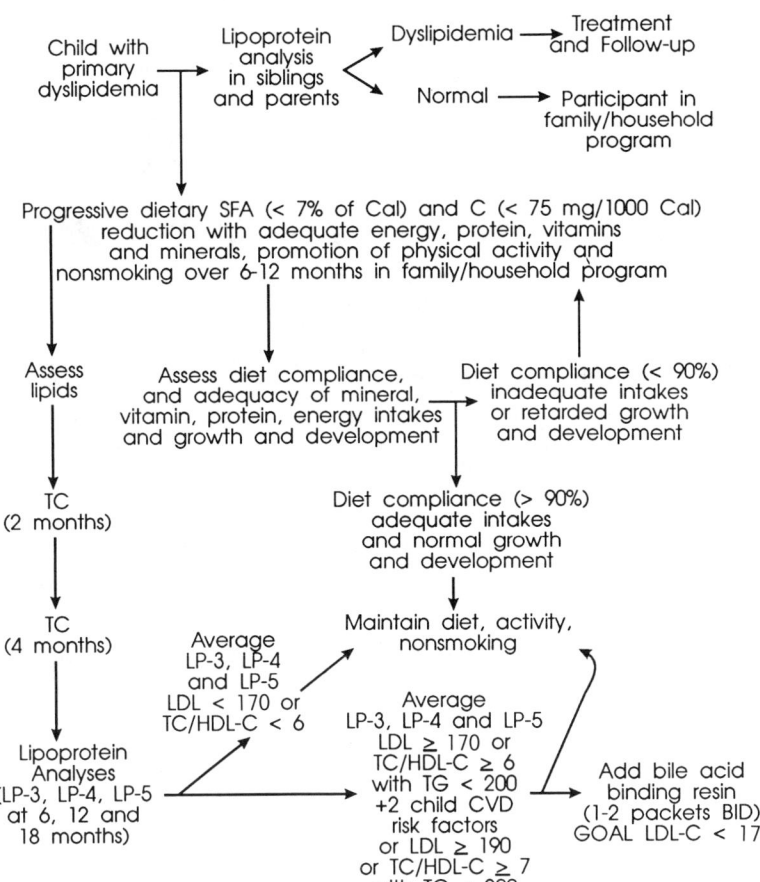

FIG. 2. Algorithm for treatment and follow-up of children with primary dyslipoproteinemia. (From ref. 139, 140, with permission.)

States children may lower TC and LDL-C approximately 20% to 25%. One problem with the protein-modified diet, however, is long-term compliance; only 50% to 60% of the children remained on a soybean diet at the 12-month follow-up.

3. Food choices and food patterns on a fat-modified diet: Universal adherence to a fat and protein-modified diet would probably require reformulation of many commercially prepared products. It is possible, however, to achieve such a diet with currently available foods by food selection that decreases SFA, maintains MUFA, and increases PUFA. In the Bogalusa Heart Study, the diet of 10-year-olds consisted of 28% of SFA from meat, primarily beef, mixed meats, and pork, and an equivalent amount of SFA from milk, with 17% coming from desserts and snacks (97). There is a tendency for the proportion of SFA from baked goods to increase during adolescence, whereas that from meat decreases (98). Analyzing individual intake patterns helps to target those foods necessary to limit in order to lower SFA intake.

4. Strategies for reducing SFA include choosing lower-fat meat and dairy products; preparing foods with less fat or choosing prepared foods that contain less fat; eating smaller portions with isocaloric substitutes for low-saturated–fatty-acid foods. It is nutritionally undesirable and/or unrealistic to consider eliminating meat, milk, and snacks completely. Meat provides 31% of the zinc and 25% of the iron in United States' children's diets (96,111). Milk and other dairy products provide 76% of children's calcium intake (96,111). Practical suggestions, however, include increasing consumption of lean red meat and lower-SFA animal flesh, such as fish and skinned (before cooking) chicken and turkey, and switching to 1% fat or skim milk. Eliminating snacks, on the other hand, would require a "cultural revolution."

PUFA can be increased by modifying eating patterns. In the Bogalusa Heart Study (97), desserts, snacks, and candy contributed 29% of the PUFA intake. This could be altered by encouraging modification of fat composition by food manufacturers or in home preparation. Poultry and fish fried in high PUFA oil are both significantly higher in PUFA than SFA. Other PUFA sources include fried vegetables, particularly potatoes and fatty breads/cereals, and salad dressing.

Because the SFA/MUFA is approximately 0.60 in meat and other animal products, MUFA may decrease more than SFA. To maintain MUFA in the diet, while decreasing SFA, it is necessary to prepare foods in low-SFA (< 20%) MUFA-rich (> 20%) oils. Acceptable oils include canola (6% and 62%), sunflower (11% and 20%), corn (13% and 25%), olive (14% and 77%), soybean (15% and 24%), peanut (18% and 49%), and many margarines

TABLE 1. *Effect of diet on lipids and lipoproteins in children*

Reference (no.)	No. of children and disorder, meal site	Study period (months)	Baseline diet	Intervention diet Cholesterol (mg/day)	Fat (%)	P/S	Protein (%)	Protein type	Change from baseline (%) TC	LDL-C	HDL-C	TG	Apo B
Stein et al. (103)	229 normal, inst	1.5	Ad libitum	575	38	1.1	13		−6	−16	NS	+36	NS
				710	38	.9	13		−11	−12	NS	+15	NS
				610	38	.3	13		−2	+1	NS	+40	NS
Ford et al. (98)	18 normal, inst	5	Fat 39% SFA 15% PUFA 30% Chol 537 mg	301	33	1.1	13		−17	NS	NS	NS	NS
Vergroesen (105)	100 normal, inst	NS	Ad libitum Fat 40–45% Chol 200–500 mg	NS	NS	2.5	NS		−20—−25	NS	NS	NS	NS
Vartiainen et al. (104)	36 normal, home	3	Fat 35% SFA 20% PUFA 3% Chol 408 mg	274	24	0.6	15		−15	−19	−17	+16	−6
		1.2		359	34	0.2	13		−6	−10	−3	+6	+2
Glueck et al. (106)	17 FH, home	6	Ad libitum	<300	NS	1.5	NS		−11	−11	NS	NS	NS
Rose et al. (101)	39 FH, home	6	Ad libitum	150–200	NS	1.5–2.0	NS		−20	NS	NS	NS	NS
Segall et al. (102)	7 FH, NS	6	Ad libitum	NS	COS	1.6	NS		−21	NS	NS	NS	NS
						4.2			−18	NS	NS	NS	NS
Stein et al. (107)	12 FH, home	3	Ad libitum	528	32	>1.5	14		−4	−6	NC	+1	NS
		3		151	35	>1.5	14		−8	−11	+2	−6	NS
		3		157	36	1.0	14		−6	−8	NC	−6	NS
		3		332	40	0.4	13		−2	−2	−4	+5	NS
Widhalm (109)	11 FH, inst	0.5	NS	180	30	1.5	15		−2	−2	−10	+9	+9
		0.5		150	30	1.5	20 S		−12	−10	−21	+13	−19
Gaddi et al. (110)	16 FH, home	1	Fat 25% P/S 1.6–1.8	NS	4	NS	NS L-TVP		−19	−19	+3	+4	NS
Fernandes et al. (108)	39 FH, home	2.5	Fat 27% P/S 1.3 Chol 109 mg	11	28	1.8	15		−10	−10	−4	NS	−10

From ref. 139, with permission.
CH, cholestyramine; Clof, clofibrate; CO, colestipol; Feno, fenofibrate; HMG-I, 3-hydroxy-3-methylglutaryl coenzyme A reductase inhibitor as 40 mg/day Simvastatin or 80 mg/day lovastatin; NC, no change; NI, niacin; NS, not specified.

(19% and 49%). Unacceptable oils include cottonseed (27% and 19%), vegetable shortening (28% and 44%), animal fat (31% to 66% and 30% to 47%) and "tropical" oils. The remaining portion of fatty acids are PUFA.

The success of a plan of modification will depend on both the nutritional changes and acceptability of those changes. This can be achieved by careful design (Table 2). Desserts and fried food should be prepared with acceptable margarines and oils. Egg whites or egg substitutes, which are excellent sources of protein, can replace eggs. No more than 1 egg yolk a week should be consumed. Vegetables and fruits could supply fiber and water-soluble vitamins. Adherence would lower SFA and cholesterol intakes, maintain MUFA, and increase PUFA intake without significant alterations in the usual diet of United States children.

5. Achieving and maintaining adherence to the fat-modified diet: In the family-based approach to diet modification, the family's knowledge of nutrition is assessed and the idea of diet as a tool for change is introduced (112–115). Foods are divided into three categories based on SFA and cholesterol content then are color-designated, on the basis of "stoplights": green—go, yellow—caution, and red—danger. During group and individual sessions, families are taught food selection and preparation skills, including label reading and restaurant ordering. There is also instruction in self-monitoring, goal setting, contracting, and rewarding. The ultimate goal is the incorporation of this information and the concomitant dietary changes, in the life of the family.

6. Adapting diets to the individual: The success of diet modification is predicated on the collaboration of the physician, the dietitian, the family, and the individual. Current diet is analyzed to assess adequacy and to help target those foods that must be modified in intake. The modification program is then designed that must incorporate a follow-up procedure to assess success.

Because the success of the child's diet is dependent on changes within the family, the eating patterns of the entire family must be assessed. This includes food preferences, usual recipes, and the income available for food. The person who purchases and prepares the food must also be identified. This and other specific information contributes to designing a regimen appropriate for each family.

The dietary assessment should also identify the major sources of SFA. This can be done through several 3-day records of a child's intake combined with an interview to determine sources of SFA consumption.

Once a plan for diet modification has been decided upon, success will depend on behavioral changes. This is best achieved by setting step-by-step priorities for the behavior/dietary modifications. Each goal should be written as a contract with a preset reward upon completion. Continuous lack of success should indicate the need for a change in design. Gradual changes in eating habits combined with realistic expectations are likely, however, to lead to long-term adherence to the diet.

Ninety percent adherence is a realistic definition of success. The final 10% does not produce much additional cholesterol-lowering, and requires significant extra effort, for example, bringing one's own food to another child's birthday party. Follow-up is important, including monitoring dietary intake (fat composition and achievement of the RDA), nutritional status (hemoglobin, serum proteins including ferritin), and growth and pubertal development, in order to prevent potential negative effects (116).

7. Diet safety: Overzealous application of a low–total fat, low-cholesterol diet resulted in growth failure in 8 of 40 children treated for hypercholesterolemia (116). Children who exhibited growth failure had been provided an average of 66% of the recommended dietary allowances (RDA) for energy and 40% of the RDA for zinc. In contrast, children with an intake of 84% of the RDA for energy and 58% of the RDA for zinc demonstrated normal growth. Three of the eight children ($\leq$10 years of age) showed stunting, whereas the remaining five demonstrated only weight loss or insufficient weight gain. Dietary fat was markedly decreased (20.5% ± 2.1% calories from fat) in the children with stunting. Intake of minerals and vitamins was markedly reduced; vitamin A, B_{12}, and niacin were less than 66% of the RDA.

Seven children, 7 to 22 months of age, evaluated for growth failure, reported an energy intake between 60% and 90% of the RDA with fat contributing 20% to 43% and protein between 9% and 23% of the total calories consumed. Nutritional rehabilitation occurred upon adequate administration of energy and nutrients (117).

Although there is not sufficient information to assess

TABLE 2. *Suggested food pattern (2000-Cal consumption) for a dyslipoproteinemic 10-year-old child*

Food group	Food recommendations	Daily consumption
Meat, fish, poultry	Lean red meat, skinless poultry, fish	7 oz
Milk, yogurt	1% or nonfat	24–32 oz
Oils and salad dressing	Low SFA (<20%)	2–10 servings
Fruits and vegetables	All except with high SFA coating	4 or more servings
Snacks and desserts	Prepared with low SFA (<20%) oils	3–4 servings
Breads, cereals, starchy food	Prepared with low SFA (<20%) oils	6 or more servings

From ref. 139, with permission.

the incidence of growth retardation following dietary fat modification, there is the suggestion that a low-energy, low–total fat diet may adversely affect children's growth. This may result from overzealous, unsupervised parents in pursuit of a healthy diet or from poorly balanced vegetarian diets (118,119). The possibility of sporadic diet abuse should not, however, be the reason for its elimination as a therapeutic tool. The potential for favorable results simply highlights the need for skilled nutrition counseling.

The Dietary Intervention Study in Children (DISC), a National Institutes of Health (NIH)-funded multicenter program, is presently evaluating the efficacy and safety of dietary treatment of hypercholesterolemia in children 8 to 10 years of age. DISC will provide a carefully controlled investigation of the frequency and severity of altered growth in children on a fat-modified diet.

Nondietary Factors

1. Physical activity and weight reduction: The development of obesity leads to a progressive increase in adverse LP patterns and diastolic hypertension. The child and family should, therefore, be encouraged to increase physical activity. Activities should combine simple energy expenditure, e.g., walking, with aerobic exercise such as jogging and bicycling that produces CV training.

Studies have illustrated the benefit of weight reduction on lipids and HDL-C. Obese adolescents on a 16-week intensive walking program, and a nondieting regimen, lost weight (mean of 6 kg) and fat (-25%), and raised both HDL-C (16%) and the HDL-C/LDL-C ratio (26%) (120). No significant change in plasma TC and TG levels was observed. Obese children on a 2-year aerobic exercise program showed 31% to 40% body fat reduction, a 16% to 19% elevation in HDL-C, a 13% to 53% decrease in free fatty acids, and a 10% to 16% decrease in triglycerides (121). Triglyceride reduction was most significant in girls. This highlights the importance of exercise in the design of any weight reduction program for children.

2. Cigarette smoking: Cigarette smoking results in devastating consequences for individuals with DLP. A child who already has one CV risk factor should be strongly counseled not to acquire the habit of smoking (92,122).

MEDICATIONS

Efficacy and Safety

There have been several investigations of drug treatment for DLP children (Table 3). Bile acid–binding resins are the most extensively studied. They produce an additional 10% to 30% decrease in TC and LDL-C beyond that which is produced by diet modification alone (123–132). The decrease in LDL-C is dose-dependent. Because of their effectiveness in lowering LDL-C and their long-term efficacy, the bile acid–binding resins are the drugs of choice, although the long-term effect appears to be less than the initial efficacy. Recommendations for initiation of bile acid–binding resin and the goal LDL-C in children are shown in Fig. 2. Although reports of safety in children are anecdotal, there is documented safety in adults (133).

Studies have shown that the fibric acid derivatives produced a 15% and 21% lowering of TC (102,134). Fenofibrate also lowered TG and LDL-C significantly (134). Long-term safety of fibric acid derivatives, however, is uncertain.

Because of the potential for high-dose resin therapy to produce fat malabsorption and alter intestinal mucosal function, there has been particular interest in the effect of resin therapy on serum fat-soluble vitamins and folate. Most hypercholesterolemic children have supernormal fat-soluble vitamin levels prior to treatment (135). After 4 months and 18 to 24 months, plasma vitamin A and E levels remained within the normal range in children on therapeutic doses of the resins (130,135). In studies of vitamin D, (25-hydroxycholecalciferol), calcium, phosphorus, alkaline phosphatase, and vitamin K (prothrombin time and partial thromboplastin time) adequacy remained unchanged (130). Serum folate was reduced significantly (10.9 ± 2.8 to 6.8 ± 2.9) after short-term resin (≤ 16 g/day) treatment only in females (7 of 11) in one study (23) and all 19 subjects (12 of 19 were females) in another study (132,136,137). Folic acid–deficient anemia did not develop. To assure safety, a multiple vitamin with iron and folic acid should be administered to children receiving bile acid–binding resins 1 hr before or at least 2 hr after the dose of resin.

The addition of nicotinic acid or a hydroxymethylglutaryl (HMG) coenzyme A (CoA) reductase inhibitor to bile acid–binding resins produced an additional lowering of LDL-C beyond the resins alone (131). Nicotinic acid produced an increase in HDL-C (131). This response is similar in adults and the combination may be utilized in children who persist with very adverse LP patterns when resins are used alone. However, the use of the HMG CoA reductase inhibitors in individuals under age 20 or in pregnant women is prohibited. Long-term safety data and the potential effects on cholesterol synthesis in the nervous system, adrenal glands, and gonads, or their potential risk to a fetus have not been established.

Adherence

Although compliance is always a potential problem, the lowest effective twice-a-day regimen of a bile acid

TABLE 3. *Drug therapy in children with familial hypercholesterolemia*

Reference (no.)	Children (no.)	Drug	Dose (g/day)	Duration (mo)	Change beyond diet (%)			
					TC	LDL-C	HDL-C	TG
Groot et al. (128)	28	CO	0.3/kg	2	−13	−16	−2	−9
Mordasini et al. (129)	12	CO	0.5/kg	2	−25	−25	NS	NC
Glueck et al. (125)	21	CO	10	7–12	−12	−19	NS	NC
Schwarz et al. (130)	10	CO	15–20	24	−13	−19	NS	NS
Farah et al. (123)	13	CH	4	.5	−11	−16	NS	NS
			8	.5	−25	−27	NS	NS
			12	.5	−29	−38	NS	NS
			16	.5	−29	−46	NS	NS
Glueck et al. (124)	20	CH	12	6	−6−−14	−4−−6	NS	NS
Glueck et al. (106)	16	CH	16	24–36	−10−−15	−10−−15	NS	NS
West and Lloyd (132)	35	CH	0.4/kg	72–96	−26−−44	NS	NS	NC
Segall et al. (102)	6	Clof	.018−.028/kg	NS	−15	NS	NS	NS
Steinmetz et al. (134)	15	Feno	0.2	3	−21	−29	NS	−37
Stein (131)	30	CH or CO	8–16 or 15–30	12–108	−15	−21	+6	+14
	6	CH + Ni or CH + Ni	8–16 + 1–3 or 15–30 + 1–3	12–108	−29	−37	+20	NS
	6	HMG-I	.04 or .08	12–108	−39	−44	−2	−14
	6	HMG-I + CH or CO	.04 or .08 + 8–24 or 15–30	12–108	−36	−45	NS	+9

From ref. 139, with permission.
CH, cholestyramine; Clof, clofibrate; CO, colestipol; Feno, fenofibrate; HMG-I, 3-hydroxy-3-methylglutaryl coenzyme A reductase inhibitor as 40 mg/day Simvastatin or 80 mg/day lovastatin; NC, no change; NI, niacin; NS, not specified.

resin is generally acceptable to children (130). Long-term, e.g., 8 years, drug compliance was better if treatment were started before age 10 (56% for <10 years vs 10% for ≥10 years) (137). When treatment was started earlier, there was some (14%) transient constipation in the first 2 months. No permanent changes in bowel habits occurred. The problem of poor palatability, which is a major reason for refusal to take the resins, should be addressed by the same strategies used for diet adherence (130,138). Children should be able to taste available resins in the physician's office and to choose the most palatable. Another important factor in compliance, especially initially, is a successful method of reminding patients to take the medication.

Management of children with severe monogenetic DLP is described elsewhere (139).

NECESSARY ELEMENTS OF AN EFFICIENT AND EFFECTIVE PROGRAM

The skill and dedication of health care professionals are the foundation of a successful program for CVD reduction in dyslipoproteinemic children. The structure of such a program must include an easily accessible screening program, including accurate TC measurements, to identify high-risk children. Screening results must be followed up with multiple high-quality measurements of LP-C to classify risk status and diagnose primary DLP.

The second step in a pediatric CVD reduction program is family-based intervention. This should include long-term follow-up in order to assess success of diet modification as well as the necessity and benefit-risk factor of drug therapy.

More universal success for CVD reduction in children necessitates carrying it beyond the individual into the society at large via a school-based health promotion program. The combination of concern for the individual child and a carefully implemented program for children, generally, should produce a major reduction in CVD when the current generation becomes adults.

REFERENCES

1. Strong JR, Newman WP III, Freedman DS, et al. Atherosclerotic disease in children and young adults: relationship to cardiovascular risk factors. In: Berenson G, ed. *Causation of cardiovascular risk factors in children.* New York: Raven Press, 1986;27.
2. Newman WP III, Freedman DS, Voors AW, et al. Relation of serum lipoprotein levels and systolic blood pressure to early atherosclerosis: the Bogalusa Heart Study. *N Engl J Med* 1986;314:138.
3. Clarke WR, Schrott HG, Leaverton PE, et al. Tracking of blood

lipids and blood pressures in school age children: the Muscatine Study. *Circulation* 1978;58:626.
4. Donahue RP, Orchard TJ, Kuller LH, et al. Lipids and lipoproteins in a young adult population: the Beaver County Lipid Study. *Am J Epidemiol* 1985;122:458.
5. Freedman DS, Shear CL, Srinivasan SR, et al. Tracking of serum lipids and lipoproteins in children over an 8-year period: the Bogalusa Heart Study. *Prev Med* 1985;14:203.
6. Frerichs RR, Webber LS, Voors AW, et al. Cardiovascular disease risk factor variables in children at two successive years—the Bogalusa Heart Study. *J Chron Dis* 1979;32:251.
7. Garn SM, Hopkins P, Block WD. Continuities (tracking) in childhood cholesterol. *Ecol Food Nutr* 1980;10:1.
8. Laskarzewski P, Morrison JA, de Groot I, et al. Lipid and lipoprotein tracking in 108 children over a four-year period. *Pediatrics* 1979;64:584.
9. Lauer RM, Lee J, Clarke WR. Factors affecting the relationship between childhood and adult cholesterol levels: the Muscatine Study. *Pediatrics* 1988;82:309.
10. Orchard TJ, Donahue RP, Kuller LH, et al. Cholesterol screening in childhood: does it predict adult hypercholesterolemia? the Beaver County Experience. *J Pediatr* 1983;103:687.
11. Webber LS, Cresanta JL, Voors AW, et al. Tracking of cardiovascular disease risk factor variables in school-age children. *J Chron Dis* 1983;36:647.
12. Wynder EL, Berenson GS, Strong WB, et al. Coronary artery disease prevention: a pediatric perspective. *Prev Med* 1989;18:323.
13. Knuiman JT, West CE, Katan MB, et al. Total cholesterol and high-density lipoprotein cholesterol levels in populations differing in fat and carbohydrate intake. *Arteriosclerosis* 1987;7:612.
14. Thompson GR, Miller JP, Breslow JL. Improved survival of patients with homozygous familial hypercholesterolemia treated with plasma exchange. *Br Med J* 1985;291:1671.
15. Moll PP, Sing CF, Weidman WH, et al. Total cholesterol and lipoproteins in school children: prediction of coronary heart disease in adult relatives. *Circulation* 1983;67:127.
16. Freedman DS, Srinivasan SR, Shear CL, et al. The relation of apolipoproteins A-I and B in children to parental myocardial infarction. *N Engl J Med* 1986;315:721.
17. Dennison BA, Kikuchi DA, Srinivasan SR, et al. Parental history of cardiovascular disease as an indication for screening for lipoprotein abnormalities in children. *J Pediatr* 1989;115:186.
18. Hunter SM, Croft JB, Parker FC. Biobehavioral studies in cardiovascular risk development. In: Berenson G, ed. *Causation of cardiovascular risk factors in children.* New York: Raven Press, 1986;223.
19. Dietz WH. Nutrition and obesity. In: Grand R, Sutphen J, Dietz W, eds. *Pediatric nutrition: theory and practice.* Stoneham, MA: Butterworth, 1987;525.
20. Epstein LH. Treatment of childhood obesity. In: Brownell KD, Foreyt JP, eds. *Handbook of eating disorders.* New York: Basic Books, 1986;159.
21. Bagdade JD, Porte D, Bierman EL. Hypertriglyceridemia: a metabolic consequence of chronic renal failure. *N Engl J Med* 1968;279:181.
22. Cress HR, Shafner RM, Laffin R, et al. Cord blood hyperlipoproteinemia and perinatal stress. *Pediatr Res* 1977;11:19.
23. Darmady JM, Fosbrooke AS, Lloyd JK. Prospective study of serum cholesterol levels during first year of life. *Br Med J* 1972;2:685.
24. Frerichs RR, Srinivasan SR, Webber LS, et al. Serum lipids and lipoproteins at birth in a biracial population: the Bogalusa Heart Study. *Pediatr Res* 1978;12:858.
25. Genzel-Bopoviczeny O, Forte TM, Austin MA. High-density lipoprotein subclass distribution and human cord blood lipid levels. *Pediatr Res* 1986;20:487.
26. Ginsburg BE, Zetterstrom R. Serum cholesterol concentrations in early infancy. *Acta Paediatr Scand* 1980;69:581.
27. Glueck CJ, Heckman F, Schoenfeld M, et al. Neonatal familial type II hyperlipoproteinemia: cord blood cholesterol in 1800 births. *Metabolism* 1971;20:597.
28. Greten H, Wengeler H, Wagner H. Early diagnosis of familial type II hyperlipoproteinemia. *Nutr Metab* 1973;15:128.
29. Hardell LI. Serum lipids and lipoproteins at birth and in early childhood. *Acta Paediatr Scand Suppl* 1981;285:
30. Klimov AN, Glueck CJ, Gartside PS, et al. Cord blood high-density lipoproteins: Leningrad and Cincinnati. *Pediatr Res* 1979;13:208.
31. Kwiterovich PO Jr, Levy RI, Fredrickson DS. Neonatal diagnosis of familial type-II hyperlipoproteinemia. *Lancet* 1973;1:118.
32. Lane DM, McConathy WJ. Changes in serum lipids and apolipoproteins in the first four weeks of life. *Pediatr Res* 1986;20:332.
33. Lindquist B, Malmcrona R. Dietary fat in relation to serum lipids in the normal infant. *Am J Dis Child* 1960;99:39.
34. Mishkel MA. Neonatal plasma lipids as measured in cord blood. *Can Med Assoc J* 1974;111:775.
35. Potter JM, Nestel PJ. Comparison of plasma lipids at birth and in second year of life. *Aust NZ J Med* 1976;6:420.
36. Van Biervliet JP, Vinaimont N, Caster H, et al. Plasma apoprotein and lipid patterns in newborns: influence of nutritional factors. *Acta Paediatr Scand* 1981;70:851.
37. Vikari J, Akerblom HK, Nikkari T, et al. Atherosclerosis precursors in Finnish children and adolescents: IV. Serum lipids in newborns, children and adolescents. *Acta Paediatr Scand Suppl* 1985;318:1035.
38. Franklin FA. The effect of infant feeding practices on lipid and lipoprotein levels and metabolism. In: Lebenthal E, ed. *Textbook of gastroenterology and nutrition in infancy.* New York: Raven Press, 1989;503.
39. Kirstein D, Johansen KB, Petersen MBV, et al. Changes in plasma lipoproteins from first day to third week of life in healthy breast-fed infants: I. Lipid and protein composition of lipoproteins. *Acta Paediatr Scand* 1985;74:733.
40. Van Biervliet JP, Rosseneu M, Caster H. Influence of dietary factors on the plasma lipoprotein composition and content in neonates. *Eur J Pediatr* 1986;144:489.
41. Ellefson RD, Elveback LR, Hodgson PA, et al. Cholesterol and triglycerides in serum lipoproteins of young persons in Rochester, Minnesota. *Mayo Clin Proc* 1978;53:307.
42. *The Lipid Research Clinics population studies data book: volume I. The prevalence study.* Lipid Metabolism Branch, Division of Heart and Vascular Diseases, National Heart, Lung, and Blood Institute: US Department of Health and Human Services, Public Health Service, National Institutes of Health: NIH Publ No 80-1527, July 1980.
43. Farris RP, Frank GC, Webber LS, et al. Influence of milk source on serum lipids and lipoproteins during the first year of life: Bogalusa Heart Study. *Am J Clin Nutr* 1982;35:42.
44. Green MS, Heiss G, Rifkind BM, et al. The ratio of plasma high-density lipoprotein cholesterol to total and low-density lipoprotein cholesterol: age-related changes and race and sex differences in selected North American populations: the Lipid Research Clinics Program Prevalence Study. *Circulation* 1985;72:93.
45. Srinivasan SR. Biologic determinants (or correlates) of serum lipoproteins in children. In: Berenson G, ed. *Causation of cardiovascular risk factors in children.* New York: Raven Press, 1986;82.
46. Srinivasan SR, Freedman DS, Webber LS, et al. Black-white differences in cholesterol levels of serum high-density lipoprotein subclasses among children: the Bogalusa Heart Study. *Circulation* 1987;76:272.
47. Berenson GS, Srinivasan SR, Wattigney W, et al. Insight into a bad omen for white men—the Bogalusa Heart Study. *Am J Cardiol* 1989;64:32C.
48. Freedman DS, Srinivasan SR, Webber LS, et al. Black-white differences in serum lipoproteins during sexual maturation: the Bogalusa Heart Study. *J Chron Dis* 1987;40:309.
49. Laskarzewski PM, Morrison JA, Kelly K, et al. Parent-child coronary heart disease risk factor associations. *Am J Epidemiol* 1981;114:827.
50. Morrison JA, Khoury P, Mellies MJ, et al. Identifying CHD risk factors in children: intrafamilial lipoprotein correlations. *Prev Med* 1980;9:484.
51. Morrison JA, Kelly K, Khoury P, et al. Parent-offspring and sibling lipid and lipoprotein associations during and after sharing of household environments: the Princeton School District Family Study. *Metabolism* 1982;31:158.

52. Dahlen G, Ericson C, de Faire U, et al. Genetic and environmental determinants of cholesterol and HDL-cholesterol concentrations in blood. *Int J Epidemiol* 1983;12:32.
53. Friedlander Y, Kark JD, Stein Y. Biological and environmental sources of variation in plasma lipids and lipoproteins: the Jerusalem Lipid Research Clinic. *Hum Hered* 1986;36:145.
54. Glueck CJ, Heiss G, Morrison JA, et al. Alcohol intake, cigarette smoking and plasma lipids and lipoproteins in 12-19-year-old children. *Circulation* 1981;64:III-48.
55. Hamsten A, Iselius L, Dahlen G, et al. Genetic and cultural inheritance of serum lipids, low and high density lipoprotein cholesterol and serum apolipoproteins A-I, A-II and B. *Atherosclerosis* 1986;60:199.
56. Namboodiri KM, Green PP, Kaplan EB, et al. Familial aggregation of high-density lipoprotein cholesterol: Collaborative Lipid Research Clinics Program Family Study. *Arteriosclerosis* 1983;3:616.
57. Namboodiri NK, Kaplan EB, Heuch I, et al. The Collaborative Lipid Research Clinics Family Study: biological and cultural determinants of familial resemblance for plasma, lipids and lipoproteins. *Genet Epidemiol* 1985;2:227.
58. Rao DC, Morton NE, Gulbrandsen CL, et al. Cultural and biological determinants of lipoprotein concentrations. *Ann Hum Genet* 1979;42:467.
59. Srinivasan SR, Freedman DS, Sundaram GS, et al. Racial (black-white) comparisons of the relationship of levels of endogenous sex hormones to serum lipoproteins during male adolescence: the Bogalusa Heart Study. *Circulation* 1986;74:1226.
60. Kirkland RT, Keenan BS, Probstfield JL, et al. Decrease in plasma high-density lipoprotein cholesterol levels at puberty in boys with delayed adolescence: correlation with plasma testosterone levels. *JAMA* 1987;257:502.
61. Johnson CC, Nicklas TA, Arbeit ML, et al. A comprehensive model for maintenance of family health behaviors: the Heart Smart Family Health Promotion Program. *Fam Commun Health* 1988;11:1.
62. Keys A, Anderson JT, Grande F. Prediction of serum cholesterol responses of man to changes in fats in the diet. *Lancet* 1957;2:959.
63. Freedman DS, Srinivasan SR, Webber LS, et al. Divergent levels of high density lipoprotein cholesterol and apolipoprotein A-I in children: the Bogalusa Heart Study. *Arteriosclerosis* 1987;7:347.
64. Dwyer T, Coonan WE, Leitch DR, et al. An investigation of the effects of daily physical activity on the health of primary school students in South Australia. *Int J Epidemiol* 1983;12:308.
65. Walberg J, Ward D. Role of physical activity in the etiology and treatment of childhood obesity. *Pediatrician* 1983;12:82.
66. Durant RH, Linder CW, Mahoney OM. Relationship between habitual physical activity and serum lipoprotein levels in white male adolescents. *J Adolesc Health Care* 1983;4:237.
67. Lauer RM, Clarke WR. Childhood risk factors for high blood pressure: the Muscatine Study. *Pediatrics* 1989;84:633.
68. Morrison JA, Kelly K, Mellies M, et al. Cigarette smoking, alcohol intake, and oral contraceptives: relationships to lipids and lipoproteins in adolescent school-children. *Metabolism* 1979;28:1166.
69. Voors AW, Srinivasan SR, Hunter SM, et al. Smoking, oral contraceptives, and serum lipid and lipoprotein levels in youths. *Prev Med* 1982;11:1.
70. Heldenberg D, Harel S, Holtzman M, et al. The effect of chronic anticonvulsant therapy on serum lipids and lipoproteins in epileptic children. *Neurology* 1983;33:510.
71. Reddy MN. Effect of anticonvulsant drugs on plasma total cholesterol, high density lipoprotein cholesterol and apolipoproteins A and B in children with epilepsy. *Proc Soc Exp Biol Med* 1985;180:359.
72. Maynert EW, Kusek JC. Phenobarbital: chemical-biophysical effects. In: Glaser GH, Woodbury DM, eds. *Antiepileptic drugs: mechanisms of action.* New York: Raven Press, 1980;541.
73. Pelkonen R, Fogelholm R, Nikkila EA. Increase in serum cholesterol during phenytoin treatment. *Br Med J* 1975;4:85.
74. Wahl P, Walden C, Knopp R, et al. Effect of estrogen/progestin potency on lipid/lipoprotein cholesterol. *N Engl J Med* 1983;15:862.
75. Morrison JA, Glueck CJ. Pediatric risk factors for adult coronary heart disease: primary atherosclerosis prevention. *Cardiovasc Rev Rep* 1981;2:1269.
76. Morrison JA, Namboodiri K, Green P, et al. Familial aggregation of lipids and lipoproteins and early identification of dyslipoproteinemia: the Collaborative Lipid Research Clinics Family Study. *JAMA* 1983;250:1860.
77. Garcia RE, Moodie DS. Routine cholesterol surveillance in childhood. *Pediatrics* 1989;84:751.
78. Kwiterovich PO Jr, Heiss G, Johnson N, et al. Assessment of plasma total cholesterol as a test to detect elevated low density (beta) lipoprotein cholesterol levels (type IIa hyperlipoproteinemia) in young subjects from a population-based sample. *Am J Epidemiol* 1982;115:192.
79. Jacobs DR Jr, Barrett-Connor E. Retest reliability of plasma cholesterol and triglyceride: the Lipid Research Clinics Prevalence Study. *Am J Epidemiol* 1982;116:878.
80. Naito HK. Reliability of lipid, lipoprotein and apolipoprotein measurements. *Clin Chem* 1988;34:B89.
81. Cooper GR, Myers GL, Smith SJ, et al. Standardization of lipid, lipoprotein and apolipoprotein measurements. *Clin Chem* 1988;34:B95-B105.
82. Laboratory Standardization Panel of the National Cholesterol Education Program. Current status of blood cholesterol measurement in clinical laboratories in the United States: a report from the Laboratory Standardization Panel of National Cholesterol Education Program. *Clin Chem* 1988;34:193.
83. Jakovcic S, Khachadurian AK, Yi-Yung Hsia D. The hyperlipidemia in glycogen storage disease. *J Lab Clin Med* 1966;68:769.
84. Merimee TJ, Hollander W, Fineberg SE. Studies of hyperlipidemia in the HGH-deficient state. *Metabolism* 1972;21:1053.
85. Papadopoulou Z, Sandler P, Leticia TU, et al. Hyperlipidemia in children with chronic renal insufficiency. *Pediatr Res* 1981;15:887.
86. Peters JP, Man EB. The significance of serum cholesterol in thyroid disease. *J Clin Invest* 1949;28:1.
87. Winter RJ, Thompson RG, Green OC. Serum cholesterol and triglycerides in children with growth hormone deficiency. *Metabolism* 1979;28:1244.
88. Hopkins PN, Williams RR, Kuida H, et al. Family history as an independent risk factor for incident coronary artery disease in a high-risk cohort in Utah. *Am J Cardiol* 1988;62:703.
89. Hopkins PN, Williams RR. Human genetics and coronary heart disease: a public health perspective. *Annu Rev Nutr* 1989;9:303.
90. Durrington PN, Ishola M, Hunt L, et al. Apolipoproteins (a), AI and B and parental history in men with early onset ischaemic heart disease. *Lancet* 1988;1:1070.
91. Sniderman A, Teng B, Genest J, et al. Familial aggregation and early expression of hyperapobeta-lipoproteinemia. *Am J Cardiol* 1985;55:291.
92. Hopkins PN, Williams RR, Hunt SC. Magnified risks from cigarette smoking for coronary prone families in Utah. *West J Med* 1984;141:196.
93. Williams RR, Hasstedt SJ, Wilson DE, et al. Evidence that men with familial hypercholesterolemia can avoid early coronary death. *JAMA* 1986;255:219.
94. Bergman AB, Stamm SJ. The morbidity of cardiac nondisease in school children. *N Engl J Med* 1967;276:1009.
95. Carroll MD, Abraham S, Dresser CM. *Dietary intake source data: United States 1976-1980.* Vital and Health Statistics Series 11, No 231, DHHS Publication No (PHS) 83-1681, US Department of Health and Human Services, 1983.
96. *Continuing survey of food intakes by individuals: women 19-50 years and their children 1-5 years, 1 day nationwide food consumption survey.* CFSII Report No 85-1, US Department of Agriculture, 1985.
97. Frank GC, Farris RP, Cresanta JL, et al. Dietary intake as a determinant of cardiovascular variables. In: Berenson G, ed. *Causation of cardiovascular risk factors in children.* New York: Raven Press, 1986;254.
98. Ford CH, McGandy RB, Stare FJ. An institutional approach to the dietary regulation of blood cholesterol in adolescent males. *Prev Med* 1972;1:426.
99. Kwiterovich PO Jr, Bachorik PS, Franklin FA, et al. Effect of

dietary treatment on the plasma levels of lipid and lipoprotein cholesterol and LDL B protein in children with type II hyperlipoproteinemia. In: Widhalm K, Naito HK, eds. *Current topics in the detection and treatment of lipid and lipoprotein disorders of childhood.* New York; Alan R Liss, 1986;123.
100. McGandy RB, Hall B, Ford C, et al. Dietary regulation of blood cholesterol in adolescent males: a pilot study. *Am J Clin Nutr* 1972;25:61.
101. Rose V, Allen DM, Pearse RG, et al. Primary hyperlipoproteinemia in childhood and adolescence: identification and treatment of persons at risk for premature atherosclerosis. *Can Med Assoc J* 1976;115:753.
102. Segall MM, Lloyd JK, Fosbrooke AS, et al. Treatment of familial hypercholesterolemia in children. *Lancet* 1990;1:641.
103. Stein EA, Mendelsohn D, Fleming M, et al. Lowering of plasma cholesterol levels in free-living adolescent males: use of natural or synthetic polyunsaturated foods to provide balanced fat diets. *Am J Clin Nutr* 1975;28:1204.
104. Vartiainen E, Puska P, Pietinen P, et al. Effects of dietary fat modifications on serum lipids and blood pressure in children. *Acta Paediatr Scand* 1986;75:396.
105. Vergroesen AJ. Dietary fat and cardiovascular disease: possible modes of action of linoleic acid. *Proc Nutr Soc* 1972;31:323.
106. Glueck CJ, Tsang RC, Fallat RW, et al. Diet in children heterozygous for familial hypercholesterolemia. *Am J Dis Child* 1977;131:162.
107. Stein EA, Shapero J, McNerney C, et al. Changes in plasma lipid and lipoprotein fractions after alternation in dietary cholesterol, polyunsaturated, saturated and total fat in free-living normal and hypercholesterolemic children. *Am J Clin Nutr* 1982;35:1375.
108. Fernandes J, Dijhuis-Stoffelsma R, Groot PHE, et al. The effect of a virtually cholesterol-free, high-linoleic acid vegetarian diet on serum lipoproteins of children with familial hypercholesterolemia. *Acta Paediatr Scand* 1981;70:677.
109. Widhalm K, Naito HK. Dietary treatment of hypercholesterolemia in children: recent aspects. In: *Recent aspects of diagnosis and treatment of lipoprotein disorders: impact on prevention of atherosclerotic diseases.* New York: Alan R Liss, 1988;219.
110. Gaddi A, Descovich GC, Noseda G, et al. Hypercholesterolemia treated by soybean protein diet. *Arch Dis Child* 1987;62:674.
111. Williams JC. Contribution of red meat to the US diet. *Food Nutr News* 1987;59:37.
112. Nicklas TA, Arbeit ML, Franklin FA, et al. A family approach to cardiovascular risk reduction through diet. *J Nutr Educ* 1987;19:302A.
113. Nicklas TA, Farris RP, Smoak CG, et al. Dietary factors relate to cardiovascular risk factors in early life: Bogalusa Heart Study. *Arteriosclerosis* 1988;8:193.
114. Nicklas TA, Johnson CC, Arbeit ML, et al. "Heart Smart" Program: a family intervention program for eating behavior of children at high risk for cardiovascular disease. *J Nutr Educ* 1988;20:128.
115. Nicklas TA, Johnson CC, Arbeit ML, et al. A dynamic family approach for prevention of cardiovascular disease. *J Am Diet Assoc* 1988;88:1438.
116. Lifshitz F, Moses N. Growth failure: a complication of dietary treatment of hypercholesterolemia. *Am J Dis Child* 1989; 143:537.
117. Publiese MT, Weyman-Daum M, Moses N, Lifshitz F. Parental health beliefs as a cause of nonorganic failure to thrive. *Pediatrics* 1987;80(2):175.
118. Dwyer JT, Andrew EM, Berkey C, et al. Growth in new vegetarian preschool children using the Jenss-Bayley curve fitting techniques. *Am J Clin Nutr* 1983;37:815.
119. Dwyer JT, Dietz WA Jr, Andrews EM, et al. Nutritional status of vegetarian children. *Am J Clin Nutr* 1982;35:204.
120. Leon AS, Conrad J, Hunninghake DB, Serfass R. Effects of a vigorous walking program on body composition, and carbohydrate, lipid metabolism of obese young men. *Am J Clin Nutr* 1979;32:1776.
121. Sasaki J, Shindo M, Tanaka H, et al. A long-term aerobic exercise program decreases the obesity index and increases the high density lipoprotein cholesterol concentration in obese children. *Int J Obes* 1987;11:339.
122. Perry CL, Silvis GL. Smoking prevention: behavioral prescriptions for the pediatrician. *Pediatrics* 1987;79:790.
123. Farah JR, Kwiterovich PO Jr, Neill CA. Dose-effect relationship of cholestyramine in children and young adults with familial hypercholesterolemia. *Lancet* 1977;1:59.
124. Glueck CJ, Fallat R, Tsang R. Pediatric familial type II hyperlipoproteinemia therapy with diet and cholestyramine resin. *Pediatrics* 1973;52:669.
125. Glueck CJ, Fallat RW, Mellies M, et al. Pediatric familial type II hyperlipoproteinemia: therapy with diet and colestipol resin. *Pediatrics* 1976;57:68.
126. Glueck CJ, Tsang RC, Fallat RW, et al. Therapy of familial hypercholesterolemia in childhood: diet and cholestyramine resin for 24–36 months. *Pediatrics* 1977;60:433.
127. Glueck CJ. Therapy of familial and acquired hyperlipoproteinemia in children and adolescents. *Prev Med* 1983;12:835.
128. Groot PHE, Dukhuis-Stoffelsma R, Grose WFA, et al. The effects of colestipol hydrochloride on serum lipoprotein lipid and apolipoprotein B and A-1 concentrations in children heterozygous for familial hypercholesterolemia. *Acta Paediatr Scand* 1983;72:81.
129. Mordasini R, Twelsick F, Oster P, et al. A comparative study of colestipol and cholestyramine in children and adolescents with familial hypercholesterolemia. *Mschr Kinderheilk* 1978;126:436.
130. Schwarz KB, Goldstein PP, Witztum JL, et al. Fat-soluble vitamin concentrations in hypercholesterolemic children treated with colestipol. *Pediatrics* 1980;65:243.
131. Stein EA. Treatment of familial hypercholesterolemia with drugs in children. *Arteriosclerosis* 1989;9(suppl I):145.
132. West RJ, Lloyd JK. Use of cholestyramine in treatment of children with familial hypercholesterolaemia. *Arch Dis Child* 1973;48:370.
133. Kwiterovich PO Jr. Bile acid sequestrant resin therapy in children. In: Fears R, ed. *Pharmacological control of hyperlipidaemia.* Barcelona: JR Prous, 1986;55.
134. Steinmetz J, Morin C, Panek E, et al. Biological variations in hyperlipidemic children and adolescents treated with fenofibrate. *Clin Chim Acta* 1981;112:42.
135. Glueck CJ, Tsang RC, Fallat RW, et al. Plasma vitamin A and E levels in children with familial type II hyperlipoproteinemia during therapy with diet and cholestyramine resin. *Pediatrics* 1974;54:51.
136. West RJ, Fosbrooke AS, Lloyd JK. Treatment of children with familial hypercholesterolemia. *Postgrad Med J* 1975;51(suppl 8):82.
137. West RJ, Lloyd JK, Leonard JV. Long-term follow-up of children with familial hypercholesterolaemia treated with cholestyramine. *Lancet* 1980;2:873.
138. Schucker BH, Goor RS. A behavioral approach for enhancing adherence to resin therapy. In: Fears R, ed. *Pharmacological control of hyperlipidemia.* Barcelona: JR Prous, 1986;91.
139. Franklin FA Jr, Brown RF, Franklin CC. Screening, diagnosis, and management of dyslipoproteinemia in children. *Endocrinol Metab Clin North Am* 1990;19(2):399.
140. National cholesterol education program coordinating committee. National cholesterol education program coordinating committee highlights of the report of the expert panel on blood cholesterol levels in children and adolescents. NHLBI information center, Bethesda, Maryland. 1991:1–12.

CHAPTER 27

Nutritional Considerations in the Therapy of the Child with Diabetes Mellitus

Allan L. Drash and Dorothy J. Becker

THE PROBLEM OF DIABETES MELLITUS IN OUR SOCIETY

Diabetes mellitus is one of the most common, serious, and chronic diseases affecting children, adolescents, and adults in the Western world. It is associated with significant morbidity and mortality rates, which are both increased and accelerated in comparison with the general population. Acute complications are generally a reflection of metabolic alterations in energy homeostasis, resulting from either hyperglycemia and insulin deficiency, or hypoglycemia from excess insulin action. The chronic complications, occurring, eventually, in over 80% of individuals with insulin-dependent diabetes mellitus, are vascular in nature, affecting both the microvasculature and the macrovasculature. Microvascular complications lead to progressive damage within the kidney, resulting in diabetic glomerulosclerosis and end-stage renal failure, damage to the vessels of the eye, resulting, initially, in background and, later, in proliferative diabetic retinopathy, which carries with it a high incidence of visual loss. The mechanism of diabetic neuropathy, both peripheral and autonomic, appears to result from both damage to the vascular supply to the nervous system as well as biochemical alterations within the peripheral nerves themselves. Atherosclerosis is a leading cause of both morbidity and mortality in the adult diabetic. The atherosclerotic process appears to be accelerated and more malignant in the diabetic individual, with significant vascular changes occurring at lower serum cholesterol levels than in the general population.

A. L. Drash: Division of Endocrinology, Metabolism, and Diabetes Mellitus, University of Pittsburgh Children's Hospital, Pittsburgh, Pennsylvania 15213.
D. J. Becker: Department of Pediatrics, University of Pittsburgh Children's Hospital, Pittsburgh, Pennsylvania 15213.

Classification and Diagnosis

Diabetes mellitus may occur as the end product of a number of somewhat dissimilar pathologic processes. Broadly speaking, diabetes mellitus in the Western world falls into two major pathologic systems. Non-insulin-dependent diabetes mellitus (NIDDM) is the form of the disease that occurs in approximately 85% of Americans with diabetes. This disorder, formerly known as maturity-onset or obesity-related diabetes, is complex, resulting from impairment of insulin action rather than primary insulin deficiency. In most cases, there is peripheral insulin resistance to normal or even elevated circulating insulin levels. This resistance may occur at the cell surface or, more often, at one of several intracellular steps of insulin action. This disorder almost always has its presentation during the adult years and is associated, in probably 80% of cases, with excess body weight.

Insulin-dependent diabetes mellitus (IDDM) is a genetically determined disease that results eventually in complete beta cell destruction and insulin deficiency. It is the primary form of diabetes seen in children and adolescents.

Our experience, in Pittsburgh, with over 2,000 diabetic children, demonstrated that greater than 97% of these children have the classical insulin-dependent form of the disease. Three percent or less have diabetes resulting from either an insulin resistant process, that is, NIDDM, usually associated with obesity, or the rarely seen, maturity-onset diabetes of youth (MODY). A very small number of patients have beta cell destruction as a consequence of a specific pathologic process such as pancreatitis or malignancy.

The diagnosis of diabetes mellitus in the child is rarely in doubt. Classification systems and their particular application to the pediatric age group clarify diagnoses on the bases of blood sugars and glucose tolerance (1–3). In the great majority of cases, children present with compelling clinical symptomatology, including a history of several days of polyuria, polydipsia, polyphagia, and weight loss. If the diagnosis is inordinately delayed, weakness, general anorexia, visual disturbances, and intellectual impairment may be noted. Severe dehydration, leading to diabetic ketoacidosis and coma, results in 3% or so of these patients at presentation. A small number of asymptomatic children will be picked up on routine pediatric evaluation, including urinalysis demonstrating glucosuria. Such patients have fasting glucose values in excess of 140 mg/dl and postprandial values exceeding 200 mg/dl. The glucose tolerance test, generally considered to be the diagnostic tool for diabetes mellitus, is rarely necessary to diagnosis the disease in children or adolescents and is usually reserved as a research tool to study insulin secretory dynamics.

The Epidemiology of IDDM in Childhood

Insulin-dependent diabetes mellitus occurs in all pediatric cultures subjected to study. However, there are major differences in the rate of expression, depending upon geographic area, cultural group, and genetic makeup. IDDM occurs with equal frequency in males and females; however, the peak incidence, in adolescents, is approximately $1\frac{1}{2}$ years earlier in girls than boys. There is a sharp decline in incidence toward the end of adolescence. IDDM ranks with cancer as one of the major chronic diseases of childhood. Both incidence and prevalence rates vary widely, both within the United States and around the world. Reported prevalence figures in the United States vary from 0.6 to 2.5 cases per 1,000 age-matched population. The prevalence figure for Allegheny County, Pennsylvania is 1.73 per 1,000; the incidence approximately 15/100,000/year. This is to be compared with an incidence of between 30 and 40/100,000/year in the Scandinavian countries, led by Finland, and approximately 1/100,000/year or less in most of the Asian nations. The remarkable geographic variations in the expression of IDDM have led to an intensive search for environmental and genetic factors that may explain these differences.

Seasonal variation in the usual time of diagnosis of IDDM is reported in essentially all countries, with peak values seen in winter months and decreased frequency of new diagnoses made in summer months. Studies of individuals who have moved from one geographic or cultural group to another have indicated that "migrants" take on the diabetes frequency of their adopted country. This has been demonstrated in Japanese moving to Hawaii as well as French, Italians, and Jews moving from Europe to Canada. Although the incidence of IDDM has remained relatively stable in the United States over the past two decades, there has been a pronounced increase in frequency of IDDM in children and adolescents in all the Scandinavian countries, particularly in Finland where the incidence rate has doubled in approximately 20 years. In addition, a number of areas have experienced apparent "epidemics" of IDDM, suggesting that changes in local environmental conditions account for provocation of the disease (4–21).

THE ETIOLOGY OF IDDM

Genetics and Autoimmunity

Insulin-dependent diabetes mellitus occurs in genetically susceptible individuals, resulting from a genetically mediated autoimmune destructive process. Islet cell antibodies (ICA) are present at the time of diagnosis in approximately 80% of IDDM patients, reflecting a preexisting inflammatory process within the islet cells of the pancreas. Although incompletely understood, the mechanism is probably chemical in nature, resulting from an immune response cascade released with the macrophage presentation of an islet cell autoantigen to helper T cells, which leads to a release of lymphokines including interleukin-1 (IL-1), tissue necrosis factor (TNF), and interferon-γ (ITF). It is likely that this process results in an accumulation of free radicals (oxides and peroxides) in the microenvironment of the beta cell. If the naturally occurring antioxidant systems are inadequate to neutralize free radicals, then direct toxic destruction of the beta cell occurs (22–24).

It has been clearly documented that susceptibility to IDDM is conferred by changes on chromosome 6 within the human leukocyte antigen (HLA) region. Increasing focus has been placed on the DR antigen complex. Approximately 90% of all IDDM patients are carriers of the HLA antigens, DR3, DR4, or both, antigens that occur commonly in the general population. The Stanford studies, which our studies confirm, have identified specific alterations in the DQ antigens, residing in the so-called codon 57 position in the beta chain of the DQ antigen. In the normal, nondiabetic individual in Western society, position 57 is occupied by aspartic acid. Susceptibility to IDDM is remarkably increased when aspartic acid is substituted by any other amino acid. The risk ratio for IDDM increases from approximately 3 in individuals with either DR3 or DR4 to 10 in those with both DR3/DR4, and to greater than 100 in individuals homozygous for nonaspartic acid at position 57 in the beta chain of the DQ antigen. This defect, however, does not represent the "diabetes gene," but rather one very important genetic susceptibility alteration. Twenty percent of the Western world population appear homozygous for nonaspartic acid. Yet, only 1 of 20 will become diabetic. One must investigate the environment for provocative events that initiate the autoimmune process (25–33).

Environmental Factors

Over 90% of the beta cell mass must be lost prior to the identification of clinical diabetes mellitus. This process probably occurs over a period of weeks, months, or, in some cases, years. It is likely that the process is discontinuous, with the inflammatory process waxing and waning with the advent of chemical damage to the beta cell followed by increased autoimmune destruction. Environmental factors that are considered of prime importance in the beta cell destructive process or the initiation and continuation of the autoimmune mechanisms include (a) viral infections, (b) environmental toxins, (c) nutrients (which in susceptible individuals act as toxic agents to the beta cell), and (d) stress-induced alterations in the endocrine and immune systems (22).

Viral infections have long been considered a major factor in the expression of IDDM. Mumps infections have had the longest connection with diabetes mellitus (34); the work of Gamble et al. (35) focused attention on the Coxsackie B group of viruses as important contributors to beta cell destruction. The most compelling evidence, linking viruses and diabetes, is the association between maternal rubella infection during pregnancy and the eventual development of IDDM in offspring. Yoon et al. (36) documented that fragments of the cytomegalovirus are frequently incorporated in the genome of individuals with IDDM. The hope of preventing IDDM by virus immunization appears unlikely (34–38).

A variety of environmental toxins are known to produce beta cell damage including alloxan and streptozotocin, which cause rapid beta cell destruction. Vacor, a commercial rodenticide, causes diabetes mellitus in the human, but not in the rat. Pentamidine, used for *Pneumocystis carinii* infection, has been reported to induce permanent beta cell destruction. Nitrosamines, a byproduct of some food preparation, particularly in the smoking of meats, are clearly beta cytotoxic in animals and probably, also, in humans.

Life-style is probably also a factor. IDDM occurs with increased frequencies in those countries most distant from the equator (both north and south) and in those countries where the mean environmental temperature is lowest. It is common in Western, affluent cultures and uncommon in the Orient, in third world countries, and in those countries with consistently warm climates. Its incidence parallels country-specific incidences of mortality from atherosclerotic cardiovascular disease. There is, therefore, the implication of diet. The rate of consumption of meat and dairy products within a country parallels the incidence of IDDM. Oriental and other countries in which the diet is predominantly carbohydrate with little protein have a very low incidence rate for IDDM. Of very special interest is the study suggesting that infants who were breast-fed had a lower incidence of diabetes. This issue is controversial and remains unresolved. It is, however, known that human breast milk provides important immunologic factors not obtained from cows' milk. Further, it is clear that cows' milk protein in certain individuals has a toxic property that may result in either acute or chronic alterations in beta cell function (39–45).

Both physical and emotional stress are known to result in alterations in the endocrine system, primarily through the hypothalamic pituitary adrenal axis. Substantial anecdotal information suggests that IDDM may be diagnosed more often following traumatic events such as the death of a parent, divorce, etc. (46–48).

THE PATHOPHYSIOLOGY OF IDDM

IDDM is a chronic, systemic disease, adversely affecting energy homeostasis. Rather than simply a disease of "sugar metabolism," insulin deficiency alters the metabolism of carbohydrates, fats, and proteins. Insulin mediates energy homeostasis, acting in concert with a group of counterregulatory hormones, including growth hormone, adrenocorticotropic hormone (ACTH), cortisone, epinephrine, norepinephrine, and glucagon. The concentration of glucose in blood is maintained within narrow limits by a balance between the production of glucose from the liver and the uptake and utilization by glucose in peripheral tissues. Insulin promotes the translocation of glucose from the intravascular to the intracellular space, effectively "opening the door" of the cell to allow glucose entry. In addition, through the stimulation of hepatic enzyme systems, insulin reduces or prevents the outflow of glucose from the liver into the general circulation when insulin is in high concentration. The net effect of a sharp rise in circulating insulin is a fall in blood glucose concentration. In terms of lipid metabolism, insulin acts to promote the synthesis and storage of triglyceride from excess dietary carbohydrates. Further, it acts to inhibit the degradation of triglycerides and the outflow of free fatty acids from adipose tissue into the circulation. In terms of protein metabolism, insulin is a growth hormone acting synergistically with pituitary growth hormone to promote the translocation of amino acids into the cell promoting cell growth and multiplication.

In the interval prior to the development of overt diabetes, as the potential diabetic moves from a state of metabolic normality through carbohydrate intolerance to overt diabetes mellitus, insulin secretion becomes blunted and postprandial glucose variation rises out of the normal range of 100 to 130 mg/dl. Eventually, the postprandial rise exceeds the renal threshold of approximately 160 mg/dl leading to glucosuria. Initial symptoms, usually polyuria, occur when the blood glucose exceeds the renal threshold continuously, promoting an osmotic diuresis. In the newly diagnosed or poorly controlled diabetic patient, as much as 1,000 calories per day may be lost in the urine.

Hyperglycemia is a hallmark of diabetes mellitus. Untreated glucose values are well in excess of 200 mg/dl. Also present is hyperlipidemia, including both elevations in total cholesterol and triglyceride. The patient may also present in a profound metabolic disequilibrium known as diabetic ketoacidosis, a result of a complete absence of insulin action. This leads to a massive outflow of free fatty acids from adipose tissue, overwhelming the ability of the TCA cycle to metabolize this energy source to CO_2 and water, resulting in the production of ketone bodies. Long-term insulin deficiency is associated with impairment in protein metabolism, reflected by poor growth preceding and during adolescence.

THERAPEUTIC OBJECTIVES

The ultimate therapeutic dream of the physician is the cure or prevention of diabetes. A therapeutic compromise is to manage the patient in such a fashion that the metabolic derangements of insulin deficiency are completely reversed and its chronic complications are prevented. Unfortunately, therapeutic programs available today are rarely effective in achieving and sustaining homeostatic normality. Consequently, optimal realistic therapeutic objectives frequently must be compromised in order to meet overriding personal, familial, and cultural requirements.

Achievable therapeutic goals include:

1. elimination of the clinical symptomatology secondary to hyperglycemia, including polyuria, polydipsia, polyphagia
2. prevention of hypoglycemia
3. prevention of diabetic ketoacidosis
4. prevention of obesity
5. promotion of normal growth and normal sexual maturation
6. achievement of a state of metabolic homeostasis as close to normal as is reasonable for the specific individual
7. promotion of optimal emotional well-being
8. prevention of the chronic micro- and macrovascular complications of diabetes
9. achievement of a fulfilling and meaningful adult life.

THE THERAPEUTIC ALLIANCE AND THERAPEUTIC TEAM APPROACH

Insulin-dependent diabetes mellitus is a complex disease. Its management is difficult and the long-term outlook for any given patient is unsatisfactory. The day-to-day demands of the therapeutic program on both the patient and other family members are greater than almost any other chronic disease. The psychological burden of the disease and its therapeutic requirements are heavy and it is not surprising that serious psychopathology occurs frequently in young patients. It is the experience of many excellent diabetologists that the management of the child or adolescent with diabetes is rarely successful when undertaken by the individual physician. Increasingly, the concept of the team approach has been endorsed by experts in the field.

The central member of the therapeutic team is the patient or, with younger children, the patient and parents. Other team members include the pediatrician-diabetologist, nurse-educator, dietitian/nutritionist, and social worker. Consulting members of the team include a psychologist and/or psychiatrist, ophthalmologist, nephrologist, and obstetrician/gynecologist for the adolescent girl. As the patient progresses into young adult life, the team pediatrician should be changed to an internist-diabetologist.

The dietitian plays a very special role. Nutritional management is key to overall therapeutic success. The most common explanation for failure to achieve blood glucose and glycosylated hemoglobin therapeutic goals is probably, in fact, dietary noncompliance. The dietitian must establish a relationship with the patient and family as soon as possible, evaluating their usual nutritional habits in order to design a nutritional plan that they will be able to understand and follow. This may take several educational sessions. Initial dietary advice must be directed toward "survival skills." Over time, optimally, experiences should help the patient and his family develop a more sophisticated knowledge of foods and their therapeutic implications. The dietitian should be available at all times for questions and should be involved, at least once a year, in helping the family update its nutritional information.

THERAPY OF THE CHILD WITH DIABETES MELLITUS

Optimal therapy for diabetes mellitus must include (a) insulin, (b) a regimen for physical fitness, (c) psychological support, and (d) nutritional management. These four therapeutic components must be properly balanced and integrated in order to approach therapeutic objectives.

Insulin

Prior to the discovery of insulin, childhood diabetes was essentially the foreshadow of impending death. Insulin, itself, has evolved from problematic to a highly purified substance that has successfully minimized the impediments of contamination and resultant allergic reactions. Recombinant DNA methodology has resulted in preparations that have the identical amino acid structure as human insulin. These, combined with methods for assessing metabolic control, including glycosylated hemoglobin and self–blood-glucose monitoring, have promoted attainment of near metabolic normality. This has lead to a number of changes in insulin therapeutics (49).

Conventional Insulin Therapy

From a long-standing regimen of one or two injections of insulin daily, conventional therapy has developed into split dosages of neutral protamine Hagedorn (NPH) and regular (or Lente plus regular or Lente plus semi-Lente) given before breakfast and the evening meal. When combined with the other components of therapy, this approach has generally been successful in eliminating the acute complications of the disease and in securing a moderate level of metabolic control. Its effect on long-term complications remains to be determined (50, 51).

Intensive Insulin Therapy

Increasingly, the serious vascular complications of diabetes mellitus are assumed to be a consequence of chronic hyperglycemia. Although conclusive evidence awaits the conclusions of the intensive collaborative research within the Diabetes Control and Complication Trial (DCCT), many physicians are managing their patients as if the glucose-complication riddle had been solved. This management concept, combined with the new tools to assess metabolic status, has initiated a therapeutic program, inaccurately referred to as "intensive insulin therapy." The specific objectives are the achievement of metabolic normality with the anticipation that all chronic vascular complications of the disease will be minimized or eliminated. Optimally, this intensive therapeutic program would involve, equally, all the components of diabetes management. Unfortunately, an excessive focus has been placed on the insulin component.

There are two approaches to intensive insulin therapy. Multiple dose insulin therapy (MDI) has received wide acceptance among diabetologists and certain patient groups. This approach involves administration of a long-acting insulin preparation (usually Ultralente) once daily and regular insulin before each meal and the bedtime snack. Typically, regular insulin is administered 30 to 40 min prior to breakfast, lunch, dinner, and bedtime snack; Ultralente, however, is added to the regular insulin prior to dinner. Variations on this theme include Ultralente administered twice daily, usually before breakfast and bedtime snack, and administered in conjunction with regular insulin. In addition, regular insulin is also given before lunch and at evening meals.

The other intensive insulin therapy includes the use of an open loop insulin infusion device. The course of the "insulin pump" has been somewhat erratic. Its measure of improved metabolic control has been predicated on the skill and motivation of the individual patient, with little indication of its successful use for the pediatric patient.

Although intensive diabetic management is founded on the hope that vascular complications can be delayed, minimized, or prevented, there are clearly identifiable risks associated with it. The frequency of severe hypoglycemia in the DCCT is approximately three times greater in the intensive group when compared with those on conventional therapy. Excessive weight gain has also occurred, indicating, perhaps, the need for improved dietary compliance when blood sugars are brought toward the normal range (52, 53).

Exercise in the Management of the Patient with IDDM

Physical exertion increases the disposal of glucose and generally leads to a drop in blood glucose concentration. A regular program of physical activity is associated with increased insulin sensitivity. Physical fitness, in the diabetic patient, appears to result in improved metabolic control at a lowered insulin dose level. Improvements in blood lipids are also characteristic. However, to be effective, physical activity must be integrated with insulin administration and dietary alterations. Exercise with inadequate caloric intake will result in hypoglycemia; intense exercise combined with marked hyperglycemia and ketonuria may result in metabolic deterioration and the precipitation of diabetic ketoacidosis (54).

However, most individuals who exercise regularly report a special feeling of well-being, with potentially decreased obesity. Our long-term studies indicate that a regular program of physical fitness during adolescence and young adulthood is associated with a decrease in both cardiovascular morbidity and mortality after several years of diabetes (55, 56).

Nutrition as a Therapeutic Component

General Principles

Dietary strategies for patients with diabetes mellitus began with the Egyptians in 1500 BC (57–59). Until the last 20 years, however, these did not differentiate between individuals with non–insulin-dependent and insulin-dependent diabetes mellitus. Recognition of the specific needs of children has been even more recent. One positive factor in this recognition is that, because diets for diabetes management are based on optimal nutritional tenets, they have the twofold advantage of being used to promote the well-being of the entire family and, simultaneously, eliminating the isolation of the diabetic child. As noted in the recommendations of the Commit-

TABLE 1. *Calculation of daily caloric requirements*

Adults
  Basal calories: desirable body weight (DBW) in pounds (lb) × 10
    Calories added for activity level
      Sedentary: DBW (lb) × 3
      Moderate: DBW (lb) × 5
      Strenuous: DBW (lb) × 10
    Added 300 to 500 cal for weight gain, pregnancy, lactation
    Subtract 500 cal for weight loss in obesity
Children
  1,000 cal + 100 cal per year to puberty
    Puberty: Females 2,400–2,800
             Males 2,600–3,400
  Caloric needs vary with rate of growth and activity
  Adjust calories to maintain normal growth (Wetzel, Iowa, or Stuart graphs)

From ref. 156.

tee on Nutrition of the American Diabetes Association, this diet must satisfy all requirements for protein, calories, and micronutrients necessary for optimal growth and maturation during the active growth phase of childhood and adolescence (Table 1) (156) (Table 2) (60).

TABLE 2. *Components of the diabetic diet based on 1986 revision of exchange lists for meal planning*

Calories	Adequate calories to reach or maintain desirable body weight
Carbohydrate	Ideally, up to 55–60% of total calories: starch/bread, vegetables, fruit, milk; natural sugars and sucrose—contingent on metabolic control and weight
Protein	Approximately 12–20% of total calories; recommended daily allowance is 0.8 g/kg of body weight for adults; elderly individuals may require more than the recommended daily allowance; reduce protein intake in patients with incipient renal disease
Fat	<30% of total calories; saturated fat should be restricted to <10% of total calories; polyunsaturated fat should be restricted to 6–8% of total calories; the remainder of fats should be supplied by monounsaturated fats
Cholesterol	<300 mg daily
Fiber	Up to 40 g daily; 25 g/1,000 Cal daily for individuals on low-calorie diets
Sodium	1,000 mg sodium per 1,000 Cal, not to exceed 3,000 mg daily; sodium should be reduced in patients with hypertension

From ref. 60.

It is important to emphasize, however, that diet is only one factor in the optimum prognosis for diabetics; other, equally important, components, including the avoidance of day-to-day problems in energy homeostasis and prevention of vascular complications, are essential.

Calories

Traditional dietary advice to diabetic patients includes specific calorie levels based on preset categories of age and average intake. It is our experience, however, that appetite level might, generally, be a better indicator of caloric need. The diet of the diabetic child or adolescent really should not be "restrictive" in terms of calorie content unless there is evidence of excessive weight gain (61).

At the time of diagnosis, the great majority of diabetic children have sustained significant weight loss with concomitant body deficits that must be repleted. An initial diet prescription of approximately 25% more calories than would be calculated based on age and sex alone will allow for rapid weight gain and replenishment of losses. In most cases, as the child returns to his ideal body weight, appetite declines and both child and parent become aware that the prior caloric intake is now excessive. This can be adjusted during subsequent sessions with the dietitian.

Carbohydrates

For many years, there has been concern that a diet in which a large number of calories were derived from carbohydrates would result in hyperglycemia. However, nutritional research from many centers has, in general, failed to substantiate this position. It is now well accepted that 55% to 60% of total calories should be derived from carbohydrate sources. Further, the recommendations are that the carbohydrate sources should be predominantly naturally occurring complex carbohydrates, including whole-grain breads and cereals, pastas, potatoes, beans or peas and other starches, as well as fruits and vegetables.

Although refined sugars should be used sparingly, recent studies suggest that isocaloric substitution of sucrose for complex carbohydrates may not result in a significant increase in blood glucose variation, if the substitution is for less than 5% of total daily calories. Although hyperglycemia and lipid alterations will probably result when intake reaches 10%, 5% appears to be a safe proportion to provide patients with natural dietary sweetening.

Dairy products with the disaccharide lactose are digested and metabolized to the monosaccharides galactose and glucose. Despite these readily available free su-

TABLE 3. *Mean glycemic indexes (MGI) of some foods proportionally adjusted to the glycemic index of white bread = 100*

Food	MGI[a]	Food	MGI
Starch/bread[b]		Dried legumes[b]	
Rye crisp	95	Baked beans (canned)	60
White (wheat)	100	Butter beans	52
Whole-grain rye	58	Chick peas	49
Whole-meal wheat	99	Green peas	56
Cereal products		Haricot beans	45
Buckwheat	74	Kidney beans	54
Millet	103	Red lentils	43
Rice (brown)	96	Soybeans (dried)	22
Rice (white)	83	Soybeans (canned)	20
Spaghetti (white)	66	Fruit	
Spaghetti (whole wheat)	61	Apple	53
Sweet corn	97	Banana	79
Breakfast cereals		Cherries	32
All-bran	73	Grapefruit	36
Cornflakes	119	Grapes	62
Meusli	96	Orange	66
Porridge oats	85	Orange juice	67
Shredded wheat	97	Peach	40
Weetabix	109	Pear	47
Biscuits		Plum	34
Digestive	82	Raisins	93
Oatmeal	78	Sugars	
Rich tea	80	Fructose	30
Water	91	Glucose	138
Vegetables		Honey	126
Frozen peas	74	Maltose	152
Root vegetables		Sucrose	86
Potato (instant)	116	Dairy products	
Potato (new, boiled)	81	Ice cream	52
Potato (russet, baked)	135	Skim milk	46
Potato (sweet)	70	Whole milk	49
Yam	74	Yogurt	52

Adapted from ref. 157, with permission.

[a] Glycemic index: amount of glucose absorbed from each food expressed as a percentage of the rise in blood glucose resulting from an equal amount of carbohydrate ingested as starch/white bread.

[b] Higher glucose rises are seen with potatoes, cereals, and starch/breads; lower responses are seen with pasta and dried legumes. Differences may be related to fiber content, to intrinsic enzymatic inhibitors, or to variations in digestive processing. Until conclusive data are accumulated, patients with diabetes can observe the effects of various carbohydrate sources by using self-monitoring of blood glucose to test the effects of these foods on glucose levels following meals.

gars, dairy product ingestion is rarely associated with significant hyperglycemia because of the fat and protein that is digested with the carbohydrate component. Fruit juices, however, although generally felt to be of nutritional value, may be of some concern. The primary carbohydrate of most fruits is the monosaccharide fructose, which is efficiently converted by the liver to glucose and may result in a hyperglycemic response. In addition, some studies suggest that fructose is more readily metabolized to triglyceride, resulting, after high intake, in hypertriglyceridemia. Neither of these problems appears to be significant when fruit intake is part of a well-balanced, well-regulated nutritional program. Ingestion of whole fruit, as opposed to fruit juices, is probably preferable (62–64).

Glycemic Index

For many years, it was assumed that the effect of comparable quantities of carbohydrate on blood glucose variation resulted primarily from the degree of complexity of the carbohydrate molecule. That is, naturally occurring complex carbohydrates, such as grains and potatoes, would be expected to provide a glycemic excursion appreciably below that of a comparable quantity of sucrose, glucose, or fructose. Surprisingly, careful studies, including those of Jenkins et al., have not confirmed these suppositions (Table 3). In the Jenkins study, a glycemic index of 100 is assigned to white bread. In comparison, baked potatoes have a glycemic index of 135; baked beans, 60; an orange, 66; sucrose, 86; and ice cream, 52. The glycemic excursion of a particular food, however, will be dependent on a variety of factors, including whether it is ingested alone or with other foods, such as protein and fats, which generally slow the digestive process and block the glycemic rise. The presence of fiber, either soluble or insoluble, will also alter the rate of digestion and generally reduce the glycemic index. Absorption rate is also affected by preparation, including methods and duration of cooking, and preservation.

Despite these major variables, it appears that there is consistency in glycemic excursion within the same individual for specific foods. As a result, although the glycemic index data may presently be too complex for routine application in patient dietary prescriptions, individual patients can and should evaluate their individual glucose responses to different foods in order to discover which result in excessive blood glucose elevations and which can be ingested with impunity, despite the similarity in apparent carbohydrate content (65–70).

Fiber

Although a multitude of commercial enterprises are actively promoting foods high in fiber as the key element in the control of blood cholesterol concentration, attempts to scientifically document such beneficial effects have been disappointing (71–77).

Fiber, which is derived from plant sources, is not hydrolyzed by the human gastrointestinal tract. It may be soluble or insoluble. Soluble fiber, found in fruits, legumes, lentils, roots, tubers, oats, and oat bran, has been observed to lower blood glucose as well as reduce cholesterol and triglyceride levels. Insoluble fiber is found in cellulose, lignin, bran, and most hemicellulose. Food sources include whole grain breads, cereals, and wheat bran. High intake has both positive and negative effects (Table 4).

Initially, Kiehm et al. reported dramatic improvement in NIDDM patients placed on high-carbohydrate, high-fiber diets, with a metabolic improvement in glucose and lipid metabolism and a decreasing need for oral agents (78). Later studies suggested similar benefits in insulin-dependent patients with a decrease in insulin requirements. Adverse side effects, however, included abdominal distention and discomfort, flatulence, increased defecation frequency, diarrhea and, in a small number of subjects, phytobezoar formation secondary to gastric hypotony. Although there is a potential for vitamin and mineral loss due to malabsorption, this has not been frequently documented (78–81).

TABLE 4. *Characteristics of the high-fiber diet (30–40 g)*

Dietary fiber
  Soluble fiber
    Pectins, plant polysaccharides, guar gum, mucilage, and a few hemicelluloses
  Insoluble fiber
    Cellulose, lignin, bran, and most hemicelluloses
Effects of fiber enrichment of diet
  Delayed gastric emptying
  Prolonged intestinal transit (depends on fiber constituents)
  Decreased glucose, cholesterol, and triglyceride absorption
  Reduced insulin and sulfonylurea requirements
Adverse effects
  Flatulence, abdominal discomfort
  Increased defecation, diarrhea
  Phytobezoar formation with gastric hypotony
  Potential for vitamin-mineral losses

From ref. 158.

There are few studies on the use of high-fiber diets in children (82–85). Our own have been unsatisfactory because the children had difficulty in consuming the full high-fiber meals. Kinmonth succeeded in carrying out a 6-week crossover trial of ten diabetic children, comparing an unrefined high-fiber diet with a refined low-fiber diet (82). He concluded that mean 24-hr blood glucose values and 24-hr urine excretion were lower with the high-fiber diet. Lindsay, in a 10-day study of diabetic children, found no significant blood glucose differences as a result of high- versus low-fiber diets (83).

The average American diet contains between 10 and 30 g of fiber per day. Current recommendations of the American Diabetes Association are to increase this gradually (86) to 35 to 40 g per day of both soluble and insoluble fiber. Gradual introduction is necessary to minimize the gastrointestinal side effects. In addition, careful blood glucose monitoring is important, particularly during an increase in fiber intake, because of the possibility of hypoglycemia secondary to delayed carbohydrate absorption.

Considerably more research is needed on the effects of high-fiber diets on both the normal population as well as individuals with disease states, including diabetes mellitus. Although such studies are especially difficult in children and adolescence, they are of particular importance (87–89).

Protein

High-quality dietary protein in the amount of 1.5 g/kg/day is recommended to ensure optimal growth in the growing child and adolescent. Because of increasing evidence of a relationship between fatty meat intake and atherosclerotic heart disease, the traditional recommendation for protein source has shifted from beef toward chicken, fish, and grains.

The degradation products of dietary protein result in obligatory work for the kidneys to excrete nitrogenous compounds. The hyperfiltration and renal hypertrophy characterizing the early onset of diabetes mellitus is felt to result primarily from hyperglycemia. However, the renal changes may be further aggravated by an increased nitrogenous load from dietary protein. There is increasing interest in reducing dietary protein in an attempt to reduce renal damage. However, although there is evidence that placing diabetic patients with microalbuminuria on a low-protein diet is associated with a decrease in albumin excretion, there is little evidence that the rate of renal functional decline is altered in these individuals prior to overt renal disease. In addition, there is clearly no evidence that protein restriction in the completely normal diabetic patient will have any beneficial long-term effect (90–91).

It is certainly improper to consider significant protein restriction in the child with diabetes who still has growth potential. On the other hand, the older adolescent, at the end of the growth phase with long-standing diabetes mellitus and significant microalbuminuria, may be an appropriate participant in the study of long-term consequences of dietary protein restriction. Until more convincing evidence is available, however, it seems reasonable to continue the recommendation that 15% to 20% of total daily calories be derived from good-quality protein in the child and adolescent with diabetes mellitus.

Fats

The recent dietary revolution in the United States, which has led to a reduction of fat intake from approximately 45% of total calories to less than 35% of a different source, resulted from increasing evidence linking atherosclerotic cardiovascular disease to saturated fat and cholesterol intake. The American Heart Association (AHA) deserves much of the credit for the public awareness and acceptance of the AHA "prudent diet" approach. Many of its principles have been incorporated into the recommendations of the American Diabetes Association. These include the suggestion that fat make up less than 30% of the diet equally divided into saturated, polyunsaturated, and monounsaturated.

In the debate over the merits of the various fatty acids, some concern has been expressed that polyunsaturated fat suppresses the immune system and possibly stimulates carcinogenesis in animal models. Monounsaturated fats, however, appear to lower low-density lipoprotein (LDL) cholesterol with no apparent adverse side effects on laboratory animals. The Mediterranean diet, composed heavily of monounsaturated fatty acids derived from olive oil, appears to be associated with a decreased frequency of vascular disease. Peanut and rapeseed oil are other excellent sources of monounsaturated fats (92–105).

Dietary Sweeteners

Although traditionally, individuals with diabetes mellitus were cautioned against intake of high sucrose-containing foods, recent studies indicate that complete avoidance of sucrose is unnecessary. It is now felt that up to 5% of total daily calories may be safely consumed if the remaining calories are well-balanced from complex carbohydrates, adequate fiber, protein, and fat. The commonly more extensive "sweet tooth," however, has resulted in the long and expensive search for food additives to provide sweetness without the adverse side effects of sugar.

Sweeteners are classified as either nutritive or nonnutritive. Nutritive sweeteners include sucrose, fructose, sorbitol, mannitol, and xylitol. Each of these carbohydrates contains approximately 4 cal per gram, which can augment daily caloric consumption appreciably. Fructose has been recommended as a substitute for sucrose in the diet of diabetic individuals because it does not stimulate insulin release and does not directly increase blood glucose. However, fructose is efficiently converted to glucose by the liver and may indirectly lead to a rise in circulating glucose concentration. Concerns about its excessive conversion to triglycerides and induction of hypertriglyceridemia have apparently not been substantiated in long-term chronic studies. It seems reasonable to allow a moderate amount of fructose, primarily through fruits and fruit products. Sorbitol, which is digested and absorbed very slowly, is widely used in dietetic foods. Following absorption, it is rapidly converted to fructose in the liver, from which glucose may be derived. Although this rise in blood glucose concentration is modest, GI complications may result from the slow absorption and induction of osmotic diarrhea. We do not recommend the routine use of foods with sorbitol (106–114).

There are two Food and Drug Administration (FDA)-approved nonnutrient sweeteners. Saccharin is a coal tar derivative that was initially synthesized in 1879. It is approximately 500 times as sweet as sucrose and is stable under cooking conditions. There continues to be concern about the possibility of bladder carcinoma resulting from chronic saccharin ingestion. However, human studies have failed to confirm animal studies. Saccharin is packaged with dextrose and contains approximately 4 cal per packet. It is sold as Sweet'n Low and Sugar Twin. Aspartame is a protein produced from phenylalanine and aspartic acid. Although it has a calorie content of 4 kilocalories (Cal) per gram, it has a sweetness factor 200 times that of sucrose. Consequently, the amount needed to add sweetness to food is not calorically significant. Unlike saccharin, aspartame has no bitter aftertaste. It is quite stable in solid form, but decomposes in solution or when heated. It cannot, therefore, be used for cooking, but is stable in acidic solutions such as soft drinks. No carefully done studies have confirmed concerns of toxic reaction to aspartame-containing foods. It is, presently, the major nonnutritive sweetener being used. It is marketed as NutraSweet in prepared foods and as Equal for individual use. Although clinical studies appear to provide a wide safety margin for the ingestion of both saccharin and aspartame, it seems reasonable to recommend moderate inclusion in the diet of the diabetic child (115–120).

Sodium, Micronutrients, and Vitamins

The poorly controlled diabetic patient has excessive urinary losses of electrolytes, micronutrients, and vitamins. Insulin deficiency is associated with failure of sodium reabsorption by the distal renal tubule, leading to large sodium losses in the urine in patients with diabetic ketoacidosis. However, reasonable insulinization results in reversal of excess electrolyte losses (121). Of greater concern than sodium depletion is the chronic effect of excess sodium intake resulting in or exacerbating the increased tendency toward hypertension in diabetic individuals. The development of hypertension causes an increased acceleration of both micro- and macrovascular disease. This is particularly true in terms of diabetic nephropathy. The rate of loss of renal function can be effectively blunted by reduction of hypertension. Consequently, moderate sodium restriction seems to be prudent, with a sodium intake of 1,000 mg/1,000 Cal ingested, not to exceed 3 g daily. Further restriction should occur in the presence of hypertension (122).

Mooradian and Morley have recently reviewed the micronutrient status in patients with diabetes (123). Micronutrients such as zinc, calcium, magnesium, and manganese have been reported to be decreased in IDDM patients (124–130). These losses are accentuated in the presence of diabetic ketoacidosis. Zinc and chromium have been implicated in the pathogenesis of carbohydrate intolerance, but appear to have no role in the etiology of IDDM. Micronutrient supplementation has been said to improve carbohydrate tolerance in NIDDM patients. There are no studies suggesting benefits of micronutrient supplementation in children with IDDM.

The chronically, poorly controlled IDDM patient may be subject to vitamin deficiencies. However, there is no evidence of clinically significant vitamin deficiencies in IDDM patients under average or good metabolic control. There is consequently no rationale for routine vitamin supplementation unless patients are on grossly aberrant diets.

Integrating the Nutrition Plan into Diabetes Therapy

The child with diabetes mellitus should be placed on a calorically adequate diet containing 55% to 60% of total calories from carbohydrate, 30% from fat, and the remainder from protein. The carbohydrate should be primarily derived from complex starches; fat sources should include a significant proportion of calories from meats, chicken, fish, and vegetable oils; protein should be derived from both animal and vegetable sources. Cholesterol should be restricted to less than 300 mg/day. Meal plans should be appropriate to the entire family; appetite and life-style should help the dietitian determine total caloric intake and distribution of meals. In the younger child, total calories should be divided among three meals and three snacks, with somewhat lesser calories associated with breakfast and more with the evening meal. In the older child, the midmorning snack is frequently eliminated, whereas the midafternoon and bedtime snacks are retained. Calorie restrictions are appropriate only if the child is gaining weight excessively.

Routine patient monitoring should include accurate determination of height and weight, three or four times per year, with the plotting of this information on standard growth grids. Decline in height or weight percentile should lead to a full inquiry as to the adequacy of diabetes management or to provide some other explanation for the failure to thrive. Excessive weight gain should

TABLE 5. *Activity factor affecting energy requirements*

Light activity (100–200 cal/hr[a])	Moderate activity (200–350 cal/hr)	Vigorous activity (400–900 cal/hr)
Driving an automobile	Active housework	Aerobic exercise
Fishing	Bicycling	Bicycling
Laboratory work	Bowling	Climbing
Light housework	Brisk walking	Dancing (fast)
Dusting	Dancing (slow)	Ice skating
Cooking	Factory work	Labor, unskilled
Secretarial work	Gardening	Outdoor sports
Typing	Golf	Running
Filing	Roller skating	Soccer
Operating computer	Truck driving	Tennis (single)
Teaching		Wood chopping
Walking casually		

Adapted from ref. 159, with permission.
[a] Time needed to expend calories varies with level of activity.

lead to a review with appropriate restriction of calories or increase in physical activity.

Insulin administration, in most patients, will include NPH and regular insulin given 30 min before breakfast and before the evening meal. Insulin dosage should be adjusted to achieve essentially normal fasting blood glucose values (80 to 120 mg/dl in the older child), with a moderate increase in those obtained at other times of the day (80 to 180 mg/dl). Ideally, daily exercise should be for approximately 60 min and vigorous enough to increase the heart rate. This may occur in either a physical education class or during after-school play. Dietary adjustments need to be made, of course, for those times when changes in physical activity are anticipated or during weekends when there is generally a later administration of the morning insulin and increased physical activity (Table 5) (159).

Sick-Day Management

Acute illnesses such as respiratory infections with fever, flu-like illnesses, and gastroenteritis may result in rapid metabolic alterations in the diabetic patient. The initial response, in the febrile, anorectic diabetic child, is to defer insulin administration until adequacy of caloric intake is established. This is almost always the wrong decision. Illness is regularly associated with insulin resistance; the sick child, despite reduced caloric intake, will need the usual dose of insulin and, in many cases, supplemental doses of regular insulin during the day, in order to maintain reasonable blood glucose levels and prevent the development of diabetic ketoacidosis. If the child is reluctant to take a normal diet, substitutes must be provided. A variety of alternate foodstuffs may be utilized (Table 6). Maintaining fluid intake, along with a moderate caloric consumption, is extremely important. Vomiting that lasts for more than a few hours may necessitate intravenous fluid therapy in either an emergency room or following hospitalization. This is usually prevented by the early introduction of alternate calorie sources combined, if needed, with vigorous insulin therapy.

Emotional-Behavioral Components of Diabetes and Their Management

Understanding the physical and psychological demands of diabetes mellitus is important to successful management (131). One of the major problems, particularly in the adolescent diabetic, is therapeutic noncompliance. This may constitute rejection of a specific aspect of the management program to wholesale rejection of the idea of diabetes and its management. Refusal to carry out monitoring requirements and/or falsification of blood glucose records is seen frequently. Rejection of the dietary program is also common. In fact, the inability to achieve blood glucose and glycosylated hemoglobin goals is usually attributable to excess caloric intake. Obesity, seen generally in teenage girls, occurs with increased frequency in the female adolescent diabetic, whose approach to weight loss may be reduction in the insulin dose in order to induce caloric loss through the urine.

Approximately 50% of adolescent diabetics experience significant psychopathology by young adult life. Usually, this is seen as depression, although character disorders, destructive acting out, daredevil-type behavior as well as overt psychosis are also seen (132, 133).

Pathologic eating disorders are of special concern (134–143). The common, relatively mild eating disturbances are particularly common in diabetic adolescent girls. In addition, anorexia nervosa and bulimia are possibly two or three times more common than in the general adolescent and young adult population. These eating disturbances are especially serious in the diabetic and can result in death of the patient. Psychiatric counseling is crucial and hospitalization may be needed. Careful collaboration between the members of the diabetes therapeutic team and the psychiatric professionals is key to a successful outcome.

TABLE 6. *Food suggestions for carbohydrate replacement during illness*[a]

Foods	Quantity for carbohydrate values	
	10 g	15 g
Carbohydrate beverages containing sugar (ginger ale, Coke, Pepsi)	½ cup (4 oz)	¾ cup (6 oz)
Corn syrup or honey	2 tsp	3 tsp (1 tbsp)
Cooked cereal		½ cup
Custard		½ cup
Eggnog, commercial		½ cup
Granulated sugar	2½ tsp	
Grape juice, unsweetened		⅓ cup
Grapefruit or orange juice		½ cup (4 oz)
Ice cream		½ cup
Milk		1¼ cup (10 oz)
Popsicle	½ twin bar	
Saltine cracker squares	4	6
Sherbet		¼ cup
Soup (broth base with vegetables, noodles, rice, or cream soup diluted with water)		1 cup (8 oz)
Sugar-sweetened gelatin	¼ cup	⅓ cup
Yogurt, plain		1 cup

Adapted from ref. 160, with permission.

[a] 50 g of carbohydrate should be consumed every 3 to 4 hours in small, frequent feedings.

The term *brittle diabetic* refers to patients who have had a clinical course characterized by episodes of recurrent diabetic ketoacidosis and/or severe hypoglycemic attacks. Close observation has defined this problem as essentially psychosocial in nature, involving both the patient and the patient's family (144–153). The variations in control seem to result from improper manipulation of both insulin and diet. Long-term counseling is usually advised. However, the problem seems to resolve spontaneously at the end of adolescence.

THE SUCCESS OF THERAPY: OUTCOME MEASURES

The ultimate success of diabetes management is associated with the ability of the diabetic patient to fulfill his or her potential socially, psychologically, and intellectually as well as preventing the serious vascular complications associated with this disorder. Patient monitoring is an essential part of this success.

Glycosylated Hemoglobin

Glycosylated hemoglobin determination assesses the quantity of glucose irreversibly attached to the hemoglobin molecule (glycosylated hemoglobin, HbA_1c, HbA_1). Results are used to help guide the patient and family toward moving their metabolic status, continuously and safely, closer to the normal range.

Self–Blood-Glucose Monitoring

The glucose determinations, when done with care, provide blood glucose measures that are generally ±10% of laboratory glucose determinations done on the same specimen. Because of concern with hypoglycemia and its adverse effects on the central nervous system, particularly in the younger child, our blood glucose recommendations are somewhat higher than normal, with fasting blood glucoses in the range of 100 to 140 mg/dl and all others in the range of 100 to 200 mg/dl. When values are either consistently above or below this range, adjustments must be made.

Blood Lipids

Blood lipid analysis, total cholesterol, HDL cholesterol, and triglyceride levels are recommended annually. Significant elevations are usually secondary to poor diabetes control although familial hyperlipidemia may occur in patients with diabetes mellitus. Pharmacologic therapy may be necessary.

Thyroid Function

Approximately 40% of our patients develop Hashimoto's thyroiditis with goiter and positive thyroid antibodies. About one-third of these children will become hypothyroid. A smaller number will have associated hyperthyroidism. Because of this, we recommend routine annual testing of thyroid function.

Renal Function

Approximately 40% of diabetic patients eventually develop significant diabetic glomerulosclerosis, leading, in many cases, to end-stage renal disease. The first detectable abnormality in renal function is the development of proteinuria. We recommend that all patients have routine urinary protein checked by the "dipstick" techniques at each clinic visit although we, and others, are moving toward routine microalbumin assessment, as well. The presence of significant proteinuria and/or declining renal function should lead to a full evaluation with the possibility of placing the patient on a protein- and salt-restricted diet and the possible use of antihypertensive agents.

Growth and Development

Inadequate insulin results in delayed growth and sexual maturation. Diabetic children should be screened for factors both within the disease as well as other determinants that may be affecting growth or development.

Other Diabetes Complications

Before adolescence, examination of the retina by the diabetologist should be part of the routine care. With adolescence, annual examinations by an ophthalmologist skilled in diabetic vascular disease should probably be supplemented with a fluorescein angiogram or stereo color photography to provide a baseline for future comparison.

Although clinically apparent diabetic neuropathy is uncommon in diabetic children and adolescents, the presence of symptoms should lead to prompt referral to a neurologist.

SUMMARY AND CONCLUSIONS

The child with diabetes mellitus presents an extraordinary therapeutic challenge. The demands on the therapeutic team, the patient, and the family are great. Nutrition plays a central role in the success, or failure, of the management program. A critical member of the diabetes therapy team is the dietitian. The importance of good nutrition and dietary management must be reinforced, however, by all members of the team.

There is great anticipation that scientific advances in the next decade will lead to means of preventing or curing diabetes in its early stages. The possibility of more physiologic insulin delivery systems, as well as pharmacologic means of impeding the progression of vascular complications, also offer great hope for future. Nutrition, however, will remain a cornerstone to good therapy (154, 155).

REFERENCES

1. National Diabetes Data Group. Classification and diagnosis of diabetes mellitus and other categories of glucose intolerance. *Diabetes* 1979;28:1039–1057.
2. Drash AL. The classification of diabetes mellitus in children and adolescents. *Acta Paediatr Jpn* 1987;29:325–334.
3. Drash AL. *Clinical care of the diabetic child.* Chicago, IL: Yearbook Medical Publishers, 1987.
4. Cruickshanks KJ, LaPorte RE, Dorman JS, et al. The epidemiology of insulin-dependent diabetes mellitus: etiology and prognosis. In: Ahmad PI, Ahmad N, eds. *Coping with juvenile diabetes.* Springfield, IL: Charles C. Thomas, 1985;332–357.
5. Drash AL. Diabetes mellitus in the child and adolescent. In: Galloway JA, Potvin JH, Shuman CR, eds. *Diabetes mellitus,* 9th ed. Indianapolis: Eli Lilly, 1988;200–212.
6. LaPorte RE, Tajima N, Akerblom HR, et al. Geographic differences in the risk of insulin dependent diabetes mellitus: the importance of registries. *Diabetes Care* 1985;8(suppl):101–107.
7. Diabetes Epidemiology Research International Group. Geographic patterns of childhood insulin dependent diabetes mellitus. *Diabetes* 1988;37:1113–1119.
8. LaPorte RE, Fishbein HA, Kuller LH, et al. The Pittsburgh insulin-dependent (IDDM) registry: the incidence of insulin-dependent diabetes mellitus in Allegheny County, Pennsylvania (1965–1976). *Diabetes* 1981;30:279–284.
9. Adams SF. Seasonal variation in the onset of acute diabetes: age and sex factors in 1000 diabetic patients. *Arch Intern Med* 1926;37:861–864.
10. Fleegler FM, Rogers KD, Drash AL, et al. Age, sex and seasonal onset of juvenile diabetes in different geographical areas. *Pediatrics* 1979;63:374–379.
11. Siemiatycki J, Colle E, Aubert D, Campbell S, Belmonti MM. The distribution of type I (insulin-dependent) diabetes mellitus by age, sex, secular trend, seasonality, time clusters and space time clusters: evidence from Montreal, (1971–1983). *Am J Epidemiol* 1986;124:546–560.
12. Mimura G. Present status and future view of the genetics of diabetes in Japan. In: Mimura G, Baba S, Goto W, Kobberling J, eds. *Clinical genetics of diabetes mellitus.* International Congress Series 597. Amsterdam: Excepta Medica, 1982;13–18.
13. Kitagawa T, Fujita H, Hibi I, Aagenaes O, Laron Z, LaPorte RE, Tajima N, Drash AL. A comparative study of the epidemiology of IDDM between Japan, Norway, Israel and the United States. *Acta Paediatr Jpn* 1984;26:275–281.
14. Siemiatycki J, Colle E, Campbell S, Dewar R, Aubert D, Bellmonti MM. Incidence of IDDM in Montreal by ethnic group and by social class and comparisons with ethnic groups living elsewhere. *Diabetes* 1988;37:1096–1112.
15. Laron Z, Karp M, Modan M. The incidence of insulin dependent diabetes mellitus in Israeli children and adolescents 0–20 years of age: a retrospective study, 1971–1980. *Diabetes Care* 1985; 8(suppl):24–28.
16. Rewers M, LaPorte RE, Walczak M, Dmochowski K, Bojaczynska E. Apparent epidemic of insulin dependent diabetes mellitus in midwestern Poland. *Diabetes* 1987;36:106–113.
17. Patterson CC, Thorogood M, Smith PG, Heasman MA, Clarke JA, Mann JI. Epidemiology of type I (insulin-dependent) diabetes in Scotland, 1968–1976: evidence of an increasing incidence. *Diabetologia* 1983;24:238–243.
18. Mann JI, Thorogood M, Smith PG. Space clustering of juvenile onset diabetes. *Lancet* 1978;1:1369–1370.
19. LaPorte RE, Orchard TJ, Kuller LH, Wagoner DK, Drash AL, Snyder BB, Fishbein HA. The Pittsburgh insulin-dependent diabetes mellitus registry. The relationship of insulin-dependent diabetes mellitus incidence to social class. *Am J Epidemiol* 1981;114:379–384.
20. DeBono J, Johnson C, Betts P. Juvenile diabetes and social class. *Lancet* 1983;1:1113–1114.
21. Tarn AC, Gorsuch AN, Spencer KM, Bottazzo GF, Lister J. Diabetes and social class. *Lancet* 1983;2:631–632.
22. Orchard TJ, Dorman JS, LaPorte RE, Ferrell RE, Drash AL. Host and environmental interactions in diabetes mellitus. *J Chron Dis* 1986;39:979–999.
23. Cahill JF, Jr, McDevitt HO. Insulin dependent diabetes mellitus: the initial lesion. *N Engl J Med* 1981;304:1454–1464.
24. Eisenbarth GS. Type I diabetes mellitus. A chronic autoimmune disease. *N Engl J Med* 1986;314:1360–1368.
25. Nerup J, Platz P, Anderson OO, et al. HLA antigens and diabetes mellitus. *Lancet* 1984;2:864–867.
26. Cavender BE, Wagener DK, Rabin BS, et al. The Pittsburgh insulin dependent diabetes mellitus (IDDM) study: HLA antigens and haplotypes as risk factors for development of IDDM in IDDM patients and their siblings. *J Chron Dis* 1984;37:555–568.
27. Todd JA, Bell JI, McDevitt HO. HLA-DQ beta gene contributes to susceptibility and resistance to insulin dependent diabetes mellitus. *Nature* 1987;329:599–604.
28. Morell PA, Dorman JS, Todd JA, McDevitt HO, Trucco M. Aspartic acid at position 57 of the DQ beta chain protects against type I diabetes. A family study. *Proc Natl Acad Sci USA* 1988;85:8111–8115.
29. Arslanian SA, Becker DJ, Rabin B, et al. Correlates of insulin antibodies in newly diagnosed children with insulin dependent diabetes prior to therapy. *Diabetes* 1985;34:926–930.
30. Bottazzo GF. B cell damage in diabetic insulitis: are we approaching a solution? *Diabetologia* 1984;26:241–249.
31. Bottazzo GF. Death of a beta cell: homicide or suicide? *Diabetic Med* 1986;3:119–130.
32. Drell DW, Notkins AL. Multiple immunological abnormalities in patients with type I (insulin-dependent) diabetes mellitus. *Diabetologia* 1987;30:132–143.
33. Trucco M, Dorman JS. Immunogenetics of insulin dependent diabetes mellitus in humans. *Crit Rev Immunol* 1989;9:201–245.
34. Sultz HA, Hart BA, Zielezny M, et al. Is mumps virus an etiologic factor in juvenile diabetes mellitus? *J Pediatr* 1975;86:654–656.
35. Gamble DR, Taylor KW, Cumming H. Coxsackie viruses in diabetes mellitus. *Br Med J* 1984;4:260–262.
36. Yoon JW, Austin M, Ondera T, et al. Virus induced diabetes mellitus: isolation of a virus from the pancreas of a child with diabetic ketoacidosis. *N Engl J Med* 1979;300:1173–1179.
37. Ginsberg-Fellner F, Witt ME, Fedun B, et al. Diabetes mellitus and autoimmunity in patients with the congenital rubella syndrome. *Rev Infect Dis* 1985;7(suppl):170–176.
38. Pak CY, McArthur RG, Eun HM, Yoon JW. Association of cytomegalovirus infection with autoimmune type I diabetes. *Lancet* 1988;2:1–4.
39. Elliott RB, Martin JM. Dietary protein: a trigger of insulin dependent diabetes in the BB rat? *Diabetologia* 1984;26:297–299.
40. Elliott RB, Reddy SN, Bibby NJ, Kidda K. Dietary prevention of diabetes in the nonobese diabetic mouse. *Diabetologia* 1988;31:62–64.
41. Skordis N, Atchison M, Beppu H, et al. The effect of diet on incidence and time of onset of insulin dependent diabetes in the BB rat. In: *Immunology of diabetes: Sixth International Congress of Immunology.* 1986;717:319–324.
42. Scott FW. Alterations in single diet constituents and diabetes expression in the BB rat. In: *Immunology of diabetes: Sixth International Congress of Immunology.* 1986;717:307–312.
43. Drash AL, Rudert WA, Borquaye S, Wang R, Lieberman I. Effect

of probucol on the development of diabetes mellitus in BB rats. *Am J Cardiol* 1988;62(3):27–31.
44. Negro G, Campea L, DeNovellis A, et al. Breast feeding and insulin-dependent diabetes mellitus. *Lancet* 1985;1:467.
45. Fort P, Lanes R, Dahlem S, et al. Breast feeding and insulin dependent diabetes mellitus in children. *J Am Coll Nutr* 1986;5:435–441.
46. Bateman A, Singh A, Kral T, Solomon S. *Endocr Rev* 1989;10:92–112.
47. Leaverton DR, White CA, MacCormick CR, et al. Parental loss antecedent to childhood diabetes mellitus. *J Am Acad Child Psychiatry* 1980;19:678–698.
48. Drash AL. Insulin dependent diabetes mellitus in children and adolescents: genetics and etiology. *Curr Opinions Pediatr* 1989;1:61–73.
49. Galloway JA. Chemistry and clinical use of insulin. In: Galloway JA, Potvin JH, Shuman CR, eds. *Diabetes mellitus,* 9th ed. Indianapolis: Eli Lilly, 1988;105–138.
50. Baum JD, Kinmonth AL. *Care of the child with diabetes.* London: Churchill Livingstone, 1985.
51. Brink ST. *Pediatric and adolescent diabetes mellitus.* Chicago: Yearbook Medical Publishers, 1987.
52. Schade DS, Santiago JV, Skyler JS, Rizza RA. *Intensive insulin therapy.* Amsterdam: Excerpta Medica, 1983.
53. Becker DJ, Kerensky KM, Transue D, Gutai JP, Nathan S, Wolfson D, Drash A. Current status of pump therapy in childhood. *Acta Pediatr Jpn* 1984;6:347–358.
54. Zinman B. Exercise in the patient with diabetes mellitus. In: Galloway JA, Potvin JH, Shuman CR, eds. *Diabetes mellitus,* 9th ed. Indianapolis: Eli Lilly, 1988;215–224.
55. LaPorte RE, Dorman JS, Tajima N, et al. Pittsburgh insulin-dependent diabetes mellitus morbidity and mortality study: physical activity and diabetic complications. *Pediatrics* 1986;78:1027–1033.
56. Moy CS, LaPorte RE, Dorman J, Songer T, Orchard T, Becker D, Drash A. Physical activity, insulin dependent diabetes mellitus and death. (In press).
57. Wylie-Rossett J, Rifkin H. The history of nutrition and diabetes. In: Jovanovic L, Peterson C, eds. *Nutrition and diabetes.* New York: Alan L. Liss, 1985;1–13.
58. Arky RA. Nutritional management of the diabetic. In: Ellenberg M, Rifkin H, eds. *Diabetes mellitus.* New Hyde Park, NY: Medical Examination Publishing, 1983;539–566.
59. McKenzie M, Korczowski M. Dietary control of diabetes: reality or myth? *South Med J* 1985;78:979–986.
60. American Diabetes Association Task Force on Nutrition. Nutritional recommendations and principles for individuals with diabetes mellitus: 1986. *Diabetes Care* 1987;10:126–132.
61. Diabetes Task Force, American Academy of Pediatrics Committee on Nutrition. In: Brink SJ, ed. Elk Grove Village, IL: American Academy Pediatrics, 1985.
62. Schauberger G, Brinck VC, et al. Exchange of carbohydrates according to their effect on blood glucose. *Diabetes* 1978;26:415–417.
63. Crapo PA, Reaven G, Olefsky J. Post-prandial plasma-glucose and insulin responses to different complex carbohydrates. *Diabetes* 1977;26:1178–1183.
64. Crapo PA, Insel J, Sperling M, Kolterman OG. Serum glucose insulin and glucagon responses to different types of complex carbohydrate in noninsulin-dependent diabetic patients. *Am J Clin Nutr* 1981;34:184–190.
65. Jenkins DJA, Wolever MMS, Jenkins AL. Starchy foods and glycemic index. *Diabetes Care* 1988;11:149–159.
66. Jenkins DJA, Wolever TMS, Taylor RH, et al. Glycemic index of foods: a physiological basis for carbohydrate exchange. *Am J Clin Nutr* 1981;34:262–266.
67. Jenkins DJA, Wolever TMS, Taylor RH, et al. Lack of effect of refining on the glycemic response to cereals. *Diabetes Care* 1981;4:509–513.
68. Jenkins DJA, Wolever TMS, Taylor RH, et al. The glycemic index of foods tested in diabetic patients: a new basis for carbohydrate exchange favoring the use of legumes. *Diabetologia* 1983;24:257–264.
69. Jenkins DJA, Wolever TMS, Taylor RH, et al. Exceptionally low blood glucose response to dried beans: comparison with other carbohydrate foods. *Br Med J* 1980;2:578–560.
70. Jenkins DJA, Taylor RH, Wolever TMS. The diabetic diet: dietary carbohydrate and differences in digestibility. *Diabetologia* 1982;23:477–484.
71. Eastwood MA, Passmore R. Dietary fibre. *Lancet* 1983;2:202–205.
72. Jenkins DJA, Wolever TMS, Leeds AR, et al. Dietary fibres, fibre analogues and glucose tolerance: importance of viscosity. *Br Med J* 1978;1:1392–1394.
73. Morgan LM, Gondler TJ, Tsiolakis D, Marks V, Alberta KGMM. The effect of unabsorbable carbohydrate on gut hormones: modification of postprandial GIP secretion by guar. *Diabetologia* 1979;17:85–89.
74. Jenkins DJA, Wolever TMS, Bacon S, et al. Diabetic diets: high carbohydrate combined with high fibre. *Am J Clin Nutr* 1980;33:1729–1733.
75. Jenkins DJA. Lente carbohydrate: a newer approach to the dietary management of diabetes. *Diabetes Care* 1982;5:634–641.
76. Jenkins DJA, Wolever TMS, Jenkins AL, Taylor RH. Dietary fibre, carbohydrate metabolism and diabetes. *Mol Aspects Med* 1987;9:97–112.
77. Wolever TMS, Jenkins DJA, Vuksan V, Josse RJ, Wong GS, Jenkins AL. Glycemic index of foods in individual subjects. *Diabetes Care* 1990;13:126–132.
78. Kiehm TD, Anderson JW, Ward K. Beneficial effects of a high carbohydrate, high fiber diet in hyperglycemic men. *Am J Clin Nutr* 1976;29:895–899.
79. Anderson JW, Midgley WR, Wedman B. Fiber and diabetes. *Diabetes Care* 1979;2:369–379.
80. Anderson JW, Ward K. High-carbohydrate, high-fiber diets for insulin-treated men with diabetes mellitus. *Am J Clin Nutr* 1979;32:2312–2321.
81. Anderson JW, Ferguson SK, Karounos D, et al. Mineral and vitamin status on high-fiber diets: long term study of diabetic patients. *Diabetes Care* 1980;3:38–40.
82. Kinmonth AL, Angus RM, Jenkins PA, Smith MA, Baum JD. Whole foods and increased dietary fibre improve blood glucose control in diabetic children. *Arch Dis Child* 1982;57(1):87–94.
83. Lindsay AN, Hardy S, Jarrett L, Rallison M. High carbohydrate, high-fiber diet in children with type I diabetes mellitus. *Diabetes Care* 1984;7:63–67.
84. Collier GR, Giudici S, Kalmusky J, et al. Low glycemic index starchy foods improve glucose control and lower serum cholesterol in diabetic children. *Diabetes Nutr Metab* 1988;1:11–19.
85. Weyman-Daum M, Fort P, Recker B, Lanes R, Lifshitz F. Glycemic response in children with insulin-dependent diabetes mellitus after high or low glycemic index breakfast. *Am J Clin Nutr* 1987;46:798–803.
86. Position Statement of the American Diabetes Association. Nutritional recommendations and principles for individuals with diabetes mellitus. *Diabetes Care* 1990;13(suppl 1):18–25.
87. O'Dea K, Nestel PJ, Antonoff L. Physical factors influencing postprandial glucose and insulin responses to starch. *Am J Clin Nutr* 1980;33:760–765.
88. Vaaler S, Hanssen K, Aagenaes O. The effect of cooking upon the blood glucose response to ingested carrots and potatoes. *Diabetes Care* 1984;7:221–223.
89. O'Dea K, Snow P, Nestel P. Rate of starch hydrolysis in vitro as a predictor of metabolic responses to complex carbohydrate in vivo.
90. Wiseman MJ, Bognetti E, Dodds R, Keen H, Viberti GC. Changes in renal function in response to protein restricted diet in Type I (insulin dependent) diabetic patients. *Diabetologia* 1987;30:154–159.
91. Brodsy IG, Robbins DC. Safety of low protein diets: where's the beef? *Diabetes Care* 1989;12:435–437.
92. Drash AL. Hyperlipidemia and the control of diabetes mellitus. *Am J Dis Child* 1976;130:1057–1058.
93. Mann JI, Hugson WG, Holman RR, et al. Serum lipids in treated diabetic children and their families. *Clin Endocr* 1978;8:27–33.

94. Chase HP, Glasgow AM. Juvenile diabetes mellitus and serum lipids and lipoprotein levels. *Am J Dis Child* 1976;30:113–117.
95. Kenien A, Hengstenberg F, Drash AL. Lipids in children and adolescents with juvenile diabetes mellitus. *Diabetes* 1977;26(suppl):365.
96. Kauffmann RL, Assal JP, Soeldner JS, et al. Plasma lipid levels in diabetic children. *Diabetes* 1975;24:672–679.
97. Blanc MH, Ganda OP, Gleason RE, et al. Improvement of lipid status in diabetic boys: the 1971 and 1979 Joslin camp lipid levels. *Diabetes Care* 1983;6:64–66.
98. Wylie-Rosett J, Engel S, guest eds. Hyperlipidemia and diabetes: the controversy continues. *Diabetes Spectrum* 1989;2:358–376.
99. Nuttall FQ, Hollenbeck CB, eds. Nutrition and metabolism: symposium highlights. Part 1. *Diabetes Spectrum* 1989;2:123–131.
100. Borkman M, Chisolm DJ, Furler SM, Storlien LH, Kraegen EW, Simmons LA, Chesterman CN. Effects of fish oil supplementation on glucose and lipid metabolism in NIDDM. *Diabetes* 1989;38:1314–1319.
101. Hollenbeck C, Coulston AM, Reaven GM. Effects of sucrose on carbohydrate and lipid metabolism in NIDDM patients. *Diabetes Care* 1989;12:62–66.
102. Bierman EL, Brunzell JD. Diet low in saturated fat and cholesterol for diabetes. *Diabetes Care* 1989;12:162–163.
103. Friday KE, Childs MT, Tsunehara CH, Fujimoto WY, Bierman EL, Ensing JW. Elevated plasma glucose and lowered triglyceride levels with omega-3 fatty acid supplementation in type II diabetes. *Diabetes Care* 1989;12:276–281.
104. Sorisky A, Robbins DC. Fish oil and diabetes: the net effect. *Diabetes Care* 1989;12:302–304.
105. Garg A, Grundy SM. Management of dyslipidemia in NIDDM. *Diabetes Care* 1990;13:153–169.
106. Bantle JP, Laine DC, Thomas W. Metabolic effects of dietary fructose and sucrose in type I and II diabetic subjects. *JAMA* 1986;256:3241–3246.
107. Brunzell JD. Use of fructose, xylitol or sorbitol as a sweetener in diabetes mellitus. *Diabetes Care* 1978;1:223–230.
108. Akerblom HK, Siltaren I, Kallio AK. Does dietary fructose affect the control of diabetes in children? *Acta Med Scand* 1972;542:195.
109. Forster M. Comparative metabolism of xylitol, sorbitol, fructose. In: Sipple HL, McNutt KW, eds. *Sugar and nutrition.* New York: Academic Press, 1975;259–280.
110. Bantle J. Clinical aspects of sucrose and fructose metabolism. *Diabetes Care* 1989;12:56–61.
111. Forlani G, Galuppi V, Cantacorsi G, Braione AF, Giangiulio S, Ciavarella A, Vannini P. Hyperglycemic effect of sucrose ingestion in IDDM patients controlled by artificial pancreas. *Diabetes Care* 1989;12:296–297.
112. Wise JW, Keim JS, Huisinga JL, Willmann PA. Effect of sucrose containing snacks on blood glucose control. *Diabetes Care* 1989;12:423–426.
113. Halfon P, Belkhadir J, Slama G. Correlation between amount of carbohydrate in mixed meals and insulin delivery by artificial pancreas in seven IDDM subjects. *Diabetes Care* 1989;12:427–429.
114. Anderson JW, Story LJ, Zettwoch NC, Gustafson NJ, Jefferson BS. Metabolic effects of fructose supplementation in diabetic patients. *Diabetes Care* 1989;12:337–344.
115. Heller A, Jovanovic L. Artificial sweeteners: safety and utility in the treatment of diabetes mellitus. In: Jovanovic L, Peterson C, eds. *Nutrition and diabetes.* New York: Alan L. Liss, 1985;37–49.
116. Council on Scientific Affairs. Aspartame: review of safety issues. *JAMA* 1985;254:400–402.
117. Spraul M, Chantelau E, Schonbach AM, Berger M. Glycemic effects of beer in IDDM patients: studies with constant insulin delivery. *Diabetes Care* 1988;11:659–661.
118. Colling S. Metabolism of cyclamate and its conversion to cyclohexylamine. *Diabetes Care* 1989;12:50–55.
119. Filer LJ Jr, Stegink LD. Aspartame metabolism in normal adults, phenyl ketonuric heterozygotes and diabetic subjects. *Diabetes Care* 1989;12:67–74.
120. Miller SA, Frattali VP. Saccharin. *Diabetes Care* 1989;12:75–80.
121. DeFranzo RA. The effect of insulin on renal sodium metabolism. *Diabetologia* 1981;21:165–171.
122. Ingelfinger JR. Salt intake in infancy and childhood. Does it have a role in adult hypertension? In: *Proceedings from a symposium,* Anaheim, California, 13 Nov. 1983. New York: Biomed Inform, 1984;1–32.
123. Mooradian AD, Morley JE. Micronutrient status in diabetes mellitus. *Am J Clin Nutr* 1987;45:877–895.
124. Hagglof B, Hallmans G, Holmgren G, Ludvigsson J, Falkmer S. Prospective and retrospective studies of zinc concentrations in serum, blood clots, hair and urine in young patients with insulin-dependent diabetes mellitus. *Acta Endocr* 1983;102:88–95.
125. Ewald U, Gebre-Medhin M, Tuvemo T. Hypomagnesemia in diabetic children. *Acta Paediatr Scand* 1983;72:367–371.
126. Canfield WK, Hambridge KM, Johnson LK. Zinc nutritive in type I diabetes mellitus: relationship to growth measures and metabolic control. *J Pediatr Gastroenterol Nutr* 1984;3:577–584.
127. Gebre-Medhin M, Kylberg E, Ewald U, Tuvemo T. Dietary intake: trace elements and serum protein status in young diabetics. *Acta Paediatr Scand* 1985;320:38–43.
128. Hambidge KM, Rodgerson DO, O'Brien D. Concentration of chromium in the hair of normal children and children with juvenile diabetes mellitus. *Diabetes* 1968;17:517–519.
129. Gebre-Medhin M, Ewald U, Plantin L, Tuvemo T. Elevated serum selenuim in diabetic children. *Acta Paediatr Scand* 1984;73:109–114.
130. McNair P, Christiansen C, Masbad S, et al. Hypomagnesemia: a risk factor in diabetic retinopathy. *Diabetes* 1978;27:1075–1077.
131. Drash AL, Becker DJ. Behavioral issues in patients with diabetes mellitus. In: Rifkin H, Porte D, eds. *Diabetes mellitus,* 4th ed. New York: Elsevier, 1989;922–934.
132. Kovacs M, Feinberg TL, Paulauskas S, Finkelstein R, Pollock M, Crouse-Novak M. Initial coping responses and psychosocial characteristics of children with insulin dependent diabetes mellitus. *J Pediatr* 1985;8:568–575.
133. Kovacs M, Brent D, Steinberg TF, Paulauskas S, Reid J. Children's self reports of psychologic adjustment in coping strategies during first year of insulin dependent diabetes mellitus. *Diabetes Care* 1986;9:472–479.
134. Adin I, Nelkin L. Juvenile diabetes with anorexia nervosa. *Harefuah* 1978;94:326–327.
135. O'Gorman EC, Eyre DG. A case of anorexia nervosa and diabetes mellitus. *Br J Psychiatry* 1980;137:103.
136. Roland JM, Bhanji A. Anorexia nervosa occurring in patients with diabetes mellitus. *Postgrad Med J* 1982;58:354–356.
137. Hudson JI, Wentworth SM, Hudson MS, Pope HG. Prevalence of anorexia nervosa and bulimia among young diabetic women. *J Clin Psychiatry* 1985;46:88–89.
138. Rodin GM, Danneman D, Johnson LE, Kenshole A, Garfinkel P. Anorexia nervosa and bulimia in female adolescents with insulin dependent diabetes mellitus: a systemic study. *J Psychiatr Res* 1985;19:381–384.
139. Hillard JR, Hillard PJ. Bulimia, anorexia and diabetes. Deadly combination. *Psychiatr Clin North Am* 1984;7:367–379.
140. Nielsen S, Berner H, Kabel M. Anorexia nervosa/bulimia in diabetes mellitus: a review and a presentation of 5 cases. *Acta Psychiatr Scand* 1987;75:464–479.
141. Rosmark B, Berne C, Holngren S, Lago C, Renholm G, Sohlberg S. Eating disorders in patients with insulin dependent diabetes mellitus. *J Clin Psychiatry* 1986;47:547–550.
142. Wing RR, Nowalk MP, Marcus MD, Koeske R, Finegold DN. Subclinical eating disorders and glycemic control in adolescents with type I diabetes. *Diabetes Care* 1986;9:162–167.
143. Stancin T, Link DL, Reuter JM. Binge eating and purging in young women with IDDM. *Diabetes Care* 1989;12:601–603.
144. Tattersall RB. Brittle diabetes. *Clin Endocrinol Metab* 1977;6:403–419.
145. Santiago JV. Another facet of brittle diabetes. *JAMA* 1986;256:3263–3264.
146. Schade DS, Drumm DA, Duckworth WC, Eaton RP. The etiology of incapacitating brittle diabetes. *Diabetes Care* 1985;8:12–20.
147. Schade DS, Eaton RP, Drumm DA, Duckworth WC. A clinical

algorithm to determine the etiology of brittle diabetes. *Diabetes Care* 1985;8:5–11.
148. Rizza RA, Zimmerman BR, Service FJ. Brittle diabetes. *Diabetes Care* 1985;8:93–96.
149. Tattersall RB. Brittle diabetes. *Br Med J* 1985;291:555–556.
150. White K, Kolman ML, Wexler P, Polin G, Winter RJ. Unstable diabetes in unstable families: a psychosocial evaluation of diabetic children with recurrent ketoacidosis. *Pediatrics* 1984;73:749–755.
151. Nathan SW. Psychological aspects of recurrent diabetic ketoacidosis in preadolescent boys. *Am J Psychother* 1985;39:193–205.
152. Chapman J, Wright AD, Nattrass M, Fitzgerald MG. Recurrent diabetic ketoacidosis. *Diabetic Med* 1988;5:659–661.
153. Orr DP, Eccles T, Lawlor R, Golden M. Surreptitious insulin administration in adolescents with insulin dependent diabetes mellitus. *JAMA* 1986;256:3227–3230.
154. Norris JM, Dorman JS, Orchard TJ, Becker DJ, Ohki Y, Ellis D, Doft BH, Lobes LA, LaPorte RE, Drash AL. Contribution of diabetes duration before puberty to development of microvascular complications in IDDM subjects. *Diabetes Care* 1989;12(10):686–693.
155. Becker DJ, Drash AL. Nutrition in the child and adolescent with insulin dependent diabetes mellitus. In: Lebenthal E, ed. *Textbook of gastroenterology and nutrition in infancy,* 2nd ed. New York: Raven Press, 1989;677–688.
156. American Diabetes Association and American Dietetic Association. *A guide for professionals: the effective application of exchange lists for meal planning.* New York: American Diabetes Association, 1977;17.
157. Jenkins DJA. The glycemic response to carbohydrate foods. *Lancet* 1984;2:388–391.
158. American Diabetes Association. Fiber and the patient with diabetes mellitus. 1986 supplement to nutritional recommendation and principles for individuals with diabetes mellitus.
159. Franz MJ. *Diabetes and exercise.* Wayzota, MN: Diabetes Center, 1988.
160. Franz MJ, Joynes JO. *Diabetes and brief illness.* Wayzota, MN: Diabetes Center, 1987.

CHAPTER 28

Nutritional Considerations in the Treatment of Acute and Chronic Diarrhea

Shimon Reif and Emanuel Lebenthal

Diarrhea is one of the major causes of infant morbidity and mortality worldwide. In recent years, significant advances have been made in the understanding of its pathophysiology and, consequently, its treatment. Analysis of the absorptive and secretory functions of the intestine has provided insight into the mechanism of diarrhea, with implications for fluid and electrolyte management during acute episodes. Furthermore, understanding specific absorption impairments, and specific nutrient, vitamin, and trace element requirements when diarrhea is accompanied by mucosal damage has led to the design of improved enteral formulas and parenteral solutions. New data about intestinal cell metabolism and luminal energy requirements have also promoted the use of specific nutrient sources. These advances have enhanced the outlook for millions of infants, especially in developing countries.

It is well accepted that diarrhea of infancy is associated with malnutrition and is primarily a nutritional disease. Thus, the main objective of treatment is immediate and adequate nutritional support. Appropriate nutrient supply during the acute stage can also prevent progression to the protracted diarrhea of infancy. Actual management, however, depends on whether the diarrhea is acute or chronic.

This chapter outlines the recent developments in the pathophysiology of diarrhea and formulates a rationale for nutritional therapy. Acute and chronic diarrhea are presented separately and the following topics are discussed: (a) the advantages and future potential of the super–oral rehydration solution (ORS), (b) the use of short polymers of glucose as the ideal carbohydrate source, (c) the need for specific nutrients such as carnitine and nucleotides, and (d) the need for intraluminal nutrition for the specific energy requirements of the enterocytes and colonocytes.

ACUTE DIARRHEA

Etiology

Infection is the major cause of acute diarrhea. The most common pathogens are listed in Table 1. Despite improved microbiological techniques, specific organisms can be detected in only 70% of the cases (1,2). The remaining 30% are attributed to a wide range of unrecognized organisms (3).

Human rotavirus (HRV) is the most common and the most studied viral enteropathogen (4,5). It mainly affects infants younger than 2 years of age and is usually sporadic. Vomiting and mild fever often precede the diarrhea. The disease can vary from an asymptomatic to a severe form with water and electrolyte loss leading to mucosal injury. HRV infection can be prolonged and even fatal. Diagnosis within 24 hr can be done by using the enzyme-linked immunosorbent assay (ELISA) test kit known as Rotazyme (6).

Like HRV, Norwalk virus seems to invade the villus epithelium of the small intestine (7,8). However, it is a milder disease, more often affecting older children, and is usually epidemic (9).

Escherichia coli is a major cause of infant diarrhea. It is classified into five groups (enteropathogenic, enterotoxigenic, enteroinvasive, enteroadherent, and enterohemorrhagic) (10), according to the mechanism by which the pathogens cause the diarrhea (Table 2).

S. Reif: Department of Pediatrics, Tel Aviv University, Tel Aviv, Israel.
E. Lebenthal: Department of Pediatrics, International Institute for Infant Nutrition and Gastrointestinal Disease, Hahnemann University Hospital, Philadelphia, Pennsylvania 19102.

TABLE 1. *The most common human enteric pathogens*

Viral agents
  Human rotavirus
  Small round virus (SRV)
    Norwalk
    Taunton
    Morin County
    Snow Mountain
    Astrovirus
    Cockle
    Wollan
    Ditchins
  Enteric adenoviruses
  Coronaviruses
Bacterial pathogens
  Escherichia coli
  Campylobacter
  Salmonella
  Shigella
  Vibrio cholera
  Yersinia enterocolitica
  Clostridium difficile
Parasitic pathogens
  Protozoa
    Giardia lamblia
    Cryptosporidium
    Entamoeba histolytica
    Balantidium coli
  Helminthic
    Nematodes
      Ancylostoma duodenale
      Strongyloides stercoralis
      Necator americanus
      Trichuris trichiura
    Trematodes
      Schistosoma
    Cestodes
      Taenia solium
      Taenia saginata
      Diphyllobothrium latum

Other bacteria that cause acute diarrhea include *Shigella, Salmonella, Campylobacter jejuni, Yersinia enterocolitica,* and *Clostridium difficle.* Their prevalence and importance in causing diarrhea vary geographically.

The most common parasite causing acute diarrhea is *Giardia lamblia* (11). However, *Cryptosporidium,* a common pathogen in the compromised immune system (12, 13), has recently been identified in day-care centers (14).

Food poisoning occurs by contamination of food with bacteria such as *Salmonella* or by bacterial toxins from such pathogens as enterotoxigenic *Staphylococcus.* Another mechanism may be the ingestion of poisonous foods such as mushrooms.

In infants, nonenteric infections such as pneumonia and otitis media are commonly accompanied by diarrhea.

TABLE 2. *Pathogenic mechanisms*

Colonization
  Adherence to bowel structures
  Pili
  Flagellar adhesions
  Other adhesions
Motility
  Penetration of mucous gel
  Chemotaxis
Toxin production
  Cytotoxins
  Enterotoxins
  Invasiveness

Pathogenesis of Acute Diarrhea

Diarrhea results when the net intestinal fecal loss of fluid and salt exceeds the absorbed amount. There are at least five forms of diarrhea.

1. *Toxigenic diarrhea:* Toxins from bacteria, like enterotoxigenic *E. coli* or *Vibrio cholerae,* bind to specific receptors. Labile toxin (LT) raises the level of cyclic guanosine monophosphate (cGMP) in the intestinal mucosa, whereas stable toxin (ST) increases the adenasine 3':5'-cyclic monophosphate (cAMP). However, eventually both toxins block the absorption of Na^+ and Cl^- ions into the villous enterocytes. At the same time, LT and, to a lesser degree, ST, induce the secretion of Cl^- and HCO_3^- ions by crypt cells (15).

2. *Osmotic diarrhea:* Characterized by a positive osmotic gap of the stool: $(Na^+ + K^+) \times 2$ is less than the osmolality of the fecal fluid. Clinically, osmotic diarrhea is distinguished by the fact that the diarrhea diminishes when the patient fasts or stops eating the poorly ingested solute (16).

3. *Secretory diarrhea:* Under normal physiologic conditions, the absorption rate of small intestinal cells is greater than the secretion rate (17). The net absorption process can be reduced in two ways: (a) by inhibition of absorption, and (b) by stimulation of secretion. In reality, most episodes of diarrhea result from a combination of these two mechanisms.

There are three major characteristics of secretory diarrhea. First, in contrast to osmotic diarrhea, there is no positive osmotic gap and the stool osmolality is equal to the ionic constituents. The equation is

$$(Na^+ + K^+) \times 2 = \text{stool osmolality}.$$

Second, food ingestion does not usually affect the stool volume. Third, the stool is watery without blood or pus and is characterized by very high volume and ion output (Table 3) (18). Accurate diagnosis of secretory diarrhea can be done by intestinal perfusion studies, a method that is not practical for clinical purposes.

4. *Invasive diarrhea:* Caused by direct mucosal damage by the invasive organism (19), this diarrhea is similar

TABLE 3. *Differential diagnosis of osmotic and secretory diarrhea*

Stools	Osmotic diarrhea	Secretory diarrhea
Electrolytes	Na < 70 mEq/l	Na > 70 mEq/l
Osmolality	>(Na$^+$ + K$^+$) × 2	=(Na$^+$ + K$^+$) × 2
pH	<5	>6
Reducing substances	Positive	Negative
Volume	<200 ml/day	>200 ml/day

to colitis and is usually associated with blood and mucous. The common organisms are *Shigella, Salmonella, Campylobacter,* and invasive type *E. coli.* Human rotavirus (HRV) also invades the small intestinal epithelium. This organism disturbs ion transport, not through an enterotoxin, but by affecting the normal renewal process of the small bowel epithelium (20,21). Thus, HRV diarrhea is caused not so much by the initial viral damage as by the later repair process. The villi become populated with less mature cells, leading to a possible deficiency of disaccharidases such as lactase. The brush border enzyme deficiency causes impaired carbohydrate absorption. The unabsorbed sugar is metabolized by the colonic bacteria first to monosaccharides and then to short-chain fatty acids and finally to CO_2, H_2, and CH_4. These breakdown products increase the intestinal osmotic load and cause diarrhea (22).

5. *Motility disorders:* Hypermotility can cause diarrhea by reduction of contact time between intestinal mucosa and its contents, despite normal absorption function of the cell. Hypermotility can result from endocrinopathy (hyperthyroidism) or tumor secretion hormones such as vasoactive intestinal polypeptide (VIP).

Hypomotility or dysmotility can be primary, as in idiopathic intestinal pseudo-obstruction syndrome (IIPOS). It can also be secondary to neuronal disorders such as diabetes neuropathy (23) or muscle disorders like scleroderma. Finally, one must remember that in a vast majority of the cases, diarrhea is not caused by a single mechanism but rather by a combination of several factors.

Treatment

Management of acute diarrhea has two objectives. The first is restoration and maintenance of adequate hydration and electrolyte balance. The second is providing nutrition adequate to prevent protracted diarrhea and malnutrition, particularly in early infancy and in the malnourished child. In about 30% of patients no specific cause can be found (24,25). Moreover, most of the isolated pathogenic organisms are viral (26). The majority of the bacterial pathogens are self-limiting. In some cases, antimicrobial therapy prolongs the infection duration. Antibiotics should be used only in young infants, in the immunocompromised, or when a systemic bacteremia is suspected. The specific persisting enteric infections that do need antibiotic therapy include *Yersinia, Campylobacter,* and *Giardia.* An important point is that antibiotic therapy has no effect on fluid transport nor on nutritional rehabilitation.

Oral Rehydration Solution (ORS)

Management of diarrhea has improved with recognition of the pathophysiologic events associated with it. Intravenous therapy is now indicated only when severe dehydration, shock, or severe electrolyte imbalance exists. Oral rehydration therapy, on the other hand, has become a universally practical and beneficial treatment of acute diarrhea (27).

The rationale for the use of ORS is based on recognition of the intestinal transport function during diarrhea. First, because during diarrhea, the normal mechanism for water and sodium absorption is impaired, replacement of water or saline fluids alone will only lead to more diarrhea. On the other hand, the sodium-glucose-coupled transport generally remains intact. This mechanism stimulates water transport by solvent drag.

The basic components of ORS are glucose and electrolytes in an isotonic solution (28–30). Optimal glucose concentration balances caloric adequacy with the acute stage, the glucose functions more as a sodium absorption facilitator than as a caloric supplier; it is, therefore, advantageous to keep equimolar ratios of sodium and glucose. In the World Health Organization (WHO) formula the glucose concentration is 2%. This is sufficient to prevent hypoglycemia, while still preventing the induction of an osmotic diarrhea secondary to the osmotic load (31).

Determining the ideal sodium concentration is more difficult. Original WHO recommendations were for a sodium concentration of 90 mEq/l, essentially for treatment of cholera. Many physicians feared iatrogenic hypernatremia if such a high concentration were used in developed countries where cholera is not a concern and the stool sodium concentration in diarrheal illness is much lower (32). Sodium concentration in ORS for developed countries is, therefore, generally much less, about 30 to 60 mEq/l (33–36). However, in many studies, the WHO solution (90 mEq/l Na$^+$) has been shown to be safe and effective, with a smaller incidence of hypernatremia than expected (27–29,37–39). One exception occurs in neonates up to 2 months of age whose kidneys have less capacity to excrete excess amounts of fluid and salt. In this population, strictly supervised administration of a solution containing sodium, 60 mmol/l, seems much more appropriate (40). It is important to recognize that the ORS serves only the function of rehydration; it does not alter the disease course and it may even increase fecal loss. The composition of some solutions is shown in Table 4.

Finally, it must be emphasized that most of the sweet "clear liquid" solutions are disadvantageous because they contain a high carbohydrate and low sodium content (Table 5).

Super–ORS

Recent studies demonstrate the advantage of short glucose polymers as the carbohydrate source in ORS (41–42). Our studies have shown that glucose absorption is optimized when the source is short polymers of glucose (G2-G9) made from a hydrolysate of rice (43). In comparison to D-glucose solution, these polymers provide a higher caloric density and increased moles of glucose, yet present a smaller osmotic load. In addition, the high resistance of glucoamylase activity, the key enzyme for short polymers of glucose absorption, in comparison to other intestinal disaccharidases during intestinal mucosal injury, is further rationale for their use (44). It is interesting that many developing countries have traditionally used rice water as a rehydration solution; only recently has "science" documented its biological advantage (45–47).

Organic nonelectrolytes have also been introduced in an attempt to improve the ORS composition. Alanine, for example, stimulated sodium-coupled water absorption independent of glucose (48–50). In contrast, glycine was less effective in water absorption and caused osmotic diarrhea and diuresis (51,52). In animal models it has been shown that the addition of 15 or 30 mM alanine led to a greater absorption of water and sodium (50,53). This effect was not only relevant to secretory diarrhea but was also found in a model of cathartic diarrhea. Furthermore, optimal water absorption was achieved when the alanine sodium molar ratio was 1:1, similar to the glucose sodium ratio. Encouraging preliminary data have been obtained from Bangladesh, where adult patients with cholera were treated with alanine 90 mM/l (8 gm/l) ORS.

Recently, it was found that acute diarrhea may be associated with zinc deficiency and that zinc supplementation decreased the diarrheal intensity and duration (54,55). This may open a new area for a "super–ORS" that may include trace elements such as zinc.

In addition, improving the taste of the solutions may encourage increased intake in infants.

Nutritional Therapy

The objective of the recovery stage of diarrhea, after the fluid and electrolyte imbalance has been corrected, is to provide adequate and balanced nutrients. Opinions differ, however, concerning optimal nutritional management. "Bowel rest" versus "early feeding" is still controversial (56–60). Recent studies support the continuation of the infant's regular feeding during acute diarrhea. These studies suggest that the early reintroduction of full feeding after rehydration results in better weight gain without causing prolongation of the diarrhea (56,61–64). Other studies have shown that prolonged bowel rest is associated with increased intestinal permeability, possibly allowing for increased absorption of allergens (65–67). We believe that continuing feeding with regular diet applies only to mild cases. We adhere to the American Academy of Pediatrics' recommendation that formula feeding "should be reintroduced gradually by starting with dilute mixtures" (68). Considerations in this approach include the child's age, the severity of the disease, and the previous diet. In general, refeeding can start gradually after 24 hr of only fluid intake, i.e., "bowel rest" (69). This approach attempts to restore the child's nutritional status and promotes repair of the intestinal mucosa.

An exception, however, is made for nursing infants, who should continue their regular feedings. Although human milk contains high amounts of lactose, it usually is fairly well tolerated. Human milk is advantageous because it has anti-infective factors such as lactoferrin, lysozyme, and secretory IgA (71–73). It also includes several known growth factors: epithelial growth factor (EGF), nerve growth factor (NGF), transforming growth factor (TGF) (74,75), and insulin-like growth factor (76). These factors may have a role in mucosal repair by their trophic effect (77,78). Surprisingly, studies by Shulman et al. (79) indicate that human milk had no effect on the functional rate of recovery of the small intestinal mu-

TABLE 5. Composition of "clear liquid" solutions[a]

	Na^+	K^+	CHO (%)
Pepsi Cola	1–2	0.1	10.9
Coca Cola	1–2	0.1	10
Ginger ale	2	0.6	9.2
Jell-O	24–27	1.3	16
Club soda	12	0.6	—
Root beer	6	0.6	10.6
Popsicles	1–4	0.5	18

[a] Concentrations are in mEq/l.

TABLE 4. Composition of oral electrolyte solutions[a]

	Na^+	K^+	Cl^-	Other anion	CHO (%)
WHO solution	90	20	80	30	2
Gastrolyte	90	20	80	30	2
Pedialyte	45	20	35	30	2.5
Rehydralyte	75	20	65	30	2.5
Lytren	50	25	45	30	2.0
Infalyte	50	20	40	30	2.0
Gatorade	23	3	17	—	5.9

WHO, World Health Organization.
[a] Concentrations are in mEq/l.

cosa as measured by water and glucose absorptive capacity and disaccharidase activities.

In contrast to human milk, cow's milk and lactose-containing formulas may not be as well tolerated during and immediately following an acute diarrheal episode because their high lactose content might exceed the reduced intestinal lactase capacity (80–86). Another major disadvantage of cow's milk is its possibly antigenic hyperallergenic capacity (87). Walker-Smith (88,89) demonstrated increased absorption of these hyperallergenic proteins during and after gastroenteritis. This may be a crucial mechanism for postenteritis diarrhea. Although acidified milk has been recommended for its inhibition of enteropathogenic growth, it does not effect milk digestion (90). It seems appropriate in non–breast-fed infants with moderate to severe diarrhea to avoid the use of lactose-containing milk for several days. Milk feedings should then be resumed gradually starting with dilute milk. Soy-based formula is not recommended because of reports of sensitivity to soy protein in the intestinal mucosa of young infants recovering from acute gastroenteritis (91–95). Furthermore, as with cow's milk, feeding soy protein in the postgastroenteritis period might increase the risk of developing soy protein enteropathy. A semi-elemental diet in this period has no advantage over a lactose-free diet, is more expensive, and may be continued beyond actual need by parents (96,97).

Infants and children already on solid foods are easier to handle. Food with a high content of disaccharides and monosaccharides (fruits, sweets) should be withheld or limited in the convalescent period. On the other hand, foods with starch carbohydrates (cereal, rice, noodles, bananas, and potatoes) should be encouraged.

In conclusion, during acute diarrhea, there is possible damage to the intestinal mucosa particularly in young and/or malnourished infants, and with specific pathogens. Generally infants require only 24 hr of rehydration before returning to their previous diets. In specific patients, however, the extent of intestinal mucosal damage and enzyme loss are key factors. Patients with more severe mucosal damage should either return more gradually to a regular diet or be treated more aggressively with semi-elemental formulas. Unfortunately, the optimal dietary approach for the postenteritis period is not yet well established. The early use of a balanced and appropriate diet in the acute stage of diarrhea should restore the child's nutritional state and enhance mucosal repair. This approach will prevent further mucosal injury that could lead to chronic diarrhea and malabsorption.

CHRONIC DIARRHEA

Etiology

Chronic or protracted diarrhea of infancy has been defined as an illness with excessive stool water lasting at least 2 weeks (98). Chronic diarrhea with prolonged mucosal injury is always associated with malabsorption. Toddler's diarrhea (chronic nonspecific diarrhea), although the most common cause of prolonged diarrhea, is not associated with malabsorption and is benign and transient.

Chronic diarrhea accompanied by malabsorption has an extensive list of specific etiologies (Table 6). The majority of cases, however, are secondary to an acute episode of diarrhea with mucosal injury. The process that eventually results in protracted diarrhea includes malabsorption of specific nutrients, decreased availability of enteric hormones, bile acid malabsorption, increased absorption of native foreign proteins, and bacterial overgrowth (99,100). This self-perpetuating cycle can be broken only by appropriate nutritional rehabilitation. The objective is to supply nutrients that can be absorbed by the damaged intestine and to restore the mucosa.

An initial, extensive workup should include a small bowel biopsy. This workup should determine etiology and assess the enzymes that are affected and the degree of mucosal injury. Determining the etiology aids in designing an effective nutritional therapy [e.g., gluten-free diet in gluten-sensitive enteropathy, or medium-chain triglycerides (MCT) supplement in abetalipoproteinemia and intestinal lymphangiectasia].

If an enteropathy is diagnosed, careful morphologic analysis should be done. For example, a patchy enteropathy with an increase in intraepithelial lymphocyte and depression of disaccharidase activity is consistent with cow's milk–sensitive enteropathy (101,102). More uniform mucosal damage with very low disaccharidase activity is suggestive of secondary mucosal injury (44,103). Of course, when diarrhea occurs with severe malnutrition, the nutritional treatment begins before the diagnostic procedures (104).

Most infants with chronic diarrhea exhibit small intestinal mucosal injury reflective of both functional and anatomic disruption of the brush border membrane (105–108). Formulas consisting of complex carbohydrates, fats, and proteins require intact absorptive epithelial cells. Thus, the specific aim of the nutritional therapy is to provide a high caloric, elemental, isosmolar, and hypoallergenic formula that is easily absorbed and minimally dependent on digestive enzymes and active transport mechanisms. The specially designed formulas contain amino acids, short-chain polypeptides, glucose, short-chain glucose polymers, medium-chain triglycerides, and unsaturated fatty acids. These nutrient components require minimal intraluminal and mucosal surface digestion.

Initial feedings for a child with chronic diarrhea should consist of diluted cow's milk or cow's milk–based formula. If diarrhea continues, soy-based formula is introduced. If diarrhea still does not abate, a semi-elemental (Pregestimil, Nutramigen) or elemental diet (Vivonex) is introduced. Parenteral alimentation is the last resort.

TABLE 6. *Disorders identified with intractable diarrhea of infancy listed by groups according to pathophysiology*

Disorders associated with villous atrophy
    Viral gastroenteritis
    Secondary disaccharidase deficiency
    Secondary monosaccharide malabsorption
    Cow's milk protein enteropathy
    Soy protein enteropathy
    Egg protein enteropathy
    Eosinophilic gastroenteropathy
    Congenital crypt hypoplasia
    Tropical sprue
    Celiac disease
    Dermatitis herpetiformis
    Immunodeficiency syndromes
    Bacterial overgrowth
    Pathogenic *Escherichia coli*
    Giardia lamblia
    Hirschsprung's disease
    Malnutrition
Disorders associated with secretory diarrhea
    Familial chloride diarrhea
    Bacterial toxins
        Escherichia coli
        Vibrio cholerae
    Hormones elaborated by tumors
        VIP-oma
        Zollinger-Ellison syndrome
        Medullary carcinoma of the thyroid
        Basophilic leukemia
        Systemic mastocytosis
    Inflammatory lesions of the colon
    Bile acid–induced secretory diarrhea
Anatomic problems
    Short bowel syndrome
    Hirschsprung's disease
    Gastroschisis
    Malrotation
    Ileal atresia
    Intestinal lymphangiectasia
    Congenital crypt hypoplasia
Metabolic entities
    Acrodermatitis enteropathica
    Abetalipoproteinemia
    Wolman disease
    Hypoparathyroidism
    Hyperthyroidism
    Adrenal insufficiency
Congenital lack of an enzyme or protein carrier in intestine
    Glucose-galactose malabsorption
    Sucrase-isomaltase deficiency
    Primary lactase deficiency
        Developmental
        Congenital
        Adult type
    Enterokinase deficiency
Pancreatic insufficiency
    Cystic fibrosis
    Shwachman-Diamond syndrome
    Congenital lipase deficiency
    Congenital trypsinogen deficiency

Predicting specific formula outcome or duration is difficult. The appropriate modality of treatment depends on the severity of the mucosal injury, the nutritional status of the child, the etiology, the age of the child, and the socioeconomic status of the family. The mucosal function is determined by the histology as well as disaccharidase activities or indirect tests such as the hydrogen breath test, D-xylose, stool pH, and reducing substance assays. Mucosal integrity can be measured by another indirect test, the lactulose/mannitol recovery ratio. This test is currently used for research purposes (109–111).

In healthy infants, the standard humanized formula may be tried first. If diarrhea persists for more than 2 weeks in early infancy, an elemental or semi-elemental diet should be attempted, especially in the face of severe disaccharidase deficiencies and villous atrophy. Multiple formula changes should be avoided. Parenteral nutrition should be instituted only when other methods have failed.

Patients must be monitored carefully for worsening of the diarrhea and failure to gain adequate weight. These indicate a need to reevaluate the nutritional therapy.

Nutrient Malabsorption and Special Requirements

Carbohydrate

During mucosal injury, lactase is the first enzyme to be affected and the last to recover (85,111–114). Infants less than 6 months of age are more prone to secondary lactose malabsorption during mucosal damage (86). In addition, malnourished infants and those with rotavirus infection may have a more severe lactose malabsorption (115–116).

α-Glucosidase activities, such as sucrase, are affected to a lesser degree, unless there is severe mucosal injury and diarrhea (117,118). In contrast to the maximal localization in the proximal small intestine of the disaccharidase activities, glucoamylase is distributed throughout the small intestinal mucosa and tends to be more resistant to injury than the disaccharidases (44). Furthermore, during the first 4 to 6 months of life the key enzyme for starch digestion, pancreatic amylase, is very low and thus the glucoamylase plays the major role in glucose polymers digestion (119–121). This is the rationale for the use of short-chain polymers of glucose (GPs). Evidence from our laboratory suggests that rice GPs are more rapidly hydrolyzed and absorbed than commercially available corn GP in infants with chronic diarrhea (122). These data have important implications in the developing world where chronic diarrhea of infancy is most prevalent, since rice may be the locally available carbohydrate source (123). An *in vitro* study demonstrated better absorption of short-chain rice GP (G2-G9) compared to isocaloric D-glucose. The benefit of using short-chain GP is that it has much less osmolarity for the same calorie content of D-glucose (124). Secondly, GP, due to incorporation of water during hydrolysis, will yield more moles of hexose than the D-glucose solution of the same weight concentration.

Fat

Fat malabsorption associated with chronic diarrhea is due to several factors in addition to mucosal injury, including bile acid deficiency secondary to fecal loss of bile acids (125–127). In short bowel syndrome, for example, fecal loss of unabsorbed bile acids is one of the main mechanisms of fat malabsorption (128). In conditions of pancreatic insufficiency, such as cystic fibrosis, the impairment of fat absorption is caused by lipase deficiency (129). In young infants, physiologic fat malabsorption is a common finding since pancreatic lipase remains low in the first 6 months of life (119). Chronic diarrhea associated with malnutrition, which may result in secondary pancreatic insufficiency, can further reduce lipase activity (130–132).

Medium-chain triglyceride (MCT)—fatty acids vary from 6 to 12 carbons in length—has been shown to be preferable to long-chain triglyceride (LCT) in steatorrhea; MCT is more soluble than LCT, hydrolyzes faster, and does not require bile-acid micelle formation for absorption (133). Finally, the MCT hydrolysis products are absorbed directly into the portal vein instead of the lymphatics, and are oxidized rapidly in the liver (134–136). However, MCT has some disadvantages: poor palatability and, in large doses, cathartic effects (136–138). In comparison with LCT, it has a lower molecular weight and therefore a higher osmolarity. MCT provides 8.3 cal per gram, slightly less than the caloric density of LCT. In addition, MCT has a lower content of some essential fatty acids, especially linoleic and arachidonic acids. Therefore, although MCT is advantageous, especially in conditions with fat malabsorption, it is only recommended in combination with LCT, to prevent essential fatty acid deficiency (usually 60:40 ratio). This can be accomplished by including 1% to 3% of total calories as linoleic acid. A good source is safflower oil, which contains 70% linoleic acid (139). Because pathologic steatorrhea is frequently superimposed on the physiologic steatorrhea of infancy, it is often presumed that infant formulas designed for treatment of protracted diarrhea should maintain a fat content of less than 6 g/kg. We have demonstrated that formula containing 8 g/kg of fat (48% of the calories) including 60% MCT with 20% unsaturated fatty acids was well tolerated and was better absorbed than lower-fat formulas (140). Providing a higher fat semi-elemental diet may be the most appropriate way to supply adequate caloric intake.

Protein

After the initial luminal phase of protein digestion, amino acids and oligopeptides are absorbed through the brush border membrane of the mature epithelial cell. The transport mechanism is characterized by a carrier-mediated process that is not energized by Na^+ or H^+ gradients (141,142). In light of this data and the competitive inhibition of neutral amino acids, it is preferable to add short polypeptides rather than free amino acids.

Allergy to cow's milk protein occurs in 1% to 2% of infants fed with cow's milk or cow's milk–based formula (143–145). Gastrointestinal manifestations vary from diarrhea and vomiting to intestinal blood loss or protein-losing enteropathy with hypoproteinemia and edema (146–150). Despite the availability of immunologic tests including skin tests, antibodies to cow's milk protein and reaginic antigen stimulation test (RAST), the diagnosis is based mainly on a positive challenge test with cow's milk as well as on a favorable response to milk protein elimination (150,151). Because chronic diarrhea produces an increased intestinal permeability to proteins that can cause hypersensitivity to cow's milk or soy protein, exclusion is recommended (89,152–156).

Nucleotides

Nucleotides play a major role in cellular function. They act as precursors of nucleic acid synthesis (DNA and RNA) and are fundamental to cell metabolism [adenosine triphosphate (ATP), nicotinamide-adenine dinucleotide (NAD), and nicotinamide-adenine dinucleotide phosphate (NADP)]. Nucleotides are essential to rapidly growing tissue such as intestinal epithelium and to regenerating tissue that requires the constant formation of DNA and RNA (157–160).

Nucleotides are now considered to be semiessential elements, especially in early life. It is suggested that they modulate the immune system by affecting the lymphocyte proliferation. In nucleotide deficiency states, increased susceptibility to infections has been noted (161–163). The nucleotide abundance in human versus cow's milk (164–166) may promote the bifidobacteria growth in the intestine of breast-fed infants (167,168). Nucleotides have a major effect on lipid metabolism, increasing the high-density/low-density lipoprotein (HDL/LDL) ratio (169). They also play a role in elongation and desaturation of essential fatty acids to long-chain polyunsaturated fatty acids. These functions are important for the structure and function of membrane tissue, for prostaglandin synthesis, and for brain maturation (170–172). Research is needed to determine the potential effects of nucleotide-enriched formulas on mucosal repair and to establish optimum dosages.

Carnitine

Carnitine is a quaternary amine required for the oxidation of long-chain triglycerides, enabling their transfer across the inner mitochondrial membrane (173,174). It is synthesized mainly in the liver and kidney from the essential amino acids lysine and methionine. Its synthesis requires vitamin C and iron as cofactors. It has been shown that prolonged carnitine-free parenteral nutrition can result in low blood and tissue levels of carnitine (175,176). Moreover, although cow's milk formulas have similar or even higher carnitine concentrations than human milk, little or no carnitine is provided in unsupplemented soy formula and in semi-elemental formulas (177,178). Therefore, several companies have supplemented their formulas with L-carnitine. An intravenous preparation of L-carnitine is currently under study.

Vitamins and Trace Elements

Requirements and recommended dietary allowances (RDA) for vitamin and trace elements, discussed in another chapter, may be increased for the child with prolonged diarrhea. Specific deficiencies, such as zinc in patients with acrodermatitis enteropathica, may occur. Evaluation should include a search for clinical signs of vitamin and trace element deficiency, e.g., dermatitis, changes in hair structure, and rickets. Vitamin blood levels can determine both the deficiency and response to treatment.

Iron should not be avoided during the nutritional supplementation of chronic diarrhea (179). Well-controlled studies have found no increase in the prevalence of diarrhea, loose stools, vomiting, or colic with iron fortified formulas or with therapeutic doses of iron.

Zinc, essential for DNA, RNA, and protein synthesis, is important to the rapidly developing intestinal epithelial cell. Animal experiments have shown that intestinal water and sodium absorption is significantly diminished in zinc deficiency. This finding may be related to zinc's role in maintaining membrane integrity (180,181). Chronic diarrhea may well be associated with zinc depletion (182). It has also been suggested that there is zinc deficiency in acute diarrhea and that oral zinc administration shortens the diarrheal duration (54,55). Furthermore, since zinc affects cell division, it can have a potential effect on intestinal mucosal repair.

INTRALUMINAL NUTRITION AND ENERGY

The concept of intraluminal nutrition and organ-specific malnutrition must be considered. It has been proposed that because of a lack of energy, the intestinal mucosa is not able to function normally in its handling of nutrients, water, and electrolytes (183–185). In addition, the exacerbation of diarrhea seen with oral feeding after severe malnutrition may be partly due to the inability of the intestinal mucosa to salvage ions because of a local cellular energy deficit (186). There is, therefore, a simultaneous need for intraluminal energy for metabolism and function. Furthermore, the rapid turnover and constant maturation of the intestinal epithelial cells require substantial energy. Studies have shown that infusing single nutrients into the small bowel lumen while nourishing the animal with total parenteral nutrition results in cell proliferation and mucosal repair. The suggested mechanism is that oral feeding stimulates release of enteric hormones and pancreatobiliary secretions, which act as trophic factors (187–192).

Because of the indirect action of the luminal nutrients, little attention has been paid to the nutrient's sources. It is clear, however, that there are organ-specific nutrients (193). Glutamine is considered to be the main respiratory fuel for the enterocyte (194–196). Furthermore, glutamine may have a direct role on mucosal regeneration, and was found to inhibit bacterial growth (197,198). There is now evidence that in catabolic and stress states, glucagon and glucocorticosteroids accelerate glutamine uptake by the enterocytes (199–201).

In contrast to the enterocyte, short-chain fatty acids are the major energy source of the colonocyte. The colon salvages ions as well as the calories that have been produced from undigested carbohydrates spilling over from the small intestine and converted by bacterial fermentation to short-chain fatty acids. This salvage route may play an important role in carbohydrate malabsorption resulting from small intestinal mucosal injury (202–205). Antibiotic treatment may interfere with this salvage mechanism (206).

Harig et al. (207) recently described the successful treatment of diversion colitis by intraluminal perfusion of the affected segment with short-chain fatty acid. There is clinical evidence supporting the hypothesis that local malnutrition of the intestine mucosa can cause disease that is treatable by specific nutrient repletion (207). Providing mucosal-specific nutrients represents a potential therapeutic modality for the future by supporting intestinal metabolism, structure, and function.

Specific Gastrointestinal Diseases with Nutritional Considerations

Inflammatory Bowel Disease

Chronic diarrhea, malnutrition, and growth failure are common characteristics of inflammatory bowel disease (IBD) and are more common in Crohn's disease than in ulcerative colitis (208–214). Nutritional support can help control disease activity, supply unique nutrients, and/or accelerate normal growth and development (213). Cases must be individually analyzed to determine which of these points needs to be addressed.

Each IBD patient needs an estimate of nutritional status. Appropriate measures include weight, height, bone age, weight-for-height ratio, and a determination of lean body mass (skeletal muscle and viscera). In addition, serum albumin, prealbumin, hemoglobin, red cell indices, folate, vitamin B_{12}, vitamin A, carotene, zinc, calcium, and phosphorus levels must be elevated. Dynamic tests include somatomedin-C, procollagen III, and fibronectin levels in response to nutritional therapy (Table 7).

There are multiple causes for the malnutrition and growth failure in patients with IBD. Anorexia and poor intake are the main factors (213,214). Malabsorption

TABLE 7. *Laboratory monitoring of nutritional status during nutritional therapy*

Hemoglobin
Mean corpuscular volume (MCV)
Albumin
Ferritin and iron
Electrolytes
Calcium
Phosphorus
Magnesium
Zinc
Folate
Vitamin B_{12}
Vitamins A, D, E, and K
Fibronectin

and secondary mucosal inflammation as well as the increased nutrient requirements resulting from the chronic inflammatory process also contribute (215,216). Nutrient deficiencies may include vitamin B_{12}, as in ileitis, or zinc, due to the changes in active transport in the mucosa. Successful nutritional treatment of the child with IBD is dependent, therefore, on the provision of a high-calorie diet with appropriate specific nutrient supplementation. A low-fiber diet is not optimum if it results in a nonbeneficial reduction in caloric intake.

The route of feeding depends on factors such as the severity of the disease and the involved part of the intestine. In Crohn's disease, for example, it should generally be more aggressive (217). During remission, patients may have normal, relatively high-calorie, intake. This may necessitate a high caloric density formula. Some studies have found an elemental diet successful in inducing remission in Crohn's disease (218,219). There is no advantage to an elemental diet over a high calorie and complex formula unless there is extensive disease with mucosal damage accompanied by malabsorption. When oral intake is poor, nasogastric feeding is recommended and can be accomplished by nocturnal infusion. Because of the risk of fistula formation, gastrostomy feeding is not the ideal solution in Crohn's patients.

Several reports demonstrate the effectiveness of total parenteral nutrition in producing remission in pediatric patients with Crohn's disease. Less success has been demonstrated with ulcerative colitis or with Crohn's disease, which is limited to the colon (219–221). Use of total parenteral nutrition (TPN) has also been shown to reduce the dosage of corticosteroids (222). Prolonged use of TPN, however, is needed only with severe disease when oral feeding is not tolerated or with enterocutaneous fistula. There is also evidence from animal models that lack of luminal nutrients can be a factor in the inflammatory process. Conversely, intraluminal administration of specific luminal nutrients such as short-chain fatty acids has a trophic and healing effect that can be beneficial. Future studies should help determine tissue levels of nutrient requirements and the relationship of potential nutrient deficiencies to disease activity.

Celiac Disease

Celiac disease or gluten-sensitive enteropathy is an intestinal intolerance to gliadin that produces specific small intestinal mucosal lesions in the susceptible individual. The wide spectrum of presentation includes a protuberant abdomen, lack of subcutaneous tissue, muscle wasting, steatorrhea, specific nutrient deficiency, and growth retardation. The clinical features and the small intestinal lesions improve after complete elimination of gluten from the diet and reoccur with the reintroduction of gluten.

Increased understanding of the pathogenesis, diagnosis, and epidemiology of this disease has shifted the potential time of diagnosis to a younger age, but, in many cases, partial treatment before accurate diagnosis is made delays definitive diagnosis until the child is much older. The prevalence, however, has not changed. Short stature and failure to thrive appear to be more frequent presenting symptoms (223–225). Three intestinal biopsies are required for the diagnosis: one at the time of presentation, a second after 6 months of gluten elimination, and a third after gluten reintroduction. The new immunologic markers used for follow-up include IgG antigliadin, IgA antigliadin (226,227), and antireticulin antibodies, which are less specific but more sensitive (228,229). We find serum antiendomysial antibodies highly specific and sensitive (230).

Therapy, essentially a gluten-free diet, has not changed, however. There is some controversy as to whether this diet must be continued for a lifetime or if, in some patients, gluten sensitivity may be transient. There is also a suggestion that in some cases, where the mechanism is by toxic effect rather than an immunologic process, gluten damage may be dose dependent (231,232). Holmes et al. (233) emphasize the importance of maintaining a gluten-free diet. They followed patients with celiac disease for two decades and found that patients with diets containing gluten had an increased risk of developing intestinal malignancy over the gluten-free diet group.

The general consensus is that children with proven celiac disease require a permanent gluten-free diet. This includes elimination of all foods containing flour or cereal derived from wheat, rye, barley, and oats. Replacements are corn, rice, and potato flour. A gluten-free diet is not easy to follow. This creates a compliance problem, particularly among adolescents (234). Compliance is also complicated by the lack of immediate adverse effects in most patients beyond infancy. Jackson et al. (235) demonstrated that only 20 of 50 parents reported strict compliance. In addition, many parents who think they enforce strict diets actually do not because of inaccurate comprehension. In the end, however, strict compliance is absolutely necessary in order to maintain a normal intestinal mucosa.

As with other malabsorptive disorders, in the initial phase of celiac disease therapy, a lactose-free diet is indicated due to the low lactase activity in the damaged mucosa. In cases with severe mucosal injury, the intestinal disaccharidase level has to be assessed to provide a more restrictive carbohydrate diet. Vitamins, especially fat-soluble, should be added early. Anemic children should receive supplemental iron, folate, or vitamin B_{12}, depending on the specific deficiency. In infants with celiac crisis, IV replacement of fluid and electrolytes is essential. Hypokalemia should be corrected promptly and hypoalbuminemia should be treated with salt-free albumin and Lasix administration. Corticosteroids may also be used in celiac crisis. Finally, despite the dietary restrictions, the diet should supply adequate calories and proteins to avoid the small intestine and pancreatic enzyme deficiencies that occur in conjunction with protein malnutrition.

Chronic Nonspecific Diarrhea

Despite increased specificity in identifying distinct diarrheal entities, most diarrhea in young children is diagnosed as chronic nonspecific diarrhea, or "toddler diarrhea." This syndrome usually begins at about age 2 and has a high rate of spontaneous resolution. Patients with nonspecific diarrhea show no evidence of malabsorptive disorder; they gain weight and grow normally (236–238).

Many of these patients eventually have adult-type lactase deficiency. This deficiency is an evolutionary process with geographic distribution. In cultures without domesticated dairy animals, e.g., Chinese, Japanese, Native-American, and Native-Alaskan, the prevalence can be as high as 70% to 100%. In contrast, only 20% of United States Caucasians have hypolactasia (239–241). It usually starts after the second year of life with the enzyme diminishing as the clinical symptoms gradually appear (242). This disorder can be diagnosed by a lactose hydrogen breath test. Rarely is an intestinal biopsy needed to determine the enzyme level and to rule out other entities (243,245). Lactose should be eliminated from the diet. In some patients, however, there is a residual activity of brush border lactase that permits limited lactose ingestion.

Lactose can be hydrolyzed into glucose and galactose by adding commercially available lactase (Lactaid) to milk. A ready-to-drink pretreated milk is also available. The *in vitro* hydrolysis of lactose enables lactase-deficient persons to consume lactose without gastrointestinal disturbances.

The diagnosis of nonspecific diarrhea can be made after excluding any malabsorption or adult-type hypolactasia syndrome and when normal growth is evident (236,238). There is little agreement regarding etiology or pathogens. Treatment is mainly empirical, designed to address the most common known causes (245). Initially, a good history should include dietary habits. When an excessive amount of fluid is found to be consumed, limiting fluid intake may be indicated (246). Parents often give apple juice, believing it to have antidiarrheal properties. Apple juice differs from most fruit juices, however, in that it contains an excess of fructose as compared to glucose (247). In addition, unlike apples, apple juice does not contain pectin. The high amount of fructose may not be tolerated in some of these children. This can be demonstrated either by fructose hydrogen breath test, or simply by reducing the amount consumed (248).

When no dietary component can be blamed, many nutritional maneuvers are available (245). Increasing the amount of fat intake slows intestinal motility (249). Eliminating chilled food is advised because intake of cold food stimulates colonic motility. Increasing fiber intake usually will firm the stool (250). In some individuals, however, fiber can increase diarrhea or even induce it with overload flow (251).

Ultimately, the symptoms often resolve spontaneously. The main obligation of the physician is to limit the therapeutic trials and to reassure parents that the condition is benign and has an excellent prognosis.

REFERENCES

1. Hamilton JR. The pathogenesis of infectious diarrhea. In: Thomson ABR, DaCosta LR, Watson WC, ed. *Modern concepts in gastroenterology*, vol 1. New York: Plenum, 1986;335–355.
2. *Manual for the treatment of acute diarrhea*. World Health Organization: Diarrhea Disease Control Program: 80.2 Rev. 1. 1984.
3. Tallet S, MacKenzie C, Middleton P, et al. Clinical laboratory and epidemiologic features of viral gastroenteritis in infants and children. *Pediatrics* 1977;60:217–221.
4. Davidson GP. Viral diarrhea. *Clin Gastroenterol* 1986;15:30–53.
5. Rodriguez WJ, Kim HW, Arrobiro JO, et al. Clinical features of acute gastroenteritis associated with human reo-virus like agents in infants and young children. *J Pediatr* 1977;91:188–193.
6. Volken RH, Miotti P, Viscidi R. Immunoassay for the diagnosis and study of viral gastroenteritis. *Pediatr Infect Dis J* 1986;5:546–552.
7. Dolin R, Treanor JJ, Madore PH. Novel agents of viral enteritis in humans. *J Infect Dis* 1987;15:365–376.
8. Schreiber DS, Blacklow NR, Trier JS. The mucosal lesion of the proximal small intestine in acute infectious nonbacterial gastroenteritis. *N Engl J Med* 1973;288:1318.
9. Greenberg HB, Valdesuso J, Yolken RH, et al. Role of Norwalk virus in outbreaks of nonbacterial gastroenteritis. *J Infect Dis* 1979;139:564–568.
10. Gracey M, Burke V. Infective diarrhea: mechanism of diarrhea pathogenesis and clinical features. In: Anderson CM, Burke V, Gracey M, eds. *Pediatric gastroenterology*, 2nd ed. Oxford: Blackwell Scientific Publications, 1987;284–291.
11. Farthing MJG. Giardiasis. *Adv Med* 1987;23:287–301.
12. Navin TR, Juranek DD. Cryptosporidiosis: clinical, epidemiologic and parasitologic review. *Rev Infect Dis* 1984;6:313–327.
13. Isaacs D, Hunt GH, Phillips AD, Price EH, Raafat F, Walker-Smith JA. Cryptosporidiosis in immunocompetent children. *J Clin Pathol* 1985;38:76–81.

14. Mathan MM, George R, Venkatesan S, Mathew M, Methan VI. Cryptosporidium and diarrhea in Southern Indian children. *Lancet* 1985;2:1172–1175.
15. Sack RB. Enterotoxigenic *Escherichia coli* identification and characterization. *J Infect Dis* 1980;142–279.
16. Powell DW. Ion and water transport in the intestine. In: Adreoli TE, Hoffman JF, Fanestil DD, Schultz SG, eds. *Physiology of membrane disorders.* New York: Plenum, 1986;559.
17. Donowitz M, Welsh MJ. Regulation of mammalian small intestinal electrolyte secretion. In: Johnson L, ed. *Physiology of the gastrointestinal tract.* New York: Raven Press, 1987;1351.
18. Shepherd RW, Gall DB, Butler DG, Hamilton JR. Determination of diarrhea in viral enteritis. The role of ion transport and epithelial changes in the ileum in transmissible gastroenteritis in piglets. *Gastroenterology* 1979;76:20–24.
19. Gordtran JS. Speculations on the pathogenesis of diarrhea. *Fed Proc* 1967;26:1405–1414.
20. Davidson GP, Gall DG, Butler DB, Petric M, Hamilton JR. Human rotavirus enteritis induced in unconventional piglets. Intestinal structure and transport. *J Clin Invest* 1977;60:1402–1409.
21. Wolf JL, Schreiber DS. Viral gastroenteritis. *Med Clin North Am* 1982;66:575–595.
22. Bond JH, Currier BE, Buchwald H, Levitt MD. Colonic conservation of malabsorbed carbohydrate. *Gastroenterology* 1980;78:444–447.
23. Whalen GE, Soergel KH, Green JE. Diabetic diarrhea. *Gastroenterology* 1969;56:1021–1032.
24. Edelman R, Levine MM. Acute diarrhea infections in infants. I: bacterial and viral causes. *Hosp Pract* 1980;15:97–103.
25. Guerrant RL, Shields DS, Thorson SM, et al. Evaluation and diagnosis of acute infectious diarrhea. *Am J Med* 1985;78(suppl 71–72 6B):91–96.
26. Uhnoo I, Wadell G, Sevensson L, et al. Aetiology and epidemiology of acute gastroenteritis in Swedish children. *J Infect Dis* 1986;13:73–84.
27. Hirschoren N. The treatment of acute diarrhea in children: a historical and physiological perspective. *Am J Clin Nutr* 1980;33:636–663.
28. Santosham M, Daum RS, Dillman L, et al. Oral rehydration therapy of infantile diarrhea. A controlled study of well-nourished children hospitalized in the United States and Panama. *N Engl J Med* 1982;101:497–499.
29. Finberg L, Harper PA, Harrison HE, Sack RB. Oral rehydration for diarrhea. *J Pediatr* 1982;101:497–499.
30. Listernick R, Zieserl E, Davis T. Oral glucose-electrolyte solutions as maintenance of acute diarrhea. *Am J Dis Child* 1985;139:571–574.
31. Meeuwisse GE. High sugar worse than high sodium in oral rehydration solutions. *Acta Paediatr Scand* 1983;72:161–166.
32. Tripp JH, Harries JT. UNISEF/WHO glucose-electrolyte solution not always appropriate. *Lancet* 1980;2:793.
33. Sokuco S, Marin S, Gunoz H, Aperia A, Neyzi O, Zetterstrom R. Oral rehydration therapy in infectious diarrhea: comparison of rehydration solutions with 60 and 90 mmol sodium per liter. *Acta Paediatr Scand* 1985;74:489–494.
34. Molla MA, Rehamn M, Sarker SA, Sach DA, Molla A. Stool electrolyte content and purging rates in diarrhea caused by rotavirus, enterotoxigenic *E. coli* and *V. cholera* in children. *J Pediatr* 1981;98:835–838.
35. MacKenzie A, Barens G. Oral rehydration in infantile diarrhea in the developed world. *Drugs* 1988;36(suppl 4):48–60.
36. Cleary TG, Cleary KR, DuPont HL, El-Malih GS, et al. The relationship of oral rehydration solution to hypernatremia diarrhea. *J Pediatr* 1981;99:739–741.
37. Santosham M, Burns B, Nadkarni V. Oral rehydration therapy for acute diarrhea in ambulatory children in the United States: a double-blind comparison of four different solutions. *Pediatrics* 1985;76:159–166.
38. Guzman C, Pizarro D, Castilo P. Hypernatremic dehydration treated with oral glucose-electrolyte solution containing 20 or 75 mEq/l of sodium. *J Pediatr Gastroenterol Nutr* 1988;7:694–698.
39. Delucchi MA, Guiraldes C, Hirsh T, Nunez N, Schele C, Gutierrez H, Torres-Pereyra J. The use of oral rehydration in the treatment of children with acute diarrhea in primary care. *J Pediatr Gastroenterol Nutr* 1989;9:328–334.
40. Marin L, Saner G, Sokuco S, Gunoz H, Neyzi O, Zetterstrom R. Oral rehydration therapy in neonates and young infants with infectious diarrhea. *Acta Paediatr Scand* 1987;76:431–437.
41. Pizarro D, Posada G, Mata LJ. Treatment of 242 neonates with dehydrating diarrhea with an oral glucose-electrolyte solution. *J Pediatr* 1983;102:153–156.
42. Jones BJM, Brown BE, Loran JS, Edgerton D, et al. Glucose absorption from starch hydrolysate in the human jejunum. *Gut* 1983;24:1152–1160.
43. Azad MAK, Lebenthal E. Role of intestinal glucoamylase in glucose polymer hydrolysis and absorption. *Ped Res* 1990;28:166–170.
44. Lebenthal E, Lee PC. Glucoamylase and disaccharidase activity in normal subjects and in patients with mucosal injury of the small intestine. *J Pediatr* 1980;97:389–393.
45. Patra FC, Mahalanabias D, Jalan KN, Sen A, Banerjee P. Is oral rice electrolyte solution superior to glucose electrolyte solution in infantile diarrhea? *Arch Dis Child* 1982;57:910–912.
46. Mehta MM, Subramania S. Comparison of rice water, rice electrolyte solution in the management of infantile diarrhea. *Lancet* 1986;1:843–845.
47. Mohan M, Sethi JS, Daral TS, Sharama MB, Hargva SK, Sachdev HPS. Controlled trial of rice powder and glucose rehydration solutions as oral therapy for acute dehydrating diarrhea in infants. *J Pediatr Gastroenterol Nutr* 1986;5:423–427.
48. Wapnir RA, Zdanowicz MM, Teichberg ST, Lifshitz F. Alanine stimulation of water and sodium absorption in a model of secretory diarrhea. *J Pediatr Gastroenterol Nutr* 1990;10:213–221.
49. Rhoads JM, MacLeod RJ, Hamilton JR. Alanine enhances jejunal sodium absorption in the presence of glucose: studies in piglet viral diarrhea. *Pediatr Res* 1986;20:879–883.
50. Wapiner RA, Lifshitz F. Osmolality and solute concentration—their relationship with oral hydration solution effectiveness: an experimental assessment. *Pediatr Res* 1985;19:894–898.
51. Vesikari T, Isolauri E. Glycine supplemented oral rehydration solutions for diarrhea. *Arch Dis Child* 1986;61:372–376.
52. Vesikari T, Isolaur E, Marnela KM. Glycinuria following administration of glycine-supplemented oral rehydration solution in rotavirus diarrhea. *Acta Paediatr Scand* 1988;77:165–166.
53. Wapiner RA, Zdanowicz M, Teichberg S, Lifshitz F. Oral rehydration solutions in experimental osmotic diarrhea; enhancement by alanine and other amino acids and oligopeptides. *Am J Clin Nutr* 1988;47:84–90.
54. Wapiner PA. Diarrhea disease and zinc supplementation. *J Pediatr Gastroenterol Nutr* 1980;7:793–794.
55. Sachdev HPS, Mittal NK, Mittal SK, Yadov HSA. Controlled trial on utility of oral zinc supplementation in acute dehydrating diarrhea in infants. *J Pediatr Gastroenterol Nutr* 1988;7:877–881.
56. Chung AH, Viscorova B. The effect of early oral feeding versus early oral starvation on the course of infantile diarrhea. *J Pediatr* 1948;33:14–22.
57. Dugdale A, Lovell S, Gibbs V, et al. Refeeding after acute gastroenteritis: a control study. *Arch Dis Child* 1982;57:76–78.
58. Rees L, Brooke CGD. Gradual reintroduction of full-strength milk after gastroenteritis in children. *Lancet* 1979;1:770–771.
59. Brown KH, Black RE, Lopez de Romana G, Kanashiro HC. Infant feeding practices and other disease in Huascar, (Lima) Peru. *Pediatrics* 1989;83:31–40.
60. Plaszek M, Walker-Smith JA. Comparison of two feeding regimens following acute gastroenteritis in infancy. *J Pediatr Gastroenterol Nutr* 1984;3:245–248.
61. Mitchell JE, Donald WD, Birdson M. A review of 396 cases of acute diarrhea in which early oral feeding was employed in treatment. *Pediatrics* 1949;35:529–539.
62. Ransome OJ, Roode H. Early introduction of milk feeds in acute infantile gastro-enteritis. *S Afr Med J* 1984;65:127–128.
63. Brown KH, Gastafladuy AS, Saavedra JM, et al. Effect of continued oral feeding on clinical and nutritional outcomes of acute diarrhea in children. *J Pediatr* 1988;112:191–200.
64. Butzner D, Butler DG, Miniates P, Hamilton JR. Impact of chronic protein-calorie malnutrition on small intestinal repair

after acute viral enteritis: a study in gnotobiotic piglets. *Pediatr Res* 1985;19:476–481.
65. Knudsen KB, Bradley EM, Lecocq FR, Bellamy HM, Welsh JD. Effect of fasting and refeeding on the histology and disaccharidase activity of the human intestine. *Gastroenterology* 1968;55:46–51.
66. Levine GM, Deren JJ, Steiger E, Zinno R. Role of oral intake in maintenance of gut mass and disaccharidase activity. *Gastroenterology* 1974;67:975–982.
67. Isolauri E, Juntunene M, Wiren S, Vuorinen P, Koivula T. Intestinal permeability changes in acute gastroenteritis: effects of clinical factors and nutritional management. *J Pediatr Gastroenterol Nutr* 1989;8:466–473.
68. *Nutritional management of chronic diarrhea and/or malabsorption.* Subcommittee on chronic diarrhea. American Academy of Pediatrics, 1989.
69. Rajah R, Pettifor JM, Noormohamad M, Venter A, Rosen EV, Rabinowitz L, Stein H. The effect of feeding of four different formulae on stool weights in prolonged dehydrating infantile gastroenteritis. *J Pediatr Gastroenterol Nutr* 1988;7:202–207.
70. Wharton BA, Pugh RE, Taitz LS, Walker-Smith JA, Booth IW. Dietary management of gastroenteritis in Britain. *Br Med J* 1988;296:450–452.
71. Macfarlana PI, Miller V. Human milk in management of protracted diarrhea of infancy. *Arch Dis Child* 1984;59:260–265.
72. Welsh JK, May JT. Anti-infective properties of human milk. *J Pediatr* 1979;94:1–9.
73. Goldman AS, Goldblum C. Immunologic system in human milk: characteristics and effects. In: Lebenthal E, ed. *Textbook of gastroenterology and nutrition in infancy.* New York: Raven Press, 1989;135–142.
74. Read LC, Francis GL, Wallace JC, Ballard FJ. Growth factor of concentration and growth-promoting activity in human milk following premature birth. *J Dev Physiol* 1985;7:135–145.
75. Read LC, Upton FC, Francis GL, Wallace JC, Dahelnberg GW, Ballard FG. Changes in the growth-promoting activity of human milk during lactation. *Pediatr Res* 1984;18:133–139.
76. Koldovsky O, Thornburg W. Hormones in milk. *J Pediatr Gastroenterol Nutr* 1987;6:172–196.
77. Berseth CL. Human-milk-enhanced intestinal and somatic growth in neonatal rates. *Biol Neonate* 1987;51:53–59.
78. Carpenter G. Epidermal growth factor is a major growth-promoting agent in human milk. *Science* 1980;210:198–199.
79. Shulman RJ, Lifschitz CH, Langston C, Gapalakrishna GS, Nichols BL. Human milk and the rate of small intestinal mucosal recovery in protracted diarrhea. *J Pediatr* 1989;114:218–223.
80. Davison GP, Goodwin D, Robb TA. Incidence and duration of lactose malabsorption in children hospitalized with acute enteritis: study in a well-nourished urban population. *J Pediatr* 1984;105:587–590.
81. Chandrasekaran R, Kumar V, Walia BNS, Moorthy B. Carbohydrate intolerance in infant with acute diarrhea and its complications. *Acta Paediatr Scand* 1975;64:483–488.
82. Dewit O, Boudraa G, Touhami M, Desjeux JF. Breath hydrogen test and stool characteristics after ingestion of milk and yoghurt in malnourished children with chronic diarrhea and lactase deficiency. *J Trop Pediatr* 1987;33:177–180.
83. Hyams JS, Kraus PJ, Gleason PA. Lactose malabsorption following rotavirus infection in young children. *J Pediatr* 1981;89:916–918.
84. Penny ME, Paredes P, Brown KH. Clinical and nutritional consequences of lactose feeding during persistent postenteritis diarrhea. *Pediatrics* 1989;84:835–844.
85. Kumar V, Chandrasekaran R, Bhaskar R. Carbohydrate intolerance associated with acute gastroenteritis. *Clin Pediatr* 1977;16:1123–1127.
86. Bartrop RW, Hull D. Transient lactose intolerance in infancy. *Arch Dis Child* 1973;48:963–966.
87. Iyngkaran N, Davis K, Robinson MJ, et al. Cows milk protein-sensitive enteropathy. *Arch Dis Child* 1979;54:39–43.
88. Walker-Smith JA. Interrelationship between cow's milk protein intolerance and lactose intolerance. In: Lifshitz F, ed. *Carbohydrate intolerance in infancy.* New York: Marcel Dekker, 1982;155–173.

89. Walker-Smith JA. Cow's milk intolerance as a cause of postenteritis diarrhea. *J Pediatr Gastroenterol Nutr* 1982;1:163–173.
90. Brunser O, Araya M, Espinoza J, Guesry PR, Secretin MC, Pacheco I. Effect of an acidified milk on diarrhea and the carrier state in infants of low socio-economic status. *Acta Paediatr Scand* 1989;78:259–264.
91. Whitington PF, Gibson R. Soy protein intolerance: four patients with concomitant cows' milk intolerance. *Pediatrics* 1977;59:730–732.
92. Goel K, Lifschitz F, Kahn E, Teicberg S. Monosaccharide intolerance and soy protein hypersensitivity in an infant with diarrhea. *J Pediatr* 1978;93:617–619.
93. Amet ME, Ruben CE. Soy protein—another cause of flat intestinal lesion. *Gastroenterology* 1972;62:227–234.
94. Cook CD. Probable gastrointestinal reaction to soy bean. *N Engl J Med* 1960;263:1076–1077.
95. Halpin TC, Byrne WJ, Ament ME. Colitis, persistent diarrhea, and soy protein intolerance. *J Pediatr* 1977;91:404–407.
96. Maclean WC, Lopez C, de Romana G, Massa E, Graham G. Nutritional management of chronic diarrhea and malnutrition: primary reliance on oral feeding. *J Pediatr* 1980;97:316–323.
97. Galeano NF, Lepage G, Lorey C, Belli D, Levy E, Roy CC. Comparison of two special infant formulas designed for the treatment of protracted diarrhea. *J Pediatr Gastroenterol Nutr* 1988;7:76–83.
98. Avery GB, Villavicencio O, Lilly JR, Randolph JG. Intractable diarrhea in early infancy. *Pediatrics* 1968;41:712–722.
99. Lebenthal E. Prolonged small intestinal mucosal injury as a primary cause of intractable diarrhea of infancy. In: Lebenthal E, ed. *Chronic diarrhea in children.* New York: Raven Press, 1984;5–29.
100. Lebenthal E. Intractable diarrhea of infancy. In: Lebenthal E, ed. *Textbook of gastroenterology and nutrition in infancy.* New York: Raven Press, 1989;1077–1092.
101. Walker-Smith JA. Temporary syndrome of food intolerance: pathology and mechanism of food allergy. In: Walker-Smith JA, McNiesh AS, eds. *Diarrhea and malnutrition in childhood.* London: Butterworths, 1986;185–193.
102. Maluenda C, Philips AD, Briddon A, Walker-Smith JA. Quantitative analysis of small intestinal mucosa in cow's milk-sensitive enteropathy. *J Pediatr Gastroenterol Nutr* 1984;3:349–357.
103. Rossi TM, Lebenthal E, Nord KS, Fazili RR. Extent and duration of small intestinal mucosal injury in intractable diarrhea of infancy. *Pediatrics* 1980;66:730–735.
104. Greene HL, McCabe DR, Merenslein GB. Protracted diarrhea and malnutrition in infancy: changes in intestinal morphology and disaccharidase activities during treatment with total intravenous nutrition or oral elemental diets. *J Pediatr* 1976;87:695–704.
105. Webb JD, Poley JR, Bhatia M, Stevenson DE. Intestinal disaccharidase activities in relation to age, race, and mucosal damage. *Gastroenterology* 1978;75:847–855.
106. Schneider RE, Viteri FE. Morphological aspects of the duodeno-jejunal mucosa in protein-calorie malnourished children and during recovery. *Am J Clin Nutr* 1972;25:1092–1102.
107. Larcher VF, Shephard R, Harries JT, Harries DE. Protracted diarrhea in infancy: analysis of 82 cases with particular reference to diagnosis and management. *Arch Dis Child* 1977;52:597–605.
108. Davidson GP, Barens GL. Structural and functional abnormalities of the small intestine in infants and young children with rotavirus enteritis. *Acta Paediatr Scand* 1979;68:181–186.
109. Lifschitz C, Polanco I, Mahoney D, Loob KW, Nichols BL. Specific changes in intestinal permeability. *Pediatr Res* 1986;20:244A.
110. Lifschitz CH, Irving CS, Marks LM, Klein PD, Finegold MJ, Nichols BL. Polyethylene glycol polmers of low molecular weight as probes of intestinal permeability. II. Application to infants and children with intestinal disease. *Lab Clin Med* 1986;108:37–43.
111. Weaver LT, Champman PD, Madeley CR. Intestinal permeability changes and excretion of micro-organism in stools of infants with rotavirus enteritis. *Arch Dis Child* 1985;60:326–336.
112. Lebenthal E. Lactose malabsorption and milk consumption in infants and children. *Am J Dis Child* 1979;133:21–24.

113. Lifschitz CH, Irving CS, Gopalkrishna GS, et al. Carbohydrate malabsorption in infants with diarrhea studied with the breath hydrogen test. *J Pediatr* 1983;102:371–373.
114. Lifshitz F, Colleo-Ramirez P, Gutierrez-Topete G, et al. Carbohydrate malabsorption in infant with diarrhea. *J Pediatr* 1971;79:760–767.
115. Hyams JS, Krause PJ, Gleason PA. Lactose malabsorption following rotavirus infection in young children. *J Pediatr* 1981;99:916–918.
116. Bowie MD, Brinkman GL, Hansen JDL. Acquired disaccharide intolerance in malnutrition. *J Pediatr* 1965;66:1083.
117. Prinsloog JG, Wittmann W, Pretorius PJ, et al. Effect of different sugar on diarrhea of acute kwashiorkor. *Arch Dis Child* 1969;44:593–599.
118. Shwachman H, Lloyed-Still JD, Khaw KT, Antonowicz I. Protracted diarrhea of infancy treated by intravenous alimentation. II. Studies of small intestinal biopsy results. *Am J Dis Child* 1973;125:365–368.
119. Lebenthal E, Lee PC. Development of functional response in human exocrine pancreas. *Pediatrics* 1980;66:556–560.
120. Lebenthal E. Pancreatic functions and disease in infancy and childhood. *Adv Pediatr* 1978;25:223–261.
121. Zoppi G, Andreotti G, Pajno-Ferrara F, Mjai DM, Gaburro DM. Exocrine pancreas function in premature and full term neonates. *Pediatr Res* 1972;6:880–886.
122. Sloven DG, Jirapinyo P, Lebenthal E. The hydrolysis and absorption of glucose polymers from rice compared to corn in chronic diarrhea. *J Pediatr* 1990;116(6);876–881.
123. Bhan MK, Ghai OP, Khoshoo V, et al. Efficacy of mung bean (lentil) and poop rice based rehydrolate solutions in comparison with the standard glucose electrolyte solutions. *J Pediatr Gastroenterol Nutr* 1987;6:392–399.
124. Rahm GG, Klein GL, Cordano A, Graham GG. Nutritive value of elemental formula with reduced osmolality. *Am J Dis Child* 1979;133:795–797.
125. Jonas A, Avigad S, Diver-Haber C, et al. Disturbed fat absorption following infectious gastroenteritis in children. *J Pediatr* 1979;95:366–372.
126. Heubi JE, Balistreri WF. Bile salt metabolism in infant and children after diarrhea. *Pediatr Res* 1980;14:943–946.
127. Heubi JE, Balistreri WF, Partin JC. Refractory infantile diarrhea due to primary bile acid malabsorption. *J Pediatr* 1979;94:546–551.
128. Zurier RB, Campbell RG, Hashim SA, et al. Use of medium chain triglyceride in management of patients with massive resection of small intestine. *N Engl J Med* 1966;274:490–493.
129. Roy CC, Weber AM, Lepage G, Smith LS, Vevy EM. Digestive and absorptive phase anomalies associated with the exocrine pancreatic insufficiency of cystic fibrosis. *J Pediatr Gastroenterol Nutr* 1988;7(Suppl 1):s1–s7.
130. Schneider RE, Viteri FE. Luminal events of lipid absorption in protein calorie malnourished children: relationship with nutritional recovery and diarrhea: II. Alterations in bile acid content of duodenal aspirates. *Am J Clin Nutr* 1974;27:788–796.
131. Mann MD, Hill ID, Peat GM, Bowie MD. Protein and fat absorption in prolonged diarrhea in infancy. *Arch Dis Child* 1982;57:268–273.
132. Barbezat GO, Hansen JDH. The exocrine pancreas and protein calorie malnutrition. *Pediatrics* 1968;42:77–92.
133. Playoust MR, Isselbacher KJ. Studies on the intestinal absorption and intramucosa lipolyse of a medium chain triglycerine. *J Clin Invest* 1964;43:870–885.
134. Greenberger NJ, Rodgers JB, Isselbacher KJ. Absorption of medium and long chain triglycerides: factors influencing their hydrolysis and transport. *J Clin Invest* 1966;2:217–227.
135. Ror CC, Ste-Marie M, Chartrand L, et al. Correction of the malabsorption of the preterm infant with a medium-chain triglyceride formula. *J Pediatr* 1975;86:446–450.
136. Bach AC, Babayan VK. Medium-chain triglycerides: an update. *Am J Clin Nutr* 1982;36:950–962.
137. Weinsier RL, Heimburger DC, Butterworth CE. *Handbook of clinical nutrition*, 2nd ed. St. Louis: CV Mosby, 1989;96,180,302.
138. Wooif GM, Jeejeebhoy KN. Dietary management of short bowel syndrome. *Gastroenterology* 1983;85:218–219.
139. MacBurney M, Jacobs D, Apelgrenk KN, et al. Modular feeding. In: Rombeau J, Caldwell M, eds. *Enternal and tube feeding*. Philadelphia: WB Saunders, 1984;199–211.
140. Jiraphinyo P, Young C, Srimaruta N, Cordano A, Lebenthal E., Rossi TM. High fat semi-elemental diet in the treatment of protracted diarrhea of infancy. *Pediatrics* 1990;86(6):902–908.
141. Silk DBA, Grimble GK, Rees, RG. Protein digestion and amino acid and peptide absorption. *Proc Nutr Soc* 1985;44:63–68.
142. Rinderknecht H. Pancreatic secretory enzymes. In: Go VLW, Gardner JD, Brooks FP, et al., eds. *The exocrine pancreas: biology, pathology, and diseases*. New York: Raven Press, 1986;163.
143. Stintzing G, Zetterstrom R. Cow's milk allergy, incidence and pathogenic role of early exposure to cow's milk formula. *Acta Paediatr Scand* 1979;68:383–387.
144. Jakobsson I, Lindberg T. A prospective study of cow's milk protein intolerance in Swedish infants. *Acta Paediatr Scand* 1979;68:853–859.
145. Freier S, Kletter B. Milk allergy in infants and young children. *Clin Pediatr* 1970;9:449–454.
146. Gerrard JW, MacKenzie JWA, Goluboff N, Garson JZ, Maningas CS. Cow's milk allergy: prevalence and manifestations in an unselected series of newborns. *Acta Paediatr Scand* 1973;(suppl 234):1–21.
147. Hill DJ, Firer MA, Hoskin CS. Manifestation of milk allergy in infancy: clinical and immunologic findings. *J Pediatr* 1986;109:270–276.
148. Kuitunen P, Visakorpi JK, Savilahti E, Pelknonem P. Malabsorption syndrome with cow's milk intolerance. Clinical findings and course in 54 cases. *Arch Dis Child* 1975;50:351–356.
149. Iyngkaran N, Robinsin MJ, Sumithran E, et al. Cow's milk protein-sensitive enteropathy. *Arch Dis Child* 1978;53:150–153.
150. Danneaus A, Johansson SGO. A follow-up of infants with adverse reactions to cow's milk. I. Serum IgE, skin test reactions and RAST in relation to clinical course. *Acta Paediatr Scand* 1979;68:377–382.
151. Sampson HA, Albergo R. Comparison of results of skin tests, RAST and double-blind, placebo-controlled food challenges in children with atopic dermatitis. *J Allergy Clin Immunol* 1984;74:26–33.
152. Jackson D, Walker-Smith JA, Phillips AD. Macromolecular absorption by histologically normal and abnormal small intestine mucosa in childhood: an in vitro study using organ culture. *J Pediatr Gastroenterol Nutr* 1983;2:235–240.
153. Firer MA, Kosking CS, Hill DJ. Possible role for rotavirus in the development of cow's milk enteropathy in infants. *Clin Allergy* 1988;18:53–61.
154. Walker-Smith JA, Harrison M, Kilby A, Phillips A, France NE. Cow's milk sensitive enteropathy. *Arch Dis Child* 1978;53:375.
155. Walker WA, Isselbacher KJ. Uptake and transport of macromolecules by the intestine. Possible role in clinical disorders. *Gastroenterology* 1974;67:531–550.
156. Udall JN, Walker WA. The physiologic and pathogenic basis for the transport of macromolecules across the intestinal tract. *J Pediatr Gastroenterol Nutr* 1981;3:295–301.
157. Henderson JF, Patterson ARP. *Nucleotide metabolism: an introduction. I.* New York: Academic Press, 1973.
158. LeLeiko NS, Bronstien AD, Baligia S, Munro NH. De novo purine nucleotides in the rat small and large intestinal mucosa. *J Pediatr Gastroenterol Nutr* 1983;2:313–319.
159. Savaianoo DA, Clifford AJ. Adenine, the precursor of nucleic acids in intestinal cells unable to synthesize purines de novo. *J Nutr* 1981;111:1816–1822.
160. Ogoshi S, Iwasa M, Yonezawa T, Tamiya T. Effect of nucleotide and nucleoside mixture on rats given total parenteral nutrition after 70% hepatectomy. *JPEN J Parenter Enteral Nutr* 1985;9:339–342.
161. Van Buren CT, Kulkarini AD, Schandle VB, Rudolph FB. Effects of dietary nucleotides on cell-mediated immunity. *Transplantation* 1983;36:350–352.
162. Rudolph FB, Kulkarini AD, Schandle VB, Van Buren CT. In-

volvement of dietary nucleotides in T lymphocytes function. *Exp Med Biol* 1984;165:175–178.
163. Kulkavini AD, Fanslow WC, Rudolph FB, Van Buren CT. Effect of dietary nucleotides on response to bacterial infections. *JPEN J Parenter Enteral Nutr* 1986;10:169–171.
164. Kobata A, Ziro S, Kida M. The acid-soluble nucleotides of milk. I. Quantitative differences and qualitative differences of nucleotides constituents in human and cow's milk. *J Biochem (Tokyo)* 1962;51:277–287.
165. Janas ML, Piccian MF. The nucleotide profile of human milk. *Pediatr Res* 1982;16:659–662.
166. Skala JP, Koldovksy O, Hahn P. Cyclic nucleotides in breast milk. *Am J Clin Nutr* 1981;34:343–350.
167. Braun HO. Effect of consumption of human milk and other formula on intestinal bacterial flora in infants. In: Lebenthal E, ed. *Textbook of gastroenterology and nutrition in infancy.* New York: Raven Press, 1982;1:247–253.
168. Tanaka R, Mutai M. Improved medium for selective isolation and enumeration of bifidobacterium. *Appl Environ Microbiol* 1980;40:866–869.
169. Sanchez-Pozo A, Pita ML, Martinex A, Molina JA, Sanchez-Medina F, Gil A. Effect of dietary nucleotides upon lipoprotein pattern of newborn infants. *Nutr Res* 1986;6:763–771.
170. Putnam JC, Carlson SE, De Voe PW, Barness LA. The effect of variations in dietary fatty acid composition of erythrocyte phosphatidylcholine and phosphatidylethanolamine in human infants. *Am J Clin Nutr* 1982;36:106–114.
171. Crawford MA, Hassan AG, Hall BM. Metabolism of essential fatty acids in the human fetus and neonate. *Nutr Metab* 1977;21:187–190.
172. Johnson M, Carey F, McMillan RM. Alternative pathways of arachidonate metabolism: prostaglandins, thromboxane and leukotrienes. *Essays Biochem* 1983;19:140–141.
173. Schmidt-Sommerfeld E, Penn D, Novak M, Wolf H. Carnitine in human perinatal fat metabolism. *J Pediatr Med* 1985;13:107–116.
174. Frinz IR, Marquis NR. The role of acylcarnitine esters and carnitine palmitoyltransferase in the transport of fatty acylgroups across the mitochondrial membranes. *Proc Natl Acad Sci USA* 1965;54:1226–1233.
175. Penn D, Ludwig B, Schmidt-Sommerfeld E, Pascu F. Effect of gestation age and nutrition on carnitine tissue concentration in infants. *Biol Neonate* 1985;47:130–135.
176. Schiff D, Chan G, Seccombe D, Hahan P. Plasma carnitine levels during intravenous feeding of the neonate. *J Pediatr* 1979;95:1043–1046.
177. Norum PR, York CM, Broquiost HP. Carnitine content of liquid formulas and special diets. *Am Clin Nutr* 1979;32:2272–2276.
178. Penn D, Dolderer M, Schmidt-Sommerfeld E. Carnitine concentrations in the milk of different species formulas. *Biol Neonate* 1987;52:70–79.
179. Committee on Nutrition. Iron-fortified infant formulas. *Pediatrics* 1989;84:1114.
180. Hambridge KM, Casey CE, Kerbs NF. Zinc. In: Mertz W, ed. *Trace elements in human and animal nutrition,* 5th ed. Orlando, FL: Academic Press, 1986;2:1–137.
181. Hambidge KM, Krebs NF, Walravens PA. Growth velocity of young children receiving zinc supplement. *Nutr Res* 1985;1(suppl):306–316.
182. McClain CJ. Zinc metabolism in malabsorption syndrome. *J Am Clin Nutr* 1985;4:49–64.
183. Penn D, Lebenthal E. Intestinal mucosal energy metabolism—a new approach to therapy of gastrointestinal disease. *J Pediatr Gastroenterol Nutr* 1990;10:1–4.
184. Morin CL, Ling V, VanCaillie M. Role of oral intake on intestinal adaptation after small bowel resection in growing rates. *Pediatr Res* 1978;12:268–271.
185. Williamson RCN. Medical progress. Intestinal adaptation. Part 1: Structural, functional, and cytokinetic changes. *N Engl J Med* 1978;293:1383–1402.
186. Roediger WEW. Metabolic basis of starvation diarrhea: implication for treatment. *Lancet* 1986;1:1082–1084.
187. Weser E, Heller R, Tawill T. Stimulation of mucosal growth in the rat ileum and pancreatic secretions after jejunal resection. *Gastroenterology* 1977;73:524–529.
188. Williamson RCN, Chir M, Buchholtz TW, Malt RA. Humoral stimulation of cell proliferation in small bowel after transection and resection in rats. *Gastroenterology* 1978;75:249–254.
189. Weser E, Bell D, Tawill T. Effects of octopeptide-cholecystokinin, secretin, and glucagon on intestinal mucosal growth in parenterally nourished rats. *Dig Dis Sci* 1981;26:409–416.
190. Niotk AJ, Crispin JS. The ability of an elemental diet to support nutrition and adaptation in the short gut syndrome. *Ann Surg* 1975;181:200–225.
191. Levin GM, Deren JJ, Stieger E, Zinno R. Role of oral intake in maintenance and disaccharidase activity. *Gastroenterology* 1974;67:975–982.
192. Adel S, Al-Jurf M, Younoszai K, Cahmpman-Furr F. Effect of nutritional method on adaptation of the intestinal remnant after massive bowel resection. *J Pediatr Gastroenterol Nutr* 1985;4:245–252.
193. Firmansyah A, Penn D, Lebenthal E. Isolated colonocyte metabolism of glucose, glutamin, N-butyrate, and β-hydroxybutyrate in malnutrition. *Gastroenterology* 1989;97:622–629.
194. Souba WW, Smith RJ, Wilmore DW. Glutamine metabolism by the intestinal tract. *JPEN J Parenter Enteral Nutr* 1985;9:608–617.
195. Windmueller HG, Spaeth AE. Respiratory fuels and nitrogen metabolism in vivo in small intestine of fed rats. *J Biol Chem* 1980;255:107–112.
196. Kimura RF. Glutamine is the preferred oxidative substrate for small intestine of suckling rat. *Pediatr Res* 1984;18:295A.
197. Mochinzuki C, Hyrocki O, Dominioni L, et al. Mechanism of prevention of post burn hypermetabolism and catabolism by early enteral feeding. *Ann Surg* 1984;200:297–310.
198. Border JR, Hassett J, LaDuca J, et al. The gut origin septic states in blunt multiple trauma (ISS40) in the ICU. *Ann Surg* 1987;206:427–448.
199. Jacobs DO, Evans DA, Meaty K, O'Dwyer ST, Smith RJ, Wilmore DW. Combined effects of glutamine and epidermal growth factor on the rat intestine. *Surgery* 1988;104:358–364.
200. Sauba WW, Smith RJ, Wilmore DW. Effects of glucocorticoids on glutamine metabolism in visceral organs. *Metabolism* 1985;34:450–456.
201. Geer J, Williams PE, Lairmore T, et al. Glucagon: an important stimulator of gut and hepatic glutamine metabolism. *Surg Forum* 1987;38:27–29.
202. Fox AD, Kripke SA, Berman JM, et al. Dexamethasone administration induces increased glutaminase specific activity in the jejunum and colon. *J Surg Res* 1988;44:391–396.
203. Sakata T. Stimulatory effect of short-chain fatty acids on epithelial cell proliferation in rat intestine: a possible explanation for trophic effects of fermentable fibre, gut microbes, and luminal trophic factors. *Br J Nutr* 1987;58:95–103.
204. Roediger WEW. Bacterial short-chain fatty acid and mucosal disease of the colon. *Br J Surg* 1988;75:346–348.
205. Rolandelli RH, Horuda MJ, Settel RH, Rombeau JL. Effects of intraluminal infusion of short-chain fatty acid on the healing of colonic anastomosis in the rat. *Surgery* 1986;100:198–204.
206. Bhatia J, Prihoda AR, Richardson J. Parenteral antibiotics and carbohydrate intolerance in term neonates. *Am J Dis Child* 1986;140:111–113.
207. Harig JM, Soergel KH, Komorwoski RA, Wood CM. Treatment of diversion colitis with short-chain fatty acid irrigation. *N Engl J Med* 1989;320:23–28.
208. McCaffery JF, Nasar K, Lawrence AM, et al. Severe growth retardation in children with inflammatory bowel disease. *Pediatrics* 1970;45:386–393.
209. Kirschner BS, Vinochet O, Rosenberg IH. Growth retardation in inflammatory bowel disease. *Gastroenterology* 1978;75:504–511.
210. Burbidge EJ, Huang S, Bayless TM. Clinical manifestations of Crohn's disease in children and adolescents. *Pediatrics* 1975;55:866–871.
211. Castille RG, Telander RL, Cooney DR, et al. Crohn's disease in children: assessment of the progression of the disease, growth and prognosis. *J Pediatr Surg* 1980;15:462–469.

212. Rosenthal SR, Snyder JD, Hendricks KM, Walker WA. Growth failure and inflammatory bowel disease: approach to treatment of a complicated adolescent problem. *Pediatrics* 1983;72:481–490.
213. Motil KJ, Grand R, Davis-Kraft E. The epidemiology of growth failure in children and adolescents inflammatory bowel disease. *Gastroenterology* 1983;84:1254.
214. Kelts DG, Grand RG, Shen G, et al. Nutritional basis of growth failure in children and adolescents with Crohn's disease. *Gastroenterology* 1979;76:720–727.
215. Smith AN, Balfur TW. Malabsorption in Crohn's disease. *Clin Gastroenterol* 1972;1:433–438.
216. Motil KJ, Grand RJ, Maletskos CJ, et al. The effect of disease, drugs and diet on whole body protein metabolism in adolescents with Crohn's disease and growth failure. *J Pediatr* 1982;101:345–351.
217. Elson CO, Layden TJ, Nemchausky BA, et al. An evaluation of total parenteral nutrition in the management of inflammatory bowel. *Dig Dis Sci* 1980;25(1):42–48.
218. Seidman EG, Bouthillier L, Weber AM, Roy CC, Morin CL. Elemental diet versus prednisone as primary treatment of Crohn's disease (abstr). *Gastroenterology* 1986;90:1625.
219. Belli DC, Seidman E, Bouthiller L, et al. Chronic intermittent elemental diet improves growth failure in children with Crohn's disease. *Gastroenterology* 1988;94:603–610.
220. Discroll RH, Rosenberg IH. Total parenteral nutrition in inflammatory bowel disease. *Med Clin North Am* 1978;62:185–201.
221. Ostro MJ, Greenberg GR, Jeejeebhoy KN. Total parenteral nutrition and complete bowel rest in the management of Crohn's disease. *J Parenter Nutr* 1985;9:280–287.
222. Strobel CT, Byrne WJ, Ament ME. Home parenteral nutrition in children with Crohn's disease—an effective management alternative. *Gastroenterology* 1979;77:272–279.
223. Langman MJS. Can epidemiology help us prevent celiac disease? *Gastroenterology* 1986;90:489–491.
224. Logan RGA, Rifkind EA, Busutti A, Gilmour HM, Ferguson A. Prevalence and "incidence" of celiac disease in Edinburgh and the Lothian region of Scotland. *Gastroenterology* 1986;90:334–342.
225. Langman MJS, McConnell TH, Spiegelhalter DJ, McConell RB. Changing patterns of celiac disease frequency: an analysis of celiac society membership. *Gut* 1985;26:175–178.
226. Burgin-Wolf A, Bertele RM, Berger R, et al. A reliable screening test for childhood celiac disease: fluorescent immunoabsorbent test for gliadin antibodies. *Pediatrics* 1983;102:651–680.
227. Stenhammer L, Kilander AF, Nilsson LA, Stromberg LT, Kowski A. Serum gliadin antibodies for detection and control of childhood celiac disease. *Acta Paediatr Scand* 1984;73:657–663.
228. Eade DE, Lloyd RS, Lang C, Wright R. IgA and IgG reticulin antibodies in celiac and nonceliac patients. *Gut* 1977;18:991–993.
229. Maki M, Hallstrom O, Vesikari T, Visakorpi JK. Evaluation of serum IgA-class reticulin antibody test for the detection of childhood celiac disease. *J Pediatr* 1984;105:901–905.
230. Rossi TM, Kumar V, Lerner A, Heitlinger LA, Tucker N, Fisher J. Relationship of endomysial antibodies to jejunal mucosal pathology: specificity towards both symptomatic and asymptomatic celiacs. *J Pediatr Gastroenterol Nutr* 1988;7:858–863.
231. McNeigh AS. Celiac disease duration of gluten free diet. *Arch Dis Child* 1980;55:110–111.
232. Kumar PG, Harris J, Colyer J, et al. Is a gluten free diet necessary for the treatment of coeliac disease? (abstr). *Gastroenterology* 1985;88:1459.
233. Holmes GKT, Prior P, Lane MR, et al. Malignancy in coeliac disease: effect of a gluten free diet. *Gut* 1989;30:333–335.
234. Colacon J, Eagen-Mitchell B, Stevens FM, et al. Compliance with gluten-free diet in celiac disease. *Arch Dis Child* 1987;62:706–708.
235. Jackson PT, Glasgow JFT, Thom R. Parents understanding of celiac disease and diet. *Arch Dis Child* 1985;60:672–674.
236. Davidson M, Wasserman R. The irritable colon of childhood (chronic nonspecific diarrhea syndrome). *J Pediatr* 1966;69:1027–1038.
237. Davidson M. Functional problems associated with colonic dysfunction. The irritable bowel syndrome. *Pediatr Ann* 1987;16:776–795.
238. Walker-Smith JA. Toddler's diarrhea. *Arch Dis Child* 1981;56:705–707.
239. Simonns FJ. Progress report. New light on ethnic differences in adult lactose intolerance. *Am J Dig Dis* 1973;18:595–611.
240. Chang MH, Hus Hym Chen CJ, Lee Ch, Hus JY. Lactose malabsorption and small-intestinal lactase in normal Chinese children. *J Pediatr Gastroenterol Nutr* 1987;6:369–372.
241. Ferguson A, MacDonald DM, Brydon WG. Prevalence of lactase deficiency in British adults. *Gut* 1984;25:163–167.
242. Douwes AC, Fernandez J, Degenhart HJ. Improved accuracy of lactose intolerance test in children, using expired H2 measurement. *Arch Dis Child* 1978;53:939–942.
243. Alliet P, Kretchmer N, Lebenthal E. Lactase deficiency, lactose malabsorption, and lactose intolerance. In: Lebenthal E, ed. Textbook of gastroenterology and nutrition in infancy. New York: Raven Press 1982;1:459–472.
244. Forget P, Lombet J, Grandils C, Dandrifosse G, Geubelle F. Lactose insufficiency revisited. *J Pediatr Gastroenterol Nutr* 1985;4:868–872.
245. Cohen SA, Hendricks KM, Mathias RK, et al. Chronic nonspecific diarrhea: dietary relationships. *Pediatrics* 1979;64:402–407.
246. Greene HL, Ghishan FK. Excessive fluid as a cause of chronic diarrhea in young children. *J Pediatr* 1983;102:836–840.
247. Hyams JS, Leichtner AM. Apple juice. An unappreciated cause of chronic diarrhea. *Am J Dis Child* 1985;139:503–505.
248. Kneepkens CMF, Jakobs C, Douwes AC. Apple juice, fructose, and chronic nonspecific diarrhea. *Eur J Pediatr* 1989;148:571–572.
249. Cohen SA, Hendricks KM, Eastham EJ, Mathias RK, Walker WA. Chronic nonspecific diarrhea. A complication of dietary fat restriction. *Am J Dis Child* 1979;133:490–492.
250. Jenkins DJA, Wolever TMS, Leeds AR. Dietary fibers, fiber analogues, and glucose tolerance: importance of viscosity. *Br Med J* 1978;1:1392–1394.
251. Saibil F. Diarrhea due to fiber overload (letter). *N Engl J Med* 1989;9:599.

CHAPTER 29

Nutritional Treatment of Growth Failure and Disease Activity in Children with Inflammatory Bowel Disease

Ernest Seidman

Inflammatory bowel disease (IBD) exists in two principal forms: ulcerative colitis and Crohn's disease. Ulcerative colitis is an idiopathic inflammatory disease characterized by continuous involvement of the rectal and colonic mucosa. Crohn's disease, a chronic inflammatory disorder of unknown etiology, can affect any part of the gastrointestinal tract from the mouth to the anus, and is typified by transmural inflammation.

Although originally described in adults, about 25% of IBD cases are diagnosed in the pediatric age group. The symptoms, signs, and overall prognosis in children generally mirror those seen in adults (1). Malnutrition is a major complication in patients of all ages. The nutritional impact is particularly severe in the prepubertal patient, in whom the added macro- and micronutrient costs for growth are unlikely to be met. Growth failure thus represents a common, serious complication unique to the pediatric age group.

Nutritional support, administered by enteral or parenteral routes, is increasingly utilized to treat patients with IBD (2). In this chapter, nutrition, as an adjunctive therapy to prevent or reverse malnutrition, is described. Subsequently, primary nutritional management of the disease activity of IBD is reviewed, including the use of diets or total parenteral nutrition (TPN) to induce remission, reverse complications, and prevent relapses.

MALNUTRITION IN IBD

At the time of first diagnosis, about 85% of pediatric Crohn's, and 65% of pediatric ulcerative colitis, patients have lost weight. As the disease progresses, particularly during the first few years, undernutrition becomes increasingly apparent. As symptoms increase, the patient's nutritional status progressively deteriorates. This is particularly true in the young Crohn's patient, where upper gastrointestinal and small bowel involvement are frequently accompanied by anorexia, even in the absence of other symptoms or signs of active disease (1,3). Undernutrition and its associated complications may become more debilitating than the underlying IBD.

Management goals are to ascertain and correct nutritional deficits, as well as to control symptoms. An initial, accurate assessment of the impact of IBD on the nutritional status of the patient will aid in designing a case-specific nutritional support program to meet management goals (4).

Assessment of Macronutrient Status of Children with IBD

Both clinical and research techniques are available to assess the protein and energy status of the child with IBD (5). Variables may be measured once to provide static data. More valuable, however, is the evaluation of dynamic changes over time, before and after alterations in disease activity or intervention strategies.

Parameters of protein and energy status include linear growth, weight, and nutritional and inflammatory markers. Height and weight can either indicate acute nutritional status, i.e., weight-for-height, or chronic nutritional status, i.e., height-for-age. Each of these converts individual measurements into percentiles when compared to an appropriate population standard. Using Wa-

E. Seidman: Department of Pediatrics and Nutrition, University of Montreal, Montreal, Québec, H3T IC5 Canada.

TABLE 1. *Nutritional assessment of the pediatric IBD patient*

Subjective nutritional assessment
    Detailed history
    Complete physical examination, pubertal staging
    Diet evaluation (3-day diary)
Anthropometry
    Height, weight
    Growth velocity
    Height-for-age, weight-for-height %
    Midarm circumference
    Tricipital skin-fold thickness
Laboratory data
    CBC, morphology
    Serum albumin
    Folic acid, B_{12}
    Serum Fe, TIBC, ferritin
    Calcium, magnesium, alkaline phosphatase
    Bone age
Additional tests if growth failure or significant malnutrition is present
    Vitamins A, D, E
    PT, PTT
    Zinc
    Retinol-binding protein
    24-hr urinary magnesium
    Phosphorus

From ref. 5, with permission.
PT, prothrombin time; PTT, partial thromboplastin time; TIBC, total iron binding capacity.

terlow's criteria, an initial determination of the severity of acute and chronic malnutrition can be ascertained (4).

Height and weight velocities, that is, the rate of growth over time, demonstrate growth patterns as compared to a norm, and are sensitive indicators of growth failure. Because growth occurs in spurts, velocities derived from intervals of less than 1 year may be inaccurate (6,7). The care and the quality of the instruments with which the measurements are taken are extremely important to their accuracy. Optimally, growth measurements should be recorded by the same individual each time (4).

Midarm muscle circumference (MAMC) and triceps skin-fold thickness (TSF) measurements, when compared to standards for age, are a reflection of protein and energy stores, respectively (4). Urinary creatinine/height index and/or 3-methylhistidine/creatinine excretion provide more sensitive measures of lean body muscle mass than MAMC. Stable isotopes, underwater weighing, total body electromagnetic conductance, and bioimpedance analysis are additional methods used for assessment of body composition (4,5). These methods are relatively unavailable and lack normative values for children. They are, therefore, often impractical outside of the research setting.

Various biochemical measurements estimate the functional aspects of body protein stores. Serum proteins that document acute or chronic protein depletion in the child with IBD include albumin, prealbumin, transferrin, and retinol-binding protein. In the research setting, one can measure basal metabolic rates, or use balance techniques or indirect calorimetry to assess the adaptive metabolic responses to IBD or to nutritional therapies (4,5).

Qualitative aspects of the inflammatory process may also be evaluated in the IBD patient using acute-phase reactant proteins (orosomucoid, α_1- and α_2-macroglobulins, transferrin, C-reactive protein, complement levels, and erythrocyte sedimentation rate). A serum protein electrophoresis, revealing hypoalbuminemia, with increased acute-phase reactant proteins (α_1- and α_2-macroglobulins) is an excellent indicator of increased inflammatory activity and protein-losing enteropathy. We have found this test superior to fecal α_1-antitrypsin determination in following a patient's inflammation and nutritional status (8).

A variety of growth, anthropometric, biochemical, and metabolic measurements have been declared to be useful (5) in the serial evaluation of each pediatric patient with IBD (Table 1).

Definition of Growth Failure in IBD

Growth failure implies a pathologic deviation from normal growth rate and must be differentiated from genetically determined short stature. Height measurements alone, therefore, do not reliably indicate growth failure (Table 2). Both disease-related growth failure and constitutionally delayed growth are associated with delayed puberty. Bone age determination, therefore, will also be delayed in both cases.

Normal growth is illustrated by the predictable curve of an infant's first 2 years of life in which birth parameters "channel" to childhood growth percentiles. Growth failure is a progressive deviation downward from this established growth curve, reflecting a fall in height velocity.

On standard growth velocity curves, prepubertal girls in the 3rd percentile increase their height by a minimum

TABLE 2. *Evaluation of short stature in IBD*

Cause of short stature	Height below 5th percentile	Bone age/pubertal delay	Height velocity abnormal
Genetic	+	−	−
Constitutionally delayed	+	+	−
IBD-related	±	+	+

From ref. 5, with permission.

of 4.2 cm/year; boys increase by 3.7 cm/year. Females growing less than 4 cm/year and males less than 3.5 cm/year are growing more than two standard deviations below the mean. This can be described as growth failure (5). Because this status is often associated with pubertal and bone age delay (Table 2), the height velocity must be interpreted in the context of bone, not chronological, age. An increase in growth velocity subsequent to therapeutic intervention indicates the initiation of catch-up growth.

A change in weight is generally indicative of an acute nutritional insult. In the child with IBD, alterations in weight may be influenced by hydration status, use of steroids, as well as disease, and is not, therefore, used as an index of growth failure (5).

Growth Failure in IBD Patients

At the time of diagnosis, 56% of our Crohn's patients were below the 3rd percentile for weight-for-age. Weight loss averaged 6 kg (1) per patient. Growth failure, defined as a height velocity greater than 2 SD below mean for bone age, is seen in almost one-half of our Crohn's and one-tenth of our ulcerative colitis patients (1,8). Severe impairment of linear growth may precede clinical evidence of bowel disease, and growth failure often continues even when IBD appears to be in clinical remission (1,9).

Micronutrient deficiencies (Table 3) as discussed below, commonly coexist with IBD and tend to be associated with extensive disease and macronutrient deficiency. Although data is primarily from pediatric Crohn's disease, the same considerations probably apply to pediatric ulcerative colitis. Numerous mechanisms contribute to the malnutrition and micronutrient deficiencies of IBD (Table 4), but inadequate caloric intake is probably the primary cause (2,9,10). Eating often brings on painful symptoms or diarrhea. Thus, malnutrition tends to be more common in patients with

TABLE 3. *Prevalence of common nutritional deficiencies in pediatric inflammatory bowel disease*

	Crohn's disease[a] (%)	Ulcerative colitis[b] (%)
Iron	83	58
Anemia	87	60
Weight loss	83	33
Hypoalbuminemia	75	35
Growth failure	47	10
Pubertal delay	30	20
Zinc	30	rare
Vitamin B_{12}	<5	<5
Calcium	10	rare
Folic acid	5	30

[a] Adapted from ref. 8.
[b] Adapted from ref. 1.

TABLE 4. *Causes of malnutrition in children with inflammatory bowel disease*

Decreased nutrient intake
  Disease-induced
  Iatrogenic
Malabsorption
  Diminished absorptive surface (disease, fistulae, resection)
  Bacterial overgrowth
  Bile salt deficiency
Increased gut losses
  Protein-losing enteropathy
  Electrolytes, minerals, trace metals (diarrhea and fistula)
  Bleeding
Drug-nutrient interactions
  Corticosteroids (calcium, protein)
  Sulfasalazine (folate)
  Cholestyramine (fat, vitamins)
Increased requirements
  Sepsis, fever
  Increased cell turnover
  Replace losses: catch-up growth

From ref. 5, with permission.

Crohn's disease involving proximal segments of small intestine because pain associated with food intake, and malabsorption, are more prominent in these patients. Iatrogenic dietary restrictions can further reduce caloric intake, often unnecessarily.

Extensive disease, surgical resection, and bacterial overgrowth contribute to malabsorption. Nutrient losses also occur because of protein exudation from the inflamed gut, iron loss by bleeding, and mineral loss through diarrhea. Other potential contributors to malnutrition (2) include steroid therapy and increased nutritional requirements caused by fever, internal fistulae, or inflammatory activity. Studies have shown, however, that most Crohn's disease patients without fever or sepsis do not have increased basal energy expenditure (11,12). Thus, chronic inflammation, itself, does not impose additional energy requirements. Drugs associated with malnutrition include sulfasalazine, which interferes with folate absorption; corticosteroids, which suppress calcium absorption; and cholestyramine, which impairs the absorption of fat and fat-soluble vitamins (Table 4).

In early IBD, as the gut becomes inflamed, patients often ingest less food. Progressive ulceration and inflammation result in cramping pains and/or diarrhea subsequent to food intake. Partial bowel obstruction or lactose intolerance may also cause acute postprandial symptoms. At this juncture, restricting lactose or fiber intake may transiently control symptoms. It is essential to supplement, rather than merely modify, the diet of the patient with weight loss. Polymeric formulas are available (2) that supply essential nutrients, restore weight, and improve symptoms. As symptoms increase, however, nutritional status generally worsens and polymeric supplements may no longer help. When that occurs, more intensive nutritional support, either concurrent with drug therapy or as a primary therapeutic approach, is indicated. The modality of choice is enteral elemental nutrition, which is almost entirely absorbed in the proximal small bowel (2).

Indications that management goals are not being met include progressive weight loss, diarrhea and pain, recurrent fever, increased abdominal mass, fistulae, anemia, and increasing hypoalbuminemia. In the past, total parenteral nutrition (TPN) was commonly employed to induce remission and improve nutritional status in such patients (13). Short-term TPN may, in fact, be useful as preparation for surgery, or to improve the nutritional status of the anorectic or malnourished patient with IBD. The only other circumstances to favor TPN in IBD are limited to the patient with a very short gut (less than 60 cm of functional small bowel), when there is a high-volume fistula that tube placement cannot bypass, or when there is near-complete obstruction.

For the most part, the cost and the risks of TPN substantiate the use of enteral nutrition, when possible, in patients with Crohn's disease. This is especially true in colonic or distal ileal Crohn's disease associated with normal jejunal and proximal ileal function. Enteral elemental nutrition is also appropriate in the malnourished Crohn's disease patient who is either steroid-dependent or -resistant (14). Enteral elemental nutrition, at 70 to 80 kilocalories per kilogram body weight per day, may not only reverse the malnutrition but, as discussed later, may induce remission as well (9).

Studies confirm that elemental diet therapy is a safe, well-tolerated, and effective treatment for acute Crohn's disease (2,15). In preoperative Crohn's disease patients, it appears to alleviate disease activity and to improve nutritional status (16). As with TPN, the mechanisms for improvement are not yet clear (5). Possible mechanisms are discussed later in this chapter.

Nutritional Therapy of Growth Failure in Children with IBD

The etiology of malnutrition and growth failure in IBD is multifactorial (Table 4). Inadequate nutrient intake is the most important factor leading to altered body composition and growth arrest in IBD (2,9,10). Motil et al. (11) have demonstrated that young Crohn's disease patients and normal controls have similar whole-body nitrogen flux, rates of protein synthesis and breakdown, and net protein retention. Thus, the key in managing growth failure is adequate, long-term renutrition.

In the prepubertal adolescent, the potential for growth is limited because of bone maturation and eventual epiphyseal fusion. This occurs concomitantly with sexual development. Early and aggressive intervention is, therefore, important in IBD complicated by growth failure.

The aim of therapy is to supply nutritional support adequate to reverse growth arrest, to permit "catch-up" growth, and to achieve the premorbid growth curve of the patient. Reinitiation of growth will only begin when weight becomes appropriate for height. The necessary caloric intake for catch-up growth, then, must be estimated according to the child's ideal weight for his age or calculated at approximately 150% of actual weight for age.

Although intestinal and systemic symptoms respond favorably to corticosteroids, severe growth impairment often persists, even in the absence of significant disease activity (9). Thirty-one percent of our Crohn's patients were below the 3rd percentile for height at the time of diagnosis (17). Despite therapy that included oral polymeric caloric supplementation, 28% remained growth retarded after a mean of $3\frac{1}{2}$ years follow-up. Of those patients initially presenting with growth failure, 50% failed to achieve any catch-up growth (1,17). Recent data from our multicentered study also suggest that chronic malnutrition and growth failure often persist in pediatric patients followed for Crohn's disease (8).

Surgical resection of diseased segments has been considered an alternative in the management of growth failure. Our experience is that less than half of these patients achieve significant "catch-up" growth postoperatively (1,17). In fact, long-term follow-up of a large series of growth-retarded Crohn's patients revealed that, whether medically or surgically treated, patients achieved an adult height significantly less than the normal population (18). Surgery, therefore, should only be considered for growth failure in the prepubertal Crohn's disease patients when extensive medical and nutritional therapy has failed.

The success of nutritional therapy in reversing growth failure in IBD is convincing evidence of malnutrition as a primary etiologic factor. Initially, total parenteral nutrition (TPN) was shown to induce weight gain and to reverse growth arrest in Crohn's disease. Its use is limited, however, by metabolic and infectious complications, as well as cost considerations. The enteral route, on the other hand, may be used to achieve nutritional rehabilitation even in the presence of disease (9,19). Our experience utilizing polymeric oral nutritional supplements yielded disappointing long-term growth results (1,17). Patients may regain weight initially, but disease-induced anorexia and a lack of long-term patient compliance, greatly limit the growth achieved by this simple method. A study of the effect of oral supplements in adult Crohn's patients showed that the compliance was as low as 20% at 6 months (20). These poor results were attributed to unpalatability, abdominal cramps, and diarrhea.

In 1982, our group reported that an elemental diet for 6 weeks improved linear and ponderal growth rates in adolescents with Crohn's disease and growth failure (21).

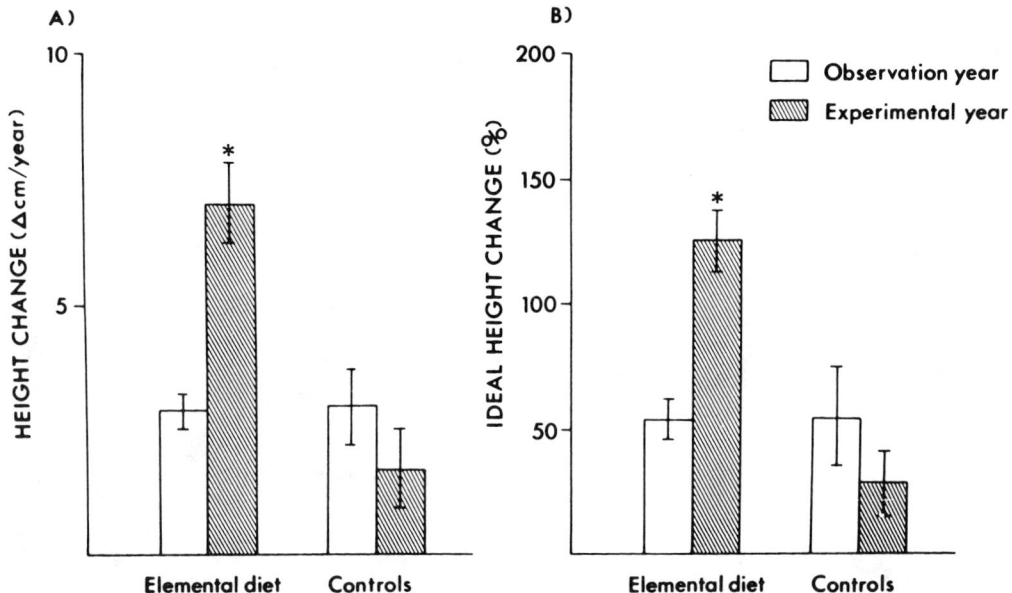

FIG. 1. Absolute (*A*) and ideal (*B*) height changes (Δ cm measured/Δ cm predicted for the 50th percentile according to bone age × 100) in the elemental diet (ED) and control groups during both observation and experimental years (*$p < .01$ vs observation year of ED group and vs experimental year of controls). (From ref. 9, with permission.)

This was achieved by providing 70 to 80 Cal/kg of an elemental formula (Vivonex, Norwich Eaton) via continuous nasogastric infusion.

More recently, we examined the possibility that intermittent courses of elemental diet therapy may reverse growth failure as well as improve the clinical course in Crohn's disease (9). The elemental formula was administered nocturnally at home by continuous nasogastric infusion, allowing patients to resume normal daily activities, including attendance at school. Patients in the treatment group received Vivonex therapy 1 month out of every 4 for 1 year. Anthropometric measurements demonstrated significant height (Fig. 1) and weight (Fig. 2) gains in patients given an elemental diet compared to controls receiving standard medical therapy. There was also a decrease in Crohn's disease activity (Fig. 3) and

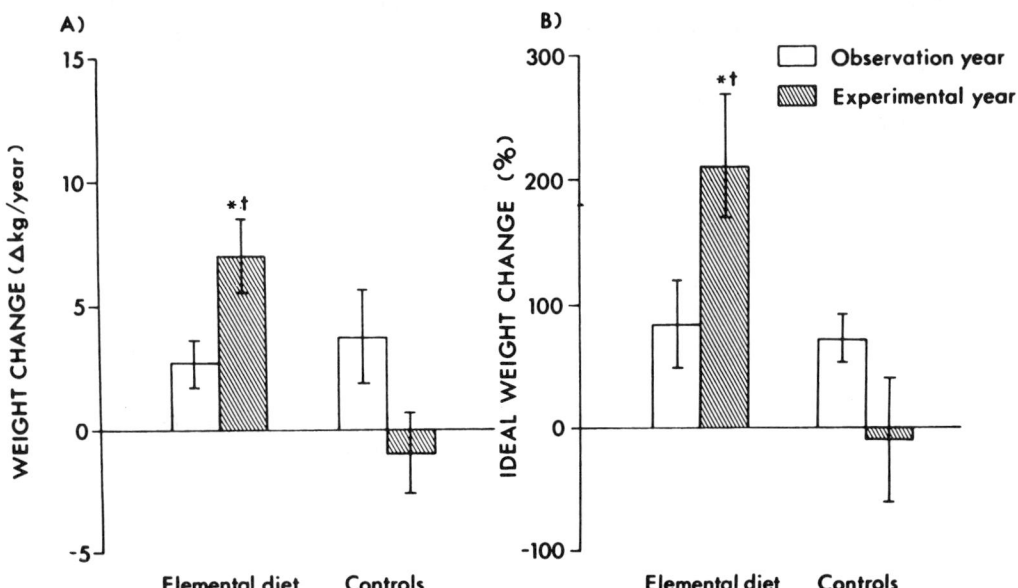

FIG. 2. Absolute (*A*) and ideal (*B*) weight changes (Δ kg measured/Δ kg predicted for the 50th percentile according to bone age × 100) in the ED and control groups during both observation and experimental years (*$p < .05$ vs observation year of ED group; †$p < .01$ vs experimental year of controls). (From ref. 9, with permission.)

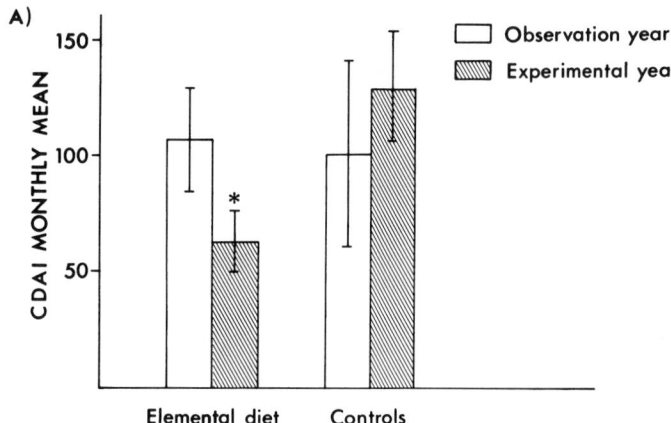

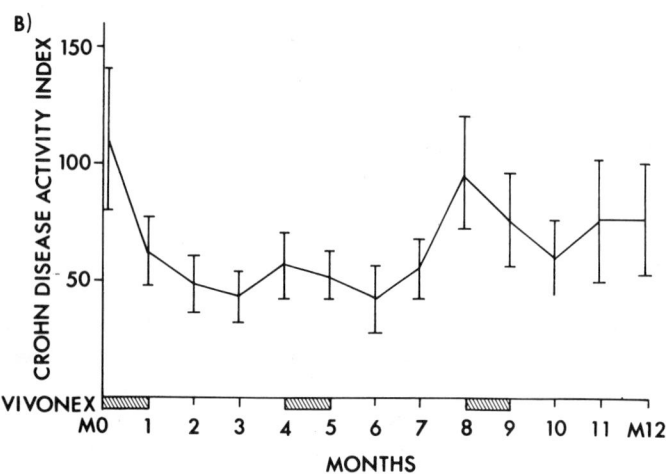

FIG. 3. (A) Monthly mean Crohn's disease activity index (CDAI) in the ED and control groups during observation and experimental years (*$p < .05$ vs observation year of ED group and vs experimental year of controls). (B) Modification of CDAI in the ED group during the experimental year. (From ref. 9, with permission.)

prednisone requirements (Fig. 4) in patients receiving the elemental diet therapy (9).

Adequate nutrient intake will, over time, permit correction of growth retardation. Optimum catch-up is more likely via a nocturnal nasogastric infusion route rather than high-calorie oral supplements (9,19). Nasogastric infusion also has the advantage of interfering less with normal daily dietary habits and may be used as a supplement in those patients in whom growth failure dominates the clinical picture.

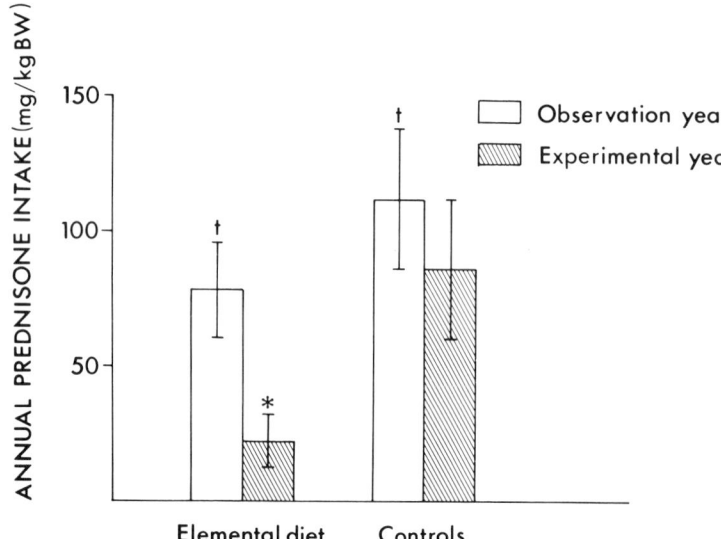

FIG. 4. Total annual prednisone intake (milligrams per kilogram body weight) in the ED and control groups during both the observation and the experimental years (*$p < .05$ vs observation year of ED group and vs experimental year of controls; †no significant difference between the two groups during observation year). (From ref. 9, with permission.)

Nocturnal administration of a polymeric formula can also reverse growth failure (19). However, Crohn's disease patients who are growth retarded and in relapse, or those with intestinal fistula or steroid dependence or resistance, probably constitute a group requiring an elemental enteral diet to the exclusion of other food intake in order to achieve "bowel rest" (22).

We generally recommend gavage feedings three times a year, once every 4 months (9). Administration continually for longer consecutive periods (19) does not appear to be have an advantage unless the patient's bone age suggests imminent epiphyseal closure.

On nocturnal Vivonex administration, once every 4 months, our patients had a mean annual growth of 7 cm, or 126% of the ideal growth rate for normal children of the same age (9). Prior to elemental diet supplementation, the growth rate for this group had only been 2.9 cm or 54% of ideal; the growth rate for medically treated controls, as well, was only 1.7 cm or 29% of ideal (Fig. 1).

Similarly, weight gain in the elemental diet group during the experimental year (6.9 ± 1.5 kg) was significantly higher than during the same group's observation year (2.7 ± 1 kg, $p < .05$), as well as compared to the control group (-0.9 ± 1.6 kg, $p < .001$) (Fig. 2).

Contraindications are less than 5% and generally limited to surgical complications (perforation, bowel obstruction, toxic megacolon) or patient nonacceptance. The child must be closely followed, ideally by a dietitian, to assure that caloric intake meets or exceeds the requirements for the 50th percentile of weight-for-age. Malnourished patients should receive 70 to 80 Cal/kg ideal weight/day. Supplementation should include vitamin K (5 mg twice weekly), folic acid (2.5 mg twice weekly), and elemental iron (1.5 mg/kg/day). Prednisone tapering by 5 mg per week may also be attempted. The diet ends with a 5-day period during which the diet is progressively replaced, as is described elsewhere (9,15).

There is an advantage to the pubertal and bone age delay in the growth-retarded adolescent with Crohn's disease because it allows time for nutritional intervention. When pubertal development and bone maturation are advanced, nocturnal supplementation must be instituted immediately and continually over several months. Unfortunately, nutritional therapy is often begun too close to epiphyseal maturation because the growth failure that results from minimal disease activity may go unnoticed.

MICRONUTRIENT DEFICIENCIES IN THE PEDIATRIC IBD PATIENT

The pathophysiologic mechanisms resulting in micronutrient deficiencies are similar to those that lead to macronutrient deficiencies (Table 4). Most studies, however, have examined adult IBD patients (23,24), and their conclusions cannot all be extrapolated to the pediatric age group. Furthermore, although they refer to IBD populations in general, the results often pertain specifically to Crohn's disease. Our recent multicentered study (8) suggests that several micronutrients deserve particular attention in the young IBD patient (Table 3).

Water-Soluble Vitamins

Folic acid is absorbed along the small bowel; 50% is stored within the liver. Overall storage capacity is relatively low and deficiencies may occur within several months. Our recent study suggests that only 5% of pediatric Crohn patients have abnormal folate levels (8). Harries and Heatley (25) reported low serum folate in 38% of Crohn's patients. Another report found deficiencies in 59% of ulcerative colitis patients (26). Inadequate intake of folate, which has been found in three-quarters of Crohn's disease patients, may be a cause of deficiency (27). Other causes include sulfasalazine intake, which interferes with absorption and/or malabsorption due to bowel inflammation or resection. This may explain the higher prevalence of folate deficiency in colitis patients (Table 3). Low serum folate levels may also be predictive of other vitamin deficiencies, including B_6, B_{12}, and C (28).

Vitamin B_{12} deficiency has been reported to occur in about one-fifth of Crohn's disease patients (25). Our recent analysis suggests that the pediatric prevalence is relatively low (8). B_{12} deficiency can be caused by ileitis or resection, gastritis, and bacterial overgrowth. Decreased intake is found in about one-third of patients (27,28).

Vitamin B_6 intake is also often inadequate in Crohn's disease (28), but sideroblastic anemia has not been described. Deficient dietary intake of thiamine (vitamin B_1), riboflavin (vitamin B_2), and pantothenic acid is also common (28).

Vitamin C deficiency in Crohn's disease has been described (29). A controversy exists as to whether abnormal tissue vitamin C levels are a contributing factor to fistula formation in Crohn's disease (30,31).

Niacin (32) and biotin (33) deficiencies have also been reported in Crohn's disease.

Fat-Soluble Vitamins

Vitamin A deficiency is most often associated with low levels of retinol-binding protein due to a decrease in visceral protein synthesis. When the diagnosis was confirmed by abnormal dark adaptation tests, the incidence of vitamin A deficiency in Crohn's patients was only 5% (34). Patients with severe acute malnutrition appeared to be at high risk.

Vitamin D deficiency has been reported in as many as two-thirds of Crohn's patients. Deficiency correlates well with anthropometric evidence of protein and energy malnutrition (25). Pathogenic mechanisms primarily include fat malabsorption, and bile acid loss leading to reduced enterohepatic circulation (35). Patients with previous ileal resection are at particularly high risk for osteomalacia (36,37).

Vitamin E levels have been reported to be lower in patients with extensive Crohn's disease (38). The consequences of this deficiency, in view of its role as a free radical scavenger, on tissue healing and inflammation are still unknown.

Vitamin K deficiency is relatively common in both Crohn's disease and ulcerative colitis (39). Potential causes include malabsorption and antibiotic use.

Minerals and Trace Elements

Iron deficiency and associated anemias are the most common abnormalities (Table 3). Measures of serum iron, however, may reflect alterations in serum proteins due to the acute phase response or to a protein-losing enteropathy. Serum ferritin correlates well with total body iron stores (25,30). Deficiency is multifactorial, related to gut losses and inadequate intake.

Zinc deficiency in pediatric IBD remains controversial in terms of measurement and significance (40). Low serum values often reflect hypoalbuminemia (41). Malabsorption and excessive urinary losses during catabolism are important factors in hypozincemia (42,43). The potential role of zinc deficiency in growth failure also warrants special attention (44–46). Almost one-third of pediatric Crohn's disease patients in disease relapse are deficient (Table 3).

Calcium deficiency, although common, is often indicative of hypoalbuminemia rather than reflecting a true deficit (25). Nevertheless, abnormal calcium metabolism in association with corticosteroid therapy places pediatric IBD patients at high risk for the development of calcium phosphate kidney stones (47).

Magnesium (Mg) deficiency occurs in IBD and may cause symptoms such as muscle cramps and bone pain (48). Intestinal losses, decreased intake, and malabsorption all play a role (48); small bowel resection is also an important risk factor (49). Periodic 24-hr urine collections are preferable to screening with serum Mg levels (48–50).

Deficiencies in copper, chromium, iodine, manganese, molybdenum, and selenium are rare and generally associated with long-term TPN (51).

Recommendations for Screening in IBD

Clinical variables that help determine screening for nutritional deficits in pediatric IBD include, but are not limited to, the type, location, and severity of the disease, the presence of resections, medication use, and diet and nutritional status.

In addition to a complete physical examination and routine anthropometric measurements (Table 1), a CBC with erythrocyte morphology, serum iron, ferritin, folic acid, B_{12}, and albumin are routine. Other determinations, including serum alkaline phosphatase to screen for zinc and vitamin D deficiency, serum vitamin A, calcium, and urinary Mg, should be monitored in patients with growth failure or significant acute malnutrition (5).

NUTRITIONAL MANAGEMENT OF DISEASE ACTIVITY IN INFLAMMATORY BOWEL DISEASE

Demonstration of the effectiveness of TPN in controlling the disease activity and complications of Crohn's disease (52,53) has been influential in the consideration of nutritional therapy as a primary therapy of IBD (53).

Some uncontrolled studies have suggested that clinical remission in Crohn's disease can be achieved using an elemental diet (2,53). These encouraging results have been substantiated by several controlled trials comparing corticosteroids (54–57) or TPN (58) with an elemental diet in acute Crohn's disease (Table 5). Results suggest that an elemental diet induces remission in Crohn's

TABLE 5. *Controlled trials utilizing elemental diets in active Crohn's disease*

Study (ref.)	Patients randomized (N)	Treatment period (weeks)	% Success rate Diet group	% Success rate Control group	Statistical difference
O'Morain et al. (54)	21	4	(E) 81.8	(P) 80	None
Saverymuttu et al. (55)	32	1.5	(E) 93.7	(P) 100	None
Seidman et al. (56)	19	3	(E) 77.8	(P) 66.7	None
Sanderson et al. (57)	17	6	(S-E) 87.5	(P) 85.7	None
Alun Jones (58)	36	2	(E) 84.6	(TPN) 87.5	None
Lochs et al. (59)	107	6	(S-E) 52.7	(P) 78.8	$p < .001$
Giaffer et al. (60)	30	4	(E) 75	(N-E) 36	$p < .03$

From ref. 5, with permission.
E, elemental diet; S-E, semi-elemental; N-E, nonelemental, polymeric; P, prednisone or prednisolone; TPN, total parenteral nutrition.

with the efficacy and rapidity of standard medical management. Improvement in symptoms and decreased disease activity index scores have also been associated with weight gain, diminished sedimentation rate, and reduced fecal granulocyte and protein losses. Only a study in which a semi-elemental diet was used suggested that steroids induced remission with greater efficacy and rapidity (59). A controlled study comparing elemental and nonelemental diets, administered isocalorically, clearly showed that an elemental formula was superior in inducing remission of active Crohn's disease (60). These results illustrate the importance of specifying the nature of the nutritional therapy (i.e., elemental vs semi-elemental or defined-formula diet). In addition, factors such as the severity, duration, and, particularly, the localization of Crohn's disease, may largely influence response to any therapy. In general, distal disease (colon, perianal) responds less favorably to nutritional treatment (61,62).

Elemental diet to induce remission of Crohn's disease (Table 6) is advantageous because of the virtual absence of side effects, the avoidance of drugs that stunt growth, and the improved growth in children resulting from nutritional repletion. It is also simpler, safer, and less expensive than TPN. Finally, the elemental formula can be administered nocturnally, at home, without necessitating lengthy hospitalization, permitting resumption of normal daytime activities.

When an elemental diet is used to treat disease activity in Crohn's disease, no other intake may be allowed. Patients and families must understand that, for a 1-month trial period, food intake will be limited to daytime clear fluids plus flavored elemental diet supplements, and nocturnal gavage (9,22). Reassurance should be given that hunger will not be a problem and that this treatment will improve symptoms and probably result in a substantial weight gain. The encouragement of the clinician is undoubtedly a key to acceptance of this diet.

The major disadvantage of elemental diets is their unpalatability, although this problem may be easily overcome by nasogastric infusion. Other disadvantages (Table 6) include the earlier relapse rate when discontinued (56,63), and the lower efficiency in distal (colonic/perianal) disease (62). Although the routine use of elemental diets to induce remission in pediatric Crohn's disease cannot yet be recommended, there is a definite role in selected cases, particularly in children with severe growth failure, when steroids may prevent catch-up growth.

Maintenance of Remission in IBD Using Nutritional Management

Diets that attempt to maintain remission in IBD are generally not effective (64). These include both "low-residue" and "high-fiber, low–refined sugar" diets (65,66). Although nutritional therapy (elemental diet or TPN) induces remission in Crohn's disease, its use for the maintenance of long-term remission is unclear. Reports suggest that most patients on TPN relapse promptly when they return to a normal diet (13,53). Furthermore, significant infectious and metabolic complications, as well as a nonnegligible mortality rate, have been associated with home TPN.

Chronic use of oligopeptide solution appears to effect long-term remission of pediatric Crohn's disease patients (63). Relapse did occur, however, once the elemental diet was discontinued. Except for highly selected cases, one could not ethically recommend maintaining a young patient on an elemental diet for more than a few months per year.

Using intermittent courses of elemental diet, we found an improved clinical outcome and catch-up growth in pediatric Crohn patients (9). The Crohn's disease activity index remained lower (Fig. 3), and the requirement for corticosteroids was significantly lower for patients in the elemental diet–treated group (Fig. 4).

Jones et al. (67) have provided provocative evidence that exclusion of specific foods on the basis of clinical intolerance dramatically improves the clinical course of Crohn's disease. These encouraging results await future corroborative studies.

Nutritional Management of Severe Crohn's Disease

Steroid dependence and resistance constitute two other potential indications for the use of elemental diet in Crohn's disease (Table 7). Seven of nine steroid-dependent adult patients studied anecdotally achieved remission with elemental diet; five of these remained in remission without steroids for 6 to 16 months (14). Only four of the ten steroid-resistant patients entered into sustained remission with nutritional therapy. In two steroid-resistant patients, TPN did not improve symptoms and surgery was required. TPN use in particularly severe, steroid-resistant Crohn's disease resulted in a

TABLE 6. *Elemental diet in treating active Crohn's disease*

Advantages
    Improved nutrition (nitrogen balance) and growth (vs prednisone)
    Nocturnal administration
    Excellent compliance
    Few complications (vs TPN)
    Steroid sparing
    Less costly (vs TPN)
    Short hospitalization (vs TPN)
Disadvantages
    Unpalatable
    Cost (vs prednisone)
    Less effective in colitis (vs prednisone)
    Significant early relapse rate when discontinued
    Fistula may reopen when discontinued

TABLE 7. *Indications for the use of elemental diet in pediatric Crohn's disease*

Proven indications
   Reversing growth failure and malnutrition
   Induction of remission
   Steroid-dependent/resistant cases
   Preoperative preparation (if malnourished)
Potential indications
   Closing fistulae (postoperative)
   Maintenance of remission
   Strictures (without obstruction)

From ref. 5, with permission.

TABLE 8. *Hypothetical mechanisms of nutritional therapy in inflammatory bowel disease*

"Bowel rest" adaptive response
   Decreased gut metabolic activity
   Altered motility, blood flow
   Induction of distal small-bowel atrophy
   Decreased pancreaticobiliary secretion
   Altered gut hormones/trophic factors
   Essential fatty acid deficiency
   Availability of glutamine
   Altered availability of short-chain fatty acids
Immunologic effects
   Decreased macromolecular (dietary, bacterial) antigen uptake
   Alteration of fecal flora
   Improved cell-mediated immunity
   Decreased gut lymphocyte recirculation owing to diminished lymphatic flow
   Decreased lymphocyte losses via gut
   Altered synthesis of inflammatory mediators (eicosanoids)
   Absence of purines, nucleotides
Nutritional effects
   Improved nitrogen/caloric intake
   Correction of micronutrient deficiencies (vitamins, trace elements)
   Decreased enteric losses (protein, trace elements)
   Altered fat and fiber intake

From ref. 5, with permission.

rapid and highly efficacious improvement in 90% of cases in one uncontrolled observation (68).

We have found elemental diet therapy to be of substantial benefit in steroid-dependent patients, particularly if growth failure or malnutrition is present. Nutritional therapy is less effective, however, whether enteral or parenteral, when steroid dependence involves the colon alone. A trial of elemental diet therapy in corticodependent patients is definitely worthwhile prior to considering additional immunosuppression or surgery. Nutritional therapy should also be considered for patients who are corticoresistant.

Both TPN and elemental diets have been utilized for Crohn's disease complicated by strictures and fistulae. Although controlled series are lacking, the majority of patients will eventually require surgery once "bowel rest" is replaced by a low-residue diet (62). A possible exception might be fistulae that occur postoperatively, in which case long-term closure can usually be achieved using nutritional therapy alone. Use of an elemental diet in perianal disease does not seem to have long-term success (62). Preoperative elemental diet therapy is useful in surgical cases such as fistulae, abscess, or fibrotic stricture (Table 7). Nasogastric Vivonex reduced symptoms in all 11 pediatric patients preoperatively, 7 of whom were weaned completely off steroids, whereas the remainder were able to reduce the dose substantially (16). In carefully selected cases, elemental diet therapy can effectively reduce Crohn's disease activity and may be considered as part of the current therapeutic arsenal of a patient with severe Crohn's disease.

Nutritional Management of Disease Activity in IBD: Future Research Considerations

The success of nutritional therapy in the treatment of acute Crohn's disease is interesting in terms of determining an etiology for IBD (5,22). The mechanisms by which elemental diet therapy improves Crohn's disease are, however, unknown. The beneficial effects are presumed to result from "bowel rest" combined with adequate nutrition. Demonstrations that a nonelemental diet is inferior to an elemental diet fed isocalorically supports a mechanism other than improved nutrition alone (60). There are three potential mechanisms to explain the response to elemental diets: "bowel rest", immunologic effects, and nutritional effects (Table 8). These mechanisms are discussed in detail elsewhere (5).

Future research will probably focus on the role of specific nutritional factors, especially glutamine, in maintaining gut mucosal homeostasis (69,70). The role of dietary purines and pyramidines in modulating mucosal immunity and stricture formation should also be investigated (71). Studying dietary fatty acids and the mucosal immune response (72) may reveal whether essential fatty acid deficient diets can reduce intestinal eicosanoid synthesis and, thereby, improve chronic IBD. Preliminary studies have suggested that fish oil supplementation (eicosapentenoic acid) improves disease activity in IBD (73–75). Further investigations on the potential role of polyunsaturated fatty acids, as found in fish oils, on disease activity in pediatric IBD, is essential. Research of this type will increase our understanding of the mechanisms that initiate and perpetuate the chronic inflammatory lesions of IBD and help to develop new therapeutic modalities to successfully treat them.

REFERENCES

1. Seidman EG, Weber AM, Morin CL, Roy CC. Inflammatory bowel disease in childhood. In: Freeman HJ, ed. *Inflammatory bowel disease,* Vol 2. Boca Raton: CRC Press, 1989;217–247.

2. Seidman EG. Nutritional management of inflammatory bowel disease. *Gastroenterol Clin North Am* 1989;18:129–155.
3. Lenaerts C, Roy CC, Vaillancourt M, Weber AM, Morin CL, Seidman E. High incidence of upper GI tract involvement in children with Crohn's disease. *Pediatrics* 1989;83:777–781.
4. Atlan P, Seidman E. Nutritional considerations in pediatric patients. *Can J Gastroenterol* 1990;4:41A–47A.
5. Seidman E, LeLeiko N, Ament M, Berman W, Caplan D, Evans J, Kocoshis S, Lake A, Motil K, Sutphen J, Thomas D. Nutritional issues in pediatric inflammatory bowel disease. *J Pediatr Gastroenterol Nutr* 1991;12:424–438.
6. World Health Organization. Use and interpretation of anthropometric indicators of nutritional status. *WHO bulletin,* number 64(6). Geneva: WHO, 1986;924–941.
7. Kien CL. Failure to thrive. In: Walker WA, Watkins JB, eds. *Nutrition in pediatrics.* Boston: Little, Brown, 1985;757–768.
8. Seidman E, Bagnell P, Griffiths AM, Issenman R, Jones A. Growth failure and nutritional deficiencies in pediatric patients with active Crohn's disease. *Gastroenterology* 1991;100:A249.
9. Belli D, Seidman EG, Bouthillier L, et al. Chronic intermittent elemental diet improves growth failure in children with Crohn's disease. *Gastroenterology* 1988;94:603–610.
10. Motil KJ, Grand RJ. Inflammatory bowel disease. In: Walker WA, Watkins JB, eds. *Nutrition in pediatrics.* Boston: Little, Brown, 1985;445–462.
11. Motil KJ, Grand RJ, Maletskos CJ, Young VR. The effect of disease, drug and diet on whole body protein metabolism in adolescents with Crohn's disease and growth failure. *J Pediatr* 1982;101:345–351.
12. Chan ATH, Fleming R, O'Fallon WM, Huizenga KA. Estimated versus measured basal energy requirements in patients with Crohn's disease. *Gastroenterology* 1986;91:75–78.
13. Ostro MJ, Greenberg CR, Jeejeebhoy KN. Total parenteral nutrition and complete bowel rest in the management of Crohn's disease. *J Parenter Enteral Nutr* 1985;9:280–287.
14. Le Quintrec Y, Cosnes J, Le Quintrec M, et al. L'alimentation entérale élémentaire exclusive dans les formes corticorésistantes et corticodépendantes de la maladie de Crohn. *Gastroenterol Clin Biol* 1987;11:447–482.
15. Sabbah S, Seidman EG. Dietary management of Crohn's disease. In: Bayless T, ed. *Current management of inflammatory bowel disease.* Burlington, Ontario: BC Decker, 1989;230–236.
16. Blair GK, Yaman M, Wesson DE. Preoperative home enteral nutrition in children with inflammatory bowel disease. *J Pediatr Surg* 1986;21:769–771.
17. Sabbah S, Seidman E. Nutritional therapy of children with inflammatory bowel disease. *Can J Gastroenterol* 1988;2:13A–17A.
18. Castile RG, Telander RL, Cooney DR, et al. Crohn's disease in children: assessment of the progression of disease, growth, and prognosis. *J Pediatr Surg* 1980;15:462–469.
19. Aiges H, Markowitz J, Rosa J, Daum F. Home nocturnal supplemental nasogastric feedings in growth-retarded adolescents with Crohn's disease. *Gastroenterology* 1989;97:905–910.
20. Imes S, Pinchbeck B, Dimwoodie K, Thomson ABR. Effect of Ensure, a defined formula diet, in patients with Crohn's disease. *Digestion* 1986;35:158–169.
21. Morin CL, Roulet M, Roy CC, Weber A, Lapointe N. Continuous elemental enteral alimentation in the treatment of children and adolescents with Crohn's disease. *J Parenter Enteral Nutr* 1982;6:194–199.
22. Seidman E, Sabbah S, Atlan P, Grey VL, Morin CL. Elemental diet in inflammatory bowel disease. *Can J Gastroenterol* 1988;2:26A–34A.
23. Goldschmidt S, Graham M. Trace element deficiencies in inflammatory bowel disease. *Gastroenterol Clin North Am* 1989;18:579–587.
24. Perkal MF, Seashore JH. Nutrition and inflammatory bowel disease. *Gastroenterol Clin North Am* 1989;18:567–578.
25. Harries AD, Heatley RV. Nutritional disturbances in Crohn's disease. *Postgrad Med J* 1983;59:690–697.
26. Elsborg L, Larsen L. Folate deficiency in chronic inflammatory bowel diseases. *Scand J Gastroenterol* 1979;14:1019–1024.
27. Imes S, Pinchbeck BR, Dinwoodie A, Walker K, Thomson AB. Iron, folate, vitamin B12, zinc and copper status in outpatients with Crohn's disease: effect of diet counseling. *J Am Diet Assoc* 1987;87:928–930.
28. Hodges P, Gee M, Grace M, Thomson AB. Vitamin and iron intake in patients with Crohn's disease. *J Am Diet Assoc* 1984;84:52–58.
29. Linaker BD. Scurvy and vitamin C deficiency in Crohn's disease. *Postgrad Med J* 1979;55:26–29.
30. Gerson CD, Fabry EM. Ascorbic deficiency and fistula formation in regional enteritis. *Gastroenterology* 1974;67:428–433.
31. Pettit SH, Irving MH. Does local intestinal ascorbate deficiency predispose to fistula formation in Crohn's disease. *Dis Colon Rectum* 1987;30:552–557.
32. Pollack S, Enat R, Haim S, Zinder O, Barzilai D. Pellagra as the presenting manifestation of Crohn's disease. *Gastroenterology* 1982;82:948–952.
33. Okabe N, Urabe K, Fujita K, Yamamoto T, Yao T, Doi S. Biotin effects in Crohn's disease. *Dig Dis Sci* 1988;33:1495–1496.
34. Main AN, Mills PR, Russell RI, et al. Vitamin A deficiency in Crohn's disease. *Gut* 1983;24:1169–1175.
35. Harries AD, Brown R, Heatley RV, Williams LA, Woodhead S, Rhodes J. Vitamin D status in Crohn's disease: association with disease activity and nutrition. *Gut* 1985;26:1197–1203.
36. Compston JE, Ayers AB, Horton LW, Tighe JR, Creamer B. Osteomalacia after small-intestinal resection. *Lancet* 1978;1:9–12.
37. Driscoll RH, Meredith SC, Sitrin M, Rosenberg IH. Vitamin D deficiency and bone disease in patients with Crohn's disease. *Gastroenterology* 1982;83:1252–1258.
38. Fernandez-Banares F, Abad-Lacruz A, Xiol X, et al. Vitamin status in patients with inflammatory bowel disease. *Am J Gastroenterol* 1989;84:744–748.
39. Krasinski SD, Russell RM, Furie BC, Kruger SF, Jacques PF, Furie B. The prevalence of vitamin K deficiency in chronic gastrointestinal disorders. *Am J Clin Nutr* 1985;41:639–643.
40. Kirschner BS. Medical management of inflammatory bowel disease in children. In: Kirsner JB, Shorter RG, eds. *Inflammatory bowel disease.* Philadelphia: Lea & Febiger, 1988.
41. Ainley CC, Cason J, Carlsson LK, Slavin BM, Thompson RP. Zinc status in inflammatory bowel disease. *Clin Sci* 1988;75:277–283.
42. Fleming CR, Huizenga KA, McCall JT, Gildea J, Dennis R. Zinc nutrition in Crohn's disease. *Dig Dis Sci* 1981;26:865–870.
43. Hambidge KM. Trace elements in human nutrition. In: Walker WA, Watkins JB, eds. *Nutrition in pediatrics.* Boston: Little, Brown, 1985:21–28.
44. Motil KJ, Altchuler SI, Grand RJ. Mineral balance during nutritional supplementation in adolescents with Crohn's disease and growth failure. *J Pediatr* 1985;107:473–479.
45. Motil KJ, Grand RJ, Davis-Kraft E. Risk factors associated with growth failure in inflammatory bowel disease. *Gastroenterology* 1983;84:1254.
46. Nishi Y, Lifshitz F, Bayne MA, Daum F, Silverberg M, Aiges H. Zinc status and its relation to growth retardation in children with chronic inflammatory bowel disease. *Am J Clin Nutr* 1980;33:2613–2621.
47. Clark JH, Fitzgerald JF, Bergstein JM. Nephrolithiasis in childhood inflammatory bowel disease. *J Pediatr Gastroenterol Nutr* 1985;4:829–834.
48. Galland L. Magnesium and inflammatory bowel disease. *Magnesium* 1988;7:78–83.
49. Hessov I, Hasselblad C, Fasth S, Hulten L. Magnesium deficiency after ileal resections for Crohn's disease. *Scand J Gastroenterol* 1983;18:643–649.
50. LaSala MA, Lifshitz F, Silverberg M, Wapnir RA, Carrera E. Magnesium metabolism studies in children with chronic inflammatory disease of the bowel. *J Pediatr Gastroenterol Nutr* 1985;4:75–81.
51. Jeejeebhoy KN, Ostro MJ. Nutritional consequences and therapy in inflammatory bowel disease. In: Kirsner JB, Shorter RG, eds. *Inflammatory bowel disease.* Philadelphia: Lea & Febiger, 1988.
52. Matuchansky C. Parenteral nutrition in inflammatory bowel disease. *Gut* 1986;27:81–84.
53. Seidman EG, Roy CC, Weber AM, Morin CL. Nutritional therapy of Crohn's disease in childhood. *Dig Dis Sci* 1987;32:825–855.
54. O'Morain C, Segal AW, Levi AJ. Elemental diet as primary treat-

ment of acute Crohn's disease: a controlled trial. *Br Med J* 1984;288:1859–1862.
55. Saverymuttu S, Hodgson HJF, Chadwick VS. Controlled trial comparing prednisolone with an elemental diet plus nonabsorbable antibiotics in active Crohn's disease. *Gut* 1985;26:944–948.
56. Seidman EG, Lohoues MJ, Turgeon J, Bouthillier L, Morin CL. Elemental diet versus prednisone as initial therapy in Crohn's disease: early and long term results. *Gastroenterology* 1991; 100:A250.
57. Sanderson IR, Udeen S, Davies PS, Savage MO, Walker-Smith JA. Remission induced by an elemental diet in small bowel Crohn's disease. *Arch Dis Child* 1987;62:123–127.
58. Alun Jones V. Comparison of total parenteral nutrition and elemental diet in induction of remission of Crohn's disease. *Dig Dis Sci* 1987;32:100S–107S.
59. Lochs H, Steinhardt HJ, Klaus-Wenz B, Bauer P, Malchow H. Enteral nutrition versus drug treatment for the acute phase of Crohn's disease. Results of the European Cooperative Crohn's Disease Study IV. *Gastroenterology* 1988;94:A267.
60. Giaffer MH, North G, Holdsworth CD. Controlled trial of polymeric versus elemental diet in treatment of active Crohn's disease. *Lancet* 1990;335:816–819.
61. Lochs H, Egger-Schodl M, Schuh R, et al. Is tube feeding with elemental diets a primary therapy of Crohn's disease? *Klin Wochenschr* 1984;62:821–825.
62. Teahon K, Levi J. Dietary management. In: Bayless T, ed. *Current management of inflammatory bowel disease.* Burlington, Ontario: BC Decker, 1989;223–230.
63. Navarro J, Vargas J, Cezard JP, Charritat JL, Polonovski C. Prolonged constant rate elemental enteral nutrition in Crohn's disease. *J Pediatr Gastroenterol Nutr* 1982;1:541–546.
64. Levi AJ. Diet in the management of Crohn's disease. *Gut* 1985;26:985–988.
65. Levenstein S, Prantera C, Luzi C, D'Ubaldi A. A low residue or normal diet in Crohn's disease. A prospective controlled study in Italian patients. *Gut* 1985;26:989–993.
66. Ritchie JK, Wadsworth J, Lennard-Jones JE, Rogers E. Controlled multicentre therapeutic trial of an unrefined carbohydrate, fibre rich diet in Crohn's disease. *Br Med J* 1987;295:517–520.
67. Jones VA, Dickinson RJ, Workman E, Wilson AJ, Freeman AH, Hunter JO. Crohn's disease: maintenance of remission by diet. *Lancet* 1985;2:177–180.
68. Lerebours E, Messing B, Chevalier B, Bories C, Colin R, Bernier JJ. An evaluation of total parenteral nutrition in the management of steroid-dependent and steroid-resistant patients with Crohn's disease. *J Parenter Enteral Nutr* 1986;10:274–278.
69. Lacey JM, Wilmore DW. Is glutamine a conditionally essential amino acid? *Nutr Rev* 1990;48:297–309.
70. Burke DJ, Alverdy JC, Aoys E, Moss GS. Glutamine-supplemented total parenteral nutrition improves gut immune function. *Arch Surg* 1989;124:1396–1399.
71. LeLeiko NS, Martin BA, Walsh M, Kazlow P, Rabinowitz S, Sterling K. Tissue-specific gene expression results from a purine- and pyrimidine-free diet and 6-mercaptopurine in the rat small intestine and colon. *Gastroenterology* 1987;93:1014–1020.
72. Kinsella JE, Lokesh B, Broughton S, Whelan J. Dietary polyunsaturated fatty acids and eicosanoids. Potential effects on the modulation of inflammatory and immune cells. An overview. *Nutrition* 1990;6:24–44.
73. O'Morain C. Nutritional treatment of inflammatory bowel disease including EPA. In: Goebell H, Peskar BM, Malchow H, eds. *Inflammatory bowel diseases—basic research and clinical implications.* Falk Symposium 46. Lancaster, England: MTP Press, 1988;315–319.
74. Lorenz R, Weber PC, Szimnau P, Heldwein W, Strasser T, Loeschke K. Supplementation with n-3 fatty acids from fish oil in chronic inflammatory bowel disease—a randomized, placebo-controlled, double-blind cross-over trial. *J Intern Med* 1989;225(731)(suppl):225–232.
75. Salomon P, Kornbluth AA, Janowitz HD. Treatment of ulcerative colitis with fish oil n-3 fatty acid: an open trial. *J Clin Gastroenterol* 1990;12:157–161.

CHAPTER 30

Nutritional Considerations in the Prognosis and Treatment of Liver Disease in Children

John B. Watkins

The liver is central to establishing nutritional homeostasis; consequently, nutritional deficiencies are common in pediatric chronic liver disease, particularly in cholestasis, where the liver disease has its onset early in infancy (1–3). Deficiencies develop from several factors. Protein and energy intake are often inadequate because of anorexia, unpalatable diets, altered taste sensation, or early satiety caused by impingement of viscera by an enlarged liver and spleen or ascites (4). Malabsorption, particularly of fat and fat-soluble vitamins, occurs as a consequence of decreased bile flow, decreased intraluminal bile acid concentrations, or therapeutic endeavors (e.g., neomycin/cholestyramine) that produce changes in mucosal transport or the intraluminal phase of lipid solubilization. In addition, altered metabolic processes, particularly in glucose and amino acid metabolism, (5) result from characteristic changes in the hormonal milieu (6). These factors contribute to the increased energy requirements (7,8), suboptimal energy utilization (4,8), decreased protein synthesis (9), and diminished growth of children with liver failure (10,11).

This chapter describes the role of the liver in establishing normal metabolic homeostasis and defines possible mechanisms responsible for some of the altered metabolic states observed in children with chronic liver failure. It also outlines appropriate methods of nutritional assessment using anthropometric and metabolic criteria. Finally, the goals of nutritional intervention and an approach for nutritional therapy are discussed, particularly in terms of the new opportunities accorded by the success of pediatric liver transplantation.

This chapter also examines the interactions between liver and muscle in the metabolism of carbohydrate, protein, and fat in chronic pediatric liver disease, and considers possible nutritional intervention strategies.

INITIAL ASSESSMENT OF THE CHILD WITH CHRONIC LIVER DISEASE

The medical history is critical to the initial nutritional evaluation of the child with chronic liver disease. It should provide information that identifies the pathophysiology responsible for the hepatic injury as well as an assessment of the degree of hepatic dysfunction. This makes it possible to address the specific nutritional risks for the patient and to fashion appropriate intervention (Table 1).

ASSESSMENT OF HEPATIC DYSFUNCTION

A quantitative assessment of hepatic function is essential, especially because of the potential for successful liver transplantation. Although tests for evaluating functional hepatic reserve in terms of metabolic capacity, excretory function, and the capacity to detoxify potentially toxic metabolites or pharmacologic agents hold promise for the future, these approaches are still in the developmental stage.

Clinically, the initial assessment of hepatic function of the child with known chronic liver disease should include an estimate of the size of the liver by physical examination. In children being considered for liver transplantation, an imaging modality, such as ultrasound, computerized axial tomography (CAT) scan, or magnetic resonance imaging (MRI), may provide a more precise estimate of hepatic volume or liver iron and cop-

---

J. B. Watkins: Department of Pediatrics, Washington University School of Medicine, St. Louis Children's Hospital, St. Louis, Missouri 63110.

TABLE 1. Nutritional risks associated with chronic liver disease

Nutritional risks	Methods of assessment/etiology	Nutritional risks	Methods of assessment/etiology
Anorexia	Nutritional history		Biochemical evidence for vitamin E deficiency
	Unpalatable diet		Ethane excretion
	Sodium restriction		Malonyldialdehyde excretion
	Protein restriction		Abnormal peroxide hemolysis
	Early satiety		Clinical evidence for vitamin E deficiency
	Ascites		
	Organomegaly		Neurological dysfunction
	Altered taste sensation		DTRs diminished
	Frequent infections/antibiotics		Wide-based gait
Growth failure	Growth velocity curve		Occular palsy
	Anthropometric measurement		Spinocerebellar degeneration
	Triceps skin-fold thickness		Anemia/hemolysis
	Midarm circumference	Vitamin D	Assessment of dietary intake of vitamin D and calcium
	Midarm muscle mass area (MAMA)		
	Fat malabsorption		Adequacy of vitamin D supplementation
	72-hr fecal fat		Determine serum 25-OH vitamin D level, absorption study
	History of drugs that bind bile acids or interfere with mucosal function		
			Increased requirements due to interaction with pharmacologic agents (e.g., phenobarbital, neomycin, cholestyramine)
Hypoproteinemia	Assess nutritional intake and distributions of calories, carbohydrates, protein, and fat		
			Radiographic studies of bone/bone densitometry
	Evaluate therapeutic maneuvers to control ascites (e.g., fluid withdrawal)		Serum alkaline phosphatase determination/bone fraction
			Determine 25-OH vitamin D level
	Clinical examination to determine the presence of edema, ascites, muscle wasting	Vitamin K	Prothrombin time/vitamin K challenge
			Clotting factor levels
	Anthropometrics		Use of antibiotics (neomycin, bile sequestering acids)
	GI protein loss		
	Fecal α_1-antitrypsin excretion and/or clearance	Mineral deficiency (iron, magnesium, and zinc)	Document adequate supplementation
	Increased catabolism, decreased synthesis due to infection, hepatic dysfunction		Use of bile acid sequestering agents
Fat-soluble vitamin deficiency			Determination of serum magnesium level/urinary excretion
Vitamin A	Serum vitamin A and retinol ester determinations (HPLC)		Serum iron, total iron-binding capacity, ferritin levels
	Retinol-binding protein, transthyretin (prealbumin) concentrations		Plasma zinc determination
			Serum alkaline phosphatase level
	Functional assessment, dark field adaptation studies (difficult to perform in children)		Urinary excretion
			Clinical evidence of deficiency
Vitamin E	Serum vitamin E level (HPLC)		Rash, skin lesions
	Vitamin E/total lipid ratio		
	Vitamin E absorption test		

Adapted from refs. 34 and 35.
HPLC, high-performance liquid chromatography.

per content, and possibly quantify the existence of portal hypertension with an estimate regarding the direction of blood flow.

Initial assessment should also ascertain the integrity of the extrahepatic biliary tree and define the degree of cholestasis. The latter may be estimated by the nuclear imaging agents (Technetium 99 IDA studies) or by the serum bilirubin concentration, including a fractionation of the direct and indirect component. Prognostically, the fractionation of bilirubin has some significance, since elevation of indirect bilirubin is now recognized as a serious prognostic sign in children with chronic liver disease. Serum bile acid concentrations provide a sensitive indicator of hepatic dysfunction, although serum bile acid levels have not proven useful in determining prognosis or in quantifying the degree of cholestasis. The presence of cirrhosis with hepatic failure is, at best, a histopathological diagnosis, and must be addressed in light of other functional considerations, including the degree of portal hypertension, the presence or absence of hepatic encephalopathy, and biochemical estimates of hepatic synthetic function.

ANTHROPOMETRIC ASSESSMENT OF NUTRITIONAL STATUS IN CHILDREN WITH LIVER DISEASE

In children and adults with chronic liver disease, both acute and chronic malnutrition are nearly universal (12). There are, however, few studies that have characterized, in a prospective, chronological fashion, anthropometric information defining the nutritional status in children with differing types of liver disease. Several excellent studies do provide general information about nutritional risks in various types of pediatric liver disease and improve the accuracy of interpreting anthropometric assessment results.

Sokol and Stall (1) studied a group of children with chronic liver disease, where onset was clinically apparent before the age of 6 months. Children were compared with an age-matched, normal control population. Cirrhosis was present in the majority of patients, although all were clinically stable, and none was considered to be an active candidate for liver transplantation at the time of evaluation. Normalized z scores were used to analyze the data sets. The data demonstrated that both acute (wasting) and chronic (stunting) malnutrition are nearly universal consequences of early childhood liver disease. A comparison of z scores for weight and height erroneously suggested that although children with chronic liver disease are stunted in linear growth, they are well nourished. This misinterpretation probably results from the increased body weight due to the organomegaly and/or ascites, which may exist even when not detected clinically. Reconfirmation of the imprecision of using a weight/height index versus a triceps skin-fold (TSF) measurement for nutritional assessments comes from a study, done within a month of transplantation, of adult patients with end-stage liver disease (13).

Acute malnutrition, therefore, is best estimated by a triceps skin-fold determination. Although weight-for-height is generally used to ascertain acute malnutrition, in children with chronic liver disease the increase in body weight resulting from the enlargement of the liver and the spleen may mask the extent of weight loss. Chronic malnutrition (stunting), which occurs over time, is best determined by a height/age index.

Nearly all nutritional studies have been cross-sectional or prevalence rather than longitudinal. Future studies are needed to confirm the possible immediate benefit of nutritional intervention in children with chronic liver disease.

NUTRITIONAL ABNORMALITIES IN LIVER DISEASE: INTERACTIONS BETWEEN LIVER AND MUSCLE

The liver is essential to regulating the distribution of most nutrients absorbed from the intestine. The compo-

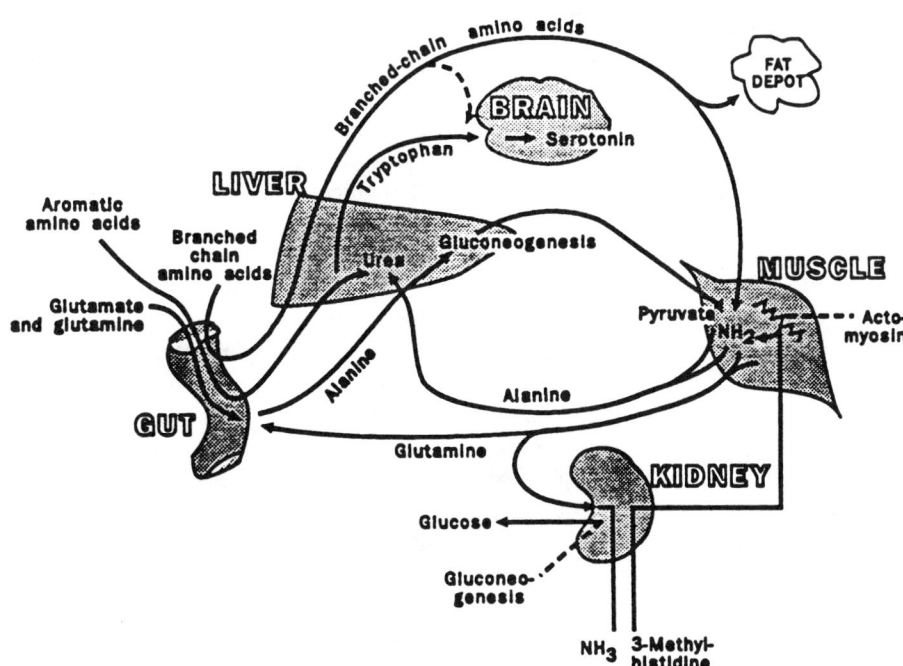

FIG. 1. The components of the regulation of liver and muscle in the metabolism.

nents of this regulation are inherently interdependent (Fig. 1) (12). Both the liver and the skeletal muscle are important in establishing nutritional homeostasis. Understanding this interrelationship is essential in determining if the gradual increase in the muscle mass to total body weight ratio, which occurs normally from infancy through adolescence, is important in the nutritional assessment of the child with chronic liver disease.

Hellerstein and Munro (12) have estimated that in the nonobese young adult the skeletal musculature represents nearly 45% of body weight. This proportion, however, is not constant throughout life. At birth, skeletal muscle mass comprises only 20% of body weight. It increases to 35% by early adolescence and reaches 45% by the end of the second decade. This is followed by a slow decline to 27% in the elderly, as judged by both ^{40}K determination and total nitrogen content.

The relative size and metabolic roles of the liver and skeletal musculature are directly related to the metabolic requirements and metabolic intensity of the organism. In humans, for example, the basal metabolic rate expressed in kilocalories (Cal) per kilogram body weight undergoes nearly a fourfold reduction from birth to adult life. Total body protein synthesis per kilogram is similarly reduced. Using total body RNA content of liver and skeletal musculature as an index of the intensity of protein synthesis by each organ, Hellerstein and Munro concluded that, with increasing body size, the reduction in the amount of protein synthesized in the liver per gram body weight is proportionately greater than in the skeletal musculature.

NUTRITIONAL ABNORMALITIES IN CHRONIC LIVER DISEASE

Carbohydrates

Due to its central anatomic location, the liver is afforded the first pass for utilization of the glucose absorbed from the intestine and the insulin secreted by the pancreas. There is increasing evidence that following a fast, glucose bypasses the liver to be glycolytically degraded to the triose level in the peripheral extrahepatic tissues and that the lactate, alanine, and pyruvates so generated are then returned to the liver to form glucose, phosphates, and sugar nucleotides through the gluconeogenesis. Since muscle represents a large portion of the extrahepatic body mass and is the major site for glucose uptake and for alanine and lactate output, the glucose recycling pathways are generally accepted to occur in muscle (12,14). Quantification of the relative importance of this pathway under different nutritional conditions indicates that the glucose recycling pathways predominate in the fasted state and during refeeding, becoming diminished in direct proportion to the degree of glycogen depletion obtained in the liver. The locus for the precise regulatory events will not be reviewed. It should be clear, however, that the integration of metabolic status of extrahepatic tissues into hepatic glucose and lipid metabolism (regulation of ketogenesis) are achieved by the sequence of peripheral uptake and glycolysis of ingested glucose followed by utilization in the liver of the triose generated. The metabolic state of the peripheral tissues are, in turn, affected by diet, exercise, the hormonal milieu, and disease (15). Thus, the liver is able to respond to the changing hormonal environment and the metabolic state of the organs, and is able to utilize a number of different substrates generated in the periphery, rather than being patterned solely for the first-pass class clearance of the glucose entering the liver through the portal vein (16). A similar organization has been noted for the utilization of dietary lipid in the chylomicrons first bypassing the liver by entering the circulation via the lymph and remetabolized in peripheral tissue before the liver removes the chylomicron remnant particles (16).

The child with chronic liver disease often demonstrates profound abnormalities of carbohydrate metabolism. These children are commonly intolerant of an oral carbohydrate load, and clinically demonstrate insulin resistance; yet they also have an inability to withstand a prolonged fast (16). The mechanism for the carbohydrate intolerance is multifactorial. In liver disease, both fasting and postprandial insulin concentrations are often elevated (12,17). The high levels are attributed both to a portosystemic shunting of insulin and to reduced insulin degradation (6,18). The insulin resistance is postulated to be due primarily to a defect in the hepatic insulin receptor (19). Studies to examine this hypothesis, and to differentiate between impaired glucose utilization and glucose production, have been performed under euglycemic conditions in adult patients with stable cirrhosis and clinically demonstrated impaired glucose tolerance (16). Resistance to insulin was demonstrated by the fact that glucose use (in milligrams per kilogram per minute) was significantly lower than controls at three plasma insulin levels tested, whereas endogenous glucose production remained unchanged. To evaluate the mechanisms for the observed insulin resistance, insulin binding and 3-orthomethyl glucose transport studies were then performed *in vitro*, using monocytes and adipocytes (19). In these tissues, both insulin binding and glucose transport were significantly diminished in the cirrhotic population compared to the normal controls, suggesting that glucose intolerance in human cirrhosis is more the result of diminished peripheral glucose utilization than to increased endogenous production. Insulin resistance appears to be the result of a defect in the insulin receptor, which is expressed by a decrease in the insulin receptor (20) number or in its binding affinity. A proposed mechanism for the decrease in insulin receptor number may best be explained by a down-regulation in the expression of insulin receptors, which would then result in a secondary decrease in insulin binding. Finally, the potential for deficit in the intracellular processing or postreceptor modulation of insulin has been postulated, but remains to be demonstrated.

Protein

Protein digestion and absorption is generally unaffected by liver disease; however, amino acid metabolism is significantly altered. In general, amino acids are utilized in three different ways: (a) they are essential precursors for protein synthesis; (b) they are precursors for essential nitrogenous molecules; and (c) when present in excess, they may be degraded to provide an energy source. New protein synthesis in the adult has been estimated to be in the range of 250 to 300 g/day (12). This is two to three times the amino acid intake and/or synthetic rate and indicates that under steady-state conditions there is considerable breakdown of tissue protein and reutilization of constituent amino acids. From recent studies of albumin synthesis and turnover rates these fluxes may be several times greater in preterm and newborn infants (21). The relative rates of protein synthesis in the liver, either retained and/or secreted, may be estimated by turnover studies to be in the range of 20 to 25 g/day, about one-half the amount synthesized by the musculature (Fig. 1). Data from isolated perfused liver techniques demonstrate that the nonessential amino acids and seven of the essential amino acids are oxidized principally in the liver. By contrast, oxidation of the branched-chain amino acids leucine, isoleucine, and valine readily occurs in the periphery, as demonstrated by limb perfusion studies. The degradative enzymes for these three branched-chain amino acids are most active in muscle, kidney, brain, and adipose tissue. This is best demonstrated by the body's response to a meal containing proteins (Fig. 1). During the meal, amino acids and some peptides are absorbed into the intestinal mucosal cells. The small peptides are subsequently degraded further by intracellular peptidases so that only free amino acids pass into the portal vein for delivery to the liver. Within the intestinal mucosal cell, there is some metabolism of amino acids, particularly glutamine and glutamic acid. These are subsequently transaminated with pyruvate to form alanine, which then provides the carbons for gluconeogenesis and for urea biogenesis. Glutamine derived from peripheral tissues (e.g., muscle) is degraded in a similar manner. The regulation of the levels of amino acids in the serum is, in general, accomplished with fine precision by the liver according to the needs of the body (22). When tryptophan intake, for example, exceeds the daily requirements, the degradative enzyme, tryptophan oxygenase, is induced, thereby directly influencing the amount of tryptophan available for the synthesis of the neurotransmitter, such as serotonin. Branched-chain amino acids, by contrast, demonstrate very little hepatic uptake and undergo minor degradation in the liver; following a meal they pass directly into the peripheral circulation for metabolism in the muscle. This accounts for their proposed utility as a nutrient source in liver disease and their potential role in the treatment of hepatic encephalopathy (23,24).

Fat

Fat digestion and absorption is a complex process, involving intraluminal lipolysis and solubilization of the hydrolyzed lipids followed by the mucosal uptake and absorption of the products of lipolysis. The majority of the biologically significant lipids are then reesterified and packaged into chylomicrons for delivery into the lymphatics before entering the general circulation. The intraluminal hydrolytic processes and micellar solubilization of nonpolar lipids are critically dependent on adequate bile salt concentrations which must remain above the critical micellar concentration. In liver disease, bile acid metabolism is altered in ways that interfere with nutritional homeostasis, limiting the absorption of nonpolar, poorly soluble lipids, such as the fat-soluble vitamins and cholesterol. Furthermore, the inefficiency of the enterohepatic circulation of bile acids, because of the diminished hepatic uptake of bile acids, results in elevated serum bile acid concentrations and in increased losses of bile acids by urinary excretion. The bile acid conjugation patterns also change to favor urinary excretion. Hepatic bile acid synthesis, which normally is increased in response to fecal and urinary losses, appears diminished, most likely due to either an alteration in regulatory processes, altered feedback regulation, or hepatic injury.

Treatment protocols, particularly those designed to relieve pruritus in cholestatic disorders using cholestyramine to bind intraluminal bile acids, may further accelerate bile acid loss and vitamin malabsorption. Calcium malabsorption occurs as a consequence of the resulting steatorrhea and, together with vitamin D deficiency, often complicates nutrition, with poor growth and rickets being a common finding. Essential fatty acid deficiency may also be biochemically evident (2,4,25).

In children with portal hypertension and cirrhosis, hepatic and intestinal lymph flow is compromised by higher pressure in the abdominal lymphatics. Bowel wall edema and poor uptake of chylomicrons contribute to the fat malabsorption and accelerate the gastrointestinal protein loss. These deficits may be addressed in part through the judicious addition of medium-chain triglycerides to the diet. These specially prepared dietary lipids possess high aqueous solubility, and are readily hydrolyzed by lipases present in both the stomach and the intestine. They do not require bile salts for solubilization in the aqueous intraluminal environment and they are readily absorbed from the intestine. In contrast to long-chain fatty acids, medium-chain fatty acids do not require chylomicron formation for transport to the periphery but are bound to albumin for direct transport to the liver, where they are quickly metabolized.

Vitamin E Deficiency

Vitamin E occurs normally in nature in as many as eight different tocopherols, with D-α-tocopherol being the most biologically active. These compounds protect the cellular components, particularly membrane phospholipids and unsaturated fatty acids, from peroxidative degradation. Dietary vitamin E occurs principally in the esterified form, which requires hydrolysis by bile acid–dependent esterases and micellar solubilization for efficient absorption. This dependence on bile acids for effective absorption has been demonstrated clinically, both in normal preterm infants and in cholestatic infants and children, all of whom characteristically exhibit reduced intraluminal bile acid concentrations. Normally, approximately 25% to 40% of ingested vitamin E are absorbed and, like most nonpolar lipids, are transported within the chylomicron fraction by lymphatics to the general circulation. In circulation, vitamin E is generally distributed between the low-density lipoprotein fraction and the chylomicron remnants for distribution to peripheral tissues and for uptake in the liver, which is the site of the immediate reserve stores.

In infants with cholestasis, vitamin E deficiency is a well-recognized entity. It may result in a hemolytic anemia, altered prostaglandin synthesis, and a distinctive neurological syndrome, characterized by a neuroaxonal degeneration, which may be clinically apparent in a child with cholestasis and depleted vitamin E reserves as early as 18 months of age. The clinical correlates of the neuroaxonal degeneration include hypo- or areflexia, truncal and limb ataxia, peripheral neuropathy, and ophthalmoplegia (2). The histopathological findings exhibited in the sural nerve and muscle biopsies are characteristic and similar to those observed in experimental vitamin E deficiency. The high prevalence of vitamin E deficiency syndrome in children compared with adults who exhibit cholestasis suggests an increased sensitivity to these neurologic complications in children.

The exact biochemical definition of vitamin E status has been elusive. This is partly due to the ready distribution of vitamin E within the lipid phase of serum. For example, hyperlipidemia, common in children with cholestasis, may cause increased concentration of vitamin E in the serum, but not in the tissue. One recommendation has been, therefore, to express the vitamin E serum concentration of hyperlipidemic infants as a ratio of the vitamin E value to serum lipid concentration (4). In the absence of hyperlipidemia, however, this may have no advantage over absolute serum concentrations. Regardless of the method, the serum concentration may not be an adequate reflection of tissue levels or a true measure of the deficiency state. Various functional tests may, more accurately, reflect vitamin E status. Oxidant stress, for example, can be assessed by determining the resistance of erythrocytes to hydrogen peroxide oxidation. Serum malonyldialdehyde concentration and breath ethane excretion, recognized by-products of the lipid peroxidation, hold promise as more sensitive indicators of the deficiency state. Direct estimates of neurological dysfunction by an electroretinogram or nerve conduction studies, though relatively specific, are difficult to perform with reliability in small infants and are usually conducted within the research setting.

Treatment protocols designed to redress the deficiency state illustrate the refractory nature of the deficiency syndrome and demonstrate that massive doses of an oral preparation are often needed. The water-soluble preparation, D-α-tocopherol polyethylene glycol-1000 succinate (TPGS), has been reported to be successful in the correction of vitamin E deficiency with an oral dose of 15 to 25 IU/kg/day (4). Studies are underway to further define the safety and efficacy of this preparation.

Vitamin A Deficiency

Vitamin A, or retinol, is required for the initiation of noncolor vision and the synthesis of light-sensitive pigments in the retina. It is also important for cellular proliferation, glycoprotein synthesis, maintenance of cellular integrity, and mucous production. Deficiency of vitamin A results in the symptoms of night blindness, xerophthalmia, and keratomalacia, with conjunctival and corneal drying (xerosis). Associated findings include decreased immune competence, increased intracranial pressure, growth failure, and reproductive failure.

Dietary vitamin A is present as the retinol ester, which is hydrolyzed intraluminally by a bile salt–dependent lipase present in human milk and/or by a pancreatic ester hydrolase. The role played by putative brush border or intracellular hydrolytic processes is more controversial. Retinol esters are solubilized within the bile salt micelle, which maximizes absorption rates. Inhibition of absorption and stability of the vitamin compound may be influenced by long-chain fatty acids and by vitamin E. Within the enterocyte, vitamin A is reesterified and enters the peripheral circulation in chylomicrons with some distribution to other lipoprotein fractions. Storage of the vitamin occurs in the liver, localized to tissue specific cells. Release from the liver occurs as a soluble complex of the retinol, retinol-binding protein, and prealbumin (transthyretin).

Serum levels of vitamin A are generally in the normal range until the liver stores are depleted. Low levels are demonstrated in hypoproteinemic states due to reduced synthesis and release of the transport protein. Deficiency states may be assessed by direct measurement of the serum concentration by high-performance liquid chromatography (HPLC) and adequacy of stores and/or toxicity by liver concentrations. In children with chronic liver disease, serum levels are often low. Abnormal dark adaptation has been reported, and has been shown to respond to supplementation with retinol-palmitate.

Zinc deficiency, common in liver disease, is also important for maintenance of visual function. It is a necessary cofactor for retinal alcohol dehydrogenase, an enzyme necessary for the regeneration of retinol in the retina. Supplementation of both zinc and vitamin A may, therefore, be required.

Vitamin D Deficiency

Vitamin D is a prohormone, not a vitamin. It is present in the diet (vitamin D_2) and synthesized in the skin by a photochemical isomerization (vitamin D_3). In the skin, the vitamin is tightly bound to vitamin D–binding protein prior to transport to the liver for one of the subsequent hydroxylation steps. Activation of vitamin D is initiated by 25-hydroxylation in the liver, followed by 1-hydroxylation in the kidneys. Dietary vitamin D is possibly absorbed in the intestine without modification. This process, which is facilitated by bile salts and an enterohepatic circulation of vitamin D and its metabolites, has been demonstrated, so that some conservation of the molecule may exist. Vitamin D absorption can be studied clinically by quantifying the serum levels that peak in serum 4 to 12 hr after an oral dose. Following absorption and transport in the chylomicron fraction, vitamin D is initially concentrated in the liver, where it undergoes 25-hydroxylation. Both vitamin D_2 and vitamin D_3 are thought to be equally well recognized by the hepatic vitamin D–25-hydroxylase, although some differences in the efficiency of the conversion between the two forms may exist. Following hydroxylation, 25-OH vitamin D is released from the liver, bound to a vitamin D–binding protein with storage occurring principally in the adipose tissue and muscle. Thus, 25-OH vitamin D, calcidiol, is the major circulating form of the vitamin, and is the metabolite most commonly assayed to assess the adequacy of vitamin D supplementation.

Children with chronic liver disease have both impaired absorption of vitamin D and decreased 25-hydroxylation rates. Some medications prescribed to relieve the pruritus of cholestatic liver disease may augment the deficiency of intraluminal bile acids (e.g., cholestyramine) or promote the synthesis of more polar, less biologically active metabolites (e.g., phenobarbital). Treating with exogenous vitamin D and/or sunlight with normalization of serum 25-OH vitamin D concentrations most effectively corrects the mineralization defect (rickets), but has less effect on the osteomalacia.

Trace Elements

Copper, zinc, and iron serve as cofactors for enzyme activation or as prosthetic groups for numerous enzymes and are, therefore, essential for liver function. Examples include cytochrome oxidase (an iron and copper enzyme), alcohol dehydrogenase, and alkaline phosphatase (zinc), and superoxide dismutase (which contains both copper and zinc). Zinc is also central in the metabolism of DNA and polyribosomes. Deficiency states are uncommon and rarely occur without the coexistence of dietary restrictions as might exist in parenteral alimentation, isolated transport defects, or due to excessive losses. The liver plays a central, though remarkably different, role in both the metabolism and as a target of the toxic effects of copper and zinc.

The liver has a remarkable capacity to conserve copper; therefore, hepatic dysfunction due to copper deficiency is unknown. Toxicity to the liver and other organs from copper excess is well characterized. Copper is absorbed from the intestine through a process that involves competition with intraluminal ligands and an intestinal transport protein. Following absorption, it is transported in plasma predominantly bound to albumin (80% to 90%), and is avidly cleared by the liver. The half-life in serum of the albumin-copper complex is in the range of 10 min. Mobilization and release of the copper from the liver takes place by two routes. The first involves the incorporation into ceruloplasmin during hepatic synthesis with its subsequent release into the peripheral circulation. The major route for the excretion of copper occurs via the biliary route in the adult (1.5 mg/day) with minimal excretion occurring via the urine (0.5 mg/day) (26).

There are remarkable variations in hepatic copper concentration among different species and during development. Neonate hepatic copper concentrations exceed those found even in Wilson's disease, with no evidence of functional or morphological alterations. Preliminary data suggest that biliary excretion is diminished. The developmentally associated mechanisms responsible for the intracellular storage of copper have not been examined in detail, although hepatic toxicity is not an apparent problem. The same concentrations (250 μg/g dry liver, or higher) in an adult liver are associated with either hepatotoxicity or with a pathological process such as cholestasis or Wilson's disease.

Wilson's disease is an example of abnormal copper accumulation resulting in acute hepatic toxicity, with steatosis progressing to a more insidious chronic active disease leading to cirrhosis and few distinguishing morphological features. In the early stage of the disease, hepatic copper moves from prelysosomes to become distributed diffusely throughout the cytoplasm. The process responsible for the change in distribution as well as the mechanisms of toxicity are currently under active investigation (26).

Copper toxicity involving other organs occurs when the hepatic storage capacity for copper is overwhelmed and copper is released unbound into the circulation.

Zinc

Zinc, another essential element, is one of the most abundant metals in the human body. Many enzymes in the liver require zinc for their catalytic activity, and zinc is believed to protect by inhibiting lipid peroxidation and stabilizing lysosomal membranes.

Zinc is absorbed principally in the upper small intestine. Prostaglandins may facilitate absorption and an excess of either copper or zinc inhibits the absorption of the other. Nearly two-thirds of the zinc in human plasma is bound to albumin; only 3% of the total body zinc is stored in the liver compared to 10% to 15% of total body copper. An important route for zinc excretion is pancreatic juice, with bile contributing relatively small amounts to the fecal losses.

Neither deficiency nor excess of zinc has been demonstrated to cause liver disease although liver disease may influence zinc homeostasis. Zinc deficiency has been associated with poor growth, hypogeusia, night blindness unresponsive to vitamin A administration, decreased vitamin A release from the liver, and altered drug metabolism. Although many of these findings are associated with or noted in children with liver disease, a poor correlation exists with zinc status and improvement is only occasionally associated with zinc supplementation.

Iron

Iron metabolism in pediatric liver disease is poorly understood. The description of possible neonatal forms of iron storage disease (27) and the ability to identify through molecular or linkage analysis the familial forms of hemochromatosis before they become clinically apparent has, however, heightened clinical interest.

The mechanism of injury in iron overload states has focused on iron-induced membrane lipid peroxidation of subcellular organelles. The possible interrelationships with vitamin E metabolism and correlations with ethane, or malonyldialdehyde excretion are, as yet, preliminary. Deficiency states occur primarily as a consequence of excessive losses that might occur through blood losses with variceal bleeding or portal hypertension. Iron deficiency is rarely the principal factor or clinical determinant in the treatment of hepatic injury.

GOAL AND STRATEGIES FOR NUTRITIONAL INTERVENTION

The ultimate goals of nutritional intervention in children with chronic liver disease are nutritional homeostasis, deposition of lean body mass, and enhanced growth. This is accomplished by (a) nutritional supplementation, which corrects existing deficits and meets ongoing losses; and (b) establishing nitrogen deposition while decreasing hepatic encephalopathy. Special attention must be directed toward infants and young children, the largest group of young patients requiring liver transplantation (1). The unique requirements and excessive losses of children with metabolic liver disease (e.g., tyrosinemia) are discussed more fully in other texts (28).

Nutritional formulas adequate to promote catch-up growth must contain approximately 150% of the recommended dietary allowances (RDA) for height and age (Table 1). Infant formulas, such as Pregestamil (Mead Johnson), which contain a balanced lipid composition to maximize absorption in the face of cholestasis and deficient lipolysis (e.g., 40% of lipid calories as medium-chain triglycerides) and yet have sufficient linoleic acid to prevent essential fatty acid deficiency, have been recommended (4). Protein intake adequate to promote growth and to maintain positive nitrogen balance is essential.

Studies that have examined nitrogen balance while reducing hepatic encephalopathy through the use of branch-chain amino acids have conflicting results (29,30). The use of branch-chain amino acids in children with liver failure has been recommended, the potential benefits being an increased utilization rate of branch-chain amino acids by skeletal muscle, which would promote net energy uptake and possibly reduce the potential for hepatic encephalopathy. To date, the high cost of these formulations and limited information demonstrating efficacy preclude their routine use in children with cholestasis and/or liver disease. Chronic malabsorption and deficiency of fat-soluble vitamins are nearly universal in children with chronic liver disease (15). Careful assessment of current status and monitoring of vitamin intake to avoid toxicity are essential (Table 2).

TABLE 2. Recommendations for vitamin supplementation and monitoring in liver disease

Vitamin	Deficiency	Drug	Dose	Monitoring
Vitamin A	Night blindness degeneration of the retina, xerophthalmia, poor growth, and hyperkeratosis	Emulsified vitamin A (may also require zinc)	5,000–15,000 IU	Serum levels 400–500 mcg/l
Vitamin D	Rickets, osteoporosis, osteomalacia, cranial bossing, epiphyseal enlargement, persistently open anterior fontanelle in infants	25-OH D	20–50 mg/day	Serum level 25–30 ng/ml (or higher), serum and phosphate, parathyroid hormone
Vitamin E	Peripheral neuropathy, ataxia, impaired intestinal absorption of vitamin E, neuroaxonal degeneration	α-tocopherol or TPGS	50–400 IU/day up to 200 IU/kg/day. 25 IU/kg/day	Serum level > 5 mg/l vitamin E; total lipid ratio 0.6 to 0.8 mg/g
Vitamin K	Coagulopathy, hemorrhagic manifestations such as bruising	Vitamin K_3	2.5–5.0 mg/day	Prothrombin time factor activities

Adapted from ref. 4.

Method of Feeding

In early liver disease, formula fed by mouth generally insures adequate intake and weight gain. When, however, chronic liver dysfunction leads to chronic malnutrition and anorexia, nasal gastric feeding, with the modern narrow gauge silicone-rubber tube and/or gastrostomy tube, is well tolerated without complications. Nasogastric feeding tubes also simplify administration of medications and do not appear to compromise oral intake. In most cases, feeding should be administered continuously rather than by bolus feeding. This appears to promote energy balance and lessen the frequency of regurgitation. Depending on the degree of malnutrition, nighttime infusions alone may be sufficient to maintain growth (4).

SUMMARY

Malnutrition is a nearly universal component of chronic liver disease in children. Causal factors are multifactorial so that careful nutritional assessment, identification of important risk factors, and specific deficiency states and/or excessive losses are essential to good management and for achievement of nutritional rehabilitation (34,35). Attention to the limited ability of the child with chronic liver disease to withstand a prolonged fast, plus alleviation and treatment of ascites or infection, which may increase energy expenditure or precipitate nutritional deficiencies, are essential (31). The increased success of programs for pediatric liver transplantation has demonstrated the importance of good nutritional rehabilitation prior to transplantation: the pretransplant nutritional status appears to impact on postoperative morbidity, expense, time in hospital, and, most importantly, survival (32,33).

ACKNOWLEDGMENTS

Supported by grant #NS-17752 awarded by the National Institutes of Health, and by the Howard Heinz Foundation. The author would like to express thanks to Julie Giordano for secretarial support and to Richard J. Grand, M.D. and Kathy Calanda, M.D., who provided much of the original background material for the oral presentation.

REFERENCES

1. Sokol RJ, Stall C. Anthropometric evaluation of children with chronic liver disease. *Am J Clin Nutr* 1990;52:203–208.
2. Balistreri WF. Neonatal cholestasis. *J Pediatr* 1985;106:171–184.
3. Balistreri WF, Schubert WK. Liver disease in infancy and childhood. In: Schiff L, Schiff E, eds. *Diseases of the liver*. Philadelphia: Lippincott, 1987;1337–1426.
4. Kaufman SS, Murray ND, Wood P, Shaw BW, Vanderhoof JA. Nutritional support for the infant with extrahepatic biliary atresia. *J Pediatr* 1987;110:679–686.
5. Cascino A, Cangiano C, Calcaterra V, Rossi-Fanelli F, Capoccia L. Plasma amino acids imbalance in patients with liver disease. *Am J Dig Dis* 1978;23:591–598.
6. Johnston DG, Alberti KGMM, Faber OK, Binder C, Wright R. Hyperinsulinism of hepatic cirrhosis: diminished degradation or hypersecretion? *Lancet* 1977;1:10–12.
7. Schneeweiss B, Graninger W, Ferenci P, Eichinger S, Grimm G, Schneider B, Laggner AN, Lenz K, Kleinberger G. Energy metabolism in patients with acute and chronic liver disease. *Hepatology* 1990;11:387–393.
8. Nosadini R, Avogaro A, Mollo F, Marescotti C, Tiengo A, Duner E, Merkel C, Gatta A, Zuin R, de Kreutzenberg S, Trevisan R, Crepaldi G. Carbohydrate and lipid metabolism in cirrhosis. Evidence that hepatic uptake of gluconeogenic precursors and of free

fatty acids depends on effective hepatic flow. *J Clin Endocrinol Metab* 1984;58:1125–1132.
9. Munro HN, Crim MC. The proteins and amino acids. In: Shils ME, Young VR, eds. *Modern nutrition in health and disease.* Philadelphia: Lea and Febiger, 1988;1–35.
10. DiCecco SR, Wieners EJ, Wiesner RH, Southorn PA, Plevak DV, Krom RAF. Assessment of nutritional status of patients with end-stage liver disease undergoing liver transplantation. *Mayo Clin Proc* 1989;64:95–102.
11. Spolidoro JVN, Berquist WE, Pehlivanoglu E, Busuttil R, Saluski I, Vargas J, Ament ME. Growth acceleration in children after orthotopic liver transplantation. *J Pediatr* 1988;112:41–43.
12. Hellerstein MK, Munro HN. Interaction of liver and muscle in the regulation of metabolism in response to nutritional and other factors. In: Arias IM, Jacoby WB, Popper H, Schacter D, Schafritz DA, eds. *The liver, biology and pathobiology,* 2nd ed. New York: Raven Press, 1988.
13. Hehir DJ, Jenkins RL, Bistrian BR, Blackburn GL. Nutrition in patients undergoing orthotopic liver transplant. *J Parenter Enteral Nutr* 1985;9:695–700.
14. MacDonald I. Carbohydrates. In: Shils ME, Young VR, eds. *Modern nutrition in health and disease.* Philadelphia: Lea and Febiger, 1988;38–71.
15. Linscheer WG, Vergroesen AJ. Lipids. In: Shils ME, Young VR, eds. *Modern nutrition in health and disease.* Philadelphia: Lea and Febiger, 1988;72–107.
16. Romijn JA, Endert E, Sauerwein HP. Glucose and fat metabolism during short-term starvation in cirrhosis. *Gastroenterology* 1991;100:731–737.
17. Marchesini G, Bianchi G, Zoli M, Dondi C, Forlani G, Melli A, Bua V, Vannini P, Pisi E. Plasma amino acid response to protein ingestion in patients with liver cirrhosis. *Gastroenterology* 1983;85:283–290.
18. Owen OE, Trapp VE, Reichard GA, Morrdi MA, Moctezuma J, Paul P, Skutches CL, Boden G. Nature and quantity of fuels consumed in patients with cirrhosis. *J Clin Invest* 1983;72:1821–1832.
19. Cavallo-Perin P, Cassder M, Bozzo C, Bruno A, Nuccio P, Dall'omo AM, Marocci M, Pagano G. Mechanism of insulin resistance in human liver cirrhosis. *J Clin Invest* 1985;75:1659–1665.
20. Blei AT, Robbins DC, Drobny E, Baumann G, Rubenstein AH. Insulin resistance and insulin receptors in hepatic cirrhosis. *Gastroenterology* 1982;83:1191–1199.
21. Eisenberg LD, Merritt RJ, Sinatra FR. Nutrition in hepatic disorders. In: Grand RJ, Sutphen JL, Dietz WH, eds. *Pediatric nutrition: theory and practice.* Boston: Butterworth, 1987;513–524.
22. Meredith CN. Nutritional biochemistry of protein and amino acids. In: Grand RJ, Sutphen JL, Dietz WH, eds. *Pediatric nutrition: theory and practice.* Boston: Butterworth, 1987;36–50.
23. Horst D, Grace ND, Conn HO, Schiff E, Schenker S, Viteri A, Law D, Atterbury CE. Comparison of dietary protein with an oral, branched chain-enriched amino acid supplement in chronic portal-systemic encephalopathy: a randomized controlled trial. *Hepatology* 1984;4:279–287.
24. Fischer JE, Rosen HM, Ebeid AM, Jones JH, Keane JM, Soeters PB. The effect of normalization of plasma amino acids on hepatic encephalopathy in man. *Surgery* 1976;80:77–91.
25. Franklin FA. Nutritional biochemistry of lipids. In: Grand RJ, Sutphen JL, Dietz WH, eds. *Pediatric nutrition: theory and practice.* Boston: Butterworth, 1987;2–18.
26. Sternlieb I. Copper and zinc. In: Arias IM, Jacoby WB, Popper H, Schacter D, Schafritz DA, eds. *The liver, biology and pathobiology.* New York: Raven Press, 1988;525–534.
27. Piccoli DA, Witzelben CL, Watkins JB, Neonatal iron storage disease. In: Walker WA, Durie PA, Hamilton JR, Walker-Smith JA, Watkins JB, eds. *Pediatric gastrointestinal disease, pathophysiology diagnosis management.* Philadelphia, Toronto: BC Decker, 1991;1063–1065.
28. Berry GT. Disorders of amino acid metabolism. In: Walker WA, Durie PA, Hamilton JR, Walker-Smith JA, Watkins JB, eds. *Pediatric gastrointestinal disease pathophysiology, diagnosis and management,* vol 2. Philadelphia, Toronto: BC Decker, 1991;943–957.
29. Weber FL, Bagby BS, Licate L, Kelsen SG. Effects of branched-chain amino acids on nitrogen metabolism in patients with cirrhosis. *Hepatology* 1990;11:942–950.
30. Wahren J, Denis J, Desurmont P, Eriksson LS, Escoffier JM, Gauthier AP, Hegenfeldt L, Michel H, Opolon P, Paris JC, Veyrac M. Is intravenous administration of branched chain amino acids effective in the treatment of hepatic encephalopathy? A multicenter study. *Hepatology* 1983;3:475–480.
31. Dolz C, Raurich JM, Ibanex J, Obrador A, Marse P, Gaya J. Ascites increases the resting energy expenditure in liver cirrhosis. *Gastroenterology* 1991;100:738–744.
32. Delafosse B, Faure JL, Bouffard Y, Viale JP, Goudable J, Annat G, Neidecker J, Bertrand O, Motin J. Liver transplantation-energy expenditure, nitrogen loss, and substrate oxidation rate in the first two postoperative days. *Transplant Proc* 1989;21:2453–2454.
33. Reilly J, Mehta R, Teperman L, Cemaj S, Tzakis A, Katsuhiko Y, Ritter P, Rezak A, Makowka L. Nutritional support after liver transplantation: a randomized prospective study. *JPEN J Parenter Enteral Nutr* 1990;14:386–391.
34. Dietz WH. Nutritional requirements and feeding of the handicapped child. In: Grand RJ, Sutphen JL, Dietz WH, eds. *Pediatric nutrition: theory and practice.* Boston: Butterworth, 1987; 387–392.
35. Merritt RJ. Nutritional requirements. In: Walker WA, et al., eds. *Pediatric gastrointestinal disease, pathophysiology, diagnosis, management,* vol 2. Philadelphia, Toronto: BC Decker 1991; 1579–1596.

CHAPTER 31

Nutritional Considerations in the Prognosis and Treatment of Children with Pancreatic Disease

J. Armando Madrazo–de la Garza and Emanuel Lebenthal

The human exocrine pancreas undergoes rapid developmental changes at the subcellular and molecular levels during fetal and immediate postnatal life. The gene expression of the zymogen enzymes, amylase, lipase, and the proteases occurs in different periods during ontogeny. Proteolytic enzyme accumulation and secretion precede those of lipolytic and amylolytic during fetal life. At birth, the human pancreas amylolytic activity is nonexistent; lipolytic activity is available to a limited extent (1–4). Alternate digestive enzymes, such as lingual lipase, salivary amylase, and intestinal glucoamylase have been described (4–8). Physiologic pancreatic insufficiency in the premature and small-for-dates infant affects digestion and absorption capabilities. The ideal formula for premature infants would be designed with an awareness of the infant's limited digestive capabilities as well as its need for rapid maturation.

Human and animal studies support the premise that variation of diet during development results in modification of pancreatic enzyme synthesis and secretory responses (9–22). In addition, the administration of thyroid or glucocorticoid hormones during development promotes early maturation of pancreatic exocrine function in animals (23–27).

Digestion of fats, proteins and starches in infants depends, to a large extent, on the degree of maturation of exocrine pancreatic function. Since the maturation processes are modifiable by exogenous factors, attempts to develop procedures to enhance these processes, during critical periods of infant development, may be of particular importance for future investigation. Adaptation of future technologies, specifically in molecular biology, will help us (a) discover genetic sequences and their molecular diversity, (b) learn about the expression of a particular gene and its dimensions, and (c) discover the sequencing of genetic material that may prove to be diagnostic of a disease or a causative agent.

Among diseases that cause pancreatic insufficiency in pediatrics, cystic fibrosis (CF) is the most prevalent. Cystic fibrosis patients suffer from pancreatic insufficiency, a decreased bile acid pool, inability of the duodenum to buffer gastric acidity, a thicker and more viscous unstirred layer in the small intestine that limits diffusion of nutrients, and, at times, secondary mucosal injury of the small intestine. Other rare causes of pancreatic insufficiency, such as Shwachman-Diamond syndrome, pancreatitis, and congenital pancreatic enzyme deficiencies combine maldigestion with an inability to assimilate complex nutrients.

Nutritional deficiencies affect pancreatic function. Nutritional deprivation leads to decreased exocrine enzyme secretion with normal volume output and preserved ability to raise pH in the duodenum (28–36). Obesity is associated with lower levels of enzyme secretion and accumulation of fat in pancreatic acinar cells (37–40).

This chapter is a review of the relationship between pancreatic disease in childhood and nutrition. It emphasizes physiologic pancreatic insufficiency in the premature and compromised infant, the nutritional aspects of pancreatic insufficiency, and the difficulty of providing enzyme supplements to relieve the steatorrhea.

ONTOGENY OF THE EXOCRINE PANCREATIC FUNCTION

Despite the relatively mature morphologic appearance of the pancreas at term, the newborn infant does

---

J. A. Madrazo–de la Garza: Departments of Gastroenterology and Ophthalmology, Hospital de Pediatria, Mexico City, Mexico 06725.

E. Lebenthal: Department of Pediatrics, International Institute for Infant Nutrition and Gastrointestinal Disease, Hahnemann University Hospital, Philadelphia, Pennsylvania 19102-1192.

not show full secretory pancreatic function in response to food, nor a full range of tissue enzymes (1). Proteolytic activity of the pancreatic tissue appears as early as 20 to 24 weeks of gestation and increases slowly until 32 weeks. After this period, there is a dramatic increase of this activity until birth (2–4). Trypsinogen-specific activity at 80% to 90% of adult values has been found in autopsy material from term infants. Full maturation of proteolytic specific activity is not reached until 18 to 24 months of age (1).

Lipase, colipase, and phospholipase A_2 are present at 16 weeks' gestation. At birth, the lipolytic-specific activity is 20% to 25% of adult values; full maturation is accomplished at 18 to 24 months of age (41).

Amylase is detectable from 16 weeks of gestation, but its activity is very low or nonexistent, remaining so until 3 months after birth. Salivary and mammary amylase compensate for complex carbohydrate digestion at this stage (8,42–46).

Pancreatic exocrine secretion into the duodenum occurs during gestation. It is not, however, until the second year of life that adult levels of all pancreatic enzymes are found in the duodenum (1). Pancreatic response to secretagogues occurs only after 1 month of postnatal life. This delayed response seems to be related to lower intracellular mediators or receptor components present in the cell membrane (47,48). Enterokinase activates trypsinogen in the duodenal lumen and indirectly activates the rest of the pancreatic proteases. At term, only 20% of adult enterokinase activity is found; this is possibly a limiting factor for proteolytic activity during the first month of life (49,50).

DIETARY AND ENVIRONMENTAL EFFECT ON EXOCRINE PANCREATIC FUNCTION

Pancreatic function is known to be altered by a number of nutritional factors, including changes in dietary components, caloric content, and patterns of food intake. The ability of the pancreas to adapt to changes in dietary constituents has been widely described (9–15). A high-carbohydrate diet results in high pancreatic amylase and low lipase activities; diets containing high levels of unsaturated fatty acids, on the other hand, promote lipase activity (51). Diets that have high protein content, a high concentration of a single amino acid, or both, evoke more complex responses. Casein increases amylase more that it increases trypsinogen or chymotrypsinogen (52). In contrast, whole egg protein seems to increase the synthesis of chymotrypsinogen more than it increases amylase (53). Supplements of methionine increase lipase and protease contents, whereas phenylalanine and isoleucine increase only protease (52).

Studies in humans seem to confirm the results in animal experimentation. Premature infants fed a high-starch diet exhibited a tenfold increase in amylase content in duodenal fluids (19). It is not clear from this early study, however, whether the amylase is of salivary or pancreatic origin. In addition, a high-protein diet fed to infants increased trypsin and chymotrypsin concentrations (19). Premature infants fed a soy protein formula had greater specific activities, following cholecystokinin (CCK) administration, of trypsin and lipase, than a group of infants fed a milk-based formula (20).

Weaning studies in rats have indicated that the appearance of pancreatic amylase is governed by both exogenous (dietary) and endogenous (hormones) factors. During premature weaning in rat pups, an early increase in amylase levels was noted (22). In contrast, when nursing was continued for longer periods of time, amylase activity increased slowly despite the absence of changes in dietary carbohydrates (22). In the latter case, changes in blood levels of corticosteroids were believed to be important in the expression of amylase in the neonatal period (54).

Short-term fasting in adult rats led to a decrease in the size of the pancreas (55,56), loss of zymogen granules (57), and changes in activities of pancreatic enzymes. Amylase activity was found to be markedly reduced, whereas lipase activity was doubled following fasting (55,58).

HORMONAL INFLUENCES ON PANCREATIC FUNCTION

It is known from animal studies that pancreatic tissue responds to exogenous hormones through specific receptors. Cholecystokinin (CCK) receptors are present at birth and rise to adult levels on day 18 in the rat pancreas. Exogenous administration of CCK during development, especially when combined with secretin, causes marked increase in pancreatic weight, DNA, RNA, and protein content in the rat. However, in children, a significant increase in enzyme concentration in the duodenal fluid is not seen until 2 years of age. This secretory response is potentiated by insulin and glucocorticoids (59–63).

Secretin stimulates water and bicarbonate secretion from the pancreas, whereas it has a slight effect on pancreatic enzyme secretion. Significant synergism occurs when secretin and CCK are given together (5,19).

Glucocorticoids are known to induce precocious maturation of enzyme synthesis in the rat pancreas during development. Specific receptors mediate this response. Also, thyroxine has an effect on glucocorticoid receptors, independent of adrenal function, modulating the rate of secretion of pancreatic juice and the content of enzymes in normal animals (64–68). After the weaning period, this effect is no longer possible, suggesting that variability of gene expression occurs during development.

Other hormones are known to inhibit the exocrine function of the pancreas. Somatostatin inhibits DNA, RNA, and protein synthesis, whereas bicarbonate secretion is not affected (69,70). Glucagon exerts its effect on the secretory apparatus, especially on bicarbonate response to duodenal acidification (70,71).

PANCREATIC DISEASE IN CHILDREN

Children with pancreatic disease manifest a wide range of clinical signs. The most significant picture is pancreatic insufficiency (PI), which only affects digestion, growth, and development in severe cases (Table 1).

Cystic Fibrosis

Cystic fibrosis is the primary cause of PI in children. Its three main characteristics are pulmonary disease, elevated sweat electrolytes, and pancreatic insufficiency. It is transmitted as an autosomal recessive disorder and the underlying genetic lesion is located in the long arm of chromosome 7 (72–74). CF has an estimated incidence of 1 in 2,000 live births in the American Caucasian population, and 1 in 17,000 in the African-American population. The pathology of cystic fibrosis is found in almost every organ (75,76); the manifestations are obstructive bronchopulmonary disease, fibrosis and ductal dilation of the pancreas, meconium ileus, and focal biliary cirrhosis. The primary, most consistent, characteristic changes are found in the exocrine glands. Their secretions may form eosinophilic precipitates or coagulates in pancreatic ducts, intestinal glands, and sublingual salivary glands. In other cases, the gland may appear to be hypersecreting, often with some distention of the ducts, but without the formation of solid casts as seen in glands from the upper respiratory tract and Brunner's glands in the duodenum (76).

The pancreas in cystic fibrosis shows progressive loss of exocrine acinar tissue at or before birth, with gradual regression in infancy characterized by a decrease in acinar to connective tissue ratios. Fibrosis accompanies the gradual acinar degeneration. Luminal dilatation is a common early change in the acinar lobules, which also affects the ducts of the pancreas in CF (77).

The pathophysiology of CF is not as yet well understood. It has been shown, however, that the primary defect involves the transport system in the epithelial cells, primarily that of chloride reabsorption (78). The cystic fibrosis transmembrane conductance regulator (CFTR), product of the defective gene in CF, is believed to function in ion conductants and to play the key role in the pathophysiology of CF (74). Increased calcium and protein concentrations in secretions may contribute to the formations of precipitates that block exocrine gland ducts. Consequently, less bicarbonate and water are secreted to the duodenum, causing failure to raise the pH of the acidic gastric product (1).

The clinical picture is variable. Approximately 12% of patients present first with meconium ileus. Cystic fibrosis accounts for 80% of cases of meconium ileus, and 50% of meconium peritonitis, in newborns (79,80). Consequently, it is recommended that every neonate with intestinal obstruction have a sweat test performed to exclude the disease.

Approximately 57% of patients with CF present with a combination of pulmonary and gastrointestinal symptoms (81). These symptoms usually include failure to thrive, chronic diarrhea, and chronic respiratory problems; 18% present with purely respiratory symptoms that may include hyperinflation, bronchiectasis, empyema, pneumonia, and nasal polyps. Children in the latter group have no evidence of pancreatic insufficiency, thus growth failure is rarely present unless recurrent infections and lung disease are advanced. Another 17% present with symptoms related exclusively to the gastrointestinal tract; 5% present with hypoproteinemia and anemia. It is important to note that because of the diversity of clinical features, and because symptoms may be so minimal, CF should never be excluded because of a normal growth pattern, absence of lung disease, or normal pancreatic function (82).

The age at which diagnosis is made varies; urban children are generally diagnosed earlier than those from rural areas (83). The diagnosis is based on a positive sweat test, although false positives and negatives have been described (84–87). Pancreatic function is usually found to be abnormal. The duodenal fluids demonstrate increased viscosity and markedly reduced secretion of bicarbonate, water, and electrolytes; in 85% to 90% of affected patients, enzymes are decreased or absent (88–

TABLE 1. *Pancreatic insufficiency in childhood*

Generalized pancreatic insufficiency
  Primary
    Cystic fibrosis
    Shwachman-Diamond syndrome
    Johanson-Blizzard syndrome
  Secondary
    Congenital rubella syndrome
    Pancreatitis
    Protein-energy malnutrition
    Obesity
  Developmental
    Prematurity
    Small for gestational age
    Neonatal period
Isolated enzyme deficiency
  Lipase
  Trypsinogen
  Enterokinase
  Amylase

Adapted from ref. 199.

94). Increased stool fat and protein are common, depending on the severity of pancreatic lesion. Stool trypsin and chymotrypsin activity will be low or absent. Serum amylase may be normal, but isoamylase evaluation will reveal that the salivary form is predominant. Similarly, serum lipase will be predominantly of the pharyngeal type (95).

Although other laboratory and radiologic parameters may help establish the diagnosis of CF, none is sensitive enough to be used alone (Table 2).

The goal of nutritional therapy for an infant or child with CF is to maintain growth velocity by correcting nutritional deficiencies. This is done by prescribing a high-caloric intake [150% of the recommended dietary allowance (RDA)] in conjunction with pancreatic exocrine enzyme replacement.

Schwachman-Diamond Syndrome

Schwachman-Diamond syndrome is the second-most common condition of primary pancreatic insufficiency in children (96,97). Its estimated incidence is 1 in 20,000 births, equally distributed between sexes. It has been attributed to an autosomal recessive genetic pattern (98).

Characteristics of Schwachman-Diamond syndrome include pancreatic insufficiency, bone marrow dysfunction, and severe growth retardation. Associated pathologies include diabetes mellitus, Hirschsprung's disease, and testicular fibrosis (96,98–103).

Steatorrhea, growth failure, and frequent infections secondary to neutropenia are the most important clinical features of this syndrome. Diagnosis is usually made by the presence of repeatedly normal sweat electrolytes in combination with an abnormal pancreatic stimulation test. Enzyme response is generally markedly reduced; bicarbonate secretion is less severely affected. In contrast to CF, the total volume and the viscosity are within the normal range (104,105). At autopsy, the pancreas typically shows replacement of acini by fat and fibrous tissue (97).

Johanson-Blizzard Syndrome

The Johanson-Blizzard syndrome is a rare disorder, with autosomal recessive inheritance, characterized by congenital aplasia of the nasal alae, deafness, microcephaly, hypothyroidism, mental retardation, absence of permanent teeth, and pancreatic insufficiency. Trypsinogen, in particular, seems to be the most severely affected enzyme (106,107). Autopsy findings include a small thyroid filled with colloid, an adipose pancreas, and a cortical developmental defect in the brain consisting of abnormalities of gyral formation and of cortical neuronal organization (108).

Sideroblastic Anemia

Sideroblastic anemia and exocrine pancreatic insufficiency is a syndrome described by Pearson et al. (109) in 1979 in which there are vacuolization of bone marrow precursors and exocrine pancreatic dysfunction.

Isolated Enzyme Deficiencies

Few cases of isolated enzyme deficiencies have been described. In most of these, it is unclear whether patients have a congenital, permanent deficiency of the enzyme, or transient developmental or acquired defects.

Congenital deficiency of pancreatic lipase is rare (110–112); the suggested mode of inheritance is autosomal recessive. It typically begins shortly after birth. Primary clinical features include severe steatorrhea, with offensive, foul smelling, bulky, pale stools. Diagnosis is made through the pancreozymin-secretin test showing solitary low or absent lipase activity but otherwise normal results. Affected individuals continue to gain weight well.

Trypsinogen deficiency results in a lack of proteolytic enzymes, since trypsin, in addition to enterokinase, is required to activate the other proteases that are secreted in an inactive form. These patients have severe malabsorption, anemia, hypoproteinemia, edema, and growth failure (113,114).

Enterokinase is produced in the intestine. Because its function is to activate trypsinogen in the duodenal lumen, its deficiency resembles trypsinogen deficiency. Clinically, it presents with diarrhea and failure to thrive. Laboratory exams report hypoproteinemia and creatorrhea. The diagnosis is made by the presence of proteolytic activity in duodenal fluid after the addition of exogenous enterokinase (115–120).

TABLE 2. *Laboratory evaluation of digestive function in cystic fibrosis*

Meconium tests
    Albumin by test strip
Stool tests
    Microscopic exam (fat droplets, undigested meat fibers)
Serological tests
    Amylase
    Lipase
    Immunoreactive trypsin
    N-Benzoyl, L-tyrosyl, p-aminobenzoic acid test
Radiology
    CAT
    Endoscopic retrograde cholangiopancreatography (ERCP)
    Sonography
Pancreatic stimulation
    Lipase, amylase, proteases
    Bicarbonate assay
    pH determination
    Protein

Adapted from ref. 95.

Isolated amylase deficiency most often seems to be a developmental defect. Selective deficiency, not related to development has, however, been reported in two cases, although one of these cases probably had other pancreatic enzyme deficiencies (121).

There is only one reported case of congenital lipase-colipase deficiency (122), and two cases of isolated colipase deficiency (123).

Pancreatitis

Acute pancreatitis is a rare disorder in pediatrics, and differs from acute pancreatitis in adults in the incidence, etiology, and clinical presentation.

The incidence in pediatrics is low; the main etiologic factors are trauma, infection, and drug intake. More rarely, association with metabolic or hereditary diseases may be detected. A high percentage of acute pancreatitis in children (19% to 25%) remains idiopathic (124,125).

The pathophysiology of pancreatitis is not well understood. The most widely accepted theory is of pancreatic ductal hypertension, which is explained by pancreatic secretion into a previously obstructed duct. Obstruction may be produced by a stone, edema, spasm, or from an acquired or congenital anomaly. This results in activation of pancreatic enzymes leading to pancreatic autodigestion (126,127). Pathologic changes range from pancreatic edema to necrosis, hemorrhage, thrombosis, ischemia, and inflammation (128).

The clinical picture is less predictable in children than in adults. Abdominal pain occurs in most cases, but the onset may be slow or sudden, with variable intensity and duration. Only the older pediatric age group presents the classic abdominal, intense, continuous, knife-like, food-related, epigastric pain. This pain frequently radiates to the back and is associated with nausea, vomiting, and fever (124,129–134).

Diagnosis of pancreatitis is made by laboratory parameters; serum and urine amylase and lipase remain the most reliable diagnostic method. Serum immunoreactive trypsin complexed to α_2-macroglobulin and α_1-protease inhibitor correlates with the histologic severity of the condition (135).

Although imaging procedures are not sensitive enough to diagnose acute pancreatitis, they are useful in confirming clinical and laboratory diagnoses.

The goals of treatment are to relieve pain, by putting the pancreas at rest, to correct fluid and electrolyte abnormalities, and to prevent complications. Stimulation of pancreatic secretion should be minimized by fasting the patient and starting an intravenous infusion to supply maintenance fluids and electrolytes. If the patient is vomiting, or has an ileus, a nasogastric tube is required. Feeding should not be resumed until abdominal tenderness has disappeared, bowel sounds are normal, and there is no biochemical evidence of inflammatory activity. Total parenteral nutrition is required when fasting needs to be prolonged more than 5 days (124,136,137). Pain is relieved with the use of meperidine 1 mg/kg IM or IV. Anticholinergics and antibiotics do not have significant benefit in this disease.

Once clinical improvement occurs, a high-carbohydrate low-fat diet is recommended (138).

Undernutrition

Protein-energy malnutrition (PEM) is the most significant public health problem in developing countries. Mild to moderate PEM is reported to affect almost two-thirds of the children in the third world (139,140). Because the pancreas, along with the liver and small intestine, demonstrates the highest rates of protein synthesis and turnover (141), abnormalities of exocrine pancreatic function and structure are expected in PEM (28,141). Examination of the pancreas in children dying of kwashiorkor shows a generalized reduction in size (31–36,142). On light microscopy, extreme atrophy, with disorganization and loss of the acinar pattern, is also seen, but with little evidence of inflammation or necrosis. Acinar cells contain few zymogen granules, appear vacuolated, and, in many instances, show hyaline masses. As might be expected, these changes are accompanied by fat degeneration in the liver and atrophy of the small intestinal mucosa.

Functional changes in the pancreas in PEM closely reflect the structural abnormalities. Steatorrhea and creatorrhea have been reported (143,144). Deterioration in basal pancreatic function seems to progress serially, lipase being the first enzyme to be affected, followed by amylase (145). In advanced cases, enzyme secretion almost completely ceases. Extensive fibrosis of the pancreas may be demonstrated and correlated with the marked suppression in function.

Little is known of the effects of malnutrition in the fetal, neonatal, and early-infancy periods in humans. In animal studies, rapid changes were observed in pancreatic function during the onset of malnutrition, probably because of the increased nutritional requirements of early growth. The decreased production of pancreatic enzymes, and the histological changes, with the exception of fibrosis, were similar to what has been observed in children and adults (146,147). In rats, pups born to dams receiving a protein-deficient diet during pregnancy had lower tissue levels of pancreatic enzymes. They recovered, following breast-feeding by dams fed adequate protein diets, or after weaning onto regular chow (146). Similar results were reported with sows fed a protein-free diet during pregnancy (148). Rat pups, malnourished from birth to weaning, have shown markedly reduced pancreatic weights and enzyme contents (29,149). Nutritional rehabilitation, following weaning, resulted in recovery of pancreatic enzymes, to control levels, within 2 weeks (29).

Obesity

Secretin stimulation tests, performed in five obese patients, revealed that obesity in humans led to pancreatic hypofunction (37). Total amylase secretion was abnormally low in three of the five, and the amylase secretion per kilogram of body weight was low in four of five. The relative pancreatic insufficiency revealed in the laboratory did not, however, lead to clinical malabsorption, the onset of which would benefit the obese. After weight reduction, there was a relative absolute increase in the rate of enzyme secretion, regardless of whether amylase secretion before weight reduction had been normal or abnormal.

At autopsy, obese subjects have demonstrated marked accumulation of fat in pancreatic acinar cells, a structural alteration that may contribute to the pancreatic hypofunction observed in obese patients (37,150). Complete reversal function following weight reduction indicates the absence of permanent structural damage.

NUTRITIONAL MANAGEMENT OF PANCREATIC INSUFFICIENCY

The chronic undernutrition of pancreatic insufficiency, with the consequential failure to thrive, is the result of a combination of inadequate caloric intake, maldigestion, malabsorption, abnormal nutrient losses, and increased requirements. Success in treatment is dependent on a complete evaluation of each patient's nutritional status in order to individualize management.

Because cystic fibrosis accounts for more than 90% of pancreatic insufficiency in children, discussion of treatment appropriately begins with this disease. Specific issues of other diseases are important to note, as well.

Caloric intake in cystic fibrosis varies widely from patient to patient. It is probably true, however, that actual intake is usually considerably lower than recommended levels (151–154). One major cause is anorexia, which may persist despite nutritional supplementation and high-energy diets. Intake also deteriorates as a result of the frequently present acute pulmonary infections (152).

The result of the decreased intake is an unfavorable energy balance and failure to grow. Recent studies demonstrate that children with CF do not grow until the percentage of energy absorbed exceeds 100% to 110% that of RDA (155); thus, a caloric intake between 120% and 150% of RDA is currently recommended (156).

Composition of the recommended diet has changed in recent years. The Toronto group suggested that, as a result of not restricting dietary fat, an improvement in weight, height, and mean survival occurred in their CF population (157,158).

Patients with CF have low circulating levels of linoleic acid and elevated palmitic, palmitoleic, and oleic acids (159–161). All four plasma lipid fractions (triglycerides, phospholipids, free fatty acids, and cholesterol esters) are reportedly abnormal in CF patients with malabsorption. Medium-chain triglyceride malabsorption was documented in CF and improved with pancreatic enzyme supplementation (162). Although low-fat diets had previously been recommended in an attempt to reduce the abdominal symptoms of malabsorption, dietary fat is now recognized as an important high-density source of calories which improves the palatability of food, and provides essential fatty acids that are unable to be synthesized by the individual. Essential fatty acid deficiency may result in major impairments, such as growth, the production of biological membranes, and the functioning of essential metabolic pathways, especially those involved with prostaglandin synthesis. Long-term consumption of supplemental linoleic acid, in addition to adequate caloric intake, should improve the linoleic acid status of most, if not all, CF patients (163).

Protein intake, in cystic fibrosis, should provide 15% to 20% of total daily caloric intake (RDA). The major risk of protein deficiency in pancreatic insufficiency occurs during the first year of life when the requirements are high.

Vitamin deficiencies have been reported in pancreatic insufficiency (164–168). Decreased vitamin A status causes night blindness, xerophthalmia, and, occasionally, keratomalacia. CF patients have been shown to have decreased plasma vitamin A concentrations, in spite of adequate supplementation with 10,000 units/day, but significantly increased hepatic stores (169,170). Explanations for the decreased serum vitamin A levels include a defect in the mobilization and transport system due to liver disease in CF, zinc deficiency, and malnutrition with decreased visceral proteins. A supplementation of 5,000 to 10,000 units of vitamin A per day is recommended (171).

Decreased vitamin D status, with bone demineralization and normal levels of circulating calcium, are also seen. Some authors, however, have reported that all CF patients under 10 years of age had normal bone mineral content, and that females suffered demineralization more than males (172). Vitamin D absorption in patients is not well known, but there are several reports on serum vitamin D metabolites. The mean serum levels of 25-OH-vitamin D have been reported as low to normal (164,165). Currently, administration of 400 to 800 IU of vitamin D per day is recommended (173).

Vitamin E is known to function as a biological antioxidant, protecting the polyunsaturated fatty acids of membrane phospholipids from oxidation (174). Deficiency of vitamin E produces changes in the hematological system associated with decreased vitamin E levels (175). A neurologic syndrome that includes areflexia, ataxia, posterior column dysfunction, peripheral neuropathy, and ophthalmoplegia has been described in vitamin E deficiency (176). Supplementation with vitamin E, ideally using a water-soluble preparation, is required to prevent tocopherol deficiency (177). In contrast to vitamin A, blood levels of vitamin E do reflect tissue concentrations, since no abnormality in tocopherol transport has been described (170). The supplements usually prescribed range from 50 IU for infants to 200 IU for adults (173).

In older CF patients, hypoprothrombinemia occurrence may be attributable to several factors. Malabsorption of vitamin K may occur, especially in the presence of steatorrhea and antibiotic intake, which can alter the bacterial flora of the intestinal tract and possibly decrease synthesis of vitamin K. It is known that vitamin K deficiency may produce hemorrhagic tendencies in patients under 4 months of age. Sources of this vitamin are green leafy vegetables, cheese, butter, and beef liver. The other 50% comes from bacterial synthesis in the intestinal tract. Recommended doses are 5 mg twice weekly (177).

Vitamin B_{12} requires pancreatic enzymes for normal absorption. The Schilling test may be abnormal, but it returns to normal with pancreatic enzyme supplements or sodium bicarbonate (178,179). The average values for vitamin B_1 (thiamine), vitamin B_2 (riboflavin), vitamin B_6 (pyridoxine), folate, and vitamin C (ascorbic acid) are similar in CF and control populations (180,181).

PANCREATIC ENZYME SUPPLEMENTATION

Pancreatic enzyme supplementation has evolved very recently. Formerly, less effective pancreas extracts had been given. With these, only 8% of ingested lipase and 22% of ingested trypsin could circumvent inactivation by gastric acidity with a 10% to 15% maximum increase in fat absorption and the risk of hyperuricosuria. This treatment did, however, correct lipid-soluble vitamin deficiency and improved growth in 50% of the patients (182,183). Adding antiacids, such as sodium bicarbonate, cimetidine, or aluminum hydroxide, to pancreatic extracts improved fat absorption by no more than 10% (95). Coating of the enzymes did not produce any advantage and, in some cases, steatorrhea increased because the tablets passed intact through the entire small bowel.

Enteric-coated encapsulated microspheres have become a useful therapeutic tool in the last 20 years. They have an acid-resistant coat and pH-dependent enzyme release which allows a higher rate of fat absorption by the patient (184–190). Velocity of enzyme release and availability of microspheres varies with commercial preparations (188). Addition of taurine has proved to be advantageous only in severe cases of steatorrhea; in such cases an increase in serum levels of triglycerides, linoleic acid, and cholesterol has been observed (191,192).

Meyer et al. (193) have concluded that size and density of microspheres are very important factors in maximizing the efficacy of therapy. They have shown faster gastric emptying with 1-mm, or smaller, microspheres. It has been demonstrated, in addition, that individualization of dosage, timing, and quantity of fat intake improves the coefficient of fat absorption in CF patients (194,195).

Administration of the enzyme supplements should be at the time of meals regardless of the pH of the food. For infants and small children, the pancreatic microspheres are mixed with food. The time between mixing the food and enzymes, and the beginning of the digestive process, must not exceed 30 min, in order to avoid inactivation by low pH (95,196). Some authors recommend starting pediatric therapy with nine to ten capsules of Pancrease MT-4 (McNeil 36,000 to 40,000 IU of lipase) a day (153,189). Bouquet et al. (197), however, as well as other groups, have shown that maximal fat absorption can be seen with only six capsules (24,000 IU of lipase). This smaller dosage of Pancrease supplies adequate proteases and amylase to maximize protein and carbohydrate digestion (197).

Acid-stable lipases, derived from fungal source or through recombinant DNA techniques, have been proposed recently as advantageous preparations in the treatment of CF. Although no conclusive data are available, it seems that smaller doses of this preparation are needed, in comparison to microsphere preparations, to achieve similar fat absorption (198).

Side effects of pancreatic enzyme preparations available in the United States include mouth soreness, perianal irritation, abdominal pain, mild diarrhea, constipation in infants, hyperuricosuria with high doses, allergic reactions to pork proteins, and immediate hypersensitivity reactions from inhaling the powder during preparation (95).

Nutritional support and pancreatic enzyme supplementation remain cornerstones of therapy for pancreatic insufficiency. Rational, individually designed use of available therapeutic resources is required to mitigate problems, although steatorrhea has not been completely corrected. Most essential, further research is necessary to continue to develop methods for optimizing digestion and absorption of nutrients.

TREATMENT OF ISOLATED ENZYME DEFICIENCIES

Isolated enzyme deficiencies are treated with replacement of pancreatic enzymes, and if required, with semielemental diets. In congenital trypsinogen and enterokinase deficiencies, protein absorption is improved by protein hydrolysate administration. Medium-chain triglycerides, on the other hand, have been shown to be advantageous in bypassing pancreatic lipase and colipase deficiency (107). Close surveillance of growth is advised for assessment of adequate nutrition.

SUMMARY

The human exocrine pancreas undergoes rapid developmental changes at the subcellular and molecular levels during fetal and immediate postnatal life. Proteolytic enzyme accumulation and secretion precede those of lipolytic and amylolytic during fetal life. At birth, the human pancreas amylolytic activity is nonexistent, whereas lipolytic activity is available to a limited extent. Alternate digestive enzymes such as lingual lipase, salivary amylase and intestinal glycoamylase were described in early life.

Disorders of pancreatic function are associated with malnutrition in the pediatric age group. The most common cause of exocrine pancreatic insufficiency in pediatrics is cystic fibrosis. It also involves lower bile acid secretion, decreased buffering capacity of the acid present in the duodenum and a thicker and more viscous unstirred layer in the small intestine that limits diffusion of nutrients.

The treatment of pancreatic insufficiency is focused on the provision of sufficient essential nutrients and the improvement of digestive capabilities by the administration of pancreatic extracts. Acid-resistant enteric-coated microsphere preparations of pancreatic extracts improved the coefficient of fat absorption to 90%. Recently, acid-stable lipases derived from fungal sources or DNA recombinant techniques have been proposed as better preparations. Finally, the development of semi-elemental formulas has greatly facilitated therapy in these patients.

REFERENCES

1. Lebenthal E, Lev R, Lee PC. Prenatal and postnatal development of the human exocrine pancreas. In: Go VLW, et al., eds. *The exocrine pancreas: biology, pathobiology and diseases.* New York: Raven Press, 1986;33–43.
2. Keene MF, Hewer EE. Digestive enzymes of the human fetus. *Lancet* 1929;1:767–769.
3. Lieberman J. Proteolytic enzyme activity in fetal pancreas and meconium: demonstration of plasminogen and trypsinogen activators in pancreatic tissue. *Gastroenterology* 1966;50:183–190.
4. Track NS, Creutzfeldt C, Bokermann M. Enzymatic, functional and ultrastructural development of the exocrine pancreas. II: The Human Pancreas. *Comp Biochem Physiol* A: Comparative Physiology 1975;51:95–100.
5. Lebenthal E, Lee PC. Development of functional response in human exocrine pancreas. *Pediatrics* 1980;66:556–560.
6. Lebenthal E, Heitlinger LA. Starch intolerance in infancy: factors involved in a controversial area. In: Lifshitz F, ed. *Carbohydrate intolerance in infancy.* New York: Marcel Dekker, 1982;213–222.
7. Lebenthal E, Lee PC. Alternate pathways of digestion and absorption in early infancy. *J Pediatr Gastroenterol Nutr* 1984;3:1–3.
8. Lee PC. Alternate pathways in starch digestion. In: Lifshitz F, ed. *Carbohydrate intolerance in infancy.* New York: Marcel Dekker, 1982;223–236.
9. Ben-Abdeljlil A, Visani AM, Desnvelle P. Adaptation of the exocrine secretion of rat pancreas to the composition of the diet. *Biochem Biophys Res Commun* 1963;10:112–116.
10. Deschodt-Lanekman M, Robberecht P, Camus H, Christophe J. Short-term adaptation of pancreatic hydrolases to nutritional and physiological stimuli in adult rats. *Biochimie* 1971;53:789–796.
11. Gidez LI. Effect of dietary fat on pancreatic lipase levels in the rat. *J Lipid Res* 1973;14:169–177.
12. Grossman MI, Greengard H, Ivy AC. The effect of dietary composition on pancreatic enzymes. *Am J Physiol* 1942;138:676–682.
13. Grossman MI, Greengard H, Ivy AC. On the mechanism of the adaptation of pancreatic enzymes to dietary composition. *Am J Physiol* 1944;141:38–41.
14. Houghton MR, Morgan RGH, Gracey M. Effects of long term dietary modifications on pancreatic enzyme activity. *J Pediatr Gastroenterol Nutr* 1983;2:548–554.
15. Snook JT. Dietary regulation of pancreatic enzyme in the rat with emphasis on carbohydrate. *Am J Physiol* 1971;221:1383–1387.
16. Desnuelle J, Reboud JP, Ben-Abdeljlil A. Influence of the composition of the diet on the enzyme content of the rat pancreas. In: CIBA Foundation Symposium. *The exocrine pancreas.* London: Churchill, 1962;90–107.
17. Dagorn JC, Lahaie RG. Dietary regulation of pancreatic protein synthesis. I. Rapid and specific modulation of enzyme synthesis by changes in dietary composition. *Biochim Biophys Acta* 1981;654:111–118.
18. Lahaie RG, Dagorn JC. Dietary regulation of pancreatic protein synthesis. Kinetics of adaptation of protein synthesis and its effect on enzyme content. *Biochim Biophys Acta* 1980;654:119–123.
19. Zoppi G, Andreotti G, Pajno-Ferrasa F, Njai DM, Gaborro D. Exocrine pancreas function in premature and full term neonates. *Pediatr Res* 1972;6:880–886.
20. Lebenthal E, Choi TS, Lee PC. The development of pancreatic function in premature infants after milk based and soy-based formulas. *Pediatr Res* 1981;15:1240–1244.
21. Adler G, Kern HF. Regulation of exocrine pancreatic secretory process by insulin in vivo. *Horm Metab Res* 1975;7:290–296.
22. Lee PC, Kimm O, Lebenthal E. Effect of early weaning and prolonged nursing on development of the rat pancreas. *Pediatr Res* 1982;16:470–473.
23. Deschodt-Lanekman M, Robberecht P, Camus J, Baya C, Christophe J. Hormonal and dietary adaptation of rat pancreas hydrolases before and after weaning. *Am J Physiol* 1974;226:39–44.
24. Morisset J, Jolicoeur L. Effect of hydrocortisone on pancreatic growth in rats. *Am J Physiol* 1980;239:G95–G98.
25. Sesso A. Effet de la thyroxine et de la cortisone sur les grains de secretion, les acides nucleiques et les activities amylolytique et proteolytique du pancreas chez la jeune rat. *C R Acad Sci Paris* 1962;254:569–570.
26. Morisset J, Jolicoeur L, Genik P, Lord A. Interaction of hydrocortisone and caerulein on pancreatic size and composition in the rat. *Am J Physiol* 1981;241:G37–G42.
27. Alliet PH, Lu RB, Madrazo-de la Garza JA, Santer R, Lebenthal E, and Lee PC. Response of exocrine pancreas to corticosterone and aldosterone after adrenalectomy. *J Steroid Biochem* 1989;33:1097–1102.
28. Slot JW, Strous GJAM, Geugz JJ. Effect of fasting and feeding on synthesis and intracellular transport of proteins in the frog exocrine pancreas. *Gastroenterology* 1979;80:708–714.
29. Rossi TM, Lee PC, Lebenthal E. Effect of feeding regimens on the functional recovery of pancreatic enzymes in postnatally malnourished weanling rats. *Pediatr Res* 1983;17:806–809.
30. Robinson LK, Hurley LS. Effect of maternal zinc deficiency or food restriction on rat fetal pancreas. I. Procarboxy peptidase A and chymotrypsinogen. *J Nutr* 1981;111:869–877.
31. Blackburn WR, Vinijchaikul K. The pancreas in kwashiorkor in electron microscopic study. *Lab Invest* 1969;20:305–318.

32. Bras G, Waterlow JC, DePass E. Further observations on the liver, pancreas, and kidney in malnourished infants and children. The relation of certain histopathological changes in the pancreas and those in liver and kidney. *West Indian Med J* 1975;6:33–42.
33. Shaper AG. Chronic pancreatic disease and protein malnutrition. *Lancet* 1960;1:1223–1224.
34. Shaper AG. Aetiology of chronic pancreatic fibrosis with calcification seen in Uganda. *Br Med J* 1964;1:1607–1609.
35. Thompson MD, Trowell HC. Pancreatic enzyme activity in duodenal contents of children with a type of kwashiorkor. *Lancet* 1951;1:1031–1035.
36. Veghelyi PV, Kemeny TT, Pozsonyi J, Sos J. Dietary lesions of the pancreas. *Am J Dis Child* 1950;79:658–665.
37. Drieling DA, Elsbach P, Schaffner F, Schwartz IL. The effect of reduction of protein and total calories on pancreatic function in obese patients. *Gastroenterology* 1961;46:686–690.
38. McGuinness EF, Morgan RG, Levinson DA, Frape DL, Hopwood D, Wormsley KG. The effects of long-term feeding of soy flour on the rat pancreas. *Scand J Gastroenterol* 1980;15:497–502.
39. Praissman M, Izzo RS. Pancreatic CCK receptors in genetically obese rats. Diminished numbers of binding sites with increased affinity compared to lean rats. *Gastroenterology* 1983;84:1276.
40. Lee PC, Bernardis LL, Brooks S, McEwen G, Lebenthal E. Effect of ventral medical hypothalamic nuclei lesions on pancreatic development in postweanling rats. *Newsletter Natl Pancreatic Cancer Proj* 1981;6:33.
41. Bokermann M, Track NS, et al. Biochemical and ultrastructural changes in human pancreas during fetal development. In: Kaiser D, eds. *Approaches to cystic fibrosis.* Heilbronn, Germany: Thunert and Bofinger GmbH, 1983;221–229.
42. Gillard BK, Simbala JA, Feig SA. Serum amylase isoenzymes in cystic fibrosis patient. *Pediatr Res* 1980;14:1168.
43. Jones JB, Mehta NR, Hamosh M. Alpha-amylase in preterm human milk. *J Pediatr Gastroenterol Nutr* 1982;1:43.
44. Lindberg T, Skude G. Amylase in human milk. *Pediatrics* 1982;70:235.
45. Heitlinger LA, Lee PC, Dillon WP, Lebenthal E. Mammary amylase: a possible alternate pathway of carbohydrate digestion in infancy. *Pediatr Res* 1982;17:15.
46. Lebenthal E, Lee PC. Glucoamylase and disaccharidase activities in normal subjects and in patients with mucosal injury of the small intestine. *J Pediatr* 1980;97:389.
47. Doyle CM, Jamieson JD. Development of secretagogue response in rat pancreatic acinar cells. *Dev Biol* 1978;65:11–27.
48. Larose L, Morisset J. Acinar cell responsiveness to urecholine with rat pancreas during fetal and early postnatal growth. *Gastroenterology* 1974;75:530–533.
49. Antonowicz I, Lebenthal E. Development pattern of small intestinal enterokinase and disaccharidase activities in the human fetus. *Gastroenterology* 1977;2:1299–1303.
50. Lebenthal E, Lee PC. Effect of pancreozymin and secretin on intraluminal enterokinase, trypsin, and chymotrypsin activities of cystic fibrosis and control children. *Digestion* 1982;23:39–47.
51. Benzonara C, Desnuelle P. Etude cinctique de l'action de la lipase pancreatique sur des triglycerides en emulsion. *Biochim Biophys Acta* 1965;105:21.
52. Snook JT. Dietary regulation of pancreatic enzyme synthesis, secretion and inactivation in the rat. *J Nutr* 1965;87:297.
53. DeVizia B, Ciccimarra F, DeCicco N, Auricchio S. Digestibility of starches in infants and children. *J Pediatr* 1975;86:50.
54. Lee PC, Lebenthal E. Role of corticoids independent of food intake in premature increase of pancreatic enzyme activities following early weaning in rats. *J Nutr* 1983;113:1381–1387.
55. Lee PC, Brooks S, Lebenthal E. Effect of fasting and refeeding on pancreatic enzymes and secretagogue responsiveness in rats. *Am J Physiol* 1982;242:G215–G221.
56. Webster PD, Singh M, Tucker PC, Black O. Effects of fasting and feeding on the pancreas. *Gastroenterology* 1972;62:600–605.
57. Carazzuti F, Paradisi R, Coppo N. Experimental pancreatic damage deficient nutrition. In: Recent advances in gastroenterology. Basel, Karger, 1966;4:345–347.
58. Christophe J, Comus J, Deschodt-Lanckman M, Rathe J, Robberecht P, Vandermeers-Piret MC, Vandermeers A. Factors regulating biosynthesis, intracellular transport, and secretion of amylase and lipase in the rat exocrine pancreas. *Horm Metab Res* 1971;3:393–403.
59. Werlin SL. Ontogeny of secretory function and cholecystokinin binding capacity in immature rat pancreas. *Life Sci* 1987;40:2237–2245.
60. Leung YK, Lee PC, Lebenthal E. Maturation of cholecystokinin receptors in pancreatic acini of rats. *Am J Physiol* 1986;250:G594–G597.
61. Chang A, Jamieson JD. Stimulus-secretion coupling in the developing exocrine pancreas: secretory responsiveness to cholecystokinin. *J Cell Biol* 1986;103:2353–2365.
62. Leung YK, Jirapinyo P, Lebenthal E, Lee PC. Effect of hydrocortisone on the maturation of cholecystokinin (CCK) binding and acini of neonatal rats. *Pancreas* 1987;2:73–78.
63. Githens S. Differentiation and development of the exocrine pancreas in animals. In: Go VLW, et al., eds. *The exocrine pancreas: biology, pathobiology, and diseases.* New York: Raven Press, 1986;21–32.
64. Lu RB, Lebenthal E, Lee PC. Developmental changes of glucocorticoid receptors in the rat pancreas. *J Steroid Biochem* 1987;26:213–218.
65. Madrazo-de la Garza JA, Yoon Y, Lu RB, Lee PC, Lebenthal E. Down and up-regulation of glucocosticoid (GC) receptors by dexamethasone (DX) in rat pancreas during different developmental stages. *Pancreas* 1989;4:629.
66. Lu RB, Lebenthal E, Lee PC. Regulation of rat pancreatic glucocosticoid receptors by thyroxine during development. *Endocrinology* 1988;123:2235–2241.
67. Lu RB, Chaichanwatanakul C, Lin CH, Lebenthal E, Lee PC. Thyroxine effect on exocrine pancreatic development in rats. *Am J Physiol* 1988;254:G315–G321.
68. Lee JT, Lebenthal E, Lee PC. Rat pancreatic nuclear thyroid hormone receptor: characterization and postnatal development. *Gastroenterology* 1989;96:1151–1157.
69. Morisset J, Genik P, Lord A, Solomon T. Effects of chronic administration of somatostatin on rat exocrine pancreas. *Regul Pept* 1982;4:49–58.
70. Leung YK, Lebenthal E. Gastrointestinal peptides: physiology, ontogeny, and clinical significance. In: Lebenthal E, ed. *Human gastrointestinal development.* New York: Raven Press, 1989;41–98.
71. Konturek S, Tasler J, Obtulowicz W. Characteristics of inhibition of pancreatic secretion by glucagon. *Digestion* 1974;10:138–149.
72. Kevem B, Rommens JM, Buchanan JA, Markiewicz D, Cox TK, Aravinda CH, Buchwald M, Tsui L.CH. Identification of the cystic fibrosis gene: genetic analysis. *Science* 1989;245:1073–1080.
73. Rommens JM, Iannuzzi MC, Kerem B, Drumm ML, Melmer G, Dean M, Rozmahel R, et al. Identification of the cystic fibrosis gene: chromosome walking and jumping. *Science* 1989;245:1059–1065.
74. Riordan JR, Rommens JM, Kerem B, Alon N, Rozmahel R, Grzelczak Z, Zielenski J, et al. Identification of the cystic fibrosis gene: cloning and characterization of complementary DNA. *Science* 1989;245:1066–1072.
75. Vawter GF, Shwachman H. Cystic fibrosis in adults: an autopsy study. *Pathol Annu* 1979;14:357–382.
76. Anderson DH. Pathology of cystic fibrosis. *Ann NY Acad Sci* 1962;95:500–517.
77. Lebenthal E. Pancreatic insufficiency in cystic fibrosis: result of defect in ontogenesis of the exocrine pancreas. *J Pediatr Gastroenterol Nutr* 1984;3:S51–S54.
78. Quinton PM, Bijman J. Higher bioelectric potentials due to decreased chloride absorption in the sweat glands of patients with cystic fibrosis. *N Engl J Med* 1983;308:1185–1189.
79. Olsen M, Luck S, Lloyd-Still JD. The spectrum of meconium disease in infancy. *J Pediatr Surg* 1982;17:479–482.
80. Hardy JD, Davison SHH, Higgins MV. Sweat test in the newborn period. *Arch Dis Child* 1973;48:316–318.
81. Gurwitz D, Corey M, Francis PWJ. Perspectives in cystic fibrosis. *Pediatr Clin North Am* 1979;26:603–615.
82. Lloyd-Still JD. Cystic fibrosis. In: Lebenthal E, ed. *Textbook of gastroenterology and nutrition in infancy,* 2nd ed. New York: Raven Press, 1989;831–876.

83. Mischler E, Rock M, Farrell P, et al. Wisconsin experience with screening and common psychosocial description of parents with false positive screen. 1987 North American Cystic Fibrosis Congress, Toronto. *Pediatr Pulmonol* 1987;1:81–83.
84. Davis PB, Hubbard VS, di Sant'Agnese PA. Low sweat electrolytes in a patient with cystic fibrosis. *Am J Med* 1980;69:643–646.
85. Sarsfield JK, Davies JM. Negative sweat test and cystic fibrosis. *Arch Dis Child* 1975;50:463–466.
86. Ruddy RM, Scanlin TF. Abnormal sweat electrolytes in a case of celiac disease and a case of psychosocial failure to thrive. Review of other reported causes. *Clin Pediatr* 1987;26:83–89.
87. Rosenstein BJ, Langbaum TS. Misdiagnosis of cystic fibrosis. Need for continuing follow-up and re-evaluation. *Clin Pediatr* 1987;26:78–82.
88. Brooks F. Testing pancreatic function. *N Engl J Med* 1972;286:300–303.
89. Dreiling DA, Janowitz HD. The measurement of pancreatic secretory function. In: deReuch ANS, Comeron MP, eds. *Ciba Foundation symposium on the exocrine pancreas.* Boston: Little, Brown, 1961;225–253.
90. Haddorn B, Zoppi G, Shmerling DH, Prader A, McIntyre I, Anderson C. Quantitative assessment of exocrine pancreatic function in infants and children. *J Pediatr* 1968;73:39–50.
91. Howat HT, Braganza JM. Assessment of pancreatic dysfunction in man. In: Howat HT, Braganza JM. *The exocrine pancreas.* Philadelphia: WB Saunders, 1979;129–175.
92. Lebenthal E. The development aspects of pancreatic exocrine function. In: Lebenthal E, ed. *Digestive diseases in children.* New York: Grune and Stratton, 1978;489–498.
93. Shwachman H, Lebenthal E, Khat KT. Recurrent acute pancreatitis in patients with normal pancreatic enzymes. *Pediatrics* 1975;55:86–95.
94. Zoppi G, Andreotti G, Pajno-Ferrera F, Bellini P, Gaburro D. The development of specific responses of the exocrine pancreas to pancreozymin and secretin stimulation in newborn infants. *Pediatr Res* 1973;7:198–203.
95. Lebenthal E, Lerner A, Heitlinger L. The pancreas in cystic fibrosis. In: Go VLW, et al., eds. *The exocrine pancreas: biology, pathobiology, and diseases.* New York: Raven Press, 1986.
96. Shwachman H, Diamond LK, Oski FA, Khaw Kon T. The syndrome of pancreatic insufficiency and bone marrow dysfunction. *J Pediatr* 1964;65:645–663.
97. Bodian M, Sheldon W, Lightwood R. Congenital hypoplasia of the exocrine pancreas. *Acta Pediatr* 1964;53:282–293.
98. Hadorn B, Thaler M. Diseases of the pancreas in childhood. In: Sleisinger M, Fordtran J, eds. *Gastrointestinal disease,* 2nd ed. Philadelphia: WB Saunders, 1978;1488.
99. Fringle EM, Young WF, Haworth EM. Syndrome of pancreatic insufficiency, blood dyscrasia and metaphyseal dysostosis. *Proc R Soc Med* 1968;61:776.
100. Schmerling DH, et al. The syndrome of exocrine pancreatic insufficiency, neutropenia, metaphyseal dysostosis and dwarfism. *Helv Paediatr Acta* 1969;24:547.
101. Shwachman H, Diamond LK, Oski FA, Khaw KT. Pancreatic insufficiency and bone marrow dysfunction. A new clinical entity. *Pediatrics* 1963;63:835.
102. Shwachman H, Holsclaw D. Some clinical observations on the Shwachman syndrome. *Birth Defects* 1972;8:46.
103. Graham AR, Watson PD, Paplanus SH, Payne CM. Testicular fibrosis and cardiomegaly in Shwachman's syndrome. *Arch Pathol Lab Med* 1980;104:242.
104. Hadorn B, Johansen PG, Anderson CM. Pancreozymin secretin test of exocrine pancreatic function in cystic fibrosis and the significance of the result for the pathogenesis of the disease. *Can Med Assoc J* 1968;98(8):377–385.
105. Hadorn B. The exocrine pancreas. In: Anderson CM, Burke V, eds. *Pediatric gastroenterology.* Oxford: Blackwell, 1975;289.
106. Johanson A, Blizzard R. A syndrome of congenital aplasia of the alae nasi, deafness, hypothyroidism, dwarfism, absent permanent teeth and malabsorption. *J Pediatr* 1971;79:982.
107. Lerner A. Hereditary abnormalities of the pancreas. In: Lebenthal E, ed. *Textbook of gastroenterology and nutrition in infancy,* 2nd ed. New York: Raven Press, 1989;877–883.
108. Daenthl DL, Frias JL, Gilbert EF, Opiz JM. The Johanson-Blizzard syndrome case report and autopsy findings. *Am J Med Genet* 1979;3:129–135.
109. Pearson HA, Lobel JS, Kocoshis SA, et al. A new syndrome of refractory sideroblastic anemia with vacuolization of marrow precursors and exocrine pancreatic dysfunction. *J Pediatr* 1979;95:978–984.
110. Sheldon W. Congenital pancreatic lipase deficiency. *Arch Dis Child* 1964;39:268–271.
111. Figarella C, DeCaro A, Deprez P, Bouvry H, Bevnier J. Un nouveau cas de deficience congenitale en lipase pancreatique avec presence de colipase. *Gastroenterol Clin Biol* 1979;3:43–46.
112. Figarella C, DeCaro A, Leopold D, Poley J. Congenital pancreatic lipase deficiency. *J Pediatr* 1980;96:412–416.
113. Townes PL. Trypsinogen deficiency disease. *J Pediatr* 1965;66:271–275.
114. Townes PL, Bryson MF, Miller G. Further observation on trypsinogen deficiency disease. Report of a second case. *J Pediatr* 1967;71:220–224.
115. Hadorn B, Tarlow M, Lloyd JK, Wolff OH. Intestinal enterokinase deficiency. *Lancet* 1969;1:812–813.
116. Tarlton MJ, Hadorn B, Arthurton MW, Lloyd JK. Intestinal enterokinase deficiency, a newly recognized disorder of protein digestion. *Arch Dis Child* 1970;45:651–655.
117. Polonvoski C, Laplane R, Alison F, Navarro J. Pseudo-deficit in trypsinogene par deficite congenital enterokinase. Etude clinique. *Arch Fr Pediatr* 1970;27:677–688.
118. Haworth JC, Gourley B, Hadorn B, Sumida E. Malabsorption and growth failure due to intestinal enterokinase deficiency. *J Pediatr* 1971;78:481–490.
119. Ghishan FK, Lee PC, Lebenthal E, Johnson P, Bradley CA, Greene HL. Isolated congenital enterokinase deficiency. Recent findings and review of the literature. *Gastroenterology* 1983;85:727–731.
120. Lebenthal E, Antonowicz I, Shwachman H. Enterokinase and trypsin activities in pancreatic insufficiency and diseases of the small intestine. *Gastroenterology* 1976;70:508–512.
121. Lowe CV, May DC. Selective pancreatic deficiency: absent amylase, diminished trypsin and normal lipase. *Am J Dis Child* 1951;82:459.
122. Gishahn FK, Moran JR, Durie PR, Green HL. Isolated congenital lipase colipase deficiency. *Gastroenterology* 1984;86: 1580–1582.
123. Hildebrand H, Borgstrom B, Bekassy A, Erlanson-Albertson C, Helin I. Isolated colipase deficiency in two brothers. *Gut* 1982;23:243–246.
124. Jordan SC, Ament MD. Pancreatitis in children and adolescents. *J Pediatr* 1977;91:211–216.
125. Weizman Z, Durie PR. Acute pancreatitis in childhood. *J Pediatr* 1988;113:24–29.
126. Lott JA. Inflammatory disease of the pancreas. *CRC Crit Rev Clin Lab Sci* 1982;17:201–228.
127. Balart LA, Ferrante WA. Pathophysiology of acute and chronic pancreatitis. *Arch Intern Med* 1982;42:113–117.
128. Lerner A. Acute pancreatitis in children and adolescents. In: Lebenthal E, ed. *Textbook of gastroenterology and nutrition in infancy,* 2nd ed. New York: Raven Press, 1989;897–906.
129. Lerner A, Lebenthal E. Acute pancreatitis in children. An update. In: Mass AJ, eds. *Pediatric update.* New York: Elsevier, 1986;257–279.
130. Hendren WH, Green JM, Patton AS. Pancreatitis in childhood: experience with 15 cases. *Arch Dis Child* 1965;40:132–145.
131. Buntain WL, Wood JB, Woolley MM. Pancreatitis in childhood. *J Pediatr Surg* 1978;13:143–149.
132. Rubin SZ, Ein SH. The unusual presentation of pancreatitis in infancy. *J Pediatr Surg* 1979;14:146–148.
133. Sibert JR. Pancreatitis in childhood. *Postgrad Med J* 1979;55:171–175.
134. Tom PKH, Saing H, Irving IM, Lister J. Acute pancreatitis in children. *J Pediatr Surg* 1985;20:58–60.
135. Durie PR, Gaskin KJ, Ogilvie JE, Smith CR, Forstner GG, Largman C. Serial alterations in the forms of immunoreactive pancreatic cationic trypsin in plasma from patients with acute pancreatitis. *J Pediatr Gastroenterol Nutr* 1985;4:199–207.

136. Regan PT. Medical treatment of acute pancreatitis. *Mayo Clin Proc* 1979;54:432–434.
137. Pellegrini CA. The treatment of acute pancreatitis: a continuing challenge. *N Engl J Med* 1985;312:436–438.
138. Keith RG. Effect of a low-fat elemental diet on pancreatic secretion during pancreatitis. *Surg Gynecol Obstet* 1980;151:337–343.
139. Jeliffe DB. *The assessment of the nutritional status of the community.* Geneva: World Health Organization, 1980.
140. Jeliffe DB. *Infant nutrition in the subtropics and tropics,* 2nd WHO Monograph, Series 29. Geneva: World Health Organization, 1968.
141. Wheeler JE, Lukens FDW, Gyorgi P. Studies on the localization of tagged methionine within the pancreas. *Proc Soc Exp Biol Med* 1949;70:187–191.
142. Davies JNP. The essential pathology of kwashiorkor. *Lancet* 1948;1:317–320.
143. Kerpel-Fronius E. *The pathophysiology of infantile malnutrition. Protein energy malnutrition and failure to thrive.* Budapest: Akademai Kiado Press, 1983.
144. Pitchumoni CS. Pancreas in primary malnutrition disorders. *Am J Clin Nutr* 1983;26:374–379.
145. Veghelyi PV. Pancreatic function in different clinical conditions. *Acta Pediatr* 1948;36:483–490.
146. Klotz AP, Murdock AL, Svoboda DJ. The effect of protein deprivation on pancreatic function in young animals in utero. *Dig Dis* 1972;17:399–406.
147. Weisblum B, Herman L, Fitzgerald PJ. Changes in pancreatic acinar cells during protein deprivation. *J Cell Biol* 1962;12:313–327.
148. Shields RG Jr, Mahan DC, Ekstrom KE. Effect of moderate or severe protein restriction during pregnancy on sow and progeny digestive enzymes. *J Nutr* 1980;110:1506–1516.
149. Hatch TF, Lebenthal E, Krasner H, Branski D. Effect of postnatal malnutrition in pancreatic zymogen enzymes in the rat. *Am J Clin Nutr* 1979;32:1224–1230.
150. Pitchumoni CS, Scheele G, Lee PC, Lebenthal E. Effects of nutrition on the exocrine pancreas. In: Go VLW, ed. *The exocrine pancreas: biology, pathology, and diseases.* New York: Raven Press, 1986;387–406.
151. Hubbard VS, Mangrum PJ. Energy intake and nutritional counseling in cystic fibrosis. *J Am Diet Assoc* 1982;80:127–131.
152. Shepherd RW, Holt TL, Thomas BJ, Ward LC, Isles A, Frances PJ. Malnutrition in cystic fibrosis: the nature of the nutritional deficit and optimal management. In: *Nutrition abstract and reviews,* vol 54, no 12. John Wiley: Commonwealth Agricultural Bureaux, 1984.
153. Dodge JA. Nutritional requirements in cystic fibrosis: a review. *J Pediatr Gastroenterol Nutr* 1988;7(Suppl 1):S8–S11.
154. Dodge JA, Yassa JG. Food intake and supplement feeding programs. In: Sturgess JM, ed. *Perspectives in cystic fibrosis.* Toronto: Imperial Press, 1980;125–136.
155. Dodge JA. Gastrointestinal tract and nutrition in cystic fibrosis: pathophysiology. *J R Soc Med* 1986;79(Suppl 12):S27–S31.
156. George DE, Mangos JA. Nutritional management and pancreatic enzyme therapy in cystic fibrosis patients: state of the art in 1987 and projections into the future. *J Pediatr Gastroenterol Nutr* 1988;7(Suppl 1):549–557.
157. Levy LD, Durie PR, Pencharz PB, et al. Effect of long-term nutritional rehabilitation on body composition and clinical status in malnourished children and adolescents with cystic fibrosis. *J Pediatr* 1985;107:225–230.
158. Corey M, McLaughlin F, Williams M, Levinson H. A comparison of survival, growth, and pulmonary function in patients with cystic fibrosis in Boston and Toronto. *J Clin Epidemiol* 1988;41:583–591.
159. Farrel PM, Mischler EH, Engle MJ, Brown DJ, Lav SM. Fatty acid abnormalities in cystic fibrosis. *Pediatr Res* 1985;19:104–109.
160. Kuo PT, Huang NN. The effect of medium chain triglyceride upon fat absorption and plasma lipid and depot fat of children with cystic fibrosis of the pancreas. *J Clin Invest* 1965;44:1924–1933.
161. Lester LA, Rothenberg RM, Dawson G, Lopez AL, Corpuz Z. Supplemental parenteral nutrition in cystic fibrosis. *JPEN J Parenter Enteral Nutr* 1986;10:289–295.
162. Durie PR, Newth CJ, Forstner GG, et al. Malabsorption of medium chain triglycerides in infants with cystic fibrosis: correction with pancreatic enzyme supplements. *J Pediatr* 1980;96:862–864.
163. Mischler EH, Powell SW, Farrell PM, Raynor WJ, Lemen RJ. Correction of linoleic acid deficiency in cystic fibrosis. *Pediatr Res* 1986;20:36–41.
164. Weisman Y, Reiter E, Stern R, Root A. Serum concentrations of 25 hydroxy vitamin D and 24-25 hydroxy vitamin D in patients with cystic fibrosis. *J Pediatr* 1979;95:416–418.
165. Hahn TJ, Squires AE, Halstead LR, et al. Reduced serum 25 hydroxy vitamin D concentration and disordered mineral metabolism in patients with cystic fibrosis. *J Pediatr* 1979;94:38–42.
166. Tomasi LG. Neurological complications in cystic fibrosis. In: Lloyd-Still JD, ed. *Textbook of cystic fibrosis.* Boston: John Wright, 1983;383–408.
167. Jacob RA, Sandstead HH, Solomons NW, et al. Zinc status and vitamin A transport in cystic fibrosis. *Am J Clin Nutr* 1978;31:638–644.
168. Derer JJ, Arora B, Toskes PP, et al. Malabsorption of crystalline vitamin B12 in cystic fibrosis. *N Engl J Med* 1973;288:949–950.
169. Underwood BA, Denning CR. Correlations between plasma and liver concentrations of vitamins A and E in children with cystic fibrosis. *Bull NY Acad Med* 1971;47:34–50.
170. Underwood BA, Denning CR. Blood and liver concentration of vitamins A and E in children with cystic fibrosis of the pancreas. *Pediatr Res* 1972;6:26–31.
171. Lloyd Still JD. Cystic fibrosis. In: Lebenthal E, ed. *Textbook of gastroenterology and nutrition in infancy.* New York: Raven Press, 1989;851–876.
172. Mischler EH, Chesney PJ, Chesney RW, et al. Demineralization in cystic fibrosis detected by direct photon absorptiometry. *Am J Dis Child* 1979;133:632–635.
173. Congden PJ, Bruce G, Rothburn MM, et al. Vitamin status in treated patients with cystic fibrosis. *Arch Dis Child* 1981;56(9):708–714.
174. McKay PB, King MM. Vitamin E: its role as biological free radical scavenger and its relationship to the microsomal mixed-function oxidase system. In: Machlin LJ, ed. *Vitamin E: a comprehensive treatise.* New York: Marcel Dekker, 1980.
175. Dolan TF. Hemolytic anemia and edema as initial signs in infants with cystic fibrosis. *Clin Pediatr* 1976;15:597–600.
176. Cynamon HA, Milov DE, Valenstein E, Wagner M. Effect of vitamin E deficiency on neurologic function in patients with cystic fibrosis. *J Pediatr* 1988;113:637–640.
177. Harries JT, Muller DPE. Absorption of different doses of fat soluble and water miscible preparations of vitamin E in children with cystic fibrosis. *Arch Dis Child* 1971;46:341–344.
178. Farrell PM, Hubbard VS. Nutrition in cystic fibrosis: vitamins, fatty acids and minerals. In: Lloyd-Still JD, ed. *Textbook of cystic fibrosis.* Boston: John Wright, 1983;263–293.
179. Deven JJ, Arora B, Toskes PP, et al. Malabsorption of crystalline vitamin B12 in cystic fibrosis. *N Engl J Med* 1973;288:949–950.
180. Tortenson OL, Humphrey GB, Edson JR, et al. Cystic fibrosis presenting with severe hemorrhage due to vitamin K malabsorption: a report of three cases. *Pediatrics* 1970;45:857–860.
181. Congden PJ, Bruce G, Rothburn MM, et al. Vitamin status in treated patients with cystic fibrosis. *Arch Dis Child* 1981;56:708–714.
182. DiMagno EP, Malagelada JR, Go VLM, Moertel CG. Fate of orally ingested enzyme in pancreatic insufficiency. *N Engl J Med* 1977;298:1318–1322.
183. Graham DY, Sackman JW. Mechanism of increase in steatorrhea with calcium and magnesium in exocrine pancreatic insufficiency. An animal model. *Gastroenterology* 1982;83:638–644.
184. Mischler EH, Parrell S, Farrell PM, Odell GB. Comparison of effectiveness of pancreatic enzyme preparations in cystic fibrosis. *Am J Dis Child* 1982;136:1060–1063.
185. Gow R, Bradbear R, Francis P, Shepherd R. Comparative study of varying regimens to improve steatorrhea and creatorrhea in cystic fibrosis. Effectiveness of an enteric coated preparation with and without antiacids and cimetidine. *Lancet* 1981;2:1071–1074.

186. Nassif EG, Younoszai MK, Einberger MM, Nassif CM. Comparative effects of antiacids, enteric coating, and bile salts on the effects of oral pancreatic enzyme therapy in cystic fibrosis. *J Pediatr* 1981;98:320–323.
187. Laenerte C, Beroud N, Castaigne JP. Pancreas gastroresistance: in vitro evaluation of pH-determined dissolution. *J Pediatr Gastroenterol Nutr* 1988;7(Suppl 1):S18–S21.
188. Littlewood JM, Kelleher J, Walters MP, Johnson AW. In vivo and in vitro studies of microsphere pancreatic supplements. *J Pediatr Gastroenterol Nutr* 1988;7(Suppl 1):S22–S29.
189. Ansaldi-Balocco N, Santini B, Sarchi C. Efficacy of pancreatic enzyme supplementation in children with cystic fibrosis: comparison of two preparations by random crossover study and retrospective study of the same patients at two different ages. *J Pediatr Gastroenterol Nutr* 1988;7(Suppl 1):S40–S45.
190. Chazalette JP, Dain MP, Costaigne JP. Efficacy of pancreas: crossover comparative study versus eurobiol in cystic fibrosis. *J Pediatr Gastroenterol Nutr* 1988;7(Suppl 1):S46–S48.
191. Thompson G, Robb T, David G. Taurine supplementation, fat absorption, and growth in cystic fibrosis. *J Pediatr* 1987;11:501–506.
192. Belli DC, Levy E, Darling P, Leroy C, Lepage G, Guiguere R, Roy CC. Taurine improves the absorption of a fat meal in patients with cystic fibrosis. *Pediatrics* 1987;80:17–23.
193. Meyer JH, Elashoff J, Porter-Fink V, Dressman J, Amidon G. What should be the size of pancreatic microspheres? *Gastroenterology* 1987;92:1533.
194. Roy CC, Weber A, Lepage G, Smith L, Levy E. Digestive and absorptive phase anomalies associated with the exocrine pancreatic insufficiency in cystic fibrosis. *J Pediatr Gastroenterol Nutr* 1988;7(Suppl 1):S1–S7.
195. Costantini D, Padoan R, Curcio L, Giunta A. The management of enzymatic therapy in cystic fibrosis by an individualized approach. *J Pediatr Gastroenterol Nutr* 1988;7(Suppl 1):S36–S39.
196. Graham DY. Pancreatic enzyme replacement; the effects of antiacids or cimetidine. *Dig Dis Sci* 1982;27:485–490.
197. Bouquet J, Sinaasappel M, Neijens HJ. Malabsorption in CF: mechanism and treatment. *J Pediatr Gastroenterol Nutr* 1988;7(Suppl 1):S30–S35.
198. Roberts IM. Enzyme therapy for malabsorption in exocrine pancreatic insufficiency. *Pancreas* 1989;4:496–503.
199. Lebenthal E, George DE. Pancreatic diseases. In: Lebenthal E, ed. *Textbook of gastroenterology and nutrition in infancy*. New York: Raven Press, 1981.

CHAPTER 32

Nutritional Management of Children with Cystic Fibrosis

Robert L. Hopkins

Cystic fibrosis (CF), first described in 1935, is the most commonly inherited fatal disease in the Caucasian population (1). The mode of inheritance is autosomal recessive. There is a gene carrier frequency of 1/20 and an occurrence of 1/2,000 live Caucasian births.

The etiology of cystic fibrosis is still not clear. Current theories include a defect in tubular ion secretion, resulting in secretions that are thick and viscid due to decreased water content (2). These secretions result in obstructive lesions in the lungs, pancreas, and liver.

A significant step toward elucidating the etiology of CF was the localization of the CF locus to chromosome 7 (3). This will aid in carrier detection, antenatal diagnosis, and ultimately isolation of the CF gene.

The diagnosis of CF is based on clinical and laboratory data. However, the demonstration of an elevated sweat chloride concentration is the only *acceptable* diagnostic test for CF (4). The sweat sample should weigh at least 50 mg and preferably 100 mg. Sweating is induced by iontophoresis of pilocarpine. The determination of sweat chloride concentrations is reliable even in the newborn period; however, the low sweating rate in neonates makes collection of an adequate sample difficult. A chloride concentration of greater than 60 mEq/l is compatible with the diagnosis of cystic fibrosis. Other diseases associated with elevated sweat chloride concentrations include adrenal insufficiency, hypothyroidism, malnutrition, and hypoparathyroidism. Clinical evidence of cystic fibrosis is related to its impact on the respiratory and gastrointestinal systems (Table 1). This evidence changes with the age of the patient.

The clinical problems experienced by CF patients mainly involve the respiratory and gastrointestinal systems. Respiratory dysfunction is caused by chronic infection and destructive lung disease that follows obstruction of the small airways by thick, viscid secretions. The gastrointestinal manifestations are also due to obstruction of organ ductules by abnormal secretions, especially in the pancreas, leading to pancreatic insufficiency and malabsorption.

The major cause of mortality in CF is progressive destructive lung disease. The initial defect is obstruction and inflammation of the bronchioles. This obstruction by thick abnormal secretions is followed by infection. Important organisms causing this pulmonary infection include *Staphylococcus aureus* and mucoid *Pseudomonas aeruginosa*. Progressive destruction of airways and parenchyma is characterized by bronchiectasis, bronchopneumonia, and emphysema. This destructive process is also associated with pulmonary hypertension and cor pulmonale. Death is usually caused by combined cardiopulmonary failure.

The prognosis for CF is improving rapidly. Median survival since 1970 has almost *doubled* (Table 2). This favorable change is due to several factors: (a) improved antibiotics, (b) enhanced respiratory care techniques, and (c) improved nutritional support regimens including enteral feeding methods. Transplantation of the heart and lungs and gene manipulation may enhance these figures in the future.

GASTROINTESTINAL PATHOLOGY

Pancreas

Approximately 85% to 90% of CF patients have pancreatic insufficiency. The pancreatic ductules are ob-

---

R. L. Hopkins: Department of Pediatrics, Section of Critical Care, Tulane University School of Medicine, New Orleans, Louisiana 70112.

TABLE 1. Clinical signs of cystic fibrosis

	Neonate	Infancy	Child	Adult
Respiratory		Bronchiolitis	Nasal polyps	Pneumothorax
		Wheezing	Sinusitis	Hemoptysis
		Pneumonia	Chronic infection	Chronic infection
Gastrointestinal	Jaundice	Rectal prolapse	Malnutrition	Malnutrition
	Meconium ileus	Malnutrition	Steatorrhea	Portal hypertension
	Steatorrhea	Steatorrhea	Intestinal	Gallstones
	Low birth weight		obstruction	Diabetes mellitus

TABLE 2. Median survival in cystic fibrosis (both sexes)

Years	Survival
1970	16 years
1976	18 years
1982	21 years
1988	22 years

structed with secretions, leading to inflammation and acinar atrophy. This obstruction is probably present at birth. Even in the newborn period there can be clinical signs of malabsorption, and trypsin in duodenal contents can be markedly decreased. These findings exist in spite of barely recognizable pathologic changes in the pancreas of the newborn with cystic fibrosis. There is gradual replacement of this organ by fat and fibrous tissue, a progressive process that can ultimately involve the endocrine structures of the pancreas, leading to diabetes mellitus in adolescence and sometimes earlier.

Liver

The classic hepatic lesion in CF is focal biliary cirrhosis that occurs in a patchy pattern. Autopsy results reveal that 10% to 20% of deceased CF patients have this finding and its frequency apparently increases with age. Because of its patchy distribution, as the name implies, significant hepatic dysfunction is unusual (<5%) (5). However, progressive evolution of the cirrhosis can lead to fibrosis, loss of portal tracts, and eventually portal hypertension. Older patients develop gallstones (about 25%) caused by excessive loss of bile salts and the subsequent generation of lithogenic bile.

Small and Large Intestines

Intestinal pathology includes dilation of Brunner's glands and stringy mucous secretions in the bowel lumen. There is a thick mucinous surface cover of the large and small bowel. Peroral biopsy reveals normal villi, villus-crypt ratio, and relatively normal cellularity in the lamina propria (6).

NUTRITIONAL ABNORMALITIES

Pancreas and Malabsorption

Normally less than 5% of total pancreatic function is necessary for normal digestion and absorption of fat and protein. Despite this tremendous reserve, fat and protein malabsorption is present in most CF patients. The less than 2% of total exocrine pancreatic capacity in cystic fibrosis results in decreased secretion of lipase, proteases, and bicarbonate. A spectrum of pancreatic insufficiency exists: (a) 55% to 60% of CF patients have complete achylia, (b) 40% to 45% have variable pancreatic involvement, and (c) 3% to 5% have no pancreatic insufficiency.

Because of the decrease in pancreatic bicarbonate secretion, gastric acid entering the small bowel is not neutralized. This large volume of gastric acid may not be neutralized until it reaches the midjejunum. Lipase is less active in this acidic milieu and bile acids may precipitate in this low pH environment. Bile salt concentration will then fall to a level that will inhibit micelle formation and worsen the steatorrhea already present due to decreased lipase activity.

Increased Energy Needs

Estimates have placed caloric requirements for CF patients at 110% to 150% of the recommended dietary allowance (RDA) to achieve growth. Parsons (7) refined these early estimates by measures of dietary energy (gross energy content of macronutrients) and stool energy content (oxygen bomb calorimetry). The difference between these measures was *absorbed energy*. Normal growth was demonstrated when absorbed energy reached 100% to 110% of requirements. Measurements using indirect calorimetry also substantiated these earlier estimates of increased energy needs. Vaisman and his coworkers (8) demonstrated energy needs at 95% to 150% of values predicted by the Harris-Benedict equation. These energy needs were inversely correlated with pulmonary function and nutritional status. Nutritional status, however, was directly correlated with pulmonary status.

A number of factors contribute to the increased energy needs in cystic fibrosis. Vaisman et al. (8) demonstrated

TABLE 3. *Energy balance in cystic fibrosis*

Factors increasing energy needs	Factors opposing energy balance
Fever	Fat malabsorption
Increased work of breathing	Anorexia
Coughing	Esophagitis
Synthesis of acute-phase reactants	Dyspnea and cough
	Chronic malaise

an increase in energy needs as pulmonary function deteriorated. This decrease in pulmonary function would imply an increase in obstructive lung disease with an increase in the work of breathing. Increased coughing also would lead to increased work and energy needs. The decrease in pulmonary function also implies a worsening of pulmonary infection. Synthesis of acute-phase reactants because of this infection will increase protein and energy needs. Low-grade fever will also increase energy requirements. Complicating these increased energy needs are several factors that impede energy intake: (a) fat malabsorption, (b) anorexia, (c) esophagitis, (d) dyspnea and cough, and (e) malaise (Table 3).

Sophisticated studies using double-labeled water techniques have shown increased energy requirements even in healthy, well-nourished infants with CF. This would seem to indicate a basic defect in energy expenditure (9).

SPECIFIC NUTRITIONAL DEFICIENCIES

Fat Malabsorption

Pancreatic insufficiency, present in 85% to 90% of CF patients, results in fat malabsorption. There are several interrelated reasons why fat malabsorption is such a major problem in CF. The pancreatic insufficiency results in excretion of up to 80% of ingested fat in CF patients with untreated pancreatic insufficiency. Loss of lipase, colipase, bicarbonate, and bile salts leads to the severe steatorrhea seen in CF patients. A decrease in pancreatic bicarbonate secretion results in a large amount of gastric acid not being neutralized in the duodenum. The resulting acidic environment causes decreased lipase activity and precipitation and loss of bile acids. This loss, combined with the decreased pancreatic lipase secretion and activity, leads to severe steatorrhea, fecal loss of energy, and essential fatty acid deficiency.

Clinical evidence of essential fatty acid deficiency is rare; biochemical abnormalities of blood and tissue lipids, however, are common. These abnormalities include decreased serum linoleic acid and elevated serum levels of palmitoleic acid and oleic acid. Etiology of these abnormalities is probably due to fat malabsorption and decreased intake of fat containing linoleic acid and not to a basic error of metabolism. Abnormalities in the levels of these fatty acids persist despite treatment with pancreatic enzyme supplementation. Additional causes of essential fatty acid deficiency include prolonged use of low-fat elemental diets or intravenous nutrition without lipids.

Protein Malabsorption

Protein absorption in CF has not been extensively studied. In untreated patients protein loss is very high, approaching 50% of ingested protein (10). There are reduced quantities of trypsin, chymotrypsin, and carboxypeptidases. All these pancreatic enzymes are necessary for digestion and subsequent absorption of dietary protein. In addition to pancreatic insufficiency, decreased colonic transit time and antibiotic usage contribute to these losses. Antibiotic usage may decrease the proteolytic activity of stool bacteria. These stool nitrogen losses are significantly decreased by pancreatic enzyme supplementation (11).

Carbohydrate Malabsorption

Carbohydrate absorption in CF is well-preserved despite low pancreatic amylase activity. There is probably increased salivary amylase activity as evidenced by increased circulating salivary isoamylase (12). A second compensation for decreased pancreatic amylase is intestinal enzymes with amylase-like function: brush-border maltase and glucoamylase as well as lysosomal maltase-glucoamylase (13).

Fat-Soluble Vitamins

Steatorrhea is associated with malabsorption of the fat-soluble vitamins (A, D, K, and E). Biochemical evidence of this malabsorption is well documented (14) and clinical deficiencies of these vitamins also have been described (15).

Vitamin A

Clinical signs of vitamin A deficiency including night blindness, xerophthalmia, and intracranial hypertension are unusual. However, untreated or treated patients occasionally exhibit these problems. More commonly seen is biochemical evidence of decreased vitamin A stores. Treated patients, despite multivitamin supplementation, still have low serum vitamin A levels in conjunction with liver concentrations five times greater than unsupplemented control patients (16). These low serum vitamin A levels are probably due to several factors: (a) malabsorption of vitamin A, which is made up of esters of long-chain fatty acids; (b) reduced synthesis of retinol-binding protein, the carrier protein for vitamin A; and (c) zinc deficiency. Adequate zinc status is necessary for retinol-binding protein synthesis and adequate vitamin A transport from the liver.

Vitamin D

Rickets is unusual in CF. It usually occurs in association with severe liver disease (17). A decrease in cortical thickness of the long bones has been more commonly reported (18). Levels of 25-hydroxycalciferol are low to normal in patients receiving 400 to 800 units of vitamin D daily (19).

Vitamin E

There is a consistent biochemical deficiency of vitamin E in unsupplemented CF patients (20). There are two well-described entities related to this deficiency: (a) a hemolytic anemia in infants (21), and (b) a neurologic syndrome resulting in areflexia, ataxia, and proprioceptive loss (22). This neurologic syndrome is progressive over time.

Vitamin K

Vitamin K deficiency has been described in newly diagnosed infants with CF (23). The presentation is a hemorrhagic diathesis. Suppression of endogenous bacterial vitamin K production by antibiotics is a risk factor in older children.

Water-Soluble Vitamins

Water-soluble vitamins, with the exception of vitamin B_{12}, are well absorbed in CF. Vitamin-supplemented CF patients have adequate levels of vitamins B_1, B_2, B_6, and folic acid (15).

Vitamin B_{12} malabsorption, however, has been well documented (24). Pancreatic proteases are needed to complete the transfer of cobalamin from the R protein to intrinsic factor. In untreated patients, decreased proteases and duodenal hyperacidity act to prevent this transfer. The rarity of clinically evident vitamin B_{12} deficiency is probably due to the wide distribution of vitamin B_{12} in food (25).

Minerals

Iron

Iron deficiency in CF is more common than is usually appreciated (26) although iron absorption is probably normal in CF. The lack of hypoxia-induced polycythemia may be due to iron deficiency associated with low ferritin levels (27). Ferritin levels, however, may sometimes be elevated in CF despite iron deficiency. This is because ferritin is an acute-phase reactant that may be elevated in association with pulmonary infections. The anemia of iron deficiency in CF patients does respond to oral iron therapy (26).

Sodium

Both chronic and acute hyponatremia can occur in CF. Chronic hyponatremia may result in anorexia and subsequent poor growth. A more acute situation, hypoelectrolytemia and metabolic alkalosis, occurs in young infants. This results from decreased dietary sodium intake and is exacerbated by hot weather and sweating (28,29).

Calcium

Despite dependence on normal fat absorption and vitamin D for intestinal transport of calcium, there are few reports of rickets or tetany in CF patients. However, decreased cortical thickness in long bones has been described (30).

Magnesium

The common symptoms in CF of weakness, muscle fatigue, and fatigue may be due in part to hypomagnesemia associated with fat malabsorption. Green et al. (31) have documented hypomagnesemia in CF patients treated with aminoglycoside antibiotics. These drugs cause an increased renal tubular loss of magnesium.

Trace Elements

Zinc

Zinc levels, measured in hair or serum of CF patients, are variable; part of this variability is due to large, but inconsistent stool losses (32). Hair measurements of zinc show more normal levels in adolescents with CF (33). Zinc has important functions in both normal somatic growth and vitamin A transport and low zinc levels have been documented in CF patients with growth retardation (34).

Copper

There is little data regarding copper and CF. Plasma levels of copper and ceruloplasmin may be elevated in CF patients (14). This elevation in copper may be due to an increase in ceruloplasmin, which is an acute-phase reactant. Infection in the CF patient will lead to a rise in acute-phase reactants, including ceruloplasmin.

Selenium

Low selenium levels have been reported in CF and are associated with increased stool losses. However, an adequate nutritional regimen will prevent this deficiency (35).

CLINICAL ASPECTS OF NUTRITION AND CYSTIC FIBROSIS

Growth Failure

Sproul and Huang (36) first reported growth patterns in CF in 1964. Children under 2 years of age with CF had *average* weights and heights between the 3rd and 10th percentiles. Females fell below the 3rd percentile for weight at 6 years; males fell to that percentile at 11 years. Height percentiles decreased steadily during childhood to between the 3rd and 10th percentile and then reached a plateau during early adolescence (36). These investigators also demonstrated a close association of poor growth and worsening pulmonary status.

Although the decline in growth parameters seemed to be inevitable, data from Toronto clearly showed that this is not an intrinsic part of CF (37). The Toronto investigators demonstrated that a high-fat diet combined with liberal doses of pancreatic enzyme supplementation produced nearly normal growth. Subsequent studies indicated that growth failure in CF is partially nutritional in origin and amenable to nutritional supplementation (38–40). Supplementation was long-term in these studies and supplied by either gastrostomy or by jejunostomy. Elemental or nonelemental formulas were used. There were significant changes in weight and a stabilization in previously declining pulmonary function tests.

NUTRITIONAL ASSESSMENT

Optimal care for the CF patient is predicated on continuing assessment at a regional CF center. Psychosocial issues, respiratory status, and nutritional status must be monitored, and treatment plans initiated and modified as needed. Frequency of visits will depend on local protocols and the acuity of problems.

Nutritional monitoring should include dietary histories, anthropometry, biochemical indices of nutritional status, and careful correlation of growth patterns with pulmonary status.

Anthropometry should include height, weight, and skin-fold measurements. Height and weight should be recorded on percentile charts. Observation of any devia-

TABLE 4. *Biochemical indices for nutritional assessment in cystic fibrosis*

Essential fatty acids
Plasma vitamin A
Plasma zinc
Prothrombin time
Plasma vitamin E
Plasma electrolytes

tion from the norm should precipitate a meticulous search for cause. Such deviations may be caused by (a) pulmonary disease, (b) deviation from recommended nutritional regimen, (c) inadequate pancreatic enzyme replacement therapy, (d) gastroesophageal reflux, (e) distal intestinal obstruction syndrome, or (f) depression.

The biochemical evaluation should be most thorough on the initial diagnostic visit and on annual "birthday" visits (Table 4). Additional monitoring will be determined by the patient's clinical status.

Serum albumin is useful in the nutritional assessment of the newly diagnosed infant. Older patients can have low albumin levels either as a result of decreased visceral protein synthesis or an expanded plasma volume (41).

NUTRITIONAL STRATEGIES FOR CF

The goal in the nutritional management of CF is to optimize growth with a relatively normal diet.

Pancreatic Enzyme Replacement

Supplementation with pancreatic enzymes is one of the cornerstones of nutritional management in CF. Newer preparations consisting of acid-resistant microspheres (Pancrease and Creon) have made this therapy simpler and more efficient (42–44).

Enzyme replacement should be administered to patients with clinical or biochemical evidence of pancreatic insufficiency. Because of the increased energy needs in the CF patient, these supplements should be used if there is *any suspicion* of pancreatic insufficiency. This will help to prevent large fecal losses of energy and protein.

The object of pancreatic enzyme replacement therapy is to markedly decrease steatorrhea with a therapeutic regimen that does not distinguish the CF patient from his peers. Fat absorption can be increased to 80% to 90% of ingested fat with appropriate supplementation.

Infants are usually begun on powdered enzyme preparations. The powder should be mixed with a small amount of milk at the beginning of a meal. Enzymes should *not* be added to the bottle. Care should be taken to ensure that the enzymes are completely washed away during a feeding since they can cause severe inflammation of the buccal mucosa.

Inadequate dosage of pancreatic enzymes is often a

problem. This may be the result of acceptance of gastrointestinal symptoms such as bloating, cramping, and flatulence, low dosage recommendations by manufacturers, as well as failure to recognize inadequate pancreatic enzyme dosage as a cause of persistent steatorrhea.

Dosage should begin at one to three capsules per meal and at least one capsule with snacks. This dose should be increased daily until complete control of gastrointestinal symptoms, including flatulence, bloating, cramps, large stools, and diarrhea, is achieved. Five capsules per meal is a common dose; however, 10 to 12 capsules per meal are occasionally needed. Newer preparations have increased lipase concentrations per capsule and dosing will depend on capsule strength. Close cooperation with the CF center nutritionist can help dose selection. Stool fat analysis may be necessary to monitor therapy. Constipation is occasionally reported as a possible consequence of overdosage, although this is very uncommon. Cautious reduction of the dosage should relieve this problem.

Fat

Earlier regimens of nutritional management recommended fat restriction to control steatorrhea. Fat, however, is an appetizing and efficient source of energy and newer forms of pancreatic enzyme supplements can produce enhanced (>80%) fat absorption, thereby fostering a calorically adequate and tasteful diet. Fat should compose about 40% of energy intake. This is of prime importance since inadequate caloric intake may be the major factor in the growth failure of CF.

Vitamins

Fat-soluble vitamins in a water-miscible form should be given in large daily dosages. Although water-soluble vitamins are usually given in large doses, i.e., twice minimum daily requirements, there is no evidence that extra supplementation is necessary (Table 5). Vitamin B_{12} supplementation may be required after resection of the ileum.

TABLE 5. *Recommended vitamin doses in cystic fibrosis*

Vitamins	Dose
Fat-soluble	
A	5,000–10,000 IU/day
D	400–800 IU/day
K	5 mg every 3 days
E	100–300 IU/day
Water-soluble	
B	2 × RDA
C	2 × RDA
B_{12}	100 mg IM/month (after ileal resection)

TABLE 6. *Nutritional support techniques in cystic fibrosis*

Nasoenteral feeding
Gastrostomy feeding
Jejunostomy feeding
Parenteral nutrition

Supplements

More aggressive and invasive means of nutritional support have been attempted because of the continuing problems of growth failure and malnutrition (Table 6). Dependence on daily *oral* intake of supplements is not effective in achieving increased weight gain.

Nasoenteral feeds, delivered at night, resulted in weight gain, but no improvement in pulmonary function (45–47). Caloric intake that resulted in growth had to be greater than 120% of RDA; however, these gains were not maintained once supplemental feedings stopped.

Gastrostomy feeding, monitored for 1 year, enhanced growth velocity with no decline in pulmonary function (39). This method is more easily accepted than nasoenteral feeds since no daily tube insertion is required, and gastrostomies can be converted to a capped stoma to relieve cosmetic concerns.

Boland and coinvestigators (48) in Ottawa have reported successful use of *jejunostomy feedings* in CF. Nonelemental formula was used and all patients showed weight gain. Enzymes were added to the feedings with no complications.

All *parenteral nutrition* trials have been short-term and included parenteral support in addition to usual therapy (49,50). All studies demonstrated weight gain; improvement in pulmonary function was observed in two studies (49,50).

Complications of long-term parenteral nutritional support include sepsis, venous thrombosis, and catheter placement accidents. Long-term parenteral support of CF patients has not been attempted and these complications must be considered.

NUTRITION AND PULMONARY FUNCTION

There is increasing evidence that pulmonary disease and malnutrition are interrelated (51): (a) the work of breathing with chronic obstructive lung disease appears to increase energy needs, (b) Vaisman et al. (8) showed an inverse relation between energy needs and pulmonary function with a positive relationship between nutritional status and pulmonary status, (c) an infectious exacerbation of the chronic lung disease in cystic fibrosis is associated with a decrease in whole-body protein synthesis, and (d) malnourished CF patients with chronic lung disease appear to exist in a state of chronic catabolism (52).

Malnutrition can also negatively affect the pulmonary system. One study showed a severe decrease in respiratory muscle size in malnourished CF patients with chronic obstructive lung disease. The sternocleidomastoid muscle in malnourished CF patients was severely reduced in size despite an increased work load due to obstructive lung disease (53). Several studies of nutritional supplementation have demonstrated fewer exacerbations of chronic obstructive lung disease and a stabilization of pulmonary functions (39,49). CF patients without steatorrhea appear to have less severe pulmonary disease, lower mean sweat chloride values, and perhaps a better prognosis than their counterparts with steatorrhea. There is no explanation for this provocative relationship at present; however, it suggests a close relationship between pancreatic and pulmonary function in CF (54).

NUTRITION AND PROGNOSIS

Studies are needed to more clearly define the relationship between nutritional support and improved survival in CF patients. The Toronto studies have shown that survival was superior in patients who had near-normal growth (54) in contrast to earlier studies that had demonstrated being underweight was associated with a poor prognosis (36). Further work is needed to more clearly show the interrelationship of pulmonary function, nutritional status, and ultimate prognosis.

REFERENCES

1. Anderson DH. Cystic fibrosis of the pancreas and its relation to celiac disease; a clinical and pathological study. *Am J Dis Child* 1938;56:344–399.
2. Wesley A, Forstner J, Quereshi R, Mantle M, Forstner G. Human intestinal mucin in cystic fibrosis. *Pediatr Res* 1983;17:65–69.
3. Wainwright BJ, Scambler PJ, Schmidtke J, Watson EA, Law H, Farrall M, Cooke HJ, Eiberg H, Williamson R. Localization of cystic fibrosis locus to human chromosome 7cen-q22. *Nature* 1985;318:384–385.
4. Gibson LE, Cooke RE. A test for concentration of electrolytes in sweat in cystic fibrosis of the pancreas utilizing pilocarpine by iontophoresis. *Pediatrics* 1959;23:545–559.
5. Stern P, Stevens D, Boat T, Doershuk C, Izant R, Matthews L. Symptomatic hepatic disease in cystic fibrosis. *Gastroenterology* 1976;70:645–649.
6. Antonowicz I, Lebenthal E, Shwachman H. Disaccharidase activities in small intestinal mucosa in patients with cystic fibrosis. *J Pediatr* 1978;92:214–219.
7. Parsons HD, Beaudry P, Dumas A, Pencharz PB. Energy needs and growth in children with cystic fibrosis. *J Pediatr Gastroenterol Nutr* 1983;2:44–49.
8. Vaisman N, Pencharz PB, Corey M, Canny GJ, Hahn E. Energy expenditure of patients with cystic fibrosis. *J Pediatr* 1987;111:496–500.
9. Shepherd RW, Cleghorn GJ. Etiology and pathogenesis of malnutrition in cystic fibrosis. In: *Cystic fibrosis: nutritional and intestinal disorders*. Boca Raton, FL: CRC Press, 1989;38–39.
10. Forstner GG, Gall DG, Corey M. Digestion and absorption of nutrients in cystic fibrosis. In: Sturgess JM, ed. *Perspectives in cystic fibrosis*. Toronto: Imperial Press, 1980;137–148.
11. Gow R, Bradbear R, Francis P, Shepherd RW. Comparative study varying regimens to improve steatorrhea and creatorrhea in cystic fibrosis. *Lancet* 1981;2:1071–1074.
12. Davidson G, Koheil A, Forstner G. Salivary amylase in cystic fibrosis: a marker of disordered autonomic function. *Pediatr Res* 1978;12:967–970.
13. Galand G, Forstner G. Soluble neutral and acid maltase in suckling rat intestine. *Biochem J* 1974;144:281–292.
14. Solomons NW, Wagonfeld JB, Riger C, Jacob RA, Bolt N, Vander-Horst J, Rothberg R, Sandstead H. Some biochemical indices of nutrition in treated CF patients. *Am J Clin Nutr* 1981;34:462–474.
15. Congden PJ, Bruce G, Rothburn MM, Clarke PCN, Littlewood JM, Kelleher J, Losowsky MS. Vitamin status in treated patients with CF. *Arch Dis Child* 1981;56:708–714.
16. Underwood BA, Denning CR. Correlations between plasma and liver concentrations of vitamin A and E in children with CF. *Bull NY Acad Med* 1971;47:34–39.
17. Scott J, Elias E, Moult PJA, Barnes S, Wills MR. Rickets in CF adults with myopathy, pancreatic insufficiency, and proximal renal tubular dysfunction. *Am J Med* 1977;63:488–492.
18. Hubbard V, Farrell P, di Santagnese P. 25 hydroxycaliferol levels in patients with CF. *J Pediatr* 1979;94:84–86.
19. Hann PJ, Squires AE, Halstead LR, Strominger DB. Reduced serum 25 vitamin D concentration and disordered mineral metabolism in patients with CF. *J Pediatr* 1979;94:38–42.
20. Harrier J, Muller D. Absorption of different doses of fat soluble and water miscible preparations of vitamin E in children with cystic fibrosis. *Arch Dis Child* 1971;46:341–344.
21. Dolan TF. Hemolytic anemia and edema as initial signs in an infant with cystic fibrosis. *Clin Pediatr* 1976;15:597–600.
22. Elias E, Muller D, Scott J. Spinocerebellar disorders in association with cystic fibrosis or chronic childhood cholestasis and virtually undetectable serum concentrations of vitamin E. *Lancet* 1981;2:1319–1321.
23. Walters TR, Koch HF. Hemorrhagic diathesis and cystic fibrosis in infancy. *Am J Dis Child* 1972;124:641–642.
24. Lindemans J, Neijens HJ, Kerrebijn KF, Abels J. Vitamin B12 absorption in cystic fibrosis. *Acta Paediatr Scand* 1984;73:537–540.
25. Deren JJ, Arorad D, Toskes PP, Hansell J, Sibinga M. Malabsorption of crystalline vitamin B12 in cystic fibrosis. *N Engl J Med* 1973;288:949–950.
26. Ater JL, Herbst JJ, Landaw SA, O'Brien RT. Relative anemia and iron deficiency in CF. *Pediatrics* 1983;71:810–814.
27. Ehrhardt P, Miller MG, Littlewood JM. Iron deficiency in CF. *Arch Dis Child* 1987;62:185–187.
28. Beckerman RC, Taussig LM. Hypoelectrolytemia and metabolic alkalosis in infants with cystic fibrosis. *Pediatrics* 1979;63:580–583.
29. Laughlin JJ, Brady MS, Eigen H. Changing feeding trends as a cause of electrolyte depletion in infants with cystic fibrosis. *Pediatrics* 1981;68:203–207.
30. Mischler EH, Chesney PJ, Chesney RW, Mazess RB. Demineralization in CF detected by direct photoabsorptiometry. *Am J Dis Child* 1979;133:632–635.
31. Green CJ, Doershuk CF, Stern RC. Symptomatic hypomagnesemia in CF. *J Pediatr* 1985;107:425–428.
32. Palin HD, Underwood BA, Denning CR. The effect of oral zinc supplementation on plasma levels on vitamin A and retinol-binding protein in cystic fibrosis. *Pediatr Res* 1976;10:358.
33. Holt TL, Thomas BJ, Ward CC, Shepherd RW. Hair analysis in CF. *IRCS—Med Sci* 1985;12:990–993.
34. Hamilton RM, Billespie CR, Cook HW. Relationships between levels of essential fatty acids and zinc in plasma in cystic fibrosis patients. *Lipids* 1981;16:374–376.
35. Ward KP, Arthur JR, Russell G. Blood selenium content and glutathione peroxidase activity in children with CF, coeliac disease, asthma, and epilepsy. *Eur J Paediatr* 1984;142:21–24.
36. Sproul A, Huang H. Growth patterns in children with cystic fibrosis. *J Pediatr* 1964;65:664–676.

37. Berry HK, Kellog FW, Hunt MM, Ingberg RL, Richter L, Gutjahr C. Dietary supplement and nutrition in children with cystic fibrosis. *Am J Dis Child* 1975;129:165–171.
38. Crozier DN. Cystic fibrosis, a not so fatal disease. *Pediatr Clin North Am* 1974;21:935–960.
39. Boland MP, Stoski DS, MacDonald NE, Soucy P, Patrick J. Chronic jejunostomy feeding with a non-elemental formula in undernourished patients with cystic fibrosis. *Lancet* 1986;1:232–234.
40. Levy LD, Durie PR, Pencharz PB, Corey M. Effects of long-term nutritional rehabilitation on body composition and clinical status in malnourished children and adolescents with cystic fibrosis. *J Pediatr* 1985;107:225–230.
41. Rosenthal A, Button LN, Khaw KT. Blood volume changes in patients with cystic fibrosis. *Pediatrics* 1977;59:588–594.
42. Khaw KT, Adeniyi-Jones S, Gordon D. Comparative effectiveness of viokase, cotazym, and pancrease in children with cystic fibrosis. *Cystic Fibrosis Club Abstr* 1977;18:57.
43. Holsclaw DS, Fahl JC, Keith HH. Enhancement of enzyme replacement therapy in cystic fibrosis. *Cystic Fibrosis Club Abstr* 1979;20:19.
44. Mischler EH, Parrel S, Farrell P, Odell GB. Comparison of effectiveness of pancreatic enzyme preparations in cystic fibrosis. *Am J Dis Child* 1982;136:1060–1063.
45. O'Loughlin E, Forbes D, Parsons H, Scott B, Cooper D, Gall G. Nutritional rehabilitation of malnourished patients with cystic fibrosis. *Am J Clin Nutr* 1986;43:732–737.
46. Moore MC, Greene HL, Donald WD, Dunn GD. Enteral tube feeding as adjunct therapy in malnourished patients with cystic fibrosis: a clinical study and literature review. *Am J Clin Nutr* 1986;44:33–41.
47. Bertrand JM, Morin CL, Lasalle R, Patrick J, Coates AL. Short-term clinical nutritional and functional effects of continuous enteral alimentation in children with cystic fibrosis. *J Pediatr* 1984;104:41–46.
48. Boland MP, Patrick J, Stoski DS, Soucy P. Permanent enteral feeding in cystic fibrosis: advantages of a replaceable jejunostomy tube. *J Pediatr Surg* 1987;22:843–847.
49. Mansell AL, Andersen JC, Muttant CR, Nores C, Loeff DS, Levy JS, Heird WC. Short-term pulmonary effects of total parenteral nutrition in children with cystic fibrosis. *J Pediatr* 1984;104:700–705.
50. Shepherd RW, Cooksley WGE, Cooke WD. Improved growth and clinical, nutritional, and respiratory changes in response to nutritional therapy in cystic fibrosis. *J Pediatr* 1980;97:351–357.
51. Hopkins RL. Malnutrition and the respiratory system. In: Suskind R, Lewinter-Suskind L, eds. *The malnourished child,* vol 19, Nestle Nutrition Workshop Series. New York: Raven Press, 1990;245–259.
52. Shepherd RW, Holt TL, Thomas BJ, Kay L, Isles A, Francis PJ, Ward LC. Nutritional rehabilitation in cystic fibrosis: controlled studies of effects on nutritional growth retardation, body protein turnover and the course of pulmonary disease. *J Pediatr* 1986;109:788–794.
53. Hopkins RL. Respiratory muscle size in cystic fibrosis. *Chest* 194;86:303.
54. Gaskin K, Gurwitz D, Durie P, Corey M, Levison H, Forstner G. Improved respiratory prognosis in patients with cystic fibrosis and normal fat absorption. *J Pediatr* 1982;100:857–862.

CHAPTER 33

Nutritional Considerations in the Prognosis and Treatment of Children with Congenital Heart Disease

Amnon Rosenthal

Although children with mild congenital heart disease generally have normal growth and development (1), those with hemodynamically significant heart disease are at high risk for becoming nutritionally depleted, often exhibiting poor weight gain and delayed growth (2–5). Malnutrition secondary to cardiac disease is the major cause of failure to thrive in these children. Approximately 60% to 70% of infants hospitalized in our institution with congenital heart disease exhibit failure to thrive as a result of insufficient nutrient intake and/or absorption.

Congenital heart disease makes up 12% of major congenital anomalies. The incidence of congenital heart disease is approximately 7 per 1,000 live births, with about half of these (3.5 per 1,000 live births) considered to have "critical" heart disease, i.e., heart disease that requires intervention prior to 1 year of age. Although previous management of cardiac disease was limited, today nearly half of all cardiac surgery for congenital heart disease is performed in infancy, 25% in the neonatal period. Moreover, at least 80% of the operations are reparative, not palliative. In addition, all the common lesions presenting in the first year of life are treatable by surgery, and all, except those in infants with hypoplastic left heart or heterotaxy, are usually completely repaired at the initial procedure (Table 1) (6). Early intervention also helps mitigate the nutritional problems prevalent in pediatric heart disease.

Many of the problems observed in infants and children with congenital heart disease are similar to those of children with other congenital defects or chronic illness. Without, and occasionally even with, appropriate surgical and medical management, cardiac disease is associated with delayed growth as well as physical and emotional disabilities that may prevent integration of the child into the physical, emotional, and social environment in which he or she lives.

Cardiac cachexia refers to a syndrome of protein-energy malnutrition seen in patients with chronic cardiac disease. The three most common pediatric clinical states associated with cardiac cachexia are chronic congestive heart failure, chronic shunt hypoxemia, and nosocomial postoperative acute and chronic states. Any one or a combination of these clinical states may exist in association with one or more of the common cardiovascular lesions (Table 1). Cardiac cachexia is most prevalent in infancy, may be mild or severe, and is largely amenable to medical and surgical therapy. Classical cardiac cachexia due to congestive heart failure may develop in infants over a period of months. The more acute nosocomial cachexia (7), resulting from inadequate intake of calories and protein, may develop in the postoperative state over a period of weeks. Advances in nutritional support therapy have markedly improved the prognosis of critically ill infants with congenital heart disease. Advances in pharmacologic therapy, intensive care unit monitoring and respiratory care, and surgical techniques, including cardiac transplantation, have also resulted, however, in a small but significant population of children with chronic cardiac illness.

It is important, in the management of congenital heart disease, especially hemodynamically significant heart disease, to understand the effect of the cardiac disease on nutritional status and, to a lesser extent, the effect of nutritional status on cardiac function.

A. Rosenthal: Department of Pediatrics, University of Michigan School of Medicine, C. S. Mott Children's Hospital, Ann Arbor, Michigan 48109.

TABLE 1. *Diagnostic categories of infants with congenital heart disease*

Diagnosis	Percent
Ventricular septal defect	17
D-transposition of the great arteries	11
Tetralogy of Fallot	9
Coarctation of aorta	8
Hypoplastic left ventricle	8
Patent ductus arteriosus	7
Atrioventricular septal defect	5
Heterotaxy syndrome	4
Others	31
Total	100

Adapted from ref. 6.

ETIOLOGY

The precise etiology of growth failure in infants with congenital heart disease, with or without hemodynamic abnormalities, remains unclear. It is difficult to separate prenatal from postnatal factors; many infants presenting with congenital heart disease exhibit intrauterine growth retardation, prematurity, or extracardiac abnormalities. Morphologic evidence indicates that reduced organ and cell size in patients dying of chronic congenital heart disease is similar in distribution to infants with protein-energy malnutrition (8). Hemodynamic factors clearly influence the nutritional state of the child with congenital heart disease (Table 2). Volume overload is usually the result of a significant left-to-right intracardiac shunt (e.g., in ventricular septal defect, patent ductus arteriosus or atrial septal defect), atrioventricular valve (mitral or tricuspid) regurgitation, or, less commonly in childhood, semilunar (aortic or pulmonary) valve regurgitation. Infants with ventricular septal defect or patent ductus arteriosus and a large left-to-right shunt are more prone to delayed height and weight maturation than those with a small shunt and less left ventricular volume overload. In the presence of a large left-to-right shunt there is increased pulmonary blood flow, increased left atrial pressure and size, and increased left ventricular dimension.

Congestive heart failure is the dominant physiologic and hemodynamic handicap that affects growth in children with congenital heart disease. Primary myocardial disease, such as cardiomyopathy or secondary myocardial dysfunction due to prolonged volume or pressure overload, leads to congestive heart failure and stunted growth. Acyanotic lesions (e.g., aortic stenosis, coarctation, pulmonary stenosis) are infrequently associated with undernutrition unless congestive heart failure supervenes.

In the absence of congestive heart failure, cyanotic congenital heart lesions (e.g., tetralogy of Fallot or tricuspid atresia) are also associated with poor growth (1). The chronic hypoxemia in patients with cyanotic heart disease is due to an intracardiac right-to-left shunt. There is a direct relationship between growth and the duration, in years, of hypoxemia. There is no direct relationship, however, to severity. Growth is most affected when the hypoxemia is associated with congestive heart failure (e.g., transposition of the great arteries or single ventricle). Hypoxemia does not necessarily imply tissue hypoxia or anoxia since oxygen consumption and tissue metabolism decrease only when arterial PO_2 falls below 30 mm Hg (9). Pulmonary artery hypertension and pulmonary vascular disease are often associated with other serious cardiovascular defects and may thus directly or indirectly influence the nutritional state. A National Institutes of Health (NIH)-sponsored study of children with ventricular septal defect related stunted height to the presence or persistence of pulmonary artery hypertension (10).

The relationship between growth failure and abnormal hemodynamics is not clearly understood. Inadequate caloric intake is probably one major factor (9,11). Studies that discounted intake as a major contributor to growth failure in pediatric cardiac patients often used weight-for-height rather than height-for-age as the primary criterion (1,12). In fact, the roles of increased energy requirements associated with a greater metabolic rate per unit of body weight, smaller energy reserves of fat and somatic protein, and malabsorption, cellular hypoxemia, or hypoxia are poorly understood and are probably quite complex. Inadequate caloric intake, especially in infants, may be the result of poor appetite, fatigue with feeding, interference of tachypnea or dyspnea with deglutition, or the result of recurrent pulmonary infections. Infants with congestive heart failure are usually hungry and begin feeding avidly, but tire quickly. Feeding time tends to increase as caloric intake decreases. Inadequate feeding may result from abdominal discomfort or distention associated with hepatomegaly or hypomotility of the gut secondary to edema or hypoxia. In adults, hepatomegaly may compress the stomach, decreasing hunger contractions and resulting in an early feeling of satiety (13,14). Children may find the restricted sodium diet unpalatable.

The increased metabolic rate in malnourished cardiac disease patients may be related to the increased work of respiratory muscles necessary for ventilation in the presence of decreased lung compliance, increased oxygen

TABLE 2. *Hemodynamic factors that may influence nutritional status in congenital heart disease*

Volume overload, right or left heart
Myocardial dysfunction
Congestive heart failure
Chronic hypoxemia
Pulmonary artery hypertension and vascular disease

consumption of the dilated or hypertrophic heart, and/or increased overall sympathetic nervous system tone (13). Evaporative water loss may also require additional expenditures of energy. Increased oxygen consumption has been demonstrated in infants with congenital heart disease and congestive failure (15). There is a direct relationship between increased oxygen consumption and the severity of failure as well as the overall caloric intake. However, when basal metabolic rate is related to lean body mass, the basal metabolic rate in children and infants with congenital heart disease is reported to be normal (16).

Inadequate absorption and excessive nutrient loss through the gastrointestinal tract may also contribute to the pathophysiology of malnutrition in these patients. Slightly decreased amino acid absorption (17) and increased fecal fat (18) possibly due to edema of the bowel or reduced pancreatic enzymes (14) have been demonstrated in adults. However, positive nitrogen balance and normal fecal fat have been demonstrated in children with congenital heart disease (19,20).

Cellular hypoxia or "stagnant anoxia" results most often from a sluggish capillary flow as in congestive heart failure. It disrupts biosynthetic function, which leads to cellular undersupply or underutilization of substrates and possible interference with cell multiplication. Growth disturbance is, in fact, most pronounced in children with both congestive heart failure and severe hypoxemia.

In addition, growth is also influenced by genetic, prenatal, and noncardiac postnatal abnormalities (Table 3) (6,16,21–23). In many children, these factors may be the determining ones influencing catch-up growth and development (24). For example, when the congenital heart disease is part of an autosomal trisomy, underdevelopment may be related to the chromosomal abnormality. Patients with Down (25) or Turner (26) syndrome exhibit delayed growth with no cardiac disease.

Growth delays may be caused by the hemodynamic disturbance caused by the cardiac defect. In addition, they may occur as a result of the extracardiac anomalies seen in nearly 25% of patients under a year of age (21,22). Extracardiac anomalies occur in 25% or more of infants with endocardial cushion defect, patent ductus arteriosus, atrioventricular septal defect, ventricular septal defect, tetralogy of Fallot, complex coarctation, and malpositions (21). In infants with congenital heart disease, the most frequent anomalies are in the musculoskeletal system, followed by those in the central nervous system, renal and gastrointestinal tracts. Among 3,357 infants admitted to the New England Regional Infant Cardiac Program between 1968 and 1977, major gastrointestinal malformations were reported in 8.3% (23). Infants with symptomatic cardiac disease showed a subnormal birth weight distribution; intrauterine growth retardation was observed in 6.1% of these infants (22). The incidence of extracardiac abnormalities among small for gestational age infants with heart disease is 28% (22).

Growth is also negatively influenced by recurrent infections, especially severe respiratory infections, adverse psychosocial components, and, in infants, gastroesophageal reflux (27). Occasionally, a specific nutrient deficiency, such as cardiomyopathies caused by a deficiency of carnitine, thiamine, or selenium, exists.

NUTRITIONAL ASSESSMENT

Accurate assessment of nutritional status is essential in the examination of infants and children with congenital heart disease. This is accomplished through parental interviews, physical examination, and laboratory procedures.

Interviews should cover appetite, dietary and nutrient intake, significant weight changes, and problems with feedings. It will generally be revealed that, in infants with more severe circulatory compromise, the volume of formula per feeding will tend to be smaller and the duration of each feeding longer. This is because infants with congestive heart failure initially feed avidly, but quickly fatigue, taking as long as 45 to 60 min to finish. These infants also perspire profusely during feeding because of the increased release of catecholamines to the circulation. Other exacerbating factors may include difficulties with swallowing and/or chewing. Adverse socioeconomic factors include low income, inexperience of the care-giver, parental drug or alcohol abuse, unstable marital status, and/or teenage parents.

Physical examination is the most important part of the nutritional assessment. Weight and height are routinely measured in our cardiology clinic; head circumference is taken in all children under the age of 3. Values are routinely plotted on appropriate growth curves for ongoing comparison. Special charts are utilized for preterm infants and Down or Turner syndrome patients (25,26). Signs of protein-energy malnutrition include a loss of subcutaneous tissue and muscle mass, small stature, or edema. At highest risk are infants with clinical signs and symptoms of congestive heart failure, cyanosis, anemia, or any combination of these factors.

Skin-fold thickness to assess adipose tissue and/or arm circumference measurement to assess skeletal muscle

TABLE 3. *Common noncirculatory factors associated with growth retardation in patients with congenital heart disease*

Congenital heart disease as part of a recognizable syndrome
Associated extracardiac anomalies
Intrauterine growth retardation/prematurity
Recurrent respiratory infections
Adverse psychosocial conditions
Gastroesophageal reflux

mass are not commonly utilized, although they may be appropriate in special circumstances.

The most useful office laboratory procedures and biochemical tests are hemoglobin determination, measurement of systemic oxygen saturation, serum proteins, and electrolytes. Hemoglobin provides a reliable estimate of blood oxygen-carrying capacity. An accurate arterial blood oxygen saturation can be measured noninvasively by the pulse volume oximeter. Blood oxygen content may thus be calculated from the hemoglobin and oxygen saturation. Serum albumin or prealbumin may be utilized as an estimate of the severity of the malnutrition, extent of liver disease, and gastrointestinal or urinary loss of protein. Prealbumin has been shown to be a sensitive indicator of protein-energy malnutrition (28). Decreased serum albumin is most common in infants or children with systemic venous hypertension associated with marked congestive heart failure, constrictive pericardial disease, restrictive cardiac disease, or post-Fontan operation (direct atrial or systemic venous anastomosis to the pulmonary artery) (29). When diuretics are used for congestive heart failure, the resulting loss of electrolytes, especially potassium, may result in digitalis toxicity and reduced renal clearance. Significant reduction in serum sodium may be accompanied by decreased gastric motility. The creatinine-height index—24-hr creatinine excretion divided by the expected 24-hr creatinine excretion of a normal child of the same height—is rarely utilized.

The calculation of approximate caloric intake versus caloric requirement, the estimated fluid and solute load, and assessment of electrolyte balance are paramount in defining treatment. Maintenance and normal growth require, for infants, 90 to 120 kilocalories per kilogram (Cal/kg) and, for young children, 75 to 90 Cal/kg. Caloric requirements increase 20% to 30% with major surgery; 50% to 100% with long-term growth failure (30). Evaluation for possible impairment of the cellular immunity is important in preoperative patients, particularly those who are malnourished, including candidates for cardiac transplantation.

Inadequate growth in infants with congenital heart disease can be established in a preliminary office visit (Table 4). Weight-for-height is an accurate indication of the acute nutrient state; a flat or declining weight percentile may signal wasting. Height-for-age, on the other hand, indicates a more long-term problem. When both height-for-age and weight-for-height are below the 3rd percentile, it is likely that severe undernutrition has been present for a prolonged period and still exists.

The brain is particularly vulnerable to nutritional deficits in infancy and early childhood. Decreasing head size indicates structural alterations in brain size (31). In infants with congestive heart failure or hypoxemia, this decline in circumference signals the presence of malnutrition.

MANAGEMENT

The ultimate goal in the care of the child with congenital heart disease is the development of a physically, intellectually, and socially mature adult. Considerations include potential medical, surgical, developmental, psychosocial, and nutritional problems. Nutritional management involves enhancement of caloric and protein intake, appropriate restriction of fluid and sodium, and supplementation of vitamins and minerals, especially iron and calcium. Nutrients must be adequate without overburdening the circulation and/or disturbing the delicate water balance. Increased caloric needs may be met by increasing the quantity or volume of feeding, increasing the density of feeding, or by attempting to reduce the metabolic demands (32). In the infant, placement in an incubator may reduce metabolic/caloric needs.

Caloric requirements for children with hemodynamically significant cardiac disease have not been established; the recommended daily allowances are not accurate for the special needs of these infants and children. Adequate intake for infants has been estimated at threefold the basal metabolic rate or nearly 175 to 180 Cal/kg per day. Infants who are malnourished may also require 175 Cal/kg for catch-up and sustained growth.

Management of the nutritionally deficient child with congenital heart disease is medical and frequently surgical. Medical-pharmacologic management may include inotropic drugs, preload reduction with diuretics, or afterload reduction in children with congestive heart failure, pulmonary edema, and/or significant myocardial dysfunction. Pulmonary vasodilator drugs or oxygen therapy may be necessary in patients with pulmonary artery hypertension and pulmonary vascular disease. Prevention of infections is paramount and includes antimicrobial prophylaxis for the prevention of infective endocarditis at times of predictable risk. In children with cyanotic heart disease, antimicrobial prophylaxis is also important for prevention of brain abscess. Routine immunizations, including HIB-conjugate, should be administered according to the American Academy of Pediatrics guidelines (33). Pneumovax vaccination and continuous antibiotic prophylaxis is necessary in children with the asplenia syndrome.

Children with large left-to-right shunts, pulmonary

TABLE 4. *Office criteria for growth failure in infants with congenital heart disease*

Disproportionate low weight-for-height percentile
Flattening or declining weight percentile
Weight and/or height less than 5th percentile
Weight gain less than $\frac{1}{2}$ oz/day in early infancy
Flattening or declining head circumference percentile

edema, or congestive heart failure from any cause are at increased risk of pulmonary infections, atelectasis, and bronchospasm. Influenza virus immunization is important prior to an anticipated epidemic. Pulmonary infections require vigorous antibiotic therapy, often in hospital. In addition, respiratory syncytial virus is associated with a high morbidity and mortality in infants with large left-to-right shunts and pulmonary artery hypertension.

Providing sufficient, but not excessive, nutrients for maintenance and growth of the child with hemodynamically significant congenital heart disease is a challenge. The ultimate plan depends on the type and severity of the cardiovascular disease and the nutritional condition of the individual child.

An appropriate formula should be provided that maximizes caloric intake (30,34). Enteral feedings are more physiologic and are preferable to parenteral alimentation when gastrointestinal function is adequate. Standard infant formula may be used with no restriction of total fluid intake. Nursing mothers may express milk before feeding in order to accurately assess intake and the need for supplementation. It is not necessary to restrict the quantity of formula to infants with congestive heart failure or severe cyanosis who are able to feed voluntarily; such restriction may well lead to malnutrition. When a larger volume of feeding is anticipated, it is preferable to be more aggressive with diuretic therapy. If, however, intolerance to volume is the limiting factor in satisfying nutritional needs, caloric density may be increased by concentrating a formula to 1 Cal/ml. Cow's milk formulas are available in concentrations of 20, 24, and 27 Cal/oz (0.67, 0.8, and 0.9 Cal/ml). If this is not feasible because of the concomitant increase in solute load, feedings may be supplemented with carbohydrates (e.g., polycose) or fats [e.g., medium-chain triglycerides (MCT) or long-chain corn oil].

Increasing the caloric density of a formula may lead to reduction of free water, and increased osmolality and solute load, including electrolytes, minerals and, most critically, sodium load. In older infants and children, formula may replace solid foods in order to achieve the necessary caloric density. Synthetic feeding mixtures should be avoided because of the associated side effects, such as abdominal distention or diarrhea.

Critically ill infants with marked tachypnea (respiratory rate >80 per min) or on ventilatory support require tube feeding, intermittent or continuous. Formula is infused via a flexible feeding tube into the stomach; quantity and duration are regulated by an intravenous drip chamber. Continuous infusion is preferable since it lessens the effects of a large volume load and increased osmolality on stomach emptying and digestive enzymes. Both PM 60/40 and SMA can be concentrated to 1 Cal/ml with a relatively low sodium content of approximately 10 mEq/l (35). The volume of feedings is generally advanced to the threshold tolerated and, if necessary, the density is then increased. When the caloric and nutrient density of intake is increased, solute load, sodium and protein, urine, and formula osmolalities should be monitored.

There are indications and contraindications to nasogastric feeding in infants and children with congenital heart disease (Table 5). Feedings via nasogastric or orogastric tube, if nasal insertion is undesirable or not feasible, is frequently utilized in severely ill infants without gastrointestinal abnormalities. Most of the complications inherent with tube feeding can be prevented by aspiration of contents every 6 hr, flushing after all medications, and slowly increasing tonicity and volume of the feeding.

Parenteral nutrition is generally used in pediatric cardiac patients with marginal nutritional reserves and/or when oral feedings will not be received for more than 3 to 5 days. This includes children with cardiac cachexia associated with chronic congestive failure, those with marked malnutrition prior to surgery, postoperative patients with or without prolonged mechanical ventilatory support, low birth weight infants, and/or infants with associated gastrointestinal anomalies.

Carbohydrates, predominantly glucose, are the main source of calories. Lipids may be added when higher caloric intakes are required, particularly in low birth weight infants, or when infused glucose concentration leads to significant hyperglycemia. Infusing glucose-amino acid solutions simultaneously with lipid emulsion via the peripheral intravenous route usually supplies sufficient nutrients and reduces the medical, technical, metabolic, and psychological complications of a central catheter placement (32). Sepsis and thrombosis are of particular concern. A central venous line may be necessary in patients who require fluid restriction or in infants with limited peripheral vein access. A Broviac catheter is preferable for prolonged nutritional support at home or in the hospital.

Peripheral hyperalimentation solution generally consists of 10% dextrose, 10% intralipids, and 1.5% amino acids. Fat should not exceed 4 g/kg/day or approximately 50% of total calories; essential fatty acids, supplied by linoleic acid, total 4% of daily calories (30). An appropriate nutrient balance usually contains 1 Cal/ml. When fluid restriction prevents peripheral hyperalimen-

TABLE 5. *Nasogastric feedings in infants with congenital heart disease*

Indications
Intractable congestive heart failure
Prematurity (<34 weeks)
Abnormal or weak swallowing mechanism
Contraindications
Gastroesophageal reflux
Intractable emesis
Umbilical artery line

tation from supplying sufficient calories, partial enteral feedings, if feasible, may be used. In fluid-restricted patients in the critical care setting, however, a high caloric density (1.5 Cal/ml) parenteral solution may be more appropriate (7). This will require a central line, usually inserted via the subclavian vein. Although both peripheral and central parenteral nutrition solutions may be infused alone, they are generally administered concomitantly with intravenous fat in order to reduce the osmolality of the final solution.

There is always the danger of congestive heart failure during parenteral nutrition (Table 6). An increased ventricular end diastolic volume or preload by excessive fluid or solute load may cause or aggravate pulmonary congestion, thereby reducing ventricular performance and cardiac output. Metabolic rate increases and mineral deficiencies, including magnesium depletion, may develop. Arrhythmia from electrolyte imbalance or catheter irritation of the atrial wall may precipitate pulmonary edema and further decrease myocardial contractility; sepsis and endocarditis are also common complications causing or increasing failure in children receiving parenteral nutrition by central venous line. Complications are usually avoidable, especially in infants, by meticulous monitoring of physical condition and biochemical values.

In patients with more acute cardiac decompensation, use of concentrated parenteral solutions should be delayed because of the obligate fluid load involved. In such cases, a glucose-insulin-potassium infusion may prove useful as an initial nutritional intervention. Use of heparin (1 to 2 units/ml) is advisable to avoid venous thrombosis, especially in patients with low cardiac output or polycythemia. Various solutions are described in our parenteral and enteral nutrition manual (30,34).

Persistent growth failure is a common indication for cardiac surgery in the infant and child with congenital heart disease. The type of surgery is lesion-specific and, to a lesser extent, related to age. Congenital anomalies, such as complete transposition of the great arteries, are generally completely reparable during the neonatal period. Defects such as tetralogy of Fallot, endocardial cushion defect, and ventricular septal defect with pulmonary artery hypertension may all be repaired during infancy. Palliative surgery is reserved for a few complex congenital heart lesions such as hypoplastic left heart syndrome, tricuspid atresia, pulmonary atresia, or single ventricle. Cardiovascular disease, and/or the surgery required for its treatment, increases the need to meet the quantitative-qualitative nitrogen and energy requirements for growth and the reparative process. Decreased postoperative mortality and morbidity are observed in patients receiving appropriate nutritional support, especially patients who were malnourished prior to surgery.

Enteral feedings can usually be resumed 2 to 3 days after simple heart surgery. Parenteral nutrition, on the other hand, may be indicated after more complex surgery, in the presence of protracted postoperative complications or an anticipated delayed recovery.

Gastrointestinal surgery, particularly gastrostomy or fundoplication, is often performed in infants with congenital heart disease because of the increased incidence of associated gastrointestinal anomalies, gastrointestinal reflux, or persistent cardiac cachexia. Gastrostomy or, less often, jejunostomy feedings are indicated when severely ill infants and children require prolonged tube feedings, have undesirable side effects from tube feedings, or have associated upper gastrointestinal abnormalities.

Cardiac disease has psychosocial as well as medical components. Successful management is predicated on communication between the cardiologist and primary physician as well as support and guidance for parents. Procedures such as cardiac catheterization and surgery have profound psychological effects on the infant or child which may result in behavioral problems. Parents must learn how to comfort the child in distress while still encouraging the development of strengths. Health professionals are important in helping the parents understand the child in order to develop techniques that avert long-term behavioral problems.

SPECIAL PROBLEMS

A number of special nutritional problems are frequent or specific to children with congenital heart disease. Prescribed drugs may lead to iatrogenic malnutrition. Drug-nutrient interaction may have adverse effects, especially in malnourished patients, in patients taking multiple and/or large doses of medication, in patients on long-term pharmacologic therapy, and in patients with compromised ability to metabolize or utilize drugs or nutrients. Maximal drug activity for some cardiovascular drugs may be achieved by administering the drug on an empty stomach (e.g., captopril, atenolol). In others, maximal activity is achieved when administered with food (e.g., propranolol, hydralazine, spironolactone, hydrochlorothiazide). Nutrients can influence drug bioavailability and therapeutic results. Absorption of phenytoin is increased by carbohydrate and reduced by protein; high carbohydrate intakes increase serum levels of theophylline, whereas a high protein intake reduces them.

TABLE 6. *Factors that may contribute to congestive heart failure during parenteral nutrition*

Increased ventricular volume
Excessive sodium retention
Increased metabolic rate
Relative deficiencies in vitamins/minerals
Alteration of electrical excitation
Sepsis, endocarditis

Children with prosthetic valves, chronic atrial flutter, or severe cardiomyopathy often require anticoagulant therapy with Coumadin. Vitamin supplements or a high intake of dietary vitamin K, such as from green leafy vegetables, decreases the anticoagulant effect. This places the child at increased risk for a mural thrombus or embolization. Highly plasma protein-bound drugs such as phenytoin or propranolol are often used in malnourished infants and children with hypoproteinemia associated with systemic venous hypertension [e.g., post-Fontan operation (29)], and restrictive myocardial or constrictive pericardial disease for therapy of arrhythmias. The reduced protein-binding sites will lead to reduced total serum drug levels, whereas free drug levels are normal. In assessing treatment, one should therefore consider adjustment of serum level for reduced protein or measure the level of free drug. Altered clearance of the drug by the liver may also occur in malnourished patients with systemic venous hypertension. Inadequate enzyme activity may influence clearance of propranolol, theophylline, or nitroprusside, leading to unexpected drug level or toxicity. In critical care, a prolonged infusion of nitroprusside in the presence of hepatic disease may lead to a high level of thiocyanate or cyanide.

Some electrolyte imbalance is inevitable when diuresis is achieved. Excessive diuresis, especially in patients with severe edema, is commonly followed by hyponatremia. Hyponatremia is more severe when the patient is on a low-salt diet or drinks excessive fluids while on prolonged diuretic therapy. Because thiazides reduce urinary calcium excretion, hypercalcemia tends to result from their use. Hypokalemia is likely to develop from multiple or high doses of diuretics, and diuretics with a longer duration of action. Hypokalemia is also more common in patients with high salt intake, in the presence of metabolic alkalosis or when high fluid intake results in large urinary volume. The hypokalemia may in turn result in cardiac arrhythmias, hypomagnesemia, negative nitrogen balance, or orthostatic hypotension. Potassium depletion may be avoided by simultaneous use of potassium-sparing drugs such as spironolactone. Potassium supplements are effective but less palatable to small children; potassium-rich foods may be a useful alternative. Bananas contain approximately 14 mEq of potassium; a glass of orange juice contains 12 mEq.

Cardiac transplants in infants and children have been associated with hyperlipidemia (hypertriglyceridemia and hypercholesterolemia), early atherogenesis, and delayed growth. Coronary atherosclerosis is a significant cause of late mortality (36). Coronary atherosclerosis appears to result from immune endothelial injury, subsequent thrombus formation, and intra-arterial deposition of lipid. Delayed growth in cardiac transplant patients is related to the use of large doses of corticosteroids. Nutritional goals in the immediate posttransplant period include a high-caloric moderate-protein diet to enhance wound healing. Long-term goals include maintaining linear growth by reducing or eliminating the need for corticosteroids, maintaining appropriate weight-for-height, and modification of fat intake to prevent early coronary atherosclerosis. Niacin supplementation may be indicated for children over 2 years of age with significant hyperlipidemia.

Anemia, regardless of its etiology, has serious, sometimes lethal consequences for the patient with congenital heart disease. A reduced hemoglobin and thereby blood oxygen-carrying capacity may result in tissue and organ hypoxia in patients with ventricular pressure overload, volume overload, congestive heart failure, or hypoxemia. In a child with moderate or severe aortic valve stenosis, anemia may lead to subendocardial ischemia and angina or a life-threatening arrhythmia. In the infant with a large ventricular septal defect, physiologic anemia of infancy may result in progressive congestive heart failure due to a decrease in blood viscosity and pulmonary vascular resistance. The change in pulmonary resistance increases the left-to-right shunt via the septal defect and consequently the pulmonary blood flow. In the child with congestive heart failure from any cause, tissue hypoxia will increase because reduced oxygen transport associated with low cardiac output will be further compromised by the diminished oxygen-carrying capacity. Anemia associated with cyanotic cardiac defects will invariably reduce total oxygen transport to the tissues. Children with chronic shunt hypoxemia (e.g., tetralogy of Fallot) require a higher than normal blood hemoglobin level to compensate for the decreased blood oxygen saturation. The infant with cyanosis and relative anemia (relative to the level of oxygen saturation) is at high risk of hyperpneic or cyanotic spells, cerebrovascular accident, or death. In older children, fatigue, exercise intolerance, and dyspnea on exertion are common. The most common etiology of the anemia is iron deficiency, but folic acid deficiency may coexist (37).

Other specific nutrient, mineral, or vitamin deficiencies exist in children with cardiac disease and recognized patterns of malformations. DiGeorge syndrome is frequently accompanied by congenital cardiac defects such as conotruncal abnormalities and aortic arch anomalies. Absence or hypoplasia of the parathyroid glands leads to hypocalcemia, resulting in the need for calcium supplementation. Nearly 50% of children with Down syndrome have associated cardiac defects. The increased frequency of thyroid disorders in this syndrome, especially hypothyroidism, may mask or complicate the effect of cardiovascular disease on the nutritional status and growth.

PROGNOSIS

Failure-to-thrive identifies infants with congenital heart disease who are at risk for persistent abnormalities in growth, cognition, and social and psychological function. A study of 173 infants indicated that congestive heart failure was significantly associated with both mental and motor developmental delay. Hypoxemia and hospitalization were also associated with delayed motor development; some delays were apparent as early as 2 months of age (38). Multiple factors, including prenatal, teratogenic, and abnormal hemodynamics, contribute to these problems (9,22,24).

Prognosis for patients with optimum management is excellent. Nutritional repletion in the pre- and postoperative child is associated with reduction in sepsis and enhanced wound healing. Deep hypothermia and circulatory arrest, utilized in the repair of congenital heart disease, do not appear to significantly influence subsequent growth or the incidence of central nervous system deficits (39,40). Following surgery, weight is restored more rapidly than height. Catch-up linear growth is more likely with corrective than palliative surgery and when repair is performed in earlier childhood (24,39,41). Decreased growth velocity was reversed in 47 infants operated on before 1 year of age for ventricular septal defect, tetralogy of Fallot, and transposition of the great arteries. Within 12 to 18 months, most infants had regained at least their birth weight percentile, and the group with ventricular septal defect exceeded it (41).

Many factors may be responsible for persistent nutritional and growth retardation in postoperative patients (Table 7). Palliative surgery may improve, but not eliminate, congestive heart failure, hypoxemia, or myocardial dysfunction (24). For example, aortopulmonary anastomosis (Blalock-Taussig shunt), a palliative operation for increasing pulmonary blood flow, reduces but does not eliminate hypoxemia. Growth and measurements of tissue development such as lean body mass, total body fat, lean/fat ratio, cellular lipid content, or lipid-containing fat cells remain unaffected despite increased oxygenation and symptomatic improvement after surgery (42). The Norwood operation is a palliative procedure performed in neonates with hypoplastic left heart syndrome. Its residua and sequelae include moderate to severe hypoxemia and/or congestive heart failure. Malnutrition and failure to thrive are common outcomes. Corrective surgery may also be accompanied by serious sequelae that lead to persistent nutritional or developmental abnormalities. Failure to achieve a normal growth pattern after the Mustard operation for transposition of the great arteries may be secondary to significant residual lesions such as pulmonary stenosis or superior vena cava obstruction (39).

The age at which surgical repair is performed may influence psychologic development as well as growth. Children who had cyanosis and transposition of the great arteries repaired in infancy showed an inverse relationship between the age at surgery and cognitive functioning (43). Preoperative psychological testing of cyanotic children with tetralogy of Fallot, repaired at a mean age of 8.7 years, correlate positively with the intellectual and psychosocial status of the postoperative adult at a mean age of 30.3 years (44).

Further research is necessary to determine the relationship between failure-to-thrive and hemodynamically significant cardiovascular disease. Additional study is warranted on the role of tissue hypoxia, hypoxemia, and gastrointestinal absorption as well as the influence of aggressive preoperative medical nutritional management, the response to different operative procedures in early infancy, and the effect of specific nutrients on growth potential. The effect of heart or heart/lung transplantation in children on long-term nutritional status and growth also remains to be fully explored.

TABLE 7. *Factors that may be responsible for persistent growth retardation in postoperative children with congenital heart disease*

Hemodynamically significant residual lesions
Sequelae or complication of surgery
Associated cardiac or extracardiac anomalies
Intrauterine growth retardation
Age at operation
Hereditary or genetic constitution

REFERENCES

1. Strangway A, et al. Diet and growth in congenital heart disease. *Pediatrics* 1976;57:75–86.
2. Linde LM, et al. Physical and emotional aspects of congenital heart disease in children. *Am J Cardiol* 1971;27:712–713.
3. Angelov G, et al. Physical development and body structure of children with congenital heart disease. *Hum Biol* 1980;52:413–421.
4. White RI Jr, et al. Delayed skeletal growth and maturation in adolescent congenital heart disease. *Invest Radiol* 1971;6:326–332.
5. Ehlers KH. Growth failure in association with congenital heart disease. *Pediatr Ann* 1978;7:750–759.
6. Report of the New England Regional Infant Cardiac Program. *Pediatrics* 1980(Feb);65(2, Suppl).
7. Quinn T, Askanaz J. Nutrition and cardiac disease. *Crit Care Clin* 1987;3(1):167–184.
8. Naeye RL. Anatomic features of growth failure in congenital heart disease. *Pediatrics* 1967;39:433–440.
9. Nadas AS, et al. Nutritional considerations in the prognosis and treatment of children with congenital heart disease. In: Suskind RM, ed. *Textbook of pediatric nutrition.* New York: Raven Press, 1981;537–544.
10. Levy RJ, et al. Determinants of growth in patients with ventricular septal defect. *Circulation* 1978;57:793–797.
11. Krieger I, Chen YC. Calorie requirements for weight gain in infants with growth failure due to maternal deprivation, undernutrition, and congenital heart disease. A correlation analysis. *Pediatrics* 1969;44:647–654.
12. Salzer HR, et al. Growth and nutritional intake of infants with congenital heart disease. *Pediatr Cardiol* 1989;10:17–23.
13. Pittman JG, Cohen P. The pathogenesis of cardiac cachexia. *N Engl J Med* 1964;271:403.
14. Pittman JG, Cohen P. The pathogenesis of cardiac cachexia (concluded). *N Engl J Med* 1964;271:453.
15. Stocker FP, et al. Oxygen consumption in infants with heart disease. Relationship to severity of congestive failure, relative weight, and caloric intake. *J Pediatr* 1972;80:43–51.
16. Krieger I. Adrenocortical and thyroid function in the deprivation

syndrome. Comparison with growth failure due to undernutrition, congenital heart disease, or prenatal influences. *Am J Dis Child* 1970;120:95–102.
17. Hardy JD, Schultz J. Jejunal absorption of amino acid mixture in normal and hypoproteinemic subjects. *J Physiol* 1952;4:789.
18. Hakkila J, et al. Absorption of I-131 triolein in congestive heart failure. *Am J Cardiol* 1962;5:295.
19. Iber FL, et al. Nitrogen metabolism in children with congenital cardiac defects and severe growth retardation. *Am J Clin Nutr* 1967;20:1166–1170.
20. Krieger I. Growth failure and congenital heart disease. Energy and nitrogen balance in infants. *Am J Dis Child* 1970;120:497–502.
21. Greenwood RD, et al. Extracardiac abnormalities in infants with congenital heart disease. *Pediatrics* 1975;55:485–491.
22. Levy RJ, Rosenthal A. Birthweight of infants with congenital heart disease. *Am J Dis Child* 1978;132:249–254.
23. Rosenthal A. Congenital cardiac anomalies and gastrointestinal malformations. In: Pierpont ME, Moller JH, eds. *Genetics of cardiovascular disease.* Boston: Martinus Nijhoff, 1986;113–126.
24. Rosenthal A, Castaneda AR. Growth and development after cardiovascular surgery in infants and children. *Prog Cardiovasc Dis* 1975;18:27–37.
25. Cronk LE. Growth of children with Down's syndrome—birth to age 3 years. *Pediatrics* 1978;61:564–568.
26. Lyon AJ, et al. Growth curve for girls with Turner syndrome. *Arch Dis Child* 1985;60:932–935.
27. Weesner KM, Rosenthal A. Gastroesophageal reflux in association with congenital heart disease. *Clin Pediatr* 1983;22:424–426.
28. Rettner R, Labbe R. Monitoring total parenteral nutrition. *Lab Med* 1985;16:476–479.
29. Behrendt DM, Rosenthal A. Cardiovascular status after repair by Fontan procedure. *Ann Thorac Surg* 1980;29:322–330.
30. *Parenteral and enteral nutrition manual,* 5th ed. Ann Arbor, MI: University of Michigan Medical Center, 1988.
31. Stoch M, et al. Psychosocial outcome and CT findings after gross undernourishment during infancy: a 20-year developmental study. *Dev Med Child Neurol* 1982;24:419–436.
32. Reimer SL, et al. Nutritional support of the critically ill child. *Pediatr Clin North Am* 1980;27:647–660.
33. Uzark K, et al. Primary preventive health care in children with heart disease. *Pediatr Cardiol* 1983;4:259–264.
34. *Physician's handbook of nutrition support, maternal and pediatric,* 1st ed. Ann Arbor, MI: Department of Dietetics, The University of Michigan Hospitals, 1988.
35. Lake AM, et al. *Enteric alimentation in specialized gastrointestinal problems: an alternative to total parenteral nutrition.* Year Book Medical Publishers, 1981;319–339.
36. Addomzio LJ, et al. Late complications in pediatric cardiac transplant recipients (abstract). *Circulation* 1989;80(Suppl):4.
37. Rook GD, et al. Folic acid deficiency in infants and children with heart disease. *Br Heart J* 1973;35:87–92.
38. Aisenberg RB, et al. Hypoxemia, congestive failure and developmental delay in infants with congenital heart disease. *Pediatr Cardiol* 1982;3:133–137.
39. Levy RJ, et al. Growth after surgical repair of simple D-transposition of the great arteries. *Ann Thorac Surg* 1978;25:225–230.
40. Stevenson GJ, et al. Intellectual development of children subjected to prolonged circulatory arrest during hypothermic heart surgery in infancy. *Circulation* 1974;50(Suppl):11.
41. Sholler GF, Celermajer JM. Cardiac surgery in the first year of life: the effect on weight gains of infants with congenital heart disease. *Aust Paediatr J* 1986;22:305–308.
42. Baum D, et al. Growth and tissue abnormalities in young people with cyanotic congenital heart disease receiving systemic-pulmonary artery shunts. *Am J Cardiol* 1982;52:349–352.
43. Newburger JW, et al. Cognitive function and age of repair of transposition of the great arteries in children. *N Engl J Med* 1984;310:1495.
44. Lon Shampaine E, et al. Longitudinal psychological assessment in tetralogy of Fallot. *Pediatr Cardiol* 1990;10:135–140.

CHAPTER 34

Nutritional Considerations in the Prognosis and Treatment of Children with Renal Disease

Warren E. Grupe

The kidneys are the primary organs responsible for the regulation of the volume and composition of the body fluids. Excretion is only one facet of their regulatory function. Because the amount and composition of ingested nutrients are major contributors to the kidney's work load, an understanding of nutritional concepts is important for understanding renal disease and its successful management. This chapter describes (a) the influence of the malnourished state on normal kidney function, (b) the influence of nutrient intake on renal growth and functional maturation, and (c) nutritional considerations in the failing kidney.

EFFECTS OF MALNUTRITION ON RENAL FUNCTION

Reports of renal function in malnourished children (1–4) indicate significant functional alterations which are unexplained by hypoproteinemia, edema, or specific morphologic lesions. These changes are also not dependent on the etiology of the malnutrition; renal changes are quite similar whether the nutritional problem is primary protein-energy malnutrition, iatrogenic malnutrition, anorexia nervosa, or secondary to another disease state. Most data indicate a physiologic, functional, and reversible effect on the kidney (4).

Protein-energy malnutrition leads to decreases in glomerular filtration rate (GFR), renal plasma flow, concentrating ability, sodium excretion, and excretion of acid (1,2,4,5). There is no consistent difference between edematous and nonedematous children, and all parameters improve with correction of the malnourished state. In well-hydrated, malnourished children, clearances are about one-half normal, whereas in the dehydrated and malnourished child, they may be as low as one-fifth of normal (2).

Both GFR and renal plasma flow vary normally with protein intake in humans, dogs, and rats (6). When normal adults are fed a low-protein diet (0.1 to 0.4 mg/kg/day) they also show a fall in both GFR and renal plasma flow, which increases toward normal on a high-protein diet (2.3 to 3 g/kg/day) (7). A calorie-deficient diet also produces a reduction in creatinine clearance in normal adults, irrespective of the proportion of calories from protein, carbohydrates, or fat (8).

The mechanism producing the decrease in GFR has been finely dissected using micropuncture techniques in the rat (9). The sequence suggested by these studies is that the low glomerular filtration rate results from an increase in arteriolar resistance, which produces a decrease in glomerular plasma flow followed by glomerular collapse, which presents a smaller surface area for filtration (4,9). The functional changes that appear despite isocaloric intake indicate that low protein intake, rather than caloric deficiency, is probably the effector for the reduction in both renal perfusion and filtration (9).

An alternative explanation is indicated in studies of patients with anorexia nervosa (10,11). Increased permeability of the capillary wall itself is postulated to increase water permeability, thereby reducing fluid absorption from the interstitium (11). The resulting fall in plasma volume is followed by a decrease in renal plasma flow and glomerular filtration rate. It has also been suggested that the dietary restriction of phosphate, rather than protein, changes intrarenal hemodynamics (12).

Malnutrition also affects the clinical measurement of glomerular filtration. Simultaneous measurements of in-

W. E. Grupe: Division of Medical and Health Sciences Education, Project HOPE Health Sciences Education Center, Millwood, Virginia 22646.

ulin and creatinine clearances in protein-energy malnutrition show excellent agreement. Urea clearances, however, may be 25% or more below a simultaneous inulin clearance (4). Several factors can contribute to this discrepancy between urea clearance and true GFR, including low urine flow rates, low protein intake, low urea production, and active tubular transport of urea (4). In any event, urea clearances provide an inadequate means of measuring glomerular filtration in the malnourished patient.

The same problem exists for blood levels of urea and creatinine as measures of renal function. The plasma levels of both tend to be low in patients with protein malnutrition, despite a demonstrated reduction in GFR. The relatively low plasma levels appear to be the result of decreased production. The decreased creatinine production is the result of decreased muscle mass, whereas the low urea levels reflect the decreased protein intake. Children recovering from malnutrition may show a rise of blood urea above normal levels, despite an increasing GFR, as a reflection of their increased protein intake.

A renal concentrating defect has been described in the malnourished state, which improves following protein-calorie repletion (1,13–15). Urine osmolality may not exceed 600 mOsm, even after severe water deprivation (4). The cause of the concentrating defect is probably a lack of urea in the renal interstitium. Administration of urea to malnourished subjects is regularly followed by an increased urine osmolality concomitant with an increase in blood urea levels and increased urinary nitrogen excretion (4,16). Rats receiving a low-protein diet and exogenously administered vasopressin will increase urinary concentration further if given urea (17). In both the immature infant and the malnourished subject, there is a positive correlation between the urinary concentrating ability and urinary nitrogen excretion. Elevating urea nitrogen excretion either rapidly by urea administration or more slowly by increased protein intake has the same effect (4).

A lack of antidiuretic hormone cannot be implicated as a cause of the concentrating defect (4,14,15,18). Administration of vasopressin to malnourished subjects decreases urine volume, lowers free-water clearance, and increases urine osmolality, indicating that the end-organ response is qualitatively intact. Intravenous nicotine provokes release of endogenous antidiuretic hormone (ADH), indicating the neurohypophysis is responsive. The response after administration of hypertonic saline demonstrates that the osmoreceptor-hypothalamus-posterior pituitary sequence is adequate. Minimal urine osmolality and free-water clearance is normal in protein-energy malnutrition. Free-water reabsorption (i.e., negative free-water clearance) is decreased in malnutrition and increases after protein repletion proportionately greater than the increase in GFR. Hence, the qualitative mechanisms for the renal handling of water appear intact (14).

Other explanations, such as transport of sodium in the loop of Henle, augmented renal blood flow in the vasa recta, and severe potassium depletion, have insufficient support (10,11,14,15). Thus, the best explanation for the concentrating defect still remains a functional abnormality related to the decreased urea concentration in the renal medulla (4).

The renal handling of sodium is also limited in malnutrition. This is immediately evident in the edematous state that may accompany malnutrition. Balance studies in the nonedematous state also show an impaired ability to handle sodium loads in the presence of malnutrition (4,15). The most reasonable explanation rests with hypovolemia, decreased renal plasma flow, and decreased GFR. The low GFR decreases the filtered load of sodium, whereas elevation of hormonal factors increases sodium reabsorption. As with the other abnormal functions, the renal handling of sodium returns to normal following correction of the malnourished state.

Acid excretion is also reduced in malnutrition (19). Metabolic acidosis is not a part of uncomplicated malnutrition, suggesting that endogenous acid production is reduced. Malnourished patients, however, do not have a normal capacity to excrete an acid load, largely due to a decreased capacity to generate titratable acid (1). Nevertheless, malnutrition does not alter the ability to produce an acid urine indicating that the hydrogen ion excretion mechanism is intact (19). The reduced ability to produce titratable acid is due to a decreased availability of intraluminal phosphate buffer. Infusion of phosphate into ammonium chloride–loaded malnourished adults has led to an increase in titratable acidity (20).

NUTRITIONAL EFFECTS ON RENAL MATURATION AND GROWTH

The fetal kidney produces urine at about 12 weeks' gestation. Nephrogenesis continues until 35 to 36 weeks of gestation, followed by continued glomerular and tubular growth postnatally. The factors that control renal growth and determine final renal size are not fully understood. The fetal kidney has little or no excretory requirement, since the placenta effectively maintains the fetal internal milieu even in the presence of bilateral renal agenesis. Therefore, the stimulus for renal growth is probably autonomous and not related to functional demands. In the human, compensatory growth does not occur until after delivery with the first demands of extrauterine life (21). This would suggest that renal growth is related at least in part to functional requirements (22). Nutrition has been one of the more thoroughly investigated factors in the renal growth response.

There is no predetermined size or functional capacity granted to the newborn kidney (21). Demands made on the developing kidney by the nutrients ingested by the infant appear to play a role. Restriction of intake retards renal growth, and starvation abolishes it (23). Conversely, a high-protein diet enhances renal growth (24–28). This appears to be more complex than a simple "work-load" effect since substituting urea for protein in the diet does not stimulate renal growth (29). Although the initial response to unilateral nephrectomy in both the mature and immature animal is hypertrophy, it is only the immature animal that is capable of hyperplasia (30).

Since most energy consumption by the kidney is devoted to the regulation of sodium, it would seem reasonable to implicate sodium as an important stimulus. Supplementing the diet with sodium chloride, however, has not had a consistent effect of renal growth (21). Water could also be an important stimulus, since its regulation constitutes an appreciable part of renal work (21). The combined effect of a balance between sodium and water has not been investigated.

Using compensatory hypertrophy as a model, functional adaptation and growth occur even during periods when the solute load remains essentially unchanged. Diets high in urea or salt fail to produce compensatory hypertrophy. When the ureter of one kidney is diverted into the peritoneal cavity, no compensatory growth occurs in the undiverted kidney which now must perform the effective work load of two kidneys (31). This suggests that a humoral factor could be responsible for compensatory growth quite separate from the solute demand (31). More recently, it has been suggested that hemodynamic changes contribute to compensatory growth (31).

There is strong evidence that the demands created by nutrient intake are related to the alteration of renal vascular resistance in the rapid improvement of renal function during the immediate postnatal period (21,32). Prematures fed a high-protein diet will increase GFR faster than control infants (27). One can produce the same effect in animals with the addition of albumin, globulin, casein, and glycine, but, interestingly enough, not with urea (21). Although high protein intake enhances renal growth and activates the renin angiotensin system, pharmacologic blockade of the angiotensin II receptors does not appear to influence this growth response. Thus, neither whole kidney nor glomerular growth appears dependent on the direct vascular change produced by angiotensin II action (33). It is interesting to note that if the protein content of the diet is too high, one can produce metabolic acidosis, failure to thrive, and irritation to the renal parenchyma as evidenced by urinary casts and proteinuria (34).

The concentrating capacity of the newborn kidney is more limited than that of the adult. Although a part of this may be explained by the incomplete penetration of the immature loop of Henle into the renal medulla (35), an appreciable portion of the limited ability appears related to nutrient intake.

In human infants, who increase urine osmolality and decrease free-water excretion with a high protein intake (36), the maturational increase in concentration capacity can be attributed almost completely to an increase in the urinary urea concentration (37). Thus, the inability to maintain the medullary osmotic gradient is not limited by immaturity alone, but by a decreased availability of osmotically active substances in the medullary interstitium, presumably the result of the profound anabolic state of the infant. In the immature infant there is a good correlation between urinary concentrating capability and urinary nitrogen excretion (36).

Since renal growth and functional maturation seem to be appropriate to the metabolic demands of the infant, and since those demands are related in part to the nutritional intake, the diet appears to be one of the stimuli for renal maturation. This is not to imply that stimulating the system with nutrient intake is necessarily good for the infant. Rather, the apparent poor functional capability of the "immature" kidney may have a nutritional component contributing to its developmental physiologic changes. Indeed, the kidney, at term, appears able to perform qualitatively all functions asked of it (21,22). Functional demands, dictated by nutrient intake, may be part of the reason a premature infant, by the time he reaches "term" weight, has renal function that exceeds the function of the term infant.

The nutritional elements that stimulate maturation are only partially apparent, however. It is also unclear whether renal functional growth is predetermined or responds to continuing metabolic challenges that imperceptibly exceed an infant's current functional capabilities. Proprietary formulas with three times the sodium load and half again as much protein as human milk challenge but do not overwhelm the normal newborn infant. The normal infant is capable of defending against a sodium load ten times that of human milk. Since nutrient intake is probably an important factor for renal growth and functional maturation, an overzealous elimination of nutrient and solutes from the infant diet could conceivably delay the attainment of maximal functional capacity.

NUTRITIONAL ISSUES IN GLOMERULAR DAMAGE

The nephrotic syndrome is a prime example of glomerular damage, accompanied by normal or increased glomerular filtration (38). It is characterized by hyperlipidemia, anasarca, and avid salt retention. Although fluid restriction is often prescribed during periods of anasarca, the major contributor to thirst and weight gain in these children is related to the sodium intake. Each positive balance of 3 g of salt, for example, results in the retention of 1 kg of fluid as edema. Sodium restriction may be the only required limitation, with sodium intake often less than 0.5 mEq/kg/day (38).

With anasarca, the children develop anorexia (38), possibly because taste function is diminished (39). Dietary intake levels appropriate to the child's height are often difficult to achieve. However, there is no evidence that dietary supplements help the patient or alter the course of the disease (38). Nitrogen retention in experimental nephrotic animals appears related to a reduced amino acid oxidation and a decrease in urinary urea nitrogen excretion. Proteinuria appears to be the stimulus that decreases the amino acid oxidation (40). Treatment with prednisone usually reverses anorexia, particularly with resolution of anasarca (38).

There are no data to document clinical improvement from a high protein intake (38). Evidence in animals, in fact, suggests benefit from a low protein intake (41), whereas a sustained high protein intake might even contribute to further glomerular damage (6,42). Diets that are high in protein increase the glomerular filtration rate (7,8,43–46), in both normal humans and experimental animals. Conversely, during periods of starvation the rates of glomerular filtration, renal plasma flow, and urine flow decrease to the sustained low levels present during protein-energy malnutrition (4,9). The mediator of these protein-related changes in renal hemodynamics and filtration may be the liver hormone, glomerulopressin, a glucuronide whose release is stimulated by the hepatic uptake of amino acids (47,48).

A dietary enhancement of renal functional capacity in glomerular disease is an attractive theory. However, the suggestion that diet-related, sustained glomerular hypertension might accelerate or perpetuate glomerular damage limits enthusiasm (42). Progressive glomerulosclerosis in experimental animals can be retarded by limiting the amount of food available or the frequency of the feedings (49,50). Conversely, glomerular damage is hastened by hyperphagia (51–53). Reports that progression to uremia can be slowed through a restriction of protein intake is consistent with the animal data (54,55).

The therapeutic implications in the treatment of infants and children with glomerular diseases is unclear. Reduction, rather than encouragement, of protein intake early in the course of the nephrotic syndrome may be appropriate. The reduction in proteinuria induced by a low-protein diet is also accompanied by a reduction in glomerular filtration rates. Converting enzyme inhibition, together with a low-protein diet, decreases proteinuria still further while returning GFR toward normal (56). Since the proteinuria in children approximates 2 g/M^2/day, the major reason for hypoproteinemia is not the urinary losses, but rather alterations in protein metabolism (38). It is unlikely that a synthetic defect can be reversed by merely increasing intake. A protein intake that approximates those levels recommended for normal growth might be more appropriate (38). For most children in the United States, this would represent a reduction in protein intake (57). It is not yet clear, however, that such restriction is beneficial to the patient or to the course of glomerular diseases.

NUTRITIONAL ISSUES IN ACUTE RENAL INSUFFICIENCY

A sudden loss of renal function produces profound electrolyte and metabolic disturbances resulting in fluid retention, acidosis, hyperkalemia, hyperphosphatemia, nitrogen retention, hypocalcemia, and hyperuricemia, often at a rate that exceeds the body's ability to compensate (58). Additionally, acute renal insufficiency, itself catastrophic, often occurs in concert with primary medical or surgical conditions that are themselves potentially fatal (58,59). The net effect is a hypercatabolic state in which attempts at repair are restricted by both the primary illness and the renal capacity to regulate and excrete. Therefore, the provision of adequate and appropriate nutrition is a fundamental part of the nondialytic therapy of acute renal failure, regardless of the etiology.

For many patients, enteral nutrition is not possible. Hope that a rapid resolution of the renal failure will occur before significant malnutrition supervenes has been a common strategy. However, for the child with a severe primary illness compounded by undernutrition and hypercatabolism, such temporization is most often counterproductive.

There are several reasons why vigorous attention to nutrition should be a central element in the management of acute renal failure. Starvation contributes to catabolism, which increases the endogenous load of water, potassium, nitrogen, phosphorus, and acid (58). In humans with postoperative acute renal failure, improved nutrition has reportedly decreased mortality, improved nitrogen metabolism, and accelerated recovery (60–62). In acute uremia, urea generation, as a reflection of net protein catabolism, has been reported to be 45% higher, and the amount of nitrogen required to produce neutral nitrogen balance is 37% higher, than in stable uremic patients undergoing chronic hemodialysis (63).

The popularity of parenteral nutrition in the management of these patients, with an emphasis on amino acids (64,65), is not evidence for the superiority of either the parenteral route or the nitrogen source. It does recognize, however, that the catabolic state deserves more direct attention than is provided by supportive care alone. Generally, enteral nutrition is preferred, either by oral intake or gastric tube, since such feedings can provide more nutrients with less fluid, are less costly, and present fewer complications. Enteral feedings through a percutaneously placed gastrostomy tube make the enteral route available to even the severely ill or obtunded child (66).

The ultimate goal of therapy is to provide sufficient nutrients to restrain the catabolic response and to hasten renal recovery, all within the restrictions demanded by limited renal capacity. Dialysis is an adjunct designed to correct fluid and electrolyte imbalances, remove nitrogenous excesses, and stabilize the extracellular milieu. The inadequacy of dialysis alone is demonstrated by the continued high mortality and morbidity in children with acute renal failure (58,59,67,68).

Traditional carbohydrate alone has been given as a "protein-sparing" energy source (69). Recent evidence suggests that the addition of essential amino acids to dextrose reduces the rise of blood urea, improves wound healing, and lessens hyperkalemia and hyperphosphatemia, even when nitrogen balance remains negative (60–62,70–73). An improvement in the rate of recovery and/or survival has not been consistently observed, however (71–75).

The role of energy intake has been variably investigated. It does not appear that the energy requirements are increased by acute renal insufficiency alone; total energy requirements seem more dependent on the primary disease process. Understandably, when available energy is not sufficient to meet the demand created by hypercatabolism, any nitrogen source, endogenous or exogenous, will become a fuel, adding to the azotemia. Investigations in undernourished anuric children found that raising the energy intake from 20 to 70 Cal/kg/day improved nitrogen balance; adding essential amino acids (including histidine and arginine in some patients) to the infusate produced a neutral or slightly positive balance (76). Carbohydrate may be a better energy source than lipid in the hypercatabolic patient (77). Effective therapy may require even larger amounts of protein and energy than traditionally prescribed, despite an effect on urea generation and dialysis requirements (63,65,73,74,78). In adults, it has been suggested that neutral nitrogen balance is approached when energy intake is above 40 or 50 Cal/kg/day, and nitrogen intake, as essential and nonessential amino acids, is as high as 1 g/kg/day (63,74,79). In children, energy intake in excess of 70 Cal/kg/day, and amino acid intake above 2 g/kg/day may be necessary (76).

Unrestrained escalation of energy and amino acid intake to overcome metabolic defects is to be avoided, particularly when essential amino acids are the sole nitrogen source. First, it is unclear that acutely uremic and catabolic infants can adequately synthesize nonessential amino acids from essential amino acids. It is also known that both histidine and arginine behave as essential amino acids in the uremic individual; the behavior of other amino acids is ill-defined (80,81). In addition, abnormal shifts in serum levels of specific amino acids have suggested that synthesis is aberrant in uremia (82). Finally, the elevated plasma ammonia and methionine concentrations that occur after intravenous treatment with large quantities of essential amino acids are completely corrected by an isocaloric isonitrogenous combination of essential and nonessential amino acids (83).

The optimal composition for parenteral amino acid solutions has not been defined, despite the availability of commercial products specifically marketed for renal failure therapy (84,85). Although some data suggest that the keto analogues of essential amino acids effectively spare nitrogen in uremia, data for acute renal failure is sparse and in children is virtually nonexistent (86–88).

Dialysis itself is a catabolic event. Hemodialysis is associated with a loss of both amino acids and glucose, whereas peritoneal dialysis results in large losses of protein and amino acids (89–92). However, both dialytic modalities relieve some of the restrictions placed on fluid, electrolyte, and nitrogen intake, and peritoneal dialysis, because of the absorption of glucose across the peritoneal membrane, adds to energy intake (89–92). The nitrogen losses, in particular, can be large and, thus, influence considerably decisions made about nutritional requirements.

Very few data are available concerning enteral nutrition in acute renal failure. The traditional prescription of 0.5 g/kg/day of "high biologic value" protein, is clearly inadequate (93). A minimum of 20 to 40 Cal/kg/day is needed to minimize tissue breakdown, and as much as 60% of the usual daily requirement for age group may be necessary to thwart net protein catabolism (58,76). When energy intake is adequate, 1 to 1.5 g/kg/day of protein may be required to attain neutral or positive protein balance (58,76).

NUTRITIONAL ISSUES IN CHRONIC RENAL INSUFFICIENCY

Few studies in children have addressed the possibility that diet directly influences the progression of chronic renal disease. Nevertheless, a known relationship exists between nutrient intake and the progressive loss of renal function (94,95). When there is an insufficient number of functioning nephrons, remaining nephrons can develop segmental sclerosis even in pure congenital renal hypoplasia. Although constituents of the diet have been incriminated (42,96–98), which components contribute to this effect is not clear. Experimental evidence has implicated protein, carbohydrate, phosphorus, and sodium.

Protein intake has been the most widely studied nutrient in renal disease in animals (99–103). In rats with renal damage created by subtotal nephrectomy, mortality increased with the protein content of the diet, and was greater with casein than with an equal amount of mixed animal-vegetable protein (104). Using isocaloric diets, the cumulative survival of animals with renal insufficiency decreases as the protein content of the diet increases; a protein content above 14 g per 100-g diet results in anorexia, poor growth, and an accelerated deterioration of renal function (105–107). In the subtotally nephrectomized rat, the progression of renal death induced by a high-protein diet appears to be prevented by parathyroidectomy.

Several laboratory studies have suggested a relationship between phosphorus intake and the progression of renal insufficiency (12,97,108). Others, however, have proposed that the lower mortality was linked to a reduction in total nutrient intake rather than just to the amount of phosphorus ingested (108). Although a role for phosphorus cannot be completely excluded, most studies suggest it is a minor one.

In some human adult studies, dietary protein and/or phosphate restriction have been reported to retard progression to renal failure (55,109–114), although the results have not been consistent (115–117). Children on unrestricted diets progress to end-stage renal insufficiency in 16 months, whereas in those adhering to a restricted diet, end-stage disease was delayed for 5 to 11 years (110). Other adult studies have also described a reduction in the rate of progression with protein/phosphorus restriction, often with amino acid or keto acid supplementation (54,55,111–114). These studies imply that dietary management might postpone dialytic therapy for those with moderate renal insufficiency.

A few studies have implicated carbohydrates (103,118). Nonetheless, even though carbohydrate intake can apparently adversely influence the renal parenchyma, the influence of severe hypertension cannot be excluded in studies done so far (118).

Sodium has also been thought to influence renal damage. The direct effect of sodium intake on the deterioration of renal function, however, has not been wholly explored (100,119). There is some indication that the damaging effects of sodium supplementation are more pronounced than the putative protective effects of sodium restriction (120).

How dietary changes produce or prevent nephron damage is not completely clear. A loss of renal mass provokes both a physical and a functional nephron hypertrophy (121). Each remaining glomerulus, then, has increased filtration, plasma flow, and transcapillary pressure (42,122). These are the same changes that normally result in the rapid improvement in glomerular filtration and renal plasma flow seen in the normal newborn period (32). Such adaptive phenomena necessary to increase glomerular filtration could lead to progressive destruction of the renal parenchyma. Theoretically, lowering the amount of protein, phosphate, or salt in the diet should reduce the filtered solute load, or change the glomerular hemodynamics to protect the nephron.

Regardless of the mechanisms involved, the dietary prescription for the child with moderate renal insufficiency must satisfy competing goals. In experimental animals, for example, maximal preservation of renal function through protein restriction is not compatible with either optimal growth or a satisfactory nutritional status (106). The microvascular hemodynamic effects noted in protein malnutrition are qualitatively and quantitatively similar to that seen in low-protein-fed, renal-ablated animals (6,9). The preservation of renal function at the expense of the entire child is of concern since this was an unsuccessful, though common, practice before dialytic therapy became widespread. However, it does seem prudent to avoid unnecessary excesses of protein, carbohydrate, phosphorus, and salt. This is particularly important in countries, such as the United States, where the spontaneous intake is generally in excess of the recommended daily allowances (57).

Appetite is generally reduced very early in chronic renal insufficiency. In this light, energy supplementation must be considered with caution, since even carbohydrates per se have been implicated in progressive renal damage (102,118).

Although a reduction in sodium intake may appear reasonable, many renal injuries are associated with an obligatory sodium chloride loss (123). Salt depletion is a well-known reason for a sudden deterioration of renal function in patients with mild renal insufficiency. Conversely, high salt usage produces positive sodium balance accompanied by fluid retention, edema, hypertension, and reduced renal function. Generally, families must be counseled to reduce salt intake, adjusting to a body weight that corresponds to the lowest serum creatinine. It is unusual for children with mild renal insufficiency to require more than 2 mEq/kg/day of sodium (124,125).

Two studies showed that the most efficient nitrogen retention occurred when energy intake ranged between 6 and 11.9 Cal/cm of height, and protein intake represented 5% to 7% of the total calories. When protein intake was above 0.15 g/cm, the ingested nitrogen appeared to be converted almost entirely to urea (125,126). There is little additional research on this topic.

Potassium retention is generally not a problem until glomerular filtration is less than 5% of normal. A sudden shift in potassium availability, either through diet or from acidosis or catabolism, can rapidly overwhelm the kidneys' capacity to excrete potassium. Elimination of high potassium-containing fruits and vegetables may be required to control serum potassium levels. Usually, restriction need not be beyond 1 mEq/kg/day (125,126).

Abnormalities of bone mineral metabolism can appear with only moderate evidence of chronic renal insufficiency (127,128). Likewise, a modest reduction in the glomerular filtration rate can be associated with significantly lower levels of 1,25-vitamin D_3 (129). Hyperphosphatemia may not occur until abnormalities of bone mineral metabolism are quite advanced (128). Restriction of high phosphorus-containing foods, coupled with aluminum hydroxide or calcium carbonate to inhibit phosphorus absorption, is a most important dietary manipulation early in the development of impaired excretory function (125,126).

NUTRITIONAL ASPECTS OF CHRONIC RENAL FAILURE

The extent of nutritional manipulation in end-stage renal failure is dictated by the degree, not the etiology, of the renal insufficiency. At this stage of disease, optimal nutritional management cannot reverse metabolic abnormalities nor restore body composition to normal. The goal of therapy is to maintain adequate nutrition within the margins imposed by limited renal excretory and regulatory capacity.

The emergence of multiple therapeutic modalities, including prolonged conservative management, hemodialysis, peritoneal dialysis (both intermittent and continuous), and transplantation, have broadened and complicated nutritional management (89,130,131). Elements that must be restricted at one point in therapy might require supplementation during a subsequent phase. The management of the child with cachexia is very different from the child with equal renal functional deterioration, who has a normal or elevated weight-for-height. The nutritional needs during continuous peritoneal dialysis differ considerably from those during intermittent hemodialysis. Thus, a routine "renal failure" diet, applicable to all situations, does not exist. Nutritional management must be individualized to the emotional, metabolic, and functional limitations of each child and adjusted during each therapeutic phase (125,132).

It makes intuitive sense that the teleologically advantageous response, as uremia progresses, is to reduce the intake of fluid and solute in order to avoid the retention of toxic metabolic products, a spontaneously poor dietary intake, not surprisingly, in children with end-stage disease (125,132). Undernutrition is the obvious end point of this adaptive response, so the many similarities between protein-energy malnutrition and the uremic state are to be expected (125,132) (Table 1).

Furthermore, if exogenous nutrients decrease below the actual metabolic requirements, endogenous catabolism must increase. This leads to an increase in the endogenous production of excretable toxins and their associated metabolic abnormalities. Thus, a point is reached where further restriction of protein and energy intake

TABLE 1. *Similarities between renal insufficiency and protein-energy malnutrition*

	Uremia	Protein-energy malnutrition
Cell mass	↓	↓
ECF	↑	↑
TBW	↑	↑
Body sodium	↑	↑
Body fat	↓	↓
Fat-free solids	↓	↓
Lean body mass	↓	↓
Growth hormone	↑	↑
Somatomedin	↓	↓
Cortisol	↑	↑
Glucose intolerance	+	+
Insulin	↑	↓
Serum zinc	↓	↓
Serum copper	↓	↓
Serum protein	↓	↓
Serum amino acids	↓	↓
Essential/nonessential amino acids	↓	↓
Valine/glycine	↓	↓

ECF, extracellular fluid; TBW, total body water; ↓, parameter decreased; ↑, parameter increased; +, parameter present.

becomes totally self-defeating; that "cachexia" is commonly listed as a contributing cause of death in uremia is not unexpected in this light (133).

Children on hemodialysis, with caloric intakes below 67% of the recommended daily allowances, have been reported to grow at a rate of 30% of normal, whereas those with higher intakes grow at 117% of normal (134). Similar improvement in growth rates has been noted when energy supplements are used (135). Energy supplementation, however, does not always improve the growth rate and may not even increase total energy intake (136). A consistent relationship between caloric intake and altered growth in renal failure has not been found (135–138).

Animal data also suggest that the altered intake produced by renal insufficiency may be related to growth failure (139,140). Thus, the growth alteration could be completely explained on the basis of decreased energy intake.

A decreased weight gain per ingested calorie in uremic animals suggests an inefficiency in the utilization of nutrient intake, which could also influence energy needs (139,140). However, oxygen consumption corrected for weight was no different in uremic animals than in normal animals, which suggests that inefficiency per se is not a major component. Other studies have failed to show a consistent relationship between calorie deficit and growth in renal insufficiency (136,138,141). Other authors have also found little evidence for malnutrition; in fact, the converse was more frequent (137). Nevertheless, the suggestion that renal insufficiency may lead to increased energy requirements requires further investigation.

Caloric intake can remain inadequate even when families receive considerable nutritional counseling. Extensive evaluation of patients with established end-stage renal disease on stable hemodialysis demonstrated an average daily intake of only 51 cal/kg/day (142). Eighty-five percent had energy intakes below the 50th percentile for height age and 31% had intakes less than the 10th percentile (142). Energy intake was clearly less than optimal and considerably less than needed for catch-up growth. Other investigators with established interests in nutrition have regularly commented on the poor results of encouraging adequate energy intake in these children (135,141,143).

When evaluated by weight-for-height or height-for-age criteria, 54% of patients had an appropriate weight-for-height as compared to 65% of their siblings. Conversely, 38% of the uremic patients had an appropriate height-for-age as compared to 76% in the control group. This suggests that stature is affected more than weight in uremic children, which differs from results with experimental rats (139,140).

Even though most studies have shown growth failure (134–136,142), not all have shown evidence of undernutrition, and some have even shown a weight that was actually higher than expected for the height (125,137,138,143). A low weight-for-height seems more frequent in older children with acquired disease, whereas normal weight-for-height is more probable in those with anomalies, long-term renal insufficiency, and a long history of poor growth (138,142). The height deficit, therefore, seems more related to the duration of the disease than the current extent of nutritional deficit (137,138,142).

Once malnutrition is established, the nutrient demands for repair are generally quite high in both normal and uremic children. It is not uncommon, for example, for normal children recovering from malnutrition to need energy intakes considerably above resting requirements; some of these children may spontaneously take more than 200 Cal/kg/day (144,145). Children with chronic uremia do not even approach such levels of intake despite appropriate incentives and energy supplementation (134,135,142).

Why uremic children fail to attain a dietary intake sufficient for "compensatory" repair is not totally known. Spontaneously, these children do seem to eat enough to maintain their current body mass, since weight-for-height is often normal (135,142,146). It can be inferred that some signal controls hunger in those children whose renal function is barely enough to sustain life. However, the factors that restrain appetite are not yet defined.

Altered ability to taste is relatively common in uremia (147–151). Taste acuity for one or more of the four primary tastes was abnormal in children receiving chronic hemodialysis therapy (147). Elevated thresholds to sweet (sucrose) and sour (HCL) were present in half of the children, often when the ability to taste bitter (urea) was intact (147). Such dysgeusia could significantly alter food preferences. Taste acuity improved immediately postdialysis, accompanied by a subjective increase in hunger and an increased food intake (147). The improvement was not sustained between dialyses, however (147). This rapid, repetitive, and unsustained recovery suggests that the taste abnormality in renal failure is functional and related to the control of uremia. Improved taste perception has followed zinc supplementation in some (150), but not all (151), children with chronic renal failure. Although plasma zinc levels are often reduced in uremic children, it is not clear that a true deficit exists (152).

The quantitative requirements of energy and protein for the children with chronic renal failure are still unclear. Standards derived from metabolically normal children with normal body composition, normal activity, and normal growth may not be applicable to children with renal failure (124,134,141,143,153,154). Growth, or its arrest, may not be an appropriate outcome variable (136–138); growth changes are not an irrefutable function of energy or protein intake (136–138), and supplementation does not necessarily repair body muscle mass (135).

Nonetheless, measurement of other outcome variables may be just as insensitive. For example, body weight can be maintained or even increased in the presence of negative nitrogen balance (155,156), whereas efficient use of nitrogen need not correlate with net nitrogen balance (155–157). Serum albumin levels may remain low in peritoneally dialyzed children despite large protein intakes (158). Unfortunately, in many studies there has been limited effort to control for those metabolic variables introduced by dialytic therapy or uremia itself (130).

Few studies have attempted to measure directly the actual needs of uremic children using outcome measurements other than growth. Conley et al. (159), using N15-lysine enrichment, noticed a decreased protein flux, which reverted toward normal with dialysis, suggesting a role for abnormal excretion. However, similar improvement was produced in both the dialyzed and nondialyzed children by increasing both the energy and nitrogen intake, suggesting an equally important role for nutrition (159). The three patients in their study whose protein flux approached that of normal children had average daily intakes of 48 Cal/kg and 2.2 g/kg of protein (159).

Some have proposed that nondialyzed uremic children receive energy intakes above 70% of the recommended daily allowances for their height, and 2 g/100

Cal of protein (134,141,160). Others have suggested that calorie intake vary from 42 to 120 Cal/kg, depending upon age and sex, and that protein intake vary from 0.6 to 1.7 g/kg, likewise depending on age and sex (161,162). One source has advocated that the diet include 75% of the calories as carbohydrate, 20% as fat, and only 5% as protein (161). Another has noted that growth is retarded at energy intakes below 80% of the recommended daily allowances (141).

The type of dialytic therapy influences the focus for nutritional management, although the general principles are similar for all modes of therapy. Glucose is absorbed during peritoneal dialysis, whereas glucose uptake during hemodialysis is minimal, even when glucose is added to the dialysate (89–92). Protein and amino acid losses are significant with both forms of dialysis and inversely proportional to body weight (163,165).

Using kinetically determined urea appearance in hemodialyzed children (166), Grupe et al. (142,167–169) found a linear relationship between protein balance and nutrient intake, with neutral protein balance occurring at 10 Cal and 0.3 g protein per centimeter of height per day (142), which is a slope similar to that noted in normal adults on marginal protein intakes (155,156). The net protein catabolic rate diminished as protein balance increased, suggesting that the production of positive protein balance, despite increasing protein intake, reduced urea generation when protein represented 12% of the total energy intake (142). Furthermore, for any given protein intake, the net protein catabolic rate was uniformly lower in those children in positive protein balance (142,169). Thus, these patients did not require additional hemodialysis despite their higher protein intake (142,169). In addition, the amount of energy required to attain neutral balance when protein intake was inadequate could be as much as 20% higher than when protein intakes above 0.3 g/cm/day were given (162,169). This apparent requirement for additional energy could conceivably exceed the appetite of any uremic children.

These data offer more indication that severe protein restriction may be counterproductive in advance renal failure. Particularly during renourishment, these children may require a protein intake of at least 8% to 10% of the total caloric intake. Children on hemodialysis probably require relatively normal protein-to-energy ratios and little, if any, protein restriction when energy levels are maintained (142). Energy intakes above 12 Cal/cm/day and protein intakes approximating 12% of the total energy seem to produce positive protein balance (142), improved protein flux (159), and increased lean body mass (162).

The nutritional requirements during peritoneal dialysis are not completely determined. Salusky et al. (131,170) found that children treated with continuous ambulatory peritoneal dialysis (CAPD) had a caloric intake that averaged 75% of the recommended daily allowance (RDA) for height. Total calories acquired by the absorption of glucose from the peritoneal dialysate amounted to 8 Cal/kg/day. The protein intake was between 100% and 150% of RDA but protein losses in the dialysate were not subtracted and protein balance was not determined (131,170). In a parallel study by Baum et al. (89), total caloric intake averaged 60 Cal/kg/day including 7.5 Cal/kg/day from absorption of dialysate glucose; the total energy intake was 79% of the RDA for height. Protein intake averaged 2.0 g/kg/day, from which 0.16 g/kg/day of protein was lost in the dialysate (89). Although both of these studies describe only the spontaneous dietary intake of these children, without any measure of actual needs, positive nitrogen balance has been reported in children undergoing CAPD (171), with neutral balance attained when dietary protein intake approaches 75% RDA and caloric intake is 35% RDA (172).

When aggressive nutritional management was added to intensive peritoneal dialysis, half of the treated children grew. Although the mean height standard deviation score for the group did not change significantly, serum albumin levels remained low and several infants became obese (158). Another report documented efficient nitrogen utilization, positive nitrogen balance, and improvements in height, weight, and midarm muscle circumference over a 14-month period from an average caloric intake of 93 Cal/kg/day, where protein represented 8% of the total energy (173a). Other suggestions for diet goals have ranged as high as 3.5 to 4.0 g/kg/day for protein, with energy intakes above 75% of the RDA for height (117,173).

The absorption of carbohydrate from the peritoneal dialysate, combined with significant protein losses through the peritoneal cavity (89–91,117,164,165), contributes to the problem of obesity, particularly when the additional energy serves to decrease the spontaneous ingestion of conventional foods (89,125) and/or a lower protein-to-energy ratio. High energy relative to protein produces an increase in fat deposition (156). Whatever lean mass accumulates appears to be related to the support of the increased fat mass. An increase predominantly in energy intake would be expected to replete only one-fourth of the lean mass lost during periods of undernutrition (156). Restoration of the major portion of the loss, therefore, requires changes in nitrogen intake independent of energy. Obesity is a common occurrence in peritoneally dialyzed children (125). Even with careful nutritional management, triceps skin-fold thickness often increases without a significant change in either midarm circumference or midarm muscle circumference. Obesity does not seem to be a valid goal in the therapy of uremic children. Although some have suggested that this propensity toward obesity is evidence of altered intermediary metabolism, it seems more likely to be the result of relative energy excess, similar to that noted in normal subjects (156).

How one maintains appropriate levels of energy and protein intake is a formidable challenge in children on dialysis. Supplements may improve nutrition for the undernourished child whose intake is inadequate (124). When nutritional intake is already adequate and the weight is appropriate for the height, energy supplementation alone may be deleterious by inciting a reduction in the spontaneous intake of all foods, especially protein (175). Carbohydrate supplements additionally may aggravate hypertriglyceridemia and lead to obesity without an increase in lean mass or linear growth (124,175). Although many authors advocate high-quality protein in the diet, the importance of the "biologic value" has not been established in uremia. For children especially, the palatability of the diet may be at least as important as the content (152,174–177).

The tolerance of the uremic patient for starvation appears poor. For example, nitrogen balance rapidly regresses during stress in uremic adults, whereas rats with renal insufficiency have an exaggerated catabolic response between meals (178). This suggests that frequent or even continuous feedings have a considered place in management. Success with continuous nasogastric feedings in both adults and children may relate as much to the avoidance of prolonged fast as to the increase in total intake (143,179,180).

An increasing number of studies have explored the value of synthetic diets in infants and children (76,83,87,88,146,153,177). The child with chronic renal failure can utilize both essential and complete amino acid mixtures (83). Although urea generation can be higher when a complete amino acid mixture is administered, nitrogen retention is also greater, producing a more positive nitrogen balance than when essential amino acids alone are used (83). Using short-term changes in weight, complete amino acid mixtures appear better utilized than their keto acid analogues. However, a longer study in undialyzed children found significant increases in growth velocity, upper arm circumference, cell mass, serum transferrin, and plasma calcium in children maintained on a protein-restricted diet supplemented with essential and calcium keto acids over a 0.4 to 1 year treatment period (146). The addition of ketoisocaproic acid, the analogue of leucine, had no demonstrable effect on growth (125).

No study has documented that these contrived diets offer more than a theoretical advantage over an appropriately designed conventional diet (153,175–177,181). Concern over long-term toxicity, even with newly formulated diets, demand continued caution in these uremic children (82,83,87,112,146). With few exceptions, the promise of good results is still dampened by severe metabolic complications and/or poor patient compliance (82,83,153,177,180).

For some children the maintenance of adequate nutrition may require an earlier institution of dialysis than might otherwise occur if protein were severely restricted. Even though synthetic diets have maintained uremic adults for extended periods (97), no advantage to this approach has been claimed for children. Excess energy alone is generally an inefficient way to promote nitrogen sparing and a poor way to promote the replenishment of lean body mass (155,156,174). Thus, early initiation of dialysis may have individual benefits, particularly in the anorectic child (175).

It is difficult to persuade children to remain on a low-protein diet with or without synthetic nutritional supplements (143,153). With the exception of one study (146), such diets have been successful only via nasogastric or parenteral feedings (76,143,179,180). No study has shown that the form or quality of any nutrient source has a demonstrated advantage over a properly designed conventional diet. For many children, standard diets with a normal protein-to-energy ratio seem more palatable and, therefore, more likely to maintain adequate nutrition over the longer term (136,142,159,163). Ultimately, however, success is usually predicated on a patient, supportive team willing to recognize each child's individuality. Simply prescribing a diet for the child in renal failure, no matter how potentially therapeutic, is the least effective therapy of all (132).

REFERENCES

1. Alleyne GAO. The effect of severe protein-calorie malnutrition on the renal function of Jamaican children. *Pediatrics* 1967;39:400.
2. Gordillo G, et al. Intracellular composition and homeostatic mechanisms in severe chronic infantile malnutrition: III. Renal adjustments. *Pediatrics* 1957;20:303.
3. Kerpel-Fronius E, Varga F, Ken K, Vonoczky J. The relationship between circulation and kidney function in infantile dehydration and malnutrition. *Acta Med Acad Sci Hung* 1954;5:27.
4. Klahr S, Alleyne GAO. Effects of chronic protein-calorie malnutrition on the kidney. *Kidney Int* 1973;3:129.
5. Klahr S, Tripathy K. Evaluation of renal function in malnutrition. *Arch Intern Med* 1966;118:323.
6. Brenner BM, Meyer TW, Hostetter TH. Dietary protein intake and the progressive nature of kidney disease. *N Engl J Med* 1982;307:652.
7. Pullman TN, Alving AS, Dern RJ, Lansdowne M. The influence of dietary protein intake on specific renal function in normal man. *J Lab Clin Med* 1954;44:320.
8. Sargent F, Johnson RE. The effects of diet on renal function in healthy men. *Am J Clin Nutr* 1956;4:466.
9. Ichikawa I, et al. Mechanism of reduced glomerular filtration rate in chronic malnutrition. *J Clin Invest* 1980;65:982.
10. Fohlin L. Body composition, cardiovascular and renal function in adolescent patients with anorexia nervosa. *Acta Paediatr Scand Suppl* 1977;6:268.
11. Aperia A, Broberger O, Fohlin L. Renal function in anorexia nervosa. *Acta Paediatr Scand* 1978;67:219.
12. Ibels LS, Alfrey AC, Haut L, Huffer WE. Preservation of function

in experimental renal disease by dietary restriction of phosphate. *N Engl J Med* 1978;298:122.
13. McCance RA, Crowne RS, Hall TS. The effect of malnutrition and food habits on the concentration power of the kidney. *Clin Sci* 1969;37:471.
14. Klahr S, et al. On the nature of the renal concentrating defect in malnutrition. *Am J Med* 1967;43:84.
15. Zilleruelo G, Strauss J. Water and electrolytes in malnourished and uremic children. In: Strauss J, ed. *Pediatric nephrology.* New York: Plenum Press, 1981;245.
16. Epstein FH, Kleeman CR, Pursel S, Hendriks A. The effect of feeding protein and urea on the renal concentrating process. *J Clin Invest* 1957;36:635.
17. Crawford JD, Coyle AP, Probst JH. Service of urea in renal water conservation. *Am J Physiol* 1959;196:545.
18. Macaron C, Schneider G, Ertel NH. The starved kidney: a defect in renal concentrating ability. *Metabolism* 1975;24:457.
19. Smith R. Urinary acidification defect in chronic infantile malnutrition. *Lancet* 1959;1:764.
20. Klahr S, Tripathy K, Lotero H. Renal regulation of acid base balance in malnourished man. *Am J Med* 1970;48:325.
21. Nash MA, Edelmann CM. The developing kidney: immature function or inappropriate standard? *Nephron* 1973;11:71.
22. Arant BS. Developmental patterns of renal functional maturation compared in the human neonate. *J Pediatr* 1978;92:705.
23. Goldman JK. Compensatory renal hypertrophy in fasted and fasted-refed rats. *Proc Soc Exp Biol Med* 1971;138:589.
24. Halliburton IW, Thomson RY. Chemical aspects of compensatory renal hypertrophy. *Cancer Res* 1965;25:1882.
25. MacKay LL, MacKay EM, Addis T. Do high protein diets increase weight of kidney because they increase nitrogen excretion? *Proc Soc Exp Biol Med* 1927;24:336.
26. MacKay EM, MacKay LL, Addis T. Factors which determine renal weight: V. The protein intake. *Am J Physiol* 1928;86:459.
27. Edelmann CM Jr, Wolfish NM. Dietary influence on renal maturation in premature infants. *Pediatr Res* 1968;2:421.
28. Cochran ST, Pagani JJ, Barbaric ZL. Nephromegaly in hyperalimentation. *Radiology* 1979;130:603.
29. MacKay LL, MacKay EM, Addis T. Influence of age on degree of renal hypertrophy produced by high protein diets. *Proc Soc Exp Biol Med* 1927;24:335.
30. Karp R, Brasel JA, Winick M. Compensatory kidney growth after uninephrectomy in adult and infant rats. *Am J Dis Child* 1971;121:186.
31. Effmann EL, Ablow RC, Siegel NJ. Renal growth. *Radiol Clin North Am* 1977;15:3.
32. Ichikawa I, Maddox DA, Brenner BM. Maturational development of glomerular ultrafiltration in the rat. *Am J Physiol* 1979;236:F465.
33. Smith LJ, Rosenberg ME, Hostetter TH. Effect of angiotensin II blockade on dietary protein induced renal growth. *J Am Soc Nephrol* 1991;2:445.
34. McCann ML, Schwartz R. The effects of milk solutes on urinary cast excretion in premature infants. *Pediatrics* 1966;38:555.
35. Edwards BR, et al. Postnatal development of urinary concentrating ability in rats. In: Spitzer A, ed. *The kidney during development, morphology and function.* Paris: Mason, 1982;233.
36. Edelmann CM Jr, Barnett HL, Troupkou V. Renal concentrating mechanisms in new born infants. Effect of dietary protein and water content, role of urea and responsiveness to antidiuretic hormone. *J Clin Invest* 1960;39:1062.
37. Spitzer A. Renal physiology and functional development. In: Edelmann CM Jr, Ed. *Pediatric kidney disease.* Boston: Little, Brown, 1978;25.
38. Grupe WE. Primary nephrotic syndrome in childhood. *Adv Pediatr* 1979;26:163.
39. Mahajan S, Speck J, Varghese G, Abu-Hamdan D, Migdal S, Briggs W, Prasad A, McDonald F. Zinc metabolism in nephrotic syndrome. *Kidney Int* 1983;23:129.
40. Choi E-J, May RC, Bailey J, Masud T, Dixon A, Maroni BJ. The effect of nephrotic syndrome on whole body protein turnover and nitrogen balance. *J Am Soc Nephrol* 1991;2:676.
41. Farr LE, Smadel JE. The effect of dietary protein on the course of nephrotoxic nephritis. *J Exp Med* 1939;70:615.
42. Hostetter TH, Olson JL, Rennke HG, et al. Hyperfiltration in remnant nephrons: a potential adverse response to renal ablation. *Am J Physiol* 1981;241:F85.
43. Hiatt EP, Hiatt RB. The effect of food on the glomerular filtration rate and renal blood flow in the harbor seal (Phoco Vitulina L.). *J Cell Comp Physiol* 1942;19:221.
44. Schoolwerth AG, Sandler RS, Hoffman PM, Klahr S. Effects of nephron reduction and dietary protein content on renal ammoniagenesis in the rat. *Kidney Int* 1975;7:397.
45. O'Connor WJ, Summerill RA. The effect of a meal of meat on glomerular filtration rate in dogs at normal urine flows. *J Physiol* 1976;256:81.
46. Bosch JP, Saccagi A, Lauer A, Belledonne M, Glabman S. Effect of diet on glomerular filtration rate: functional reserve of the normal kidney. *Kidney Int* 1983;23:118.
47. Alvestrand A, Bergstrom J. Glomerular hyperfiltration after protein ingestion, during glucagon infusion, and in insulin-dependent diabetes is induced by a liver hormone: deficient production of this hormone in hepatic failure causes hepatorenal syndrome. *Lancet* 1984;1:195.
48. Uranga J. Effect of glomerulopressin, oxytocin and norepinephrine on glomerular pressure in the toad. *Gen Comp Endocrinol* 1973;20:515.
49. Tucker SM, Mason RL, Beauchene RE. Influence of diet and feed restriction on kidney function of aging male rats. *J Gerontol* 1976;31:264.
50. Johnson JE, Barrows CH. Effects of age and dietary restrictions on the kidney glomeruli of mice: observations by scanning electron microscopy. *Anat Res* 1980;196:145.
51. Kennedy GC. Effects of old age and over-nutrition on the kidney. *Br Med Bull* 1957;13:67.
52. Shimamura T. Relationship of dietary intake to the development of glomerulosclerosis in obese Zucker rats. *Exp Mol Pathol* 1982;36:423.
53. Weisinger JR, Kempson RL, Eldridge FL, Swenson RS. The nephrotic syndrome: a complication of massive obesity. *Ann Intern Med* 1974;81:440.
54. Editorial: Diet and the progression of chronic renal failure. *Lancet* 1982;2:1314.
55. Mitch WE, Walser M, Steinman TE, Hill S, Zeger S, Tungsanga K. The effect of a keto acid–amino acid supplement to a restricted diet on the progression of chronic renal failure. *N Engl J Med* 1984;311:623.
56. Ruilope LM, Casal MC, Praga M, Alcazar JM, Lahera V, Decap G, Rodicio JL. Additive antiproteinuric effect of converting enzyme inhibition and low protein diet. *J Am Soc Nephrol* 1991;2:243.
57. McCammon RW. *Human growth and development.* Springfield, IL: Charles C. Thomas, 1979;63.
58. Harmon WE, Grupe WE. Acute renal insufficiency. In: Welch KJ, ed. *Complications of pediatric surgery.* Philadelphia: WB Saunders, 1982;54.
59. Counahan R, Cameron JS, Ogg CS, et al. Presentation, management, complication and outcome of acute renal failure in childhood: 5 years' experience. *Br Med J* 1977;1:599.
60. Dudrick SJ, Steiger E, Long JM. Renal failure in surgical patients: treatment with intravenous essential amino acids and hypertonic glucose. *Surgery* 1970;68:180.
61. Abel RM, Abbott WM, Fisher JE. Intravenous essential L-amino acids and hypertonic dextrose in patients with acute renal failure. Effects on serum potassium phosphate and magnesium. *Am J Surg* 1972;123:632.
62. Abel RM, Beck CH Jr, Abbott WM, et al. Improved survival from acute renal failure after treatment with intravenous essential L-amino acids and glucose. Results of a prospective double-blind study. *N Engl J Med* 1973;288:695.
63. Spreiter SC, Myers BD, Swenson RS. Protein-energy requirements in subjects with acute renal failure receiving intermittent hemodialysis. *Am J Clin Nutr* 1980;33:1433.
64. Blumenkrantz MJ, Kopple JD, Koffler A, et al. Total parenteral

nutrition in the management of acute renal failure. *Am J Clin Nutr* 1978;31:1831.
65. Blackburn GL, Etter G, Mackenzie T. Criteria for choosing amino acid therapy in acute renal failure. *Am J Clin Nutr* 1978;31:1841.
66. Andrassy RJ, Mahour GH, Harrison MR, Muenchow SK, Mishalany HG, Woolley MN. The role and safety of early postoperative feeding in the pediatric surgical patient. *J Pediatr Surg* 1979;14:381.
67. Chesney RW, Kaplan BS, Freedom RM, et al. Acute renal failure: an important complication of cardiac surgery. *J Pediatr* 1975;87:381.
68. Hodson EM, Kjellstrand CM, Mauer S. Acute renal failure in infants and children: outcome of 53 patients requiring hemodialysis treatment. *J Pediatr* 1978;93:756.
69. Blagg CR, Parson FM, Young GA. Effect of dietary glucose and protein in acute renal failure. *Lancet* 1962;1:608.
70. Baek SM, Makabali GG, Bryan-Brown CW, Kusek J, Shoemaker WC. The influence of parenteral nutrition on the course of acute renal failure. *Surg Gynecol Obstet* 1975;141:405.
71. Leonard CD, Luke RG, Siegel RR. Parenteral essential amino acids in acute renal failure. *Urology* 1976;6:154.
72. Abel RM, Abbott WM, Beck CH Jr, Ryan JA Jr, Fischer JE. Essential L-amino acids for hyperalimentation in patients with disordered nitrogen metabolism. *Am J Surg* 1974;128:317.
73. Rainford DJ. Nutritional management of acute renal failure. *Acta Chem Scand* 1980;507(Suppl):327.
74. Feinstein EI, Blumenkrantz MJ, Healy M, et al. Clinical and metabolic responses to parenteral nutrition in acute renal failure—a controlled double blind study. *Medicine* 1981;60:124.
75. Freund H, Harmian S, Fischer JE. Comparative studies of parenteral nutrition in renal failure using essential and non-essential amino acid containing solutions. *Surg Gynecol Obstet* 1980;151:652.
76. Abitbol CL, Holliday MA. Total parenteral nutrition in anuric children. *Clin Nephrol* 1976;5:153.
77. Woolfson AMJ, Heatley RV, Allison SP. Insulin to inhibit protein catabolism after injury. *N Engl J Med* 1979;300:14.
78. McMurray SD, Luft FC, Maxwell DR, et al. Prevailing patterns and predictor variables in patients with acute tubular necrosis. *Arch Intern Med* 1978;139:950.
79. Feinstein EI, Kopple JD, Silberman H, et al. Total parenteral nutrition with high or low nitrogen intake in patients with acute renal failure. *Kidney Int* 1983;16:S319.
80. Heird WC, Nicholson JF, Driscoll JM, Schullinger JN, Winters RW. Hyperammonemia resulting from intravenous alimentation using a mixture of synthetic L-amino acids. A preliminary report. *J Pediatr* 1972;81:162.
81. Kopple JD, Swendseid ME. Evidence that histidine is an essential amino acid in normal and chronically uremic man. *J Clin Invest* 1975;55:881.
82. Alvestrand A, Bergstrom J, Furst P, Germais G, Widstam U. Effects of essential amino acid supplementation on muscle and plasma free amino acids in chronic uremia. *Kidney Int* 1978;14:323.
83. Motil KJ, Harmon WE, Grupe WE. Complications of essential amino acid hyperalimentation in children with acute renal failure. *J Parenter Enteral Nutr* 1980;4:32.
84. Blackburn GL, Desai SP, Keenan RA, et al. Clinical use of branched chain amino acid enriched solutions in the stressed and injured patient. In: Walser M, Williamson JR, eds. *Metabolism and clinical implications of branched chain amino and ketoacids.* Elsevier/North Holland, 1981;18:521.
85. Freund HR, Lapidot A, Fischer JE. The use of branched chain amino acids in the injured septic patient. In: Walser M, Williamson JR, eds. *Metabolism and clinical implications of branched chain amino and ketoacids.* Elsevier/North Holland, 1981;18:527.
86. Alvestrand A, Ahlberg M, Furst P, Bergstrom J. Clinical experience with amino acid and keto acid diets. *Am J Clin Nutr* 1980;33:1654.
87. Giordano C, DeSanto NG, DiToro R, Pluvio M, Perrone L. The imbalance effect of amino acid and keto acid diet for growth of the uremic infant. In: *Proceedings of the VIIth International Congress of Nephrology.* Basel: S. Karger, 1978;477.
88. Giordano C. Amino acids and keto acids—advantages and pitfalls. *Am J Clin Nutr* 1980;33:1649.
89. Baum M, Powell D, Calvin S, McDaid T, McHenry K, Mar H, Potter D. Continuous ambulatory peritoneal dialysis in children: comparison with hemodialysis. *N Engl J Med* 1982;307:1537.
90. Salusky IB, Kopple JD, Fine RN. Continuous ambulatory peritoneal dialysis in pediatric patients. A 20-month experience. *Kidney Int* 1983;24:S101.
91. Broyer M, Niaudet P, Champion G, Jean G, Chopin N, Czernichow P. Nutritional and metabolic studies in children on continuous ambulatory peritoneal dialysis. *Kidney Int* 1983;24:S106.
92. Tepper T, VanderHem GK, Tuma GJ, Arisz L, Donker AJM. Loss of amino acids during hemodialysis: quantitative and qualitative investigations. *Clin Nephrol* 1978;10:16.
93. Kopple JD, Coburn JW. Metabolic studies of low protein diets in uremia. I. Nitrogen and potassium. *Medicine* 1973;52:583.
94. Addis T. *Glomerular nephritis. Diagnosis and treatment.* New York: Macmillan, 1950;265.
95. KacKay EM, Oliver J. Renal damage following the ingestion of a diet containing an excess of inorganic phosphate. *J Exp Med* 1935;61:319.
96. Mitch WE. The influence of the diet on the progression of renal insufficiency. *Annu Rev Med* 1984;35:249.
97. Walser M, Mitch WE, Collier VU. The effect of nutritional therapy on the course of chronic renal failure. *Clin Nephrol* 1979;11:66.
98. Nolen GA. Effect of various restricted dietary regimens on the growth, health and longevity of albino rats. *J Nutr* 1972;102:1477.
99. Moise TS, Smith AH. The effect of high protein diet on the kidneys. An experimental study. *Arch Pathol* 1927;4:530.
100. Lalich JJ, Burkholder PM, Paik WCW. Protein overload nephropathy in rats with unilateral nephrectomy. *Arch Pathol* 1975;99:72.
101. Bovee KC, Kronfeld DS, Ramberg C, et al. Long-term measurement of renal function in partially nephrectomized dogs fed 56, 27, or 19% protein. *Invest Urol* 1979;16:378.
102. Blatherwick NR, Medlar EM. Chronic nephritis in rats fed high protein diets. *Arch Intern Med* 1937;59:572.
103. Bras G, Ross MH. Kidney disease and nutrition in the rat. *Toxicol Appl Pharmacol* 1964;6:247.
104. Swenseid ME, Wang M, Vyhmeister P, et al. Amino acid metabolism in the chronically uremic rat. *Clin Nephrol* 1975;3:240.
105. Kleinknecht C, Salusky I, Broyer M, Gubler MC. Effect of various protein diets on growth, renal function and survival of uremic rats. *Kidney Int* 1979;15:534.
106. Salusky I, Kleinknecht C, Broyer M, Gubler MC. Prolonged renal survival and stunting with protein-deficient diets in experimental uremia. *J Lab Clin Med* 1981;97:21.
107. Laouari D, Kleinknecht C, Gubler MC, Ravet V, Broyer MC. Importance of proteins in the deterioration of the remnant kidneys, independently of other nutrients. *Int J Pediatr Nephrol* 1982;3:263.
108. Laouari D, Kleinknecht C, Cournot-Witmer G, et al. Beneficial effect of low phosphorus diet in uremic rats: a reappraisal. *Clin Sci* 1978;63:539.
109. Maschio G, Oldrizzi L, Tessitore N, D'Angelo A, Valvo E, Lupo A, Loschiavo C, Fabris A, Gammaro L, Rugiu C, Panzetta G. Effects of dietary protein and phosphorus restriction on the progression of early renal failure. *Kidney Int* 1982;22:371.
110. Giordano C. Early diet to slow the course of chronic renal disease. In: *Proceedings of the 8th International Congress of Nephrology.* Athens: Karger 1981;71.
111. Heidland A, Kult J, Rockel A, Heidbreder E. Evaluation of essential amino acids and keto acids in uremic patients on low-protein diet. *Am J Clin Nutr* 1978;31:1784.
112. Alvestrand A, Ahlberg M, Furst P, Bergstrom J. Clinical results of long-term treatment with a low protein diet and a new amino acid preparation in patients with chronic uremia. *Clin Nephrol* 1982;19:67.
113. Gretz N, Korb E, Strauch M. Low protein diet supplemented by

keto-acids in chronic renal failure: a prospective controlled study. *Kidney Int* 1983;16:S263(Suppl):12.
114. Barsotti G, Morelli E, Giannoni A, Guiducci A, Lupetti S, Giovanetti S. Restricted phosphorus and nitrogen intake to slow the progression of chronic renal failure: a controlled trial. *Kidney Int* 1983;16:S278(Suppl):24.
115. Bergstrom J, Alvestrand A, Bucht H, Guiterrez A. Progression of chronic renal failure in man is retarded with more frequent clinical followups and better BP control. *Clin Nephrol* 1986;25:1.
116. Grupe WE. Nutritional factors which may influence the rate of progression to chronic renal insufficiency in children. In: Strauss J, ed. *Renal-genitourinary disorders: progression, replacement therapy, growth.* Coral Gables, FL: University of Miami Press, 1987;61.
117. Hellerstein S, Holliday MA, Grupe WE, Fine RN, Fennell RS, Chesney RW, Chan JCM. Nutritional management of children with chronic renal failure. *Pediatr Nephrol* 1987;1:195.
118. Laouari D, Kleinknecht C, Dodu D, et al. Role of glucides in the progression of experimental renal disease. *Eur J Pediatr* 1983;140:202.
119. Koletsky S, Goodstitt AM. Natural history and pathogenesis of renal ablation hypertension. *Arch Pathol* 1960;69:654.
120. Purkerson ML, Hoffsten PE, Klahr S. Pathogenesis of the glomerulopathy associated with renal infarction in rats. *Kidney Int* 1976;9:407.
121. Kaufman JM, DiMedla HJ, Siegel NJ, et al. Compensatory adaptation of structure and function following progressive renal ablation. *Kidney Int* 1974;6:10.
122. Olson JL, Hostetter TH, Rennke HG, et al. Altered glomerular permeability and progressive sclerosis following extreme ablation of renal mass. *Kidney Int* 1982;22:112.
123. Danovich GM, Bourgoinie J, Bricker NS. Reversibility of the "salt-losing" tendency of chronic renal failure. *N Engl J Med* 1977;296:14.
124. Wassner SJ. The role of nutrition in the care of children with renal insufficiency. *Pediatr Clin North Am* 1982;29:973.
125. Wassner SJ, Abitbol C, Alexander S, Conley S, Grupe WE, Holliday MA, Rigden S, Salusky IB. Nutritional requirements for infants with renal failure. *Am J Kidney Dis* 1986;7:300.
126. Harmon WE, Grupe WE, Spinozzi NS. Nutritional management of infants with chronic renal failure without dialysis. *Kidney Int* 1988;33:193.
127. Norman ME, Mazur AT, Borden S, et al. Early diagnosis of juvenile renal osteodystrophy. *J Pediatr* 1980;97:226.
128. Krensky AM, Harmon WE, Ingelfinger JR, Kirkpatrick JA, Grupe WE. Elevated nephrogenous cyclic adenosine monophosphate to monitor early renal osteodystrophy. *Clin Nephrol* 1981;16:245.
129. Portale AA, Booth BE, Tsai MC, et al. Reduced plasma concentration of 1,25 $(OH)_2$ D in children with moderate renal insufficiency. *Kidney Int* 1982;21:627.
130. Harmon WE, Ingelfinger JR. Dialytic management of end-stage renal disease. In: Mendoza SA, Tune BM, eds. *Contemporary issues in nephrology,* vol 12. New York: Churchill Livingstone, 1984;343.
131. Salusky IB, Lucullo L, Nelson P, Fine RN. Continuous ambulatory peritoneal dialysis in children. *Pediatr Clin North Am* 1982;29:1005.
132. Spinozzi NS, Grupe WE. Nutritional implications of renal disease. *J Am Diet Assoc* 1977;70:493.
133. Donkerwolcke RA, Chantler C, Broyer M, et al. Combined report on regular dialysis and transplantation in Europe. *Eur Dial Transplant Assoc* 1980;17:94.
134. Simmons JM, Wilson CJ, Potter DE, et al. Relation of calorie deficiency to growth failure in children on hemodialysis and the growth response to calorie supplementation. *N Engl J Med* 1971;285:653.
135. Arnold WC, Danford D, Holliday MC. Effects of calorie supplementation on growth in children with uremia. *Kidney Int* 1983;24:205.
136. Broyer M. Growth in children with renal insufficiency. *Pediatr Clin North Am* 1982;29:991.
137. Bergstrom WH, deLeon AS, vanGemund JJ. Growth aberrations in renal disease. *Pediatr Clin North Am* 1964;11:563.
138. Stickler GB, Berger BJ. A review: short stature in renal disease. *Pediatr Res* 1973;7:978.
139. Chantler C, Lieberman E, Holliday MA. A rat model for the study of growth failure in uremia. *Pediatr Res* 1974;8:109.
140. Diaz M, Kleinknecht C, Broyer M. Growth in experimental renal failure: role of calorie and amino acid intake. *Kidney Int* 1975;8:349.
141. Betts PR, Macgrath G. Growth pattern and dietary intake of children with chronic renal insufficiency. *Br Med J* 1974;2:189.
142. Grupe WE, Harmon WE, Spinozzi NS. Protein and energy requirements in children receiving chronic hemodialysis. *Kidney Int* 1983;24:S6.
143. Chantler C, ElBishti M, Counahan R. Nutritional therapy in children with chronic renal failure. *Am J Clin Nutr* 1980;33:1682.
144. Ashworth A. Energy balance and growth: experience in treating children with malnutrition. *Kidney Int* 1978;14:301.
145. Spady DW, Payne PR, Picou D, Waterlow JC. Energy balance during recovery from malnutrition. *Am J Clin Nutr* 1976;29:1073.
146. Jones R, Dalton N, Turner C, Start K, Haycock G, Chantler C. Oral essential amino acid and keto acid supplements in children with chronic renal failure. *Kidney Int* 1983;24:95.
147. Spinozzi NS, Murray CL, Grupe WE. Altered taste acuity in children with end-stage renal disease (ESRD). *Pediatr Res* 1978;12:442.
148. Burge JC, Parks HS, Whitlock CP, Schemmel RA. Taste acuity in patients undergoing long term hemodialysis. *Kidney Int* 1979;15:49.
149. Ciechanover M, Peresecenschi G, Aviram A, et al. Malrecognition of taste in uremia. *Nephron* 1980;26:20.
150. Mahajan SK, Prasad AS, Lambujon J, Abbasi AA, Briggs WA, McDonald FD. Improvement of uremic hypogeusia by zinc: a double-blind study. *Am J Clin Nutr* 1980;33:1517.
151. Arbus GS, Wolffe E, Williams W, et al. Zinc supplementation in predialysis patients. In: Gruskin AB, Normal ME, eds. *Pediatric nephrology.* Boston: Martimus Nijhoff, 1981;495.
152. Grupe WE, Kopito LE, Lazarus JM, Brown JA. Copper and zinc depletion in end-stage renal disease. *Pediatr Res* 1976;10:439.
153. Jones RWA, Dalton N, Start K, ElBishti MM, Chantler C. Oral essential amino acid supplements in children with advanced chronic renal failure. *Am J Clin Nutr* 1980;33:1696.
154. Abitbol CL, Holliday MA. Effect of energy and nitrogen intake upon urea production in children with uremia and undernutrition. *Clin Nephrol* 1978;10:9.
155. Garza C, Scrimshaw NS, Young VR. Human protein requirements: the effect of variations in energy intake within the maintenance range. *Am J Clin Nutr* 1976;29:280.
156. Garza C, Scrimshaw NS, Young VR. Human protein requirements: evaluation of the 1973 FAO/WHO safe level of protein intake for young men at high energy intakes. *Br J Nutr* 1977;37:403.
157. Wassner SJ, Orloff S, Sanders R, et al. Determination of essential and total amino acid nitrogen requirements in protein deprived patients receiving parenteral alimination. *Am J Clin Nutr* 1979;32:1497.
158. Conley SB, Brewer ED, Gandy S, et al. Normal growth in very small children on peritoneal dialysis: 18 months experience. *Am J Kidney Dis* 1982; Nov (suppl):8.
159. Conley SB, Rose GM, Robson AM, Bier DM. Effects of dietary intake and hemodialysis on protein turnover in uremic children. *Kidney Int* 1980;17:837.
160. Wilson CJ, Potter DE, Holliday MA. Treatment of the uremic child. In: Winters RW, ed. *The body fluids in pediatrics.* Boston: Little, Brown, 1973;579.
161. Schoeneman M. Dietary and pharmacologic treatment of chronic renal failure. In: Edelmann CM Jr, ed. *Pediatric kidney disease.* Boston: Little, Brown, 1978;475.
162. Harmon WE, Grupe WE. Urea kinetics in the clinical management of children on chronic hemodialysis. In: Fine RN, Gruskin AB, eds. *End-stage renal disease in children.* Philadelphia: WB Saunders, 1984;54.

163. Broyer M. Chronic renal failure. In: Royer P, Habib R, Mathieu H, Broyer M, Walsh A, eds. *Pediatric nephrology.* Philadelphia: WB Saunders, 1974;358.
164. Giordano C, DeSanto NG, Capodicasa G. Amino acid losses of children on CAPD. *Int J Pediatr Nephrol* 1981;2:85.
165. Blumenkranz MG, Gahl GM, Kopple JD, Kamdar AV, Jones MR, Kessel M, Coburn JW. Protein losses during peritoneal dialysis. *Kidney Int* 1981;19:593.
166. Sargent J, Gotch F, Borah M, Piercy L, Spinozzi N, Schoenfeld P, Humphreys M. Urea kinetics: a guide to nutritional management of renal failure. *Am J Clin Nutr* 1978;31:1696.
167. Harmon WE, Spinozzi N, Meyer A, Grupe WE. The use of protein catabolic rate to monitor pediatric hemodialysis. *Dial Transplant* 1981;10:324.
168. Harmon WE, Spinozzi NS, Sargent JR, Grupe WE. Determination of protein catabolic rate (PCR) in children on hemodialysis by urea kinetic modeling. *Pediatr Res* 1979;13:513.
169. Grupe WE, Spinozzi NS, Harmon WE. Protein balance more dependent on protein intake than on energy intake in hemodialyzed children. *Kidney Int* 1983;23:149.
170. Salusky IB, Fine RN, Nelson P, et al. Nutritional status of children undergoing continuous ambulatory peritoneal dialysis. *Am J Clin Nutr* 1983;38:599.
171. De Santo NG, Capodicasa G, Pluvia M, Gilli G, Giordano C. Nitrogen balance and growth in children on CAPD. In: Gahl GM, Kessel M, Nolph KD, eds. *Advances in peritoneal dialysis.* Amsterdam: Excerpta Medica, 1981;397.
172. Edefonti A, Picca M, Guez S, Bassi S, Cattarelli D, Montini G, Zacchello G. Use of nitrogen balance to determine protein and calorie requirements of children treated with chronic peritoneal dialysis. *J Am Soc Nephrol* 1991;2:360.
173. Warren S, Conley SB. Nutritional considerations in infants on continuous peritoneal dialysis (CPD). *Dial Transplant* 1983;12:263.
173a. Alexander SR, Corneil AT, Pavlinac J, et al. Accelerated growth in an anuric infant treated for 14 months with conventional CAPD and tube feedings providing only the RDA for energy and protein. *Am J Kidney Dis* 1984;4:294.
174. Grupe WE, Spinozzi NS, Harmon WE. Protein utilization in chronic renal insufficiency in children. In: Cummings N, Klahr S, eds. *Chronic renal disease: causes, complications, and treatment.* New York: Plenum, 1985;309.
175. Grupe WE. Nutrition in renal diseases. In: Grand RJ, Sutphen JL, Dietz WH, eds. *Pediatric nutrition: theory and practice.* Boston: Butterworths, 1987;579.
176. Hegsted DM. Assessment of nitrogen requirements. *Am J Clin Nutr* 1978;31:1669.
177. Counahan R, El Bishti M, Chantler C. Oral essential amino acids in children or regular hemodialysis. *Clin Nephrol* 1978;9:11.
178. Grodstein GP, Blumenkrantz MJ, Kopple JD. Nutritional and metabolic response to catabolic stress in uremia. *Am Clin Nutr* 1980;33:1411.
179. Guillot M, Broyer M, Cathelineau L, Boulegue D, Dartois AM, Folio D, Guimbaud P. Nutrition enterale a debit constant en nephrologie pediatrique: resultats a long terme de son utilisation dans les nephroses congenitales, les cystinoses graves et les insuffisances renales. *Arch Fr Pediatr* 1980;37:497.
180. Abras E, Walser M. Nitrogen utilization in uremic patients fed by continuous nasogastric infusion. *Kidney Int* 1982;22:392.
181. Bergstrom J, Ahlberg M, Alvestrand A, Furst P. Metabolic studies with keto acids in uremia. *Am J Clin Nutr* 1978;31:1761.

CHAPTER 35

Nutritional Considerations in the Diagnosis and Treatment of Children with Juvenile Arthritis

Daniel J. Lovell

Nutritional concerns are important in the care of children with juvenile rheumatic diseases. Food allergy has been cited as a cause of chronic arthritis; chronic malnutrition may contribute to the growth failure observed in adults who had juvenile rheumatoid arthritis (JRA) during childhood.

Chronic arthritis in childhood is not an uncommon problem; approximately 200,000 children in the United States are estimated to have arthritis related to a rheumatic disease (1). Current prevalence rates (2) establish JRA as one of the more common chronic diseases of childhood (Table 1). In addition, it is the most common pediatric rheumatic disease, representing approximately 50% of the cases seen in pediatric rheumatology centers (Fig. 1) (3). JRA is the pediatric rheumatic disease in which the bulk of work related to nutrition has been performed.

The diagnosis of JRA is established entirely on clinical grounds. It is based on the observation of (a) persistent arthritis of one or more joints of at least 6 weeks' duration (b) in a patient 16 years or less, (c) with the exclusion of all other causes of chronic arthritis in childhood (4). The peak age of onset is between 1 and 3 years, although a substantial number of cases begin later in childhood (5). Onset before 6 months of age is unusual.

Common constitutional symptoms of JRA include joint stiffness in the morning or after a period of inactivity. A very common presentation in the younger child is increased irritability and assumption of guarded posture or refusal to walk. Fever, fatigue, anorexia, weight loss, and failure to grow may occur in all subtypes (5).

Three distinct subtypes of juvenile rheumatoid arthritis have been described (Table 2). Systemic JRA patients manifest spiking fevers greater than 103°F once or twice daily as well as the appearance of a characteristic fleeting erythematous rash. These patients commonly develop pericarditis, pleuritis, hepatosplenomegaly, and generalized lymphadenopathy, but are at low risk for development of chronic iritis, i.e., inflammation of the anterior chamber of the eye. Polyarticular JRA, arthritis in five joints or more, occurs in slightly less than half of the cases of JRA and carries an increased risk for chronic iritis. Most patients have pauci- or oligoarticular JRA, four joints or less involved, which carries the greatest risk for the development of iritis. All of the pediatric rheumatic diseases can be accurately characterized as chronic inflammatory conditions with multisystem involvement either primarily or as a consequence of added effects from medications used in treatment.

JRA has served as the stimulus for the development of a health care team approach to address the broad spectrum of medical and psychosocial problems that arise as a result of the problems of inflammatory chronic arthrop-

TABLE 1. *Prevalence estimates for selected childhood chronic diseases*

Disease	Rate (cases/1,000 children)
Asthma (moderate or severe)	10.00
Congenital heart disease	7.00
Diabetes mellitus	1.80
Cleft lip/palate	1.50
Juvenile rheumatoid arthritis	1.0
Sickle-cell anemia	.28
Cystic fibrosis	.20
Hemophilia	.15
Acute lymphocytic leukemia	.11
Chronic renal failure	.08
Muscular dystrophy	.06

From ref. 2.

D. J. Lovell: Department of Pediatrics, University of Cincinnati Children's Hospital Medical Center, Cincinnati, Ohio 45229-2899.

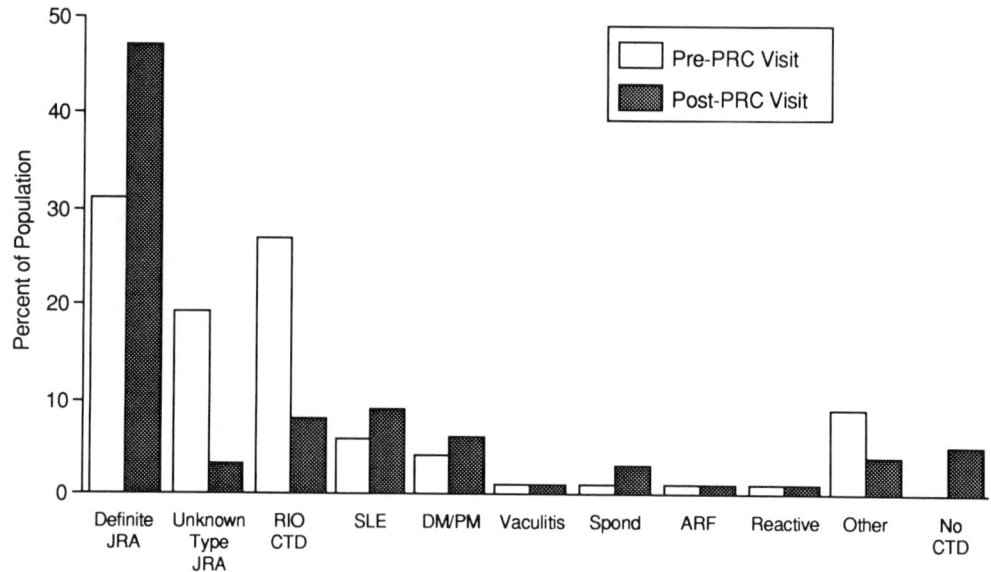

FIG. 1. Pre- and post–pediatric rheumatology centers (PRC) visit diagnoses. JRA, juvenile rheumatoid arthritis; CTD, connective tissue disease; SLE, systemic lupus erythematosus; DM/PM, dermatomyositis/polymyositis; Spond, spondyloarthropathy; ARF, acute rheumatic fever; Reactive, postinfectious reactive arthritis.

athy in childhood. The necessity of this concern is apparent when one considers that, despite growing evidence that a significant proportion of JRA patients have nutritional problems, less than 8% of the patients with JRA had been seen by dietitians, as data from two recent national surveys have demonstrated (2,6). This lack of professional guidance is not the result of patient or parent apathy. In a recent survey of families of JRA patients, 86% of the respondents indicated that nutrition was the topic about which they would most strongly like information (7). Other studies (8,9) have shown that 66% to 70% of JRA patients have used unconventional therapies, approximately 45% of those being unprescribed dietary alterations.

FOOD ALLERGY AND ARTHRITIS

Chronic arthritis associated with intake of certain foods, primarily dairy products, has been reported in adults (10–13) and one pediatric patient (14). The patients all had objective arthritis of sufficient severity and chronicity to have been diagnosed as rheumatoid arthritis in the adults and JRA in the pediatric patient. Some of the adult patients had experienced chronic debilitating synovitis with destructive joint changes present on radiographs for over 10 years and had been treated with some of the most potent arthritis medications, including gold, penicillamine, azathioprine, and prednisone. The elimination of associated foods, however, began a sustained remission. This was followed by exacerbation when the foods were reintroduced and improvement with subsequent omission.

One patient, studied under the controlled conditions of a clinical research center (CRC), had an 11-year history of exacerbations associated with the ingestion of meat, milk, and beans. After 6 days in the CRC, on a regular diet, she was found to have nine tender and three swollen joints. Five days later, after being placed on an

TABLE 2. *Juvenile rheumatoid arthritis (JRA)*

	Course subtypes		
	Systemic	Polyarticular	Pauciarticular
Percent of cases	10%	40%	50%
Sex (F:M)	1:1	2:1	2:1
Number of joints involved	variable	≥5	≤4
Chronic eye disease	<2%	5%	20%
Prolonged fever	100%	30%	0%
Hepatosplenomegaly	85%	10%	0%
Lymphadenopathy	70%	5%	0%
Functional status (10 years after onset)			
No limitations	25%	50%	40%
Mild to moderate	60%	25%	60%
Wheelchair/crutches	15%	25%	0%

elemental Vivonex diet, examination showed one tender joint and no swollen joints. For the next month, the patient was maintained on a Vivonex diet with blinded intermittent ingestion of food capsules. Following ingestion of capsules containing evaporated milk, the patient was noted to develop 14 tender joints, 4 swollen joints, and circulating IgG immune complexes (13).

The pediatric patient reported had a 6-year history of bouts of intermittent high fevers, rash, and objective arthritis involving large and small joints. All symptoms ceased with the elimination of cow's milk from the diet, returning with dietary provocation on four occasions, two inadvertent. This patient was noted to have milk-specific IgM and IgG, but not IgE, antibodies (14). In cases of milk-related arthritis, periods of up to 2 months without milk products have been necessary to demonstrate complete resolution of symptoms.

In the absence of studies designed to assess the prevalence of food-related chronic arthritis, strong recommendations are impossible. But, as a result of the excellent clinical results gained from milk elimination, one investigator suggested that patients with possible JRA who are negative for rheumatoid factor and antinuclear antibodies and who are lactase-deficient or have a family history of milk allergy should be given a 3-week trial of a diet completely free of cow's milk protein (14).

NUTRITIONAL ASSESSMENT IN JUVENILE ARTHRITIS

JRA patients with significant nutritional problems have been described (15–18) and several recent studies have assessed the nutritional status of JRA patients by carefully monitoring growth and body composition.

Studies that enroll patients consecutively, as they appear in clinic, tend to overestimate the severity of the disease since they do not study the significant numbers in remission who are less likely to be attending clinic. This problem was obviated in one university-based pediatric rheumatology center by the use of randomized sampling (19). The average age of the subjects was 12.6 years, average disease duration 6.7 years; 15 were female; 6 had active JRA and 13 were in partial or total remission. Study results showed that 21% were less than the 5th percentile for height, 21% were less than the 5th percentile for weight, 37% weighed less than 80% of the recommended weight-for-height (adjusted height-for-weight index); 16% were less than the 5th percentile for arm circumference, 53% were below the 5th percentile in both arm muscle circumference and arm muscle area. Only 5%, however, were below the 5th percentile for subcutaneous fat stores. Short half-life visceral protein stores (retinol-binding protein and prealbumin) were more than two standard deviations below age-matched norms in 37%, but longer half-life proteins (albumin and total protein) were normal in all subjects (19).

In a study of Swedish females between 11 and 16 years of age, 26 with chronic juvenile arthritis and 28 controls (20) were similar in height and weight. Arthritis patients, however, had significantly lower values for midarm and arm muscle circumference, and significantly higher levels of subcutaneous fat and lower levels of serum albumin and prealbumin. These changes were observed only in patients with polyarticular arthritis (≥5 joints) or systemic arthritis but not in those in the pauciarticular (≤4 joints) subtype. Malnutrition was reported in 19% of the arthritis patients and 0% of the controls (20).

Similar results were obtained in another study (21) of 33 JRA patients in which 18% had heights < 5th percentile, 15% had weights < 5th percentile, subcutaneous fat stores were greater than normal, and somatic muscle measures fell below normal in over 50% of the patients.

In another study, 36% of 28 JRA patients were found to be protein-energy malnourished (PEM). Of the malnourished patients, 80% had weight < 5th percentile, 30% had heights < 5th percentile, 50% had subnormal somatic proteins, but none had depletion of subcutaneous fat reserves (22). In this study, 70% of the JRA patients referred to a dietitian by the managing pediatric rheumatologist had PEM and almost 20% of the JRA patients who were screened by the nutritionist without a referral were found to have PEM (Table 3). A study performed in a Mexican-American population of JRA patients revealed similar trends in anthropometric values (23).

Despite the variable population selection methods and geographic and ethnic backgrounds, a surprisingly consistent message emerges of a high prevalence of PEM in this population, with the loss of somatic and visceral protein stores occurring prior to, and more than, the loss of overall weight or subcutaneous fat stores.

A very important factor is the difference between intake and energy requirements. A study utilizing indirect calorimetry demonstrated that measured metabolic needs for JRA patients were not greater than standard estimates based on age, sex, and height (Table 4) (19). Dietary analyses, however, have revealed that JRA pa-

TABLE 3. *Protein-energy malnutrition (PEM) in JRA*

	PEM	At risk	Not at risk
JRA onset			
Systemic (n = 7)	2	4	1
Polyarticular (n = 11)	5	4	2
Pauciarticular (n = 10)	3	0	7
Referral status			
Referred to nutritionist (n = 10)	7	3	0
Screened without referral (n = 18)	3	5	10
Overall (n = 28)			
36% Had PEM			
28% At risk for PEM			
36% Not at risk for PEM			

From ref. 22.

TABLE 4. *Caloric intake and estimates of metabolic needs in JRA patients (Cal/day)*

Method	Mean	Median	SD
Indirect calorimetry	2,096	2,227	654
Height age for actual height	2,058	2,007	336
Weight age/actual weight	2,093	2,076	452
Weight age/ideal body weight	2,344	2,410	553
Actual intake (3-day diet diary)	1,958	1,942	404

From ref. 19.

tients' mean caloric and selected nutrient (calcium, iron) intake ranged from 50% to 80% of that recommended for healthy children of comparable sex and age (23). One study (19), which analyzed a 3-day diet diary, found a median caloric intake 285 kilocalories (Cal) per day below the median measured metabolic need, based on indirect calorimetry (Table 4). Analysis of the intake of specific nutrients (24) confirmed frequent dietary deficiencies (Table 5). Bacon et al. (25) also demonstrated that systemic JRA patients had both mean caloric and mean vitamin E intakes below RDA.

In a study of adult patients with rheumatoid arthritis, Helliwell et al. (26) demonstrated that 30% had evidence of PEM. These findings should not be unexpected in JRA patients. The chronic inflammation present in juvenile arthritis results in these patients being at risk for "complicated starvation" (27) where over 50% of any weight loss comes from lean body mass (primarily somatic muscle stores). This predisposition for loss of lean body mass can make even small amounts of weight loss significant (28).

GENERALIZED GROWTH DISTURBANCE

Growth disturbances in children with JRA were noted by Still (29) and Chauffard and Raymond (30) over 90 years ago. An important early study (18) described the growth pattern of 119 JRA patients with disease onset prior to 14 years of age. It demonstrated that, during periods of active articular disease, over half of the children had heights more than 10% below normal. If remission occurred, however, growth would resume, usually normalizing height in the younger patients not on steroids. A significant decrease in overall height ($p < .001$) was also described by Laaksonen (31) in Finland, in a series of 544 juvenile arthritis patients.

A more recent study demonstrated that systemic onset JRA patients are significantly more likely than polyarticular or pauciarticular JRA patients to develop growth retardation (32). A markedly high use (85%) of corticosteroids in systemic patients, as compared to 0% in polyarticular/pauciarticular patients, however, complicates the interpretation of the growth data in this study. Longitudinal analysis of the study population revealed that 53% were below the 3rd percentile for height after 7.5 years of follow-up (32). A more recent study demonstrated heights less than the 5th percentile in 9 of 28 JRA patients (32%) with a mean disease duration of 3.7 years (22). A similar study demonstrated height less than the 5th percentile in 25% of the polyarticular onset, 22% of the systemic onset, and none of the pauciarticular onset JRA patients (21).

One provocative observation is that 33% of the children, at the time of diagnosis, had documented heights below the 3rd percentile, suggesting that growth and/or nutritional problems may be very early involved in the development of the disease process.

In a randomly selected population of JRA patients ($n = 56$), the mean heights for age were below the 35th percentile for the polyarticular and systemic onset groups but normal for the pauciarticular onset JRA patients (Table 6). The polyarticular JRA patients demonstrated statistically significantly ($p < .01$) lower weight-for-height measurements (mean = 32nd percentile) as compared to systemic (mean = 70th percentile) and pauciarticular (mean = 56th percentile) onset groups (25).

What is the effect of JRA on adult heights? Do the observed growth problems reported in these studies persist into adulthood? Preliminary results of a longitudinal project (24) involving 156 JRA patients followed past 18 years of age identify clear-cut differences from normal adult heights. Fifty percent of the systemic onset group, 16% of the polyarticular onset, and 11% of the pauciarticular onset patients had adult heights below the 5th

TABLE 5. *Dietary intake in JRA patients (3-day diet diary)*

Nutrient	Mean % RDA	Median % RDA	% of group <80% of RDA
Vitamin A	120	113	28
Vitamin C	213	132	21
Thiamin	147	126	14
Riboflavin	179	179	0
Niacin	133	132	21
Phosphorus	120	115	21
Calcium	100	84	50
Zinc	77	69	57
Iron	106	116	28

From ref. 19.
RDA, recommended dietary allowance.

TABLE 6. *Comparison of height and weight by JRA (n = 56)*

	Mean height percentile	Mean weight percentile	Mean weight-for-height percentile
Systemic ($n = 15$)	31.5	41.5	70
Polyarticular ($n = 26$)	34.9	28.6	32
Pauciarticular ($n = 15$)	46.2	49.6	56

From ref. 92.

percentile for normal adults. None of the systemic onset and only 12% of the polyarticular onset patients had heights above the 75th percentile for adult normals. It is important to note that only 42% of the growth failure group had ever used corticosteroids. This study indicates that growth failure does persist into adulthood in a significant proportion of JRA patients, primarily those with systemic onset, and occurs most often without a history of steroid use (24).

Several investigators have demonstrated that JRA patients with growth failure have normal baseline serum growth hormone levels and normal growth hormone secretion responses to pharmacologic stimulation (33–36). Growth hormone is thought to exert its influence by acting through secondary messengers. These secondary messengers (somatomedins, also called insulin-like growth factors) (37) have been noted to be low in growth hormone deficiency (38), idiopathic growth retardation (39–63), all three JRA types (64), and malnutrition (65). Bennett et al. (37) studied JRA patients and demonstrated serum levels of insulin-like growth factors I and II that on average were 46% to 64% of age-matched normal controls and negatively correlated with the sedimentation rate (37). Allen et al. (64) reported a patient with a 1-year period of catch-up growth following spontaneous remission of systemic JRA (erythrocyte sedimentation rate 106 to 3 mm/hr). During this period of rapid growth, serum somatomedin levels increased fivefold and growth hormone levels tripled (64).

Human growth hormone treatment in JRA patients with severe growth failure resulted in normalized growth in 17 of 30 patients (33–35,66) despite normal pretreatment basal and stimulated growth hormone levels (Table 7). Unfortunately, studies relating to growth hormone and somatomedins in JRA patients have failed to comprehensively assess the nutritional status of patients in determining the impact of nutritional factors on growth failure and on the individual's response to growth hormone therapy.

Recent studies demonstrate very encouraging results on the effect of recombinant growth hormone on non–growth-hormone-deficient but growth-retarded children (39–46,48,49,53). A very high proportion of these patients demonstrated accelerated linear growth, with many maintaining improved growth velocity after termination of exogenous growth hormone therapy. Longitudinal growth gains were accomplished while skeletal maturation continued at a normal rate, so that eventual adult height was at least maintained and likely improved. This has added significance in light of studies demonstrating that growth hormone has certain anabolic effects such as decreasing subcutaneous fat stores and lipogenesis (67,68), increasing muscle mass (69), and conserving lean body mass during massive weight loss due to dietary restriction (70).

ANEMIA

Anemia in juvenile arthritis is usually in concert with the level of underlying inflammation—the anemia of chronic disease. Patients may present with a normocytic hypochromic anemia, a hemoglobin in the range of 7 to 10 g/dl with low serum iron, low iron binding capacity, and adequate or elevated hemosiderin stores (71). Serum ferritin in JRA patients most closely reflects the inflammatory state and is an unreliable indicator of iron stores (72–74). Iron deficiency may also develop due to poor dietary intake, gastrointestinal blood loss secondary to medications, or preferential uptake of iron by inflamed synovial tissue (75,76). The observation that 13 of 15 anemic JRA patients responded to a 6-month trial of supplemental iron therapy with a rise in hemoglobin of 1 g/dl or more, combined with the difficulty of distinguishing the anemia of chronic disease from iron deficiency, have lead some investigators to recommend a trial of iron therapy for any JRA patient with a low hemoglobin and mean corpuscular volume (MCV) for age (77). The use of therapeutic iron in JRA is not, however, without risk, and should be instituted with caution and clinical follow-up to assess the effect on synovial inflammation. This is because iron deposits in synovial membranes promote production of oxygen free radicals and the release of lysosomal enzymes contributing to synovial inflammation (78). Treatment of arthritis patients with active arthritis and anemia with desferrioxamine has resulted in increased hemoglobin and serum iron and a decreased level of articular inflammation (79).

IMPACT OF DRUG THERAPY ON NUTRITION

Virtually all patients with juvenile arthritis are treated with a variety of medications (Table 8) (80). Salicylates

TABLE 7. Treatment with human growth hormone (n = 30)

	Number of patients	Percent
Growth rate normalized	17	57
Mild improvement	1	3
No improvement	12	40

From refs. 33, 35, and 66.

TABLE 8. Drug therapy and nutrition in JRA patients: percent of population on drug with side effect

Drug	Nausea	Abdominal pain	Mouth ulcers
Aspirin	5%	20%	0%
Other NSAIDs	5%	2–9%	0%
IM gold	5%	5%	10%
Oral gold	17%	30%	10%
D-penicillamine	7%	7%	2%
Methotrexate	7–18%	10–20%	5–10%

NSAID, nonsteroidal anti-inflammatory drug.

and the other nonsteroidal anti-inflammatory drugs (NSAIDs) form the foundation of pharmacologic management of most forms of arthritis. Side effects of the NSAIDs include drowsiness, nausea, vomiting, irritability, abdominal pain, gastritis, and gastrointestinal ulceration. Gastrointestinal complications can be minimized by taking the medication with meals (80).

Approximately 20% to 40% of JRA patients fail to improve sufficiently on NSAIDs and require additional medications (71). Penicillamine may cause an unpleasant change in taste and, unlike other arthritis medications, must be taken on an empty stomach to facilitate absorption (71).

Corticosteroid use in juvenile arthritis should be reserved for life-threatening systemic disease, severe chronic uveitis unresponsive to local therapy, and intraarticular injections. It should be emphasized that systemic steroid therapy in chronic arthritis, while excellent in decreasing symptoms and physical findings of articular inflammation, has never been shown to limit the duration of active disease, decrease or prevent the development of bony or cartilaginous damage, or improve long-term functional outcome (71,81–86). Systemic steroids are, however, part of standard, accepted therapy for the more severe rheumatic diseases such as systemic lupus erythematosus (SLE), dermatomyositis, and systemic vasculitis. Although an in-depth review of the literature related to desired and undesired effects of steroids is outside the scope of this topic, the following effects are germane to nutritional concerns: Corticosteroids contribute to the development of catabolism (80). Patients with severe inflammation, those most likely to receive corticosteroids, are also the ones most likely to have PEM with compromised somatic and visceral protein stores. Steroids contribute to the development of osteopenia (86–88). This effect is additive to the bone demineralization that has been observed (89) in up to 50% of non–steroid-treated JRA patients studied by single photon densitometry (bone density greater than 2 standard deviations below age- and sex-matched norms). Corticosteroids also contribute to the growth retardation associated with the underlying disease (24,32).

ANOREXIA IN JUVENILE ARTHRITIS

Anorexia is a problem in active juvenile arthritis. Although many factors are contributory, the inflammatory cytokines, interleukin-1 and tumor necrosis factor, have been shown to cause profound anorexia in experimental animals and humans (90) and to be present in elevated amounts in JRA patients (91). This anorexia can be severe enough to thwart all efforts to increase volitional oral intake. In the pediatric rheumatology center at the Cincinnati Children's Hospital Medical Center, seven children have received aggressive nutritional intervention to counteract the chronic growth failure and profound PEM that occurred despite heroic efforts by family members and nutritionists to increase the patients' volitional oral intake. Patients were nutritionally repleted through outpatient nocturnal nasogastric tube feedings of standard commercial products in combination with daily volitional intake. The initial caloric intake necessary for repletion, based on indirect calorimetry, was about 1.5 times the estimated metabolic need. This was subsequently adjusted to match weight gain velocity with height velocity.

TABLE 9. Results of nocturnal enteral feeding in JRA (n = 7)

Parameter	6 months before	6 months after
Height velocity (mean)	0.15 cm/month	1.62 cm/month
Weight velocity (mean)	−0.22 kg/month	0.8 kg/month

During the 6 months prior to the initiation of the nocturnal nasogastric drip feedings, the average growth velocity for these seven patients was 0.15 cm/month; weight gain velocity was −0.22 kg/month (Table 9). During the 6 months following initiation of feedings, the average growth velocity was 1.62 cm/month and weight gain velocity was 0.8 kg/month. In all seven patients, repletion resulted in normalization of retinol-binding protein, and prealbumin and albumin within a time frame consistent with the serum half-lives of the proteins. All patients also demonstrated more gradual normalization in anthropometric measurements of somatic protein stores. This improvement occurred despite continuation of very severe arthritis. However, these patients have generally required nocturnal drip feedings for prolonged periods of time (months to years) until the underlying inflammatory process remits spontaneously or is controlled with drug therapy. Although these patients represent an extreme of the spectrum, anorexia in varying degrees is a very common finding in systemic and polyarticular JRA patients.

MECHANICAL PROBLEMS

A variety of mechanical problems can impact on dietary intake. Arthritis of the temporomandibular joint, which develops in 18% to 30% of JRA patients, can be associated with pain with jaw movement, limitation in mouth opening, or chronic facial pain. Patients with painful temporomandibular joints often benefit from physical or occupational therapists with expertise in this area. Hypoplasia of the mandible occurs in 20% to 25% of JRA patients and can result in malocclusion and difficulty in swallowing (7). Arthritis of the upper extremities can make food preparation and handling of eating utensils difficult, painful, embarrassing, or even impossible.

Occupational therapists should be consulted for evaluation of a patient's particular deficits and for developing appropriate measures designed to improve functional independence and decrease pain either through the use of alternative movements that relieve unnecessary mechanical stress on the joints or through the use of adaptive equipment (7).

ROLE OF THE NUTRITIONIST ON THE ARTHRITIS TEAM

Clearly a large proportion of juvenile arthritis patients are at risk for developing a variety of nutritional problems. These problems may occur at any time during the course of the disease and, since rheumatic diseases are characterized by frequent fluctuations in the severity of the inflammatory process, may vary in severity in the same patient. Dietitians need to be aware of these changes in the patient's overall disease status in order to be able to identify potential nutritional deficits. Early recognition of these problems prior to significant decline in growth or depletion of body stores requires ongoing periodic rescreening of all patients in the clinic. The nutritionist, along with other rheumatology team members, should be involved in the initial evaluation of all new patients. This is essential not only for nutritional screening but for establishing the relationship for ongoing nutritional dialogue with the family. The combination of early education regarding a low-sodium/low-caloric diet, begun on the very day that corticosteroids are prescribed, coupled with ongoing, frequent support and new dietary suggestions, has been very effective in minimizing weight gain. In those patients developing PEM, the nutritionist is instrumental in instructing the family in methods of increasing the protein and caloric density of the child's diet and in directing nocturnal enteral feeding, if instituted. In short, the nutritionist should be an integrated member of the interdisciplinary team providing care for children with rheumatic diseases.

SUMMARY

Nutritional considerations are important in arthritis, from the time of development of arthritis to the determination of permanent residua. A nutritionist should be part of interdisciplinary pediatric rheumatology teams; nutritional support of the rheumatology patient is essential to the optimal care of the underlying disease. There is a need for further research in this area.

ACKNOWLEDGMENTS

The author wishes to thank Ms. Carolyn Haun for her patience and timely help in preparation of the manuscript. This work was partially supported by a Maternal and Child Health Services grant H5-7-38. Computational assistance was provided in part by the CLINFO Project (supported by grant RR-00350 from the Division of Research Resources, National Institutes of Health).

REFERENCES

1. Cassidy JT, Nelson AM. The frequency of juvenile arthritis. *Arthritis Rheum* 1988;15:535–536.
2. Gortmaker SL, Sappenfield W. Chronic childhood disorders: prevalence and impact. *Pediatr Clin North Am* 1974;31:3.
3. Lovell DJ, Levinson JE, Lindsley C, and Members of the SPRANS Centers. Pediatric rheumatology as a special project of regional and national significance. *J Rheumatol* 1986;13:978.
4. Brewer EJ, Bass JC, Cassidy JT, Fink C, Jacobs J, Hanson V, Levinson JE, Schaller J, Stillman JS. Current proposed revision of JRA criteria. *Arthritis Rheum* 1977;20:195–199.
5. Cassidy JT. Juvenile rheumatoid arthritis. In: Kelley WN, Harris ED, Ruddy S, Sledge CB, eds. *Textbook of rheumatology*, 2nd ed. Philadelphia: WB Saunders, 1985.
6. Lovell DJ. Health care services, school performance and needs in pediatric rheumatology. *Arthritis Rheum* 1987;30(Suppl):S35.
7. Lovell D, Henderson C, Warady B, Roth J. Role of nutrition in juvenile rheumatoid arthritis. In: Ekvall S, Wheby E, eds. *Nutritional needs of the child with a handicap or a chronic illness*. Cincinnati: University Affiliated Cincinnati Center for Development Disorders, 1988.
8. Southwood TR, Malleson PN, Roberts-Thomson PJ, Mahy M. Unconventional remedies used for patients with juvenile arthritis. *Pediatrics* 1990;85:150–153.
9. Hoyeraal HM, Brewer EJ, Giannini EH, et al. Unconventional therapies in pediatric rheumatology. *Scand J Rheumatol* 1984;53(Suppl):113.
10. Parke AL, Hughes GR. Rheumatoid arthritis and food: a case study. *Br Med J* 1981;282:2027–2029.
11. Williams R. Rheumatoid arthritis and food: a case study (letter to the editor). *Br Med J* 1981;283:563.
12. Ziff M. Diet in the treatment of rheumatoid arthritis. *Arthritis Rheum* 1983;26:457–461.
13. Panush RS, Stroud RM, Webster EM, Endo LP, Nauman J. Food-induced (allergic) arthritis. *Arthritis Rheum* 1985;28(Suppl):S14.
14. Ratner D, Eshel E, Vigder K. Juvenile rheumatoid arthritis and milk allergy. *J R Soc Med* 1985;78:410–413.
15. Coss JA, Botts RH. Juvenile rheumatoid arthritis. A study of fifty-six cases with a note on skeletal changes. *J Pediatr* 1946;29:143–156.
16. Kuhns JG, Swaim LT. Disturbances of growth in chronic arthritis in children. *Am J Dis Child* 1932;43:1118–1133.
17. Lockie LM, Norcross BM. Juvenile rheumatoid arthritis. *Pediatrics* 1948;2:694–698.
18. Ansell BM, Bywaters EG. Growth in Still's disease. *Ann Rheum Dis* 1956;15:295–318.
19. Lovell DJ, Gregg D, Heubi J, Levinson JE. Nutritional status in juvenile rheumatoid arthritis (JRA)—an interim report. *Arthritis Rheum* 1986;29:567.
20. Johnansson V, Portinsson S, Akesson A, Svantesson H, Ockerman PA, Akesson B. Nutritional status in girls with juvenile chronic arthritis. *Hum Nutr Clin Nutr* 1986;40:57–67.
21. Warady BD, McCammon SP, Lindsley CB. Anthropometric assessment of patients with juvenile rheumatoid arthritis. *Top Clin Nutr* 1989;4:7–14.
22. Henderson CJ, Lovell DJ. Assessment of protein-energy malnutrition in children and adolescents with juvenile rheumatoid arthritis (JRA). *Arthritis Care Res* 1989;2:108–113.
23. Miller ML, Chacko JA, Young EA. Dietary deficiencies in children with juvenile rheumatoid arthritis. *Arthritis Care Res* 1989;2:22–24.
24. Lovell DJ, White PH. Growth and nutrition in juvenile rheuma-

toid arthritis. In: Woo P, White P, Ansell B, eds. *Pediatric rheumatology update.* Oxford: Oxford University Press, 1990;47–56.
25. Bacon MC, Raiten DJ, Sami S, White PH. Nutritional status and its relationship to growth among children with JRA. *Arthritis Care Res* 1989;2:S14.
26. Helliwell M, Coombes EJ, Moody BJ, Batstone GF, Robertson JC. Nutritional status in patients with rheumatoid arthritis. *Ann Rheum Dis* 1984;43:386–390.
27. Mascioli EA, Blackburn GL. Nutrition and rheumatic diseases. In: Kelley WN, Harris ED, Ruddy S, Sledge CB, eds. *Textbook of rheumatology.* Philadelphia: WB Saunders, 1985;352–360.
28. Lovell DJ, Henderson CJ. Juvenile rheumatoid arthritis. In: Eckvall S, ed. *Pediatric nutrition in chronic and developmental diseases/disorders,* 2nd ed. Springfield: Charles C. Thomas, 1990; (in press).
29. Still GF. On a form of chronic joint disease in children. *Trans R Med Chir Soc* 1897;80:47–59. (Reprinted in *Arch Dis Child* 1941;16:156.)
30. Chauffard A, Raymond F. Adenopathies in chronic infectious rheumatism. *Rev Med* 1897;16:345–359.
31. Laaksonen AL. A prognostic study of juvenile rheumatoid arthritis: analysis of 544 cases. *Acta Paediatr Scand* 1966;166(Suppl):49–55.
32. Bernstein BH, Stobie D, Singsen BH, Koster-King K, Kornreich HK, Hanson V. Growth retardation in juvenile rheumatoid arthritis. *Arthritis Rheum* 1977;20(Suppl):212–216.
33. Ward DJ, Hartog M, Ansell BM. Corticosteroid-induced dwarfism in Still's disease treated with human growth hormone—clinical and metabolic effects including hydroxyproline excretion in two cases. *Ann Rheum Dis* 1966;26:416.
34. Ansell BM. Cortisol and growth hormone secretion in relation to linear growth: patients with Still's disease on different therapeutic regimens. *Br Med J* 1970;3:547.
35. Butenandt O. Rheumatoid arthritis and growth retardation in children: treatment with human growth hormone. *Eur J Pediatr* 1979;130:15.
36. Allen R, Jimenez M. Cowell C. Physiologic growth hormone secretion and somatomedin levels in juvenile rheumatoid arthritis. *Arthritis Rheum* 1988;31(Suppl):S118.
37. Bennett AE, Silverman ED, Miller JJ, Hints RL. Insulin-like growth factors I and II in children with systemic onset juvenile arthritis. *J Rheumatol* 1988;15:655–658.
38. Van Wyk JJ, Underwood LE, Hintz RL, et al. The somatomedins: a family of insulin-like hormones under growth hormone control. *Recent Prog Horm Res* 1974;30:259–295.
39. Carrascoa A, Vicens-Calvet E, Audi L, Gusinye M, Albisu M, Potau N. Chronic growth retardation with normal growth hormone response to provocative stimuli and low somatomedin activity. *Acta Paediatr Scand* 1987;76:489–494.
40. Albertsson-Wikland K. Growth hormone treatment in short children—short-term and long-term effects on growth. *Acta Paediatr Scand* 1988;(Suppl 343):77–84.
41. Carrascosa A, Albisu M, Gusinye M, Potau N, Audi L, Vicens-Calvet E. Chronic delay of growth with normal response of growth hormone secretion to provocation stimuli for its liberation and decreased somatomedin activity: treatment with growth hormone over 6 months. *Ann Espanoles Pediatr* 1986;25:429–434.
42. Albertsson-Wikland K, Hall K. Growth hormone treatment in short children: relationship between growth and serum insulin-like growth factor I and II levels. *J Clin Endocrinol* 1987;65:671–678.
43. Ranke MB. Human growth hormone therapy of non-growth hormone deficient children. *Pediatrician* 1987;14:178–182.
44. Bozzola M, Cisternino M, Biscaldi I, Maghnie M, Valtorta A, Moretta A, Severi F. Effectiveness of growth hormone (GH) therapy in GH-deficient children and non-GH-deficient short children. *Eur J Pediatr* 1988;147:248–251.
45. Penny R. Growth retardation. Impaired height velocity. *Am J Dis Child* 1989;143:1269–1270.
46. Thompson RG, Conforti P, Holcombe J. Biosynthetic human growth hormone: current status and future questions. *J Endocrinol Invest* 1989;12(8 Suppl 3):35–39.
47. Bierich JR. Growth hormone therapy in short children without classical growth hormone deficiency. *J Endocrinol* 1989;12(8 Suppl 3):25–33.
48. Kaplan SL, Grumbach MM. Long-term treatment with human growth hormone in children with non-growth hormone deficient short stature. *Acta Paediatr Jpn* 1988;30(Suppl):35–38.
49. Rappaport R, Brauner R, Mugnier E. Treatment with growth hormone: results and new perspectives. *Ann Endocrinol* 1988;49:319–322.
50. Hughes IA, Preece MA. Use of growth hormone (letter). *Arch Dis Child* 1988;63:1294–1295.
51. Howrie DL. Growth hormone for the treatment of growth failure in children. *Clin Pharm* 1987;6:283–291.
52. Williams TC, Frohman LA. Potential therapeutic indications for growth hormone and growth hormone–releasing hormone in conditions other than growth retardation. *Pharmacotherapy* 1986;6:311–318.
53. Raiti S, Kaplan SL, Van Vliet G, Moore WV. Short-term treatment of short stature and subnormal growth rate with human growth hormone. *J Pediatr* 1987;110:357–361.
54. Rudman D, Kutner MH, Blackston RD, Cushman RA, Bain RP, Patterson JH. Children with normal-variant short stature: treatment with human growth hormone for six months. *N Engl J Med* 1981;305:123–131.
55. Hayek A, Peake GT. Growth and somatomedin-C responses to growth hormone in dwarfed children. *J Pediatr* 1981;99:868–872.
56. Frazer T, Gavin JR, Daughaday WH, Hillman RE, Weldon VV. Growth hormone-dependent growth failure. *J Pediatr* 1982;101:12–15.
57. Plotnick LP, Van Meter QL, Kowarsky AA. Human growth hormone treatment of children with growth failure and normal growth hormone levels by immunoassay: lack of correlation with somatomedin generation. *Pediatrics* 183;71:324–327.
58. Bright GM, Rogol AD, Hohanson AJ, Blizzard RM. Short stature associated with normal growth hormone and decreased somatomedin-C concentrations: response to exogenous growth hormone. *Pediatrics* 1983;71:576–580.
59. Van Vliet G, Styne DM, Kaplan SL, Grumbach MM. Growth hormone treatment for short stature. *N Engl J Med* 1983;309:1016–1022.
60. Gertner JM, Genel M, Gianfredi SP, et al. Prospective clinical trial of human growth hormone in short children without growth hormone deficiency. *J Pediatr* 1984;104:172–176.
61. Spilotis BE, August GP, Hung W, Sonis W, Mendelson W, Bercu BB. Growth hormone neurosecretory dysfunction. *JAMA* 1984;251:2223–2230.
62. Valenta LJ, Sigel MB, Lesniak MA, et al. Pituitary dwarfism in a patient with circulating abnormal growth hormone polymers. *N Engl J Med* 1985;312:214–217.
63. Zadik Z, Chalew SA, Raiti S, Kowarsky AA. Do short children secrete insufficient growth hormone? *Pediatrics* 1985;76:355–360.
64. Allen R, Jiminez M, Cowell C. Physiologic growth hormone (GH) secretion and somatomedin (Sm) levels in juvenile rheumatoid arthritis (JRA). *Arthritis Rheum* 1988;31:S118.
65. Daughaday WH, Herrington AC, Phillips LS. The regulation of growth by endocrines. *Annu Rev Physiol* 1975;37:211–244.
66. Haapasaari J, Perheentupa J. Growth hormone treatment in children with juvenile rheumatoid arthritis. *Scand J Rheumatol* 1984;14:37.
67. Rosenbaum M, Gertner JM, Leibel RL. Effects of systemic growth hormone (GH) administration on regional adipose tissue distribution and metabolism in GH-deficient children. *J Clin Endocrinol Metab* 1989;69:1274–1281.
68. Wit JM, van't Hof MA, Van den Brande JL. The effect of human growth hormone therapy on skinfold thickness in growth hormone-deficient children. *Eur J Pediatr* 1988;147:588–592.
69. Rutherford OM, Jones DA, Round JM, Preece MA. Changes in skeletal muscle after discontinuation of growth hormone treatment in young adults with hypopituitarism. *Acta Paediatr Scand* 1989;356:61–63.
70. Clemmons DR, Snyder DK, Williams R, Underwood LE. Growth hormone administration conserves lean body mass during dietary restriction in obese subjects. *J Clin Endocrinol Metab* 1987;64:878–883.
71. Cassidy JT, Petty RE. *Textbook of pediatric rheumatology,* 2nd ed. New York: Churchill Livingstone, 1990.
72. Bentley DP, William P. Serum ferritin concentrations as an index

73. Harvey AR, Pippard MJ, Ansell BM. Microcytic anaemia in juvenile chronic arthritis. *Scand J Rheumatol* 1987;16:53–59.
74. Pelkonen P, Swanljung K, Siimes MA. Ferritinemia as an indicator of systemic disease activity in children with systemic juvenile rheumatoid arthritis. *Acta Paediatr Scand* 1986;75:64–68.
75. Giordano N, Fioravanti A, Sancasciani S, Marcolongo R. Increased storage of iron and anaemia in rheumatoid arthritis: usefulness of desferrioxamine. *Br Med J* 1984;289:961–962.
76. Lloyd KN, Williams P. Reaction to total dose infusion of iron dextran in rheumatoid arthritis. *Br Med J* 1970;2:323–325.
77. Koerper MA, Stempel DA, Dallman PR. Anemia in patients with juvenile rheumatoid arthritis. *J Pediatr* 1978;92:930–934.
78. Blake DR, Hall ND, Bacon PA, Dieppe PA, Helliwell B, Guttenridge JMC. The importance of iron in rheumatoid disease. *Lancet* 1981;2:1142–1144.
79. Marcus RE. Treatment of rheumatoid arthritis with desferrioxamine: pilot study. *Arthritis Rheum* 1987;30:S95.
80. Garceau AO, Dwyer JT, Holland M. A practical approach to nutrition in the patient with juvenile rheumatoid arthritis. *Clin Nutr* 1989;8:55–64.
81. Brewer EJ, Giannini EH, Person DA. *Juvenile rheumatoid arthritis,* 2nd ed. Philadelphia: WB Saunders, 1982.
82. Ansell BM, Bywaters EGL, Isdale IC. Comparison of cortisone and aspirin in the treatment of juvenile rheumatoid arthritis. *Br Med J* 1956;1:1075.
83. Good RA, Vernier RL, Smith RT. Serious untoward reactions to therapy with cortisone and A.C.T.H. in pediatric practice. *Pediatrics* 1957;19:95.
84. Lindbjerg IF. Juvenile rheumatoid arthritis. A follow-up of 75 cases. *Arch Dis Child* 1964;39:576.
85. Ansell BM. Problems of corticosteroid therapy in the young. *Proc R Soc Med* 1968;61:281.
86. Schaller JG. Corticosteroids in juvenile rheumatoid arthritis. *Arthritis Rheum* 1977;20:537.
87. Williams R. *Textbook of endocrinology.* Philadelphia: WB Saunders, 1974.
88. Hahn T, Halstead L, Teitelbaum S. Altered mineral metabolism in glucocorticoid-induced osteopenia: effect of 25-hydroxyvitamin D administration. *J Clin Invest* 1979;64:655–665.
89. Lovell DJ, Gregg D, Heubi J, Levinson J. Bone mineralization in JRA patients. *Arthritis Rheum* 1984;27:1336–1343.
90. Tracey KJ, Wei H, Manogue KR. Cachectin/tumor necrosis factor induces cachexia, anemia and inflammation. *J Exp Med* 1988;167:1211.
91. Martini A, Ravelli A, Notarangelo LP. Enhanced interleukin-1 and depressed interleukin-2 production in juvenile arthritis. *J Rheumatol* 1986;13:598.
92. Bacon MC, White P. A new approach to the assessment of growth in JRA. *Arthritis Rheum* 1987;30:S192.

CHAPTER 36

Nutrition and Childhood Malignancies

Lolie C. Yu

Malnutrition, often related to the consequences and complications of therapy, is not uncommon in certain types of childhood cancer. This chapter reviews the relationship of nutrition and childhood malignancies and describes the role of nutritional intervention in averting malnutrition, thereby increasing chemotherapeutic tolerance and improving host immunity. Methods for assessing the nutritional status of children with cancer are also described.

PREVALENCE OF MALNUTRITION

Although not prevalent in all pediatric cancers, malnutrition in childhood cancer is a common, serious problem. Its incidence is related to the type of tumor and the extent of the disease, varying from 8% in newly diagnosed children to 50% in children with disseminated disease (1).

Although protein-energy malnutrition (PEM) is not uniformly found in all pediatric malignancies, it is a common occurrence in certain types of childhood cancer (Table 1). These include patients who present with tumors primarily seen in the abdomen and pelvis, such as neuroblastoma and Wilms' tumor, and patients with newly diagnosed Ewing's sarcoma (2).

PEM can also develop as a result of treatment, for example major operative procedures of the abdomen or irradiation to the head, neck, esophagus, abdomen, and pelvis (3). In addition, the intensive chemotherapy used in the advanced stages of the malignancies usually involves drugs [e.g., cytosine arabinoside (ara-C) infusion for acute nonlymphocytic leukemia] that have significant gastrointestinal toxicity, causing nausea, vomiting, and diarrhea.

THE ETIOLOGY OF MALNUTRITION IN NEOPLASTIC DISEASE

Tumors of the gastrointestinal tract affect intake both by direct mechanical interference and by the need for surgical resection and regional irradiation. Mechanical interference with food intake is the primary cause of the associated nutritional impairment and electrolyte deficiency. The steady slow growth of a cancer may cause only partial obstruction so that malnutrition is not apparent until late in the course of the disease.

Partial obstruction often results in decreased nutritional intake and may ultimately cause vomiting, with the associated fluid and electrolyte loss. This is often seen in children with rapidly progressing non-Hodgkin's lymphoma of the abdomen who appear with abdominal pain and vomiting usually associated with dehydration. Impaired GI function is also the result of head and neck cancer, which inhibits swallowing, and cancer of the head of the pancreas, which inhibits digestion.

Anorexia, a prevalent symptom in cancer, may be caused by both biological and psychological factors (4). Studies indicate the importance of noradrenergic, dopa-

TABLE 1. *Types of neoplastic diseases associated with nutritional risks*

High nutritional risk
    Advanced diseases (solid tumors)
        Stages III and IV Wilms' tumor
        Stages III and IV neuroblastoma
        Pelvic rhabdomyosarcoma
        Ewing's sarcoma
    Acute nonlymphocytic leukemia
    Multiple relapse leukemia
    Medulloblastoma
Low nutritional risk
    Nonmetastatic solid tumors
    Good prognosis acute lymphocytic leukemia
    Advanced diseases in remission

L. C. Yu: Department of Pediatrics, Louisiana State University School of Medicine, New Orleans, Louisiana 70112.

minergic, serotonergic, and, to a lesser extent, endorphinergic systems in the modulation of normal food intake (5–7). Peptides, such as cholecystokinin (CCK), insulin, and bombesin have also been found to be potent in altering food intake. This suggests that a variety of biochemical changes influences the decreased intake common in the presence of a growing tumor growth. Further studies are needed to more clearly define this phenomenon and to document effective treatment strategies (8,9).

Learned food aversion may also be a factor in the anorexia and weight loss of children with cancer. Bernstein (10) was able to rapidly induce such aversions in children receiving chemotherapy. In fact, it has often been observed that children will develop aversions to once-preferred foods while receiving gastrointestinal-toxic therapy. Such foods become associated with nausea, vomiting, and malaise.

Stress, commonly seen in teenage patients, which grows out of anxiety, depression, and fear, is another powerful force associated with a decreased food intake and malnutrition.

Finally, altered taste perception as a cause of anorexia has been documented in pediatric cancer patients (11). Children with leukemia had significantly higher recognition for all four tastes (sweet, salt, sour, bitter) than did healthy children. This results in specific rejection of certain foods as well as, generally, a craving for salty foods, such as hot dogs and pizza. Knowledge of taste changes increases the potential for improving the nutritional status of patients via anticipatory nutritional counseling.

The causes of the anorexia of cancer appear to be multifactorial, including intestinal obstruction, treatment side effects, and biochemical as well as psychological changes. As these factors become more clearly defined, potential for successful treatment becomes possible.

The inefficient metabolism of tumors results in an almost exclusive need for carbohydrates as an energy source. Generally, patients with cancer have a higher caloric expenditure than patients without cancer. Norton et al. (12) have elegantly shown that the daily glucose consumption of patients with large sarcomas may be as high as 500 g per day. This increased metabolic rate and energy consumption may also result from anemia and chronic infections in cancer patients.

Tumors increase energy consumption primarily because of their misuse of the metabolic pathways (13). They use both dietary glucose as well as that produced by gluconeogenesis and from amino acids. Glucose is transformed into lactate by the tumor. The lactate must then be reconstituted by the liver, at a large energy cost. This process, the Cori cycle, is significantly increased in patients with advanced cancer (14). It requires that muscle proteins, as well as a large proportion of amino acid intake, be used for gluconeogenesis (Fig. 1).

Studies suggest that the severe decrease in total body fat might be ascribed, at least partially, to the production of cachectin/tumor necrosis factor (TNF) by the normal macrophages in response to the tumor (15,16). Cachectin/TNF, in addition to inhibiting lipoprotein lipase and therefore the deposition of fat, also has direct effects on the tumor, including hemorrhagic necrosis and changes in vessels, synovial surfaces, and kidneys. Other monocyte mediators, such as interleukin-1 (IL-1), have also been found in patients with Hodgkin's disease and renal cell carcinoma; there is also an increased production of IL-1 in amounts not sufficient to cause fever, but enough to cause metabolic changes including an increased breakdown of proteins and a decreased synthesis of albumin (17).

Intestinal malabsorption syndromes are underestimated as a cause of malnutrition in cancer. Lymphoma-

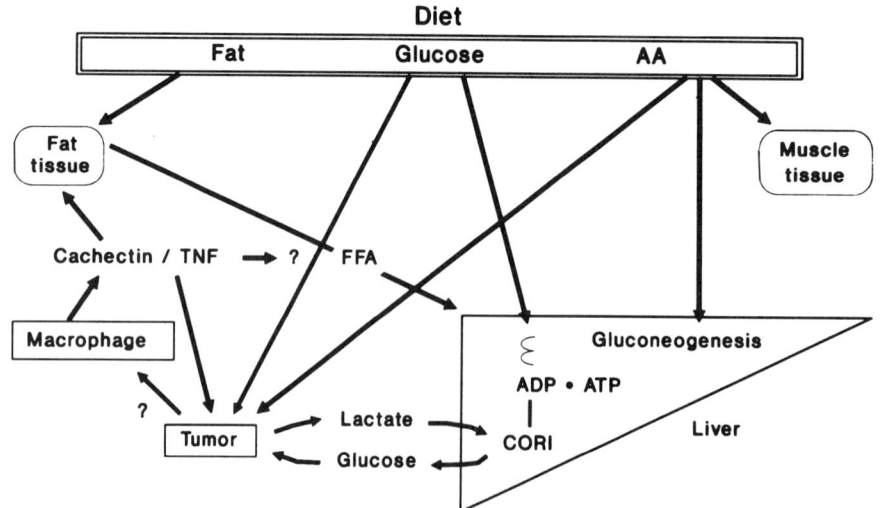

FIG. 1. Changes in the metabolism of fat, glucose, and amino acids (AA) induced by the presence of the tumor. ADP, adenosine diphosphate; ATP, adenosine triphosphate; FFA, free fatty acids; TNF, tumor necrosis factor.

tous involvement of the small intestine or its mesenteric lymphatics may induce a "celiac syndrome" (18). This could be explained by the disruption of intestinal epithelium due to generalized villous atrophy and the obstruction of mesenteric lymph glands with the resulting protein loss from dilated lymphatics within the intestinal villi (19). The ultimate clinical effect is steatorrhea and/or a protein-losing enteropathy.

Malabsorption is often the consequence of treatment, including radio- or chemotherapy. For example, the indiscriminate use of high-dose methotrexate in many childhood tumors, with its early and profound effect on the intestinal lining, constitutes a major problem (20). In addition, malnutrition, itself, may cause malabsorption. This "cancer enteropathy" may be caused by secondary changes in the small intestinal mucosa that result from a decrease in cell proliferation (21,22). The resulting reduction in intestinal enzymes produces a malabsorption state that compounds the nutritional problems that initiated it (23).

THERAPEUTIC FACTORS CONTRIBUTING TO NUTRITIONAL DEFICIENCY

Because multimodality-approach therapies for pediatric cancer may also affect normal tissues, they may contribute either directly or indirectly to nutritional deficiencies.

Chemotherapy and its consequences are potentially damaging to nutritional status and, significantly, there is evidence that nutritional status also affects the results of chemotherapy (Table 2) (24). Nearly all chemotherapeutic agents cause nausea and vomiting which may be severe, although usually brief. Rarely, patients suffer prolonged gastrointestinal toxicity. Some patients report vomiting for as long as a week following administration of cis-platinum (25). Constipation and adynamic ileus are major toxicities of vincristine that have also been observed (26). Mucosal ulceration presenting as mucositis, cheilosis, glossitis, stomatitis, and esophagitis painfully interfere with ingestion of nutrients. Actinomycin D and Adriamycin have been shown to exhibit the "recall phenomenon," i.e., the reactivation of latent radiation effects with subsequent administration of drugs (24). These reactions may affect oral intake by recreating severe irritation to the gastrointestinal mucosa.

Chemotherapy is also almost always myelosuppressive; children may well develop prolonged periods of severe neutropenia putting them at high risk of infection. The impact of this infection on nutritional status may be very damaging. The prevalent negative nitrogen balance associated with infection may result from the increased

TABLE 2. *Commonly used chemotherapeutic agents in childhood malignancies for which gastrointestinal toxicity is often seen*

Agent	Other conditions or results
Anorexia, nausea, vomiting	
Nitrogen mustard	Mucositis
Imidazole carboxamide (DTIC, DIC)	Stomatitis, hepatitis
Cis-diaminodichloroplatinum (CDDP)	Severe at doses $\geq$ 90 mg/m^2; also nephrotoxicity; ototoxicity
Adriamycin	Cardiomyopathy
Cyclophosphamide	Hemorrhagic cystitis
Mucositis	
Methotrexate	Radiation increases severity; nephrotoxicity; hepatitis; dermatitis
Vinblastine	May be accompanied by ileus, especially with high-dose schedules; myelosuppression
Bleomycin	Increases the severity with high doses and prolongs the mucositis; pulmonary fibrosis
Actinomycin D	Expected mucositis can be severe; radiation recall; hyperpigmentation
Adriamycin	Severe; radiation recall
Ileus	
Vincristine	Usually preventable with stool-softeners and laxatives; peripheral neuropathy
Vinblastine	As with vincristine; ileus rarely a problem with conventional low doses
Other significant GI toxicities	
Asparaginase	Hepatic dysfunction; coagulopathy; pancreatitis; hyperglycemia; hypersensitivity reactions
Methotrexate	Cirrhosis

caloric requirements, the decreased efficiency of the normal nitrogen-conserving mechanism, and the decreased intake (27).

The side effects from radiation therapy are usually localized, unlike those from chemotherapy. These may occur by a direct radiation effect upon the tumor or upon its surrounding normal tissue (24). Problems may be encountered acutely, during treatment, or as a delayed consequence (Table 3). Chronic radiation injury is especially likely to adversely affect nutrition. The effects on the gastrointestinal tract include mucositis with pain on deglutition, cramps, nausea, diarrhea, and malabsorption (28). The loss of taste for sucrose, hydrochloric acid, and quinine, studied before, during, and after oropharyngeal irradiation, occurs rapidly, returning to preirradiation acuity 60 to 120 days after the completion of treatment (29). These alterations probably result from radiation-induced damage to the microvilli of the taste cells or their surfaces (24).

Radiotherapy to major portions of the salivary glands results in decreased salivation and causes difficulty in eating. The volume of salivary secretion declines and the quality changes to a viscid, acid mixture with abnormally high amounts of organic minerals. Dysphagia as well as dental caries in cancer patients are often a result of this thickened saliva. This impairment of both taste and salivary secretion negatively affects food intake.

Radiation therapy also affects intestinal function. Nausea, vomiting, and diarrhea frequently result from irradiation. They may occur with the initiation of gastrointestinal irradiation and may persist throughout therapy, resulting in weight loss and malnutrition.

A delayed radiation-induced enteritis may occur at any time following a course of high-dose gastrointestinal irradiation, presenting as a chronic diarrhea or as a partial or complete obstruction (30). Its pathophysiology may be partially explained by gross morphologic changes in the bowel, alterations in the cell kinetics of intestinal mucosa, decreases in intestinal enzyme activity, and vascular abnormalities (31). Essentially, within 12 hr of the first irradiation treatment, the number of mitoses in the crypts of the bowel may be reduced significantly when compared to controlled preirradiation mitotic indices. Within several days, edema may collect in the submucosa. With progressive treatment, atrophy becomes marked, mucosal cells assume a cuboidal shape, lymphocytes diminish in the lamina propria, and polymorphonuclear leukocytes accumulate in increased numbers. The inflammatory reaction may be sufficiently severe to result in microabscess formation in some crypts. The lesions may persist for as long as 4 months after completion of therapy (32).

Malabsorption may also result from the effect of radiation on the absorptive cells and composition and concentration of enzymes in the mucosal brush border. Decrease of both disaccharidase and peptidase has been observed (32,33). The peculiar sensitivity of the bowel to radiation injury is undoubtedly due to the rapid cell turnover of the epithelium in the mucosa (34).

Thirty-eight percent of children who experience acute reactions during abdominal irradiation are prone to develop delayed radiation injury within 2 months after completion of therapy (30). Histologic appearances in the small bowel at the time of the delayed radiation injury revealed severe villous blunting, lymphatic dilatation, and moderately dense inflammatory infiltrates. Clinical improvement in all these patients, accompanied by a reversal of abnormal bowel roentgenographs and small bowel biopsies, followed the intake of a fractionated low-residue, low-fat diet, free of gluten and free of milk and milk products.

The extent of nutritional impairment resulting from combining chemo- and radiation therapy is not yet known. Fifty-five percent of the 44 children receiving aggressive combined treatment lost weight during the course of whole abdominal radiation (30). Severe acute enteritis was seen only in those patients receiving concomitant chemotherapy and radiation therapy.

Surgery is the third form of treatment for cancer, and radical surgical resection is the primary cause of malnutrition in pediatric cancer patients. Malnutrition occurs when either partial or total gastrectomy leads to problems causing malabsorption or decreased intake (35). The extent of nutritional sequelae is directly related to the extent of resection (36). In duodenal resection, nutritional impact is related more to the anatomic alteration of the pancreatic and biliary secretions than to the mechanical and absorptive functions of the duodenum itself. Studies demonstrate that although all nutrients except vitamin B_{12} are most efficiently absorbed in this segment of the intestine, in normal subjects the reserve capacity of the ileum can compensate for any functional change produced by loss of the more proximal bowel (37,38). In addition to this backup role, the distal ileum

TABLE 3. *Localized effects of radiotherapy causing GI symptoms*

Region	Acute	Chronic
Central nervous system	Nausea	
Head and neck	Sore throat	Ulcer
	Dysphagia	Xerostomia
	Xerostomia	Dental caries
	Stomatitis	
	Mucositis	
	Loss of taste	Altered taste
Thorax	Dysphagia	Fibrosis
	Fistula	Stenosis
Abdomen-pelvis	Anorexia	Ulcer
	Nausea	Malabsorption
	Vomiting	Diarrhea
	Diarrhea	Chronic enteritis
	Acute enteritis	Chronic colitis
	Acute colitis	

is also responsible for absorption of vitamin B_{12} and conjugated bowel salts. The increased absorptive capabilities of other segments of the small intestine is a major factor in preventing major clinical problems after small bowel resection except for patients whose resection is 75% or more of the total small bowel.

NUTRITIONAL ASSESSMENT OF CHILDREN WITH CANCER

Malnutrition is defined by (a) a pathological loss in total body mass, (b) a loss in lean body mass, and/or (c) a defect in the immune system (39). The various anthropometric and biochemical indices used for evaluation need further study to verify their validity for children with cancer (Table 4). Normal weight-height standards are used to assess total body mass. Children with a weight to height ratio of less than 80% of the 50th percentile for age and sex are considered malnourished. Lean body mass is usually assessed by measuring the midarm circumference corrected for subcutaneous fat, estimated by the triceps skin fold (40). A decreased serum albumin of less than 3.5 g/dl represents a state of visceral protein depletion (41–44). Immune function, as it relates to the nutritional state, is assessed by delayed hypersensitivity and total lymphocyte counts.

The problem with using normal standards for children with cancer is that although many of these children at the time of diagnosis are not overtly malnourished, many become malnourished quickly after the onset of treatment (1). These are "marginally malnourished" children who do not meet specific criteria for malnutrition, but whose body stores are depleted to the extent that overt malnutrition will follow without nutritional intervention (42). Although there are no laboratory tests that infallibly define these patients, they are most likely to present with a history of inadequate dietary intake, untreated anorexia, and/or malabsorption from ongoing treatment and specific diagnoses, including Ewing's sarcoma and neuroblastoma. Studies have investigated serum proteins, which have shorter half lives than albumin, to determine if these proteins can be used as early indicators of malnutrition in children with cancer (45–47).

One method of defining the nutritional status of pediatric cancer patients begins by determining baseline anthropometric measurements and transport proteins prior to treatment (Table 4).

Anthropometrics are calculated against standards from the National Center for Health Statistics (48). A weight-for-height of less than 90% of the standard is defined as first-degree malnutrition. Arm circumference and triceps skin fold are measured by techniques described by Grant (49). Values below the 15th percentile are considered representative of malnutrition. The lack of reliability in anthropometric data, especially for skinfold thickness and arm circumference, is due to the variation in technique and interpretation (50).

Visceral protein status is determined through radioimmunoassay by measuring serum concentrations such as prealbumin, albumin, transferrin, and retinol-binding protein (RBP).

Malnutrition is said to exist when a patient's weight-for-height is less than 90% of the standard and/or at least one abnormally low transport protein is present.

In our study of 51 newly diagnosed, untreated children with cancer (51), none had significant anthropometric deficits, but over 50% demonstrated abnormally low levels of prealbumin and retinol-binding protein. The majority of those patients who were not given nutritional intervention developed overt malnutrition while on therapy. Those who were given nutritional supplementation either maintained or improved in their nutritional status.

From this study, it is still too early to determine the effect of nutritional status on the ultimate survival of these children. There are, however, indications that favorable nutritional status has a positive prognostic effect on the outcome of children with cancer (43,52,53). In one study of 455 children, nutritional status was directly related to freedom from relapse among children with solid tumors, whether the disease was localized or nonlocalized (43). Of 18 children with stage IV neuroblastoma, the median survival of those malnourished at diagnosis was 5 months, compared with 12 months for those who had been adequately nourished (52). Van Eys (53) also reported a slightly improved survival in well-nourished patients with stage IV neuroblastoma.

Further studies are needed to corroborate the role of pediatric cancer on nutritional status and role of nutritional status on survival of the pediatric cancer patient.

CONSEQUENCES OF MALNUTRITION

Protein-energy malnutrition (PEM) in children with cancer affects major organ function, including immune competence, ability to resist infections, and bone marrow suppression (54–58).

TABLE 4. *Nutritional assessment of children with cancer*

Anthropometric
Height-for-age
Weight-for-age
Weight-for-height
Skin-fold thickness (triceps)
Arm circumference
Biochemical
Albumin
Transferrin
Prealbumin
Retinol-binding protein (RBP)

There is a strong relationship between malnutrition and immunity. Rickard et al. (3) documented anergy in 17 of 18 malnourished children with newly diagnosed advanced solid tumors and relapsed leukemia-lymphoma. Anergy was defined as the inability to respond to any one of four recall skin test antigens. Van Eys et al. (59) found significantly higher rates of infectious complications when children with metastatic disease involving bone were malnourished. In addition, an association of *Pneumocystis carinii* with protein-energy malnutrition has been found in malnourished children with cancer (60). Children with acute nonlymphocytic leukemia have also been found to have decreased ability to maintain skin test reactivity (61). Finally, bone marrow suppression may be attenuated by parenteral nutritional support in patients with stages III and IV neuroblastoma, acute nonlymphocytic leukemia, and metastatic disease involving bone (52,59,61,62).

Although the etiology of the immunologic impairment may be difficult to determine, it is likely that immune suppression in children with cancer, and the concomitant complications, are often nutritional rather than the result of treatment or the disease.

Malnutrition may also decrease tolerance to chemotherapy. Children who had optimal nutrition during the first 21 days of treatment had significantly fewer delays and fewer drug reductions throughout the first 10 weeks of treatment (52). Rickard et al. (62) also documented treatment tolerance benefits from reversal or prevention of PEM in 32 patients with Evans stage III or IV neuroblastoma.

Although the relationship between nutritional status and treatment tolerance has been corroborated in other studies (59,60,63) it is important to emphasize that ultimate survival is, nonetheless, predicated on the effectiveness of the primary oncologic treatment (53,64). The impact of nutritional support on outcome is most apparent, however, when therapy cannot be delivered because of the nutritional state of the patient.

In addition, malnutrition should be reversed in the child with cancer for the same reasons that it must be reversed for any child. Its simplest ramifications are lethargy, irritability, and a lack of interest in playing. The long-term, more serious consequences include inadequate growth and, when malnutrition occurs at an early age, the potential of delayed brain development (1). The improved prognosis for cure in pediatric cancer highlights the need to make sure that children with cancer maintain normal growth and development.

NUTRITIONAL SUPPORT

Nutritional support should consist of the simplest method that will be effective. Success will depend on the effectiveness of the team that designs and promotes it. Factors that must be considered include (a) current nutritional assessment, (b) identification of potential nutritional problems, (c) appropriate therapy, (d) monitoring of therapy, and (e) communication with patient, parents, and primary physicians (65).

For children with cancer who are at low nutritional risk, enteral nutrition is preferred (46). Children should be allowed to eat their favorite nutritious foods during treatment-free periods to prevent aversive conditioning associated with nausea and vomiting (66). Commercially available supplements that are concentrated sources of carbohydrate, protein, or fat can help satisfy nutrient requirements. It should be noted, however, that children who have the greatest need for supplements may be the least likely to accept them (46). Children who are unable to take adequate nutrition voluntarily but whose gastrointestinal tract is functional may be fed by nasogastric tube (67). Appropriate formulas are relatively low in osmolality and in residue. Patients fed by this method must be able to cooperate and have minimal gastrointestinal complaints and adequate platelet counts. There is also a need for family education and support by the oncology team.

Tube feeding, in general, however, is a less favorable method of nutritional support. There is often considerable psychological trauma resulting from the insertion and maintenance of tubes. In addition, effectiveness may be diminished by nausea and vomiting as well as decreased intestinal motility and absorption from ongoing treatment (46).

The advantages of enteral nutrition include a lower risk of infection or other catheter-related complications, normal play, economy, and a positive role for the parent and child in the child's care. Enteral feeding is also more likely to be effective in preventing malnutrition in well-nourished children who have less advanced disease or disease in remission on maintenance therapy and in children with acute lymphocytic leukemia with good prognosis. It is, however, ineffective in preventing or reversing malnutrition in most high-risk children undergoing intensive initial therapy (46).

Parenteral nutritional support may be used to supplement enteral feeding programs or to bypass a nutritionally ineffective gastrointestinal tract altogether. It is safe and effective in children with advanced neoplastic disease (68,69). The effectiveness of central parenteral nutrition (CPN) in reversing PEM and restoring immunity has been documented in a number of studies (3,62,70). All 18 malnourished children with stage III or IV solid tumors or second-relapse leukemia lymphoma who received CPN for a mean period of 24 days were able to normalize weight-for-height percentiles, subscapular skin-fold percentiles, and albumin and transferrin concentrations (3). Its efficacy, compared to enteral feeding, has also been shown in children undergoing abdominal-pelvic irradiation with or without additional chemotherapy (70). Total parenteral nutrition (TPN) has been associated with improved nutritional status during radiotherapy.

The effectiveness of hyperalimentation in reversing PEM may be dependent on its being given for not less than 10 days (3,42). CPN should be strongly considered for patients with abnormal gastrointestinal function in whom nutritional support is required for 28 days or longer. The central line would allow a greater concentration of glucose and would obviate problems with subcutaneous peripheral infiltrations. The daily complication rate appears to be no different between children fed peripherally or centrally (71). One study of 64 children with neoplastic diseases confirmed that complications (except for fever) that might be attributed to CPN were seen in the control groups, as well (69).

The value of TPN as adjunct treatment in newly diagnosed patients who are not malnourished has not been demonstrated. In addition, no nutritional support, and particularly parenteral nutrition, has demonstrated consistent therapeutic benefit to outcome, except in bone marrow transplantation (71). When nutritional support is indicated, however, the method or combination of methods chosen should be the one that is the most effective and the least risk to the patient (63).

CONCLUSION

Malnutrition occurs in up to 50% of children with cancer, including newly diagnosed patients (especially with disseminated disease), those who have suffered a relapse, and those undergoing intensive therapy. In children, the additional metabolic demands imposed by growth make it crucial to maintain adequate nutrition during therapy to prevent death either directly from starvation or from the increased susceptibility to infection. Although there is no clear evidence that nutritional support produces better outcome in children with cancer, studies indicate that some type of nutritional supplementation is important for maintaining normal growth in the young patient. There are no data, as yet, indicating that a well-nourished state prevents any form of childhood cancer.

REFERENCES

1. van Eys J. Nutrition of children with cancer. *Front Radiat Ther Oncol* 1982;16:177–183.
2. Carter P, Carr D, van Eys J, Coody D. Nutritional parameters in children with cancer. *J Am Diet Assoc* 1983;82:616.
3. Rickard KA, Grosfeld J, Kirksey A, Balantinc T, Baehner R. Reversal of protein-energy malnutrition in children during treatment of advanced neoplastic disease. *Ann Surg* 1979;190:771.
4. Bernstein IL. Etiology of anorexia in cancer. *Cancer* 1986;58:1881–1886.
5. Le Magner J. Body energy balance and food intake: a neuroendocrine regulatory mechanism. *Physiol Rev* 1983;63:314–386.
6. Kissileff HR, Van Itallie TB. Physiology of the control of food intake. *Annu Rev Nutr* 1982;2:371–418.
7. Lytle LD. Control of eating behavior. In: Wurtman RJ, Wurtman JJ, eds. *Nutrition and the brain,* vol 2. New York: Raven Press, 1977.
8. Bruera E, Carraro S, Roca E, et al. Association between malnutrition and caloric intake, emesis, psychological depression, glucose taste and tumor mass. *Cancer Treat Rep* 1984;68:873–876.
9. Dewys WD. Anorexia as a general effect of cancer. *Cancer* 1979;43:2013–2019.
10. Bernstein IL. Learned taste aversions in children receiving chemotherapy. *Science* 1978;200:1302–1303.
11. Wall DT, Gabriel LA. Alterations of taste in children with leukemia. *Cancer Nurs* 1983,Dec;447–452.
12. Norton J, Burt M, Brennan M. In vivo utilization of substrate by sarcoma bearing limbs. *Cancer* 1980;45:2934–2939.
13. Bruera E, Macdonald RN. Nutrition in cancer patients: an update and review of our experience. *J Pain Sympt Manag* 1988;3:133–140.
14. Holroyde C, Reichard G. Carbohydrate metabolism in cancer cachexia. *Cancer Treat Rep* 1981;65:55–59.
15. Torti F, Dieckman B, Beutler B, et al. A macrophage factor inhibits adipocyte gene expression: an in vitro model of cachexia. *Science* 1985;229:867–869.
16. Theologides A. Anorexins, asthenins, and cachectins in cancer. *Am J Med* 1986;81:296–298.
17. Bistrian B. Some practical and theoretical concepts in the nutritional assessment of cancer patients. *Cancer* 1986;58:1863–1866.
18. Ehrlich A, Stalder G, Geller W, Sherlock P. Gastrointestinal manifestations of malignant lymphoma. *Gastroenterology* 1968;54:1115–1121.
19. Waldman TA, Broder S, Strober W. Protein-losing enteropathies in malignancy. *Ann NY Acad Sci* 1974;230:306–317.
20. Green HL. The effects of malnutrition and cancer therapy agents on small bowel. In: van Eys J, Nichols BJ, Seelig M, eds. *Nutrition and cancer.* Spectrum Press, 1979.
21. Creamer B. Malignancy and the small intestinal mucosa. *Br Med J* 1964;2:1435–1436.
22. Hooper CS, Blair M. The effect of starvation on epithelial renewal in the rat duodenum. *Exp Cell Res* 1958;14:175–181.
23. Adibi SA, Allen ER. Impaired jejunal absorption rates of essential amino acids induced by either dietary caloric or protein deprivation in man. *Gastroenterology* 1970;59(3):404–413.
24. Donaldson SS, Lenon RA. Alterations of nutritional status: impact of chemotherapy and radiation therapy. *Cancer Suppl* 1979;43(5):2036–2052.
25. Gottlieb JA, Drewinko B. Review of the current clinical status of platinum coordination complexes in cancer chemotherapy. *Cancer Chemother Rep* 1975;59:621–628.
26. Sandler SG, Tobin W, Henderson ES. Vincristine-induced neuropathy in a clinical study of fifty leukemic patients. *Neurology* 1969;19:367–374.
27. Beisel WR, Sawyer WD, Ryll ED, Crozier D. Metabolic effects of intracellular infection in man. *Ann Intern Med* 1967;67:744–779.
28. Duncan W, Leonard JC. The malabsorption syndrome following radiotherapy. *Q J Med* 1965;34:319–329.
29. Conger AD. Loss and recovery of taste acuity in patients irradiated to the oral cavity. *Radiat Res* 1973;53:338–347.
30. Donaldson SS, Jundt S, Ricour C, Sarrazin D, Lemerle J, Schweisguth O. Radiation enteritis in children: a retrospective review, clinicopathologic correlation and dietary management. *Cancer* 1975;35:1167–1178.
31. Trier JS, Browning TH. Morphologic response of the mucosa of human small intestine to x-ray exposure. *J Clin Invest* 1966;45(2):194–204.
32. Tarpila S. Morphological and functional response of human small intestine to ionizing radiation. *Scand J Gastroenterol* 1971;6:(suppl 12): 1–52.
33. Jervis HR, Donati RM, Stromberg LR, Springz H. Histochemical investigation of the mucosa of the exteriorized small intestine of the rat exposed to x-radiation. *Strahlentherapie* 1969;137:326–343.
34. Lipkin M. Cell replication in the gastrointestinal tract in man. *Gastroenterology* 1965;48:616–624.
35. Bradley EL III, Isaacs J, Hersh T, Davidson O, Milikan W. Nutri-

tional consequences of total gastrectomy. *Ann Surg* 1975; 182:415–429.
36. Lawrence W. Effects of cancer on nutrition: impaired organ system effects. *Cancer Suppl* 1979;43(5):2020–2029.
37. Dowling RH. Compensatory changes in intestinal absorption. *Br Med Bull* 1967;23:275–278.
38. Wright HK, Tilson MD. The short gut syndrome: pathophysiology and treatment. In: *Current problems in surgery.* Chicago: Yearbook Medical Publishers, 1971.
39. van Eys J. Nutrition and neoplasia. *Nutr Rev* 1982; 40(12):353–359.
40. Blackburn GL, Schlamm HT. Nutritional assessment and treatment of hospital malnutrition. In: *Nutrition and cancer.* Van Eys J, Seelig MS, Nichols BL, eds. New York: SP Medical and Scientific Books, 1979; 1–30.
41. Lundholm K, Karlberg I, Schersten T. Albumin and hepatic protein synthesis in patients with early cancer. *Cancer* 1980;46:71–76.
42. van Eys J. Malnutrition in children with cancer: incidence and consequence. *Cancer* 1979;43:2030–2035.
43. Donaldson SS, Wesley MN, Dewys WD, et al. A study of the nutritional status of pediatric cancer patients. *Am J Dis Child* 1981;135:1107–1112.
44. Waterlow J. Classification and definition of protein calorie malnutrition. *Br Med J* 1972;3:566.
45. Coody R, Carr D, van Eys J, Carter P, Ramirez I, Taylor G. Use of thyroxine-binding prealbumin in the nutritional assessment of children with cancer. *JPEN J Parenter Enteral Nutr* 1983; 7(2):151–153.
46. Rickard K, Grosfeld J, Coates T, Weetman R, Baehner R. Advances in nutrition care of children with neoplastic diseases: a review of treatment, research, and application. *J Am Diet Assoc* 1986;86(12):1666–1676.
47. Yu LC, Kuvibidila S, Ducos R, Warrier RP. Nutritional status of children with cancer. *Clin Res* 1990;38(1):46A.
48. Hamill PV, Drizd TA, Johnson C, Reed RB, Roche AF, Moore WM. Physical growth: National Center for Health Statistics percentiles. *Am J Clin Nutr* 1979;32:607.
49. Grant A. *Nutritional assessment guideline.* Berkeley, CA: Cutter Laboratories, 1979;11–12.
50. Hall IC, O'Quigley J, Giles GR, Appleton N, Stocks H. Upper limb anthropometry: the value of measurement variance studies. *Am J Clin Nutr* 1980;33:1846.
51. Yu LC, Kuvibidila S, Warrier RP. Nutritional evaluation of pediatric patients with cancer. *Pediatr Res* 1991;29(4, part 2):154A.
52. Rickard KA, Detamore CM, Coates TD, et al. Effect of nutrition staging on treatment delays and outcome in stage IV neuroblastoma. *Cancer* 1983;52:587–598.
53. van Eys J. Effect of nutritional status on response to therapy. *Cancer Res* 1982;42(suppl):747x–753x.
54. Edelman R. Cell-mediated immune response in protein calorie malnutrition: a review. In: Suskind RM, ed. *Malnutrition and the immune response.* New York: Raven Press, 1977.
55. Chandra RK. Interaction of nutrition, infection and immune response: immunocompetence in nutritional deficiency, methological considerations and intervention strategies. *Acta Paediatr Scand* 1979;68:137.
56. Viteri FE, Schneider RE. Gastrointestinal alterations in protein calorie malnutrition. *Med Clin North Am* 1974;58:1487.
57. Finch CA. Erythropoiesis in protein calorie malnutrition. In: Olson RE, ed. *Protein calorie malnutrition.* New York: Academic Press, 1975.
58. Vilter RW. The anemia of protein calorie malnutrition. In: Olson RE, ed. *Protein calorie malnutrition.* New York: Academic Press, 1975.
59. van Eys J, Copeland EM, Cangir A, et al. A clinical trial of hyperalimentation in children with metastatic malignancies. *Med Pediatr Oncol* 1980;8:63–73.
60. Hughes WT, Price RA, Sisko F, et al. Protein-calorie malnutrition: a host determinant for *Pneumocystis carinii* infection. *Am J Dis Child* 1974;128:44–52.
61. Hays DM, Merritt RJ, White L, et al. Effect of total parenteral nutrition on marrow recovery during induction therapy for acute nonlymphocytic leukemia in childhood. *Med Pediatr Oncol* 1983;11:134–140.
62. Rickard KA, Loghmani ES, Gorsfeld JL, et al. Short- and long-term effectiveness of enteral and parenteral nutrition in reversing or preventing protein energy malnutrition in advanced neuroblastoma. A prospective randomized study. *Cancer* 1985; 56: 2881–2897.
63. Ghavimi R, Shils ME, Scott BF, et al. Comparison of morbidity in children requiring abdominal radiation and chemotherapy, with and without total parenteral nutrition. *J Pediatr* 1982; 101:530–537.
64. Mauer AM, Burgess JB, Donaldson SS, et al. Special nutritional needs of children with malignancies: a review. *JPEN J Parenter Enteral Nutr* 1990;14(3):315–324.
65. Cohen IT, Coulston AM, Ferrero CM, et al. The role of the nutritional team in the management of the child with cancer. *J Pediatr Surg* 1978;13:287–291.
66. Rickard K, Farnum S. Food for fun and thought: nutrition education in a children's hospital. *J Am Diet Assoc* 1974;65:294.
67. Lukens JN. Supportive care for children with cancer. Guidelines of the Children's Cancer Study Group. The use of nutritional therapy (review). *Am J Pediatr Hematol Oncol* 1984;6:261–265.
68. Rickard KA, Foland BB, Detamore CM, et al. Effectiveness of central parenteral nutrition vs peripheral parenteral nutrition plus enteral nutrition in reversing PEM in children with advanced neuroblastoma and Wilms' tumor: a prospective randomized study. *Am J Clin Nutr* 1983;38:445.
69. van Eys J, Wesley MN, Cnagir A, et al. Safety of intravenous hyperalimentation in children with malignancies: A Cooperative Group Trial. *JPEN J Parenter Enteral Nutr* 1982;6:291.
70. Donaldson SS, Wesley MN, Ghavimi F, et al. A prospective randomized clinical trial of total parenteral nutrition in children with cancer. *Med Pediatr Oncol* 1982;10:129–139.
71. Weisdorf SA, Lysne J, Wind D, et al. Positive effect of prophylactic total parenteral nutrition on long term outcome of bone marrow transplantation. *Transplantation* 1987;43:833–838.

CHAPTER 37

Nutritional Support of Children with Sickle-Cell Disease and Thalassemia

Solo Kuvibidila and Rajesekharan P. Warrier

SICKLE-CELL DISEASE

Sickle-cell disease (SCD), or sickle-cell anemia, is the most common genetic disease of African-Americans and of Africans south of the Sahara (1). In the United States, it affects between 0.26% and 0.35% of African-Americans (2). The disease results from a point mutation in DNA that leads to the substitution of glutamic acid by valine at the 6th position of the β-globulin chain of hemoglobin (Hb). Being a recessive trait, sickled hemoglobin (Hb S) is phenotypically expressed only when an individual is homozygous (Hb SS) or when there is a second mutation in the genes which code for Hb, as in the case of Hb C and Hb β^{thal}. The disease is characterized by hemolytic anemia caused by increased fragility of red blood cells (RBC), vaso-occlusive pain crises, increased susceptibility to bacterial infections, and delayed physical growth.

Although considerable effort has been devoted to understanding the genetic abnormalities of this disease, and the drugs that might control it, it is also important to understand the significant influence of nutritional factors on the outcome of SCD. The next section describes assessment of the nutritional status of children with sickle-cell disease, including anthropometry, transport proteins, vitamins, trace elements and minerals. The third section outlines the role of endocrine factors in the growth retardation of SCD children. The fourth section discusses cell-mediated immunity, humoral immunity, nonspecific immunity, and the responses to infections and vaccines. The fifth section describes the possible mechanisms responsible for growth retardation. The chapter concludes with a discussion of thalassemia.

Assessment of Nutritional Status

Anthropometric

Evaluation of the nutritional status of SCD children includes weight (Wt), height (Ht), and Wt/Ht (2–7). In addition, skin-fold thickness, head circumference, and somatomedin-C may also be used (3,8,9). Impaired physical growth, characterized by Wt and Ht below the 5th percentile of the NCHS growth charts (2–9), decreased levels of somatomedin-C (9), and delayed bone maturation (6,9) have been well documented in children with sickle-cell disease. Although there is no evidence of general growth retardation before, or at, 6 months of age, in some populations 17% to 22% of SCD children are below the 5th percentile for Wt and/or Ht (10).

Delayed physical growth appears after 6 months of age, at the time that the levels of fetal hemoglobin (Hb F) begin to decrease and clinical symptoms become apparent. By 2 years of age, the median Wt and Ht percentiles fall below the 50th percentile, with the deficits increasing with age (4,5). By 7 years of age, growth retardation is apparent (11). Although physical growth retardation is present in both sexes, boys seem to be more affected than girls (2,7).

The ability to achieve catch-up growth is unclear. Some investigators have reported that SCD patients who reach adulthood remain thin (2). Other studies indicate that adult SCD patients remain thin but achieve either normal or supranormal height (3). Differences in data probably reflect differences in the environmental conditions of study populations as well as differences in the

---

S. Kuvibidila, R. P. Warrier: Department of Pediatrics, Louisiana State University School of Medicine, New Orleans, Louisiana 70112.

TABLE 1. *Levels of transport proteins in sickle-cell disease children and control children*

	PA (mg/dl)	PA%[a]	RBP (mg/dl)	Tr (mg/dl)	Alb (g/dl)
SCD children					
Boys ($n = 20$)	14.4 ± 4.3	63.8 ± 28.2	2.95 ± 0.99*	242 ± 60	4.03 ± 0.41
Girls ($n = 14$)	13.3 ± 5.0	56.8 ± 18.9	3.39 ± 1.25†	254 ± 81	4.05 ± 0.42
All ($n = 34$)	14.0 ± 4.5	60.8 ± 24.6	3.13 ± 1.1**	246 ± 69	4.04 ± 0.46
Control children					
Boys ($n = 11$)	16.2 ± 5.6	62.0 ± 23.0	4.71 ± 3.1	276 ± 69	3.83 ± 0.46
Girls ($n = 12$)	16.7 ± 4.4	71.3 ± 18.3	5.70 ± 1.63	267 ± 38	4.20 ± 0.43
All ($n = 23$)	16.5 ± 4.9	67.8 ± 20.0	5.23 ± 2.44	272 ± 54	4.03 ± 0.47

Mean ± SD. PA, prealbumin; RBP, retinol-binding protein; Tr, transferrin; Alb, albumin.

[a] PA% = percent of the expected value for age and sex. The expected values for sex and age are those published by Bevenga et al. (113).

* $p < .05$; † $p < .001$; ** $p < .07$; SCD children compared to control children (ANOVA). No significant differences were found between sexes.

disease process and the secondary metabolic consequences of the disease.

Protein and Vitamin Assessment

Transport Proteins

The visceral proteins, albumin (Alb), prealbumin (PA), transferrin (Tr), retinol-binding protein (RBP), and total serum proteins, have been measured in several studies (8–10). The results of our study (Table 1) and others suggest that albumin and transferrin synthesis are not affected by the disease process (8,9). PA and RBP, which have shorter half-lives (19 hr and 8 hr, respectively) are, in contrast, decreased in both boys and girls as well as in adult patients (12). Both of these proteins are more affected in growth-retarded than in growth-normal SCD children (8).

Thus, children with SCD have decreased Wt, Ht, and body fat, a delayed bone age, decreased somatomedin-C levels, and decreased levels of RBP and PA, but normal levels of total protein, albumin, and transferrin (Table 2).

Fat-Soluble Vitamins

Vitamin A. In addition to its antioxidant function, vitamin A is required for growth, regeneration of epithelial cells, cell-mediated immunity, and for normal vision (6,13,14). Decreased plasma levels of retinol and its carrier, retinol-binding protein, have been reported in most SCD children although the mean levels are more reduced in those who are growth-retarded (8,10,15,16). Abnormal levels of plasma vitamin A precursors (β-carotene, α-carotene and cryptoxanthin) have also been reported in adult SCD patients (17).

Abnormalities associated with vitamin A deficiency such as growth retardation, impaired cell-mediated immunity, and abnormal dark adaptation (night blindness) have been described in SCD children and adults. However, since some of these functions are also altered in other nutritional disorders such as protein-energy malnutrition (PEM) and zinc deficiency, it is not known whether long-term, mild vitamin A deficiency plays an important role in these abnormalities. The effects of vitamin A supplementation at recommended dietary allowance (RDA) levels (5,000 IU) on plasma retinol and growth rate were studied in children 10 years old and older (15). After 3 months of supplementation, there was no improvement in either plasma retinol levels or growth rate. This suggests that the limiting factor for growth in these children may be inadequate caloric intake or factors other than an inadequate vitamin A intake. No data have been published on liver vitamin A stores in SCD patients. There are also no data suggesting inadequate vitamin A intake. In fact, in a study conducted by Finan et al. (8) on normal-growing and growth-retarded SCD children, vitamin A intake was reportedly more than three to four times the RDA. If vitamin A intake is more than adequate, and fat absorption is normal, the decreased levels of plasma retinol must be due to either a defect in vitamin A metabolism or a decreased synthesis of RBP occurring as a result of decreased visceral protein synthesis.

TABLE 2. *Anthropometric assessment and transport protein levels in sickle-cell disease children*

Decreased
Weight
Height
Body fat
Delayed development of bone age
Somatomedin-C
Plasma prealbumin
Plasma retinol-binding protein
Normal
Total serum protein
Albumin
Transferrin

Vitamin E. Vitamin E, or α-tocopherol, is the most studied fat-soluble vitamin in SCD patients because of its direct role in preventing lipid peroxidation of RBC membranes and cytoplasm. Lipid peroxidation causes the RBC to become more rigid, affects the RBC membrane permeability to calcium and other macromolecules and ions, increases RBC hemolysis, decreases RBC life span, and worsens the clinical severity of SCD.

Measurement of plasma levels of α-tocopherol in SCD patients has yielded controversial results. Most (15,17–22) but not all (8,9,23) studies have demonstrated abnormal plasma levels when compared to control subjects. In one study, although plasma vitamin E levels of SCD children were similar to those of non-SCD children, RBC vitamin E levels were higher in SCD children than in controls (8). The study by Chiu and Lubin (22), however, reported decreased RBC and plasma vitamin E levels in SCD.

Absorption of oral vitamin E was either normal (8) or abnormally low (17) in SCD children. Vitamin E supplementation for 1 to 2 months resulted in an increase in plasma vitamin E levels compared to pretreatment levels (15,19). Long-term double-blind studies on a large population are needed for corroboration of these positive effects.

The etiology of the low levels of plasma vitamin E in SCD patients has been ascribed to poor dietary intake, malabsorption of dietary fat, abnormal levels of plasma low-density lipoproteins (the vitamin E carrier molecules), and increased utilization and catabolism. To date, there is no evidence that dietary intake is abnormal in SCD children. In adult SCD patients, vitamin E and total fat intake are reportedly slightly higher than in control subjects (16). Malabsorption, suggested by Chiu et al. (17), is questionable, not only because of the normal fat absorption observed by other investigators (24) but also because of the normal response to an oral dose of vitamin E reported in some of the patients studied by Heyman et al. (9). In addition, the increase in plasma vitamin E levels following supplementation suggests adequate vitamin E absorption. More plausible is the suggestion by Stone et al. (20) and Adebonojo et al. (21) that abnormal levels of low-density lipoproteins may contribute to the low plasma vitamin E levels seen in SCD patients. Finally, the most important mechanism may be an increased utilization of vitamin E because of the increased sensitivity of sickled RBC to lipid peroxidation, especially in the presence of hydrogen peroxide (H_2O_2).

Water-Soluble Vitamins

Abnormal levels of ascorbic acid (vitamin C) have been reported in SCD patients, significant because of vitamin C's role as an anti-oxidant (16,25,26). Incubation of sickle cells with ascorbic acid in the presence of H_2O_2 leads to reduced lipid peroxidation, as measured by malonyl-aldehyde formation (25). Decreased leukocyte vitamin C levels have also been reported (26). There is no report suggesting poor dietary intake of vitamin C in SCD children. In adult SCD patients, ascorbic acid intake was found to be three times the RDA (16). As is true for vitamin E, low plasma and/or leukocyte vitamin C may be due to increased utilization.

Decreased plasma levels of vitamin B_6 (27), increased levels in red blood cells (28), deficiencies of riboflavin (29) and folate (28), and abnormal levels of plasma cobalamin (30) have also been reported. Increased utilization may again be the most important factor in the decrease in at least some of these factors.

In summary, SCD children appear to suffer from mild or moderate deficiencies of vitamin A, α-tocopherol, ascorbic acid, folate, riboflavin, and pyridoxine (Table 3). Because these vitamins play a role in many biochemical processes such as anti-oxidant activity (vitamins A, C, and E), and in the detoxification of free radicals (lipid peroxides) or hemoglobin biosynthesis (folate), even mild deficiencies of these nutrients may worsen the severity of SCD.

Trace Elements and Mineral Assessment

Selenium and Zinc

Selenium and zinc are the two most important trace elements that have been studied in SCD. Selenium is a cofactor of glutathione peroxidase, an enzyme required for detoxification of H_2O_2 and other peroxides (32). As previously noted, red cell membranes of sickled cells are more sensitive to lipid peroxidation than those of normal RBC, and sickled RBC produce more H_2O_2 than normal RBC (31). Removal of both hydrogen peroxide and hydroperoxides is required to sustain the normal RBC and increase the life span of sickled RBC.

Data on glutathione peroxidase (GPx) activity in SCD RBC are controversial. Although some studies have suggested no significant change in GPx activity compared to non-SCD subjects (33), others have suggested either an

TABLE 3. *Fat- and water-soluble vitamin status of children with sickle-cell disease*

Vitamins	Response
Fat Soluble	
Plasma retinol (vitamin A)	Decreased
α-Tocopherol (vitamin E)	Decreased
Water Soluble	
1. Riboflavin (vitamin B_2)	Decreased
2. Pyridoxine (vitamin B_6)	Decreased
3. Cobalamin (vitamin B_{12})	Decreased
4. Ascorbic acid (vitamin C)	Decreased
5. Folate	Decreased

increase (21) or a decrease (22). In one study, plasma selenium levels were lower in SCD patients than in normal controls (22). It is, however, still unclear whether selenium deficiency actually exists in SCD children and how important it is. In addition, the activity of glutathionine peroxidase is influenced by several other nutrients or factors, such as vitamin B_6 and riboflavin. Deficiencies of both of these vitamins have been reported in SCD children (27,29).

Zinc, the most studied trace element, is required for normal physical growth, control of vision through vitamin A metabolism, gonadal development, and cell-mediated immunity. Some studies (15,34–38) have suggested zinc deficiency in SCD patients, whereas others have not (8,39,40). Even in studies in which zinc deficiency was demonstrated, not all SCD patients were affected. However, it has been clearly shown that following zinc supplementation, several abnormal functions, including dark adaptation, physical growth, natural killer cell activity, and sexual maturation, return to normal (34,38,41).

As with other nutrients, studies on zinc supplementation have not resulted in uniform results. For example, in a study by Heyman et al. (9), SCD children supplemented with trace elements, including zinc, but without increased caloric intake did not have an increase in height, weight or body fat.

The lack of consistent data may be partially due to the fact that plasma zinc was used in some studies. Plasma zinc is a poor indicator of zinc status, in part because of contamination with RBC zinc which is 14-fold greater than that of plasma zinc. Zinc deficiency in SCD patients has been attributed to urinary losses. Until zinc deficiency is demonstrated in all populations of SCD patients, it will remain uncertain whether zinc supplementation should be generally recommended.

Iron

Iron deficiency, as determined by decreased bone marrow iron stores, has been demonstrated in SCD children and adults, especially pregnant women (42). An increased prevalence of iron deficiency has been reported in SCD children (36% to 47%) and pregnant women (63% to 80%) in Africa and Jamaica but not in the United States (43). In general, little attention has been paid to the prevalence of iron deficiency in SCD patients because of the influence of both iron deficiency and SCD on some of the most frequently measured indicators of iron status, such as hemoglobin and mean corpuscular volume. Serum ferritin, the most sensitive indicator of iron status, is useful in the diagnosis of iron deficiency in SCD children and/or adults only when they are in a stable state and not infected. Following pain crisis, serum ferritin levels are falsely increased (42).

The most important problem associated with iron metabolism in SCD patients, however, is not iron deficiency but iron overload, especially in adults who have received multiple blood transfusions. Iron deposition in the parenchymal cells due to blood transfusion induces lipid peroxidation and causes spleen and liver dysfunction.

Splenectomy due to splenic dysfunction leads to increased susceptibility to infections. This results in the production of H_2O_2, which causes lipid peroxidation and hence RBC hemolysis. The management of iron status in these patients is, therefore, more difficult than that of other trace elements such as zinc.

Copper, Magnesium, Manganese, Chromium, and Calcium

Little information is available on either copper or magnesium status of SCD children. SCD patients have higher levels of plasma copper than normal children but their RBC copper levels are similar to those of controls (44). SCD patients have lower levels of plasma magnesium but higher RBC magnesium levels than normal individuals (44). No information is available on the manganese or chromium status of SCD patients.

Intracellular RBC levels of calcium are higher in SCD patients than in non-SCD individuals (45). The increased RBC calcium levels contribute to the formation of irreversibly sickled cells.

In summary, data available in the literature suggest that zinc deficiency exists in many SCD patients due to increased urinary excretion (Table 4). Iron deficiency in children as well as pregnant women also exists. However, with regard to iron status, iron overload, especially in older patients who have received multiple blood transfusions, is more frequent than iron deficiency. There is no evidence of copper deficiency in SCD children. Too few studies have been conducted on other trace elements such as selenium, magnesium and chromium to understand their effect on SCD.

Endocrine Assessment

In an attempt to explain the delayed physical growth and sexual maturation frequently observed in SCD children, endocrine and pituitary functions have been studied. Basal levels of growth hormone as well as growth hormone responses to insulin-induced hypoglycemia are reportedly normal in SCD children (46). Growth hormone responses to growth hormone releasing factor are

TABLE 4. *Trace elements and minerals in SCD patients*

	Plasma/Serum	RBC	WBC
Zinc	Decreased/±	Decreased	Decreased
Selenium	Decreased	–	–
Magnesium	Decreased	Increased	–
Copper	Increased	±	–
Iron	Increased/±; decreased	Increased[a]	–
Calcium	–	Increased	–

RBC, red blood cells; WBC, white blood cells; ±, normal or no change; –, information is unknown.
[a] RBC ferritin.

also not altered (47). This suggests that the abnormal growth rate is not due to a defect in the pituitary response.

In the evaluation of gonadal function, circulating plasma levels of testosterone, luteinizing hormone (LH), and follicle-stimulating hormone (FSH) have been studied in SCD adult patients from Africa (48) and the United States (49). Both studies suggest that plasma testosterone levels are decreased in SCD patients compared to control African or African-American males. The levels of LH and FSH have been reported to be decreased in African patients (48) but not in African-Americans (49). Following stimulation with gonadotropin releasing factor, the levels of LH and FSH further increase, suggesting hypogonadism in these patients (49).

Thyroid function has been studied in SCD children by Lukanmbi et al. (50). Thyroid function as assessed by serum levels of thyroxine, thyroxine-binding capacity, and the calculated thyroxine index of free thyroxine, is normal. However, the levels of thyrotropin (TSH) are significantly decreased, a function that is inconsistent with the normal thyroxine levels and thyroxine-binding capacity.

Immune Status and Response to Infections

The immune response has also been studied in SCD (Table 5). The percentage of total T cells, helper T cells, and suppressor/cytotoxic T cells, is either normal, decreased, or increased (38,51–57), and that of B cells is either normal or increased. The percentage of monocytes and neutrophils is higher in SCD patients than in controls of similar age, sex, and gender (53,58). All SCD patients consistently show an abnormal skin test response to antigens (26,58), decreased activity of killer cells and natural killer cells (26,41,57), and decreased opsonic activity to yeast (59) and/or streptococcus pneumonia (60).

Most (38,51,57,60,61,62) but not all (63,64) studies show impaired proliferative responses of blood lymphocytes to different mitogens. Although the concentration of complement components is either normal (65,66), decreased (67), or increased (68), the classical complement pathway is normal and the alternative pathway is increased, probably due to continuous stimulation by bacteria. The response to pneumococcal polysaccharide vaccines is normal (66,70), whereas total serum Ig levels are either normal (53), increased (71,72), or decreased (71). In parallel with normal responses to vaccination, the incidence of pneumococcal infection in vaccinated children is decreased (73).

TABLE 5. *Immune status of children with sickle-cell disease*

Variables	Responses
Cellular response	
Skin responses to antigens	Decreased (impaired)
T cells	Normal, decreased, or increased
Helper T cells	Normal, decreased, or increased
Suppressor T cells	Normal or increased
Proliferative response to blood lymphocytes to mitogens	Normal or decreased
B cells	Normal or increased
Neutrophils	Increased
Monocytes	Increased
Humoral response	
Immunoglobulin levels	Normal or increased
Complements levels	Normal, decreased, or increased
Classical complement pathway	Normal
Alternative complement pathway	Increased
Opsonization of yeast	Decreased (impaired)
Opsonization of strep pneumonia	Decreased (impaired)
Response to vaccination (pneumococcal polysaccharides)	Normal
Infection rate	
Incidence of pneumococcal infections before 5 years of age	Increased
Incidence of infection following vaccination	Decreased or no change

Etiology of Growth Retardation

If the abnormal physical growth observed in SCD children is not the result of a defect in the response of pituitary growth hormone to growth hormone releasing factor, then it must be ascribed to other factors such as inadequate nutrition and recurrent infections. Although the cause and effect are not always possible to separate, it is generally accepted that malnutrition, whether of single or multiple nutrients, alters resistance to infection, and that infection precipitates malnutrition by causing anorexia, and affecting nutrient absorption and utilization.

Four possible mechanisms related to nutrient status may explain the growth retardation in SCD children: (a) decreased dietary intake of energy, (b) increased requirements for energy and other nutrients, (c) malabsorption of nutrients and/or (d) increased turnover (utilization, catabolism, excretion, etc.).

Decreased Dietary Intake of Energy and Other Nutrients

Existing data on dietary intake of SCD patients remain controversial. Some investigators have found decreased dietary intakes in SCD (9), while others have found normal intake (8,16). Decreased dietary intake may result from anorexia associated with infection. Frequent pneumococcal infections, especially in children under 5 years of age, are, in fact, the most common cause of death in these patients.

Increased Nutrient Requirements

Accelerated breakdown of the RBC is one of the most important characteristics of SCD. In a normal non-SCD adult, the life span of an RBC is 120 days; in children, it is 90 days. In SCD patients, however, the RBC life span has been estimated to be only 15 to 20 days (74), due to membrane lipid peroxidation and increased permeability to different macromolecules, including minerals such as calcium. The rate of red cell destruction has been estimated to be 6 to 20 times that of a non-SCD individual. Therefore, for an SCD patient to maintain his/her RBC mass, the rate of Hb synthesis also has to increase by 6- to 20-fold. Since energy is required for the synthesis of Hb, it is likely that energy as well as protein and/or vitamin requirements must also increase.

Increased Hb SS breakdown may, in fact, also increase the requirement for specific amino acids such as histidine, glycine, valine, leucine—amino acids that are in a high concentration in hemoglobin (74). Although some of these amino acids are reabsorbed in the kidneys and reutilized, the efficiency of reabsorption may not be adequate due to impaired renal function with increasing age. This implies that RDA dietary intake may not meet actual requirements. Failure to increase energy intake may lead to decreased growth rate, in part because the intake of all other nutrients including nitrogen (protein), fat, water-soluble vitamins, minerals, and trace elements is directly related to energy intake.

Studies on energy intake in children (9) and adults (16) suggest normal or slightly above normal intake of energy when compared to the RDA. Heyman et al. (9), on the other hand, found, in two children, that increasing energy and protein intake by nasogastric feeding improved physical growth and body fat, decreased the frequency of hospitalization and pain crises, and improved health status in general. In the same study, children given only trace elements, including zinc and vitamins (folate and vitamin E), failed to show any improvement. Since the sample size was small, it is uncertain how general and important the increased energy requirement may be. Energy requirements are especially difficult to study outside of a controlled environment because of the lack of reliability of the recall method in free-living persons.

Malabsorption

Thus far, there is lack of conclusive evidence associating malabsorption with growth retardation of SCD children. Rahbar et al. (24), studying glucose tolerance and absorption of xylose, fat, and protein, found normal gastrointestinal function in all children. Jejunal biopsy was also normal. Heyman et al. (9), studying vitamin E absorption in five children, found normal absorption in three children and abnormal absorption in the other two. A study by Chiu et al. (17) on vitamin E absorption also suggested abnormal curves compared to non-SCD children. These two studies suggest impaired fat absorption in some SCD children. The studies of Sindel et al. (15) and Natta et al. (19), on the other hand, show increased plasma vitamin E levels after vitamin E supplementation for 1 to 3 months, which implies adequate fat absorption. Given the limited and controversial data on fat absorption, the association between malabsorption and delayed growth rate in SCD children is not clear.

Increased Turnover and Catabolism of Certain Nutrients

Increased Hb breakdown in SCD patients, which may cause an increase in nitrogen and energy requirements relative to non-SCD patients, has been reviewed. Several vitamins, A, B_2, B_6, B_{12}, E, C, and folate, have been studied. Vitamin A, for example, plays a crucial role in growth and defense against infections. The utilization of vitamins A, E, and C is crucial in the frequency and severity of pain crises because of their roles as antioxidants. A high rate of lipid peroxidation of RBC in SCD patients not only has been demonstrated *in vitro*, but is also responsible for accelerated RBC breakdown.

Due to the increased rate of lipid peroxidation of sickled RBC and the increased rate of production of hydrogen peroxide, children with SCD must continue utilizing their anti-oxidant pool in order to protect their RBC, thereby depleting it over time.

Thus, increased requirements resulting from increased turnover and catabolism of nutrients, relative to actual intake, are most likely the basis for the nutritional depletion of these nutrients and the associated growth retardation in SCD children.

Sickle Cell Disease: Conclusion

There is no doubt that deficiencies of several nutrients exist in SCD children. Although more studies are needed, the abnormal levels of some nutrients (vitamins A, E, and C, and zinc) do not seem to be due to poor dietary intake or to malabsorption. Increased utilization, as in the case of vitamin E and C, or increased excretion (zinc), may be responsible for deficiencies.

Energy may be the one nutrient in which intake is inadequate. Energy requirements in all children may be divided into four components: requirements for basal metabolic rate, requirements for physical activity, requirements for growth and development, and replenishment of the portion lost through the skin and other routes. Each component must be satisfied to maintain energy balance.

There is no evidence that basal metabolic rate is increased in SCD children relative to non-SCD children. However, the increased rate of RBC destruction, the increased rate of daily Hb synthesis and RBC membrane production, pain crises, and the increased incidence of infection not only alter energy metabolism through losses, poor absorption, and utilization, but also increase the metabolic rate. The result is an increased energy requirement in SCD.

Dietary intake of all nutrients is also directly related to energy intake except when vitamins and/or mineral supplements are given. The SCD child requires increased energy in order to replace the destroyed RBC and Hb. In all documented cases of nutritional deficiencies, supplementation has been recommended. However, supplementation of all nutrients may be dangerous because of possible side effects and the long-term effects of megadoses of some nutrients. Prospective studies on dietary intake, with adequate sample sizes, are required to determine which nutrients must be supplemented, for how long, and from what age.

THALASSEMIA

Thalassemias are hereditary anemias caused by decreased, or lack of, production of either the α or the β polypeptide in hemoglobin. Most α-thalassemia occurs in China and the Far East, whereas β-thalassemia occurs primarily in Mediterranean and African countries (75). The nature of the genetic defect determines the degree of red blood cell destruction and the resultant clinical picture (76). The most severe form in North America is homozygous β-thalassemia major. It presents with severe hemolysis and ineffective erythropoiesis and is characterized by severe hypochromia, target cells, organomegaly, transfusion dependency complicated by growth failure, and hemosiderosis. The severe forms of α-thalassemia with deletion of three or four loci are seen in the Far East and may result in hydrops fetalis (Bart's hemoglobin) or hemolytic anemia (Hb H disease.)

Advances in the molecular analysis of hemoglobins have improved the antenatal and neonatal diagnosis of these hemoglobinopathies. In the future, genetic engineering may completely alter the course of the disease. Bone marrow transplantation has also improved prognosis in β-thalassemia major.

Optimal nutritional status is essential in thalassemia in order to take advantage of future therapeutic modalities and to avoid growth failure, delayed sexual development, and the immune deficiency that may be associated with the secondary malnourished status of the patient.

Assessment of Nutritional Status

Folic Acid

Folic acid deficiency is frequently the cause of megaloblastic anemia in β-thalassemia major (77,78). Folic acid deficiency associated with megaloblastic anemia has also been documented in heterozygous β-thalassemia (thalassemia minor) (79–81). While the Indian and Italian studies have documented decreased folate even in β-thalassemia minor, Fromme et al. (82), in Israel, have documented normal folate levels in heterozygous thalassemia patients. Folate deficiency may well result from red cell destruction and increased needs secondary to increased erythropoiesis as well as decreased intake and absorption. Folic acid supplementation of 1 mg/day is required for patients with thalassemia major or minor. Chronically transfused patients with well-maintained hematocrits and very little active erythropoiesis do not need supplementation (76).

Vitamin B_{12}

Vitamin B_{12} deficiency is rarely diagnosed in thalassemia patients (83). However, Kumar et al. (78) observed that the diagnosis of folate and B_{12} deficiencies cannot be based solely on serum folate or B_{12} levels. They recommend a therapeutic trial to confirm the deficiencies. Jenks et al. (84) reported an unusual case of a woman who presented with two coexisting genetic disorders, thalassemia and cobalamin R. binder deficiency.

Vitamin C

The role of vitamin C in the thalassemic child with hemosiderosis has been perplexing. Hypercatabolism of vitamin C with resultant low levels has been reported in siderotic Bantus by Lynch et al. (85). The effectiveness of ascorbic acid supplementation in enhancing the chelating effect of desferrioxamine (86) should be balanced by the potential of cardiotoxicity (87). Because supplemental vitamin C may induce cardiotoxicity in chronically transfused children receiving desferrioxamine, caution is warranted (87,88). Ozzincolo et al. (89) described radiological abnormalities in long bones, comparable to rachitic and scorbutic changes, that they attributed to a possible toxicity of the chelating agent, desferrioxamine.

Vitamin E

Vitamin E acts as a potent anti-oxidant in red cell membrane lipid peroxidation (90). Very low levels of vitamin E have been reported in homozygous β-thalassemia/Hb E and α-thalassemia (91). Low levels of vitamin E also have been described in sickle-cell anemia, β-thalassemia, and other chronic hemolytic anemias. It has also been suggested that vitamin E deficiency results from increased utilization in the repair of oxidative damage to the red cell membrane and other tissues (92–94). The use of vitamin E in β-thalassemia has not resulted in a decrease in transfusion requirements, increased Hb levels, or other significant clinical benefits (95,96).

Adding canthaxanthin to vitamin E did not improve the results obtained by vitamin E alone in nine patients treated for 4 to 10 months (97). Plasma levels of vitamin E did increase with the decrease in erythrocyte lipid membrane peroxidation but there were no changes in such clinical parameters as hemoglobin levels and transfusion requirements.

Zinc

Growth retardation and delay in sexual maturation is a well-documented but unexplained phenomenon in thalassemia (98–100). Prasad et al. (100) and others have assumed that impaired growth was secondary to zinc deficiency. However, Rea et al. (101) studied 92 patients with β-thalassemia who had been treated for 2 years with hypertransfusion and desferrioxamine, which chelates both iron and zinc. In these patients, there was no apparent decrease in serum, hair, or urine zinc levels. In addition, most of the children also had normal growth.

Decreased serum zinc levels have been reported by Aracasoy et al. (102) and Vatanavicharn et al. (103). Vatanavicharn et al. studied 14 patients with Hb H disease, 34 patients with β-thalassemia/Hb E disease, and 30 control subjects. Plasma zinc levels were decreased and the plasma copper levels higher in patients than in controls. Plasma copper to zinc (cu:zn) ratio is a more sensitive index of zinc deficiency than the plasma level alone. Thalassemics with retarded growth had higher cu:zn ratios than patients with normal development (104). The increased urinary zinc levels in thalassemic children may be secondary to the chronic hemolytic state. Liver impairment secondary to hemosiderosis may also increase urinary zinc excretion.

Aracasoy et al. (105) found decreased zinc levels, increased serum copper, and iron, and normal magnesium in a study of 42 thalassemics. Growth retardation may result from the decreased production of somatomedin-A secondary to the chronic zinc deficiency. Zinc supplementation of 45 mg/day did not result in any significant growth differences in 11 thalassemic patients who were compared to unsupplemented controls over a period of 3 to 5 years. More positive results were obtained in four patients given zinc in doses adequate to achieve and maintain normal blood levels (102).

Protein-Energy Malnutrition

Few studies have looked at protein-energy malnutrition (PEM) in thalassemic patients. Rea et al. (101) found no evidence of PEM in 92 hypertransfused patients, 82 homozygous β-thalassemic patients, or 82 control subjects when weight, height, and total protein and plasma albumin levels were evaluated.

Immune Status of Patients with Acute Thalassemia

Defects in immune status ranging from defective phagocytic and bactericidal function of polymorphonuclear lymphocytes to alterations in T cell lymphocyte numbers, natural killer (NK) cell activity (106), and mitogenic responsiveness of lymphocytes and immunoglobulin production have been described (107–112). The significant effects of malnutrition on immunity may be responsible for some of the deficits in immune function found in patients with thalassemia.

SUMMARY

Children with sickle-cell disease suffer from growth retardation as determined by deficits in weight, height, body fat (skin-fold thickness), growth velocity, bone age, and sexual maturation. Growth retardation does not occur before 6 months of age, but many children at 2 years are already below the 50th percentile for weight and/or height. These deficits increase with age, boys being more affected than girls. Abnormal biochemical parameters include prealbumin, retinol-binding protein, plasma retinol, α-tocopherol, pyridoxine, riboflavin, folate, ascorbic acid, fatty acids, and zinc. Iron deficiency and iron overload exist in patients of different ages. The several impaired immune responses, including skin response to antigens, T cell numbers, lymphocyte proliferation, NK cell activity, neutrophil function, and increased susceptibility to infections, have been attributed to specific nutrient deficiencies, in addition to other factors. Increased energy requirement due to the increased turnover of red blood cells may be one of the main causes of growth retardation in SCD. Additional research on specific nutrient deficiencies and specific requirements may have significant implications regarding the treatment of the child with SCD.

The effects of nutritional deficiencies in thalassemia, and their relationship to immunity, infection, and other clinical parameters, require further study. Deficiencies are most likely detrimental to the complicated clinical course of the chronically hypertransfused child. Improved therapeutic intervention will result from an increased understanding of these problems.

REFERENCES

1. Nutritional costs of sickle cell anemia. In: Enwonwu CO, ed. *Impact of nutrition on health and disease in blacks and other minorities.* Annual Nutrition Workshop Series, vol 1, Nashville: Meharry Medical College, 1987.
2. Phebus CK, Gloninger MF, Maciak BJ. Growth patterns by age and sex in children with sickle cell disease. *J Pediatr* 1984;105(1):28–33.
3. Kramer MS, Rooks Y, Washington LR, Pearson HA. Pre- and postnatal growth and development in sickle cell anemia. *J Pediatr* 1980;96(5):857–860.
4. Grey RH. Clinical features of homozygous SS disease in Jamaican children. *West Indian Med J* 1971;20:60–68.
5. Lowry MF, Desai P, Ashcroft MT, Sergeant BE, Sergeant GR. Heights and weights of Jamaican children with homozygous sickle cell disease. *Hum Biol* 1977;49:429–436.
6. Olambiwonnu NO, Penny R, Frasier SD. Sexual maturation in subjects with sickle cell anemia. Studies of serum gonadotropin concentration, height, weight, and skeletal age. *J Pediatr* 1975;87:459–464.
7. McCormack MK, Dicken L, Katz SH, et al. Growth pattern of children with sickle cell disease. *Hum Biol* 1976;48:429–437.
8. Finan AC, Elmer MA, Sasanow SR, McKinney S, Russel MO, Gill FM. Nutritional factors and growth in children with sickle cell disease. *Am J Dis Child* 1988;142:237–240.
9. Heyman MB, Katz R, Hurst D, et al. Growth retardation in sickle cell disease treated by nutritional support. *Lancet* 1985;1:903–906.
10. Russel MO, Finan A, Moskowitz SR, Elmer MA, Gill FM. Nutrition and poor growth in pre-adolescent children with sickling disorders. *Pediatr Res* 1981;15:586(abstr 865).
11. Oberfield SE, Wethers DL, Kirkland JL, Levine LS. Growth hormone response to growth hormone releasing factor in sickle cell disease. *Am J Pediatr Hematol Oncol* 1987;9(4):331–334.
12. Haider M, Haider OS. Assessment of protein-calorie malnutrition. *Clin Chem* 1984;30:1286–1299.
13. Zile MH, Cullum ME. The function of vitamin A: current concepts. *Proc Soc Exp Biol Med* 1983;172:139–152.
14. Thurnham DI. Vitamin A deficiency and its role in infection. *Trans R Soc Trop Med Hyg* 1989;83:721–723.
15. Sindel LJ, Baliga BS, Bendich A, Mankad V. Nutritional deficiencies associated with vitamin E deficiency in sickle cell patients: the effect of vitamin supplementation. *Nutr Res* 1990;10:267–273.
16. Tangney CC, Phillips G, Bell RA, Fernandes P, Hopkins R, Wu SM. Selected indices of micronutrient status in adult patients with sickle cell anemia (SCA). *Am J Hematol* 1989;32:161–166.
17. Chiu D, Vinchinsky E, Yee M, Kleman K, Lubin B. Peroxidation, vitamin E and sickle cell anemia. *Ann NY Acad Sci* 1982;393:323–335.
18. Natta CL, Machlin L. Plasma levels of tocopherol in sickle cell anemia subjects. *Am J Clin Nutr* 1979;32:1359–1362.
19. Natta CL, Machlin LJ, Brim MA. Decrease in irreversible sickled erythrocytes in sickle cell anemia patients given vitamin E. *Am J Clin Nutr* 1980;33:968–971.
20. Stone WL, Adhikary PK, Lownes RL, Nicholas CA, Sollis CM. Vitamin E and abnormal lipoprotein cholesterol levels in sickle cell disease. *Fed Proc* 1983;42:1181.
21. Adebonojo FO, Payne P, Kheshti A, Stone WL. Vitamin E and abnormal lipoprotein levels in sickle cell disease. *J Nutr* 1986;116:101(abstr).
22. Chiu D, Lubin B. Abnormal vitamin E and glutathione peroxidase levels in sickle cell anemia. Evidence of increased susceptibility to lipid peroxidation in vivo. *J Lab Clin Med* 1979;94:542–548.
23. Muskiet FD, Muskiet AJ. Lipids fatty acids and trace elements in plasma and erythrocytes of pediatric patients with homozygous sickle cell disease. *Clin Chim Acta* 1984;142:1–10.
24. Rahbar F, Scott RB, Jilly P. Studies in sickle cell anemia: preliminary observation on gastrointestinal digestion and absorption. *J Natl Med Assoc* 1977;69(2):104–114.
25. Jain SK, Williams DM. Reduced levels of plasma ascorbic acid (vitamin C) in sickle cell disease patients: its possible role in the oxidant damage to sickle cell in vivo. *Clin Chim Acta* 1984;149:257–261.
26. Vichinsky E, Heyman M, Hurst D, Chiu D, Lubin B. Nutrition in sickle cell anemia (Hb SS). *Pediatr Res* 1984;18:251(abstr 930).
27. Natta CL, Reynold RD. Apparent vitamin B6 deficiency in sickle cell anemia. *Am J Clin Nutr* 1985;40:235–239.
28. Lin TK. Folic acid deficiency in sickle cell anemia. *Scand J Haematol* 1975;14:71–79.
29. Varma RN, Mankad VN, Phelps DD, Jenkins LD, Suskind RM. Depressed erythrocyte glutathione reductase activity in sickle cell disease. *Am J Clin Nutr* 1983;38:884–887.
30. Osifo BO, Adeyokunu A, Parmentier Y, Gerard P, Nicolas JP. Abnormalities of serum transcobalamins in sickle cell disease (HbSS) in Black Africa. *Br J Haematol* 1983;30:135–140.
31. Hebbel RP, Eaton JW, Balasingam M, Seinberg MH. Spontaneous oxygen radical generation by sickle erythrocytes. *J Clin Invest* 1982;70:1253–1259.
32. Dois SK, Nair RC. Superoxide dismutase, glutathione peroxidase catalase and lipid peroxidation of normal and sickled erythrocytes. *Br J Haematol* 1980;44:87–92.
33. Stone WL, Adebonojo FO, Enwonwu CO. Antioxidant micronutrients and sickle cell disease. In: Enwonwu CO, ed. *Impact of nutrition on health and disease in blacks and other minorities.* Annual Nutrition Workshop Series, vol 1. Nashville: Meharry Medical College, 1987;187–193.
34. Prasad A, Cossack ZT. Zinc supplementation and growth in sickle cell disease. *Ann Intern Med* 1981;100:367–371.
35. Daeschner CW III, Matustick C, Carpentier U. Zinc and growth in patients with sickle cell disease. *J Pediatr* 1981;98(5):778–780.
36. Neill HB, Leach BL, Kraus AP. Zinc metabolism in sickle cell anemia. *JAMA* 1979;242:2686–2687.
37. Carpentieri M, Smith L, Daeschner CW III, Haggard ME. Neutrophils and zinc in infection-prone children with sickle-cell disease. *Pediatrics* 1983;72:88–92.

38. Mankad VN, Ronnlund RD, Suskind RM. Increased immune function in sickle cell disease patients after zinc. *Pediatr Res* 1982;1717:237A.
39. Abshire TC, English JL, Githens JH, Hambidge KM. Zinc status in children and young adults with sickle cell disease. *Am J Dis Child* 1988;142:1356–1359.
40. Alayashi AI, Dafallah A, Al-Ouorain, Omer AHS, Wilson MT. Zinc and copper status in patients with sickle cell anemia. *Acta Haematol* 1987;77:87–89.
41. Tapazoglow E, Prasad AS, Hill G, Brewer GJ, Kaplan J. Decreased natural killer cell activity in patients with zinc deficiency with sickle cell. *J Lab Clin Med* 1985;105:19–22.
42. Brownell A, Lowson S, Brozoric M. Serum ferritin concentration in sickle cell crisis. *J Clin Pathol* 1986;39:253–255.
43. Reed JD, Redding-Lallinger R, Orringer EP. Nutrition and sickle cell disease. *Am J Hematol* 1987;24:441–455.
44. Prasad AS, Ortega J, Brewer GJ, Oberleas D, Schoomaker EB. Trace elements in sickle cell disease. *JAMA* 1976;235(22):2396–2398.
45. Nash DB, Boghossian S, Parmar J, Dormandy JA, Bevan D. Alteration of mechanical properties of sickle cells by repetitive deoxygenation: role of calcium and the effects of calcium blockers. *Br J Haematol* 1989;72:260–264.
46. Canale VC, Steinberg P, New M, Erlandson M. Endocrine function in thalassemia major. *Ann NY Acad Sci* 1974;232:333–345.
47. Oberfield SE, Wethers DL, Kirkland JL, Levine LS. Growth hormone response to growth hormone releasing factor in sickle cell disease. *Am J Pediatr Hematol Oncol* 1987;9(4):331–334.
48. Dada OA, Nduka EU. Endocrine function and haemoglobinopathies: relation between the sickle cell gene and circulating plasma levels of testosterone, luteinizing hormone (LH) and follicle stimulating hormone (FSH) in adult males. *Clin Chim Acta* 1980;105:269–273.
49. Abbasi AA, Prasad AS, Ortega J, Congco E, Oberleas D. Gonadal function abnormalities in sickle cell anemia. Studies in adult male patients. *Ann Intern Med* 1976;85:601–605.
50. Lukanmbi FA, Adeyokunnu AA, Osifo BOA, Bolodeoku JO, Dada OA. Endocrine function and haemoglobinopathies: biochemical assessment of thyroid function in children with sickle cell disease. *Am J Med Sci* 1986;15:25–28.
51. Glassman AR, Bennett CE. B and T lymphocytes: quantitation, function and clinical applicability. *Ann Clin Lab Sci* 1980;10(6):455–462.
52. Ronnlund RD, Mankad VN, Phelphs DD, Suskind RM. Assessment of cellular and humoral immunity in patients with sickle cell anemia. *Pediatr Res* 1982;16:213(abstr 806).
53. Rivero RA, Macia G, del Valle L, Larigados LC, et al. Alteraciones immunologicas en la anemia drepanocitica. *Sangre (Baro)* 1991;36:15–20.
54. Hendricks J, Deceulaer K, Williams E, Serjeant GR. Mononuclear cells in sickle cell disease: subpopulations and in vitro response to mitogens. *J Clin Lab Immunol* 1980;13:129–132.
55. Ades EW, Hinson AN, Morgan SK. Immunological studies in sickle cell disease. I. Analysis of circulating T lymphocyte subpopulations. *Clin Immunol Immunopathol* 1980;17:459–462.
56. Gill JC, Maples J, et al. Inherited absence of OH T4 lymphocyte antigen in a chronically transfused patient with homozygous sickle cell disease. *J Pediatr* 1985;107:251–253.
57. Kaplan J, Sarnaik S, Gitlin J, Lusher J. Diminished helper/suppressor lymphocyte ratios and natural killer activity in recipients of repeated blood transfusions. *Blood* 1984;64:308–310.
58. Hernandez P, Cruz C, Santos MP, Ballester JM. Immunology dysfunction in sickle cell anemia. *Acta Haematol* 1980;63:156–161.
59. Larcher VF, Wyke RJ, Davis R, Strong GE, Williams R. Defective yeast opsonization and functional deficiency of complement in sickle cell anemia. *Arch Dis Child* 1982;57:343–346.
60. Bjornson AB, Lobel JS, Magnafichi PI, Lampkin BC. Restoration by normal human immunoglobulin G of deficient serum opsonization for *Streptococcus pneumoniae* in sickle cell disease. *Infect Immun* 1981;33(2):636–640.
61. Glassman AB, Deas DV, Berlinsky FS, Bennett CE. Lymphocytic blast transformation and peripheral lymphocyte percentages in patients with sickle cell disease. *Ann Clin Lab Sci* 1980;10:9–12.
62. Escalona E, Malone I, Rodriguez E, Inati J, Arends A, Perdomo Y. Mitogen induced lymphoproliferative response and lymphocyte subpopulations in patients with sickle disease. *J Clin Lab Immunol* 1987;22:191–196.
63. Ogunge OO, Uy CG, Seagreen MN, Ballester JM. Immunological dysfunction in sickle cell anemia. *Nigerian Med J* 1979;9:33.
64. Boghossian SH, Wright G, Webster DB, Segal AW. Investigators of host defence in patients with sickle cell disease. *Br J Haematol* 1985;59:523–531.
65. DeCeulaer K, Paglinca A, Forbes M, Maude GH, Sejeant BE, Serjeant GR. Recurrent infections in sickle cell disease: haematological and immune studies. *Clin Chim Acta* 1985;148:161–165.
66. Morgan AG, Venner AM. Immunity and leg ulcers in homozygous sickle cell disease. *J Clin Lab Immunol* 1981;6:51–55.
67. DeCeulaer K, Wilson WA, Morgan AG, Serjeant GR. Plasma A haemoglobin and complement activation in sickle cell disease. *J Clin Lab Immunol* 1981;6:57–60.
68. Chudwin DS, Korenblit AD, Kingzette M, Artrip S, Kao S. Increased activation of the alternative complement pathway in sickle cell disease. *Clin Immunol Immunopathol* 1985;37:93–97.
69. Buchanan GR, Schiffman G. Antibody responses to polyvalent pneumococcal vaccine in infants with sickle cell anemia. *J Pediatr* 1980;96:264–266.
70. Omanga M, Safary A, Mulefu KM. Evaluation clinique de la vaccination anti-pneumococcique chez l'enfant drepanocytaire homozygote. *Ann Soc Belg Med Trop* 1984;64:283–289.
71. Millard D, DeCeulaer K, Vaidya S, Serjeant GR. Serum immunoglobulin levels in children with homozygous sickle cell disease. *Clin Chim Acta* 1982;125:81–87.
72. Gavrilis P, Rothenburg SP, Guy R. Correlation of low serum IgM levels with absence of functional splenic tissue in sickle cell disease syndromes. *Am J Med* 1974;57:542–545.
73. John AB, Jackson H, Maude GH, Sharma AW, Searjeant GR. Prevention of pneumococcal infection in children with homozygous sickle cell disease. *Br Med J* 1984;288:1567–1570.
74. Enwonwu CO. Nutritional support in sickle cell anemia: theoretical considerations. *J Natl Med Assoc* 1988;80:139–144.
75. Weatherall DJ, Clegg JB. *The thalassemia syndromes*, 3rd ed. Oxford Blackwell Scientific, 1981.
76. Niehaus AN, Wolfe L. In: Nathan, Oski, eds. *Hematology of infancy and childhood*, 3rd ed. Philadelphia: WB Saunders, 1987.
77. Robinson M, Watson RJ. Megaloblastic anemia complicating thalassemia major. *Am J Dis Child* 1963;165:275.
78. Kumar R, Sarya C, Chouphury VP, Sundaran KR, Kailash S, Seghal AK. Vitamin B_{12}, folate and iron studies in homozygous beta thalassemia. *Am J Clin Pathol* 1985;84:668–671.
79. Lubhy AL, Cooperman JM, et al. Folic acid deficiency as a limiting factor with anemia of thalassemia major. *Blood* 1981;18:78.
80. Saraya AK, Kumar R, Kailash S, Seghal AK. Vitamin B_{12} and folic acid deficiency in β heterozygous thalassemia. *Indian J Med Res* 1989 (June);7(9):783–788.
81. Gastaldi G, Bagni B, Trotta E, Menegale G, Cavallini AR, Piffanelli A. Folic acid deficiency in β thalassemia heterozygotes. *Scand J Haematol* 1983;30:125–129.
82. Fromme P, Agha E, Quitt MS, Yechiely H, Kahana L. Folate studies in thalassemia minor. *Isr J Med Sci* 1985(Oct);21(10):895–896.
83. Lubhy AL, Cooperman JM, Lopez R, Giorgia AJ, et al. Vitamin B_{12} metabolism in thalassemia major. *Ann NY Acad Sci* 1969;165:444–460.
84. Jenks J, Begley J, Howard L. Cobalamin R. binder deficiency in a women with thalassemia. *Nutr Rev* 1983 (Sept);41(9):277–280.
85. Lynch SR, Seftel HC, et al. Accelerated oxidative catabolism of ascorbic acid in siderotic bandu. *Am J Clin Nutr* 1967;26:641.
86. O'Brien RT. Ascorbic acid enhancement of desferrioxamine induced urinary iron excretion in thalassemia major. *Ann NY Acad Sci* 1974;232:221.
87. Nienhaus AW. Thalassemia major: molecular and clinical aspects. *Ann Intern Med* 1979;91:883.
88. Nienhaus AW. Vitamin C and iron. *N Engl J Med* 1981;304:170.
89. Ozzincolo C, Castaldi G, De Sanjisu, Scutellar PH, Ciaccio C, Vullo C. Rickets and/or scurvy-like bone lesions in beta thalassemia major. *Radiol Med (Torino)* 1990(Dec);80(6):823–829.

90. Cranfield M, Golan JL, et al. Serum antioxidant activity in normal and abnormal subject. *Ann Clin Biochem* 1979;16:299.
91. Vatanavicharn S, Yenchitsomanus P, Siddhikol C. Vitamin E in β thalassemia and α thalassemia (H_b H disease). *Acta Haematol* 1985;73:183.
92. Minerio R, Piga A, et al. Vitamin E and β thalassemia. *Hematology* 1983;68:562–566.
93. Rachmilewitz EA, Lubin BH, Shobet SB. Lipid membrane peroxidation in β thalassemia major. *Blood* 1976;47:495–505.
94. Chiu D, Lubin BH. Abnormal vitamin E and glutathione peroxidase levels in sickle cell anemia. *J Lab Clin Med* 1979;94:542–548.
95. Minerio R, Canducci DH, Sarraco P, Vullo C. Vitamin E in β thalassemia. *Acta Vitaminol Enzymol* 1982;4:21–25.
96. Rachmilewitz A, Shifter A, Kahane I. Vitamin E deficiency in β thalassemia major: changes in hematological and biochemical parameters after a therapeutic trial with α tocopherol. *Am J Clin Nutr* 1979;32:1850–1858.
97. Minerio R, David O, Ghigho D, Luzzato L, et al. Administration of vitamin E heterozygous β thalassemia—the effect on RBC survival. *Panminerva Med* 1984;26:283–286.
98. Constantoulakis M, Panagopoulous G, Augoustakio B. Stature and longitudinal growth in thalassemia major. *Clin Pediatr* 1975;14:355–368.
99. Borgna-Pignatte C, Destefano P, Zanta I, Vullo C, DeSanctis V, Melevindi C, et al. Growth and sexual maturation in thalassemia major. *J Pediatr* 1985;106(1):150–155.
100. Prasad AS, Diwany M, Gabor M, Sandstead HH, Hefny AE, et al. Biomedical studies in thalassemia. *Ann Intern Med* 1965;62:87–96.
101. Rea F, Perrone L, Mastrobuno A, Toscano G, Amico MD. Zinc levels of serum, hair, and urine in homozygous β thalassemic subjects under hyper transfusional treatment. *Acta Haematol* 1984;71:139–142.
102. Aracasoy A, Cavdar AO, Halil Ertug, Gurpinar F. Zinc treatment in homozygous thalassemia (a preliminary study). In: *Zinc deficiency in human subjects.* New York: Alan R. Liss, 1983;107–116.
103. Vatanavicharn S, Pringsulka P, Kritalugsana S, Phuapairoj P, Wasi P. Zinc and copper status in hemoglobin H disease and β thalassemia Hb E disease. *Acta Haematol* 1982;68:317–320.
104. Aracasoy A, Cavdar AO. Growth retardation in β thalassemia (editorial correspondence). *J Pediatr* 1981;99:671–672.
105. Aracasoy A, Cavdar AO. Changes of trace minerals serum iron, zinc, copper and magnesium in thalassemia. *Acta Haematol* 1979;62:42–44.
106. Skoutelis ATh, Lianou E, Papa Vassiliou Th, Karamerou A, Politi K, Bassaris HP. Defective phagocytic and bactericidal function of polymorphonuclear leukocytes in patients with β thalassemia major. *J Infect* 1984;8:118–122.
107. Giuntoli JM, Estevez MA, Sen L, Penalver JA. Defective function of the peripheral blood neutrophils in thalassemia major. *J Am Soc Pediatr Hematol Oncol* 1984;Sept:215–218.
108. Quntiliani L, Mastro Minaro A, Giuilani E, et al. Immune profile alterations in thalassemia patients. *Boll Ist Sieroter Milan* 1983;62:6.
109. Luria D, Cohen IJ, et al. Impaired immune regulation in children and adolescents with hemophilia and thalassemia in Israel. *J Am Soc Pediatr Hematol Oncol* 1984;6(4)Winter:371–378.
110. Guglielmo P, Cunsolo F, Lombardo T, Sortino G, et al. T-subset abnormalities in thalassemia intermedia. Possible evidence for a thymic functional deficiency. *Acta Haematol* 1984;72:361–367.
111. Neri A, Rugiatelli B, Iacopino P, Callia V, Konso F. Natural killer cell activity and T-subpopulations in thalassemia major. *Acta Haematol* 1984;71:263–269.
112. Munn CG, Makenson AI, Kapadia A, Desousa M. Impaired T cell mitogen responses in some patients with thalassemia intermedia. *Thymus* 1981;3:119–128.

CHAPTER 38

Nutritional Management of Immunodepressed Children

Ricardo U. Sorensen, Solo Kuvibidila, and Robert M. Suskind

Children with primary and secondary immunodeficiency diseases have an increased susceptibility to life-threatening infections that may be aggravated by malnutrition. Appropriate management of these patients includes early recognition and treatment of the immunodeficiency, as well as prevention and treatment of the malnutrition. Understanding the physiologic basis for the nutritional management of primary immunodeficiency diseases necessitates understanding basic host defense mechanisms, and the immunologic abnormalities in secondary malnourished states. These two topics have been presented in detail in chapter 12.

Malnutrition is an important determinant of morbidity and mortality due to infections in young children (1). It is also the most common cause of secondary immunodeficiency (2). Cause and effect are not always separable, however. Malnutrition increases susceptibility to infections by impairing different components of the immune response. Infections, on the other hand, induce malnutrition by interfering with food intake, by decreasing nutrient absorption, and by increasing nitrogen and other nutrient losses as a result of the catabolic state induced by infection. These processes become important when infections such as those that cause diarrhea become chronic and/or recurrent in very young children.

When immunodeficient children present with chronic infection and secondary malnutrition, the child's basic immunodeficiency may be further complicated by the nutritionally induced secondary immunodeficiency. Although the immunodeficiencies secondary to malnutrition improve with appropriate nutritional support, the patient's basic immunodeficiency state will not respond to nutritional support alone. Since immunological abnormalities caused by immunodeficiencies and by malnutrition often overlap, it is important to understand the relationship between the various immunodeficiencies and the host defense mechanisms that are affected (Table 1). It is also essential to recognize that all immunodeficiency syndromes have an increased risk of infection, gastrointestinal disease, and secondary malnutrition (3,4). In addition, specific immunodeficiencies have special nutritionally related problems.

COMPLEMENT DEFICIENCIES

There is no special association between specific complement deficiencies and nutritional deficiency states. Patients with angioedema have a deficiency of C1 esterase inhibitor. Some of these patients present mainly with recurrent abdominal pain due to recurrent episodes of edema of the intestinal wall. Although the deficient C1 esterase inhibitor production is an inherited disorder, many patients do not become symptomatic before adolescence (5). Secondary deficiencies of C1 esterase inhibitor have also been described, but are extremely rare in childhood.

DEFICIENCIES OF PHAGOCYTOSIS

Neutropenic patients sometimes develop a life-threatening enterocolitis that requires aggressive treatment and nutritional support. Although most cases have been described in adults (6), we observed one case of salmonella ileitis in a patient with autoimmune neutropenia (7). In this case the ileitis improved only after the neutro-

---

R. U. Sorensen, S. Kuvibidila, R. M. Suskind: Department of Pediatrics, Louisiana State University School of Medicine, New Orleans, Louisiana 70112.

TABLE 1. *Main primary immunodeficiency syndromes according to the host defense mechanism affected*

Complement deficiencies
  Single complement deficiencies
Deficiencies of phagocytosis
  Adherence and chemotaxis deficiencies
    Adherence glycoprotein deficiency
    Hyper-IgE syndrome
  Intracellular killing abnormalities
    Chronic granulomatous disease
    Chédiak-Higashi syndrome
Deficiencies in cell-mediated immunity
  DiGeorge syndrome
  Nezelof syndrome
  Chronic mucocutaneous candidiasis
Antibody deficiencies
  Decreased immunoglobulin levels
    X-linked agammaglobulinemia
    X-linked immunodeficiency with hyper-IgM
    Common variable hypogammaglobulinemia
    Transient hypogammaglobulinemia of infancy
    IgG subclass deficiency
    IgA deficiency
  Decreased specific antibodies with normal or elevated total immunoglobulins
Combined cellular and antibody deficiencies
  Severe combined immunodeficiencies (SCID)
    X-linked SCID
    Autosomal recessive SCID
    Adenosine deaminase deficiency
    Bare lymphocyte syndrome
  Partial combined immunodeficiencies with associated abnormalities
    Wiskott-Aldrich syndrome
    Ataxia telangiectasia
    Intestinal lymphangiectasia

penia was resolved with high dose intravenous immune globulin and corticosteroids.

DEFICIENCIES IN CELL-MEDIATED IMMUNITY

Chronic mucocutaneous candidiasis is the only deficiency of cell-mediated immunity associated with a specific nutritional deficiency. This is a heterogeneous syndrome characterized by chronic candidial infection of the skin and mucous membranes (8). Notably, there are no invasive *candida* infections in any of the forms of this syndrome. Twenty-three of 31 patients in one series had low serum iron and decreased iron stores. Most patients treated with iron showed significant clinical improvement (9). However, we have observed patients in whom oral iron was ineffective and intravenous iron infusions were necessary to normalize iron stores. The presence of anemia due to chronic infection may prevent the correction of hemoglobin levels if the candidiasis is not appropriately treated.

ANTIBODY DEFICIENCIES

X-linked agammaglobulinemia, a condition that was first described by Bruton (10) in 1952, is characterized by absence of mature B lymphocytes and absent or very low levels of all immunoglobulins including secretory IgA. Patients usually present with recurrent respiratory infections after maternal IgG has decreased below protective levels at 6 months of age. However, gastrointestinal disorders also occur. Diarrhea, steatorrhea, giardiasis, and bacterial overgrowth are well-known associations (11). A regional enteritis-like enteropathy has been described in a patient with agammaglobulinemia (12). Notably, despite the intense inflammatory reaction present in this patient's intestinal mucosa, he was asymptomatic for large periods of time. The only indication of an abnormality was the very short half-life of IgG, which made it difficult to maintain adequate IgG trough levels with intravenous immune globulin (7). No specific pathogen was identified and the patient responded well to treatment of bacterial overgrowth with metronidazole plus low-dose corticosteroids.

Common variable hypogammaglobulinemia (CVH) frequently presents with, or has gastrointestinal problems associated with, recurrent respiratory infections. CVH can present at any age; the youngest patient we observed was 19 months old at presentation. Patients with common variable hypogammaglobulinemia have mature B cells in circulation. Some IgM and IgG is usually detectable in their serum. In adult patients, achlorhydria with gastric atrophy and a pernicious anemia–like syndrome is common (11). Malabsorption, occasionally associated with celiac disease, is also frequent (13,14). We observed the development of malabsorption and failure to thrive in an 8-year-old patient who was on home treatment with intravenous immune globulin (15). Concomitantly with the development of malabsorption, his IgG trough levels dropped markedly. However, except for increased stool frequency, this patient remained asymptomatic. The malabsorption was corrected by treatment of bacterial overgrowth with metronidazole. The patient resumed normal growth and corrected IgG levels without an increase in intravenous immune globulin dose.

Patients with CVH may also develop zinc deficiency. In one series, zinc deficiency was detected in 26% of 19 adult patients with CVH (16). The two patients with the most profound zinc deficiency had a complete resolution of intractable diarrhea after zinc repletion. The possibility of a correctable zinc deficiency needs to be considered in children with CVH and chronic diarrhea.

Transient hypogammaglobulinemia of infancy is a self-limited disorder characterized by prolongation and accentuation of the physiologic decline in serum IgG concentrations normally seen during the third to sixth month of life. A high incidence of transient hypogammaglobulinemia has been observed in infants with diarrhea (17). This group of patients differed from other patients with diarrhea and normal levels of immunoglobulins in the earlier onset of diarrhea (3.1 months vs 8.2 months). Significant problems outside the gastrointestinal tract did not occur in this patient population.

Selective IgA deficiency is seen in 1 of every 886 blood donors in the United States (18). IgA deficient patients usually have deficient serum and secretory IgA. The association of selective IgA deficiency with gastrointestinal abnormalities includes chronic or recurrent *Giardia lamblia* infection, food allergy, gluten-sensitive enteropathy, increased incidence of circulating antibodies against food antigens, circulating autoantibodies to intestinal epithelial cells, and basement membrane and inflammatory bowel disease (11). Since most IgA-deficient patients are asymptomatic, it still needs to be determined why some develop gastrointestinal disease. Nutritional considerations will be most important in this regard.

SEVERE COMBINED IMMUNODEFICIENCIES (SCID)

Failure to thrive is a characteristic presentation of SCID. Intensive nutritional support can achieve some weight gain but is unlikely to normalize nutritional parameters if the basic immunologic abnormality is not corrected. The need to consider nutritional aspects in the treatment of SCID was illustrated in an evaluation of 14 patients with SCID due to adenosine deaminase deficiency receiving enzyme replacement therapy with polyethyleneglycol-treated adenosine deaminase (PEG-ADA). All patients had documented biochemical, immunological, and clinical improvement. However, 10 of the 14 patients, including the 3 patients with persistent low $CD4^+$ cells, remained below the 10th percentile for weight on PEG-ADA treatment (M. Hershfield, personal communication). A complete nutritional evaluation may explain the persistence of immunological abnormalities after correction of the biochemical abnormalities.

PARTIAL COMBINED IMMUNODEFICIENCIES WITH ASSOCIATED ABNORMALITIES

Ataxia telangiectasia patients may gradually develop nutritional deficiencies due, not directly to their immunodeficiency syndrome, but to their progressive ataxia and lack of appetite. This is a problem common to all patients who have neurological disease in addition to their immunodeficiency syndrome.

Intestinal lymphangiectasia is a complex disease entity characterized by dilated intestinal channels, chronic diarrhea, protein-losing enteropathy, hypoproteinemic edema, and lymphopenia. The accompanying immunodeficiency is thought to be secondary to intestinal immunoglobulin and lymphocyte loss. Pediatric cases of primary intestinal and generalized lymphangiectasia are rare. We have observed thymic atrophy in one patient with primary lymphangiectasia, suggesting that thymic atrophy may occur and further contribute to the development of a deficiency in cell-mediated immunity (19). Treatment with a low-fat diet designed to decrease lymphatic pressure has been of benefit in some patients (20).

NUTRITIONAL ASPECTS OF SECONDARY IMMUNODEFICIENCIES

Most chronic diseases including infections caused secondary immunodeficiencies mainly through the effects of malnutrition on the immune system. Therefore, the immunodeficiencies can be prevented to the extent that adequate nutrition and control of infection are preserved. Only malignancies and chemotherapy for malignant diseases had the potential of a direct impact on immunity. However, even in these diseases, concomitant malnutrition often played an important pathogenic role (21).

In the immunodeficiency caused by HIV infection, a set of complex interactions between immunodeficiency, infection, and malnutrition occurs. The immunologic abnormalities caused by the HIV virus overlap to a great extent with those caused by malnutrition. Although the progressive immunodeficiency caused by HIV infection increases susceptibility to infection, infections in turn may activate T lymphocytes and increase the expression of HIV, thus accelerating the progression of HIV infections toward the full expression of the acquired immunodeficiency syndrome. In children the situation is further complicated by the fact that specific immune responses still in a developmental phase may be truncated by the HIV infection. HIV infections acquired later in life cause a true secondary immunodeficiency in the individual who previously had normal immunity. For example, although adults with HIV infections may gradually lose tuberculin reactivity acquired earlier in life from bacille Calmette-Guérin (BCG) immunization or exposure to *Mycobacterium tuberculosis,* HIV-infected children with tuberculosis may never turn tuberculin positive.

Our knowledge about pediatric HIV infections stems mainly from the observations of children with AIDS (22,23). As the HIV epidemic spreads more and more through heterosexual transmission and the numbers of asymptomatic HIV-infected women of childbearing age increases, vertical transmission of the HIV virus has become the main source of HIV infections in children. The 20% to 50% of infants born to HIV-infected mothers who are, themselves, infected have clearly become a major challenge to pediatricians. Because many of these children are asymptomatic, delayed recognition may preclude early intervention.

Prospective cohort studies have begun to examine the natural history of congenital HIV. The potential importance of nutrition in determining the course of HIV infection in children makes nutrition an important component of such studies.

The major pathogenic process of HIV infection includes binding of the HIV envelope glycoprotein gp 120 on the HIV to the CD4 molecule on both T cells and monocyte/macrophages, with subsequent functional impairment and ultimate destruction of the CD4+ helper T cell and a relatively stable or raised numbers of the cytotoxic (CD8+) subset (24). *In vitro* proliferative responses to antigens are clearly depressed. Decreased IL-2 secretion, IL-2 receptor expression, and interferon (IFN)-γ production and a defective cytolytic function of natural killer (NK) cells are associated with disease progression (25).

In spite of this hypergammaglobulinemia, there is a deficient antibody response to new antigens, a particularly important problem in HIV-infected infants who are prevented from developing a normal repertoire of specific antibodies to common viral and bacterial pathogens (24).

In children, symptomatic HIV infections are an important cause of failure to thrive (26,27). Several factors may contribute to this. Because of the possibility of HIV transmission through breast milk, breast-feeding is not recommended (23,28,29). In addition, symptomatic HIV-infected women may not be able to breast-feed, especially those who are intravenous drug addicts. Adequate nutritional intake is further complicated in infected children with central nervous system involvement, and those with diarrhea and subsequent malabsorption syndromes. Acute and chronic infections and fever raise the basal energy expenditure and further deteriorate the nutritional balance in these patients.

An evaluation of older hemophiliac children with asymptomatic HIV infection showed that 40% were malnourished compared to 4.5% of the noninfected children with hemophilia (30). This indicates that nutritional deficiency may present before progression to AIDS in HIV-infected patients.

In adults with AIDS, weight loss is probably due to the combined effect of anorexia, fever, diarrhea, malabsorption, and the catabolic response to opportunistic infections (31,32).

In addition to general malnutrition, several specific nutrient deficits have been observed in patients with AIDS. Some patients have vitamin E deficiency manifested clinically as the yellow nail syndrome, which improves with vitamin E supplementation (33). Pediatric and adult patients have been found to develop zinc deficiency and acrodermatitis enteropathica (34-36). Severely diminished plasma and red cell levels of selenium have been observed independent of the presence of malabsorption or disease duration (37). Serum iron concentrations are significantly reduced and ferritin levels significantly higher in AIDS patients compared to patients with persistent generalized lymphadenopathy (38). This suggests that infectious agents draw on body iron stores and that the phagocytic cells that actively ingest these agents incorporate this iron, synthesizing and releasing ferritin. Hence, the malnutrition commonly seen in HIV-infected patients may further contribute to impair their host defense mechanisms.

Most of our information about nutritional deficiencies in HIV infection comes from adult patients with AIDS. In order to enhance the management of HIV-infected infants, evaluation of their specific nutritional needs is essential.

EVALUATION AND DIFFERENTIAL DIAGNOSIS OF IMMUNODEFICIENCY SYNDROMES

A complete diagnostic evaluation of a patient with recurrent or unusually severe infections should include appropriate indicators of both the status of the various host defense mechanisms and of nutritional status (Table 2). The diagnostic problems are somewhat different at the time of initial diagnosis of children with immunodeficiency disorders and in the follow-up of patients with identified immunodeficiency syndromes. Once the presence of an immunodeficiency syndrome is established, it is important to monitor not only the immunological response to the specific treatment of the immunological abnormality, but also the nutritional status.

In general, primary immunodeficiencies can be differentiated from immunodeficiency due to malnutrition based on inheritance patterns, onset of presentation independent of nutritional status, the specificity and severity of immunological abnormalities, and the characteristic associated abnormalities frequently present in primary immunodeficiency diseases.

SCID with failure to thrive can be differentiated from PEM based on the severity of the deficiency of cellular immunity in SCID, on the frequently low immunoglobulin levels in SCID, and on the presence of characteristic genetic or biochemical markers, e.g., X-linked inheritance or adenosine deaminase or nucleoside phosphorylase deficiency. Furthermore, nutritional treatment of SCID patients alone does not restore lymphocyte function. A profound lymphopenia and absent lymphocyte blastogenic responses to mitogens *in vitro* are suggestive of a primary immunodeficiency syndrome. *In vivo,* BCG-immunized SCID patients do not react at all to tuberculin (39), whereas even severe PEM patients may have tuberculin reactivity. Only kwashiorkor patients

TABLE 2. *Immunologic and nutritional evaluation of patients with suspected immunodeficiency and malnutrition*

Initial evaluation	Advanced evaluation
Immunological evaluation	

Cell-mediated immunity
  CBC, lymphocyte count
  PA and lateral chest x-ray to evaluate the thymus
  Delayed hypersensitivity
Antibody-mediated immunity
  Serum protein electrophoresis
  Serum immunoglobulin levels including IgG subclasses
	Lymphocyte subpopulations
	Blastogenic responses to antigens and mitogens
	Cytokines and lymphokines
	
	B lymphocyte numbers
	Specific antibody responses to proteins and polysaccharides
	In vitro immunoglobulin production

Phagocytosis Neutrophil count and smear	Chemotaxis Superoxide generation Opsonophagocytosis

Complement
  Serum hemolytic complement
  Quantitation of C3 and C4
Acute-phase reactants (chronic inflammation)
  C-reactive protein
	Individual components
	
	Inflammatory mediators, TNF
	Ceruloplasmin
	α_1-Acid glycoprotein

Nutritional evaluation	
Height and weight Total protein and albumin Hemoglobin	Prealbumin Retinol-binding protein Vitamin levels Iron and ferritin Zinc and trace elements

have consistently decreased delayed-type hypersensitivity (DTH) to tuberculin after BCG immunization (40,41).

It has become possible to measure IL-2 secretion and the effect of exogenous IL-2 on lymphocyte proliferative responses. Some forms of SCID have been found to respond *in vitro* and *in vivo* to exogenous administration of IL-2 (42,43). IL-2 deficiencies seen in HIV-infected patients (44,45) as well as in patients with chronic infections like leprosy and tuberculosis, do not improve upon exposure to IL-2 *in vitro* (46,47). It is important to establish similar data for IL-2 and other lymphokines in other forms of malnutrition and also for immunodeficiency syndromes in order to be able to differentiate various forms of immunodeficiency, each of which may require a different therapeutic approach.

Antibody deficiency syndromes with decreased immunoglobulin levels rarely present a diagnostic problem. Most forms of malnutrition, including kwashiorkor, have normal or elevated levels of immunoglobulins. Patients with primary immunoglobulin deficiencies are unable to increase immunoglobulin production even in the presence of infections. Specific antibody deficiencies with normal levels of immunoglobulins have been described (4). The clinically relevant specific antibody deficiencies involve deficient production of antibodies against bacterial polysaccharides present after 2 years of age (48). Antibody responses to polysaccharides do not seem to be altered in patients with PEM (49).

The differential diagnosis of secondary immunodeficiencies from immunological abnormalities caused by PEM and/or specific nutrient deficiencies is based on the identification of the condition causing the secondary immunodeficiency. This usually does not represent a problem in secondary immunodeficiencies caused by neoplasia and immunosuppressive and cytoreductive drugs. Regularly monitoring the nutritional status of these patients in order to prevent additional immunological impairment due to malnutrition is recommended.

Diagnosing asymptomatic HIV infection in infants who still have transplacentally transported maternal IgG in circulation is dependent on detecting viral DNA or antigens (22,23). The presence of anti-HIV antibodies after 15 months of age is indicative of infection. It is important to note, however, that some HIV infected children are seronegative (50). Asymptomatic HIV infected children with immunological abnormalities have a progressive decrease of $CD4^+$ cells and increased immunoglobulin levels. Both abnormalities are more pronounced in HIV-infected patients than in infected patients with PEM. In particular, immunoglobulin levels are significantly increased in HIV-infected children even in the absence of other secondary infections. HIV infections and PEM rarely cause the profound lymphocyte unresponsiveness to mitogens seen in patients with SCID. Symptomatic HIV-infected patients are recognized by a typical spectrum of infections and other complications (22,23).

The differential diagnosis of failure to thrive and chronic diarrhea is a frequent problem that can be caused by multiple pathologic conditions. The main immunodeficiency syndromes that need to be considered are SCID, X-linked agammaglobulinemia, CVH, IgA deficiency, and HIV infection. The presence of specific chronic intestinal infections is not pathognomonic for any given immunodeficiency. Chronic rotavirus infections have been described in patients with SCID, X-linked agammaglobulinemia, X-linked immunodeficiency with hyper-IgM, CVH, selective IgA deficiency, transient hypogammaglobulinemia, and ataxia telangiectasia (51,52). We have also observed chronic rotavirus infection in patients with congenital HIV infection and immunodeficiency. However, some special associations do exist. Severe, early gastrointestinal candidiasis is suggestive of SCID or early onset symptomatic HIV infection. Esophageal candidiasis is typical of patients with HIV infection. Later onset chronic mucocutaneous candidiasis is suggestive of the syndrome of chronic mucocutaneous candidiasis or of the Nezelof syndrome. Chronic *Cryptosporidium* diarrhea is a hallmark of HIV infections. Giardiasis is suggestive of IgA deficiency or other antibody deficiency syndromes.

Some immunological abnormalities are suggestive of specific immunodeficiencies or related immunological abnormalities. However, they are rarely pathognomonic. Elevated IgE levels can be seen in patients with food allergy, intestinal parasitoses, and in all immunodeficiencies affecting cellular immunity. These include some cases of SCID, the hyper-IgE syndrome, as well as HIV infections (53,54). Decreased IgG levels are suggestive of antibody deficiency or combined immunodeficiency syndromes with decreased IgG production. However, in malabsorption syndromes an increased gastrointestinal loss of IgG may be responsible for reduced circulating IgG levels. A primary antibody deficiency syndrome may coexist with increased IgG loss. In this case, IgG replacement will not be effective until the gastrointestinal abnormalities leading to increased IgG loss are treated.

PREVENTION OF MALNUTRITION IN IMMUNODEFICIENCY DISEASES

Optimal treatment of immunodeficiency diseases requires early recognition and immunological reconstitution. In addition, it is essential to prevent the development of additional immunodeficiency due to malnutrition and to prevent the onset of infections. In deficiencies of cell-mediated immunity, it is important to prevent graft versus host disease caused by live lymphocytes in unirradiated blood transfusions.

Treatment of Immunodeficiency Diseases

Severe or recurrent infections are best prevented by the correction of the immune defect. However, when adequate correction of the immune defect is not possible, preventive antibiotic treatment may be necessary. Immunological reconstitution of all immunodeficiency syndromes affecting IgG or specific antibody production can be achieved with monthly infusions of intravenous immune globulin (IVIG) (55). Selective IgA-deficient patients usually do not have abnormalities involving IgG, and should not receive IgG replacement therapy. Any blood product contaminated with IgA carries the risk of inducing anti-IgA antibodies and severe anaphylaxis in these patients.

Oral administration of immune globulin preparations has been successful in suppressing rotavirus excretion in patients with primary immunodeficiencies (52). We have confirmed this in an infant with AIDS and chronic rotavirus infection. Daily immune globulin administration through a gastrostomy tube stopped virus secretion and normalized the stool. This effect was not achieved with monthly IVIG infusions given concomitantly. Recently, an immunoglobulin preparation containing both IgG and IgA has been used successfully in the prevention of necrotizing enterocolitis in low birth weight infants (56). The preparation was obtained from human serum and, therefore, did not contain the more resistant secretory IgA. If such preparations become available at an acceptable cost, oral immunoglobulin therapy may be incorporated into the treatment options of gastrointestinal infections in immunodeficient patients.

Bone marrow transplantation is the treatment of choice for all patients with SCID and the Wiskott-Aldrich syndrome when an identical donor is available. When no identical donor is available, partially identical (haploidentical) bone marrow can be used after depletion of the mature T lymphocytes capable of causing graft versus host disease. For SCID patients with adenosine deaminase deficiency, enzyme replacement with polyethylene glycol–treated adenosine deaminase has become available (57). IgG replacement therapy should be given to all patients with SCID before immunological reconstitution is achieved through bone marrow transplantation or other treatment forms.

Prevention of Malnutrition in Immunodeficient Patients

Prevention of malnutrition is the most important goal of nutritional care of every immunodeficient patient. For newborns, breast-feeding reduces the incidence and severity of infections (58). The decrease of gastrointestinal infections has been attributed to secretory IgA and other antimicrobial components present in breast milk that may act locally in the gut of the newborn infant (59). Milk leukocytes are also capable of producing factors that participate in cell-mediated immunity, e.g., interferon (60). Breast milk was also found to significantly enhance spontaneous proliferation and T-cell blastogenic responses at 6 days and 6 weeks of age, suggesting a systemic effect (61).

After infancy, a balanced diet is probably adequate for most appropriately treated patients with immunodeficiencies. If chronic infections, e.g., giardiasis and diarrhea, are present, a vigorous effort to eliminate the infection needs to be made even when the infection is relatively mild. Appropriate nutritional support of patients with secondary immunodeficiencies due to debilitating diseases, lymphoreticular malignancies, or HIV infection is also important in order to help prevent a vicious cycle of secondary immunodeficiencies, infection, and further malnutrition.

Nutrition and Immunization of Immunodeficient Patients

In most patients with primary immunodeficiencies and all those on IgG replacement therapy, no immunizations should be given since no adequate response is expected. Furthermore, live immunizations involve risk of disease, e.g., polio from oral polio vaccine, or disseminated BCG-osis from BCG immunization. Childhood immunization is recommended in IgA-deficient patients who should never be treated with IgG replacement therapy. Inactivated polio vaccine should be given instead of live oral polio vaccine to patients with selective IgA deficiency, as a safety measure precaution.

In HIV-infected infants, the immunodeficiency syndrome develops gradually and some benefit may be derived from immunization before the disease becomes symptomatic (62). Inactivated oral polio should be given instead of live vaccine. Other live vaccines can be used, however, since those disease states are always worse than the effect of their vaccines.

In many countries, tuberculosis has become the main infectious complication of patients with HIV infection (63). Therefore, routine childhood or newborn BCG immunization is still recommended in many developing nations affected by a high incidence of heterosexual and congenital HIV infections. One study has suggested a more vigorous cellular response to BCG in infants breast-fed at the time of immunization (64). This adds to the dilemma of the risk of HIV transmission through, versus the beneficial effect of, breast milk. It also accents the need for infant formulas that offer maximal support for the development of immunity.

TREATMENT OF MALNUTRITION IN CHILDREN WITH IMMUNODEFICIENCY

Fluid and Electrolyte Therapy in Patients with Acute Infections

Children with immunodeficiency who are severely malnourished have a marked increase in total body water and a decrease in electrolytes (65). Normally, the patient presents with normal or low serum Na^+, low K^+, and often depressed Mg^{2+}. The use of Mg^{2+} in the treatment of children with PEM is based on the work of Caddell et al. in Thailand (66) and in East and West Africa (67).

The initial rehydrating fluid is $\frac{1}{2}$ N saline/5% glucose, which supplies 75 mEq of Na^+ per liter. Patients showing evidence of severe K^+ depletion may be given up to 6 to 7 mEq/kg of K^+. Although these children have an increase in their total body water, they often show evidence of intravascular dehydration. This is especially true of children with a history of severe diarrhea. If there is evidence of intravascular dehydration, the water deficit is replaced in the first 8 to 12 hr of therapy. For example, a 5-kg child who is 10% dehydrated will receive a total of 500 ml of fluid during this period. A severely dehydrated child may receive as much as 20 ml/kg (2% of body weight) of Ringer's lactate or normal saline during the first hour of therapy to increase intravascular volume and therefore renal blood flow. B-complex vitamins are given parenterally for the first 3 days.

Following rehydration, maintenance intravenous therapy is given using $\frac{1}{4}$ N saline/5% glucose until oral therapy is initiated. Because of the marked decrease in total body K^+, the patient is given supplemental intravenous and oral K^+ at a maintenance dose of 5 mEq/kg daily. Magnesium is given at a dose of 0.4 mEq/kg intramuscularly for 7 days followed by oral Mg^{2+} in dosage of 1.4 mEq/kg/day. Once an oral intake of 175 Cal and 4 g/kg/day of protein is reached, the requirement for Mg^{2+} at doses of 1.4 mEq/kg/day and K^+ at 5 mEq/kg/day is met by the formula alone. No further oral supplementation is usually required.

Dietary Therapy of Patients with Severe Diarrhea

When diarrhea is severe, a patient may be kept without oral intake for up to 24 to 48 hr. Problems with hypoglycemia are minimized by increasing the glucose concentration to 10%. After 24 to 48 hr, the patient may begin gradually increasing protein and energy intakes. Graham et al. (68), Waterlow (69), and others have demonstrated that optimum intake for recovery from PEM is 175 Cal and 3 to 4 g/kg/day of protein.

When children with immunodeficiency and malnutrition are offered *ad libitum* solid food, they reach an intake of 160 to 180 Cal/kg and 4 g/kg of protein by the second week of hospital treatment. This is maintained until the child reaches ideal weight-for-height, after which it gradually decreases to 120 Cal/kg.

Chronic Nutritional Support of Immunodeficient Patients

In the early stages of immunodeficiency and PEM, it is easier to give the necessary energy and protein in a milk-based formula that can be given by tube feeding when necessary. Formula is initially more readily taken than solid food (70). Prolonged lactose intolerance and some monosaccharide intolerance has, however, been observed in children with immunodeficiency and malnutrition. A nonlactose-containing milk-based formula supplemented with dextromaltose and corn oil does not appear to be associated with prolonged diarrhea. When such a formula is used, it is important to consider the addition of essential vitamins and minerals.

One of several important minerals to consider in the therapy of immunodeficiency and malnutrition is iron. Lynch et al. (71) have shown that iron absorption in immunodeficiency and PEM is decreased. The increased bone marrow stores that most patients with immunodeficiency and PEM show on admission, gradually disappear completely within 4 to 6 weeks, without supplementation.

Intramuscular iron produces an immediate increase in bone marrow stores. Because oral iron is poorly absorbed in malnutrition, the use of parenteral iron or high doses of oral iron in the range of 6 mg/kg of elemental iron per day should be considered. However, iron therapy should be initiated only if the patient is on antibiotics and/or after the threat of infection has passed, usually after 1 to 2 weeks of hospitalization.

Zinc is another important mineral to consider. Investigators in Chile found that supplementation of marasmic infants with 2 mg/kg of elemental zinc as zinc acetate had significantly positive effects on weight gain and host defense mechanisms (72).

Antibiotic Therapy of Intercurrent Infections

Infection is one of the most serious problems facing the child with immunodeficiency and PEM. Several of the host defenses against infection are affected in these children. In such cases, when immunologic defenses against overwhelming infection are inadequate, the physician must give priority to the question of localization and treatment of infection.

Antibiotics are an important factor associated with the decreased morbidity and mortality associated with immunodeficiency and PEM. This is especially true in the septic child, for whom large doses of broad-spectrum antibiotics are used. Generally this indicates a regimen of ampicillin and gentamicin, or a cephalosporin. Gentamicin is also used frequently because of the common occurrence of *Pseudomonas* sepsis (Table 3).

Colistin and Metronidazole may be considered for intestinal antisepsis against small bowel aerobic and anaerobic bacterial overgrowth. This is because of the occurrence of small bowel bacterial overgrowth in the malnourished, immunocompromised patient (73). The GI tract is one of the major sources of endotoxin production. If the GI tract is sterilized, a potential source of gram-negative sepsis and endotoxic shock may be eliminated for the few days needed to regenerate an intact GI mucosa. Gastrointestinal antisepsis should be combined with at least one broad spectrum systemic antibiotic such as Gentamycin.

CONCLUSION

The immunocompromised patient who develops secondary malnutrition as a result of recurrent infection

TABLE 3. *Antibiotics used in treating the malnourished child*

Indications	Antibiotic	Dose (mg/kg/day)
Pneumonia or otitis media	Ampicillin	50–100
	Penicillin	50–100
	Trimethoprim (TMP) and sulfamethoxazole	8–10 mg/k TMP
Staph pneumonia	Oxacillin	100–200
Genitourinary infection	Ampicillin	100
	Sulfisoxazole	150–200
Sepsis	Systemic antibiotics	
	Ampicillin and	200–300
	Gentamycin, or	3–7.5
	Cefuroxime, or	75–150
	Ceftriaxone	50–100
Gastrointestinal antisepsis	Colistin (for aerobic organisms)	5–10
	Metronidazole HCl (for anaerobic organisms)	35–50

should be as aggressively treated as the primarily malnourished child who, as a result of nutrient depletion, is at serious risk of overwhelming sepsis and death.

REFERENCES

1. Gordon JE, Scrimshaw NS. Infectious disease in the malnourished child. *Med Clin North Am* 1970;54:1495–1508.
2. Singh G, Chandra RK. Use of immunological indices for nutritional assessment and outcome. In: Sitges-Serra, Sitges-Creus, Schwartz-Riera, eds. *Clinical progress in nutrition research.* Basel: Karger, 1988;59–70.
3. Singh G, Chandra RK. Immunological effects of malnutrition. In: Sitges-Serra, Sitges-Creus, Schwartz-Riera, eds. *Clinical progress in nutrition research.* Basel: Karger, 1988;136–154.
4. Berger M, Sorensen RU. Immune defects associated with recurrent infections. *Adv Pediatr Infect Dis* 1989;4:111–138.
5. Frank MM, Gelfand JA, Atkinson JP. Hereditary angioedema: the clinical syndrome and its management. *Ann Intern Med* 1976;84:580–593.
6. Alt B, Glass NR, Sollinger H. Neutropenic enterocolitis in adults. Review of the literature and assessment of surgical intervention. *J Surg* 1985;149:405–408.
7. Sorensen RU, Kallik MD. Clinical uses of intravenous immune globulin. Immunoglobulin replacement therapy and treatment of autoimmune cytopenias. *J Clin Apheresis* 1988;4:97–103.
8. Kirkpatrick CH. Host factors in defense against fungal infections. *Am J Med* 1984;77:S1–S11.
9. Higgs JM, Wells RS. Chronic mucocutaneous candidiasis: associated abnormalities of iron metabolism. *Br J Dermatol* 1972;86:S88–102.
10. Bruton OC. Agammaglobulinemia. *Pediatrics* 1952;9:722–728.
11. Doe WF. Immunodeficiency and the gastrointestinal tract. *Clin Gastroenterol* 1983;12:839–853.
12. Abramowsky CR, Sorensen RU. Regional enteritis-like illness in a patient with agammaglobulinemia (histological and immunocytological studies). *Hum Pathol* 1988;19:483–486.
13. Hughes WS, Cerda JJ, Holtzapple P, Brooks FP. Primary hypogammaglobulinemia and malabsorption. *Ann Intern Med* 1971;74:903–910.
14. Webster ADB, Slavin G, Shiner M, Platts-Mills TA, Asherson GL. Case report: coeliac disease with severe hypogammaglobulinaemia. *Gut* 1981;22:153–157.
15. Sorensen RU, Kallik MD, Berger M. Home treatment of antibody deficiency syndromes with intravenous immune globulin. *J Allergy Clin Immunol* 1987;80:810–815.
16. Cunningham-Rundles C, Cunningham-Rundles S, Iwata T, et al. Zinc deficiency, depressed thymic hormones, and T lymphocyte dysfunction in patients with hypogammaglobulinemia. *Clin Immunol Immunopathol* 1981;21:387–396.
17. Glassman M, Grill B, Gryboski J, Dwyer J. High incidence of hypogammaglobulinemia in infants with diarrhea. *J Pediatr Gastroenterol Nutr* 1983;2:465–471.
18. Ropars C, Muller A, Paint N, Beige D, Avenard G. Large scale detection of IgA deficient blood donors. *J Immunol Methods* 1982;54:183–189.
19. Sorensen RU, Halpin TC, Abramowsky CR, Hornick DL, Miller K, Naylor P, Incefy G. Intestinal lymphangiectasia and thymic hypoplasia. *Clin Exp Immunol* 1985;59:217–226.
20. Jeffries GH, Chapman A, Sleisenger MH. Low-fat diet in intestinal lymphangiectasia: its effect on albumin metabolism. *N Engl J Med* 1984;270:761–766.
21. Rickland KA, Bachner RL, Coates TD, et al. Supportive nutritional intervention in pediatric cancer. *Cancer Res* 1982;42(suppl):766S–773S.
22. Fallon J, Eddy J, Wiener L, Pizzo PA. Human immunodeficiency virus infection in children. *J Pediatr* 1989;114:1–30.
23. Nicholas SW, Sondheimer DL, Willoughby AD, Yaffe SJ, Katz SL. Human immunodeficiency virus infection in childhood, adolescence, and pregnancy: a status report and national research agenda. *Pediatrics* 1989;83:293–308.
24. Seligmann M. Immunological features of human immunodeficiency virus disease. *Baillieres Clin Haematol* 1990;3:37–63.
25. Brenner BG, Dascal A, Margolese RG, Wainberg MA. Natural killer cell function in patients with acquired immunodeficiency syndrome and related diseases. *J Leukoc Biol* 1989;46:75–83.
26. Rubinstein A, Sicklick M, Gupta A, et al. Acquired immunodeficiency with reversed T4/T8 ratios in infants born to promiscuous and drug-addicted mothers. *JAMA* 1983;249:2350–2356.
27. Lesbordes JL, Chassignol S, Ray E, et al. Malnutrition and HIV infection in children in the Central African Republic. *Lancet* 1986;2:337–338.
28. Thyri L, Sprecher-Goldberger J, Jonckheer T, et al. Isolation of AIDS virus from cell-free breast milk of three healthy virus carriers. *Lancet* 1985;2:891–892.
29. Bucens M, Armstrong J, Stuckey M. Virological and electron microscopic evidence for postnatal HIV transmission via breast milk. Presented at Fourth International Conference on AIDS, June 12–16, 1988, Stockholm, Sweden. Abstract 5099.
30. Kuvibidila S, Warrier R, Suskind D, et al. Nutritional status of hemophiliacs with and without infection with the human immunodeficiency virus (HIV). *Nutr Res* 1989;9:1197–1206.
31. Dworkin B, Wormser GP, Rosenthal WS, et al. Gastrointestinal manifestations of the acquired immunodeficiency syndrome: a review of 22 cases. *Am J Gastroenterol* 1985;80:774–778.
32. Moseson M, Zeleniuch-Jacquotte A, Belsito DV, Shore RE, Marmor M, Pasternack B. The potential role of nutritional factors in the induction of immunologic abnormalities in HIV-positive homosexual men. *J Acquir Immun Defic Syndr* 1989;2:235–247.
33. Ayres S Jr. Yellow nail syndrome controlled by vitamin E therapy. *J Am Acad Dermatol* 1986;15:714–715.
34. Weiner RG. AIDS and zinc deficiency. *JAMA* 1984;252:1409–1410.
35. Tong TK, Andrew LR, Albert A, Mickell JJ. Childhood acquired immune deficiency syndrome manifesting as acrodermatitis enteropathica. *J Pediatr* 1986;108:426–428.
36. Falutz J, Tsoukas C, Gold P. Zinc as a cofactor in human immunodeficiency virus-induced immunosuppression. *JAMA* 1988;259:2850–2851.
37. Dworkin BM, Rosenthal SW, Wormser GP, Weiss L. Selenium deficiency in the acquired immunodeficiency syndrome. *JPEN J Parenter Enteral Nutr* 1986;10:405–407.
38. Blumberg BS, Hann HWL, Mildvan D, Mathur U, Lustbader E, London WT. Iron and iron binding proteins in persistent generalized lymphadenopathy and AIDS (letter). *Lancet* 1984;2:347.
39. Gonzalez B, Moreno S, Burdach R, et al. Clinical presentation of bacille Calmette-Guerin infections in patients with immunodeficiency syndromes. *Pediatr Infect Dis* 1989;8:201–206.
40. Satyanarayara K, Bhaskaram P, Seshu V, Reddy V. Influence of nutrition on postvaccinal tuberculin sensitivity. *Am J Clin Nutr* 1980;33:2334–2337.
41. Seth V, Kukreja N, Sundaram KR, Malaviya AN, Seth SD. *In vivo* and *in vitro* correlation of cell mediated immune response in preschool children after BCG in relation to their nutritional status. *Indian J Med Res* 1982;75:360–365.
42. Pahwa R, Chatila T, Pahwa S, et al. Recombinant interleukin-2 therapy in severe combined immunodeficiency disease. *Proc Natl Acad Sci USA* 1989;86:5069–5073.
43. Chatila T, Wong R, Young M, Miller R, Terhorst C, Geha RS. An immunodeficiency characterized by defective signal transduction in T lymphocytes. *N Engl J Med* 1989;320:696–702.
44. Rook AH, Masur H, Lane HC, et al. Interleukin-2 enhanced the depressed natural killer and CMV specific cytotoxic activities of lymphocytes from patients with acquired immune deficiency syndrome. *J Clin Invest* 1983;72:398–403.
45. Gluckman JC, Klatzmann D, Cavaille-Coll M, et al. Is there correlation of T-cell proliferative functions and surface marker phenotypes in patients with acquired immune deficiency syndrome of lymphadenopathy syndrome? *Clin Exp Immunol* 1985;60:8–16.
46. Haregewoin A, Godal AT, Mustafa AS, Belehu A, Yemaneberhan T. T-cell conditioned media reverse T-cell unresponsiveness in lepromatous leprosy. *Nature* (Lond.) 1983;303:342–344.
47. Toosi Z, Kleinhenz ME, Ellner J. Defective interleukin-2 production and responsiveness in human pulmonary tuberculosis. *J Exp Med* 1986;163:1162–1172.

48. Ambrosino DM, Siber GR, Chilmonczyle BA. An immunodeficiency characterized by impaired responses to polysaccharides. *N Engl J Med* 1987;316:790–793.
49. Neumann CG, Lawlor GI, Stiehm ER, et al. Immunologic responses in malnourished children. *Am J Clin Nutr* 1975;28:89–104.
50. Borkowsky W, Paul D, Bebenroth D, Kransinski K, Moore T, Chandwani S. Human-immunodeficiency-virus infections in infants negative for anti-HIV by enzyme-linked immunoassay. *Lancet* 1987;1:1168–1171.
51. Saulsbury FT, Winkelstein JA, Yolken RH. Chronic rotavirus infection in immunodeficiency. *J Pediatr* 1980;97(1):61–65.
52. Losonsky GA, Johnson JP, Winkelstein JA, Yolken RH. Oral administration of human serum immunoglobulin in immunodeficient patients with viral gastroenteritis. *J Clin Invest* 1985;76:2362–2367.
53. Polmar SH, Waldmann TA, Terry WD. IgE in immunodeficiency. *Am J Pathol* 1972;69(3):499–512.
54. Chren M-M, Silverman R, Sorensen RU, Elmets CA. Leukocytoclastic vasculitis in a patient infected with human immunodeficiency virus. *J Am Acad Dermatol* 1989;21:1161–1164.
55. Sorensen RU, Polmar SH. Immunoglobulin replacement therapy. *Ann Clin Res* 1987;19:293–304.
56. Eibl MM, Wolf HM, Furnkranz H, Rosenkranz A. Prevention of necrotizing enterocolitis in low-birth-weight infants by IgA-IgG feeding. *N Engl J Med* 1988;319:1–7.
57. Levy Y, Hershfield MS, Fernandez-Mejia C, et al. Adenosine deaminase deficiency with late onset of recurrent infections: response to treatment with polyethylene-glycol modified adenosine deaminase (PEG-ADA). *J Pediatr* 1988;113:312–315.
58. Cunningham AS. Morbidity in breast-fed and artificial-fed infants. II. *J Pediatr* 1979;95:685–689.
59. Welsh JK, May JT. Anti-infective properties of breast milk. *J Pediatr* 1979;94:1–9.
60. Lawton JWM, Shortridge KF, Wong RLC, Ng MH. Interferon synthesis by human colostral leukocytes. *Arch Dis Child* 1979;54:127–130.
61. Stephens S, Brenner MK, Duffy SW, Lakhani PK, Kennedy CR, Farrant J. The effect of breast-feeding on proliferation by infant lymphocytes. *Pediatr Res* 1986;20:227–231.
62. General recommendations on immunization. *MMWR* 1989;38:205–228.
63. Selwyn PA, Hartel D, Lewis VA, et al. A prospective study of the risk of tuberculosis among intravenous drug users with human immunodeficiency virus infection. *N Engl J Med* 1989;320:545–550.
64. Pabst HF, Godel J, Grace M, Cho H, Spady DW. Effect of breast feeding on immune response to BCG vaccination. *Lancet* 1989;1:295–297.
65. Garrow JS, Smith R, Ward EE. *Electrolyte metabolism in severe infantile malnutrition.* Oxford: Pergamon, 1968.
66. Caddell JL, Suskind R, Sillup H, Olson RE. Parenteral magnesium load evaluation of malnourished Thai children. *J Pediatr* 1973;83:129–135.
67. Caddell JL, Goddard DR. Studies in protein-calorie malnutrition. I. Chemical evidence for magnesium deficiency. *N Engl J Med* 1967;276:533–555.
68. Graham GG, Cordano A, Baertl JM. Studies on infantile malnutrition. II. Effect of protein and calorie intake on weight gain. *J Nutr* 1963;81:249–254.
69. Waterlow JC. The rate of recovery of malnourished infants in relation to the protein and calorie levels of the diet. *J Trop Pediatr* 1961;7:16–22.
70. Dean RFA, Swanne J. Abbreviated schedule of treatment for severe kwashiorkor. *J Trop Pediatr* 1963;8:97–98.
71. Lynch SR, Becker D, Seftel H, et al. Iron absorption in kwashiorkor. *Am J Clin Nutr* 1970;23:792–797.
72. Castillo-Duran C, Heresi G, Fisburg M, Uauy R. Controlled trial of zinc supplementation during recovery from malnutrition: effects on growth and immune function. *Am J Clin Nutr* 1987;45:602–608.
73. Suskind R. The in-patient and out-patient treatment of the child with severe protein-calorie malnutrition. In: Olson RE, ed. *Protein-calorie malnutrition.* New York: Academic Press, 1975;403–410.

CHAPTER 39

Pediatric AIDS and Nutrition

Anthony R. Mawson, Rajesekharan P. Warrier,
Solo Kuvibidila, and Robert M. Suskind

OVERVIEW OF THE AIDS EPIDEMIC

Acquired immunodeficiency syndrome (AIDS) is caused by a member of the lentivirus family, the human immunodeficiency virus (HIV) (1). This virus has been isolated in numerous body fluids but appears to be spread most commonly through sexual activity and contact with infected blood or needles. In the United States, the two groups most commonly affected are homosexual males and intravenous drug abusers.

First reported in 1981 (2), AIDS has continued to rise dramatically in incidence and prevalence. Cases have been reported from virtually every country in the world (3). Reports of its lethal effect on the immune system of infants and children first appeared in 1983 (4). By the end of January 1992, the Centers for Disease Control reported 209,693 adult/adolescent cases of AIDS in the United States, and 2,502 cases among children under age 13. At least 250,000 people are presently ill with the virus, but do not fulfill the criteria for full-blown AIDS. Probably over 1 million people in the United States (1 in 250) are thought to be carriers of the AIDS retrovirus (5). By 1992, approximately 4,000 children in the United States will have AIDS and five to eight times that number will be HIV-positive (6). By 2000, the World Health Organization projects that at least 30 million people will have been infected: 15 to 20 million adults and 10 million infants and children (7).

In addition to the cost in human suffering, the AIDS epidemic is resulting in staggering health care costs. Pediatric AIDS will be a major cause of death among infants and children around the world in the 1990s (7). Studies suggest that in the absence of effective long-term therapy, roughly 50% of HIV (+) persons will develop AIDS within 10 years, and up to 99% after 15 to 20 years (8,9). Projected costs range from $50,000 to over $150,000 per patient (10). Pediatric costs far exceed those for other childhood diseases. New Jersey estimates medical costs at $50,000 per hospitalization, with two to three hospitalizations required each year (11).

In the United States, 4% of all AIDS cases are children under age 13. Eighty percent of those are African-American or Hispanic (2). For 70%, transmission was maternal-fetal from mothers who were asymptomatic or who had mild infections (12). In 1989, one in 77 childbearing women in New York City was found to be HIV (+) (13). There is a 25% to 35% chance that an infant born to an HIV (+) mother will be infected (14,15). Although the development of AIDS occurs in 8% to 34% of adults after 3 years following seroconversion (16), AIDS develops in 50% of perinatally infected infants within 9 to 12 months and in 82% by age 3 (17). The median time of incubation is estimated at 1.9 years in children under age 5, and 8 years in adults (18). The case-fatality rate of pediatric AIDS (56%) is the same as in adult AIDS (58%).

THE CLINICAL PICTURE OF PEDIATRIC AIDS

At present it is difficult to reliably determine if a child born to an HIV-infected mother is infected without serial virologic, serologic, immunologic, and clinical assessments over a period of 15 months or longer. This

---

A. R. Mawson: Department of Ophthalmology, Louisiana State University School of Medicine, New Orleans, Louisiana 70112.
R. P. Warrier, S. Kuvibidila, and R. M. Suskind: Department of Pediatrics, Louisiana State University School of Medicine, New Orleans, Louisiana 70112.

lack of an early definitive diagnostic technology hampers the conduct of research into the epidemiologic, natural history, and therapeutic aspects of pediatric HIV disease (14).

The clinical syndrome in pediatric AIDS usually includes fever, diarrhea, anorexia, weight loss, adenopathy, developmental delay or encephalopathy, and eventually opportunistic infections (Table 1) (17,19). The latter include *Pneumocystis carinii* pneumonia, *Candida, Cryptosporidium,* toxoplasmosis *Cryptococcus,* and herpes simplex.

The characteristic wasting and significant nutritional deficiencies found in AIDS patients tend to precede the occurrence of opportunistic infections and tumors (20). Infection leads to fever and a rise in basal energy expenditure (21), often exacerbating anorexia. Reports indicate that up to 90% of AIDS children present with failure to thrive (FTT) (22,23), associated with deficiencies of nitrogen, potassium, body fat, and intracellular water volume (24,25). Malabsorption is an unlikely primary cause of this growth arrest since FTT frequently antedates changes in gastrointestinal function (26). However, both diarrhea and malabsorption are major nutritional problems in patients with AIDS and AIDS-related complex (ARC) (27). Intestinal parasites appear to play a role in the etiology of diarrhea, especially *Cryptosporidium,* a protozoan that can cause intractable, profuse, secretory diarrhea that may last for months (28) and for which no cure has been found. Diarrhea often persists despite a variety of standard antidiarrheal therapies as well as systemic treatment for fungal and mycobacterial disease and intravenous antibiotics. The cause of the diarrhea remains uncertain.

A study of 22 patients with AIDS (29) revealed diarrhea in 55% of the patients, a mean weight loss of 35 lb, hypoalbuminemia in 100%, and gastrointestinal infections in 45%. A wide range of gastrointestinal pathogens were identified. Abnormal D-xylose tests were present in 57% and fat malabsorption in 29% of patients. A retrospective review of the hospital charts of 24 patients with AIDS and *Pneumocystis carinii* pneumonia (PCP) (30) revealed a history of weight loss in 91% of patients, an average documented weight loss of 25 lb in 15 patients, abnormal albumin levels (below 3.5 g/dl) in 42% of patients at the time of admission, and a progressive decrease in albumin levels during hospitalization. Using body cell mass (determined by measuring total body potassium and adjusting for age and height—KHT) to assess the degree of wasting, Grunfeld et al. (31) found that the mean KHT value in AIDS patients was significantly lower than that of HIV (+) persons and of a control group. Fifty percent of the AIDS patients ($n = 32$) showed "wasting" (2 standard deviations below normal) versus none among the HIV (+) patients ($n = 8$) and none among the controls ($n = 17$) (31).

IMMUNOLOGIC DYSFUNCTION AND AIDS

HIV preferentially infects T lymphocyte cells containing T4 receptors, but it can also infect other cells such as peripheral blood monocytes (32) and macrophages (33). Immunological abnormalities in AIDS include a reversal in the ratio between helper (T4) and suppressor (T8) cells, a decrease in lymphokine production, and a decrease in the activity of cytotoxic cells (34). The selective depletion of helper/inducer $CD4^+$ lymphocytes (T4 cells) caused by the AIDS retrovirus results in a profound and persistent cellular immunodeficiency, rendering the patient susceptible to the growth of tumors and opportunistic infections. A comparison between the immunologic dysfunction in AIDS and that found in protein-energy malnutrition (PEM) is shown in Table 2.

MALNUTRITION AND IMMUNE DYSFUNCTION

The three principal cell types involved in immunoregulation are T and B lymphocytes and macrophages. T

TABLE 1. *Manifestations of AIDS*

Neoplasms
    Kaposi's sarcoma
    Lymphoma (non-Hodgkins)
Opportunistic infections
    Fungi
        Candida
        Cryptococcus
        Aspergillus
        Coccidiodes
        Histoplasma
        Blastomyces
    Viruses
        Cytomegalovirus (CMV)
        Herpes simplex virus
        Epstein-Barr virus (EBV)
        Varicella-zoster virus (VZV)
        Papovavirus
        Adenovirus
    Bacteria
        Atypical mycobacteria
        Mycobacterium tuberculosis
        Legionella
        Salmonella
        Listeria
        Brucella
        Shigella
        Camphylobacter
    Protozoa
        Pneumocystis carinii
        Toxoplasma
        Cryptosporidium
        Isospora belli
    Direct HIV infection
    AIDS encephalitis
    AIDS enteropathy

From ref. 77.

TABLE 2. *Immunologic dysfunction in AIDS and protein-energy malnutrition (PEM) compared*

	AIDS	PEM
Cell immunity		
Total lymphocyte condition	Decreased	Decreased
Total T cell number	Decreased	Decreased
Helper T cell number	Decreased	Decreased
Suppressor T cell number	±	±
Helper/suppressor T ratio	Decreased	Decreased
T lymphocyte proliferation	Decreased	Decreased
Cytokine production	Decreased	Decreased
Skin response to antigens	Impaired	Impaired
Humoral immunity		
B cell number	±	±
Immunoglobulin levels	Normal or increased	Normal or increased
Antibody response	Decreased	Normal or decreased
Phagocytic system		
Phagocytes or PMN number	Normal/increase	Normal or increased
PMN bone marrow reserve	?	Decreased
PMN migration	?	Normal
PMN chemotaxis	Decreased	Decreased
Monocyte migration	?	Decreased
Phagocytosis	?	Normal
Killing function	Decreased	Decreased
Complement system		
C3 levels	Decreased	Decreased
C4 levels	Decreased	Normal
CH_{50} levels (total hemolytic activity)	?	Decreased
Other immunity		
NK cell activity	Decreased	Decreased
Anatomic barriers	Altered	Altered
Mucosal immunity	Altered	Altered

PMN, polymorphonuclear neutrophil leukocytes; NK, natural killer; ±, no significant change; ?, information unavailable.

lymphocytes, derived from stem cells that migrate to the thymus from the bone marrow or from fetal liver (35), mediate the cellular immune response which includes delayed hypersensitivity, tissue rejection, and destruction of viruses, bacteria, infected cells, and tumor cells. Helper-inducer T cells (CD4$^+$ helper cells) facilitate antibody production by plasma cells, whereas cytotoxic-suppressor T cells (CD8$^+$ cells) destroy target cells, provide negative feedback to inhibit the antibody response or down-regulate the inflammatory response. The B lymphocyte is responsible for immunoglobulin production; in malnourished children the number of B cells is normal or elevated, as are circulating immunoglobulin levels (36).

Macrophages process antigens before presenting them to lymphocytes and serve as accessory cells in lymphocyte proliferation (37). Activated macrophages/monocytes produce several monokines including interleukin-1 (IL-1) and tumor necrosis factor (TNF), both of which influence T-cell functions. IL-1 induces T lymphocytes IL-2 secretion, a cytokine that plays a central role in many T-cell, B-cell, and neutrophil functions (38). TNF has been implicated as a mediator of anorexia and cachexia, the wasting syndrome usually associated with infections (39). TNF levels are elevated in patients with severe malnutrition (40) and in patients with AIDS (41).

Even mild protein-energy malnutrition (PEM) is associated with a consistent impairment of cell-mediated immunity, with a reduction in the proportion and absolute number of circulating thymus-dependent T lymphocytes (42). In particular, there is a marked numerical and functional deficiency of CD4$^+$ helper cells, whereas CD8 cytotoxic-suppressor cells are affected to a lesser extent (43). Malnourished subjects have a normal number of B lymphocytes. Malnutrition is the most common cause of acquired immune dysfunction worldwide (44). All levels of nutritional deficiencies influence specific components of the immune system. Malnutrition results in reduced numbers of T lymphocytes, as well as impaired cell-mediated immunity (45), impaired secretory immunity, reduced complement levels (46), altered phagocytic function (40), and decreased killer cell activity (47). Deficiencies in trace elements and minerals, including iron, selenium, copper, magnesium, lithium, nickel, tin, arsenic, silicon, and heavy metals (48–51) and vitamins, including A, C, E, pyridoxine, and folate (55), impair immune function. Malnutrition also affects immune function by limiting amino acid and nucleotide substrate availability to support cell proliferation (53).

The course and severity of most infectious illnesses are affected by nutritional status. Patients with acute leukemia who develop *Pneumocystis carinii* infection have lower serum albumin levels than those who do not (54). Episodes of diarrhea last two to three times longer in wasted children. Both acute and chronic starvation produce thymic involution and marked lymphopenia due to reduced cell proliferation, decreased protein synthesis, cytolysis due to increased cortisol levels, and the effects of infection (44).

Optimum functioning of the immune system is dependent on adequate vitamin and trace mineral intake (55). Zinc deficiency results in diarrhea and growth failure, serious viral, bacterial, and fungal infections, and a marked impairment of cell-mediated immunity involving a reduction in $CD4^+$ helper cells (56). Iron deficiency, the most common type of nutritional deficiency worldwide, is associated with impaired lymphocyte and neutrophil function (57). Animals deficient in copper and selenium (56) show a reduced number of antibody-producing cells compared to healthy and pair-fed controls, together with a reduction in thymic activity (56,57). Deficiencies of vitamin A, pyridoxine, folate, and vitamin C also result in impaired cell-mediated immunity (44). Vitamin A deficiency in particular is associated with an increase in the severity and frequency of viral, bacterial, and parasitic infections (58,59). Murthy et al. (60) reported that vitamin A deficiency was associated with a decreased number and percentage of T cells, particularly helper T cells, resulting in altered helper/suppressor T cell ratios. T cells from vitamin A–deficient rats also had a significantly reduced proliferative response to phytohemagglutinin and produced significantly reduced levels of IL-2 compared to controls.

IMMUNE DYSFUNCTION, MALNUTRITION, AND AIDS

The gastrointestinal manifestations of AIDS are severe and include fever, diarrhea, and wasting. It has been hypothesized that the severe weight loss seen in patients with AIDS sets up a vicious cycle in which an underlying immunologic deficit is exacerbated by the immune dysfunction associated with weight loss itself (34,61,62). In short, malnutrition produces a downward spiral of depressed immunity, leading to increased infections and complications. These in turn worsen the patient's nutritional status, which further impairs immune function (Fig. 1). Although the underlying mechanisms of this process are uncertain, immune dysfunction results in antigen and pathogen adherence and penetration of the mucosa, followed by chronic viral and bacterial infections, lymphoproliferation, and a possible autoimmune response. Histologic damage to the intestinal tract leads to malabsorption, increased losses of protein and other nutrients, and systemic immune stimulation from luminal antigens. The resulting state of malnutrition, including vitamin, mineral, and energy deficiencies is inadequate to support the immune response. A self-perpetuating cycle may ensue, leading to reduced gastrointestinal function and a terminal course (Fig. 1).

SPECIFIC NUTRIENT DEPLETION IN HIV DISEASE

In addition to generalized malnutrition, specific nutrient deficits have been observed in patients with HIV disease. These include severely decreased serum levels of selenium (29,48), independent of malabsorption or disease duration. Although decreased serum selenium levels correlate with serum albumin levels (48), selenium is transported in plasma bound to nonalbumin proteins (63). Red blood cell selenium levels are also reduced, and correlate with the activity of the selenoenzyme, glutathione peroxidase which reduces hydroperoxides and protects membrane lipids against oxidant damage.

Selenium deficiency may also have a further negative impact on an already compromised immune system (64). Diminished helper T-cell numbers responsive to selenium repletion have been reported in patients on long-term parenteral nutrition lacking selenium (29).

Several groups of investigators have reported decreased levels of vitamins B_{12} (cobalamin) and folate in patients with early HIV infection and AIDS (52,65,66). In one study (66), decreased B_{12} levels were found in 36% of patients taking transcobalamin II, supporting Kotler

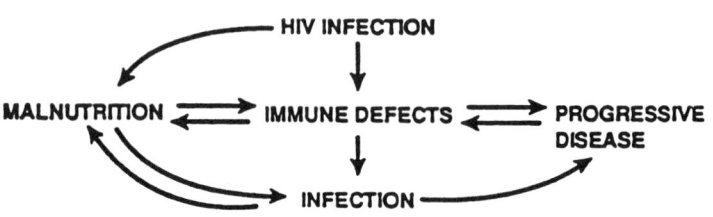

FIG. 1. Infection-immunity-nutrition interaction.

et al.'s (67) view that AIDS patients, even those without diarrhea, often have intestinal damage and malabsorption.

Several studies have shown that pediatric and adult patients with AIDS are deficient in zinc (68,69); some also develop acrodermatitis enteropathica, a zinc deficiency syndrome involving eczematous perioral and perianal lesions, alopecia, conjunctivitis, chronic diarrhea, stomatitis, intercurrent bacterial and candidal infections, growth retardation, and severe immune deficiency (68). In view of the important role of zinc in the immune response (44), it has been suggested that zinc supplementation might be useful in the prevention or correction of immune dysfunction in HIV disease (69). Some patients with AIDS also have a yellow nail syndrome (70), which has been associated with vitamin E deficiency and shown to be responsive to vitamin E supplementation (71).

CAUSES OF MALNUTRITION IN HIV DISEASE

It is well known that malnutrition increases the risk and severity of infection, whereas infection in turn, no matter how mild, negatively affects nutritional status (44,72–75). The development of PEM in HIV infection is multifactorial and not completely understood (76). Several factors hinder the patient's ability to maintain nutritional status (Table 3) (77,78).

All infections induce a degree of anorexia, which inhibits normal dietary intake. In addition, anorexia may result from fever, infection, gastrointestinal symptoms, emotional stress, and the side effects of medication. Bactrim and pentamidine, for instance, may cause nausea and vomiting (77), and pentamidine can induce hypoglycemia (79). A decrease in vitamin B_{12}, associated with bone marrow toxicity, has been reported with azidothymidine (AZT) (80). Solid food is often deliberately but unwisely withdrawn during episodes of infection, especially diarrhea, thereby contributing to clinically evident nutritional deficits (81).

Oral and esophageal pain during eating may occur in persons with *Candida* esophagitis, herpetic esophagitis, or Kaposi's sarcoma, resulting in oral or esophageal ulcers, sore gums, esophageal inflammation, and dysphagia. Neurologic complications of AIDS can result in confusion and dementia, which interfere with eating. In some cases, the patient may not remember how to eat or manipulate eating utensils. Impaired motor ability may lead to tremor, lack of coordination, dysphagia, impaired ability to eat, and decreased appetite. Additionally, depression may contribute to anorexia, further reducing food intake.

Diarrhea and malabsorption are probably the major problems affecting nutritional status and may be the most difficult to resolve. Gastrointestinal complications,

TABLE 3. *Causes of malnutrition in AIDS*

Decreased appetite	Diarrhea and malabsorption
Respiratory infections, febrile illness	Treatable causes
Medication-side effects	Kaposi's sarcoma
Gastrointestinal complications	*Candida*
Emotional stress	Herpes simplex virus
Oral and esophageal pain	*Salmonella*
Kaposi's sarcoma	*Giardia lamblia*
Candida esophagitis	Resistant to treatment
Herpetic esophagitis	Cytomegalovirus
Mechanical problems with eating	Atypical mycobacteria
Central nervous system infections	*Cryptosporidium*
AIDS encephalitis	*Isospora belli*
Dementia	Unknown etiology
Impaired motor ability	AIDS enteropathy
Dysphagia	

From ref. 77.

gastrointestinal infections, and diarrhea decrease absorptive efficiency and require an increased intake of energy and protein. Abnormal D-xylose absorption and steatorrhea are frequently seen in AIDS patients with diarrhea (77). However, as previously noted, in pediatric AIDS, FTT frequently antedates any history of gastrointestinal disturbance, suggesting that malabsorption is not the primary cause of growth arrest (26). Inadequate intake may be the main factor since appropriate weight gain is reportedly achieved with RDA levels of intake (26).

Diarrhea is associated with decreased absorption of nitrogen, fat, carbohydrate, vitamin A, vitamin B_{12}, and folate, and an extended recovery of normal absorption (44). Mechanisms include increased transit time, the direct effect of toxins produced in the lumen, bacterial overgrowth in the small intestine, and flattening of the intestinal villi and microvilli. Intestinal protozoan infections are more likely to be a cause of malabsorption than intestinal helminths, and impaired vitamin A absorption in particular occurs in the presence of *Giardia lamblia* infections in children. Systemic infections, e.g., measles and chronic intestinal infections, are also known to cause malabsorption. Infections result in negative nitrogen balance, decreases in plasma ascorbic acid and vitamin A, and increases in the urinary excretion of these vitamins. The negative nitrogen balance occurring during acute infections is associated with the increased urinary excretion of potassium, magnesium, phosphate, zinc and sulfate, weight loss, and impaired growth and development.

Malabsorption of fat, monosaccharides, disaccharides, and vitamin B_{12} is known to occur in patients with intestinal infections (e.g., Kaposi's sarcoma, *Candida*, herpes simplex virus, salmonella, and giardiasis). Some infections, e.g., cytomegalovirus, atypical mycobacteria, and cryptosporidia, are more resistant to treatment (82). Tumor necrosis factor (TNF) and interleukin-1 (cytokines that mediate the body's response to infection) have been implicated in the pathogenesis of nonspecific wasting in AIDS patients who have elevated levels of circulating TNF (83).

NUTRITIONAL STATUS OF HIV (+) CHILDREN WITH HEMOPHILIA

Because of exposure to commercial coagulation factors derived from blood, children with hemophilia are a high-risk group for infection with HIV. Our study of the nutritional status of 65 hemophiliac children, ages 1 to 18 (84), revealed that 26 (40%) were HIV (+). Using the Waterlow (85) criteria for malnutrition, 62% of the HIV (+) children were found to be malnourished, compared to 18% among the controls (Chi-square = 12.96, $p < .001$).

Recently, we investigated the nutritional status of 20 HIV (+) and HIV (−) children with hemophilia, ages 22 months to 18 years (86). None of the HIV (+) children had AIDS-associated symptoms. Nutritional measures included anthropometry—weight, height, weight-for-height; hematology—hemoglobin (Hb), white blood count (WBC), total lymphocyte count, and absolute lymphocyte count; and biochemical indices—prealbumin (PA), retinol-binding protein (RBP), transferrin (Tr), C-reactive protein (CRP), and α_1-acid glycoprotein (AGP). A significantly higher percentage of HIV (+) children were below the 5th percentile for height (40% vs 4.5%; Chi-square = 5.5, $p < .02$) but not for weight. The HIV (+) hemophiliac children also had significantly lower mean levels of RBP and PA. Since no association was found between RBP and PA and either CRP or AGP, the abnormal levels of these proteins were probably due to protein-energy malnutrition rather than to inflammation. HIV (+) subjects frequently showed abnormal levels of plasma proteins even in the absence of growth deficits or clinical symptoms. These data suggest that PEM starts very early following infection with HIV, prior to changes in weight, height, or clinical symptoms of AIDS. Measurement of these transport proteins may, therefore, be helpful in identifying HIV (+) individuals for whom dietary supplementation may be helpful in slowing the development of AIDS (34).

HIV, MALNUTRITION, AND PSYCHOLOGICAL DEFICITS

Six hemophiliac children ages 6 to 16 [three HIV (+), three HIV (−)] were evaluated psychologically and nutritionally (87). HIV (+) children had lower scores on the Wechsler Intelligence Scale for Children—revised (WISC-R) measures of verbal ability, slower finger-tapping speeds in the dominant and nondominant hands, and lower RBP and transferrin levels.

NUTRITIONAL ASSESSMENT OF HIV (+) CHILDREN

A thorough nutritional assessment should be included in the evaluation of all children with HIV, even those who are asymptomatic (88). Assessment should include anthropometry (weight- and height-for-age, weight-for-height, body mass index, total body fat) and visceral proteins (albumin, transferrin, prealbumin, retinol-binding protein). Children should be weighed at least weekly (89). Acute-phase proteins such as C-reactive protein, α_1-acid glycoprotein, and ceruloplasmin should also be measured to rule out the presence of inflammation and/or infection, which may decrease the levels of prealbumin and retinol-binding protein or elevate ferritin levels. Trace elements and minerals such as serum iron and white blood cell zinc, and selenium, vitamins, including plasma and whole blood α-tocopherol (vitamin E), vitamin B_{12}, vitamin C, and pyridoxine, should also be evaluated. Body potassium should be measured to determine the ratio (or content) of body water, fat free mass, and total body fat. Blood urea nitrogen, creatinine, and liver function should also be monitored where indicated. Determining energy and protein intake may also be useful in establishing supplementation protocols.

RECOMMENDATIONS FOR THE NUTRITIONAL SUPPORT OF HIV (+) CHILDREN

Provision of adequate calories, protein, vitamins, and minerals is essential in preventing or curtailing catabolism and weight loss. Because of their increased metabolic demands, AIDS patients have increased caloric and protein requirements and may require two to three times the recommended dietary allowance (RDA) (89–91). Caloric needs can either be calculated using the classic equations of Harris and Benedict (92), correcting for activity levels and injury factors (93).

To gain weight, a caloric intake of at least 150% of RDA for age is usually recommended. For an increase of 1 kg/week, intake should be increased above requirements by 1,000 Cal/day or 7,000 Cal/week. Protein requirements for people with AIDS are at least 2.0 to 3.0 g/kg/day to reach positive nitrogen balance and prevent continued weight loss (20). Vitamin and mineral supplementation in amounts two to three times greater than the RDA are required to offset deficits and increased metabolic needs. Meals should incorporate personal food preferences and be offered in small, frequent servings. Supplements may include high calorie/high protein snacks, e.g., peanut butter, cheese, and oral liquid supplements, which will increase total daily intake.

For patients with diarrhea associated with hypoalbuminemia and malnutrition ("osmotic diarrhea"), antidiarrheal agents or bowel rest may be helpful. Dietary modifications, including restricting lactose-containing and fatty foods, increasing intake of protein and fiber, and increasing fluid and electrolyte balance, are also recommended. When tube feeding is indicated, patients should be given isotonic lactose-free formulas or elemental formulas.

Patients with "secretory diarrhea" may have several watery stools per day (94), losing excess amounts of water, electrolytes, and nutrients. These patients often have chronic cryptosporidiosis infection that does not respond to medication, dietary intervention, or withholding food. They are very difficult to treat nutritionally.

Several case reports (20,26,77,89,95) have shown that aggressive nutritional intervention in conjunction with antibiotic therapy results in rapid normalization of nutritional indices such as total protein, albumin, and transferrin, conversion to a positive nitrogen balance, and significant improvement in the patient's sense of well-being. In one study, "meticulous attention to food intake" led to an average weight gain of 65 g/week on diets of 90 to 108 Cal/kg/day in four children ages 9 months to 42 months, leading the authors to conclude that "caloric intake within the normal range will support adequate growth velocities in a subpopulation of children with AIDS-related FTT" (26).

CONCLUSION

It is recognized that the wasting syndrome associated with HIV disease contributes to disease progression by worsening immune function and increasing host susceptibility to opportunistic infections. It is widely accepted that aggressive nutritional support should be included in the management of ARC/AIDS patients. Promoting good nutrition may prevent some of the complications of AIDS and protect against further exacerbation (34,61,62,96). Case-control studies are indicated to assess the nutritional status of children with HIV disease. Results should lead to clinical trials aimed at determining the impact of aggressive nutritional supplementation on immune function and clinical status of patients who are HIV positive or who have AIDS.

REFERENCES

1. Levy JA. Human immunodeficiency viruses and the pathogenesis of AIDS. *JAMA* 1989;261:2997-3006.
2. Centers for Disease Control. Kaposi's sarcoma and pneumocystis pneumonia among homosexual men: New York City and California. *Morbid Mortal Weekly Rep* 1981;30:305-308.
3. Chin J. Current and future dimensions of the HIV/AIDS pandemic in women and children. *Lancet* 1990;336:221-224.
4. Oleske J, Minnefor A, Cooper R, et al. Immune deficiency syndrome in children. *JAMA* 1983;249:2345-2349.
5. Morgan M, Curran JW, Berkelman RL. The future course of AIDS in the United States. *JAMA* 1990;263:1539-1540.
6. Rogers MF. Pediatric HIV infection: epidemiology, etiopathogenesis and transmission. *Pediatr Ann* 1988;17:324-331.
7. WHO predicts up to 30 million world AIDS cases by year 2000. *The Nation's Health.* 1991 (January); 1,8.
8. Liu K-J, Darrow WW, Rutherford GW III. A model based estimate of the mean incubation period for AIDS in homosexual men. *Science* 1988;240:1333-1335.
9. Goedert JJ, Kessler CM, Aledort LM, et al. A prospective study of human immunodeficiency virus type I infection and the development of AIDS in subjects with hemophilia. *N Engl J Med* 1989;321:1141-1148.
10. Scitowsky AA, Rice DP. Estimates of the direct and indirect costs of acquired immunodeficiency syndrome in the United States, 1985, 1986 and 1991. *Public Health Rep* 1987;102:5-17.
11. Oleske JM, Connor EM, Boland MG. A perspective on AIDS. *Pediatr Ann* 1988;17:319-321.
12. Guinan ME, Hardy A. Epidemiology of AIDS in women in the United States: 1981-86. *JAMA* 1987;277:2039-2042.
13. Novick LF, Berns D, Stricoff R, et al. HIV seroprevalence in newborns in New York state. *JAMA* 1989;261:1745-1750.
14. Willoughby A. Pediatric HIV infection and AIDS: Research perspectives and opportunities. *Semin Pediatr Infect Dis* 1990; 1(1):174-179.
15. Kozinetz CA, Crane MM, Reves RR. Pediatric HIV infection and AIDS: epidemiology. *Semin Pediatr Infect Dis* 1990;1(1):6-16.
16. Goedert JJ, Biggar RJ, Weiss SH, et al. Three-year incidence of AIDS in five cohorts of HTLV-III-infected risk group members. *Science* 1986;231:992-994.
17. Falloon J, Eddy J, Wiener J, Pizzo PA. Medical progress: human immunodeficiency virus infection in children. *J Pediatr* 1989;114:1-30.
18. Medley GF, Anderson RM, Cox DR, et al. Incubation period of AIDS in patients infected via blood transfusion. *Nature* 1987;328:719-721.
19. Gottlieb MS, Groopman JE, Weinstein WM, et al. The acquired immunodeficiency syndrome. *Ann Intern Med* 1983;99:208-220.
20. Hickey MS, Weaver KE. Nutritional therapy for the malnourished ARC or AIDS patient: current therapeutic concepts and basic therapy outline. *Cont Surg* 1988;33(Suppl 1A):1-32.
21. Krause MV, Mahan LR. *Food, nutrition and diet therapy,* 7th ed. Philadelphia: WB Saunders, 1984.
22. Rubinstein A, Sicklick M, Gupta A, et al. Acquired immunodeficiency with reversed t_4/t_8 ratios in infants born to promiscuous and drug addicted mothers. *JAMA* 1983;249:2350-2356.
23. Beach RS, Laura PF. Nutrition and the acquired immunodeficiency syndrome. *Ann Intern Med* 1989;99:565-566.
24. Malebranche R, Guerin J, Laroche AC, et al. Acquired immunodeficiency syndrome with severe gastrointestinal manifestations in Haiti. *Lancet* 1983;2:873-878.
25. Kotler DP, Wang J, Pierson RN. Body composition studies in patients with the acquired immunodeficiency syndrome. *Am J Clin Nutr* 1985;42:1255-1265.
26. Fennoy I, Leung J. Refeeding and subsequent growth in the child with AIDS. *Nutr Clin Pract* 1990;5:54-58.
27. Garcia ME, Collins CL, Monsell WA. The acquired immune deficiency syndrome. *Nutr Clin Pract* 1987;2:108-111.
28. Modigliani R, Bories C, Le Charpentier Y, Saleron M, Messing B, Galian A, Rambaud JC, Lavergne A, Cochand-Priollet B, Desportes I. Diarrhoea and malabsorption in acquired immune deficiency syndrome: a study of four cases with special emphasis on opportunistic protozoan infestations. *Gut* 1984;26:179-187.
29. Dworkin B, Wormser GP, Rosenthal WS, et al. Gastrointestinal manifestations of the acquired immunodeficiency syndrome: a review of 22 cases. *Am J Gastroenterol* 1985;80:774-778.

30. Chelluri L, Jastremski MS. Incidence of malnutrition in patients with acquired immunodeficiency syndrome. *Nutr Clin Pract* 1989;4:16–18.
31. Grunfeld C, Kotler DP, Hamadeh R, Tierney A, Wang J, Pierson RN Jr. Hypertriglyceridemia in the acquired immunodeficiency syndrome. *Am J Med* 1989;86:27–31.
32. Ho DD, Rota TR, Hirsch MS. Infection of monocyte/macrophages by human T lymphotropic virus type III. *J Clin Invest* 1986;77:1712–1715.
33. Gyorkey F, Nebnick J, Sinkovics J, et al. Retrovirus resembling HTLV in macrophages of patients with AIDS. *Lancet* 1985; 1:106.
34. Jain VK, Chandra RK. Hypothesis: does nutritional deficiency predispose to acquired immune deficiency syndrome? *Nutr Res* 1984;4:537–543.
35. Owen JJT, Jenkinson EJ. Embryology of the lymphoid system. *Prog Allergy* 1981;29:1–34.
36. Suskind RM, Sirisinha S, Edelman R, et al. Immunoglobulins and antibody response in Thai children with protein calorie malnutrition. In: Suskind RM, ed. *Malnutrition and the immune response.* New York: Raven Press, 1977;185–190.
37. Johnston RB. Monocytes and macrophages. *N Engl J Med* 1988;318:747–752.
38. Smith KA. Interleukin-2: inception, impact and implication. *Science* 1988;240:1169–1176.
39. Cerami A, Ibuda Y, Le Trang N, Hotez PJ, Bentler B. Weight loss associated with endotoxin-induced mediator from peritoneal macrophages: the role of cachectin (tumor necrosis factor). *Immunol Lett* 1985;11:173–177.
40. Keusch GT, Orrutia JJ, Fernandez R, et al. Humoral and cellular aspects of intracellular bacteria killing in Guatemalan children with protein-calorie malnutrition. In: Suskind RM, ed. *Malnutrition and the immune response.* Raven Press: New York, 1977;245–251.
41. Maury CPJ, Lahadevista J. Correlation of serum cytokine levels with haematological abnormalities in human immunodeficiency virus infection. *J Int Med* 1990;227:253–257.
42. Chandra RK. Lymphocyte subpopulation in human malnutrition: cytotoxic and suppressor cells. *Pediatrics* 1977;59:423–427.
43. Chandra RK, Gupta S, Singh H. Inducer and suppressor T cell subsets in protein energy malnutrition: analysis by monoclonal antibodies. *Nutr Res* 1982;2:21–26.
44. Chandra RK. Golan memorial lecture. Nutritional regulation of immunity and infection: from epidemiology to phenomenology to clinical practice. *J Pediatr Gastroenterol Nutr* 1986;5:844–852.
45. Chandra RK. Mucosal immune responses in malnutrition. *Ann NY Acad Sci* 1983;409:345–352.
46. Chandra RK. Serum complement and immunoconglutinin in malnutrition. *Arch Dis Child* 1975;50:225–229.
47. Saxena QB, Saxena RK, Adler WH. Effect of protein calories malnutrition on levels of natural and inducible cytotoxic activities in mouse spleen cells. *Immunology* 1984;51:727–733.
48. Dworkin BM, et al. Selenium deficiency in the acquired immunodeficiency syndrome. *JPEN J Parenteral Enteral Nutr* 1986; 10:405–407.
49. Goldsmith GA. Trace element regulation of immunity and infection. *J Am Coll Nutr* 1985;51:727–733.
50. Cunningham-Rundles C, et al. Zinc deficiency, depressed thymic hormones, and T lymphocyte dysfunction in patients with hypogammaglobulinemia. *Clin Immunol Immunopathol* 1981; 21:387–396.
51. Fernandes G, et al. Impairment of cell-mediated immunity functions by dietary zinc deficiency in mice. *Proc Natl Acad Sci USA* 1979;76:457–461.
52. Hutchin KC. Thiamine deficiency, Wernicke's encephalopathy and AIDS. *Lancet* 1987;1:2100.
53. Ortiz R, Bentancourt M. Cell proliferation in bone marrow cells of severely malnourished animals. *J Nutr* 1984;114:472–476.
54. Hughes WT, Price RA, Sisko F, et al. Protein-calorie malnutrition. *Am J Dis Child* 1974;128:44–52.
55. Biesel WR. Single nutrients and immunity. *Am J Clin Nutr* 1982;35:417–468.
56. Chandra RK, Dayton DH. Trace element regulation of immunity and infection. *Nutr Res* 1982;2:721–733.
57. Vyas D, Chandra RK. Functional implications of iron deficiency. In: Stekel A, ed. *Iron nutrition in infancy and childhood.* New York: Raven Press, 1984;45–49.
58. Dennert GA. Retinoids and the immune system: immunostimulation by vitamin A. In: Sporn M, ed. *The retinoids,* vol 2. New York: Academic Press, 1984.
59. Hussey GD, Klein M. A randomized, controlled trial of vitamin A in children with severe measles. *N Engl J Med* 1990;323:160–164.
60. Murthy KK, Suskind SAL, Ventatash V, et al. Decreased T lymphocyte function and interleukin-2 production associated with vitamin A deficiency (abstract and resume). *6th Int Congr Immunol* 1986;86.
61. Chlebowski RT. Significance of altered nutritional status in acquired immune deficiency syndrome (AIDS). *Nutr Cancer* 1985;7:86–89.
62. Begin ME, Das UN. A deficiency in dietary gamma-linolenic and/or eicosapentaenoic acids may determine individual susceptibility to AIDS. *Med Hypotheses* 1986;20:1–8.
63. Motsenbocker A, Tappel AL. A selenocysteine-containing selenium transport protein in rat plasma. *Biochem Biophys Acta* 1982;719:147–153.
64. Beisel WR, Edelman R, Nauss K, et al. Single-nutrient effects on immunologic functions. *JAMA* 1981;245:53–58.
65. Beach RS, Mantero-Atienza E, Eisdorfer C, et al. Altered folate metabolism in early HIV infection. *JAMA* 1988;259:519.
66. Herbert V. B_{12} deficiency in AIDS. *JAMA* 1988;260:2837.
67. Kotler D, Gaetz HP, Lange M, et al. Enteropathy associated with the acquired immune deficiency syndrome. *Ann Intern Med* 1984;101:421–428.
68. Tong TK, Andrew LR, Albert A, Mickell JJ. Childhood acquired immune deficiency syndrome manifesting as acrodermatitis enteropathica. *J Pediatr* 1986;108:426–428.
69. Fabris N, Mocchegiani E, Galli M, et al. AIDS, zinc deficiency and thymic hormone failure (letter). *JAMA* 1988;259:839–840.
70. Chernovsky ME, Finley VK. Yellow nail syndrome in patients with acquired immunodeficiency disease. *J Am Acad Dermatol* 1985;13:731–736.
71. Ayres S. Yellow nail syndrome controlled by vitamin E therapy. *J Am Acad Dermatol* 1986;15:714–715.
72. Suskind RM. Malnutrition and the immune response. In: Suskind RM, ed. *Textbook of pediatric nutrition.* New York: Raven Press, 1981;241–262.
73. Scrimshaw NS. Significance of the interactions of nutrition and infection in children. In: Suskind RM, ed. *Textbook of pediatric nutrition.* New York: Raven Press; 1981;229.
74. Keusch GT. Malnutrition, infection, and immune function. In: Suskind RM, Lewinter-Suskind L, eds. *The malnourished child.* Nestle Nutrition Workshop Series, vol 19. New York: Nestec, Vevey/Raven Press, 1990;37–55.
75. Suskind D, Murthy KK, Suskind RM. The malnourished child: an overview. In: Suskind RM, Lewinter-Suskind L, eds. *The malnourished child.* Nestle Nutrition Workshop Series, vol 19. New York: Nestec, Vevey/Raven Press, 1990;1–20.
76. Kotler DP. Protein-energy malnutrition in AIDS. *Nutr Clin Pract* 1990;5:41–42.
77. Resler SS. Nutrition care of AIDS patients. *J Am Diet Assoc* 1988;88:828–832.
78. Cuff PA. Acquired immunodeficiency syndrome and malnutrition: role of gastrointestinal pathology. *Nutr Clin Pract* 1990;5:43–53.
79. Stahl-Bayliss CM, Kalman CM, Laskin OL. Pentamidine-induced hypoglycemia in patients with acquired immunodeficiency syndrome. *Clin Pharmacol Ther* 1986;39:271.
80. Barbaro D. Nutrition for AIDS patients. *Directions Applied Nutr* 1986;1(2):4.
81. Fuchs GJ. Secondary malnutrition in children. In: Suskind RM, Lewinter-Suskind L, eds. *The malnourished child.* Nestle Nutrition Workshop Series, vol 19. New York: Nestec, Vevey/Raven Press, 1990;23–36.
82. Cone LA, Woodward DR, Potts BE, Byrd RG, Alexander RM,

Last MD. An update on the acquired immune deficiency syndrome (AIDS). Associated disorders of the alimentary tract. *Dis Colon Rectum* 1986;29:60.
83. Maury CPJ, et al. Raised levels of circulating tumor necrosis factor-alpha/cachectin in patients with acquired immunodeficiency syndrome: pathogenetic implications. Presented at the Fifth International Conference on AIDS. *The Scientific and Social Challenge* 1989; W.C.P. 114.
84. Warrier RP, Kuvibidila S, Wulfe K, Deselle B, Suskind D, Andes WA. Nutritional evaluation of children with hemophilia (abstract). *Clin Res* 1988;36(1):62A.
85. Waterlow JC. Classification and definition of protein-energy malnutrition. *Br Med J* 1974;4:566–569.
86. Kuvibidila S, Warrier R, Suskind D, Sarpong D, Desselle B, Suskind RM, Andes WA. Nutritional status of hemophiliacs with and without infection with the human immunodeficiency virus (HIV). *Nutr Res* 1989;9:1197–1206.
87. Sirois PA, Hill SD, Kuvibidila S, Warrier R, Andes WA. Psychological and nutritional profiles of hemophiliac children exposed to HIV. Paper presented at the First Meeting of the American Psychological Society, Alexandria, VA, June 12, 1989.
88. Prestridge LL, Klish WJ. Pediatric HIV infection and AIDS: nutrition and wasting. *Semin Pediatr Infect Dis* 1990;1(1):73–76.
89. Bentler M, Stanish M. Nutrition support of the pediatric patient with AIDS. *J Am Diet Assoc* 1987;87:488–491.
90. Hyman C, Kaufman S. Nutritional impact of acquired immune deficiency syndrome: a unique counseling opportunity. *J Am Diet Assoc* 1989;89(4):520–527.
91. Keithley JK, Kohn CL. Managing nutritional problems in people with AIDS. *Oncology Nursing Forum* 1990;17(1):23–27.
92. Harris JA, Benedict FG. *A biometric study of basal metabolism in man,* vol 2. Washington DC: Carnegie Institute of Washington, 1919;227.
93. Long GL. Energy and protein requirements in stress and trauma. *Crit Care Nurs Curr* 1984;2(2):7–12.
94. Weller IVD. AIDS and the gut. *Scand J Gastroenterol* 1985;20(Suppl 14):77–89.
95. Benkov KJ, Stawski C, Sirlin SM, et al. Atypical presentation of childhood acquired immune deficiency syndrome mimicking Crohn's disease: nutritional considerations and management. *Am J Gastroenterol* 1985;80:260–265.
96. Gray RH. Similarities between AIDS and PCM (letter). *Am J Public Health* 1983;73:1332.

CHAPTER 40

Food Allergy in Children

Ricardo U. Sorensen, Mary Catherine Porch, and Lan C. Tu

The subject of food hypersensitivity and the role of food and food additives as causative factors of disease have evoked considerable controversy in past years. A better understanding of pathophysiologic mechanisms of immune and nonimmune food reactions and the introduction of double-blind food challenges have clearly established the existence of immunologically mediated adverse reactions to food components. These reactions play an especially important role in pediatrics. In the first year of life there are special conditions that increase the risk for immunologic reactions to food components. At the same time, the repertoire of foods is limited and severe disturbances in nutrition can have negative consequences on growth and development. The goals of this chapter are to explain and describe the features of pediatric food allergy for a practical approach to prevention and treatment of this disorder.

Prevention is the most important primary consideration in food allergy in children. Infants at risk for food hypersensitivity can sometimes be identified before the symptoms begin. This allows preventive measures to be maintained throughout the period of increased susceptibility, averting development of a clinical problem.

When immunologically mediated adverse reactions to food do occur, they take the form of distinct clinical syndromes with characteristic pathogenic mechanisms. In order to understand these clinical presentations, some definitions and immunologic mechanisms must first be understood.

DEFINITIONS OF FOOD ALLERGY AND FOOD HYPERSENSITIVITY

By the late 19th century, scientists began to call the phenomenon of a host's reaction to toxins for which the host had been immunized, "anaphylaxis" or "supersensitivity in an immune person." At the turn of the century, Von Pirquet, a physician at the University of Vienna, was concerned about the contradiction of terms describing a supposedly immune person as supersensitive. He introduced the term *allergy* as a general term to apply to any change in reactivity, positive or negative, encompassing both immunity and hypersensitivity. Through the years, however, the definitions of the terms have changed. *Immunity* now refers to the positive, usually protective, responses that result from the introduction of foreign substances capable of activating the immune system. *Allergy*, on the other hand, describes a hypersensitivity reaction with adverse effects on the host (1).

Because the word allergy is often used to describe any adverse reaction, even those unrelated to an immune response, the American Academy of Allergy and Immunology (AAAI) Committee of Adverse Reactions to Foods and the National Institutes of Health (NIH) have published a list of definitions of terms describing all adverse reactions to foods, including immunologic and nonimmunologic mechanisms (Table 1) (2). In this listing, food hypersensitivity and food allergy are described as immunologic reactions resulting from the ingestion of food or food additives. This implies that any of several adverse immune reactions to foods may be described as hypersensitivity or allergy. In this chapter, the term *food allergy* is reserved for those reactions clearly involving IgE-mediated immune reactions. The term *food hypersensitivity* is used in a general sense to include all adverse immune reactions to foods. A brief discussion of the immunologic mechanisms involved in food hypersensitivity should clarify these concepts.

IMMUNE RESPONSES TO FOOD COMPONENTS

Immune reactions against food components differ from other immune reactions only by the presentation

---

R. U. Sorensen, M. C. Porch, L. C. Tu: Department of Pediatrics, Louisiana State University School of Medicine, New Orleans, Louisiana 70112.

TABLE 1. *Definitions of terms describing adverse reactions to foods*

Adverse reaction (sensitivity) to a food: a general term that can be applied to a clinically abnormal response attributed to an ingested food or food additive.
  Food hypersensitivity (allergy): an immunologic reaction, resulting from the ingestion of a food or food additive.
    Food anaphylaxis: a classic allergic hypersensitivity reaction to food or food additives in which the immunologic activity of IgE homocytotropic antibody and release of chemical mediation are involved.
  Food intolerance (nonimmunologic response): a general term describing an abnormal physiologic response to an ingested food or food additive; this reaction is not proved to be immunologic.
    Food toxicity (poisoning): implies an adverse effect caused by the *direct* action of a food or food additive upon the host recipient without the involvement of immune mechanisms. This type of reaction may involve nonimmune release of chemical mediators. Toxins may be either contained within food or released by microorganisms or parasites contaminating food products. On some occasions the term may be synonymous with idiosyncratic adverse reaction. When the reaction is anaphylaxis-like, it may be called "anaphylactoid."
    Food idiosyncracy: a quantitatively abnormal response to a food substance or additive; this reaction differs from its physiologic or pharmacologic effect and resembles hypersensitivity but does not involve immune mechanisms. Food idiosyncratic reactions include those that occur in specific groups of individuals who may be genetically predisposed. When the reaction is anaphylaxis-like, it may be called "anaphylactoid."
    Anaphylactoid reaction to a food: an anaphylaxis-like reaction to food or food additive as a result of nonimmune release of chemical mediators. This reaction mimics the symptoms of food hypersensitivity (allergy).
    Pharmacologic food reaction: an adverse reaction to a food or food additive as a result of a naturally derived or added chemical that produces a drug-like or pharmacologic effect in the host.
    Metabolic food reaction: an adverse reaction to a food or food additive as the result of the effect of the substance upon the metabolism of the host recipient.

Adapted from ref. 2.

of foods through the gut mucosa, and the usually high exposure to foreign material at the time of food consumption. The different host defense mechanisms and their interactions are discussed in detail in chapter 12.

Immunologic reactions pertinent to food hypersensitivity are depicted in Fig. 1. Food components that induce immune responses are called *antigens*. These food components must be small enough to cross the gut mucosa and large enough to be immunogenic, i.e., capable of eliciting an immune response. Immunogenic food

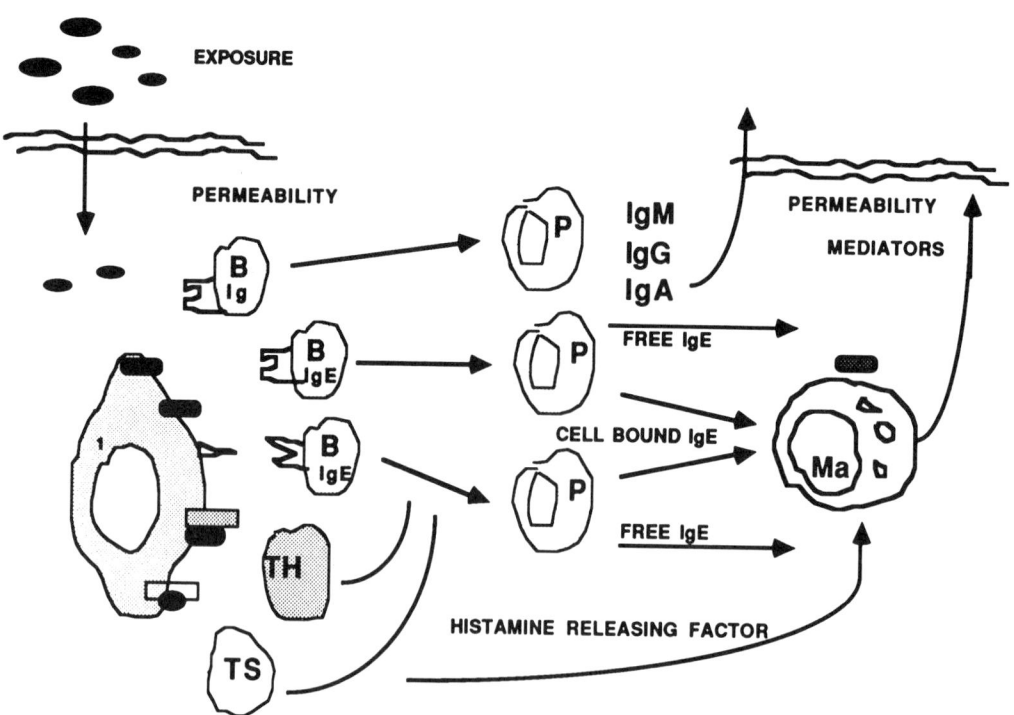

FIG. 1. Immune responses to food antigens. Immunogenic food components need to cross the intestinal mucosa and be presented to lymphocytes by antigen-presenting cells (*1*). B lymphocytes (*B*) with IgE or other immunoglobulins, Ig, on their surfaces are depicted. Different food components interact with specific receptors on B lymphocytes. Presentation of antigens to T cells occurs in conjunction with histocompatibility antigens on antigen presenting cells and lymphocytes. P, plasma cell; TH, helper T cell; TS, suppressor T cell; Ma, mast cell. See text for further explanation.

components that reach immune cells in the gut mucosa are presented by antigen-presenting cells to B and T lymphocytes with specific receptors for each particular food component. B cell clones reacting with food antigens may develop into IgM-, IgG-, IgA-, or IgE-producing plasma cells. IgG and IgM are the main antibodies in circulation. IgA is secreted into the gut lumen after combining with a secretory piece released by epithelial cells. In the gut lumen, it combines with antigenic food components and prevents their absorption and interaction with IgE. IgE will bind to a large extent to specific receptors present on basophils in the circulation and mast cells in tissues including the gastrointestinal mucosa. Only the free portion of IgE can be measured in circulation. The cell-bound fraction is evaluated only indirectly through skin reactions with specific antigens.

Food components also react with both helper T cells and suppressor T cells. These cells regulate the production of IgG and IgA antibodies (generally increased by helper T cells) and the production of IgE (generally down-regulated by suppressor T cells). The reaction of T cells with food antigens may also have an effect on the release of histamine by mast cells through the secretion of histamine releasing factor. A direct effect of T cells has been postulated in adverse reactions to foods such as in celiac disease (3).

Genetic regulation of the immune response to food components can occur at many different levels, including the antigen processing step and the interaction of food antigens with specific receptors on T and B lymphocytes. The interaction of food antigens with specific receptors will determine the predominant type of cell reacting (e.g., IgE producing B lymphocytes or helper or suppressor T cells). Further regulation may occur at the level of lymphokine secretion by T lymphocytes, some of which enhance production of IgE by B lymphocytes and determine the affinity of mast cell receptors for IgE.

Under certain conditions the same immunological mechanisms that have a protective effect react in such a way that there is an adverse effect on the host, generating a hypersensitivity reaction. Coombs and Gell (4) divided hypersensitivity reactions into four types. Types I, II, and III involve antibodies, whereas type IV is mediated by T lymphocytes. The type I, IgE-mediated reaction develops very rapidly and is called an immediate reaction. An important late phase of this hypersensitivity is discussed in the next subsection. Type II hypersensitivity is caused by cytotoxic reactions of IgG and IgM against a cell membrane after interaction with complement. It is probably not involved in food hypersensitivity and is not discussed in this chapter. Type III reactions entail the formation of deleterious antigen-antibody complexes and usually take 6 to 8 hr to develop. Type IV reactions, called delayed-type hypersensitivity (DTH) reactions, involve cellular immunity and are manifested after 48 to 72 hr.

Food allergy, as defined, always includes a type I, IgE-mediated reaction, but is not limited to this hypersensitivity type alone. IgE-mediated reactions are somewhat easier to recognize clinically, and comprise the only form of hypersensitivity for which we have supporting diagnostic tests. The other forms of food hypersensitivity may be equally important in pediatrics, but their presence is more difficult to document.

Type I Hypersensitivity

Type I hypersensitivity reactions involve both immediate and late reactions (Fig. 2). They are triggered by the cross-linking of two IgE molecules on the surface of basophils or mast cells by an allergenic molecule. This interaction activates the immediate release of mediators such as histamine, slow reacting substances (SRS), bradykinin, prostaglandins, and chemotactic factors for eosinophils and neutrophils. Histamine release results in the contraction of smooth muscle of blood vessels, dilatation of small venules, and increased capillary permeability. SRS primarily causes contraction of bronchioles and an increase in venular permeability. Bradykinin causes hypotension due to vasodilation, increases capillary permeability, and contracts bronchial smooth muscle (5). The effect of these mediators is reversible without significant tissue damage. However, the release of chemotactic factors for neutrophils and eosinophils eventually produces an inflammatory response with a rich cellular infiltrate. Enzymes and other factors released by these secondary cells will cause characteristic tissue damage in the late phase.

Antigens capable of eliciting type I reactions are also called allergens. Using double-blind placebo-controlled trials following elimination of foods incriminated in the development of symptoms, Sampson and McCaskill found that milk, eggs, peanuts, wheat, soy, shellfish, and fish cause most allergic reactions (6,7). Most of these foods have unique allergenic glycoproteins that are heat and acid stable, with molecular weights of 18,000 to 36,000 daltons.

Type III Hypersensitivity

Type III hypersensitivity is caused by antigen-antibody immune complexes usually involving precipitating IgG or IgM antibodies that combine with antigen in the presence of antigen excess and complement. The local deposition of immune complexes can cause an Arthus reaction, whereas circulating immune complexes cause serum sickness with various degrees of vasculitis and tissue damage. Circulating immune complex has been found in some individuals with food sensitivity. Frick (8) detected β-lactoglobulin in immune complexes in the sera of milk-sensitive individuals. Sandilands et al. (9) suggested that transient reduction in circulating lym-

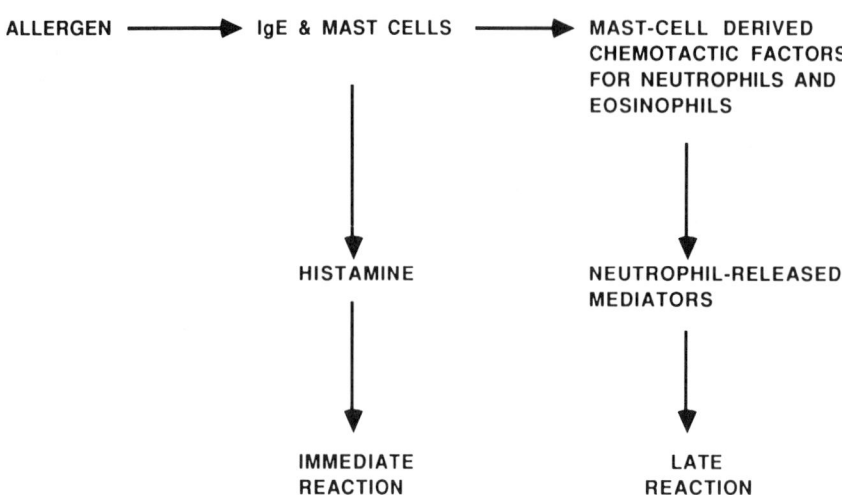

FIG. 2. Pathophysiology of immediate and late reactions mediated by IgE. See text.

phocytes that have receptors for the Fc fragment of IgG after oral milk challenge may be the result of soluble antigen-antibody complexes. Carini et al. (10) studied patients with asthma, eczema, and arthralgia by monitoring the formation of immune complexes containing IgE, IgG, and antigen after challenge with food antigens. The appearance of complexes correlated well with the production of symptoms. The resulting delayed onset of symptoms could be viewed as a form of serum sickness with few or many organs affected. However, the pathogenic role of immune complexes involving food components remains unclear. Immune complexes have been observed in both allergic and nonallergic individuals after food ingestion (11) and many individuals develop antigen-antibody complexes without developing adverse reactions.

Type IV Hypersensitivity

Type IV hypersensitivity is mediated by T lymphocytes. Following the interaction between a food antigen and sensitized T lymphocytes, the release of lymphokines activates monocytes and macrophages and may cause granulomatous formations. Clinical reactions include contact dermatitis and gastrointestinal and chronic pulmonary symptoms. Endre et al. (12) and Scheinmann et al. (13) demonstrated milk-induced lymphoblastic transformation *in vitro*. Minor et al. (14) and Ashkenazi et al. (15) have suggested that type IV cell-mediated immunity may explain delayed reactions to cow's milk and corn. Both groups of authors reported production of leukocyte inhibitory factor by peripheral blood lymphocytes *in vitro* in approximately one-half of the patients reportedly suffering delayed allergic reactions to milk and corn.

PREDISPOSING FACTORS FOR FOOD ALLERGY

The factors that predispose to the development of food allergy may be either genetic or acquired (Fig. 3). Genetic factors persist for life, whereas most acquired factors in infants and young children are transient.

In 1925, Coca and Grove (16) described the presence of genetic and acquired factors as atopy, defining atopy as a condition manifested by a group of allergic diseases with a common hereditary influence in which the atopic reagins (allergens) are often demonstrable. This group of diseases includes bronchial asthma, hay fever, and infantile eczema or atopic dermatitis. Another important feature is the multiplicity and independence of the organs

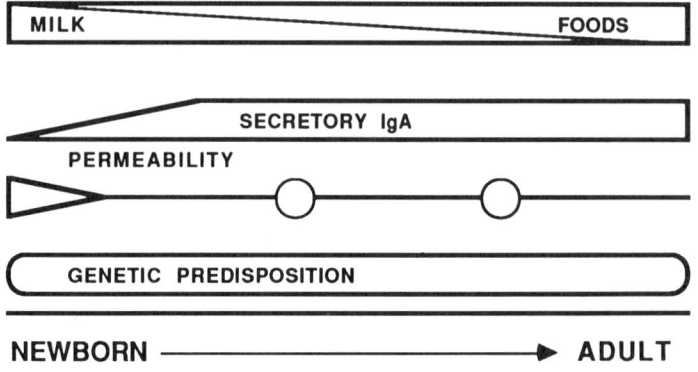

FIG. 3. Factors regulating food hypersensitivity in children and adults. The genetic predisposition to develop IgE antibodies probably remains constant throughout life. Gut permeability is increased in infancy and may increase again with gastrointestinal mucosal damage. As secretory IgA develops, it protects against food sensitization by binding food antigens in the intestinal lumen. Initially, most food antigens are milk components. The source of food antigens changes with the introduction of solid foods into the diet.

affected. The best-known genetic factors are those favoring the development of IgE antibodies and allergic manifestations due to the presence of IgE antibodies. For infants born to atopic parents, certain acquired factors may enhance the production of IgE antibodies. Notably, cow's milk or soy milk formulas and the early introduction of allergenic solid foods can elicit the production of IgE antibodies in children with a genetic predisposition to develop food allergy (17,18). Even transplacentally transmitted allergens can induce IgE production in the fetus (19,20). In such cases, elevated IgE levels can already be detected in the newborn period. Such elevations of IgE signal a risk for the development of IgE antibodies and allergic reactions to foods introduced postnatally.

IgA, like IgE and IgM, does not cross the placenta. In the first few months of life a newborn may have very low levels of IgA. It is produced in high concentrations within the lymphoid tissues lining the gastrointestinal, respiratory, and genitourinary tracts. IgA functions as an antibody to food within the external secretory system. Its presence in the lining of the gastrointestinal tract may help to control food antigen absorption. This relative deficiency in very young infants is thought to permit an increase in resorption of food antigens, which results in IgE antibody production and, possibly, allergic disease.

Increased permeability of the gastrointestinal tract in young infants may further enhance the uptake of macromolecules by the immature intestine (21–24). Factors that dictate the uptake of intact antigens across the intestinal mucosa include impairment of mucosal barrier function (21), alterations in the composition of microvillous membranes in newborns that facilitate attachment and transport of antigens (22), and decreased IgA-containing cells in the intestinal mucosa (25). The amount of antigen that crosses the intestinal barrier may also be significant. Mucosal injury by acute infectious gastroenteritis, celiac disease, inflammatory bowel disease, cystic fibrosis, achlorhydria, or food allergy may lead to increased antigenic penetration and increased formation of IgE antibodies.

CLINICAL MANIFESTATIONS OF FOOD ALLERGY

Blind food challenges have substantiated the association of certain clinical manifestations with food hypersensitivity (Table 2) (6,26–29). Symptoms often occur together in a variety of combinations and syndromes (Table 3).

In the gastrointestinal tract, manifestations of food sensitivity can be evident from the oral mucosa to the colon. Common reactions are nausea, vomiting, diarrhea, and abdominal pain. Oral pathology may be the first indication of a reaction. Symptoms include oral pruritus, pharyngeal pruritus, edema of the lips, palate and tongue,

TABLE 2. *Clinical manifestations of food allergy substantiated by blind challenges*

Gastrointestinal manifestations
  Lip, palate, and tongue swelling
  Oral, pharyngeal pruritus
  Colic (cow's milk antigens)
  Emesis
  Acute and chronic diarrhea
  Malabsorption
  Failure to thrive
Systemic manifestations
  Anaphylaxis
  Dermatologic
    Urticaria, angioedema
    Eczema
  Respiratory
    Allergic rhinitis
    Conjunctivitis
    Laryngeal edema
    Wheezing

and aphthous lesions. Oral pathology caused by food hypersensitivity is, however, believed to be rare.

The small intestine is the site most affected by food sensitivity to cow's milk, soy, and gluten. Injury to the small intestinal mucosa from cow's milk antigens may produce chronic gastrointestinal blood loss leading to iron deficiency and anemia (30), gastrointestinal protein loss, edema, and hypoalbuminemia (31), and malabsorption and chronic diarrhea. Failure to thrive may occur secondary to any of these symptoms or conditions (32,33).

The reported incidence of infantile colic is from 8% to 40% in various studies of infants from 2 to 16 weeks of age (34–36). This wide range is possibly due to the difficulty in establishing a definition of colic and parental difficulty in assessing the severity of the problem.

Generally, colic is defined by the duration, quality, and frequency of crying episodes as well as certain physical characteristics of the infant during these episodes. Wessel et al. (37) define it as crying that occurs during the first 3 months of life, lasting longer than 3 hr per day, for more than 3 days in 1 week, continuing for at least 3 weeks.

Associations between colic and familial allergy have been reported (38). A number of other studies have associated allergens in human, soy, and cow milk formula with infant colic (39,40). Caution, however, must be used in making a direct association since symptoms may

TABLE 3. *Food allergy syndromes*

Protein-induced gastroenteropathy in infants and children
Allergic eosinophilic gastroenteropathy
Gluten-sensitive enteropathy (celiac disease)
Dermatitis herpetiformis
Heiner's syndrome
Atopic dermatitis

be a result of a toxic effect of the proteins rather than a true allergic response. If a food allergy is strongly suspected as a cause of colic, accepted methods of diagnosing allergy should be applied.

Food allergy may cause respiratory conditions, such as allergic rhinitis, conjunctivitis, serous otitis media, asthma, and laryngeal edema. Food allergens have been suspected as a cause of perennial allergic rhinitis when occurring with other conditions, such as urticaria, asthma, atopic dermatitis, and gastrointestinal disturbances following food ingestion (41).

The direct association between serous otitis media and food allergy remains controversial. Serous otitis media may, however, be a result of nasal congestion brought on by food allergens.

Food allergy is an infrequent cause of asthma. When a double-blind food challenge was conducted in 38 children with severe asthma induced by foods, less than one-third responded with predominantly gastrointestinal symptoms and none reacted with asthma (26).

Skin manifestations of food hypersensitivity occur as urticaria, angioedema, and eczematous lesions. Acute urticaria is marked by lesions with raised, erythematous, serpiginous edges and blanched centers which appear on the superficial layers of the skin. The pruritic wheal lesions may be from 1 or 2 mm to 20 or 30 cm in diameter. Angioedema occurs in deeper subcutaneous layers and is marked by colorless, well-demarcated edema that may or may not be pruritic. Milk, eggs, soy, nut, peanuts, other legumes, fish, and seafood (including mollusks and crustacea) are foods most commonly implicated in causing urticaria and angioedema. In infants, milk and eggs are the foods most commonly involved. Responses due to food contact or ingestion usually take place within an hour (42). Atopic dermatitis and eczema due to food allergies will be discussed in the next section.

Anaphylactic reactions to food antigens are characterized by an immediate, severe, systemic response that can be fatal. Various combinations and degrees of symptoms occur. These may be urticaria, angioedema, dyspnea, cyanosis, chest pain, and nasal and conjunctival symptoms, or gastrointestinal disturbances that may be associated with hypotension, cardiac arrhythmias, and shock. Ingestion of certain foods has also been associated with exercise-induced anaphylaxis (43,44).

Patients who have experienced anaphylactic reaction in response to food allergens should avoid any exposure to the offending food. In severe cases of allergy, the mere aroma of particular foods or eating from food-contaminated utensils can cause an anaphylactic reaction. There is always the risk of inadvertent exposure to these food components, and the patient should carry emergency medication to treat anaphylactic shock.

Other systemic conditions are thought to be associated with food allergy but have yet to be proven. These include migraine (45), tension fatigue syndrome (46), and hyperkinesis (47). Some cases of sudden infant death syndrome are thought to occur as a result of an allergic reaction (48).

FOOD HYPERSENSITIVITY SYNDROMES

Protein-Induced Gastroenteropathy

Protein-induced gastroenteropathy in infants and young children is caused by intolerance to cow and/or soy protein. Symptoms of intolerance usually appear within the first months of life (49) and may be manifested by gastrointestinal, respiratory, skin, blood, or behavioral changes (50) with gastrointestinal changes occurring most frequently. Diarrhea is the most prominent symptom, although vomiting, abdominal distention, protein-losing enteropathy, colitis, colic, malabsorption, and steatorrhea are also possible. Dehydration and failure to thrive may result.

The most common antigenic components found in cow's milk are casein, α-lactalbumin, β-lactoglobulin, bovine serum albumin, and gamma globulin. The increased permeability of the infant intestine, the dosage and physical properties of the antigens, and physiologic deficiency in IgA in the newborn are possible causes of early sensitization. By 30 to 36 months of age, protein-induced gastroenteropathy of infancy is usually resolved and cow and soy proteins may be reintroduced in an open challenge.

Allergic Eosinophilic Gastroenteritis

Eosinophilic gastroenteritis (EGE) is characterized by protein-losing enteropathy, peripheral eosinophilia, and iron deficiency anemia secondary to gastrointestinal blood loss. The intestinal lesion is focal in distribution, affecting the stomach most often. Klein et al. (51) proposed that EGE be divided into three pathological entities: (a) primary mucosal disease leading to iron deficiency anemia from fecal blood loss and hypoproteinemia from malabsorption; (b) predominant muscle layer disease, usually characterized by features simulating regional enteritis in the small bowel and obstructive symptoms secondary to obstruction in the stomach; and (c) predominant serosal disease, a rare form presenting with ascites and marked eosinophilia in the ascitic fluid.

The association of allergic symptoms, elevated serum IgE, and response to corticosteroid therapy in some patients suggests type I hypersensitivity. Atopic cases account for only about one-half of all reported cases of EGE and among these cases food allergy is rare (52). Katz et al. (53) report a study of patients with symptoms of EGE who have food allergy confirmed by skin test and radioallergosorbent test (RAST) in which elimination of suspect foods controlled atopic symptoms but not intestinal disease. Conversely, in a second group of patients with IgE-independent disease, withdrawal of milk caused a remission of intestinal symptoms. The mechanism by which food causes disease and the immunologic relationship has yet to be elucidated.

Gluten-Sensitive Enteropathy (Celiac Disease)

Celiac disease is caused by exposure of the mucosa of the small intestine to gluten. The mechanism is not yet clear. One theory suggests that gluten interacts with immunocytes in the lamina propria causing the formation of immune products that ultimately cause lysis and premature death of the absorptive cell leading to a flat mucosa and malabsorption (3). As a compensatory measure there is an increase in crypt cell proliferation (54). The striking association of celiac disease with human leukocyte antigens (HLA) suggests a genetic regulation of the immune response to gluten. The molecular basis for this association, however, has yet to be described (55). Diarrhea and weight loss are the most common presenting symptoms. The disease may occur as early as infancy when cereal is introduced in the diet. Spontaneous remission may occur during adolescence. Growth retardation, emaciation, muscle-wasting, dehydration, hypotension, hypokalemia, and acidosis can result from severe malabsorption. Iron deficiency anemia is common, due to the malabsorption in the proximal small intestine.

Dermatitis Herpetiformis

Like celiac disease, dermatitis herpetiformis (DH) is believed to be an immunologically abnormal response to dietary gluten. The appearance of this disease exclusive of celiac disease is rare in children (56). Onset occurs at approximately 7 years of age (57) and continues, with varying severity, for life. The primary lesion is either an erythematous papule, an urticarial-like plaque, or a vesicle. The papules often evolve into vesicular groupings to form herpes-like lesions. The lesions are usually symmetrical and may involve any region (58). Reunala et al. (57) found, by jejunal biopsy, subtotal villous atrophy in 61% and partial villous atrophy in 28% of 57 children with dermatitis herpetiformis. All 18 children who stayed on a gluten-free diet for an average of 21 months had increased villous height. In addition, a gluten-free diet resulted in the disappearance of the rash in the three patients treated with diet alone for 3 to 6 months. In those treated with medication and diet, 8 of 12 children were free of the rash after 11 months (57).

Heiner's Syndrome

Heiner's syndrome is characterized by a constellation of symptoms, namely, recurrent vomiting and diarrhea, severe chronic cough, tachypnea, chronic rhinitis, recurrent fever, earache, and hemoptysis. Noninfectious pulmonary infiltrates are usually seen as a manifestation of chronic pulmonary disease. Patients with this syndrome are found to have serum precipitins to cow's milk proteins, recurrent or persistent eosinophils, and iron deficiency anemia. Failure to thrive, anorexia, colic, and wheezing are also occasionally associated with this syndrome (59).

Six of the seven children originally reported by Heiner were treated by either a change to evaporated milk or a milk-free diet. All their symptoms disappeared within a few days. When the six children were rechallenged, two had a recurrence of symptoms and four became tolerant to milk in varying degrees following a 3 to 6 month restricted milk diet (59).

Atopic Dermatitis

Atopic dermatitis affects between 1.9% and 4.3% of children (60,61). The distribution and characteristics of the lesions vary with age. Sixty percent of children are affected by the first year of life and 85% within the first 5 years (62). Symptoms rarely occur before 2 months of age. Between the third and sixth month, the infant may develop erythematous, dry lesions on the lateral aspects of the face, and pruritic, vesicular lesions on the cheeks. The common scaling of the scalp and neck makes the distinction of atopic dermatitis from seborrheic dermatitis difficult. Lesions on the extensor surfaces of the arms and legs are common. The severity of symptoms varies and the condition may occasionally disappear temporarily. Following gradual improvement, the condition may disappear permanently by 3 to 5 years of age.

Childhood atopic dermatitis usually begins between the third and sixth year. Lesions are typically pruritic papules appearing on the flexor surfaces of the extremities, neck, and perioral areas. Fissuring at the corners of the mouth is not uncommon. Secondary to scaling and itching of the lesions, lichenification may occur. The condition in childhood tends to be more constant. It may disappear before puberty or persist into adulthood. As the child reaches puberty the lesions change to those that are characteristic of the teenage and adult age groups.

Adult atopic dermatitis is marked by pruritic lesions on the flexor surfaces of the hands, feet, arms, and legs. The sides of the neck and face may also be involved. With prolongation of symptoms, pigmentation occurs at the lichenified areas. Although the disease has been known to persist throughout adulthood, symptom-free periods are not uncommon.

The etiology of atopic dermatitis is unknown and, therefore, difficult to classify as immediate or delayed hypersensitivity. Although it is often associated with type I diseases (allergic rhinitis and bronchial asthma) (63), there is no conclusive evidence that IgE has any relationship to the production of eczema (64). While Johnson et al. (65) reported elevated serum IgE concentrations in approximately 80% of children with atopic dermatitis, this is not a constant finding. Some patients with atopic dermatitis who do not exhibit the manifestations of allergic rhinitis or bronchial asthma have normal IgE levels (64).

Sampson (6) evaluated 26 children with atopic dermatitis and markedly elevated serum IgE concentrations for food hypersensitivity using double-blind placebo-controlled food challenges. There were 23 positive challenges in 15 children, 21 of which manifested primarily pruritus and erythematous macular rashes over 5% of the body within 10 min to 2 hr after challenge. This demonstrates that in some children with atopic dermatitis, immediate food hypersensitivity can provoke cutaneous pruritus and erythema, which leads to scratching and subsequent eczematoid lesions (6). Sampson also found that 84% of 113 patients with severe atopic dermatitis developed skin symptoms using double-blind placebo-controlled oral food challenges. Of this group, 94% had a positive family history of atopic disorders and 50% had both allergic rhinitis and asthma. Of 370 food challenges, 101 were positive in 56% of the patients. Among the 20 foods used in the testing, eggs, peanuts, and milk were the foods most frequently involved (7). All initial reactions occurred within 2 hr of challenge; some recurrence of pruritus 6 to 8 hr later in several patients suggested the late-phase reactions sometimes associated with type I hypersensitivity.

DIAGNOSIS OF FOOD HYPERSENSITIVITY

Because no one test confirms or denies the diagnosis of food allergy, a meticulous diagnostic approach is required in patients with suspected food hypersensitivity. The first important tools are a detailed history and comprehensive physical examination. These will help distinguish IgE-mediated food allergy from other types of hypersensitivity reactions and other types of adverse food reactions.

The medical history must include the following information: the nature and severity of the symptoms, age at onset, possible precipitating factors, the temporal relationship between the ingestion of the offending food(s) and the onset of symptoms, reproducibility of the apparent allergic response, as well as the quantity and a detailed description of the food ingested. The physical setting of the reaction, including any associated exercise and extreme heat or cold, should be described. Several cases of postprandial exercise-induced reactions have been reported after the ingestion of either a specific food, such as shrimp or celery, or with any food (43,44). The presence of other atopic illnesses such as asthma, allergic rhinitis, and atopic dermatitis should be identified. Similar problems in other family members may indicate a genetic predisposition.

The failure of a suspected food to cause an allergic reaction may be the result of the amount consumed, delayed digestion, simultaneously digested foods, method of food preparation, or the use of medications, such as antihistamines (66).

Although physical examinations may not help in the diagnosis, results may serve as a baseline for future evaluation. In addition, nutritional status and growth and development parameters should be assessed for possible chronic conditions.

In vivo tests for food allergy include skin-prick testing (SPT), intradermal testing with food allergens, and elimination diets–oral food challenges. The SPT is an excellent means of identifying food allergens when the history is not highly indicative of specific food sensitivity (67). In some cases, a false-negative reaction may occur, especially when late reactions predominate. In one study, 20% of children less than 3 years of age with late reactions had false-negative skin tests (68).

In SPT and intradermal testing, potent food antigens are used to reveal the presence of IgE antibodies by a local wheal and flare reaction. In certain situations the allergens should be fresh in order to give reliable skin test results. Ortolani et al. (69) compared the results of SPT using fresh foods, commercial food extracts, and *in vitro* testing in 100 adult patients with oral allergy syndrome (OAS). They concluded that confirmation of a history of OAS to certain alimentary allergens such as apple, orange, tomato, carrot, cherry, celery, and peach was enhanced with fresh food SPT compared to SPT with commercial food extracts or an *in vitro* test. Commercial SPT was more sensitive for peanut, pea, and walnut, and the *in vitro* test was more sensitive for hazelnut. Intradermal skin tests, it is important to note, have higher false-positive results and may produce severe anaphylactic reactions.

Skin testing requires strict adherence to proven methods. Standardization and maintenance of extracts, correct dose, proper technique for pricking or injection, plus correct location and timing are very important. The association of death with intradermal testing highlights the need for the immediate availability of medications and supplies to control severe reactions.

In vitro diagnostic tests for type I hypersensitivity are used to demonstrate elevations of total IgE levels and the presence of specific IgE antibodies to food allergens. Total IgE levels are measured by radioimmunoassay (RIA) or by enzyme-linked immunosorbent assay (ELISA). Specific IgE antibodies to food allergens are measured by radioallergosorbent test (RAST). RAST is the most commonly used test. It is especially useful in patients with severe atopic dermatitis or dermographism, those taking antihistamines, and those prone to anaphylactic or severe systemic responses following *in vivo* testing. The disadvantages of RAST are the high cost, the limited number of allergens that can be tested, variations among laboratories, a relative decrease in specificity when elevated IgE levels to other antigens are present, and less sensitivity than the SPT. One other *in vitro* test method, the basophil histamine release test, is the only test based on the indirect detection of IgE bound to basophils. This test is not routinely done because it is cumbersome, expensive, and time-consuming. Albani et al. (70) studied the diagnostic value of a lymphocyte stimulation test in cow's milk protein intolerance. They concluded that this test was useful in the diagnosis of cow's milk intolerance in patients in whom an IgE-mediated allergy could not be established.

An elimination diet may be useful when the ingestion of foods and the occurrence of symptoms do not correlate well. Its usefulness is, however, limited by the lack of double blinding and consequent psychological factors that may influence the findings. When just a few foods are suspected, simple dietary changes are possible. The stringent elimination diet required when several foods are suspected necessitates the supervision of a registered dietitian to monitor an age-appropriate diet.

The elimination diet should be maintained for 1 to 2 weeks. If improvement occurs, eliminated foods should be added, one at a time at 2 to 3 day intervals. Adequate amounts of each food need to be consumed so the reaction will occur in those patients who react only to large amounts of food allergens.

A double-blind food challenge is the "gold standard" for making or confirming the diagnosis of food hypersensitivity (71). Subjective bias is excluded by this method. A food challenge is performed after a food has been eliminated for at least 2 weeks and the patient is asymptomatic. It can be open, single-blind, or double-blind. It should be done in a hospital or an office equipped with appropriate emergency resuscitation equipment. Bock et al.'s (72) recommendations for administering the double-blind food challenge in an office setting include avoidance of the food allergen 2 to 3 weeks before the challenge, the use of dry foods when possible, and administration of the dose according to the suspected degree of hypersensitivity. Symptoms usually occur within 2 hr. If no reaction occurs within 24 hr, the dose may be doubled daily until 8 g of dried food is reached. This amount of dried food taken without problems usually implies that the food can be included in the diet. A single unequivocal positive reaction is definitive. Diagnosis can only be made when symptoms are clearly related to the antigens being challenged. The patient should be observed considerably longer than the period of time it usually takes symptoms to appear.

In complicated or confusing cases, intestinal biopsy before or after a food challenge may be needed to exclude other intestinal lesions and help quantitate mucosal injury due to ingested food. Similarly, other nonspecific measures of intestinal function such as D-xylose absorption, fecal fat smears, and serum carotene can help identify mucosal injury, although these tests cannot rule out the specific cause of the injury.

DIFFERENTIAL DIAGNOSIS

A large number of conditions must be considered in the differential diagnosis of food allergy (Table 4) (73). Presenting symptoms in gastrointestinal disorders that are similar to those in food allergy include nausea, vomiting, diarrhea, and abdominal pain. When these occur during the newborn period, food hypersensitivity is often prematurely, and erroneously, suspected. For example, aspiration during feedings can lead to coughing and wheezing. Structural abnormalities such as hiatal hernia with gastroesophageal reflux or pyloric stenosis may cause vomiting following feedings. Hirschsprung's disease, characterized by diarrhea, vomiting, tachypnea secondary to abdominal distention, and irritability, may also be responsible. Older children may need to be evaluated for peptic ulcer disease or cholecystitis/cholelithiasis if they complain of abdominal pain or vomiting after meals.

Several enzyme deficiencies cause gastrointestinal symptoms. Lactase deficiency may occur after a viral or bacterial infection or develop without a known cause. The occurrence of this deficiency is as high as 80% among African-Americans, Africans, and Asiatics (74).

Foods and food additives used in processed foods can cause a variety of symptoms including gastrointestinal, respiratory, and dermatologic problems. Additives include tartrazine, sodium metabisulfite, nitrites and nitrates, benzoates, butylated hydroxytoluene, and buty-

TABLE 4. *Differential diagnosis of food allergy*

Gastrointestinal disorders
  Structural abnormalities (reflux)
  Enzyme deficiencies (lactase)
  Cystic fibrosis, malabsorption syndromes
  Chronic infections, giardiasis
  Pharmacologic food reactions
  Food contaminants and additives
Skin disorders/atopic dermatitis
  Seborrheic dermatitis
  Gluten-sensitive enteropathy
  Other causes of eczema
    Wiskott-Aldrich syndrome
    Bruton's agammaglobulinemia
    Leiner's disease
    Histiocytosis X
    Acrodermatitis enteropathica
    Metabolic diseases
Sinopulmonary allergic manifestations
  Antibody deficiency syndromes
  Cystic fibrosis
  Immotile cilia syndrome

lated hydroxyanisole. Preservatives such as sulfites, which are used to keep food looking fresh, are found in processed foods, salad bars, and prescription drugs. Monosodium glutamate, used widely as a flavoring agent in oriental foods, canned soups, and gourmet seasoning (75), produces the "Chinese restaurant syndrome," characterized by burning sensations, facial and chest pain, and migraine headache.

Contamination and additives in foods may cause adverse reactions that appear to be food related. For example, milk from cattle may be contaminated with antibiotics such as penicillin, bacitracin, or tetracycline that are used to treat bovine diseases. These contaminants, however, are used much less frequently than in the past. Pesticides in produce and insect parts in processed foods may also cause symptoms mimicking food sensitivity.

Bacteria, fungi, and algae can produce toxins that cause severe gastrointestinal disturbances and sometimes neurological symptoms. These include *Clostridium botulinum, Staphylococcus aureus, Aspergillus flavus, Salmonella, Shigella, Escherichia coli,* and *Campylobacter.* Consumption of infected foods and water may result in exposure to infectious agents such as *Giardia lamblia* and *Trichinella spiralis.*

Pharmacologic agents in foods have also been responsible for gastrointestinal and neurological symptoms as well as general interference with normal metabolism. These agents include caffeine, theobromine, histamine, tyramine, tryptamine, serotonin, phenylethylamine, glycosidal alkaloid solanine, and alcohol.

PREVENTION

The prevention of allergic diseases is best done by early identification of high-risk individuals in order to initiate avoidance of known allergens during the time of risk for the development of allergy. Identification is based on family history and measurement of IgE levels in the newborn period.

Expression of IgE-mediated allergic disorders appears to be under genetic control. Using parental atopy as an indicator of risk, it has been established that when both parents are atopic, the infant's risk of developing allergy is 40% to 60%. If both parents are atopic with the same manifestations, the risk increases to 50% to 80%. Infants with one atopic parent have a risk of 25% to 35% (76).

In the human fetus IgE production is low, but in some fetuses IgE has been found as early as the 11th week of gestation (77–79). Since IgE does not cross the placenta, the presence of IgE in cord blood may be due to intrauterine sensitization or contamination with maternal blood. Kjellman et al. (80) reported a 7-year study of 1,651 children from infancy. Atopic disease developed in 82% of children with cord blood levels of IgE $\geq$ 0.9 IU/ml. This method of prediction resulted in fewer false-positive results than did family history alone (17.8% vs 49.8%, $p \geq$ .001). Cord blood was a better predictor than family history between atopic and nonatopic subjects but, together, cord blood and family history increased the screening accuracy (80). The predictive value of different types and severity of allergy in parents has not been explained.

Atopic-prone infants tend to develop hypersensitivity to many allergens in their environment. Nutrients are clearly the earliest, most significant potential source of allergens. In vulnerable infants the ingestion of small quantities of these substances can cause the production of IgE antibodies. Numerous measures to prevent the onset of allergic symptoms are being investigated. These preventative measures may be started while the mother is pregnant (81) or at birth in infants at risk.

Conflicting studies about the effect of breast-feeding on the development of atopy have been reported (17,61,82–87). Differences in study quality and design make comparisons difficult. In addition, the immunologic basis for protection afforded the infant by breast-feeding is not completely understood. Indeed, any exposure to deleterious allergens in breast milk from the mother's diet may result in subsequent infant sensitization (88,89). Nevertheless, breast-fed infants who are not introduced early to solid foods have been found to have significantly lower serum IgE levels at less than 4 months (90) and by 1 year (82).

Soy formula has been shown to cause hypersensitivity similar to that of milk proteins (91,92) and is no longer considered effective in preventing or delaying allergies in infants. Hydrolysate formulas offer delayed sensitization in some infants at high risk for atopy (93) but have not been proven to prevent the development of allergy later in life.

Delayed introduction of solid foods is recommended for decreasing the allergenic load in high-risk infants. Fergusson et al. (17) studied the relationship between parental atopy, breast-feeding, early solid food diet, and the rate of eczema in 1,262 two-year-old children. Children of atopic parents given solid food during the first 4 months had over $2\frac{1}{2}$ times the rate of eczema of children with nonatopic parents who had not been fed solid food. The rates of eczema increased in almost direct proportion to the number of different types of solid food that the children had been given during the first 4 months.

TREATMENT

Once the diagnosis of food allergy has been established and the food allergen identified, elimination of the incriminated food and any cross-reacting substances is the primary mode of treatment. Obtaining the patient's compliance may be difficult. Although complete elimination of the offending food is the primary goal, in selected patients a reduction of the implicated food may provide relief. If several food groups are implicated, a nutritionally adequate elimination diet must be offered. The patient or food provider should be given appropriate literature on food avoidance.

In patients with a history of proven anaphylaxis, an offending food should never be reintroduced into the diet. In addition, foods should be removed permanently from the diet when symptoms persist after a number of challenges. This is especially important in cow's milk allergy and other allergic food reactions in young infants. Sensitivity does not necessarily persist for life and the patient can be rechallenged again in the future (7). This procedure should be done in a setting where adequate preparation for treating anaphylaxis is readily available.

When food allergy results in malabsorption and poor nutrition, nutritional supplementation may be advisable. Supplementation may include the use of elemental formulas, parenteral nutrition, as well as the correction of specific nutritional deficiencies with vitamin, mineral, and trace element supplements.

Pharmacologic therapy for food allergy can be attempted in the rare patients with multiple food sensitivities who do not respond to conventional elimination dietary management. Oral cromolyn sodium appears promising in the treatment of food allergy when administered at least 30 to 60 min prior to food ingestion (94).

The role of H_1 antihistamines in food hypersensitivity is limited to food allergic reactions that involve the release of histamine. Some authors advocate using H_1 antihistamines prophylactically in young children whose gastrointestinal complaints are attributable to sensitivity to foods that are not avoidable (95).

Studies with Ketotifen suggest a potentially effective role in food hypersensitivity. Ketotifen is an oral tricyclic benzochloheptathiophene agent that blocks the release of chemical mediators from human leukocytes causing an antihistamine effect. Unlike cromolyn, Ketotifen is easily absorbed from the gastrointestinal tract.

Inhibition of the effects of histamine on gastric acid by H_2 antihistamine are well documented in animal models. The H_2 antihistamines have been used in the treatment of chronic urticaria in combination with H_1-receptor antagonists regardless of the relation with food allergy.

Corticosteroids are rarely used in the treatment of food hypersensitivity, although improvement has been found in some patients with milk-induced allergic gastroenteropathy (96). They have also been used in the treatment of eosinophilic gastroenteritis caused by food sensitivity. Although prednisone may be used to ameliorate symptoms, when prolonged use is required, only the minimal dose necessary to control symptoms should be given.

The treatment of anaphylactic symptoms due to food ingestion differs only slightly from the treatment of other anaphylactic reactions. In some patients gastric lavage may have to be added to reduce the antigen absorption and exposure. Patients at risk should be educated in self-injecting epinephrine and have an epinephrine-filled syringe and antihistamines available at all times. A Medic Alert or other identification bracelet is also highly recommended.

Unlike desensitization with inhalant allergens for respiratory allergy, there is no evidence to support the use of immunotherapy with food antigens in the treatment of food hypersensitivity.

REFERENCES

1. Bellanti JA, Kadlec JV. Introduction to immunology. In: Bellanti JA, ed. *Immunology: basic processes,* 2nd ed. Philadelphia: WB Saunders, 1985.
2. American Academy of Allergy and Immunology Committee on Adverse Reactions to Foods. National Institute of Allergy and Infectious Diseases. *Adverse reactions to foods* (NIH Publication No. 84-2442). Washington, DC: U.S. Department of Health and Human Services. Public Health Service. National Institutes of Health, July, 1984.
3. Trier JS, Falchuk M, Carey MC, Schreiber DS. Celiac sprue and refractory sprue. *Gastroenterology* 1978;75:307–316.
4. Coombs RRA, Gell PGH. Classification of allergic reactions responsible for clinical hypersensitivity and disease. In: Coombs RRA, Gell PGH, eds. *Clinical aspects of immunology.* Oxford: Blackwell Scientific Publications, 1975.
5. Crawford LV. *Pediatric allergic diseases: focus on clinical diagnosis,* 2nd ed. Garden City, NY: Medical Examination Publishing, 1982.
6. Sampson HA. Role of immediate hypersensitivity in the pathogenesis of atopic dermatitis. *J Allergy Clin Immunol* 1983;71: 473–480.
7. Sampson HA, McCaskill CM. Food hypersensitivity and atopic dermatitis: evaluation of 113 patients. *J Pediatr* 1985;107:669–675.
8. Frick OL. B-Lactoglobulin in immune complexes in milk-sensitive children (Abstract). *J Allergy Clin Immunol* 1982;69 (suppl):157.
9. Sandilands GP, Reid FM, Galbraith I, Peel MG, Lewis CJ. *In vivo* modulation of human lymphocyte FcY-receptors in response to oral antigen (cow's milk) challenge. *Int Arch Allergy Appl Immunol* 1982;67:344–350.
10. Carini C, Brostoff J, Wraith DG. IgE complexes in food allergy. *Ann Allergy* 1987;59:110–117.
11. Haddad ZH, Vetter M, Friedmann J, Sainz C, Brunner E. Detection and kinetics of antigen specific IgE and IgG immune complexes in food allergy. *Ann Allergy* 1983;51:255.
12. Endre L, Osváth P. Antigen-induced lymphoblast transformation in the diagnosis of cow's milk allergic diseases in infancy and early childhood. *Acta Allergol* 1975;30:34–42.
13. Scheinmann P, Gendrel D, Charlas J, Paupe J. Value of lymphoblast transformation test in cow's milk protein intestinal intolerance. *Clin Allergy* 1976;6:515–521.
14. Minor JD, Tolber SG, Frick OL. Leucocyte inhibition factor in delayed-onset food allergy. *J Allergy Clin Immunol* 1980;66: 314–321.
15. Ashkenazi A, Levin S, Idar D, Or A, Rosenberg I, Handzel ZT. *In vitro* cell-mediated immunologic assay for cow's milk allergy. *Pediatrics* 1980;6:399–402.
16. Coca AF, Grove EF. Classification of allergic disease. In: Coca AF, ed. *Familial nonreaginic food-allergy,* 1st ed. Springfield, IL: Charles C. Thomas, 1943.
17. Fergusson DM, Horwood LJ, Beautrias AL, Shannon FT, Taylor B. Eczema and infant diet. *Clin Allergy* 1981;11:325–331.
18. Kajosaari M, Saarinen UM. Prophylaxis of atopic disease by six

months total solid food elimination. *Arch Paediatr Scand* 1983;72:411–414.
19. Michel FB, Bousquet J, Greillier P, Robinet-Levy M, Coulomb Y. Comparison of cord blood immunoglobulin E and maternal allergy for the prediction of atopic disease in infancy. *J Allergy Clin Immunol* 1980;65:422–430.
20. Kaufman HS. Allergy in the newborn: skin test reactions confirmed by the Prausnitz-Küstner test at birth. *Clin Allergy* 1971;1:363–367.
21. Udall JN, Pang K, Fritze L, Kleinman R, Walker WA. Development of gastrointestinal mucosal barrier: I. The effect of age on intestinal permeability to macromolecules. *Pediatr Res* 1981; 15:241–244.
22. Pang KY, Bresson JL, Walker WA. Development of the gastrointestinal mucosal barrier. V. Comparative effect of calcium binding on microvillus membrane structure in newborn and adult rats. *Pediatr Res* 1983;17:856–861.
23. Stern M, Pang KY, Walker WA. Food proteins and gut mucosal barrier. II. Differential interaction of cow's milk proteins with the mucous coat and the surface membrane of adult and immature rat jejunum. *Pediatr Res* 1984;18:1252–1257.
24. Seidman EG, Hanson DG, Ely I, Udall JN, Walker WA. Macromolecular uptake from colon: effect of age on permeability in rabbits (Abstract). *Gastroenterology* 1985;88:1579.
25. Perkkio M, Savilahti E. Time of appearance of immunoglobulin-containing cells in the mucosa of the neonatal intestine. *Pediatr Res* 1980;14:953–955.
26. May CD. Objective clinical and laboratory studies of immediate hypersensitivity reactions to foods in asthmatic children. *J Allergy Clin Immunol* 1976;58:500–515.
27. Bock SA, Lee W-Y, Remigio LK, May CD. Studies of hypersensitivity reactions to foods in infants and children. *J Allergy Clin Immunol* 1978;62:327–334.
28. Bernstein M, Day JH, Welsh A. Double blind food challenge in the diagnosis of food sensitivity in the adults. *J Allergy Clin Immunol* 1982;70:205–210.
29. Atkins FM, Steinberg SS, Metcalfe DD. Evaluation of immediate adverse reactions to foods in adult patients. II. A detailed analysis of reaction patterns during oral food challenge. *J Allergy Clin Immunol* 1985;75:356–363.
30. Wilson JF, Lahey ME, Heiner DC. Studies on iron metabolism: V. Further observations on cow's milk-induced gastrointestinal bleeding in infants with iron-deficiency anemia. *J Pediatr* 1974;84:335–344.
31. Waldman TA, Wochner RD, Laster L, Gordon RS. Allergic gastroenteropathy: a cause of excessive gastrointestinal protein loss. *N Engl J Med* 1967;276:761–769.
32. Iyngkaran N, Robinson MJ, Prathap K, Sumithran E, Yadav M. Cow's milk protein-sensitive enteropathy: combined clinical and histological criteria for diagnosis. *Arch Dis Child* 1978;53:20–26.
33. Kuitunen P, Visakorpi JK, Savilahti E, Pelkonen P. Malabsorption syndrome with cow's milk intolerance: clinical findings and course in 54 cases. *Arch Dis Child* 1975;50:351–356.
34. Brazelton TB. Crying in infancy. *Pediatrics* 1962;29:579–588.
35. Illingworth R. Three-months colic. *Arch Dis Child* 1954; 29:165–174.
36. Stahlberg M. Infantile colic: occurrence and risk factors. *Eur J Pediatr* 1984;143:108–111.
37. Wessel MA, Cobb JC, Jackson EB, Harris GS, Detweiler BA. Paroxysmal fussing in infancy, sometimes called "colic." *Pediatrics* 1954;14:421–434.
38. Farran C. *Infant colic*. New York: Charles Schribner's Sons, 1983.
39. Jakobsson I, Lindberg T. Cow's milk as a cause of infantile colic in breast-fed infants. *Lancet* 1978;2:437–439.
40. Lothe L, Lindberg T. Cow's milk whey protein elicits symptoms of infantile colic in colicky formula-fed infants: a double-blind crossover study. *Pediatrics* 1989;83:262–266.
41. Ricketti AJ. Allergic rhinitis. In: Patterson R, ed. *Allergic diseases: diagnosis and management*, 3rd ed. Philadelphia: JB Lippincott, 1985;207–227.
42. Lemanske RF, Sampson HA. Adverse reactions to foods and their relationship to skin diseases in children. *Adv Pediatr* 1988; 35:189–218.
43. Maulitz RM, Pratt DS, Schocket AL. Exercise-induced anaphylactic reaction to shellfish. *J Allergy Clin Immunol* 1979;63:433–434.
44. Kidd JM III, Cohen SH, Sosman AJ, Fink JN. Food-dependent exercise-induced anaphylaxis. *J Allergy Clin Immunol* 1983; 71:407–411.
45. Egger J, Wilson J, Carter CM, Turner MW, Soothill JF. Is migraine food allergy? A double-blind controlled trial of oligoantigenic diet treatment. *Lancet* 1983;2:865–869.
46. Crook WG, Harrison WW, Crawford SE, Emerson BS. Systemic manifestations due to allergy. Report of fifty patients and a review of the literature on the subject (sometimes referred to as allergic toxemia and the allergic tension-fatigue syndrome). *Pediatrics* 1961;27:790–799.
47. Feingold B. *Why your child is hyperactive*. New York: Random House, 1975.
48. Parish WE, Barrett AM, Coombs RRA, Gunther M, Camps FE. Hypersensitivity to milk and sudden death in infancy. *Lancet* 1960;1:1106–1110.
49. Freier S. Paediatric gastrointestinal allergy. *Clin Allergy* 1973; 3(Suppl):597–618.
50. Hill DJ, Ford RPK, Shelton MJ, Hosking CS. A study of 100 infants and young children with cow's milk allergy. *Clin Rev Allergy* 1984;2:125–142.
51. Klein NC, Hargrove RL, Sleisenger MN, Jeffries GH. Eosinophilic gastroenteritis. *Medicine* 1970;49:299–319.
52. Caldwell JH, Mekhjian HS, Hurtubise PE, Beman FM. Eosinophilic gastroenteritis with obstruction: immunological studies of seven patients. *Gastroenterology* 1978;74:825–829.
53. Katz AJ, Twarog FJ, Zeiger RS, Falchuk ZM. Milk-sensitive and eosinophilic gastroenteropathy: similar clinical features with contrasting mechanisms and clinical course. *J Allergy Clin Immunol* 1984;74:72–78.
54. Trier JS, Browning TH. Epithelial cell renewal in cultured duodenal biopsies in celiac sprue. *N Engl J Med* 1970;283:1245–1250.
55. Falchuk ZM, Rogentine GN, Strober W. Predominance of histocompatibility antigen HL-A8 in patients with gluten-sensitive enteropathy. *J Clin Invest* 1972;51:1603–1605.
56. Gellis SE. Bullous diseases of childhood. *Dermatol Clin* 1986;4:89–98.
57. Reunala T, Kosnai I, Karpati S, Kuitunen P, Török E, Savilahti E. Dermatitis herpetiformis: jejunal findings and skin response to gluten free diet. *Arch Dis Child* 1984;59:517–522.
58. Duhring LA. Dermatitis herpetiformis. *JAMA* 1884;3:225–229.
59. Heiner DC. Multiple precipitins to cow's milk in chronic respiratory disease. *Am J Dis Child* 1962;103:634–654.
60. Johnson ML, Roberts J. *Prevalence of dermatologic disease among persons 1–74 years of age* (PHS no. 79-1660). Washington, DC: Department of Health, Education, and Welfare, 1979.
61. Halpern SR, Sellars WA, Johnson RB, Anderson DW, Saperstein S, Reisch MS. Development of childhood allergy in infants fed breast, soy or cow milk. *J Allergy Clin Immunol* 1973;51:139–151.
62. Rook A, ed. *Major problems in dermatology: atopic dermatitis*. Vol 3. Philadelphia: WB Saunders, 1975.
63. Pasternak B. The prediction of asthma in infantile eczema: a statistical approach. *J Pediatr* 1965;66:164–165.
64. Sparks DP. Atopic dermatitis. In: Patterson R, ed. *Allergic diseases: diagnosis and management,* 3rd ed., Philadelphia: JB Lippincott, 1985;491–504.
65. Johnson E, Irons J, Patterson R, Roberts M. Serum IgE concentration in atopic dermatitis. *J Allergy Clin Immunol* 1974;54:94–99.
66. Metcalfe DD. Food hypersensitivity. Relationship to severity of disease and resource of atopic respiratory disease. (CME) *J Allergy Clin Immunol* 1984;73:749–764.
67. Sampson HA, Albergo R. Comparison of results of skin tests, RAST, and double-blind, placebo-controlled food challenges in children with atopic dermatitis. *J Allergy Clin Immunol* 1984; 74:26–33.
68. Kravis L. Skin test in the diagnosis of allergic conditions. *Pediatr Rev* 1981;2:327–332.
69. Ortolani C, Ispano M, Pastorello EA, Ansaloni R, Magri GC. Comparison of the results of skin prick tests (with fresh foods and commercial food extracts) and RAST in 100 patients with oral allergy syndrome. *J Allergy Clin Immunol* 1989;83:683–690.

70. Albani S, Avanzini MA, Plebani A, et al. Diagnostic value of a lymphocyte stimulation test in cow milk protein intolerance. *Ann Allergy* 1989;63:489–492.
71. Bock SA, Atkins FM. Patterns of food hypersensitivity during sixteen years of double-blind, placebo-controlled food challenges. *J Pediatr* 1990;117:561–567.
72. Bock SA, Sampson HA, Atkins FM, et al. Double-blind, placebo-controlled food challenge (DBPCFC) as an office procedure: a manual. *J Allergy Clin Immunol* 1988;82:986–997.
73. Sampson HA. Differential diagnosis in adverse reactions to foods. *J Allergy Clin Immunol* 1986;78:212–219.
74. Gray GM. Maldigestion and malabsorption of carbohydrates. In: Winick M, ed. *Nutrition and gastroenterology.* New York: John Wiley, 1980.
75. Kwok RH. Chinese-restaurant syndrome (letter). *N Engl J Med* 1968;278:796.
76. Bousquet J, Kjellman N-IM. Predictive value of tests in childhood allergy. *J Allergy Clin Immunol* 1986;78:1019–1027.
77. Miller DL, Hirvonen T, Gitlin D. Synthesis of IgE by the human conceptus. *J Allergy Clin Immunol* 1973;52:182–188.
78. Levin S, Altman Y, Sela M. Penicillin and dinitrophenyl antibodies in newborns and mothers detected with chemically modified bacteriophage. *Pediatr Res* 1971;5:87–88.
79. Delespesse G, Sarfati M, Lang G, Sehon AH. Prenatal and neonatal synthesis of IgE. *Monogr Allergy* 1983;18:83–95.
80. Kjellman N-IM, Croner S. Cord blood IgE determination for allergy prediction—a follow-up to seven years of age in 1651 children. *Ann Allergy* 1984;53:167–171.
81. Chandra RK, Puri S, Suraiya C, Cheema PS. Influence of maternal food antigen avoidance during pregnancy and lactation on incidence of atopic eczema in infants. *Clin Allergy* 1986;16:563–569.
82. Chandra RK. Prospective studies of the effect of breast feeding on incidence of infection and allergy. *Acta Paediatr Scand* 1979;68:691–694.
83. Chandra RK, Puri S, Cheema PS. Predictive value of cord blood IgE in the development of atopic disease and role of breast feeding in its prevention. *Clin Allergy* 1985;15:517–522.
84. Hide DW, Guyer BM. Clinical manifestations of allergy related to breast and cows' milk feeding. *Arch Dis Child* 1981;56:172–175.
85. Gruskay FL. Comparison of breast, cow, and soy feedings in the prevention of onset of allergic disease: a 15-year prospective study. *Clin Pediatr* 1982;21:486–491.
86. Golding J, Buttler NR, Taylor B. Breast-feeding and eczema/asthma (letter). *Lancet* 1982;1:623.
87. Van Asperen PP, Kemp AS, Mellis CM. Relationship of diet in the development of atopy in infancy. *Clin Allergy* 1984;14:525–532.
88. Hemmings WA, Kulangara AC. Dietary antigens in breast milk (letter). *Lancet* 1978;2:575.
89. Van Asperen PP, Kemp AZS, Mellis CM. Immediate hypersensitivity reactions on the first known exposure to the food. *Arch Dis Child* 1983;58:253–256.
90. Saarinen UM, Backman A, Kajossari M, Simes M. Prolonged breast-feeding as prophylaxis for atopic disease. *Lancet* 1979; 2:163–166.
91. Brown EB, Josephson BM, Levine HS, Rosen M. A prospective study of allergy in a pediatric population. The role of heredity in the incidence of allergies, and experience with milk-free diet in the newborn. *Am J Dis Child* 1969;117:693–698.
92. Kjellman N-IM, Johanson SGO. Soy versus cow's milk in infants with a biparenteral history of atopic disease: development of atopic disease and immunoglobulins from birth to four years of age. *Clin Allergy* 1979;9:347–358.
93. Chandra RK, Singh G, Shridhara B. Effect of feeding whey hydrolysate, soy and conventional cow milk formulas on incidence of atopic disease in high risk infants. *Ann Allergy* 1989;63:102–106.
94. Pelikan Z, Pelikan-Filipek M. Effects of oral cromolyn on the nasal response due to food. *Arch Otolaryngol Head Neck Surg* 1989;115:1238–1243.
95. Bahna SL, Heiner DC. *Allergies to milk.* New York: Grune and Stratton, 1980.
96. Whitington PF, Whitington GL. Eosinophilic gastroenteropathy in childhood. *J Pediatr Gastroenterol Nutr* 1988;7:379–385.

CHAPTER 41

Nutritional Treatment of Children with Inborn Errors of Metabolism

Joyce M. Bradburn and Emmanuel Shapira

Inherited disorders of the urea cycle, amino acid, and organic acid metabolism, although individually rare, represent, together, a significant segment of infant and childhood morbidity and mortality. This group of disorders characterizes the two major concepts of human genetics:

1. *Variability:* The extent of expression of the very same disorder may vary markedly in different patients affected by a mutation in the same locus (1). Variability can be in age of onset (which may extend from the newborn period to adulthood), severity, and phenotypic expression. Although patients from different families may exhibit wider variability with the same disorder, significant variability is not uncommon even among affected siblings within the same family.
2. *Heterogeneity:* Different disorders, representing mutations in different loci, may well have indistinguishable phenotypic, clinical, and even laboratory manifestations (1).

Because inherited disorders are rare, their clinical presentation is variable and heterogeneous and, because of the relatively complex requirements for establishing diagnosis, they are often excluded from routine diagnostic workups. This chapter describes clinical presentations, the approach to the diagnostic workup, the concept of treatment and management, and some of the pitfalls in treatment and management. To demonstrate these, selected case histories from each category of disorder will be presented. Although a detailed description of all of the disorders and their variants is impossible within the scope of this chapter, some of the more relevant disorders are summarized (Tables 1, 2, and 3).

CLINICAL PRESENTATION

The lack of a specific phenotypic presentation constitutes a major problem in diagnosing an inborn error of the urea cycle, amino acid, and organic acid metabolism. Generally, however, patients will present with one of the following:

1. "Rule out sepsis" in a newborn or a child: This very stormy presentation is characterized by altered consciousness to coma or shock, which is very often preceded by vomiting and seizures.
2. Failure to thrive, in an infant, child, or young adult, with or without developmental delay, mental retardation, and/or seizures: Significant in these patients is an acute, disproportionate response to intercurrent infections.
3. "Near-SIDS" babies or siblings of a baby with sudden infant death syndrome (SIDS): Several SIDS babies have had an inborn error of organic acid metabolism as their underlying defect (2). Thus, all babies who have experienced an acute life-threatening episode themselves or are siblings of SIDS babies should be evaluated for the possibility of an inborn error of organic acid metabolism.

THE APPROACH TO THE DIAGNOSTIC WORKUP

Rule Out Sepsis Patients

The workup should evaluate ammonia levels, acid base status, glucose, and electrolytes. Some of the more

---

J. Bradburn, E. Shapira: Human Genetics Program, Hayward Genetics Center, Tulane University School of Medicine, New Orleans, Louisiana 70112.

TABLE 1. Urea cycle defects[a]

	Clinical presentation	Laboratory diagnostic findings
Carbamoyl phosphate synthetase deficiency	Severe MR, FTT, seizures, and exacerbations with profuse vomiting and encephalopathy. Death in infancy.	Hyperammonemia. Elevated plasma glutamine, alanine, glutamate, glycine, and lysine. Generalized aminoaciduria. DEA of carbamoyl phosphate synthetase in liver.
Ornithine carbamoyl transferase deficiency	X-linked dominant inheritance. Most common urea cycle defect. Clinically indistinguishable from carbamoyl phosphate synthetase deficiency. Males die in infancy. Variable expression in females.	Hyperammonemia and elevated levels of orotic acid in plasma and urine. Elevated plasma glutamine, glycine, and alanine. Decreased plasma arginine. Increased urinary glutamine and lysine excretion. DEA of ornithine carbamoyl transferase in liver.
Argininosuccinate synthetase deficiency (citrullinemia)	Neonatal form: hypertonicity, vomiting seizures, MR, and coma. Subacute form: MR and ataxia in older children. Exacerbations with vomiting and encephalopathy. Variants with milder clinical expressions.	Hyperammonemia. Elevated citrulline in plasma, CSF, and urine. Decreased plasma arginine. Increased urinary excretion of glutamine, glycine, proline, alanine, and lysine. Deficiency of arginosuccinate synthetase in liver, fibroblasts, lymphocytes, and CVS. Partial deficiencies in some variants.
Argininosuccinate lyase deficiency (argininosuccinic aciduria)	FTT, seizures, coma, MR, and eventually death. In older children, ataxia, trichorrhexis nodosa, and hepatomegaly. Exacerbations with vomiting and encephalopathy. Variants with milder clinical expressions.	Hyperperammonemia. Marked elevation of argininosuccinic acid in plasma, urine and CSF. Elevation of plasma glutamine, proline, glycine, alanine, and citrulline. Decreased plasma arginine and ornithine. Deficiency of L-argininosuccinate lyase in red blood cells.
Arginase deficiency (argininemia)	Extremely rare, only few patients described. MR, spasticity, ataxia, seizures, vomiting, and hepatomegaly. Exacerbations with vomiting and encephalopathy.	Moderate hyperammonemia. Elevated CSF, plasma, and urine arginine. Orotic aciduria during exacerbations. Deficiency of arginase in red blood cells, leukocytes, and liver.

From ref. 14, with permission.
CSF, cerebrospinal fluid; CVS, chorionic villus sampling; DEA, deficient enzyme activity; FTT, failure to thrive; MR, mental retardation; WBCs, white blood cells.
[a] Because of their limited scope, Tables 1, 2, and 3 include only the most common variants. They do not describe the marked variability between and within the different subtypes of each clinical entity. The mode of inheritance of all of the entities described is autosomal recessive unless otherwise specified.

common inborn errors of metabolism presenting as "rule out sepsis" include three variables: acidosis, hypoglycemia, and hyperammonemia (Fig. 1). When the underlying etiology is suspected to be an inborn error of urea cycle, amino acid, or organic acid metabolism, plasma for amino acids and urine for organic acids should be evaluated. These tests must be routinely completed in order to rule out the possibility of an underlying metabolic disorder, just as a spinal tap is routinely performed to rule out meningitis. Since treatment and management of "sepsis" is very similar to the treatment of the acute phase of many of these metabolic disorders, it is important to retain a urine specimen and preferably also a plasma specimen from the acute phase of the episode. Unfortunately, the specimens for evaluation of amino acids and organic acids are often obtained 2 to 3 days after the acute presentation, after the patient has been maintained for several days on IV fluids with no dietary intake, and when some of the more pathognomonic patterns of amino acids or organic acids might have disappeared or been altered. This precludes an accurate diagnosis.

"Failure to Thrive" Patients

Urine and plasma amino acids as well as urine organic acids should be evaluated whether or not patients exhibit developmental delay, mental retardation, and/or seizures. The ratio between the plasma and urine amino acids will rule out the possibility of proximal tubular dysfunction as well as many of the inborn errors of amino acid metabolism presenting with this clinical picture. Urinary organic acids should be evaluated, espe-

TABLE 2. Disorders of amino acid metabolism

	Clinical findings	Laboratory diagnostic findings
Arginine		
Argininemia	See Table 1.	See Table 1.
Carnosine		
Carnosinemia	MR, seizures, and progressive neurological deterioration.	Elevated levels of carnosine in blood and urine. Deficiency of carnosinase postulated.
Citrulline		
Citrullinemia	See Table 1.	See Table 1.
Cystathione		
Cystathionuria, primary	Phenotypically asymptomatic. Association with abnormal neurological findings, MR, and microcephaly is most likely secondary to biased ascertainment.	Elevation of cystathionine in plasma, urine, and CSF.
Cystathionuria, secondary	Can be found in pyridoxine deficiency, neuroblastoma, hepatoblastoma, or other tumors.	Elevation of cystathionine in urine.
Cystine		
Cystinosis	Infantile type: severe FTT, proximal renal tubular dysfunction and retinopathy. If untreated, death before puberty. Variants with later onset and milder degrees of expression have been described.	Aminoaciduria, phosphaturia, and glucosuria. Renal tubular acidosis. Marked elevation of intracellular cystine content. Cystine crystals in bone marrow, conjunctivae, kidneys, and leukocytes. Intralysosomal storage of cystine.
Cystinuria	Nephrolithiasis, nephrological complications, and MR in some patients.	Marked urinary excretion of cystine and dibasic amino acids. Normal to low-normal plasma lysine, arginine, and ornithine.
Dibasic-aminoaciduria	Short stature, malabsorption, and varying degree of MR.	Increased urinary excretion of lysine, arginine, and ornithine without cystinuria. Normal plasma amino acids.
Glycine		
Nonketotic hyperglycinemia	MR, FTT, lethargy, seizures, and coma after valine load. Death during early infancy or childhood.	No ketosis. Elevated glycine in plasma, urine, and especially CSF. Occasionally ammonia is elevated.
Histidine		
Formiminoglutamic (FIGLU) aciduria	MR, cortical atrophy, abnormal EEGs, and gastrointestinal symptoms. Asymptomatic individuals described. Can be secondary to liver disease, pregnancy, folate or B_{12} deficiency.	Urinary excretion of FIGLU. Excretion increased following histidine load. Elevated serum folic acid. Deficiency of formiminotransferase in erythrocytes and/or jejunal mucosa.
Histidinemia	Phenotypically asymptomatic. Association with MR, growth retardation, and impaired speech is most likely secondary to biased ascertainment.	Elevated levels of histidine in plasma and urine. Deficiency of histidase in liver and fibroblasts.
Homocystine		
Homocystinuria (methyltransferase deficiency)	Lethargy, seizures, feeding difficulties, and MR. Some patients are vitamin B_{12}-responsive.	Hyperammonemia. Hypoglycemia. Increased levels of homocystine and cystathionine; normal or low levels of methionine and methylmalonic acid in blood and urine.
Homocystinuria (methylenetetrahydrofolate reductase deficiency)	MR, seizures, and proximal muscle weakness. Some patients are responsive to pharmacologic doses of folic acid.	Increased levels of homocystine in blood and urine.
Homocystinuria (cystathionine β-synthase deficiency)	Marfanoid features: optic lens dislocation, MR, osteoporosis, and thromboemboli. Some patients respond to pyridoxine (vitamin B_6); others to a diet restricted in methionine and supplemented with cysteine.	Elevated homocystine and methionine; decreased cystine in urine and plasma.

continued

TABLE 2. *Continued.*

	Clinical findings	Laboratory diagnostic findings
Lysine		
Persistent hyperlysinemia	Varying degree of expression. MR, vomiting, seizures, and hypotonia.	Elevation of lysine in plasma, urine and CSF; without hyperammonemia. Deficiency of lysine 2-oxoglutarate: NADPH oxidoreductase ± saccharopine dehydrogenase.
Lysinuric protein intolerance	Diarrhea, vomiting, malnutrition, osteoporosis, and hepatomegaly. Precipitated by protein or lysine load.	Postprandial hyperammonemia. Elevation in urine and decrease in plasma of lysine, arginine, and ornithine. Elevated plasma glutamine.
Methionine		
Hypermethioninemia, primary	Phenotypically asymptomatic.	Marked elevation of methionine in blood. Minimal elevation of methionine in urine. Deficiency of methionine adenosyltransferase.
Hypermethioninemia, secondary	Secondary elevation in tyrosinemia and in homocystinemia.	Marked elevation of methionine in plasma and urine.
Ornithine		
Gyrate atrophy of the choroid and retina	Progressive chorioretinal degeneration. Myopia, night blindness, and loss of peripheral vision late in first decade; eventual blindness by third and fourth decades.	Elevated ornithine in plasma, urine, and CSF. Deficiency of L-ornithine: 2-oxoacidaminotransferase.
Hyperornithinemia-hyperammonemia-homocitrullinuria syndrome (HHH syndrome)	Feeding difficulties, protein intolerance, and MR. No retinal or gyrate atrophy.	Elevated plasma ornithine and urine homocitrulline. Hyperammonemia. Defect probably in mitochondrial ornithine transport.
Phenylalanine		
Phenylketonuria (PKU)	Incidence 1/14,000. If untreated, MR, musty odor, eczema, microcephaly, seizures, and vomiting. Treatment: dietary restriction of phenylalanine to maintain serum levels 5–9 mg/dl. Restricted dietary intake during pregnancy of PKU patients to prevent maternal hyperphe syndrome.	Plasma phenylalanine (Phe) levels greater than 20 mg/dl with normal or low normal tyrosine levels. Elevation of phenylpyruvic acid and 2-OH-phenylacetic acid in urine. Deficiency of phenylalanine hydroxylase in liver.
Persistent hyperphenylalaninemia (PHP)	Presumably normal neurological and intellectual development even without dietary restriction of Phe.	Plasma Phe levels on unrestricted protein diet lower than 17 mg/dl with normal or low normal tyrosine. Decreased Phe dydroxylase in liver. Several patients cannot be classified as either PKU or PHP and might represent compound heterozygotes.
Transient mild hyperphenylalaninemia	No clinical symptomatology. Mainly premature infants.	Transient elevation of plasma Phe levels early in life.
Dihydropteridine reductase deficiency	Initially normal; later seizures, MR, choking, eczema, and hypotonia. Deterioration despite adequate phenylalanine-restricted diet. Dopa, 5-OH-tryptophan, and carbidopa are used in treatment.	Elevated levels of phenylpyruvic acid and 2-OH-phenylacetic acid in urine. Variable plasma phenylalanine levels may be greater than 20 mg/dl. Altered neopterin/biopterin ratio in urine. Deficiency of dihydropteridine reductase in fibroblasts.
Abnormal dihydrobiopterin function	Pseudobulbar palsies, athetoid movements, and abnormal EEG. Dopa, carbidopa, and 5-OH-tryptophan used in treatment.	Plasma Phe level may be greater than 20 mg/dl. Abnormal and decreased biopterin metabolites in urine. Altered neopterin/biopterin ratio in urine. Defect in dihydrobiopterin synthesis suggested.
Alkaptonuria	Arthritis. Black discoloration of cheeks, nose, sclerae, and ears by midlife.	Elevated urine homogentisic acid. Urine turns black on standing (seen on diapers). Deficiency of homogentisic acid oxidase in tissues.

TABLE 2. Continued.

	Clinical findings	Laboratory diagnostic findings
Proline, hydroxyproline		
Hyperhydroxyprolinemia	Phenotypically asymptomatic. Association of MR most likely secondary to biased ascertainment.	Elevation of hydroxyproline in plasma and urine. Deficiency of hydroxyproline oxidase in fibroblasts.
Hyperprolinemia, type I	In some families, associated with seizures, nerve deafness, MR, nephrolithiasis, nephrotic syndrome, ichthyosis, aniridia, and ophthalmological findings.	Aminoaciduria with predominantly proline, hydroxyproline, and glycine. Elevated plasma proline. Deficiency of proline oxidase in fibroblasts.
Hyperprolinemia, type II	Phenotypically asymptomatic. Association with MR and seizures is most likely secondary to biased ascertainment.	Elevation of proline in plasma, CSF, and urine. Iminoglycinuria. Deficiency of Δ'-pyrroline-5-carboxylate dehydrogenase.
Iminoglycinuria, familial	Seizures, MR, hypotonia, and blindness/deafness.	Increased excretion of proline, hydroxyproline, and glycine in urine with normal plasma concentrations. Abnormal renal transport suggested.
Prolidase deficiency with hyperimidodipeptiduria	Peculiar facies, chronic dermatitis, and recurrent infections.	Elevation of proline and hydroxyproline dipeptides in urine. Prolidase deficiency in leukocytes and erythrocytes documented.
Sarcosine		
Sarcosinemia	FTT, MR, and hepatosplenomegaly.	Elevated levels of sarcosine in urine and blood. Deficiency of sarcosine dehydrogenase in liver.
Tryptophan		
Hartnup disease	Photosensitivity, motor abnormalities, and psychological signs. Some patients are responsive to pharmacologic doses of nicotinamide; some show spontaneous remission.	Generalized aminoaciduria and increase of indole and indoxyl derivatives (indican) in urine. Low plasma levels of tryptophan. Defect is in transport of tryptophans by intestinal mucosa and renal tubules.
Tryptophanuria	MR, dwarfism, cerebellar ataxia, and pellagra-like rash.	Isolated elevation of tryptophan in plasma and urine.
Tyrosine		
Tyrosinemia	See Table 3.	See Table 3.

From ref. 14, with permission.

TABLE 3. *Inborn errors of organic acid metabolism*

	Clinical findings	Laboratory diagnostic findings
Disorders of leucine metabolism		
Isovaleric acidemia	A. Severe form presents in the neonatal period with poor feeding, vomiting, ketoacidosis, and coma. Urine has "sweaty feet" odor. B. Chronic course has exacerbations with encephalopathy, ketoacidosis, MR, and characteristic urine odor.	Severe acidosis. Increased concentrations of blood lactate and pyruvate during ketoacidosis. Characteristic urine organic acids are isovalerylglycine and 3-hydroxyisovaleric acid. Elevated plasma levels of isovaleric acid. Pancytopenia. Deficiency of isovaleryl-CoA dehydrogenase.
3-Methylcrotonylglycinemia	FTT, erythematous rash, alopecia, developmental delay, and hypotonia. Urine has cat's urine odor.	Characteristic urine organic acids are 3-hydroxyisovaleric acid and 3-methylcrotonylglycine. Deficiency of 3-methylcrotonyl-CoA carboxylase in fibroblasts.
3-Hydroxy-3-methylglutaric acidemia	Hepatomegaly. Exacerbations with Reye's syndrome–like presentation.	Acidosis. Profound nonketotic hypoglycemia. No ketonuria. Characteristic urine organic acids are 3-hydroxy-3-methylglutaric and 3-methylglutaconic. Deficiency of hydroxymethylglutaryl-CoA lyase in fibroblasts and leukocytes.

continued

TABLE 3. *Continued.*

	Clinical findings	Laboratory diagnostic findings
Disorders of isoleucine and valine metabolism		
2-Methyl-3-hydroxybutyric acidemia (β-ketothiolase deficiency)	Ketoacidosis, FTT, encephalopathy, and MR.	Acidosis. Occasional hyperammonemia. Characteristic urine organic acid is 2-methyl-3-hydroxybutyric acid and frequently also 2-methylacetoacetic acid and tiglyglycine. Deficiency in activity of a β-ketothiolase in fibroblast.
Propionic acidemia	Acute presentation with lethargy and vomiting. Chronic presentation with FTT, hyperglycinemia, and neutropenia. Seizures and MR are common in both.	Acidosis. Hypoglycemia. Hyperammonemia. Characteristic urine organic acids are 3-hydroxypropionic and methylcitric. Deficiency of propionyl-CoA carboxylase in fibroblasts, leukocytes, and liver.
Congenital methylmalonic acidemia		
mut⁻ or mut⁰ group	Vomiting, hypotonia, upper respiratory tract infections, and FTT. Usually unresponsive to vitamin B_{12}.	Acidosis. Hypoglycemia. Hyperammonemia. Characteristic urine organic acid is methylmalonic acid. Frequently also lactic, 3-hydroxybutyric, acetoacetic, 3-hydroxy-n-valeric and 3-keto-n-valeric acids. Defects in the methylmalonyl-CoA mutase apoenzyme.
cbl C and cbl D group	Severe CNS dysfunction (seizures, hypotonia, MR, and microcephaly) and eventually megaloblastic anemia.	Acidosis. Hypoglycemia. Hyperammonemia. Characteristic urine organic acids as above. Low serum methionine and high serum and urine cystathionine. Defect is in the synthesis of both methylcobalamin and adenosylcobalamin.
cbl A and cbl B group	Vomiting, hypotonia, and FTT. Usually responsive to vitamin B_{12}.	Acidosis. Hypoglycemia. Hyperammonemia. Characteristic urine organic acids as above. Defect is in the synthesis of adenosylcobalamin.
Multiple carboxylase deficiency	Skin rash, MR, alopecia, seizures, hypotonia, and abnormal urinary odor.	Acidosis. Characteristic urine organic acids are β-methylcrotonylglycine and 3-hydroxyisovaleric. Deficient activity of β-methylcrotonyl CoA carboxylase, pyruvate carboxylase, and propionyl-CoA carboxylase in fibroblasts secondary to holocarboxylase synthetase deficiency.
Maple syrup urine disease (branched-chain ketoaciduria)		
Type I (classic)	MR, episodes of recurrent cerebellar ataxia, feeding difficulty, high-pitched cry, CNS deterioration, and seizures. Urine odor of maple syrup.	Acidosis. Hypoglycemia. Ketonuria. Characteristic urine organic acids are 2-oxoisocaproic, 2-oxo-3-methylvaleric, and 2-oxoisovaleric acids. Aminoacidemia and aminoaciduria of mainly branched-chain amino acids. Deficiency of the oxidative decarboxylation of branched-chain amino acids.
Type II (intermediate)	MR, anemia, and no obvious ketoacidotic episodes. Characteristic urine odor is variable.	Acidosis. Variable excretion of organic acids as in type I. Aminoacidemia and aminoaciduria of mainly branched-chain amino acids, but not to extent of type I. Decreased activity of the oxidative decarboxylation.
Type III (intermittent)	Acute onset of CNS symptoms, including seizures and coma. Exacerbations precipitated by infection, stress, or protein load. Characteristic urine odor during exacerbations.	Acidosis. Variable excretion of organic acids as in type I. Aminoacidemia and aminoaciduria of branched-chain amino acids when symptomatic.

TABLE 3. Continued.

	Clinical findings	Laboratory diagnostic findings
Type IV (thiamine-responsive)	MR, characteristic urine odor. No obvious ketoacidotic episodes.	Hyperuricemia. Variable excretion of organic acids as in type I. Aminoacidemia and aminoaciduria of branched-chain amino acids.
Dihydroliopoyl dehydrogenase (E3) deficiency	Floppiness and lethargy with a deteriorating course.	Acidosis. Aminoacidemia and aminoaciduria of branched-chain amino acids. 2-Ketoglutaric aciduria.
Disorders of lysine and tryptophan metabolism		
2-Ketoadipic acidemia	Varying degrees of MR, metabolic acidosis, and hypotonia.	Acidosis. Characteristic urine organic acids are 2-ketoadipic and 2-ketoglutaric. 2-Aminoadipic acidemia. Probably deficient activity of 2-oxoadipic acid dehydrogenase in fibroblasts.
Glutaric acidemia, type I	Normal early development. Exacerbation following an infection with encephalopathy, seizures, and hepatomegaly. Recovery is slow and incomplete. Deteriorating course.	Acidosis. Hypoglycemia. Characteristic urine organic acids are glutaric acid, 3-hydroxyglutaric acid, and glutaconic acid. Deficiency of glutaryl-CoA dehydrogenase in fibroblasts and leukocytes.
Glutaric acidemia, type II (multiple acyl-CoA dehydrogenase deficiency)	Hypotonia, poor weight gain, episodic vomiting, polycystic kidneys, and the "smell of sweaty feet." Death in early childhood.	Acidosis. Profound hypoglycemia. Hyperammonemia. Characteristic urine organic acids include glutaric, 2-hydroxyglutaric, ethylmalonic, and others. Defect is electron transfer flavoprotein.
Miscellaneous organic acidemias		
Lactic acidosis/aciduria	MR, FTT, lethargy, ataxia, vomiting, and hepatomegaly. Some patients have intermittent attacks.	Characteristic urine organic acids are lactic, pyruvic, and 2-hydroxybutyric acids. Elevated serum pyruvic acid and alanine. Secondary lactic acidosis should be ruled out.
D-Glyceric acidemia	Early onset of hypotonia, seizures, MR, and FTT.	Acidosis. Characteristic urine organic acid is D-glyceric acid. Enzymatic defect is unknown.
Hyperglycerolemia	Varies from normal to growth and psychomotor retardation, spasticity, esotropia, osteoporosis, and pathologic bone fractures.	Characteristic urine organic acid is glycerol. Deficiency of glycerol kinase in leukocytes, fibroblasts, and other tissues.
Proglutamic acidemia (5-oxoprolinemia)	MR, ataxia, and hemolysis.	Acidosis. Characteristic urine organic acid is pyroglutamic acid. Deficiency of glutathione synthetase. May be seen secondary to Nutramigen diet.
Dicarboxylic acidurias	Vomiting, hepatomegaly, encephalopathy, and hypotonia.	Acidosis. Hypoglycemia. Characteristic urine organic acids are adipic, suberic, and sebacic. Enzymatic defect is not known. May be seen secondary to diets containing medium-chain triglyceride supplementation.
Tyrosinemias		
Tyrosinemia I, hereditary tyrosinemia		
Acute	FTT, irritability, fever, vomiting, diarrhea, bleeding manifestations, hepatic failure, hepatomegaly, cirrhosis, and a cabbage-like odor. Rapidly progressive fetal outcome by 12 months. High frequency of the gene in the Chicoutimi-Lac St. Jean region of Quebec province.	Characteristic urine organic acids are 4-hydroxyphenyllactic and 4-hydroxyphenylpyruvic. Hypermethionimenia, mild hypertyrosinemia, and tyrosyluria. Hypoglycemia, hypoproteinemia, and hypoprothrombinemia. Tyrosine crystals in bone marrow. Variable deficiency of fumarylacetoacetate hydrolase of 4-hydroxyphenylpyruvate dioxygenase suggested.

continued

TABLE 3. *Continued.*

	Clinical findings	Laboratory diagnostic findings
Subacute or chronic	Renal tubular dysfunction, vitamin D–resistant rickets, anemia, and progressive cirrhosis associated with hepatomas. Clinical symptoms apparent after the first year of age with death by 10 years. Treatment: dietary restriction of tyrosine, methionine, and phenylalanine.	Same as for acute tyrosinemia.
Tyrosinemia II, persistent tyrosinemia (Oregon-type) (Richner-Hanhart syndrome)	Symptom complex of MR, palmar and plantar hyperkeratosis, and keratitis. Attempted therapy with tyrosine/phenylalanine–restricted diet.	Characteristic urine organic acids are 4-hydroxyphenylacetic, 4-hydroxyphenyllactic, and N-acetyltyrosine. Tyrosinemia. Severe deficiency of cytoplasmic tyrosine aminotransferase in liver.
Transient tyrosinemia of the newborn	Usually premature infants and full-term infants with hepatitis or sepsis.	Same characteristic urine organic acids as tyrosinemia II.
Secondary tyrosinemia	Secondary to hepatic dysfunction. Can be associated with galactosemia and hereditary fructose intolerance.	Same characteristic urine organic acids as tyrosinemia II.
Ketosis		
Primary	Recurrent attacks of severe ketoacidosis. Permanent ketosis both in urine and plasma, increasing from morning to night. Triggered by catabolism, intercurrent infectious diseases, fasting, and high protein intake.	Severe ketoacidosis. Characteristic urine organic acids are 3-hydroxybutyrate and acetoacetate in succinyl-CoA transferase deficiency. Characteristic urine organic acids are 3-hydroxybutyrate, 2-methyl-3-hydroxybutyrate, and tiglyglycine in methylacetoacetyl-CoA thiolase deficiency. Both can be confirmed by fibroblast culture.
Secondary	Starvation and prolonged vomiting. Also in some of the glycogen storage disorders.	Characteristic urine organic acids are acetoacetic and 3-hydroxybutyric acids.

From ref. 14, with permission.

cially among patients with a history of disproportionately severe presentation during intercurrent infections.

"Near-SIDS" Patients or Siblings of SIDS Babies

Urinary organic acids and plasma and urine carnitine should be evaluated (3). Secondary carnitine deficiency is a very common phenomenon in all of the inborn errors in which a chronic accumulation of acyl coenzyme A (acylCoA) compounds occurs (4).

PRINCIPLES OF TREATMENT AND MANAGEMENT

Dietary Restriction of a Specific Dietary Component

An approach similar to that of phenylalanine restriction in phenylketonuria (5) can be used for the treatment and management of disorders associated with inherited defects in the metabolic pathways of branched-chain amino acids (isoleucine, leucine, and valine). Examples include maple syrup urine disease (6), in which the defect involves all of the branched-chain amino acids, β-ketothiolase, which involves the isoleucine pathway (7), and 3-hydroxy-3-methylglutaryl-CoA lyase (7), which involves a defect in the pathway of one amino acid. Similarly, the restriction of total protein, lysine, ornithine, medium-chain triglycerides, and other dietary components can be used in the treatment and management of many of these disorders (Tables 2 and 3).

Inhibition of Endogenous Synthesis

Inhibition of endogenous synthesis is used in the treatment and management of the urea cycle defects by shunting the ammonia through an alternate pathway (treatment with sodium benzoate or sodium phenylacetate) or by supplementation with arginine or citrulline to "turn the cycle" once (8).

Substrate Removal

Substrate removal is used during the acute phase of the disease by either exchange transfusion, peritoneal di-

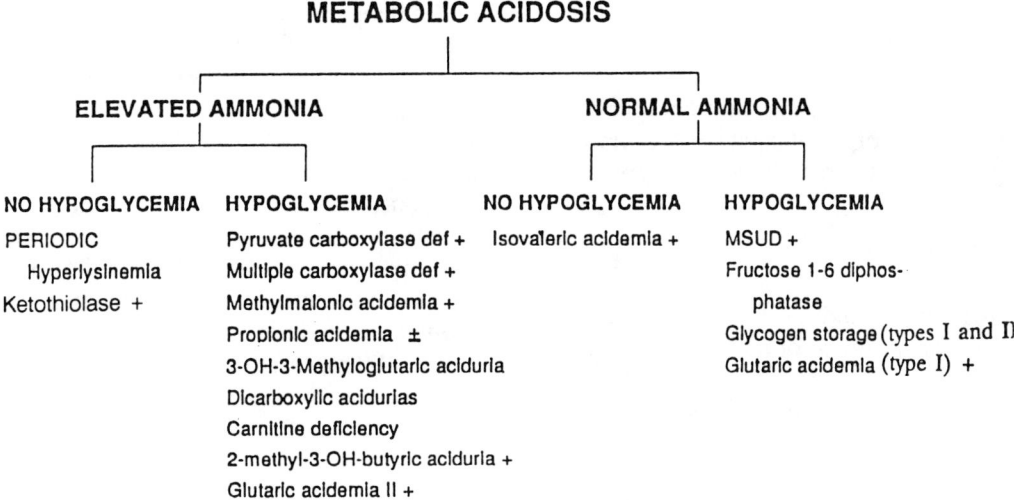

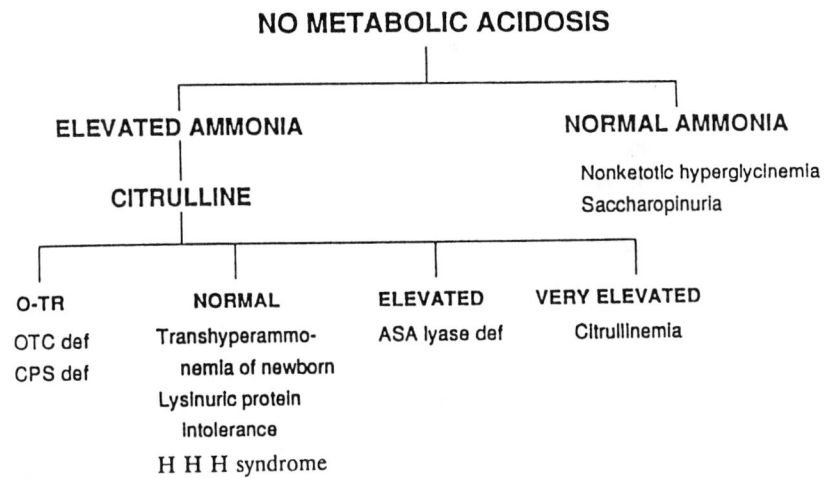

FIG. 1. A schematic flow diagram showing the relatively common inborn errors according to their typical laboratory presentation.

alysis, or hemodialysis (9). Substrate removal in the acute phase could also be achieved by using alternate pathways and supplementation of arginine and citrulline as described above. Another example of this approach is carnitine supplementation in an attempt to buffer and remove the excess of acylCoA compounds in patients who have developed secondary carnitine deficiency.

Vitamin Supplementation in Pharmacological Doses

In several of these inherited disorders, the underlying defect is in the binding affinity of the coenzyme (vitamin) to the mutant apoenzyme (10). By providing the vitamin in pharmacological quantities, the clinical sequelae of the mutations can be either ameliorated or, in many patients, completely prevented. Examples of this approach include patients with methylmalonic acidemia, multiple carboxylase deficiency, primary lactic acidosis, and biotinidase deficiency.

Enzyme Replacement

Although enzyme replacement by DNA insertion (genetic engineering) remains largely a dream of the future, successful treatment and management of some inherited disorders by liver transplantation has already been accomplished (11).

PROBLEMS IN TREATMENT AND MANAGEMENT

The most common problems in treatment and management occur as a result of insufficient education in the pathophysiology of inherited metabolic disorders.

Overlooking the Consequences of Intercurrent Infections

This is the most serious and most prevalent pitfall in the treatment and management of patients with inborn errors of metabolism. Nearly all of these patients, even with appropriate treatment and management, will tend to experience severe metabolic exacerbation during intercurrent infections or physiologic insult (trauma, surgery, starvation, heat stroke, etc.). Patients must be observed more closely, and treated more aggressively, whenever such an episode occurs. The worst and, unfortunately, most common mistake is that of prescribing antibiotics by telephone without evaluating the patient.

Delayed and/or Incomplete Management of Hyperammonemia

Regardless of whether the hyperammonemia is secondary to a urea cycle defect or an inborn error of organic acid metabolism, (Fig. 1) it is a medical emergency. It is heartbreaking to see patients carrying the sequelae of a hyperammonemic encephalopathy that occurred prior to accurate diagnosis and treatment or during a period of exacerbation.

Delayed and/or Incomplete Management of Acidosis and Hypoglycemia, Associated with Some of the Inborn Errors of Organic Acid Metabolism

Metabolic acidosis, often associated with severe hypoglycemia, occurs as a presenting symptom and again during exacerbations in many patients (Fig. 1). Most patients will require IV therapy. It is critical (especially for the hypoglycemia) that treatment is not discontinued when blood levels return to normal, but is continued for as long as the physiological insult leading to the exacerbations persists.

The Mistaken Identification of Secondary Carnitine Deficiency for the Inherited Disorder

Secondary carnitine deficiency, which may occur in patients with an inborn error of organic acid metabolism, is often phenotypically indistinguishable from the clinical presentation of the inherited disorder. Carnitine values (and especially the ratio of free carnitine to acylcarnitine) should be monitored in all of these patients.

The inherited disorders most prone to develop secondary carnitine deficiency are methylmalonic acidemia, propionic acidemia, isovaleric acidemia, glutaric acidemia types I and II, β-ketothiolase, and medium-chain acylCoA dehydrogenase deficiency (12). It is advisable to include carnitine and acylcarnitine determinations in urine and plasma as part of the diagnostic workup of patients suspected of having an inborn error of organic acid metabolism. Carnitine should also be determined periodically during management and follow-up, especially if any deterioration occurs. Carnitine supplementation (100 mg/kg/day) in patients with primary or secondary carnitine deficiency often improves motor performance and decreases susceptibility to exacerbations (13).

SELECTED PATIENT PRESENTATIONS

Inborn Errors of the Urea Cycle

Case History 1

J.D. was the first child born to a healthy nonconsanguineous couple. He was born full-term following an uneventful pregnancy via spontaneous vaginal delivery, with a birth weight of 7 lb, 9 oz. He was discharged from the hospital at the age of 3 days and readmitted the following day because of marked hypotonia, lethargy, unresponsiveness, and a seizure episode. He was treated for sepsis. Eight hours after admission, following further clinical deterioration, plasma ammonia was determined to be 700 μmol/l (normal range 30 to 50 μmol/l). A two-volume exchange transfusion was performed after which the plasma ammonia dropped to 400 μmol/l. The following morning the ammonia level increased to 1,200 μmol/l at which stage urine and plasma were referred to our laboratory for diagnostic workup. Urine organic acids revealed a normal pattern, whereas both plasma and urine amino acids revealed marked increases in glutamine, citrulline, and arginosuccinic acid (663 nmol/ml in plasma and 1,858 nmol/mg creatinine in the urine). The diagnosis of arginosuccinic acidemia (urea cycle defect type IV) was later confirmed by deficient enzymatic activity of arginosuccinate lyase in both red cells and fibroblasts. The patient was transferred from the community hospital to a central medical facility where treatment was initiated by total protein restriction, sodium benzoate (250 mg/kg/day), arginine (800 mg/kg/day), and peritoneal dialysis. Within the next 48 hr, ammonia levels gradually returned to normal. The sodium benzoate and the peritoneal dialysis were discontinued and the patient was sent home on a protein restricted diet (between 1.5 to 2 g/kg/day) and arginine supplementation of 500 mg/kg/day. The patient has been followed and managed in our clinic for the past 5 years. His ammonia levels have been maintained within the normal range except for several exacerbations during intercurrent infections (especially purulent otitis media) during which time ammonia levels increased for several days to between 100 and 150 mmol/l. Although the patient was very well controlled by dietary management and arginine supplementation, marked developmental and motor delays have been documented. In a later pregnancy, prenatal diagnosis revealed an unaffected carrier male offspring.

Case History 2

S.L. was the second child of a healthy consanguineous couple. The first son of this couple had been treated for "sepsis" 7 days after he was born. He gradually gained weight but was delayed in achieving his motor milestones. At the age of 6 months, during an episode of upper respiratory tract infection, he lapsed into coma and died within 12 hr, with the diagnosis of "sepsis." His sister, S.L., was born after an uneventful pregnancy and was sent home at the age of 48 hr. She was admitted to the community hospital at the age of 3 days with grunting respiration, tachypnea, and tachycardia. She was started on antibiotic therapy IV with a presumptive diagnosis of sepsis. She was transferred after several hours to a central medical facility following further deterioration in her clinical condition. On admission, plasma ammonia of 481 mmol/l was detected and although she underwent two volume exchange transfusions, her ammonia continued to increase to a level of 1,344 mmol/l. Urine and plasma amino acids revealed a significant increase in citrulline and a marked decrease in arginine, both of which are characteristic of type III urea cycle defect (citrullinemia). This diagnosis was further confirmed by deficient activity of arginosuccinic synthetase in fibroblasts. She was treated by peritoneal dialysis, 250 mg/kg/day of sodium benzoate, and 800 mg/kg/day of arginine. Her ammonia levels dropped to normal within the next 48 hr and the patient was placed on a diet with restricted protein intake (1.5 g/kg/day), 600 mg/kg/day of arginine, and on Ucephan (a mixture of sodium benzoate and sodium phenylacetate providing 250 mg/kg/day of each). She has been followed and managed by our clinic since that time. During the first year of life she had only one short exacerbation during an episode of viral gastroenteritis in which her ammonia levels increased for 1 day to the level of 150 mmol/l. Otherwise, her ammonia levels have been maintained between 30 and 50 μmol/l, which is within the high-normal range. By the age of 1 year she had achieved all of her developmental and motor milestones. A developmental assessment recently revealed somewhat advanced development for her age.

Discussion

These patients demonstrate the major concepts in the diagnosis and treatment of patients with urea cycle defects. In each, a stormy episode of hyperammonemic encephalopathy occurred on the third to fourth day of life. These episodes were misinterpreted as sepsis until plasma ammonia levels suggested a urea cycle defect. Diagnosis was determined within several hours by evaluating plasma and urine amino acids. Therapy in the acute phase of the hyperammonemia included exchange transfusion and peritoneal dialysis, complete restriction of protein, supplementation of arginine, and treatment with sodium benzoate. The supplementation of arginine in urea cycle defect types III and IV and supplementation of citrulline in types I and II, provides the ability to "turn" the urea cycle one time. Thus, for each mole of arginine or citrulline that the patients receive, one mole of ammonia will be converted into nontoxic compounds in the urea cycle prior to the metabolic block. The aim of treatment with sodium benzoate and sodium phenylacetate is to shunt ammonia through alternate pathways—sodium benzoate, ammonia, and glycine are converted to hippuric acid, whereas sodium phenylacetate, ammonia, and glutamine are converted to phenylacetylglutamate. The treatment with sodium benzoate and sodium phenylacetate (provided as one preparation in Ucephan) is used in the acute phase of hyperammonemia and is recommended as part of the chronic treatment and management of patients with urea cycle defect types I, II, and III.

Acute-phase presentation was similar in both patients; both reached similar levels of plasma ammonia, and both were followed and managed with no further significant exacerbations. J.D., however, is markedly developmentally delayed as a result of the initial hyperammonemic encephalopathy, whereas S.L. is developing normally.

Of interest is S.L.'s brother who had been treated for "sepsis" as a newborn, continued to show developmental delay, and died at the age of 6 months during an intercurrent infection with a similar clinical presentation of "sepsis." Recognition that an underlying inborn error might phenotypically present as "rule out sepsis" may have saved his life and provided the option of prenatal diagnosis for this couple in their next pregnancy.

Inborn Errors of Amino Acid Metabolism

Case History 3

C.R. was the first offspring born to a healthy nonconsanguineous couple following an uneventful pregnancy and delivery. The results of her newborn screening Guthrie test, obtained at the age of 48 hr, revealed an elevated plasma phenylalanine. (A quantitative determination of phenylalanine and tyrosine at the age of 11 days revealed a phenylalanine value of 41.5 mg% and a tyrosine value of 1.0 mg%.) The following day she was placed on a diet with restricted phenylalanine content (Lofenalac and Similac, containing 60 mg/kg/day of phenylalanine). Her plasma phenylalanine level dropped to 11 mg% within 5 days and to 1.6 mg% after 10 days of dietary restriction. The phenylalanine content in the diet was increased to 65 mg/kg/day and plasma phenylalanine and tyrosine values were monitored weekly at first, at biweekly intervals for several months, and then on a monthly basis. Plasma phenylalanine values were between 2.8 and 5.2 mg%, with tyrosine values between 0.7 and 1.2 mg%. The dietary intake of phenylalanine was adjusted according to the plasma phenylalanine values and by the end of her first year of life the phenylalanine intake was decreased to 20 mg/kg/day with plasma levels stabilized between 1.8 and 4.7 mg%. A phenylalanine loading test at the age of 14 months confirmed the diagnosis of "classical" phenylketonuria secondary to deficient phenylalanine hydroxylase activity. At the age of 14 months the protein supplementation with Lofenalac was replaced by a PhenylFree diet, which enabled variability in her food intake. She has achieved all of her motor and developmental milestones, and is a healthy, intelligent $3\frac{1}{2}$-year-old as documented by repeated developmental assessments.

Phenylketonuria (PKU) is an autosomal recessive inborn error of amino acid metabolism described as early as 1934. It involves a block in the pathway that converts phenylalanine to tyrosine. If untreated, patients with PKU will develop significant neurological involvement, especially mental retardation and seizure disorders between the second and fifth years of life. The neurological sequela are irreversible; thus, an appropriate diet should be initiated early in infancy to prevent neurological complications. The goal of the diet is to restrict the phenylalanine to the amount required for normal growth and development, but to prevent an excess of phenylalanine which, through the catabolic pathways, would lead to the metabolites causing the neurological complications. During the first year of life, when growth is relatively accelerated, larger quantities of phenylalanine should be provided in the diet. These are decreased between 12 and 18 months of age to maintain plasma phenylalanine levels between 2 and 8 mg%. Team approach is essential. The physician's role is primarily for determining optimum phenylalanine intake. The actual composition of the diet is the job of the nutritionist, whose expertise this is.

Case History 4

C.M. was born following an uneventful pregnancy and delivery. On her second day of life, she appeared very somnolent and on her third day of life, intractable seizures became apparent. Laboratory tests revealed moderate metabolic acidosis, mild hypoglycemia, and ketonuria. Blood and urine sent to our laboratory showed marked elevation of the branched-chain amino acids (leucine, isoleucine, and valine) in both urine and plasma. There was marked excretion of 2-oxoisocaproic, 2-oxo-3-methylvaleric, and 2-oxoisovaleric acids in her urinary organic acids. These findings were characteristic of maple syrup urine disease (MSUD). The patient was placed on a diet restricted in branched-chain amino acid content (MSUD diet) and Similac to provide the required branched-chain amino acids for growth and development. The ratio of the MSUD protein to that of the Similac protein was determined in such a way that the patient was free from ketonuria as determined by dinitrophenylhydrazine (DNPH) urine tests with minimal to moderate elevation of the branched-chain amino acids in the plasma. C.M.'s grandmother, with whom she lived, learned to perform the urine DNPH test and to modify the diet accordingly. The patient was admitted to the local hospital several times due to exacerbations occurring during intercurrent infections. She was treated by discontinuing protein intake and with IV treatment of fluids, glucose, and electrolytes. She developed very well with minimal delay in her developmental milestones. At age 3, her grandmother died and she began to live with an aunt. Unfortunately, the aunt was not able to maintain or modify her diet according to instructions. At 3 years and 8 months she developed an upper respiratory tract infection for which antibiotics were prescribed over the telephone. She became unconscious and seizures (of which she had been free since early infancy) reappeared. She was taken to the hospital on the third day of this episode, declared brain dead, and expired after 24 hr. This case is representative of the most critical danger in the treatment and management of patients with inborn errors of the urea cycle, amino acid, and organic acid metabolism. It highlights the need to recognize that any intercurrent infection in these patients, especially when associated with changes in consciousness, must be considered a medical emergency.

Inborn Errors of Organic Acid Metabolism

Case History 5

K.C. was born to a healthy mother following an uneventful pregnancy by spontaneous vaginal delivery with a birth weight of 6 lb, 6 oz. She was discharged from the hospital after 48 hr. She was readmitted at 18 days of age because of vomiting, lethargy, and dehydration. Laboratory tests revealed moderate metabolic acidosis, hypoglycemia, and marked hyperammonemia (blood ammonia 1,200 mmol/l). She was treated by IV fluids (D10 1/2 saline) and two volume exchange transfusions. Urine and plasma for amino acids and urine organic acids, which were submitted the following morning, revealed a normal pattern of urine and plasma amino acids. The urinary organic acids, however, showed huge quantities of methylmalonic acid with minimal to moderate excretion of 2-hydroxyisobutyric, 3-hydroxy-n-butyric, maleic, adipic, suberic, and methylcitric acids. This pattern is characteristic of methylmalonic acidemia. A clinical trial with vitamin B_{12} (hydroxycobalamin 1 mg/day IM) was initiated following a second exchange transfusion. The patient improved dramatically with alleviation of clinical symptoms and normalization of blood chemistry. She was sent home on the fourth day after admission and has been followed and managed by our clinic. Repeat testing of plasma and urine carnitine was within the normal range. Skin fibroblasts confirmed the diagnosis of methylmalonic acidemia secondary to a defect in the synthesis of adenosylcobalamin (complementation group cb1A). Propionic acid uptake by cultured fibroblasts was very low but was responsive to vitamin B_{12} added to the culture medium, which was similar to her clinical response to B_{12} supplementation. The patient has been maintained on B_{12} supplementation by daily IM injections and in the past 2 years has had only one exacerbation during an intercurrent infection. She has reached all of her developmental milestones properly and a developmental assessment revealed normal intelligence.

This patient is representative of patients with inborn errors of organic acid metabolism who are responsive to pharmacological doses of a cofactor vitamin. Besides some of the forms of methylmalonic acidemia, these patients include those with multiple carboxylase deficiency (responsive to biotin), type IV MSUD (thiamine), biotinidase deficiency (biotin), some forms of lactic acidosis (thiamine), and rarely, patients of glutaric acidemia type II (riboflavin). In some patients, as in the patient described above, a complete metabolic correction can be obtained by supplementing the cofactor, whereas in others only a partial response can be determined. Thus, when an inborn error of organic acids is suspected, and a stat diagnostic test for amino and organic acids is not available, a therapeutic trial with a "megavitamin cocktail" is recommended. This includes a pharmacological dosage of biotin, thiamine, riboflavin, B_{12}, and carnitine.

Case History 6

J.G. was born after an uneventful pregnancy via vaginal delivery to a healthy nonconsanguineous couple. She was first admitted to the hospital at the age of 10 days because of severe metabolic acidosis, which was treated as "sepsis." Her second admission was at the age of 11 months because of severe metabolic acidosis, ketosis, and hypoglycemia. On admission, blood pH was recorded as low as 6.7. She was treated with IV fluids, glucose, and bicarbonate, and plasma for amino acids and urine for organic acids were sent to our laboratory. Plasma amino acids revealed a normal pattern for age. The urinary organic acids revealed excessive excretion of 3-hydroxy-2-methylbutyric, 2-methyl-3-hydroxybutyrate, tiglyglycine, 2-methylacetoacetic, 4-hydroxyphenylacetic, and citric acids. This pattern is very characteristic of β-ketothiolase deficiency. The diagnosis was confirmed by skin fibroblasts that revealed a deficiency of 2-methylacetoacetic-thiolase. As this inborn error of metabolism is in the degradation of isoleucine, her diet was restricted in isoleucine content. This was achieved by using an MSUD diet supplemented with leucine and valine. The patient improved markedly and achieved normal developmental milestones with some delay in her motor milestones. Numerous exacerbations occurred during intercurrent infections that required admission and IV therapy. When she was 2 years old, we considered the possibility of secondary carnitine deficiency, and evaluated her urine and plasma carnitine. These tests revealed decreased total carnitine in the plasma and undetectable free carnitine and markedly increased excretion of acylcarnitine in the urine. Carnitine supplementation (100 mg/kg/day) was initiated and resulted in a dramatic improvement in her motor performance. According to her mother, "before carnitine supplementation she climbed one step at a time, whereas now I can hardly catch up with her." Following the carnitine supplementation, the frequency and severity of the exacerbations decreased markedly. When the patient was 5 years old, her mother became pregnant and prenatal diagnosis revealed that the fetus was also affected. The family opted to continue with the pregnancy and her brother, J.G., was born after an uneventful pregnancy. Diet restricted in isoleucine and supplementation of carnitine were initiated at birth. Her brother, at 18 months of age, had had only one episode of mild metabolic acidosis during an intercurrent infection, and was achieving all of his motor and developmental milestones.

J.G. illustrates the major role of secondary carnitine deficiency in some inborn errors of organic acid metabolism. Secondary carnitine deficiency in these patients is initiated by "buffering" acylCoA compounds from the mitochondria and excreting them as acylcarnitine according to the following formula:

$$AcylCoA + Carnitine \rightarrow Acylcarnitine + CoA.$$

Because the clinical presentation of secondary carnitine deficiency resembles that of an inherited inborn error of organic acid metabolism, secondary carnitine deficiency should be suspected in all patients in whom the underlying metabolic defect leads to an increased concentration of acylCoA compounds. These include methylmalonic acidemia, propionic acidemia, isovaleric acidemia, glutaric acidemia types I and II, medium-chain acylCoA dehydrogenase deficiency, β-ketothiolase, and others. It is important to recognize the relatively mild clinical course experienced by J.G.'s brother whose dietary management and carnitine supplementation had been initiated at birth.

CONCLUSION

Patients with inborn errors of urea cycle, amino acid, and organic acid metabolism present with nonspecific clinical findings. The diagnostic workup, therefore, depends mainly on laboratory findings. Appropriate tests include blood gases, glucose, electrolytes, ammonia, and lactate in all patients presenting as "rule out sepsis." When an inborn error is suspected, plasma amino acids and urinary organic acids should be evaluated. For patients presenting as "failure to thrive, developmental delay, and seizures," plasma and urine amino acids as well as urinary organic acids should be evaluated.

Effective treatment for many patients includes either dietary management, supplementation of cofactors in pharmacological dosage (or both), and, in others, removal of the "toxic" compounds by use of hemodialysis or alternate pathways. In many cases, prenatal diagnosis may be provided to the family during future pregnancies.

Most importantly, because of their tendency to have metabolic exacerbations during intercurrent infections, these patients must always be followed and managed as medical emergencies.

REFERENCES

1. Beaudet AL, Scriver CR, Sly WS, Valle D, Cooper DN, McKusick VA, Schmidke J. Genetics and biochemistry of variant human phenotypes. In: Scriver CR, Beaudet AL, Sly WS, Valle D, eds. *The metabolic basis of inherited disease,* vol 1. New York: McGraw-Hill, 1989;3-53.
2. Green A. Inborn errors of organic acid metabolism. *Br J Hospital Medicine* 1989;41:426-434.
3. Bennett MJ, Varlend S, Pollitt RJ. Screening siblings for inborn errors of fatty acid metabolism in families with a history of sudden infant death. *Lancet* 1986;2:1470.
4. Chalmers RA, Roe CR, Stacey TE, Hoppel CL. Urinary excretion of L-carnitine and acylcarnitines by patients with disorders of organic acid metabolism: evidence for secondary insufficiency of L-carnitine. *Pediatr Res* 1984;18:1325-1328.
5. Scriver CR, Kaufman S, Woo SL. The hyperphenylalaninemias. In: Scriver CR, Beaudet AL, Sly WS, Valle D, eds. *The metabolic basis of inherited disease,* vol 1. New York: McGraw-Hill, 1989;495-546.
6. Danner DJ, Elsas LJ II. Disorders of branched chain amino acid and keto acid metabolism. In: Scriver CR, Beaudet AL, Sly WS, Valle D, eds. *The metabolic basis of inherited disease,* vol 1. New York: McGraw-Hill, 1989;671-692.
7. Sweetman L. Branched chain organic acidurias. In: Scriver CR, Beaudet AL, Sly WS, Valle D, eds. *The metabolic basis of inherited disease,* vol 1. New York: McGraw-Hill, 1989;791-819.
8. Brusilow SW, Horwich AL. Urea cycle enzymes. In: Scriver CR, Beaudet AL, Sly WS, Valle D, eds. *The metabolic basis of inherited disease,* vol 1. New York: McGraw-Hill, 1989;629-663.
9. Benson PF, Fensom AH. *Genetic biochemical disorders,* 1st ed. Oxford: Oxford University Press, 1986.
10. Rosenberg LE. Vitamin responsive inherited metabolic disorders. In: *Advances in human genetics,* vol 6. New York: Plenum Press, 1976;1-74.
11. Malatack JJ, Iwatsuki S, Gartner JC, Roe T, Finegold DN, Shaw BW, Zitelli BJ, Starzl TE. Liver transplantation for type I glycogen storage disease. *Lancet* 1983;1:1073.
12. Stumpf DA, Parker WD Jr, Angelini C. Carnitine deficiency, organic acidemias, and Reye's syndrome. *Neurology* 1985;35:1041-1045.
13. Ashbrook DW. Carnitine supplementation in human carnitine deficiency. In: Borum PR, ed. *Clinical aspects of human carnitine deficiency.* New York: Pergamon Press, 1986;120-134.
14. Shapira E, Blitzer MG, Miller JB, Africk D. *Biochemical genetics, a laboratory manual.* New York: Oxford University Press, 1989.

CHAPTER 42

Nutritional Support of the Developmentally Disabled Child

Ann C. H. Tilton and Marilyn D. Miller

Optimum nutrition is critical for maximizing the physical and developmental potential of all children. The developmentally disabled child has problems in this realm, although the pathophysiology is not completely understood. What is acknowledged is that children with developmental disabilities are at significant risk of developing secondary nutritional deficits.

Evaluating developmentally disabled children is often difficult because they do not fit into our "normal" standards for assessment. Successful evaluation requires knowledge of nutrition and neurochemistry, of normal central nervous system development, and of the etiologies of developmental disabilities. This knowledge, combined with a detailed assessment of the individual disability, including metabolic needs and behavioral issues, will aid in accurate evaluation and appropriate intervention.

NUTRITION AND NEUROCHEMISTRY

Nervous system function is dependent on highly specific and yet interrelated chemical reactions. It is well recognized that abnormalities in glucose levels and oxygenation result in metabolic derangements. Recent studies confirm the importance of other nutrients, as well (1). Vitamins may act as cofactors to expedite neurochemical reactions. Amino acid precursors directly affect the availability of neurotransmitters that are instrumental in conveying excitatory and inhibitory information at a cellular level. This delicate balance of neurotransmitters

---

A. C. H. Tilton: Department of Pediatric Neurology, Tulane University School of Medicine, New Orleans, Louisiana 70112.
M. D. Miller: Department of Nursing, Children's Hospital, New Orleans, Louisiana 70118.

and other neuromodulators enables the central nervous system to fine-tune responses to a continuously changing environment. All functions, from learning and emotional responses to gross motor movements, are affected (2).

In the mid-1970s, only a few neurotransmitters, including acetylcholine, noradrenaline, dopamine, and serotonin, had been recognized. We are now aware of more than 60, and it is hypothesized that the actual number may be greater than 200. The majority of these neurotransmitters are peptides, containing up to 40 amino acids (3).

In addition, there are estimated to be at least 10 billion neurons, each having more than 3,000 synaptic connections with other nerve cells. Neurotransmitters affect neurons by means of pre- or postsynaptic receptors. Receptor availability may be altered by changes in pharmacologic, physiologic, or pathologic conditions. It is now recognized that several neurotransmitters and neuropeptides may be present in a single neuron (3).

Specific dietary-induced changes in neurotransmitters have been identified. The availability of serotonin is, for example, altered by increased carbohydrate loads. This occurs when the resulting increased insulin levels cause an increased relative availability of tryptophan to the brain. Tryptophan is, then, responsible for the subsequent formation of serotonin (2).

Other neurotransmitters are also very active in central nervous system function. γ-Aminobutyric acid (GABA), dopamine, acetylcholine, norepinephrine, and epinephrine, as well as serotonin, have been labeled the "classic" neurotransmitters because of their early recognition and the fact that they are the most investigated. γ-Aminobutyric acid is produced from the amino acid glutamic acid and is active in basal ganglia function. It is used as an anticonvulsant and antispasmodic agent. Dopamine, a product of the amino acid tyrosine, is implicated in movement disorders. Additionally, a major action of tranquilizers in psychiatric disorders is to block dopamine. Dopamine is also a precursor in the synthesis of such catecholamines as norepinephrine and epinephrine. Acetylcholine, a product of glucose metabolism, is active in multiple areas of neurotransmission. Clinically, it is useful in the treatment of Parkinson's disease and myasthenia gravis (2,3).

CAUSES OF DEVELOPMENTAL DISABILITIES

The most important factor determining the long-term impact on development is the timing, rather than the etiology, of an insult. In order to understand the vulnerability of the central nervous system, it is important to understand normal development.

During the first 6 weeks of gestation, dorsal and ventral induction occurs. Dorsal induction corresponds with the formation of the external structure of the brain and the spinal cord on the dorsal side of the embryo. Abnormalities in this area produce dramatic structural changes such as myelodysplasia and encephaloceles. The ventral induction phase is responsible for the formation of the face and the forebrain. The cleavages that occur during this period provide the paired optic vesicles, olfactory system, cerebral hemispheres, ventricles, and basal ganglia, as well as the thalamus and hypothalamus. At this point, the external structure of the brain is completed (4).

During the neuronal proliferative phase, the full complement of neurons are produced. This occurs between the second and fourth months of gestation. Concomitantly, the glial cells are produced. These will ultimately be involved in the migration of neurons to specific areas of the brain, fulfilling a genetic template. Microcephaly and macrocephaly are seen clinically as the consequence of abnormalities of this phase. Although there is speculation that primary proliferative abnormalities may result in a quantitatively abnormal neuron pool, this is difficult to substantiate scientifically (5).

During the migrational phase, from 3 to 5 months of gestation, the neurons migrate from the periventricular area to the cortex in a specific sequence. Malformations that result from a disruption of this process include a clinical spectrum from a brain with no gyri (lissencephaly) to a brain with too many gyri (polymicrogyria). Although major migration abnormalities generally result in significant neurological abnormalities, a very mild form of this migratory abnormality (heterotopias) may occur without major clinical significance (5).

The organizational phase occurs from 6 months of gestation to several years of life. This critical period provides the "elaborate circuitry that distinguishes the human brain" (5). It is a complex process in which the neuronal arborizations are either eliminated or expand their contacts in order to enhance their interrelationship. Physicians involved in the care of developmentally delayed or severely neurologically involved children are often perplexed by the discrepancy between the neuroimaging studies and the individual's clinical features. The subtle intracellular level of disturbance that occurs during the organizational phase may provide the most plausible explanation (5).

The sequence of myelination occurs from the second trimester to adulthood. It is during this phase that inborn errors of metabolism, i.e., aminoacidopathies and organic acidopathies, have significant impact. Phenylketonuria may also result from an abnormality during this phase.

The exact mechanism by which aminoacidopathies affect myelination remains unresolved (5). Animal, as well as human, studies confirm, however, that undernutrition has a deleterious effect on brain development, primarily impacting myelinogenesis. Fishman, et al. (6) and Fox et al. (7) demonstrated a reduction in myelination, although the myelin that was formed was of normal constitution. Martinez (8) described the forebrain as the most vulnerable area during the perinatal period.

Presumed intrapartum insults, especially ischemia and anoxia, are assumed to be a major contributor to developmental disabilities in children. Nelson, et al. (9) investigated this hypothesis in cerebral palsy patients. They reported that the leading predictors of cerebral palsy were maternal mental retardation, birth weight less than 2,001 g, and associated fetal malformations. Only 21% of the 189 children examined had a clinical marker suggestive of asphyxia.

Early nutritional deprivation has been shown to have long-term negative effects. Chase and Martin (10) studied children hospitalized with undernutrition in the first year of life. The duration of undernutrition correlated with impairment of physical and mental development; undernutrition for more than 4 months had the most deleterious impact on growth and developmental quotients (10). Another study correlated a history of early malnutrition with poor academic performance and classroom behavior (11). A prospective 20-year study confirmed the association between early undernutrition and organic brain damage (12).

Normal motor development is predicated on passing through preset sequences. Although the timing and caliber may vary, the order may not. Before sitting or crawling becomes possible, for example, all individuals must develop postural control. Motor ability progresses from rostral to caudal and from midline to the periphery. Appropriate tone and postural stability then enable the child to develop sitting balance and ultimately to crawl and to walk.

In addition, the primitive reflexes that are present in infancy, must be integrated. For example, a persistent bite reflex will preclude development of normal eating patterns. With an obligate asymmetric tonic neck reflex after 6 months, the individual will be unable to turn over because of arm extension. In addition, abnormal tone such as spasticity or hypotonia will clearly alter the normal developmental process.

DEFINING THE DEVELOPMENTALLY DISABLED

Developmental disabilities include a wide range of handicaps, both motor and cognitive. Mental retardation affects over 6 million people in the United States. More than 50% of these cases may have been prevented by nutritional intervention, immunizations, genetic counseling, and/or high-risk pregnancy identification (13). Motor disabilities range from mild, with scant impact on function, to impairment that is so severe that movement is dominated by posturing with primitive reflexes.

Although some disabled children may have an identifiable etiology, it is often difficult to ascribe an individual's disability to a single cause. Some individuals, in addition, demonstrate more than one disability. Patients with "cerebral palsy" from anoxia or congenital malformations also often have epilepsy. Mental retardation may be accompanied by autistic-like behavior that affects feeding. This exemplifies the fact that disabilities are generally complex in nature.

Studies have also shown that a large percentage of children with developmental disabilities have primary nutritional disorders (14). This is undoubtedly the result of such problems as poor intake, poor dentition, and behavior problems (2,15–17). The complexity and diversity of developmental problems, however, prevent a too-generalized approach to finding solutions to these problems. Basically, these children require the same nutrients for growth as all children. The quantity, however, will be dependent on factors such as energy expenditure, medications, physical impairment, and possible altered growth rate (3,14). Studies are needed to evaluate the role of nutritional problems on growth failure in these children.

NUTRITION AND DEVELOPMENT IN THE DEVELOPMENTALLY DISABLED

Energy intake for all children must be sufficient for expenditure as well as for providing the nutritional needs for growth and development. Special problems arise, however, when normal energy requirements and growth parameters do not apply (18,19). This is readily apparent in conditions that limit activities, such as myelodysplasia. Dramatic examples of increased calories up to 6,000 cal are reported in patients with choreoathetosis (2). Nutritional planning for children with developmental disabilities, therefore, must be individualized because of the delicate state of intake, expenditure, and complicating factors.

As with all children, linear growth is an important indication of well-being. Usual standards are difficult to apply, however, in the developmentally disabled child. Certainly weight-for-age, based on normal growth, will be irrelevant in assessing children with short stature and central nervous system deficits. Weight-for-height standards, useful for the prepubescent disabled child, regardless of chronological age, are no longer useful once the child enters puberty (18).

Standard techniques for measurement must also be adapted to the patient. Recumbent length, for example, may be used for patients who cannot stand. The technique is the same as that used with infants on an infant board. It is important to remember that recumbent length is 2.0 cm greater than standing until the age of 4 to 5 years, and thereafter the difference is approximately 1.0 cm. If this were not recognized, these children would be compared to standing height norms making them appear taller than appropriate (18).

When individuals with motor dysfunctions have contractures, it is necessary to take measurements in the flexed position. Both sides must be measured, particularly if there is unilateral disease. Spender et al. (18) particularly recommend the lower leg length, which offers a measure that does not cross a joint. Unfortunately, no anthropometric standards exist for this population.

It is very important that anthropometric data be collected in a consistent and standardized manner. In addition, using several indices, such as height, weight, arm circumference, and skin fold, improves reliability. Head circumference is debated as a consistent nutritional indicator. However, studies have documented smaller head circumferences and lower developmental quotients occurring as a result of prolonged early undernutrition (9–11).

Culley and Middleton (21) developed an approach for estimating caloric requirements in mentally retarded children that expresses caloric needs in terms of body size and motor status rather than age. They studied children with difficulties ranging from hypotonia and ataxia to choreoathetosis and spasticity. They found that ambulatory mentally retarded children without motor dysfunction had similar caloric needs per centimeter of height, which did not significantly change with height or age. A nonambulatory child, however, required fewer calories per centimeter of height. They concluded that, although motor dysfunction might affect caloric needs to some extent, the significant factor determining caloric needs was the ability to ambulate (21).

For assessment of nutritional deficiencies, Fee et al. (15) recommend documentation of caloric intake and a differential of possible difficulties in weight gain. The developmentally disabled child may have feeding difficulties including dysfunctional oral skills, behavioral problems, choking, or vomiting. The difficulties may also be family initiated including insufficient food availability, formula mixing errors, or inadequate parenting, such as an adversarial parent-child relationship. Dental problems can be both an etiology as well as an outcome of poor nutrition. Gastroenterological problems such as reflux may complicate weight gain and also be responsible for other medical issues including aspiration pneumonia and esophagitis. Calories may be consumed but not absorbed. Rumination and food intolerance may prevent the food from being available for appropriate utilization.

Pesce et al. (22) evaluated residents of a multidisciplinary intermediate care facility. They found suboptimal intake occurred more frequently in residents with behavioral or dental problems who were able to self-feed than those who were dependent on one-on-one assistance. They believed that monitoring individual growth patterns was essential for assessing both development and the need for nutritional intervention. They also recommended a multidisciplinary approach to maximize the outcome of nutritional support.

Nutritional deficiencies documented in children with developmental disabilities include deficiencies of calcium, iron, vitamin C, folic acid, vitamin A, riboflavin, and thiamine (15,17,20,21,23). In addition, a recent study of 47 children with scurvy found that 50% had severe psychomotor retardation. The mean age of diagnosis was 4 years, 4 months. The clinical presentation often paralleled that seen in the adult population i.e., significant gingival involvement. Although the diagnosis of scurvy had been made in the hospital, all of the children had been admitted for other reasons (24).

It is also clear that the developmentally disabled are at higher risk of being iron deficient. Problems such as esophagitis and reflux contribute to iron loss. In addition, iron intake may be inadequate. The earliest parameter to reflect iron deficiency is serum ferritin (22).

Another question that is often raised concerns the relationship between somatic growth and brain damage. Nutritional factors have traditionally been felt to be the reason these children are frequently lower than the 5th percentile for weight and height and often underweight for height. Increased feeding gastrostomy tube placement offers the opportunity to review the growth characteristics of children with severe neuromotor and orofacial involvement where nutritional deficits are avoided or treated.

Rempel et al. (25) studied the growth characteristics of 57 children with severe neuromuscular and oral motor involvement. Before gastrostomy placement, 80% were underweight for height. Following the gastrostomy, 33% remained underweight for height and 21% became overweight for height. Documented improvement in height was less frequent than in weight. The majority of children remained below the 5th percentile for height and weight. Improvement was correlated with placement of the gastrostomy within the first year of life. Children with gastrostomies for more than 2 years and those with fundoplications were also more likely to reach appropriate weight-for-height. In spite of the gastrostomy feedings, however, most children did not reach the 5th percentile for height. This fact, the operative risk, and the complications following surgery cause this procedure to be less than optimal (26,27). The authors, however, emphasize that the benefit of gastrostomies comes from the ability to more easily provide nutritional support for the child (28).

In an attempt to relate somatic growth with developmental disabilities, Pryor and Thelander (29) suggest the analogy of a "time clock." In the cascade of events that follows implantation, differentiation, growth, and development, the earlier the initial influence, the more substantial the deviation of growth. Chromosomal aberrations, such as Down syndrome, produce greater deviations from normal growth than abnormalities occurring later in the intrauterine period. Children with multiple congenital anomalies due to later insults, however, are less severely affected. Even less growth aberration is seen in children who sustain birth injury following an otherwise normal gestation period. Although nutrition clearly has a role in growth failure, the mechanism is yet unclear (16). Studies indicate that growth is contained within certain limitations, based on the patient's underlying disorder (22,25).

NUTRIENT/DRUG INTERACTIONS

Anticonvulsants, necessary for seizure control, deleteriously affect up to 25% of children receiving them. Phenytoin and phenobarbital, for example, may cause deficiencies in folate and vitamin B_{12}. Pathologic fractures and rickets result from disruption of bone metabolism caused by the effect of long-term use of anticonvulsants on vitamin D absorption. The pathophysiology of rickets associated with anticonvulsants may depend on the drug-induced activation of the hepatic microsomal enzymes, which increases the metabolism of 25-OH-cholecalciferol. Rickets appears to occur more often in nonambulatory institutionalized patients (2,11,13). It is hypothesized that reduced exposure to sunlight or reduced calcium or vitamin D intake may be causal. However, rickets may also occur in ambulatory patients.

Other documented abnormalities resulting from anticonvulsants include abnormal levels of zinc, copper, and pyridoxine. The gum hypertrophy associated with phenytoin may further affect dental hygiene and, potentially, food intake (1,2,13).

The tricyclic antidepressants used for hyperactivity

and behavioral problems have anticholinergic effects which cause dry mouth and eyes. In addition to being irritating, dry mouth may increase dental problems. Tranquilizers may also result in decreased activity and nutritional intake. Amphetamines, used for hyperactivity, have been linked with the suppression of growth in height and weight. Reduction of intake has been well described. Monitoring height, weight, and caloric intake is obviously a necessary component of this program.

The constipation common to children with developmental disabilities can decrease intake because of discomfort as well as early satiety. Laxatives may provide relief from the discomfort but may also inhibit the absorption of vitamins and other nutrients.

INBORN ERRORS IN METABOLISM

Appropriate diets for inborn errors of metabolism either limit intake of abnormally accumulated nutrients or increase intake in the face of deficiency. High doses of vitamins may be used to encourage a particular biochemical reaction. The risk is, therefore, of deficiencies from an inadequate diet or toxicities from oversupplementation. In aminoacidopathies, for example, protein restriction to 1.0 g/kg may well inhibit growth. Children with urea cycle defects are affected by protein restriction as well as benzoate supplementation.

Galactosemia results from a lack of galactose-1-phosphate uridyltransferase. A galactose-free diet is used to prevent physical and mental retardation, cataracts, portal hypertension, and cirrhosis. Soy-based formulas may be utilized for infants. In the older child, all milk products, as well as other galactose-containing foods, must be avoided. Nutritional supplements with calcium, vitamin D, and riboflavin are recommended (30).

FEEDING

Neurologically impaired children often have feeding difficulties due to an inability to coordinate mastication and swallowing (14,31,32). Persistence of primitive oral reflexes delay the development of normal oral motor function (14,31–33). Problems with overall development, including difficulty in maintaining proper seating alignment, also contribute to poor feeding (14,32,34). Occupational and speech therapists are important for evaluation and implementation of programs geared toward improving oral motor skills (14,32,34). Adaptive equipment and supportive seating devices may be used to promote successful feeding in these children.

Development of neural pathways for feeding begins early in fetal life. For infants, sucking and swallowing are the essentials of adequate nutrition. Later, mastication becomes the primary skill (31,32). Oral reflexes are necessary in both.

Oral motor development begins in the ninth week of gestation, when the fetus is able to move its mouth and lower jaw (31). By the 12th week, the fetus is able to swallow fluid. Sucking begins by 18 to 24 weeks, and the gag reflex appears by 26 weeks (31). At 32 to 34 weeks, the fetus is able to independently meet its nutritional needs (31).

The feeding process is innervated by cranial nerves V, VII, IX, X, and XII (31,32). The trigeminal nerve innervates the muscles of mastication and receives sensory input from the lower face. The facial nerve provides motor stimulation to the face. The glossal-pharyngeal and vagus nerves are responsible for the gag reflex. The hypoglossal nerve innervates the tongue. The nuclei of cranial nerves V, VII, IX, and X make up the sucking and swallowing centers in the rostral brainstem (31,32). Sucking and swallowing have two main components—oral motor function and epiglottal coordination. For the first 6 months, infants subsist primarily by sucking. Afterward, enough oral motor coordination is present to allow the infant to spoon-feed (31,32).

The oral and primitive reflexes are the final aspect of oral motor development (4,31,33). In normal children, the following reflexes begin at birth and disappear by 3 to 5 months: sucking, rooting, asymmetric tonic neck reflex (ATNR), tongue thrust, and bite. Feeding difficulties will result from unusual persistence of these reflexes. A weak suck and delayed tongue thrust, for example, will impair spoon-feeding (31,35).

Persistent rooting and ATNR lead to improper positioning of the head and trunk. A continued bite reflex causes the child to clamp down on any object that is placed in his mouth. Two reflexes persist throughout life: swallowing and gag (34–36). If abnormalities are present in either or both, aspiration becomes a potential threat.

Overall development will also affect feeding. Hypotonia, dystonia, and spasticity result in abnormal seating and positioning during feedings. Spasticity and dystonia will affect the disappearance of oral and primitive reflexes and cause gross uncoordination of oral motor and epiglottal function (34).

Feeding problems require evaluation in the following areas: position, oral reflexes, oral-digital, jaw control, lip and tongue movement, malocclusion, high arched palate, and breathing. In order to attain proper feeding position, the child should have 90° flexion at the hips, knees, and ankles. The trunk should be stable and the head maintained in the midline. The presence of oral reflexes is then determined. An oral digital exam is performed to assess rolling tongue movements, necessary to propel food to the back of the pharynx. Proper lip closure is ascertained by the ability to spoon-feed. The normal tongue rests in the midline position and should lateralize on command. Malocclusion and high arched palate that impair swallowing are determined by observation and digital exam. Finally, coordination of breathing and swallowing with food intake is evaluated (34,36). First, the gag reflex is observed. If the presence of the gag reflex is in question, a barium swallow is conducted to ascertain any evidence of aspiration. Children with aspiration may require gastrostomy feedings and may never be able to tolerate food by mouth.

Stability, sucking, swallowing, gag and bite reactions, and tongue movements may be improved via occupational and speech therapies in conjunction with appropriate adaptive equipment (14,34). Stability is enhanced with a chair that keeps the child in an upright position (14,34). Hip and H-straps provide truncal stability. Headrests help maintain a midline position. Lapboards assist in establishing arm and hand stability. Nonnutritive sucking and swallowing patterns are established with a pacifier. When a gag reflex exists, semisolid food is introduced first, since it is easiest to swallow (14,32). This is followed by new textured foods and, finally, liquids, since they require the most epiglottal coordination (32,34). Specific exercises may be recommended to aid in improvement of tongue movements. Ultimately, other adaptive equipment is used to aid the child in independent feeding (15). Two-handled cups and padded spoons are examples of such utensils.

Additional difficulties may also occur as a result of the caretaker. A tremendous amount of time, energy, and patience is required to meet the nutritional needs of these children. It also takes a level of understanding and discipline for implementation of prescribed diets and therapies (33). Parents of disabled children may not always have the necessary personal skills to function effectively. This may be exacerbated by negative feelings generated by the child's lack of ability to thrive or return parental affection (36,37). In addition, parents may not relate the child's neurological condition to his or her inability to feed, ascribing it, rather, to "badness" (34,37). Even love for the child may have negative ramifications when parents resort to "quick cures" in attempts to find easy answers to a complicated problem.

When parents are part of the problem, the professional must be especially sure that they learn how to be part of the solution (34,37). Parents must be provided with adequate information regarding the child's condition and dietary needs, with patient explanations until it is understood. In addition, parents should participate in occupational and speech therapy sessions with their child in order to learn the techniques that enhance oral motor and other functioning; eventually such programs should be continued at home under parental guidance (14,34).

The psychosocial effect of a disabled child on a family can be profound. Special formulas may drain already limited financial means. In addition, there may be a deterioration of self-esteem in parents whose children do not develop "normally." The resulting breakdown in the parent-child relationship can produce a nonorganic failure to thrive in a child who already has an organic feeding problem (37).

As the disabled child grows, intake may be also be negatively affected by behavioral issues such as short attention span and hyperactivity. This is especially true during school meals for school-age and adolescent children on rigid diet plans. This problem may be addressed with smaller, more frequent meals. The help of school nurses may be enlisted. Diets should be individualized to comply with religious and ethnic considerations (38).

SUMMARY

The aim of parenting is very often to have a "perfect" child. Parents of disabled children, whose ideas of perfection may come from idealized unattainable standards, can never achieve this. The goal of the professional is to help the parent understand the child, understand what realistic goals for the child are, and how those goals might be achieved. The compassion and positive reinforcement of the professional may give parents the support necessary for accepting their child.

Nutritional goals for the disabled child are, as they are for all children, aimed at maximizing growth, both physical and mental. Standards for the disabled child are less readily available. Growth must be monitored on an individual basis and diets must be designed for each child based on his or her disability and progress. Alternative methods of feeding may be utilized to enhance intake.

The combination of individualized diets, the use of alternative methods to aid intake, and the involvement of parents may make the critical difference in the growth of the developmentally disabled child.

REFERENCES

1. Grand RJ, Sutphen JL, Dietz WH. *Pediatric nutrition theory and practice.* Boston: Butterworths, 1987.
2. Howard RB, Fetters L, MacDonald DM. Nutrition in neurological disorders and in the care of the disabled. In: Howard RB, Herold N, eds. *Nutrition in clinical care.* New York: McGraw Hill, 1982;594–627.
3. Widerlou E. The future of neuropeptides in psychiatry and neurology. In: Nemeroff CB, ed. *Neuropeptides in psychiatric and neurological disorders.* Baltimore: The Johns Hopkins University Press, 1988;281–306.
4. Volpe JJ. Overview: dorsal induction and ventral induction. In: Volpe JJ, ed. *Neurology of the newborn.* Philadelphia: WB Saunders, 1987;2–32.
5. Volpe JJ. Neuronal proliferation, migration, organization, and myelinization. In: Volpe JJ, ed. *Neurology of the newborn.* Philadelphia: WB Saunders, 1987;33–68.
6. Fishman MA, Prensky AL, Dodge PR. Low content of cerebral lipids in infants suffering from malnutrition. *Nature* 1969; 221;552–553.
7. Fox JH, Fishman MA, Dodge PR, Prensky AL. The effect of malnutrition on human central nervous system myelin. *Neurology* 1972;22:1213–1216.
8. Martinez M. Myelin lipids in the developing cerebrum, cerebel-

lum, and brain stem of normal and undernourished children. *J Neurochem* 1982;39:1684–1692.
9. Nelson KB, Ellenberg JH. Antecedents of cerebral palsy: multivariants of risk. *N Engl J Med* 1986;315:81–86.
10. Chase HP, Martin HP. Undernutrition and child development. *N Engl J Med* 1970;282:933–939.
11. Galler JR, Ramsey F, Solimano G. The influence of early malnutrition on subsequent behavioral development III. Learning disabilities as a sequel to malnutrition. *Pediatr Res* 1984;18:309–313.
12. Stoch MB, Smythe PM, Moodie AD, Bradshaw D. Psychosocial outcome and CT findings after gross undernourishment during infancy: a 20 yr developmental study. *Dev Med Child Neurol* 1982;24:419–436.
13. Blyler E, Lucas B. Nutrition in comprehensive program planning for persons with developmental disabilities: technical support paper. *J Am Diet Assoc* 1987;87:1069–1074.
14. Palmer S, Horn S. Feeding problems in children. In: Palmer RD, Ekuall S, eds. *Pediatric nutrition in developmental disorders.* Springfield: Charles C. Thomas, 1978;107–129.
15. Fee MA, Charney EB, Robertson WW. Nutritional assessment of the young child with cerebral palsy. *Inf Young Child* 1988;1:33–40.
16. Shapiro BK, Green P, Krick J, Allen D, Capute AJ. Growth of severely impaired children: neurological versus nutritional factors. *Dev Med Child Neurol* 1986;28:729–733.
17. Infant and child nutrition: Concerns regarding the developmentally disabled. A statement by the American Dietetic Association. *J Am Diet Assoc* 1981;78:443–452.
18. Spender QW, Crok CE, Charney EB, Stallings VA. Assessment of linear growth of children with cerebral palsy: use of alternative measures to height or length. *Dev Med Child Neurol* 1989;31:206–214.
19. Ruby DO, Matheny WD. Comments on growth cerebral palsied children. *J Am Diet Assoc* 1961;40:525–527.
20. Phelps WM. Dietary requirements in cerebral palsy. *J Am Diet Assoc* 1951;27:869–876.
21. Culley WJ, Middleton TO. Caloric requirements of mentally retarded children with and without motor dysfunction. *J Pediatr* 1969;75:380–384.
22. Pesce KA, Wodarski LA, Wang M. Nutritional status of institutionalized children and adolescents with developmental disabilities. *Res Dev Disabil* 1989;10:33–52.
23. Berg K. Nutrition of children with reduced physical activity due to cerebral palsy. *Nutr Diet* 1973;19:12–20.
24. Garty B, Danon Y, Grunebaum M, Nitzan M. Scurvy in children with severe psychomotor retardation. *Int Pediatr* 1989;4:280–282.
25. Rempel GR, Colwell SO, Nelson RP. Growth in children with cerebral palsy fed via gastrostomy. *Pediatrics* 1988;82:857–862.
26. Wilkinson JD, Dudgeon DL, Sondheimer JM. A comparison of medical and surgical treatment of gastroesophageal reflux in severely retarded children. *J Pediatr* 1981;99:202–205.
27. Mollitt DL, Golladay S, Seibert JJ. Symptomatic gastroesophageal reflux following gastrostomy in neurologically impaired patients. *Pediatrics* 1985;75:1124–1126.
28. Krick J, Van Duyn MAS. The relationship between oral-motor involvement and growth: a pilot study in a pediatric population with cerebral palsy. *J Am Diet Assoc* 1984;84:555–559.
29. Pryor HB, Thelander HE. Growth deviations in handicapped children. *Clin Pediatr* 1967;6:501–512.
30. Escott-Stump S. *Nutrition and diagnosis related care,* 2nd ed. Philadelphia: Lea & Febiger, 1988.
31. McBride MC, Danner SC. Sucking disorders in neurologically impaired infants: assessment and facilitation of breastfeeding. *Clin Perinatol* 1987;14:109–130.
32. Hargrove R. Feeding the severely dysphagic patient. *J Neurosurg Nurs* 1980;12:102–107.
33. Sheppard JJ, Mysal ED. Ontogeny of infantile oral reflexes and emerging chewing. *Child Dev* 1984;55:831–843.
34. Pipes PL, Pritkin R. Nutrition and feeding of children with developmental delays and related problems. In: Pipes PL, ed. *Nutrition in infancy and childhood.* St. Louis: Times Mirror/Mosby, 1985;347–371.
35. Ingram TTS. Clinical significance of infantile feeding reflexes. *Dev Med Child Neurol* 1962;4:159–169.
36. Frappier PA, Marino BL, Shishmanian E. Nursing assessment of infant feeding problems. *J Pediatr Nurs* 1987;2:37–44.
37. Durand B. Failure to thrive in a child with Down syndrome. *Nurs Res* 1975;24:272–285.
38. Lowenber ME. The development of food patterns in young children. In: Pipes PL, ed. *Nutrition in infancy and childhood.* St. Louis: Times Mirror/Mosby, 1985;175–193.

CHAPTER 43

Nutritional Support for Optimizing Children's Dental-Oral Health

Kenneth C. Troutman

The nutritional needs of the dental/oral structures are similar to those of the rest of the body. Optimal maternal and neonatal nutrition are necessary to promote sound development of the primary dentition and oral structures. In addition, development of the permanent dentition and maintenance of the oral structures that support it are dependent on continued adequate nutrition. Although the etiology of dental diseases is multifactorial, nutritional and dietary factors are significant in the oral disease process. Ultimately, sound teeth will be resistant to caries, and sound periodontal structures will resist gingival and periodontal diseases (1).

ABNORMALITIES OF CALCIFICATION—ENAMEL HYPOPLASIA AND HYPOCALCIFICATION

Enamel hypoplasia, the most evident developmental defect related to nutrition, occurs as a result of a disturbance in the formation of enamel matrix, resulting in a deficient amount of matrix and subsequent deficient amount of enamel tissue. Variable in its clinical appearance, it may involve only the primary dentition, only the permanent dentition, or both. In its milder form, it may appear as a single row of pits or a horizontal groove across the surface of the crown of the tooth. The most severe form may involve the complete absence of enamel, suggesting a prolonged disturbance of the ameloblasts (2).

Hypocalcification results when an adequate amount of enamel matrix is improperly calcified during the formation of hydroxyapatite. Such enamel is usually chalky in appearance (2). Factors that adversely affect the ameloblasts and result in enamel hypoplasia or hypocalcification include the following (3–14,16,17):

1. deficiencies of vitamins A, C, and D, protein, calories, calcium, and phosphorus
2. exanthematous disease including measles, chicken pox, scarlet fever, and congenital syphilis
3. birth injury, prematurity, Rh hemolytic disease
4. local infection
5. trauma to primary teeth
6. ingestion of tetracycline or excessive fluoride
7. genetic causes (amelogenesis imperfecta and genetic syndromes)
8. endocrine disturbances including hypothyroidism, hypoparathyroidism.

CONCEPT OF THE CRITICAL PERIOD FOR NUTRIENT INTAKE

Malnutrition is extremely disruptive to the development of the lens of the eyes and the enamel of teeth. Once teeth erupt into the oral cavity, the enamel has no cellular mechanism to repair damage and defects are essentially irreversible.

Protein-energy malnutrition and low serum levels of vitamin A during gestation and the neonatal period may result in enamel hypoplasia and/or hypocalcification and increased susceptibility of the primary dentition and permanent first molars to dental caries. A linear hypoplastic enamel defect, especially common in developing countries (3,7), is often found in children who were born prematurely or suffered from neonatal infection and low levels of vitamin A during dental development. Such disturbances may be manifested from the 28th day of gesta-

---

K. C. Troutman: Department of Pediatric Dentistry, Columbia University, Columbia-Presbyterian Medical Center, New York, New York 10032.

tion until, for third molars, 16 years of age. The crown of a tooth, like the lens of the eye, may, therefore, provide a permanent record of malnutrition or systemic disturbances that occur during the course of the development of the dentition. This allows the aware clinician to do retrospective investigations as to the time and duration of suspected systemic or developmental disturbances by correlating the observation of clinical hypoplasia with the knowledge of enamel deposition, calcification, and maturation.

Nutrient deficiencies indirectly affect the dentition by inhibiting jaw growth, altering morphology, and impacting on structural integrity, size, composition, position, alignment, eruption, and resistive capability of teeth to microbial acid challenges at maturity. Smaller jaw size results in crowding, malalignment, and malocclusion. This leads to poor aesthetics and, more importantly, masticatory problems and increased susceptibility to dental caries and periodontal diseases because of the difficulty of properly removing plaque. Morphologically, decreases in salivary gland size may also reduce salivary volume output, alter the capacity of saliva to buffer a caries challenge, and reduce the amount of protective protein (antibacterial) substances present in the oral cavity (10).

NUTRIENTS CRITICAL FOR DENTAL-ORAL DEVELOPMENT

Nutrients that have a significant effect, both positively and negatively, on dentofacial development include vitamins A, D, and C, calcium, phosphorus, fluoride, protein, calories, amino acids, and a host of other minerals (3–9). Optimal protein, vitamins A and D, calcium, phosphorus, the calcium/phosphorus ratio, and fluorides in the diet during the developmental period may result in teeth more resistant to caries attack. Fluoride, especially, increases resistance of teeth to caries acid challenges.

Nutrient deficiencies, however, have a negative impact, often resulting in teeth with an increased susceptibility to caries attack (3,6–9). Low-protein diets in infants, for example, may result in smaller teeth, delayed eruption, impaired salivary function, and reduced salivary flow with subsequent increased caries susceptibility (3–9). Altered tissue development from various deficiencies may result in a reduced capacity to resist disease challenges.

THE ROLE OF NUTRITION AND DIET IN DENTAL CARIES

Dental diseases are a major public health problem. It is, however, tooth decay or caries that causes the most concern, results in the most pain, and requires the greatest expense to treat.

All dental caries result from the interaction of four factors: (a) the agent—pathologic microorganisms in the mouth, (b) the environment—fermentable carbohydrates that microorganisms utilize to produce acid, (c) the host—tooth surfaces that are susceptible to an acid challenge and dissolution, and (d) time—the acid challenge (pH 5.2 or lower must be present for at least 20 min to cause enamel decalcification) (Fig. 1) (10).

Through the synthesis of long-chain dextrans by bacteria, primarily streptococci, an insoluble gummy mass called plaque is produced that can form a matrix for the colonization of organisms on tooth surfaces. Coating of dental enamel by the dextran plaque establishes a unique local environment between the organism-laden plaque and the tooth surface. The production of acids as a consequence of energy metabolism by the bacteria lowers the pH of this environment to 5.2 or lower, past the critical level at which decalcification occurs. This destruction, the result of the loss of calcium and phosphate ions, cavitates the enamel surface.

Susceptibility

Although nutritional deficiencies during dental development may influence caries susceptibility by affecting

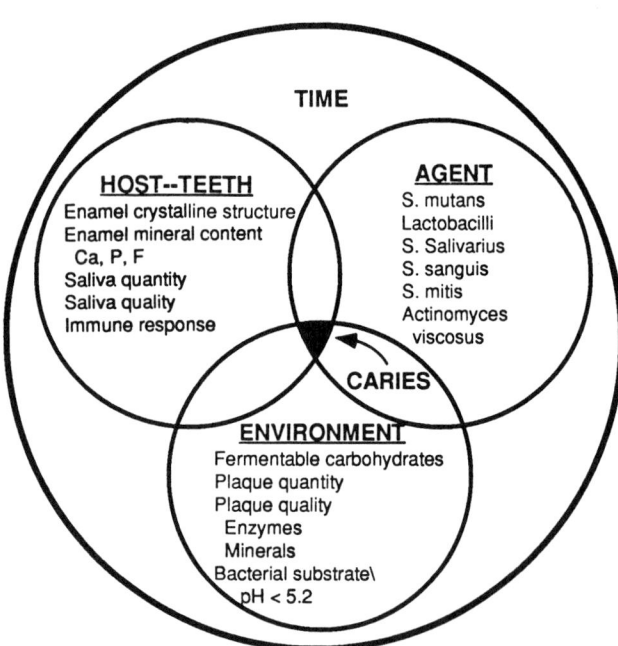

FIG. 1. Multifactorial model of dental caries, depicting the relationship between oral bacteria and the presence of an appropriate environment on susceptible teeth for an adequate period of time in the etiology of dental caries. (Adapted from ref. 10.)

enamel formation, salivary composition and function, and perhaps immunological responses, there is no evidence that nutrition in the post–dental-developmental period has any influence on caries. On the other hand, foods in the diet vary considerably in their tendency to promote tooth decay (11).

Acidogenicity

Although no test yet measures all components of a food's ability to produce dental caries, the measurement of acidogenicity by plaque pH telemetry has provided some valuable information (Table 1) (12–14).

Certain foods should be avoided, especially between meals, because of their tendency to produce a significant drop in the oral pH to below 4.5 for longer than 20 min. These are the highly acidogenic foods listed in Table 1.

Some foods produce very minimal plaque pH responses but are still not considered "safe" for teeth." These foods are moderately acidogenic (Table 1) and are probably cleared relatively rapidly from the oral cavity due to their form and the salivary flow promoted by their consumption. Although not noncariogenic, they are preferable for between-meal snacks to the highly acidogenic foods.

A third category of foods represents those low in acidogenicity (Table 1).

Cariogenicity

The development of a clinical lesion is determined not simply by the acidogenic potential of a given food or beverage but by a combination of several factors (16):

1. bacteria (oral flora)
2. structure and composition of enamel and dentin
3. morphology and alignment of teeth
4. nutritional status and infectious episodes during tooth development
5. fluoride status (available fluoride concentration in oral fluids plaque, and external layers of enamel)
6. oral hygiene habits
7. saliva flow rate and composition
8. food consumed
   a. composition
   b. form
   c. texture
   d. pH
9. dietary patterns
   a. amount
   b. combinations
   c. frequency of intake
   d. eating order.

These factors, individually and in combination, produce various degrees of susceptibility to caries, most critically when the ingested food is particularly active in promoting caries. Knowledge of the caries potential of a food is essential to planning diet modifications designed to prevent dental disease.

Role of Sugars in Caries

The focus on sucrose as a cause of dental caries has led to an erroneous belief that other sweeteners, such as fructose, high-fructose corn syrups, and so-called natural sugars such as honey, are either noncariogenic or are significantly less cariogenic than sucrose. Studies clearly demonstrate that all sweeteners, including sucrose, glucose, fructose, and honey are equally cariogenic (17). In addition, little attention is given to the substantial amounts of naturally occurring cariogenic carbohydrates in many fruits and vegetables.

Baby Bottle-Nursing Caries

Dental caries in children under 3 years of age is often a direct result of baby feeding practices. It occurs when a child is allowed to bottle feed past 18 months of age, allowed to sleep with a bottle containing liquid condu-

TABLE 1. *Categorization of foods by degree of acidogenicity*

High acidogenicity	Moderate acidogenicity	Low acidogenicity
Raisins	Pears	Broccoli
Dried apricots	Peaches	Cauliflower
		Celery
Dried apples	Apples	Cucumbers
		Dill pickles
Dried pears	Grapes	Carrots
Dates	Apple cider	Green peppers
		Ground beef
Wheat cracker	Orange juice	Beef steak
Sugar cookie	Grape juice	Ham
		Pepperoni
Soda cracker	Soft drink	Peanuts
		Almonds
Cream-filled cookie		Hazel nuts
		Filberts
Milk chocolate		Walnuts
Snack cracker		Pecans
		Walleye
Potato chips		Trout
		Red snapper
		Selected cheeses
		Popcorn

Adapted from refs. 12–15.

cive to the formation of dental caries, and when breast-fed children sleep with their mothers and feed, *ad libitum,* throughout the night (18,19). This problem, traditionally found in lower socioeconomic populations, is increasing in upper socioeconomic children as well (18–20). The prevalence is as high as 20% in United States urban populations and up to 50% in Native American or Native Alaskan preschool children. Head Start surveys estimate a prevalence of about 15% in fluoridated areas and 20% in nonfluoridated areas. The estimated United States national prevalence is about 5% (18,20).

This type of caries occurs when the milk curds formed in the acid media of the mouth are fermented, producing acids that remain in the mouth for long periods of time, causing etching (decalcification) of the enamel. The pattern is very specific. Usually the maxillary incisors and canines are affected first, exhibiting white decalcified areas (Fig. 2). In advanced cases, all four maxillary incisors are frequently destroyed completely and the primary canines and molars show evidence of facial decalcification.

Fruit juices given by bottle are equally culpable. The American Academy of Pediatrics and The American Academy of Pediatric Dentistry have stated that

> [the] marketing of juices in ready-to-use nursing bottles may tend to prolong bottle feeding and encourage the use of the bottle as a pacifier, both of which promote dental caries. The use of juices from a bottle should be discouraged and infants should be offered juice from a cup as soon as possible. (21)

Frequency of Food Consumption and Caries

Frequency of snacking between meals is associated with increased numbers of decayed, missing (extracted), and filled (DMF) teeth from infancy through adolescence. In one study, a significant DMF increase was directly related to the increased frequency of between-meal consumption of sugar-rich foods (one to six times per 24 hr) (10,22). DMF values also increased, although somewhat less, with the frequency of non–sugar-rich snack intake. The relationship between dental caries and snacking appears to be, in fact, the frequency of food consumption and the consistency of the foods themselves, rather than simply the sucrose content (10,15,22–26).

Caries-Protective Mechanisms of Foods

Sugar Alcohols

Sugar alcohols are termed nutritive sweeteners because they have a similar level of sweetness and caloric yield as sugars. These polyalcohols or polyols are formed by hydrogenating the appropriate sugar. D-Glucose, for example, yields sorbitol. The most commonly used sugar alcohols are sorbitol, mannitol, xylitol, maltitol, and lactitol. Because they ferment very slowly in the oral cavity, the acid challenge to teeth is much less than sugar. Very few plaque bacteria are capable of fermenting polyols, especially xylitol. Those that can, such as *Streptococcus mutans* and *Lactobacillus casei* which can ferment mannitol and sorbitol, have the necessary degradative enzymes present at such low levels that they cannot rapidly utilize these substrates (27–31).

Plaque pH studies in humans indicate that sugar alcohols are hypoacidogenic or nonacidogenic and noncariogenic (29). Several experimental studies have demonstrated an extremely low caries rate in a xylitol-containing diet (27). Total substitution of sucrose with xylitol resulted in caries scores comparable to or lower than those in sugar-free controls (28). This type of substitution may allow the repair (remineralization) of early subsurface carious lesions. The body of clinical evidence seems to indicate that the use of sugar alcohols may actually be anticariogenic, resulting in the reduction of dental caries.

Using xylitol chewing gum as an addition to normal caries prevention results in a significant reduction in caries (42%) without the use of occlusal fissure sealants (29,30). Chewing gum, even gum with sugar, for 10 to 20 min after a meal has been shown to prevent interproximal caries formation, much as toothbrushing and flossing do (32–35). Jensen and Wefel (34) reported that without stimulation of saliva with gum chewing and without cleaning the teeth, there was significant acid formation in plaque after any meal, the acid attack lasting significantly longer than 20 min. The benefits of chewing gum to neutralize decay-causing acids outweigh any harm that may be caused by the sugar in the gum, as long

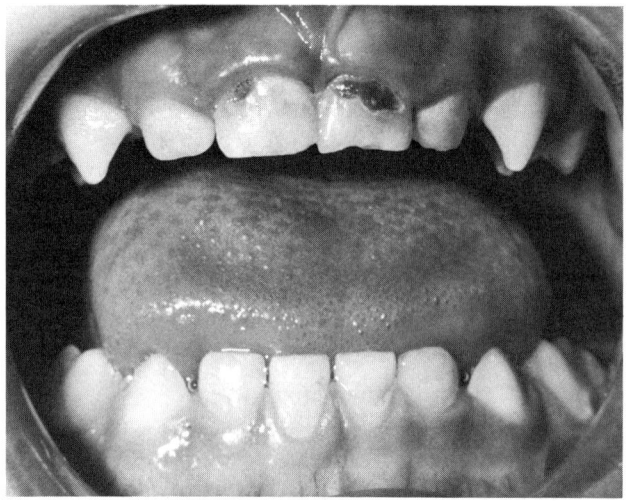

FIG. 2. Early signs of baby bottle nursing caries showing decalcified facial surfaces.

as the gum is chewed for 10 to 20 min. These benefits are lost, however, if the gum is discarded too soon (34).

"Gummi bears," a carbohydrate-containing confection, highlights the importance of the form of foods on dental decay. This candy is made with gelatin but with a carbohydrate content almost completely unavailable to plaque bacteria. Its rubber-like cohesive form, together with its flavoring and citric acid, stimulates salivary flow, neutralizing acid and increasing oral clearance. "Gummi bears" are, therefore, a nonacidogenic, if not actually a noncariogenic snack (36).

The Protective Mechanisms of Cheeses

Rosen et al. (37) and Jensen et al. (12–14) have determined the low cariogenic potential and possible cariostatic activity of cheddar and some other cheeses (37,38). These cheeses are not only nonacidogenic but have the ability to prevent a significant pH drop when consumed immediately before or shortly after highly acidogenic food. This protective effect may be related to one or more of the following mechanisms:

1. buffering of plaque pH at a safe level by cheese components and/or saliva stimulated by chewing
2. acceleration of pH rise by peptides similar to pH rise factor, occurring during aging of cheese
3. inhibition of cariogenic bacteria by fatty acids or other unidentified cheese components
4. common ion reduction of demineralization by the calcium and phosphate present in the cheese.

Cheeses that reduce the acidogenicity of other foods, and may, therefore, be considered a noncariogenic snack, include cheddar, Swiss, Gouda, Monterey Jack, and mozzarella. Other practical implications of this finding are as yet unknown.

There are no generally accepted methods for measuring cariogenic potential of most foods. Therefore, all foods must be considered in the context of an individual's total diet. For example, concluding a meal with chewing gum or cheddar cheese may nullify the cariogenicity of the meal, regardless of the other foods consumed.

FLUORIDE AND DENTAL HEALTH

Fluoride is the single most significant factor contributing to the recent decline of caries prevalence among children and young adults throughout the world.

Mechanisms of Action

There is no doubt of the anticaries effectiveness of fluoride, either taken systemically during tooth formation and mineralization or applied topically after eruption. Dental researchers have proposed several hypotheses for how fluoride works: (a) modification of the crystalline lattice (converting hydroxyapatite, the principal inorganic mineral of enamel, into partially fluoridated hydroxyapatite) which reduces solubility, improves crystallinity, and enhances remineralization of calcium-depleted mineral; (b) inhibition of dental plaque bacteria; (c) enamel surface actions that desorb proteins and bacteria or lower free surface energy; (d) alteration of tooth morphology.

Fluoride can be incorporated into the enamel during formation, mineralization, preeruptive maturation, and posteruptive maturation. The major increase in fluoride in the surface layers of enamel occurs during preeruptive maturation, but appreciable uptake also occurs immediately following eruption. Newly erupted teeth have a much greater capacity to take up fluoride than older teeth (39).

Absorption and Bioavailability

In general, the absorption of fluoride from an ingested dose of soluble fluoride salt is rapid and nearly complete (40,41) whether from liquids, tablets, gels, or dentifrices. The rate of absorption from the stomach is dependent on the acidity of the ingested solution, as well as on gastric acid secretion. Eighty percent of the fluoride ingested is absorbed within 90 min.

Fluoride supplements should be taken immediately prior to going to bed, with water, if necessary, and not milk (40–42). The bioavailability of preventative fluoride agents is 100% when given with water during fasting. Peak levels taken with milk products, on the other hand, are three to four times lower than IV (control) or oral fasting fluoride doses. Taken at mealtime, with milk, formula, or baby food, the absorption of fluoride is in the 50% to 70% range.

Drinking Water Fluoridation

The safety and efficacy of drinking water fluoridation for prevention of tooth decay have been clearly documented. In the United States, about 56% of the population having access to public water systems have natural or adjusted fluoridation (43).

The incidence of dental caries is as much as 70% higher in 5- to 17-year-old children who have never had exposure to optimally fluoridated water (0.7 to 1.2 ppm) (42). More significantly, children drinking fluoridated drinking water have 65% to 89% fewer missing teeth than those drinking nonfluoridated water (43). During the early days of water fluoridation (1950s and 1960s), caries reduction in children from 5 to 15 years of age was about 50% to 70%. Today the mean is about 18%

(44,45), a reduction largely attributable to the recent use of topical fluorides, especially fluoridated toothpastes.

The fluoridation of municipal water supplies, although effective, must be accompanied by other dental health measures for complete prevention or control of carious lesions. This includes the use of topical fluoride and, when appropriate, systemic fluoride supplements. Systemic fluorides are especially important for populations that have water supplies deficient (less than 0.3 ppm) in fluoride.

School Water Fluoridation

When water fluoridation is not possible, fluoridation of the school water supply reduces caries in schoolchildren by about 40% (46). The level of fluoridation in the school water must be approximately 4.5 times the optimum indicated for community fluoridation to adjust for the decreased number of hours children spend in schools. Thus, in an area where a fluoride level of 1 ppm is indicated, the school water supply should contain 4.5 ppm of fluoride.

School supplementation of fluoride is definitely beneficial, although it is less effective than the protection achieved from full-time optimal systemic use from birth.

Systemic Versus Topical Fluoride

Topical and systemic modes of fluoride therapy are neither separate from nor alternatives to each other. Systemically administered fluoride in fluoridated water or fluoride supplements acts both systemically and topically at the time of ingestion. Similarly, topical fluoride, administered via dentifrice, mouth rinse, or gel, may be inadvertently swallowed, becoming systemic as well as topical.

Evidence indicates that topical fluoride application will provide additional caries protection for children who have received systemic fluoride, either from drinking optimally fluoridated water or from ingesting fluoride supplements. The additional benefit from topical fluoride depends on the type and frequency of application. Topical, professionally applied, fluoride therapy applied once a year provides about 10% additional caries reduction. Twice annual therapy results in about a 20% reduction and daily topical fluoride (toothpaste and rinses) use results in a 30% reduction. Teeth erupting during periods of multiple topical fluoride therapy develop almost 50% fewer caries (42).

Clearly, it is not a question of systemic versus topical fluoride for maximum caries protection. Both forms of therapy are appropriate, and dissimilar mechanisms of action are involved. To maintain maximal caries protection, fluoride should be available systemically at low levels, both pre- and posteruptively, continuously, from birth until age 16, and topically throughout life.

Recommended Supplemental Fluoride Therapy

To assure the greatest protection for primary as well as permanent teeth in children who are not consuming fluoridated drinking water, optimal fluoride supplementation should begin as soon as possible after birth and be continued on a daily basis thereafter until about 16 years of age (47,48).

Optimum dental protection results from early initiation of fluoride supplements. Tooth decay in preschoolers receiving dietary fluoride supplements is decreased 50% to 70%. Programs initiated at 6 years of age result in a 20% to 45% decrease (42).

For optimal effectiveness, fluoride supplementation must be tailored to the specific needs of the individual patient. This requires

1. determining the fluoride content of the patient's drinking water supply
2. determining the proper dosage by age
3. selecting the appropriate type of supplement
4. teaching the patient and parents how to properly use the supplement.

Other important factors include assessing

1. the amount of fluoridated water consumed daily
2. the daily use of topical fluoride, i.e., fluoride dentifrice, oral fluoride rinses
3. the daily dietary intake of foods with high fluoride content
4. caries prevalence (in older children)
5. oral hygiene status (in older children).

It is essential to know the child's age and the fluoride concentration of the drinking water in order to determine the need for systemic fluoride supplementation. When the fluoride content of the home or school water supply is unknown, samples must be analyzed. Because of possible daily variations, water samples should be drawn on two or three separate days. Because the water in infant formula and baby foods is defluoridated to less than 0.3 ppm, this is no longer a concern (47). If children are drinking bottled water, that, too, should be analyzed because of the variable amounts of fluoride bottled water contains (49).

The American Academy of Pediatrics (AAP), the American Academy of Pediatric Dentistry (AAPD), and the American Dental Association (ADA) have designed a dose schedule for fluoride supplementation based on age and fluoride content of drinking water (Table 2) (47–

50). Doses have been calculated to not exceed the optimal dose range of 0.05 to 0.07 mg/kg/day (47).

In addition, prescriptions for dietary fluoride supplements should not exceed 120 mg fluoride ion (256 mg N_2F) to avoid accidental poisoning. Although the acute lethal dose of fluoride is about 15 mg F/kg body weight, deaths have been reported with as little as 5 mg F/kg (39).

Prenatal Fluoride Supplements

Fluoride is an essential element in the mineralization of teeth and bones, although it is unclear when fluoride supplementation should begin in order to produce maximum cariostatic benefit. Traditionally, fluoride supplements have been considered systemic agents that protect prior to the eruption of teeth. Some data suggest a possible prenatal effect in primary teeth (51). Some dentists, pediatricians, and family practitioners think that supplementation should be started prenatally (52).

However, because there is insufficient evidence to show the positive benefits of supplemental fluoride in pregnant women, the routine prescription of prenatal fluoride supplements is not recommended at this time (39,42,47,54,55). The clinical efficacy of prenatal fluoride and how it might impart cariostasis is unclear. The optimal fetal fluoride plasma level for optimal dental therapeutic benefits is not known. Sufficient fluoride is acquired from normal dietary sources and passes through the placenta to facilitate normal enamel and bone mineralization (39). In 1966, because of the lack of data, the United States Food and Drug Administration banned pharmaceutical companies from advertising that prenatal fluoride supplements inhibit dental caries (53).

Fluoride Supplements for Breast-Fed Infants

Should supplemental fluoride be prescribed to infants breast-fed by mothers who live in an optimally fluoridated area? The fluoride content of mother's milk in fluoridated areas has been shown to have a mean fluoride concentration of 0.077 ± 0.029 ppm with a range of 0.024 to 0.172 ppm (56,57). An infant consuming an average of 600 ml of mother's milk per day would, therefore, take in about 0.046 mg of fluoride daily. This is far less than the 0.25 mg recommended for children under 2 years of age.

Since breast milk contains low levels of fluoride, even when the mother consumes fluoridated water, infants in optimally fluoridated communities who are solely breast-fed should be given the same recommended fluoride supplements as infants in areas having negligible amounts of fluoride in the water supply (less than 0.3 ppm). A daily fluoride supplementation of 0.25 mg from birth until weaning is recommended for the fully breast-fed infant (56).

Selecting Appropriate Fluoride Supplements

Fluoride supplements are available as drops, solutions, lozenges, and tablets separately or combined with vitamins. Factors that determine selection include personal preference, the child's age, including the ability and willingness to chew and swallow, and the relative cost. Solutions that dispense 0.125 mg fluoride per drop are convenient for infants since the dose can be easily adjusted. Tablets containing 0.25 or 0.5 mg fluoride ion are appropriate at about 3 years of age when the child is able to chew and swallow a chewable tablet.

The effectiveness of fluoride-vitamin supplements in reducing dental caries is the same as that produced by fluoride supplementation alone (39,47,50). The determining factor should be whether a vitamin-supplement is needed. When appropriate, a combined supplement is more convenient and, because parents are often motivated to give vitamins to children, probably enhances compliance.

Most important is positive communication between the parent and the dentist and the dentist and physician to assure that supplementation is patient-appropriate and that it is clearly understood that even when vitamins are discontinued fluoride supplementation is not.

Fluorosis

Dental fluorosis is a hypoplastic or hypomineralization defect of tooth enamel produced by chronic ingestion of excessive amounts of fluoride during the period when teeth are developing. Dental fluorosis is characterized by a lusterless opaque appearance to the enamel, which may appear as barely visible white striations in the mild forms. In the more severe forms, the enamel is yellow or brown and is often mottled and pitted in varying degrees. Severity is largely dependent upon the amount

TABLE 2. *Recommended fluoride dose levels for specific ages: dietary fluoride supplementation dose schedule[a] in milligrams of fluoride ion per day[b]*

Age[c] (years)	Fluoride content of water		
	Less than 0.3 ppm	0.3 to 0.7 ppm	Greater than 0.7 ppm
Birth to 2	0.25	0	0
2–3	0.50	0.25	0
3–13 (16)	1.00	0.50	0

[a] Recommended by the American Dental Association, the American Academy of Pediatric Dentistry, and the American Academy of Pediatrics.
[b] 2.2 mg of sodium fluoride provides 1.0 mg fluoride ion.
[c] American Academy of Pediatrics (47) recommends initiation by 2 weeks of age and continuing until age 16 years.

of fluoride ingested. In its most severe form, fluorosis can grossly alter the morphology of the crown. It usually occurs symmetrically in the dental arches, but sometimes with extensive variability in hypoplastic and hypocalcific effects on the teeth. When teeth are affected by severe fluorosis, they may be aesthetically compromised or subject to fracture of unsupported enamel.

There is no evidence that the fluorosis defect occurs due to exposure to high fluoride intake during the early stages of enamel formation. On the contrary, fluorosis is most likely produced by exposure to high fluoride intake during the latter part of enamel formation, the maturation stage. If one is concerned about fluorosis, it makes more sense to reduce supplemental fluoride during the second and third years rather than during the first year of life.

No occurrences of aesthetically unacceptable fluorosis have been reported when following the use of the dosage schedule established by the AAP, AAPD, and ADA (Table 2) (39,47,57).

There are no data confirming the anecdotal reports of increasing prevalence of fluorosis in youngsters. If fluorosis is increasing, it is most likely not the result of early supplementation. Rather, it probably stems from misprescribing fluoride supplements for children whose intake via the water supply and other sources, particularly fluoride toothpaste, is already sufficient, if not excessive. Rather than advocating a reduction of fluoride in water supplies to combat this perceived problem, an educational program is necessary to teach pediatricians and dentists methods to determine accurate fluoride supplementation. Parents must also learn to supervise the use of fluoride dentifrice in preschool children. And toothpaste manufacturers should begin producing fluoride toothpaste with lower amounts of fluoride (250 to 500 ppm, instead of the conventional 1,000 ppm) specifically for preschool children.

ROLE OF NUTRITION AND DIET IN DISEASES OF THE ORAL MUCOSA

There are no identifiable mucosal signs suggestive of a subclinical nutritional deficiency state. The manifestations of the latent phase of nutritional deficiencies in infants and children are of unknown etiology, and vary greatly in intensity, frequency, and dominance from subject to subject (58,59).

The oral symptoms of malnutrition are usually represented by burning, soreness, tenderness, dryness, sialorrhea, xerostomia, and cheilosis. They may occur singly or in combination, may come and go, and may vary in severity from one subject to another. Soreness of the tongue is encountered in iron, vitamin B_{12}, folic acid, niacin, and protein-energy deficiencies. Stomatodynia is an early and prominent symptom of niacin, tryptophan, folic acid, vitamin B_{12}, and protein-energy and protein-vitamin deficiencies. Sialorrhea frequently accompanies acute nutritional stomatitis and is especially copious in acute niacin deficiency. Partial xerostomia is associated with vitamin A, riboflavin, niacin, iron, and folic acid deficiencies. Impairment of taste acuity is common in thiamin, niacin, vitamin B_{12} deficiency, and zinc deficiency. Cheilosis and cheilitis are early indications of riboflavin deficiency as well as of niacin, folic acid, vitamin B_6, and protein-energy deficiencies (7,58–62).

THE ROLE OF NUTRITION IN GINGIVAL AND PERIODONTAL DISEASES

Gingivitis

Gingivitis, an early, reversible stage of periodontal disease, is confined to the gums. Inflamed gums, irritated by plaque buildup, may look red and puffy, feel tender, and bleed easily when brushed. Pockets, formed between gums and teeth, accumulate plaque. In addition, a cement-like substance called tartar (or calculus) forms on teeth, trapping even more plaque. Tartar cannot be removed by brushing and must be scraped off by a dentist or dental hygienist using a process called scaling.

When gingivitis is not intercepted, a vicious cycle develops: plaque and tartar buildup cause deepening of tissue pockets which, in turn, trap more plaque. If untreated, gingivitis may progress to periodontitis.

Periodontitis

Periodontal disease involves progressive destruction of the gums, bone, and tooth-supporting tissues. As bone deteriorates, teeth may loosen and fall out or may need to be extracted.

Clinical signs of periodontal diseases usually do not appear until puberty. Prior to puberty, the principal expression of an irritation in the dental supporting structures is gingival inflammation at the marginal areas. Except in conjunction with systemic diseases, this inflammation is usually due to local causes, especially poor oral hygiene.

The form of gingivitis seen in young children generally occurs at the gingival margin and is characterized by prominent bulbous interproximal papillae, in contrast to the absence of papillae seen in adult Vincent's type periodontal infections. Acute gingival and periodontal disturbances in children are common, chronic periodontal disturbances are less frequent, and atrophic and degenerative disease are rare.

The most common form of gingival disease in children under 5 years of age is primary herpetic gingivostomatitis, which is of short duration (about 10 days) and is not true periodontal disease.

Atrophic and degenerative periodontal diseases, seen in a child only when severe systemic disease or nutritional deficiency is present, are not very common.

The conditions associated with gingival enlargement in children may be relatively transient, e.g., during eruption of the primary teeth in infancy, at times of primary herpetic infections, during puberty, following the use of Dilantin (phenytoin), during times of severe vitamin C deficiency, and during the period of mixed dentition (primary and permanent teeth present at the same time) when the teeth are in various stages of exfoliation and eruption (63). Drugs such as cyclosporine, nifedipine, and diltiazem, administered after organ transplants, have also been associated with gingival enlargement (hyperplasia) and inflammation, especially when administered in conjunction with prednisone (64).

Nutrition and Periodontal Diseases

It is difficult to establish a definitive relationship between malnutrition and the etiology of periodontal disease. This is essentially because of the multifactorial nature and variety of periodontal diseases as well as the difficulty in assessing nutritional status. Overall, nutritional deficiencies alter the severity of periodontal diseases by changing the repair properties of the tissues. Inadequate nutrient intake could also affect the metabolism of plaque flora in the gingival sulcular crevice, as well as systemic immunological responses to microbial antigens (63).

Animals fed protein-deficient diets may have adversely affected salivary gland development and function (3,6,59). Saliva production and the total protein concentration may also be significantly reduced. Such malnutrition may impair immunologic functions, making animals more susceptible to deficiencies of either ascorbic acid or folic acid which, in turn, can severely alter epithelial functions, particularly in the sulcular crevice areas around the teeth. The permeability of the oral epithelium to large irritating molecules may be markedly increased by early malnutrition, a condition that can persist to adulthood (63).

Protein Deficiency

Protein and amino acid deficiencies have, in some cases, been associated with increased susceptibility to periodontal disease. Protein supplementation, on the other hand, has a positive effect on the reduction of gingival and periodontal inflammation and tooth mobility, even greater than scaling and dental prophylaxis alone, a benefit that is increased when supplementation is combined with scaling and prophylaxis (65).

Folic Acid, Ascorbic Acid, and Iron

Ascorbic acid deficiency can cause alveolar bone destruction resulting in the teeth becoming loose and eventually lost.

Folic acid deficiency seems to result in a relatively high incidence of reversible changes in epithelial cells, including those in the oral mucosa. Vogel et al. (66,67) demonstrated that gingival inflammation can be decreased by supplementation of 2 mg of folic acid twice daily combined with rinsing with 5 cc of a 1 mg/cc solution of folic acid for 5 min twice daily. This process is most likely facilitated by folic acid absorption through the nonepithelialized surface of the gingival sulcus.

Folic acid supplementation also decreases the incidence and severity of phenytoin-induced gingival hyperplasia. Supplementation with 3 mg per day reduced the extent of existing hyperplasia and inhibited the occurrence of hyperplasia in several children (68). In another study, 5 mg/day for 6 months significantly decreased the extent of existing hyperplasia (69).

Studies indicate that, for periodontal health, there may be a need for greater amounts of folic acid, ascorbic acid, and iron than are normally found in human dietary intake. Although systemic levels of these nutrients in either serum or white blood cells may be within normal limits, supplementation above recommended daily allowances resulted in increased concentration within the gingival tissues, which was associated with an increase in the defense mechanisms of the tissues to local etiologic factors.

Until further studies confirm a relationship between human nutritional status and periodontal diseases, periodontal diseases can be characterized as conditional nutritional diseases. That is, nutritional status can condition an individual's susceptibility to periodontal diseases. Almost any nutritional deficiency, if sufficiently severe and long-term, might affect some component of the host defense system including the various tissue and cells of the oral mucous membranes. As is true for the body as a whole, healthy periodontal epithelium is less susceptible to disease.

CONCLUSION

The primary oral health goal is the development and maintenance of optimum oral health in infancy and childhood that can be carried into adulthood. Its success is largely predicated on a program of preventive dental care begun at a very early age. The program design must include awareness of the following:

1. Children under 1 year of age may already have caries, most of which could have been prevented with appropriate intervention.

2. Nutritional status may affect susceptibility to mucosal and periodontal diseases.
3. Optimum caries prevention is dependent on optimum fluoride levels in the diet within a few weeks following birth, continuing until age 16.
4. Topical fluorides must supplement dietary fluoride from the time the primary teeth erupt and continue throughout adulthood.
5. Pits and fissures of susceptible posterior teeth should be sealed as soon as possible after their eruption.

Optimum infant oral health care begins with a dental office visit for preventive counseling no later than 12 months of age. This dramatically increases the likelihood of a caries-free child and, done societally, may provide the United States with a caries-free generation. Three years of age, which has been traditionally recommended for a first dental visit is, by far, too late.

Nutritional deficiencies during the development of teeth, jaws, salivary glands, and the immune system may alter postdevelopmental resistive capabilities to dental-oral diseases. For this reason, the negative attention on sucrose and its deleterious effect on teeth should be expanded to include other, equally negative nutritional and environmental precursors that may predispose the host to dental caries as well as other oral diseases. For example, a susceptible tooth is essential for caries development. Those factors that affect a tooth's susceptibility include size, shape, composition, alignment, jaw size, salivary function, and immunocompetence.

Nutritional factors are important in the development of caries-resistant teeth. Although it is virtually impossible to produce a tooth that can withstand a prolonged caries challenge by highly virulent bacteria, it is possible to increase the tooth's resistance considerably with optimum nutritional status. Fluoride is, of course, the most essential of these nutrients.

Further studies are essential to delineate the importance of dietary counseling in ameliorating the prevalence of caries and mucosal and periodontal diseases. Until such studies provide conclusive data on food cariogenicity and its relationship to periodontal diseases, counseling must be done on an individual basis, taking into account individual clinical status and using a good deal of professional intuition and common sense.

REFERENCES

1. Yudkin J. Nutritional deficiency. In: Sorsby H, ed. *Systemic ophthalmology*. St. Louis: CV Mosby, 1958;287–301.
2. Stewart RE, et al. The dentition. In: Stewart RE, et al., eds. *Pediatric dentistry—scientific foundations and clinical practice*. St. Louis: CV Mosby, 1982;87–134.
3. DePaola DP. Human diet and dental caries: effect of diet in the early years. In: Hefferren JJ, Koehler HM, eds. *Foods, nutrition and dental health*, vol 1. Park Forest S., IL: Pathotox Publishers, 1981;14:35–42.
4. Glick PL. Mineralization of the teeth: prenatal and postnatal nutrient requirements. In: Wei SHY, ed. *National symposium on dental nutrition*. Iowa City: University of Iowa, 1978;87–110.
5. Weinmann JP. Bone changes related to eruption of teeth. *Angle Orthod* 1941;11:83–99.
6. DePaola DP, Kuftinec MM. Nutrition in growth and development of oral tissues. *Dent Clin North Am* 1976;20:441–460.
7. Boyle PE. Manifestations of vitamin A deficiency in a human tooth germ. *J Dent Res* 1933;13:39–50.
8. Shaw JH, Sweeney EA. Nutrition in relation in dental medicine. In: Goodhart RS, Shils ME, eds. *Modern nutrition in health and disease*. Philadelphia: Lea and Febiger, 1973.
9. Shaw JH. Preeruptive effects of nutrition on teeth. *J Dent Res* 1970;49(6, suppl):1238–1250.
10. Burt BA, Ismail AL. Diet nutrition and food cariogenicity. *J Dent Res* 1986;65(Spec. Iss.):1475–1484.
11. Bibby BG. Cariogenicity of food stuffs. In: Sweeney EA, ed. *The food that stays: update on nutrition, diet, sugar, and caries*. New York: Medcom, Inc. 1977;32.
12. Jensen ME, et al. Evaluation of the acidogenic potential of reference foods by telemetry from inter-proximal sites in the human dentition. In: Hefferren JJ, et al., eds. *Foods, nutrition and dental health*, vol. 5. Park Forest S., Pathotox Publishers, 1984;109–122.
13. Jensen ME, et al. Evaluation of the acidogenic and antacid properties in cheeses by telemetric monitoring of human dental plaque pH. In: Hefferren JJ, et al., eds. *Foods, nutrition and dental health*, vol 4. Park Forest S., Pathotox Publishers, 1984;3–31.
14. Jensen ME, Schachtele CF. The acidogenic potential of reference foods and snacks at interproximal sites in the human dentition. *J Dent Res* 1983;62:889–892.
15. Jensen ME. Dental caries: a diet-related disease. *Currents Q* 1985;1:18–21.
16. Navia JM. Models for food cariogenicity testing: report of a collaborative study using animal models. In: Hefferren JJ, et al., eds. *Foods, nutrition and dental health*, vol 3. Park Forest S., IL: Pathotox Publishers, 1981;1–13.
17. Scheinin A, Mäkinen KK, Ylitalo K. Turku sugar studies. V. Final report on the effect of sucrose, fructose, and xylitol on the caries incidence in man. *Acta Odontol Scand* 1976;34(4):179–216.
18. Ripa LW. Nursing caries: a comprehensive review. *Pediatr Dent* 1988;10:268–282.
19. Loesche WJ. Nutrition and dental decay in infants. *Am J Clin Nutr* 1985;41:423–435.
20. Johnsen DC, Nowjack-Raymer R. Baby bottle tooth decay: issues, assessment, and an opportunity for the nutritionist. *J Am Diet Assoc* 1989;89:1112–1116.
21. News and Comments: a joint statement from the American Academy of Pediatrics and the American Academy of Pediatric Dentistry. *Pediatr Dent* 1979;29:1.
22. Burt BA, Eklund SA. Sugar consumption and dental caries patterns in the United States. In: Hefferren JJ, et al. *Foods, nutrition, and dental health*, vol 3. Park Forest S., Pathotox Publishers, 1981;171–179.
23. Wei SHY, Andersan TA. Nutrition and dental health. In: Stewart, RE, et al., eds. *Pediatric dentistry—scientific foundations and clinical practice*. St. Louis: CV Mosby, 1982;561–575.
24. Geddes DAM, et al. Apples, salted peanuts, and plaque pH. *Br Dent J* 1977;142:317–319.
25. Rugg-Gunn AJ, et al. The effect of different meal patterns upon plaque pH in human subjects. *Br Dent J* 1975;139:351–356.
26. Burt BA, Eklund SA, Morgan KJ, et al. The effects of sugars intake and frequency of ingestion on dental caries increment in a three year longitudinal study. *J Dent Res* 1988;67:1422–1429.
27. Bar A. Caries preventive with xylitol: a review of the scientific evidence. *World Rev Nutr Diet* 1988;55(1):1–27.
28. Loesche WJ. The rationale for caries prevention through the use of sugar substitutes. *Int Dent J* 1985;35(1):1–8.
29. Loesche WJ, et al. The effect of chewing xylitol gum on the plaque and saliva levels of *Streptococcus mutans*. *JADA* 1984;108(4):587–592.
30. Isokangas P, et al. Xylitol chewing gum in caries prevention: a field study in children. *JADA* 1988;117:315–320.
31. Scheinin A. Sucrose substitutes. In: Stewart RE, et al., eds. *Pediatric dentistry—scientific foundations and clinical practice*. St. Louis: CV Mosby, 1982;590–597.

32. Jensen M. Responses of interproximal plaque pH to snack foods and effects of chewing sorbitol-containing gums. *JADA* 1986;113:262–266.
33. Jensen M. Effects of chewing sorbitol gum and paraffin on human interproximal plaque pH. *Caries Res* 1986;20:503–509.
34. Jensen M, Wefel JS. Human plaque pH responses to meals and the effects of chewing gum. *Br Dent J* 1989;167(6):204–208.
35. Yankell SL, Emling RC. Clinical study to evaluate the effects of three marketed sugarless chewing gum products on plaque pH, pCA and swallowing rate. *J Clin Dent* 1989;1(3):70–74.
36. Jakush J. Diet, nutrition, and oral health: a rational approach for the dental practice. *JADA* 1964;108:21–32.
37. Rosen S, et al. Effect of cheese, with and without sucrose, on dental caries and recovery of *Streptococcus mutans* in rats. *J Dent Res* 1984;63:894–896.
38. Mackay DAM. Prospects of phosphate supplementation of foods for dental purposes. In: Wei SHY, ed. *National symposium on dental nutrition.* Iowa City: University of Iowa, 1979;87–110.
39. Ekstrand J, Fejerskov O, Silverstone LM. *Fluoride in dentistry.* Chicago: Yearbook Medical Publishers, 1988.
40. Ekstrand J, et al. Pharmacokinetics of fluoride in man after single and multiple oral doses. *Eur J Clin Pharmacol* 1977;12:311.
41. Ellingsen J, Ekstrand J. Plasma fluoride levels in man following intake of SnF_2 in solution or toothpaste. *J Dent Res* 1985;64:1250–1252.
42. Wei SHY ed. Fluorides and dental health. In: Stewart RE, et al., eds. *Pediatric dentistry—scientific foundations and clinical practice.* St. Louis: CV Mosby, 1982;717–779.
43. McCann D. Fluoride and oral health—a story of achievement and challenges. *JADA* 1989;118:529–540.
44. Brunelle JA, Carlos JP. Changes in the prevalence of dental caries in US Schoolchildren, 1960–1980. *J Dent Reg* 1982;61(special issue):1346–1351.
45. Marshall E. The fluoride debate: one more time. *Science* 1990;247:276–277.
46. Horowitz HA, Heifetz SB, Law FE. Effect of school water fluoridation on dental caries: final results in Elk Lake Pennsylvania after 12 years. *JADA* 1972;84:832–838.
47. American Academy of Pediatrics Committee on Nutrition. Fluoride supplementation (RE6069). *Pediatrics* 1986;77(5):758–761.
48. American Academy of Pediatric Dentistry. *Oral health policy—Preventive Dentistry-Fluoridation,* 1978 and Protocol for Fluoride Therapy, Council on Dental Therapeutics. 1985. American Academy of Pediatric Dentistry, Chicago, 1991.
49. Nowak AJ. Primary preventive dentistry for children. *Update Pediatr Dent* 1990;3(1):1–7.
50. American Dental Association. Prescribing fluoride supplements. In: *Accepted dental therapeutics,* 39th ed. Chicago: American Dental Association 1982;347–351.
51. Glenn F. Immunity by a fluoride supplement during pregnancy. *J Dent Child* 1977;44:391–395.
52. American Dental Association, Council on Dental Therapeutics. *Value of fluoride administered to expectant mothers.* Chicago: American Dental Association, 1962.
53. Food and Drug Administration. Statements of general policy or interpretation. Oral prenatal drugs containing fluorides for human use. *Federal Register,* October 10, 1966.
54. Thylsbup A. Is there a biological rationale for prenatal fluoride administration. *J Dent Child* 1981;48:103–108.
55. Stamm JW. Perspectives on the use of prenatal fluorides: a reactor's comments. *J Dent Child* 1981;48:128–133.
56. Latifah R, Razak IA. Fluoride levels in mother's milk. *J Pedodont* 1989;13:149–154.
57. Latifah R, Duguid R. Measurements of ionic fluoride in milk. *Ann Acad Med* 1986;15(3):299–304.
58. Dreizen S. The mouth as an indicator of internal nutritional problems. *Pediatrician* 1989;16:139–146.
59. Navia JM. Nutrition and oral disease. In: Caldwell RC, Stallard RE, eds. *A textbook of preventive dentistry.* Philadelphia: WB Saunders, 1977;118–153.
60. Rosenblum LA, Jolliffe N. The oral manifestations of vitamin deficiencies. *JAMA* 1941;117:2245–2248.
61. Dinnerman M. Vitamin A deficiency in unerupted teeth of infants. *Oral Surg* 1951;4:1024–1038.
62. Boyle PE. The tooth germ in acute scurvy. *J Dent Res* 1934;14:172.
63. Vogel RI. Periodontal disease host defense mechanisms affected by nutrition: clinical trials. In: Hefferen JJ, et al. *Foods, nutrition and dental health,* vol 5. Park Forest S., Pathotox Publishers, 1984;163–179.
64. Meyers R, Guerra A. Dentistry and the pediatric cardiac transplant patient. *NY State Dent J* 1990, February;56:31–34.
65. Wei SHY, ed. Pathogenesis and prevention of dental caries and periodontal disease. In: Stewart RE, et al., eds. *Pediatric dentistry—scientific foundations and clinical practice.* St. Louis: CV Mosby, 1982;566–633.
66. Vogel R, Deasy M. The effect of folic acid on experimentally produced gingivitis. *J Prev Dent* 1978;5:30–32.
67. Vogel R, et al. The effect of topical application of folic acid on gingival health. *J Oral Med* 1978;33:20–22.
68. Vogel R. Gingival hyperplasia and folic acid deficiency from anticonvulsive drug therapy. A theoretical relationship. *J Theor Biol* 1977;67:269.
69. Inoue F, Harrison J. Folic acid and phenytoin hyperplasia. *Lancet* 1981;2:86.

CHAPTER 44

Characterizing Children's Eating Behavior

Rosanne Perlman Farris and Theresa A. Nicklas

It is widely recognized that health patterns during childhood have an impact on many chronic diseases. Epidemiologic research has focused on the associations between dietary patterns of children and young adults and cardiovascular risk factors (1,2). The knowledge of this association, coupled with dietary intake information, form the basis for nutrition counseling in clinical settings, as well as intervention program planning and nutrition education efforts for public and preventive health measures (3,4).

Studies that attempt to identify dietary patterns, either for groups or time periods, depend on dietary assessment methods that yield the highest degree of validity, fulfill study goals, are appropriate for the study population, and consider biological issues and statistical limitations (5–8). Considerations also include (a) the age and aptitude of the child; (b) knowledge of food and preparation components; (c) the ability to visualize, recall, and assess amounts; and (d) respondent burden, i.e., the perceived time and effort necessary to complete study requirements by the respondent (9–14).

DIETARY STUDY METHODS

Each dietary method has its own set of functions, advantages, and limitations. Although the validity and reliability of many techniques have been ascertained, there is a paucity of research on methods most appropriate for use with children (8–16).

It is essential to be aware of the uses and limitations of various methods and how they relate to study goals. The lack of a standardized methodology for dietary data collection, however, usually limits or eliminates the possibility of comparing studies. Although limitations such as these may be minimized by a careful selection of method coupled with a cautious interpretation of results, they highlight the need for alternative approaches.

NATIONAL FOOD AVAILABILITY

Food availability data quantify the net amount of food available to a population based upon food production and imports, excluding industrial wastage and nonhuman use. They represent estimates of food intake without consideration of specific distribution of food within a population; subtle differences in dietary intakes in subgroups or by individuals cannot be detected. The data can, however, reveal gross changes in food production and consumption patterns as well as trends over time (17–19).

A recent important change in the United States has been in the levels and sources of fat consumption (Fig. 1). General fat consumption represents over one-third of caloric intake: 40% of fat intake in the U.S. comes from fats and oils, 33% from meat, poultry, and fish, and 13% from dairy products. Changes in fat/oil consumption include (a) increased use of vegetable oils; (b) a consumer shift from butter to margarine; and (c) use of hydrogenated vegetable shortening replacing lard for frying, especially in fast-food restaurants (17). There is also increased beef and poultry consumption, a decreased consumption of pork, and an increased consumption of low-fat milk with a decreased consumption of whole milk. These changes in fat intake have changed the fatty acid content of the American diet (Table 1) (19).

There is some controversy about the total amount of fat actually ingested in the United States. Food supply disappearance data suggest that per capita consumption has, in fact, increased since the late 1970s. This may be attributed, at least partially, to the increased use of fast-

---

R. P. Farris: Department of Pediatrics, Louisiana State University School of Medicine, New Orleans, Louisiana 70112.

T. A. Nicklas: Department of Medicine, Louisiana State University School of Medicine, New Orleans, Louisiana 70112.

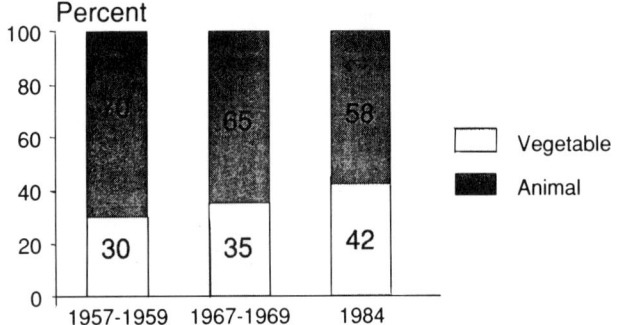

FIG. 1. Fat from animal versus vegetable sources in the United States' food supply for selected years. (Data from ref. 20.)

food restaurants, where many foods are cooked in oil (20). However, because disappearance data are not adjusted for waste, cooking loss, or spoilage, they do not indicate the amount of fat clinically consumed (17). In fact, cross-sectional surveys, which measure actual consumption, indicate that fat consumption has decreased in the United States (21–23). The surveys did, however, indicate a change in food selection; the National Research Council (NRC) reported a decrease in red meat/whole-milk consumption and an increase in poultry/low-fat milk consumption (19).

WEIGHED-FOOD RECORD

In the weighed-food record method, food is weighed before and after feedings. Specific intake is determined by estimated nutrient calculations or actual chemical analysis. A high degree of subject cooperation and a precise knowledge of the nutrient components are essential. Because this is one of the most costly and labor intensive methods, it is primarily used in metabolic studies when precise information on the relationship between specific nutrients and their metabolic effects is being investigated.

Less valid are studies in which weighed-food records are recorded by the participant, since this technique probably influences eating patterns (24).

DIET DIARY

Subjects keep a record of measured food consumption during a specific time period. Participants who are cooperative, intelligent, motivated, or rewarded will provide the most nearly complete data. This method, however, has the highest refusal rate and greatest percentage of participants with unusable data (25). The quality of diet diaries may decrease during an extended recording period, e.g., 7 days. There is also a responder tendency to subconsciously select or record a better diet.

Record keeping has become, however, a popular strategy to involve children in changing their own eating behaviors. By observing and recording information, not only about the specific foods and amounts eaten, but also about locations, times, and events associated with eating, children become aware of the best targets for change.

The goals of each study is affected by the precision required and the specific nutrient being investigated. Because of intraindividual variability of eating patterns, true correlations between nutrient intake and the physiologic characteristic of interest must be assessed (26). Estimating the true correlation coefficient between a nutrient and blood pressure, with 90% efficiency, takes from 4 to 7 days of food records. Sodium, which has large intraindividual variation, requires 7 days, whereas calories require 4 days. These estimates are conservative since, in fact, the intraindividual variation in the measurement of blood pressure itself would increase the number of days required. It is generally agreed that at least 7 days are needed to characterize an individual, whereas 1 or more days on a sample of at least 60 subjects can accurately characterize a group (27). Some nutrients, such as vitamin C, have larger intraindividual variations because of limited food sources, and may require longer study periods.

24-HOUR DIETARY RECALL

The use of 24-hr dietary recall relies on memory to recall food consumption during the preceding 24 hr; individual accuracy is predicated on multiple recalls over an extended period of time. An accurate nutrient profile of large groups may be accurately drawn, however, from a single 24-hr recall (27).

Group dietary recall yields the highest percentage of usable data. Bias is reduced when interviews are conducted unannounced. In addition, the inclusion of atypical days, such as weekends and holidays, helps to pro-

TABLE 1. *Selected fatty acids in the United States' food supply (in percent)*

	Year								
Fatty acid	1909–1913	1925–1929	1935–1939	1947–1949	1957–1959	1967–1969	1973	1980	1984
Saturated	42	42	42	40	40	37	35	34	35
Oleic	37	38	37	38	38	38	39	38	38
Linoleic	7	8	9	10	11	13	15	16	15

Adapted from ref. 20.

INSTRUCTIONS: For each food item listed below, mark an "X" in the column that best describes how often you ate each food last week (7-day period)	NEVER	NOT LAST WEEK	ONCE OR TWICE LAST WEEK	3 - 6 TIMES LAST WEEK	ONCE OR TWICE A DAY	3 OR MORE TIMES A DAY
	1	2	3	4	5	6
Margarine (all brands, such as Parkay, Chiffon, etc)	( )	( )	( )	( )	( )	( )
Butter (all brands, such as American Beauty, Land-O-Lakes, etc.)	( )	( )	( )	( )	( )	( )
Lard, vegetable fat (white)	( )	( )	( )	( )	( )	( )
Bacon, beef or pork drippings	( )	( )	( )	( )	( )	( )
Vegetable oil	( )	( )	( )	( )	( )	( )
Mayonnaise	( )	( )	( )	( )	( )	( )
Salad dressings (French, oil and vinegar, Thousand Island, etc.)	( )	( )	( )	( )	( )	( )
Gravy (pork, chicken, beef, tomato, etc.)	( )	( )	( )	( )	( )	( )

FIG. 2. Self-administered questionnaire used in the food-frequency method of diet assessment.

duce a more nearly complete picture of nutrient patterns (28). Dietary recalls relying only on weekdays may result in an underestimation of such nutrients as energy, carbohydrate, and sucrose (29).

Although there is little difference in results obtained from the less expensive 24-hr dietary recalls and 7-day food record diaries, one drawback of the single day dietary recall is the high intraindividual variance, which causes problems in associating diet with chronic disease. With a homogeneous population, the variation of a dietary factor within the same individual from day to day may be as large or larger than the variation of that factor within the group as a whole. Discerning the diet–chronic disease relationship is not possible simply by increasing the number of individuals studied; it requires increasing the number of recall periods for each person over a period of time.

Ten years of age appears to be the earliest age that reliable information can be obtained from a 24-hr dietary recall (10,13). Combining parents and children as respondents increases accuracy (30,31). Added accuracy may be obtained from weighed school lunch portions calculated from exact recipes (32).

Diet recalls may be obtained by a short, 15 to 20 min interview or by a self-administered questionnaire. Interviews are preferable for a more qualitative dietary assessment. Food models and measuring cups may help children determine quantity.

FOOD FREQUENCY

A food-frequency method attempts to discover the frequency per unit of time that specific foods are consumed. This information is usually obtained by interview or self-administered questionnaire (Fig. 2). Quantification is achieved by multiplying the estimated amount of food consumed by the frequency (Fig. 3). In this way, the long-term character of a diet can be observed, providing a basis of comparison to demonstrate trends or patterns.

There are, however, drawbacks. Estimation is a crude method of quantification. There is also the possibility of

On the average, how much of each kind of fat or oil did you eat on any one day last week? Mark an "X" in the column closest to the amount used. (See food model if needed.)				
	NONE	1-3 teaspoons	1-3 tablespoons	3 OR MORE tablespoons
	1	2	3	4
Mayonnaise	( )	( )	( )	( )
Gravy	( )	( )	( )	( )
Butter	( )	( )	( )	( )
Margarine	( )	( )	( )	( )
Salad Dressing	( )	( )	( )	( )

FIG. 3. Self-administered questionnaire used in the food-frequency method of diet assessment.

systematic bias as a result of responses that reflect attitudes and expectations toward different foods. For example, staple foods may be overestimated and sucrose-rich foods underestimated (30). Use of parents as respondents is also inappropriate since the parent may not really know what, or how much, the child is eating when he/she is away from home. Frequencies also suffer from dependence on memory ability, a problem that worsens as the study continues. Finally, the reliability and validity of food frequency decreases proportionate to the increase in the variability in the subject's eating habits (33).

In addition, although computerized food frequency questionnaires have become increasingly popular among some health professionals, their value for assessment of nutrient intake is limited because of a lack of professional input.

DIET HISTORY

Diet histories seek to draw a picture of eating patterns over an extended period of time and attempt to determine an individual's relative rank with respect to Burke's method, which includes (a) a section to discern usual eating patterns, (b) a cross-check of frequency of usual intake of specific foods, and (c) a 3-day recall or diary (34).

Although diet histories are appropriate for determining the qualitative aspects of eating behavior, and may draw a true estimate of the usual eating pattern, they have a tendency to overestimate intakes, are time-consuming, and require highly trained interviewers (34, 35). In addition, they are expensive, relying on time-consuming interviews which may take, on average, an hour to conduct (30). School-age children show just enough cooperation and intelligence to fulfill the time required for the interview.

COMPUTERIZED DIETARY ANALYSIS

Computers are playing an increasingly important role in the two major components of diet evaluation: (a) collection of information about the kinds and amounts of foods consumed, and (b) translation of that information into nutritional terms. Computer programs that store nutrient values are able to compare an individual's intake with recommended dietary allowances, point to dietary shortcomings, and make recommendations for change.

Computerized dietary analysis has improved the accuracy and efficiency of nutrient calculations in research, teaching, dietary interventions, and clinical applications (36–42). Technology, however, cannot compensate for inaccuracies in food-intake or -composition data. Taylor et al. (43) reported that many currently available data bases are incomplete and inaccurate. Comparing values derived from three separate computerized data bases, they analyzed a series of diets for energy and 18 nutrients. Differences were found in mean values for 9 of the 19 dietary components evaluated (43).

Shanklia et al. (44) studied a set of 24-hr dietary intakes of 60 women, infants, and young children, and found that the energy, protein, and fat composition of diets of children and women were significantly different when different nutrient data bases were compared.

In a study by Yarde et al. (45) the nutrient content of 100 commonly eaten food items was analyzed using three computerized nutrient data base systems: Extended Table of Nutrient Values (ETNV), Nutrition Coordinating Center (NCC), and Dennison Inventory of Nutrition Evaluation (DINE). The values obtained for energy, protein, fat, saturated fat, carbohydrate, total sugar, and sodium were compared (Table 2). Results demonstrated the possibility of sizable variations. For example, when saturated fatty acid (SFA) content was compared by calculating the mean and percent difference from the mean, differences in SFA values of up to 5 g per 100 g of meats, and up to 6 g in recipes, were found among the three data bases. Although a difference of 5 to 6 g per food may seem small, this represents 10% of the average daily SFA intake of 50 g and could potentially obscure a desired intervention effect. Other variations for SFA included dairy foods (Table 3), with less than 2 g per 100 g, and fats and oils, with up to 15 g per 100 g.

The factors that influenced this observed variability include (a) incompatible data sources, (b) manipulation of data, (c) lack of uniformity of food descriptions, and (d) lack of standards for commercial product data.

In order to select the most appropriate data base, therefore, it is essential to ascertain its ultimate use: clinical, epidemiological, research, administrative, and/or educational. Each data base has unique characteristics includ-

TABLE 2. *Comparison of nutrient values of cheese pizza (per 100 g) in three data bases*

Data base	Energy (Cal)	Protein (g)	Fat (g)	SFA (g)	Carbohydrate (g)	Sugar (g)	Sodium (mg)
ETNV	225.0	9.2	4.4	1.9	36.6	2.8	382
DINE	236.0	12.0	7.7	3.2	28.5	0.0	702
NCC	326.0	14.3	17.9	6.8	27.0	2.5	938

SFA, saturated fatty acid; ETNV, Extended Table of Nutrient Values; DINE, Dennison Inventory of Nutrition Evaluation; NCC, Nutrition Coordinating Center.

TABLE 3. *Comparison of three computerized nutrient data bases*

Dairy (per 100 g)	Saturated Fat (g)						Mean
	ETNV	%Diff	NCC	%Diff	DINE	%Diff	
Milk, whole	2.1	0.0	2.1	0.0	2.0	4.8	2.1
Milk, evaporated	4.6	0.0	4.5	−2.2	4.6	0.0	4.6
Milk, skim	0.1	0.0	0.1	0.0	0.1	0.0	0.1
Milk, chocolate whole fluid	2.1	0.0	2.1	0.0	2.1	0.0	2.1
Cheese, American pasteurized	19.7	1.0	19.7	1.0	19.1	−2.1	19.5
Cheese, cheddar	21.1	1.9	21.1	1.9	20.8	0.5	20.7
Cheese, cottage lowfat 1%	0.3	−25.0	0.3	−25.0	0.7	75.0	0.4
Cheese, cream Philadelphia	22.0	1.4	22.0	1.4	21.1	−2.8	21.7
Yogurt, plain lowfat	1.0	−28.5	2.2	71.4	0.9	−35.7	1.4
Ice cream, regular vanilla 10% fat	6.7	0.0	6.7	0.0	6.6	−1.4	6.7

ETNV, extended table of nutrient values; NCC, nutrition coordinating center; DINE, Dennison inventory of nutrition evaluation.

ing data base size, number of nutrients analyzed, type of calculations and comparisons performed, and format. Hoover and Perloff (46,47) identify six tasks to assist in the successful selection of a nutrient analysis system.

ELECTRONIC METHODS

Other innovative dietary methodology has been developed and tested for individual diet characterization (48). In order to evaluate electronic methods, telephone recall and tape recorded food records were obtained from 8- to 10-year-old children. The purpose was to decrease the respondent burden of multiple recalls or food record keeping.

Initially, face-to-face 24-hr recalls were conducted with each child-parent pair. The child was expected to contribute most of the information; parents provided missing data on brand names, preparation techniques, and ingredients. Children were instructed on procedures for documentation, use of food models as techniques for estimating portion sizes, and describing methods of preparation. Children's telephone recall and tape-recorded dietary records were then compared with parent's written records. Results indicated that preadolescent children are able to provide dietary intake data using electronic methods comparable to their parents' written records (48).

Other studies are testing the feasibility of collecting 24-hr dietary recalls on children using the Nutrient Data System Microversion developed by the Nutrition Coordinating Center (NCC) at the University of Minnesota (49). This system includes over 3,500 brand-name foods. It operates by way of 24-hr dietary recalls that are entered, via a programmed interview, directly onto a computer. Each interview is designed to solicit all necessary nutritional information, including recipe ingredients and brand names, to insure accurate and complete data information. Interviews last approximately 20 to 25 min. Present indications are that this method has many advantages for nutritional assessment.

SUMMARY OF ASSESSMENT METHODS

Assessment methods are essential tools for the health professional who must have information about a child's dietary intake. Most fall into two general groups. Those techniques that assess intake by recall, such as the 24-hr recall and food frequencies, are essentially retrospective; the subject has not been forewarned and has not modified behavior in anticipation. The second method involves ongoing record keeping. This method may elicit an increased awareness of eating behavior, such as time, place, and amount. Other techniques, such as diet histories, may be combinations of recall and record keeping.

Selection of a particular dietary assessment technique should be determined by the purpose for which it will be used. Some methods are essentially for individual evaluations, e.g., the 7-day record and dietary history; others are designed for appraisal of groups, such as the 24-hr dietary recall. Investigations into eating habits, food frequencies, or meal patterns may demand procedures other than energy and nutrient intake estimations.

There are special considerations when attempting dietary histories in children, including an awareness of possible rapid changes in eating habits and nutrient intake, variability in day-to-day intake, the limited ability of young children to cooperate or to recall food intake, and the need to decipher dietary information submitted by adults who may not be with the child the entire day. A skilled dietitian is a prerequisite.

Budget constraints are very important in the planning of epidemiological dietary studies. Some methods, such as the 24-hr recall, are quick and relatively inexpensive; others are time-consuming and, therefore, expensive, e.g., diet histories. Interview time is, however, only a minor part of the time needed for the collection and processing of dietary data. Depending on the complexity of the study, preparation of recall data for computer entry followed by the calculation and processing procedures, can vary from days to months. Methods of entering dietary information directly into the computer during the interview are being investigated.

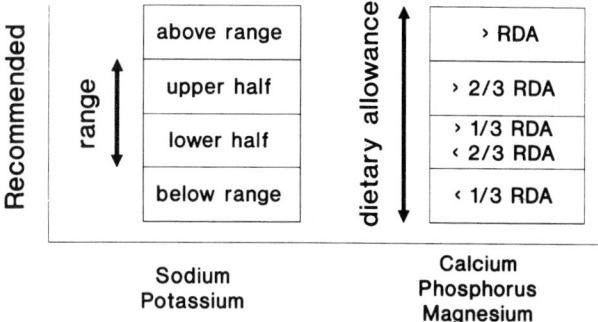

FIG. 4. Method for comparison of intake with recommended levels and ranges. The National Academy of Science's National Research Council provides the criteria for evaluating adequacy of intake.

INTERPRETATION

Once dietary nutrients have been determined, they are generally compared to some standard. The recommended dietary allowances (RDA) are the dietary standards in the United States. They prescribe levels of nutrient intake assumed to be both safe and sufficient for maintenance of good health. They also purport to take into account presumed individual variability in nutrient requirements.

There is a specific format for reporting adequacy of intakes for electrolytes and minerals using group data (Fig. 4). For determining the relationship to a range, intake is divided into the percentage of children within, below, or above the range. For establishing a relationship, intake is divided into the percentage of children less than or equal to one-third of the RDA, from one-third to two-thirds, and from two-thirds to the full RDA or greater than the RDA.

The Bogalusa Heart Study compared the electrolyte and mineral intake of study children with that of the RDA and the recommended range (Fig. 5). Results indicated that 60% to 80% of children exceeded the recommended range of sodium intake; 40% of teenagers were in the upper half of the range or higher. Intake of potassium was high in preschoolers; 60% to 70% exceeded the range. In 80% of the children who were 10 and older, however, intakes were at or below the range. The mean calcium intake appeared fairly stable. There was, however, a decrease in the percentage of teenagers exceeding

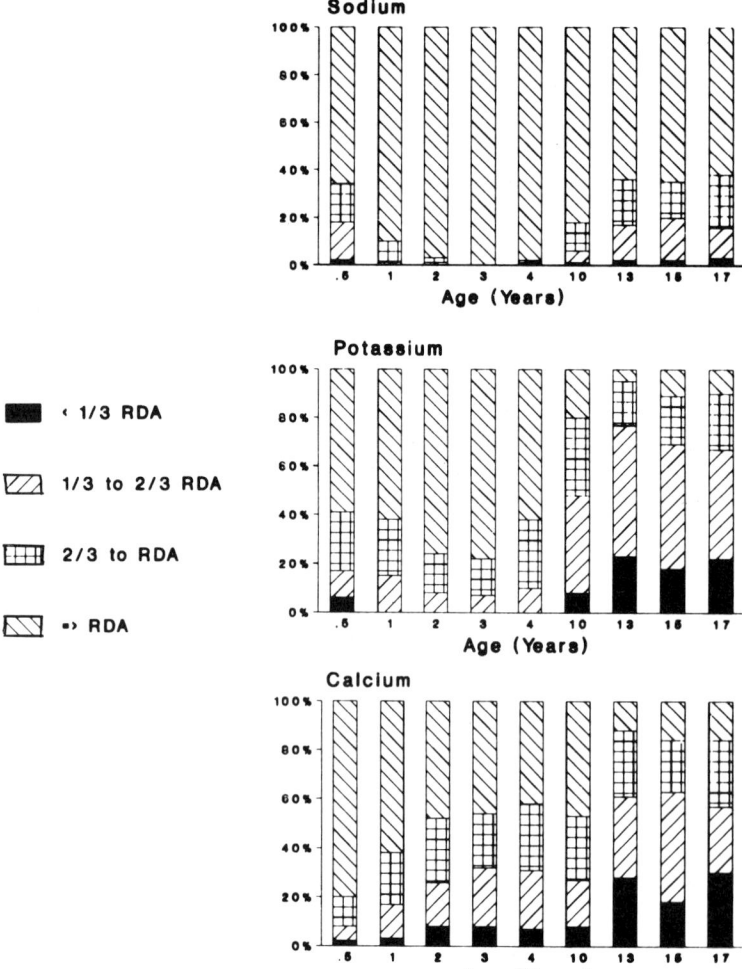

FIG. 5. Comparison of electrolyte intake with recommended dietary range. Bar graphs illustrate an exceptionally high sodium intake for all children, with approximately 65% exceeding the recommended range. In contrast, approximately 10% of adolescents exceeded the potassium recommended range and 20% the calcium RDA.

the calcium RDA: 50% to 60% of teenagers ingested two-thirds or less of the RDA for calcium.

The RDA is a useful tool for planning food allocation for population subgroups, for interpreting food consumption records of individuals and populations, and for developing strategies for nutrient intervention.

Although the RDA is most appropriately applied to groups, comparing an individual's intake to the RDA over a sufficient length of time provides an estimate of dietary adequacy. Identified deficiencies may be supplemented; excessive intakes, such as sodium, would lead to a complete dietary assessment in order to identify the foods that must be limited to reduce intake of the identified nutrient (51).

IMPLICATIONS

Understanding the strengths and limitations of the various dietary assessment methods is essential for the successful design and interpretation of dietary studies. Weaknesses can be diminished by improving standardization, refining probing tools, and more carefully training examiners. In addition, reliance on memory, which is often unreliable, is less preferable than a technique that allows ongoing assessment of intake.

DIETARY ASSESSMENT METHODS FOR CHILDREN

For more than 18 years, the Bogalusa Heart Study has collected dietary data in a biracial pediatric community. More than 3,000 24-hr dietary recalls have been analyzed to characterize the eating behavior of children and relate it to the eventual inception of heart disease (52).

The 24-hr recall method used in the Bogalusa study was especially adapted for use with children. Interviewers are carefully trained via a standardized protocol that specifies exact techniques for interviewing, recording, and calculating results. Quality controls, which improve both reliability and validity, include the following:

1. A standardized protocol, which enumerates the descriptive information to be recorded for each food, specifically (a) the name—common and/or brand; (b) the method of preparation—homemade, commercial, ready-to-eat, fried, baked, or casserole; and (c) the physical nature—color, shape, fresh, frozen, and unit size. Each food or recipe is clearly identified during the interview so that it can be assigned a proper identification number before nutritional analysis on the computer data base.
2. A snack-probing tool, the "Product Identification Notebook" (PIN), was developed to help children remember snack consumption. It groups snacks into five categories according to consistency and texture. Snacks are illustrated by pictures, product labels, or drawings, as well as labels, a color wheel, and a ruler for determining size. Each interview ends with a page-by-page review of the PIN to identify any food that may have been forgotten.
3. School lunch assessment: this information should (a) identify all school recipes and ingredients used during the 24-hr recall period, (b) determine average portions of each item on the menu, and (c) obtain measurements for each item served. With the increasing number of children eating school meals, breakfast and lunch may contribute over 56% of a child's total daily intake. Detailed school lunch information may therefore be useful in characterizing changes in children's eating behaviors (32).
4. Standardized graduated food models for quantification of foods and beverages consumed. These models are based on size, volume, or weight equivalents and do not depict specific foods.
5. A computerized nutrient data base for nutrient analysis. The Extended Table of Nutrient Values (ETNV), consisting of over 3,000 core foods and recipes, with values for 97 dietary components, is used for data analysis. Except for a slightly higher level of sucrose, nutrient content of the ETNV appears to be similar to other computerized data bases. Eight programs are available, including 24-hr recall calculations per day, per meal, and by snack period. Data can also be analyzed for the contribution of individual foods to each eating period, percentage conformity to the NRC Recommended Dietary Allowances (RDA), nutrient-to-calorie ratio, and sources, i.e., percentage of protein, fat, and carbohydrate. The advantage of the data bank is that it permits continuous updating of existing values as well as the ability to add new foods and recipes. In the case of the Bogalusa study, control over entries and nutrient calculations is maintained through strictly applied safeguards. Data are pooled to describe the mean intakes of groups of children.

EATING PATTERNS OF CHILDREN

Nutrition is one of the most important variables affecting serum lipids and lipoproteins (53). Successful deterrents to coronary artery disease and essential hypertension in adulthood may well be predicated on understanding, and changing, the nutritional habits of children. In the Bogalusa Heart Study, dietary data collected on children from infancy through adolescence help to characterize children's eating patterns and, potentially, may help in the design of appropriate intervention strategies.

GENERAL OBSERVATIONS: 2 TO 17 YEARS

The energy intake for all children, 2 to 17 years of age, exceeded the RDA. Carbohydrates provided approxi-

TABLE 4. Dietary composition of diets of young children and adolescents by age compared to current dietary recommendations: the Bogalusa Heart Study

Diet component	Age (yr)							Current dietary recommendations (after age 2)
	2	3	4	10	13	15	17	
Energy (Cal)	1,922	2,162	2,258	2,144	2,361	2,334	2,438	
Protein (% Cal)	13	12	13	13	13	14	14	15%
Carbohydrate (% Cal)	48	51	49	49	47	50	46	55%
Fat (% Cal)	41	38	39	39	41	38	40	30%
Saturated fat (% Cal)	16	14	14	15	15	13	14	10%
Cholesterol (mg/1,000 Cal)	193	164	172	138	129	146	151	100 mg/1000 Cal (not to exceed 300 mg/day)

mately 48% to 55% of total energy intake; the percent contributed by sucrose exceeded the recommended level of <10%. Although the mean percent of energy from protein, about 13%, approached the recommended level at all ages, there was an increased saturated fat intake of 14% to 16%, with 5% to 7% of total energy from polyunsaturated fat and 14% to 15% of total energy from monounsaturated fat (Table 4).

Preschoolers: 2 to 4 Years

Mean dietary cholesterol intake per 1,000 Cal was 193 mg at 2 years, decreasing slightly to 172 mg at 4 years of age. Dietary cholesterol averaged 24 mg/kg body weight for preschoolers, compared with 10 mg/kg body weight for 10-year-old children (30). In addition, the mean percent of energy from total fat exceeded the 30% recommendation at 2 years (41%), 3 years (38%), and 4 years of age (39%).

Children: 10 to 17 Years

School-age children in Bogalusa ate a typical adult American diet, characterized by high intakes of sodium, refined carbohydrates, animal protein, and animal fat, with low intakes of potassium, complex carbohydrates, vegetable protein, and vegetable fat (30).

Mean energy intake ranged from 2,144 cal at age 10 to 2,438 cal at age 17, with boys consuming more calories than girls. Thirty-nine percent to 41% of the total calories were from fat. The fatty acid composition during this period was consistent for saturated fat (14% to 16%), polyunsaturated fat (5% to 7%), and monounsaturated fat (14% to 15%). Dietary cholesterol intake increased from age 10 (302 mg) to age 17 (378 mg) and exceeded 100 mg/1,000 Cal at each age. The mean protein density of the diet remained consistent at 13% to 14% of calories; protein was mainly from animal sources. Half of the total energy intake came from carbohydrate. The sucrose-to-starch ratio, reflecting a high sucrose intake, was greater than one. Sodium intake ranged from 3.4 to 3.7 g for children in this age group.

COMPARISON WITH OTHER SURVEYS

The macronutrient intakes of Bogalusa male children, 2 to 17 years of age, have been found comparable with data reported in the second Health and Nutrition Examination Survey, a major national study (Figs. 6 and 7) (52,54).

MEAL PATTERNS

For children 2 to 4 years of age, snacks provided a significant proportion of energy, mainly from carbohydrates, whereas breakfast, lunch, and dinner each provided approximately 16%, 22%, and 23%, respectively, of the energy intake (Fig. 8). In children from 10 to 17 years of age, breakfast contributed approximately 15% of energy, whereas more than 50% of energy was derived from dinner and snacks.

Most school-age children being studied ate school

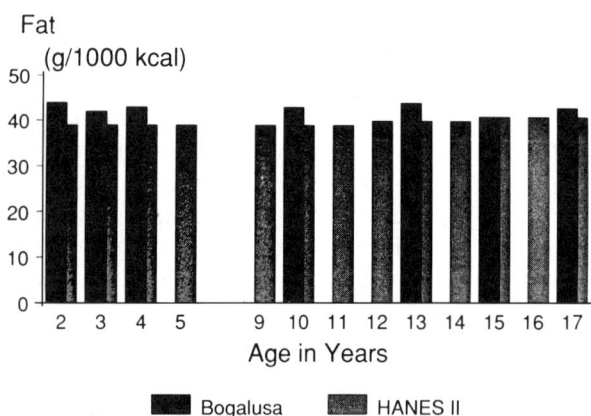

FIG. 6. Mean intakes of fat of school-age boys in the Bogalusa study and the Second Health and Nutrition Examination Survey (HANES II).

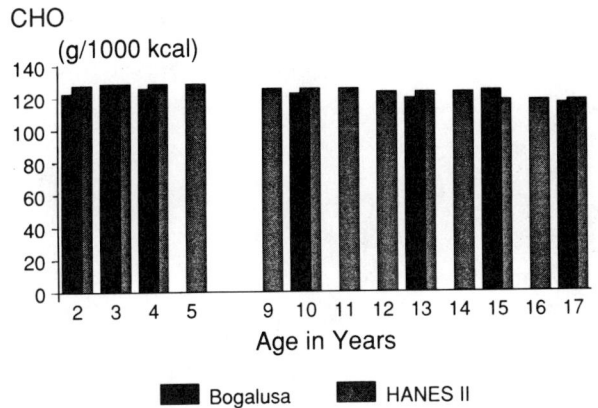

FIG. 7. Mean intakes of cholesterol of school-age boys in the Bogalusa study and the Second Health and Nutrition Examination Survey (HANES II).

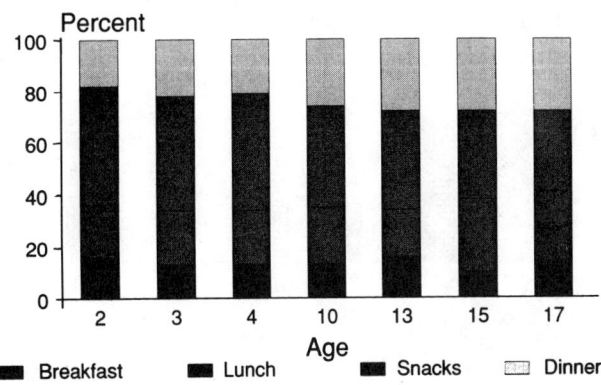

FIG. 9. Percentage of 24-hr total carbohydrate intake by meal and snack periods for children at various ages who were included in the Bogalusa Heart Study.

lunches. About 22% of total calories, 20% of total fat, 22% of protein (Fig. 8), 33% of sodium, and 20% of carbohydrate intake came from this meal (55) (Fig. 9). As children became independent, snack foods and fast food outlets accounted for a greater part of the energy intake.

FOOD SOURCES

The Bogalusa Heart Study demonstrated that the percent of total energy intake from meats increased from 14% at 2 years of age to 26% by age 17. By age 17, energy from dairy products fell, from 16% at age 2, to 12%. Vegetables, on the other hand, contributed 5% to 8% at all ages. Fruits contributed 6% of energy intake at 2 years of age and 4% at age 17. The major sources of total fat and saturated fat in rank order for preschool and school-age children were beef, milk, pork, and desserts (Fig. 10). There was a decrease in percent total fat coming from poultry and an increase in fat contribution by pork from age 2 to age 17. From ages 2 to 17, percent of cholesterol intake from the major food sources derivatives changed from milk (18% to 11%) and eggs (45% to 24%) to beef (7% to 19%). Processed breads contributed approximately one-third of the total sodium intake in school-age children; vegetables contributed approximately 19%, essentially from preservatives added to canned vegetables or as a result of salting during food preparation. The percentage of sodium ingested from processed meats increased with age (57).

Sucrose intake from fruits decreased slightly from 2 years (12%) to 17 years of age (11%); during the same period, the percent of sucrose intake from beverages increased from 22% to 30% (56).

COMPARISON WITH CURRENT DIETARY RECOMMENDATIONS

Approximately 80% to 90% of all children studied had dietary intakes of total fat greater than 30% of total energy (Fig. 11). In 80% to 94% of the children saturated fat intakes were greater than 10% of energy. The percentage with cholesterol intakes greater than 100 mg/1,000 Cal ranged from 65% to 76% (58).

SECULAR TRENDS IN DIETARY INTAKE: 1973–1985

Five groups of 10-year-old children were examined over 12 years to study changing trends in dietary intakes. Means were calculated annually for energy, macronutrients, cholesterol, and fatty acid intakes (Figs. 12 and 13) (13,23).

Total energy intakes were lower in 1981–82 than in 1976–77. No racial differences were demonstrated; boys had higher intake than girls from 1973 to 1982. Calories per kg of body weight were significantly lower, overall, in 1981–82 than previous years. Mean total protein intakes ranged from 67.4 g (1981–82) to 79.8 g (1976–77). Mean

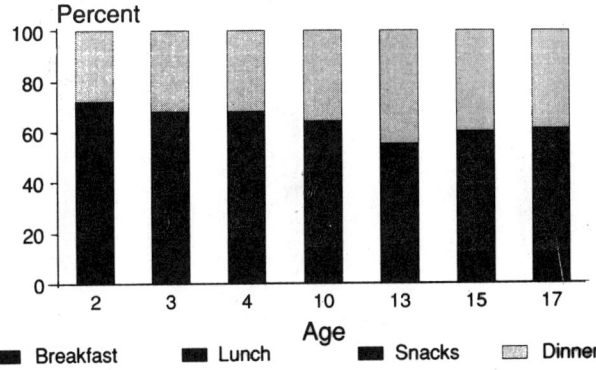

FIG. 8. Percentage of 24-hr total protein intake by meal and snack periods for children at various ages who were included in the Bogalusa Heart Study.

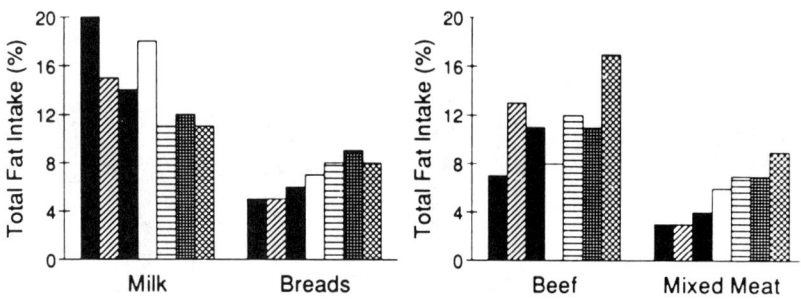
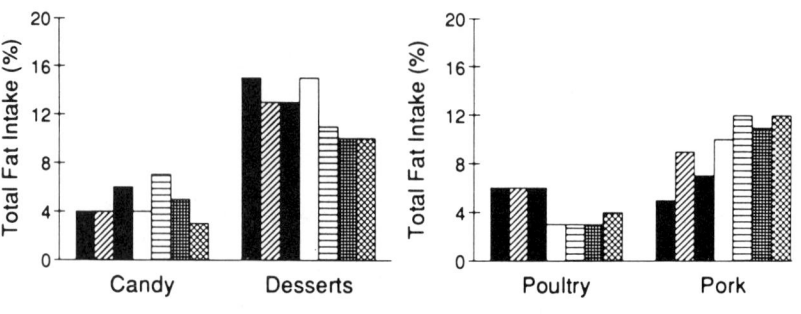
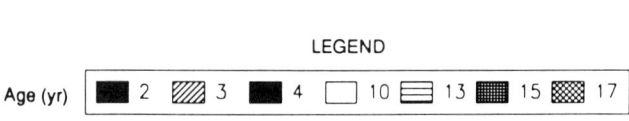

FIG. 10. Contribution of total fat intake to the diet by various food groups, as reported in the Bogalusa Heart Study.

carbohydrate intake tended to increase from 1976–77 to 1984–85.

Mean daily fat intake declined during the decade, ranging from 98 g in the 1970s to 87 g in 1984–85. There were no differences in fat intake per 1,000 Cal, but intakes per kilogram of body weight were lower in 1981–85 than in 1973–79. A shift was noted toward higher values in the polyunsaturated/saturated fat (P/S) ratio (0.31 to 0.48) from 1973 to 1985; however, the percent of calories from fat did not change during this period. This decrease in saturated fat intake and increase in polyunsaturated fat is most likely a result of an industry shift in fat-oil products.

Dietary cholesterol intake decreased from 324 mg to 256 mg between 1973 and 1985. No secular trend was noted in dietary intake of selected electrolytes and minerals. Sodium intake ranged from 3.3 to 3.7 g from 1973 to 1982, with sodium intake per 1,000 Cal only slightly higher in 1978 to 1984 (1.7 g) than reported in earlier years (1973–1977).

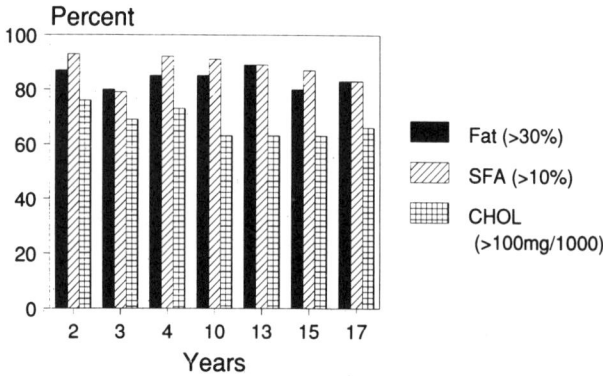

FIG. 11. The percent of children exceeding the American Heart Association's dietary recommendations. CHOL, cholesterol; SFA, saturated fatty acid.

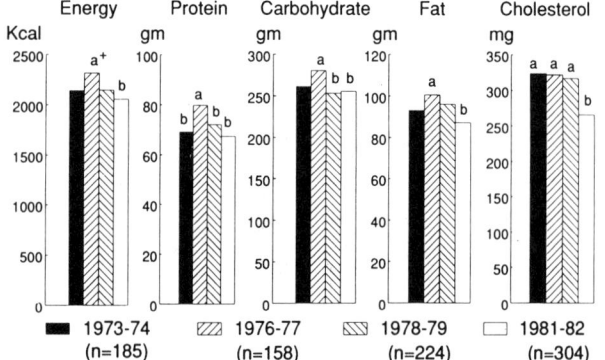

FIG. 12. Mean intakes of selected dietary components in four surveys of 10-year-olds, 1973 to 1982. +, For all comparisons, a > b, p < 0.05.

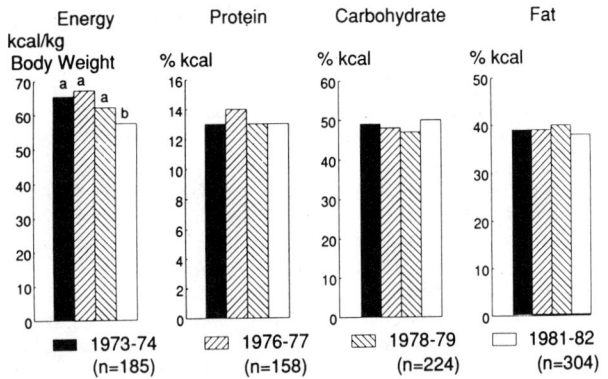

FIG. 13. Mean intakes of selected dietary components in four surveys of 10-year-olds, 1973 to 1982. $^+$ For all comparisons, a > b, p < 0.05.

SUMMARY

Diet plays a major role in chronic health problems. Studies which have described eating patterns and nutrient intakes of children have equated these findings to health status. Such observations provide the rationale for development of healthy eating habits early in life and for programs that promote such habits. Success of such programs will have a major impact on the population's overall morbidity and mortality.

ACKNOWLEDGMENTS

Thanks must be extended to the parents, teachers and particularly the children of Bogalusa for their cooperation and support over the years. Appreciation is also extended to Margaret C. Moore for the development and maintanence of the ETNV. A special thanks is given to Dr. Gerald S. Berenson, director of the Bogalusa Heart Study for the past 19 years.

REFERENCES

1. Frank GC, Farris RP, Cresanta JL, Nicklas TA. Dietary intake as a determinant of cardiovascular risk factor variables. Part A—Observations in a pediatric population. In: Berenson GS, ed. *Causation of cardiovascular risk factors in children. Perspectives on cardiovascular risk in early life.* New York: Raven Press, 1986;254–291.
2. Laskarzewski P, Morrison JA, Khoury P, Kelly K, Glatfelter L, Larsen R, Glueck CJ. Parent-child nutrient intake interrelationships in school children ages 6 to 19: The Princeton School District Study. *Am J Clin Nutr* 1980;33:371–380.
3. Grundy SM, Bilheimer D, Blackburn H, et al. AHA committee report: rationale of the diet-heart statement of the American Heart Association. *Circulation* 1982;65:839A–854A.
4. Healthy People 2000. National health promotion and disease prevention objectives. U.S. Department of Health and Human Services. Public Health Service. DHHS publication no. (PHS) 91-50213. U.S. government printing office, Washington, D.C., 1990.
5. Beaton GH, Milner J, Corey P, et al. Sources of variance in 24-hour dietary recall data: implications for nutrition study design and interpretation. *Am J Clin Nutr* 1979;32:2546–2559.
6. Liu K, Stamler J, Dyer A, McKeever J, McKeever P. Statistical methods to assess and minimize the role of intra-individual variability in obscuring the relationship between dietary lipids and serum cholesterol. *J Chronic Dis* 1978;31:399–418.
7. Gordon T, Fisher M, Rifkind BM. Some difficulties inherent in the interpretation of dietary data from free-living populations. *Am J Clin Nutr* 1984;39:152–156.
8. Medlin C, Skinner JD. Individual dietary intake methodology: a 5-year review of progress. *J Am Diet Assoc* 1988;88:1250–1254.
9. Baranowski T, Dworkin R, Henske JC, Clearman DR, Dunn JK, Nader PR, Hooks PC. The accuracy of children's self-reports of diet: Family Health Project. *J Am Diet Assoc* 1986;10:1381–1385.
10. Emmons L, Hayes M. Accuracy of 24-hour recalls of young children. *J Am Diet Assoc* 1973;62:409–415.
11. Dwyer JT, Kroll EA. The problem of memory in nutritional epidemiology research. *J Am Diet Assoc* 1987;87(11):1509–1512.
12. Klesges RC, Klesges LM, Brown G, Frank GC. Validation of the 24-hour dietary recall in preschool children. *J Am Diet Assoc* 1987;87:1383.
13. Frank GC, Berenson GS, Schilling PE, Moore MC. Adapting the 24-hour recall for epidemiologic studies of school children. *J Am Diet Assoc* 1977;71:26–30.
14. Eppright ES, Patton MB, Marlatt AL, et al. Dietary study methods. V. Some studies in collecting dietary information about groups of children. *J Am Diet Assoc* 1952;28:43–48.
15. Block G. A review of validations of dietary assessment methods. *Am J Epidemiol* 1982;115(4):492–505.
16. Sorenson AW. Assessment of nutrition in epidemiologic studies. In: Schottenfeld D, Fraumeni JF Jr, eds. *Cancer epidemiology and prevention.* Philadelphia: WB Saunders, 1982;434–474.
17. Park YK, Yetley EA. Trend changes in use and current intakes of tropical oils in the United States. *Am J Clin Nutr* 1990;51:738–748.
18. Stephen AM, Wald NJ. Trends in individual consumption of dietary fat in the United States 1920–1984. *Am J Clin Nutr* 1990;52:457–469.
19. Committee on Diet and Health; Food and Nutrition Board, Commission on Life Sciences, National Research Council. Dietary intake and nutritional status: trends in assessment. In: *Diet and health. Implications for reducing chronic disease risk.* Washington, DC: National Academy Press, 1989;3:41–84.
20. Raper NR, Marston RM. Levels and sources of fat in the U.S. food supply. In: Ip C, Birt DF, Rogers AE, Mettlin C, eds. *Dietary fat and cancer.* New York: Alan R Liss, 1988.
21. Human Nutrition Information Service, U.S. Dept. of Agriculture. *Nationwide Food Consumption Survey. Continuing Survey of Food Intakes by Individuals (CSFII).* NFCS report #86-3. Washington, DC: U.S. Government Printing Office, 1987;182.
22. Friend BL, Page L, Marston R. Food consumption patterns in the United States: 1909–13 to 1976. In: Levy R, Rifkind BL, eds. *Nutrition, lipids and heart disease.* New York: Raven Press, 1979;489–522.
23. Webber LS, Nicklas TA, Farris RP, Berenson GS. Secular trends in dietary intake of 10-year-old children 1973–1975. Presented at the 73rd Annual American Dietetic Association Meeting. Oct. 16, 1990. *J Am Diet Assoc* 1990;90(suppl 9):32.
24. Hankin JH, Huenemann R. A short dietary method for epidemiologic studies. I. Developing standard methods for interpreting seven-day measured food records. *J Am Diet Assoc* 1967;50:487–492.
25. Endozien JC, Bazzarre T. 1978 Guidebook for inclusion of dietary and anthropometric parameters in cancer epidemiology studies. School of Public Health, University of North Carolina, NCI Contract NO 1-CP-75880, 1978.
26. Sempos CT, Johnson NE, Smith EL, Gilligan C. Effect of intraindividual and interindividual variation in repeated dietary records. *Am J Epidemiol* 1985;121(1):120–130.
27. Chalmers FW, Clayton MM, Gates LO, et al. The dietary record. How many and which days? *J Am Diet Assoc* 1952;28:711–717.
28. Morgan RW, Jain M, Miller AB, et al. A comparison of dietary recall methods in epidemiologic studies. *Am J Epidemiol* 1978;107:488–498.

29. Persson LA, Carlgren G. Measuring children's diets: evaluation of dietary assessment techniques in infancy and childhood. *Int J Epidemiol* 1984;13(4):506–517.
30. Frank GC, Webber LS, Farris RP, Berenson GS, eds. *Dietary data book: quantifying dietary intakes of infants, children and adolescents—The Bogalusa Heart Study, 1973–1983.* New Orleans: Louisiana State University Medical Center, 1986.
31. Eck LH, Klesges RC, Hanson CL. Recall of a child's intake from one meal: are parents accurate? *J Am Diet Assoc* 1989;6:784–789.
32. Nicklas TA, Forcier JE, Webber LS, Berenson GS. School lunch assessment as part of a 24-hour dietary recall in children. *J Am Diet Assoc* 1991;6:711–713.
33. Willett WC, Sampson L, Stampfer MJ, Rosner B, Bain C, Witschi J, Hennekens CH, Speizer FE. Reproducibility and validity of a semiquantitative food frequency questionnaire. *Am J Epidemiol* 1985;122:51–65.
34. Burke BS. The dietary history as a tool in research. *J Am Diet Assoc* 1947;23:1014–1046.
35. Beal VA. The nutritional history in longitudinal research. *J Am Diet Assoc* 1967;51:426–432.
36. Hoover LW. Computers in dietetics: state-of-the-art. *J Am Diet Assoc* 1976;68:39–42.
37. Youngwirth J. The evolution of computers in dietetics: a review. *J Am Diet Assoc* 1983;82:62–67.
38. Hayes DB, Abraham S, Caceres CA. Computers in epidemiologic dietary studies. *J Am Diet Assoc* 1964;44:456–460.
39. Caster WO. Use of a digital computer in the study of eating habit patterns. *Am J Clin Nutr* 1962;10:98–106.
40. Williams CS, Burnet LW. Future applications of the microcomputer in dietetics. *Hum Nutr Appl Nutr* 1984;38(2):99–109.
41. McMurray P, Hoover LW. The educational use of computers: hardware, software, and strategies. *J Nutr* 1984;16(2):39–42.
42. Hoover LW. Computerized nutrient data bases: 1. Comparison of nutrient analysis systems. *J Am Diet Assoc* 1983;82(5):501–505.
43. Taylor M, Kozlowski BW, Baer MT. Energy and nutrient values from different computerized data bases. *J Am Diet Assoc* 1985;85(9):1126–1138.
44. Shanklia MS, Endves JM, Sawicki M. A comparative study of two nutrient data bases. *J Am Diet Assoc* 1985;85(3):308–313.
45. Yarde EB, Nicklas TA, Farris RP, Webber LS, Berenson GS. Nutrient comparison of foods and recipes using three computerized nutrient data bases. American Dietetic Association, 71st Annual Meeting, San Francisco, CA, 1988.
46. Hoover LW, Perloff BP. Computerized nutrient data bases: development of model for appraisal of nutrient data base system capabilities. *J Am Diet Assoc* 1983;82(5):506–508.
47. Hoover LW, Perloff BP. *Model for review of nutrient data base system capabilities.* Columbia, MO: University of Missouri, 1984;9.
48. VanHorn L, Gernhofer N, Moaq-Stahlberg A, Farris RP, et al. Dietary assessment in children using electronic methods: telephones and tape recorders. *J Am Diet Assoc* 1990;90(3):412–416.
49. Nicklas TA, Reed DB, Rupp J, Snyder P, et al. The potential of school lunch program in effecting nutrient changes in school meals. Presented at the 73rd Annual American Dietetic Assoc. Mtg. Oct. 16, 1990. *J Am Diet Assoc* 1990;90(suppl 9):39.
50. National Research Council. *Recommended dietary allowances,* 10th ed. Washington, DC: National Academy Press, 1989;285.
51. Nicklas TA, Farris RP, Srinivasan SR, Webber LS, Berenson GS. Nutritional studies in children and implications for change: The Bogalusa Heart Study. *J Adv Med* 1989;2(3):451–474.
52. Berenson GS, Strong WB, Williams C, Haley NJ, Mancini M, Nicklas TA, Spark A, Okuni M, Srinivasan SR, Tamir D, Walter H, Webber LS. Coronary artery disease prevention: cholesterol, a pediatric perspective. An American Health Foundation Monograph, Wynder EL, Barone J, Horn C, eds. *Prev Med* 1989;18(3):323–409.
53. Carroll MD, Abraham S, Dresser CM. *Dietary intake source data: United States 1976–1980.* US Department Health and Human Statistics. DHEW Publication No (PHS) 83-1681 (Vital and health statistics, series 11, no 231). Washington, DC: Government Printing Office, 1983;1–483.
54. Farris RP, Nicklas TA, Webber LS, Berenson GS. Impact of school lunch program on dietary intakes of 10-year-old children. *J Sch Health* (in press).
55. Nicklas TA, Farris RP, Johnson CC, Webber LS, Berenson GS, eds. *Food sources of nutrients: a tool for dietary management and health—The Bogalusa Heart Study, 1973–1983.* New Orleans: Louisiana State University Medical Center, Library of Congress Publication TXU 465-795, 1990.
56. Berenson GS, Srinivasan SR, Nicklas TA, Johnson CC. Prevention of adult disease beginning in the pediatric age. Chapter 2. In: Frohlich E, ed. *Cardiovascular clinics: preventive aspects of coronary heart disease.* F. A. Davis, Philadelphia: 1990;21–45.
57. Farris RP, Cresanta JL, Frank GC, Webber LS, Berenson GS. Dietary studies of children from a biracial population: intakes of fat and fatty acids in 10- and 13-year-old children. *Am J Clin Nutr* 1984;39:114–128.
58. Nicklas TA, Webber LS, Srinivasan SR, Berenson GS. Secular trends in dietary intakes and cardiovascular risk factors of 10-year-old children. *The Bogalusa Heart Study, 1973–1988.* (Submitted).

CHAPTER 45

Nutritional Surveillance and Supplemental Food Programs in the United States

David M. Paige

Nutritional assessments have critical medical, social, economic, and public health importance. Awareness of this has resulted in an increased number of programs for monitoring nutritional status and dietary practices at the local, state, national, and international level. These studies provide the basis for more accurate descriptions of the nutritional status of a population as well as helping to identify populations at risk for nutrition-related diseases. The ultimate advantage is more appropriately designed intervention strategies with better-targeted resources and better-developed tools for tracking morbidity, for evaluating and modifying programs, for long-term monitoring of health and nutrition indices, and for designing effective programs in public education (1).

NUTRITIONAL SURVEILLANCE

Nutritional surveillance has its roots in the more familiar area of disease surveillance. Recommendations from the World Food Conference of 1974 include "a global nutritional surveillance system . . . to monitor the food and nutrition conditions of populations at risk, and to provide a method of rapid and permanent assessment of all factors which influence food consumption patterns and nutritional status" (2).

Nutritional surveillance is predicated on regular, long-term rather than one-time, data collection. Household surveys are only included when they form part of the regular data collection or are designed to amplify other findings. Other single studies are not considered to be surveillance.

Data from nutritional surveillance studies are collected and analyzed for the specific purpose of decision-making in nutrition-related programs. Therefore, data must pertain to, and be interpretable for, the intended purpose. In addition, institutional links should exist between the agencies responsible for surveillance and those that determine policy.

The difference between nutritional surveillance and nutritional screening is that screening identifies individuals at risk and surveillance determines status and necessary intervention at the community, regional, national, or international level. Data collected in screening programs may be used, however, for surveillance (3).

Nutritional surveillance can be based on simple measurements such as height, weight, hemoglobin, and hematocrit obtained, often as part of routine procedures, at nutrition and health care facilities. These measurements provide relatively inexpensive monitoring of nutrition-related health problems and behavioral risk factors in designated populations (4,5). Rapid analysis permits the possibility of faster intervention, both individually and on a larger scale (6).

Surveillance methods are, however, limited. The self-selected or convenience sample of individuals in a surveillance system prevents the interpretation of these data as representative of the community at large. Multiple collection points make measurement standardization and quality control more difficult than in rigorously controlled surveys (5). In addition, project implementation must be distinguished from the effects of this implementation. Although a program may have an impact on a population, it must be determined whether some, or all, changes may have occurred irrespective of the intervention (6).

D. M. Paige: Departments of Maternal and Child Health, The Johns Hopkins University School of Public Health, Baltimore, Maryland 21205.

Surveillance Objectives

Nutritional surveillance activities may be classified as follows (3):

1. *Monitoring national and regional indicators of nutrition status.* This consists of monitoring nutritional status and trends, often within a particular socioeconomic or geographical subgroup, for planning policies and programs, and predicting future trends, often at a national level. Because collection and collation of data take considerable time, effect on policy is relatively slow. The value of an indicator may be defined by its sensitivity—the proportion of those with the condition that are actually classified as having the condition, and specificity—those without the condition who are appropriately categorized (7).
2. *Evaluating specific nutritional programs.* Changes in nutritional indicators are monitored during implementation of a specific program. The resulting information helps to redesign programs for better effectiveness. Data for program evaluation are relatively circumscribed and may be limited to anticipated outcomes and/or to program recipients. Response is more immediate than at the national or regional planning level.
3. *Predicting food consumption inadequacy for early intervention.* Data are used to prevent, or mitigate, short-term worsening of nutritional status in vulnerable populations. Information is not designed to evaluate chronic inadequacies of food consumption or malnutrition. Rather, a reliable indicator is provided for predicting potential, acute problems, so that rapid, short-term interventions can be mobilized, in advance.

SURVEYS

Nutrition surveys, in contrast to nutritional surveillances, provide a valid, statistical estimate of the prevalence of nutrition-related health problems or risk factors in a study population at a single point in time. When studies employ standardized, comparable methods, findings can be compared to define trends (8–11).

It is essential that surveys are conducted by well-trained, supervised, interviewers; assessment methods and equipment must be standardized and controlled. Data may be collected in specially equipped mobile vans or through house-to-house interviews (12,13). Recent surveys have used random-digit dial telephone methods, an advantage in terms of speed and cost (6).

Surveys are generally more comprehensive in terms of scope and sophistication. The cost of field surveys is high, however, and the analysis and reporting of findings can take several years to complete (6).

METHODS OF ASSESSMENT

Nutritional assessment methods include anthropometric measurements, clinical evaluation, laboratory assessment, and dietary evaluation. Each method has strengths and limitations; no single measure provides a comprehensive assessment of nutritional health. Selection of a specific indicator is determined after assessing the specific characteristics of each method and the needs of the intended study (14).

Sensitivity and Specificity

Nutritional indicators may (a) predict future events; (b) reflect current status; or (c) follow a specific parameter, e.g., head circumference. Each test will also specify the point at which an individual is determined to be at risk, or to already have the condition of interest. No diagnostic measure can, however, precisely reflect the true absence or presence of a particular state; misclassifications will occur (15). For example, hemoglobin and hematocrit cutoff levels may fail to indicate a condition that actually exists. This misclassification is referred to as a false negative; the reverse, nonexistent problems described by a test are referred to as false positives. The ideal methods result in the least false positives or false negatives (16). Sensitivity and specificity of any indicator are inversely related. Factors that determine which is the more appropriate measures include field conditions, expense, level of staff training, precision of information needed, and intended use (Fig. 1) (16).

Anthropometry

Anthropometry is considered the most useful tool for assessing the nutritional status of children. Deficits in a

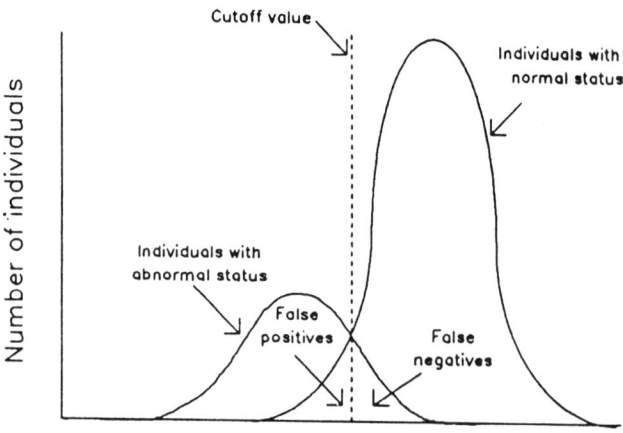

FIG. 1. Effect of applying a cutoff value for an indicator of nutritional status to the distributions of values for individuals with normal status and individuals with abnormal status.

child's growth generally reflects inadequate food intake, illness, and/or metabolic disorders.

Impaired growth is not, however, always the most sensitive indicator of inadequate nutrition. For example, a marginally inadequate energy intake may cause a reduction in physical activity before there is any discernible impairment of growth. Genetics is another unavoidable influence. Although these factors do not eliminate anthropometry's important role in nutritional assessment, they are important considerations in presentation, analysis, and interpretation of the data (16).

In addition, other tests, such as biochemical and immunological, are increasingly being used in clinical practice.

Interpretation of Anthropometric Data

The most commonly used anthropometric measurements are weight and height. An individual measurement has no meaning, however, unless it is related to another, e.g., weight compared to height or age. Combinations of measurements are referred to as indices.

Indices are necessary for grouping and interpreting measurements. For example, the relationship of weight to height may be expressed arithmetically, e.g., by the body mass index (BMI) or (Wt/Ht^2), or by relating the weight to that of a reference subject of the same height.

The indicator is often constructed from population indices and used to discern broader indications of health status. Thus the proportion of children below a certain level of weight-for-age may be used as an indicator of community status. Sometimes an index and an indicator may be the same. For example, the infant mortality rate is an index (ratio of deaths to births), but it is also used as an indicator of the state of public health (17).

Growth Charts

Because of the prevalent use of growth charts, it is important to distinguish between references and standards. A reference population suggests a pattern of growth to be used for comparative analysis. A standard, on the other hand, suggests the desired pattern of growth to be achieved. The latter approach is not appropriate for populations unrelated to the one from which the data is drawn.

Growth in a reference population, when cautiously used, may be helpful in assessing patterns of growth in diverse populations. In principle, it does not matter what set of reference data is used, provided that it is large enough to contain adequate statistical information and the population is reasonably healthy and appropriately nourished to avoid major distortions. It is also clearly desirable, for comparative purposes, that there be a common reference (18). The World Health Organization (WHO) has adopted the National Center for Health Statistics (NCHS) population growth pattern as a reference for international use (19).

Developing local standards of growth may be the most appropriate method to assess the adequacy of growth of an indigenous population. These may help governments identify the extremes of the distribution and design more effective intervention programs. Further, at-risk populations could be identified and support services designated to mitigate the possibility of more serious problems. Indigenous growth charts must, however, often separate data derived from a privileged socioeconomic elite, which may be anthropologically different from the indigenous populations. In addition, the international growth chart may be used, when appropriate, for reference and background comparison (15).

The NCHS–Centers for Disease Control (CDC)–WHO reference growth charts are drawn from different, dissimilar populations. Children under 2 years of age were part of the Fels Yellow Springs study. Data for the 2 to 6 years of age category are from the first Health and Nutrition Examination Survey, conducted between 1971 and 1974 (20). Length measurements in the former are longer than those in the NCHS population. The CDC is currently revising the growth curves in the under-2-years-of-age category, to reduce this discrepancy. These revisions will be available, on diskette, for analytical and research purposes. No changes will be made on growth charts because of the negligible effect on clinical tracking of individual children. A complete revision of the growth references will be made over the next several years, following the completion of the National Health and Nutrition Examination Survey (NHANES)–III (21).

Interpretation of Growth Patterns

Growth data may be presented in two ways: (a) by describing the population distribution, and (b) by providing an estimate of the number or proportion outside the reference distribution. The approaches are complementary and the analytical objective will determine which is preferred. An observed measurement may be related to the reference population in one of three ways: (a) its position within the percentile distribution of the reference, (b) as a standard deviation score (Z score), or (c) as a percentage of the reference median (17,18).

The population distribution may be represented in percentiles. Statistical methods, such as the chi-square test, can be used for comparing distributions. However, using percentiles for cutoff points has the disadvantage that the number at the extreme degrees of risk cannot be quantified, since percentiles below the 3rd or above the 97th cannot be defined from the reference population except by back-calculation from the standard deviations.

The presentation and statistical treatment of the numbers are the same, whether they represent Z scores or percentages of the reference median. The simplest description of the whole distribution is the mean Z score with the SD, or the mean percentage of the reference median with the SD. Standard statistical tests can be applied to these numbers.

It is in the choice of cutoffs that the difference between Z scores and percentage of the median becomes important. For example, on surveys of weight-for-height of children between 1 and 2 years old, 27% had Z scores of -2 or below, whereas only 15% were below 80% of the reference median. This discrepancy cannot be eliminated simply by adjusting one or the other cutoff, because the coefficient of measurement variation varies with age. By definition, Z-score cutoffs take this into account; percentage of the median cutoffs do not.

Velocity of Growth

Weight and height velocities are calculated from serial measurements. The significance of a change depends on the time over which that change is observed; different time intervals will, however, be appropriate for different situations. Appropriateness of time intervals will depend on different factors, including the age of the children, whether weight or height is being observed, and whether the process being studied is of short or long duration. A reduction in velocity is an earlier and more sensitive index of growth failure than a deficit in attained weight or height. Yet it is uncertain when the degree or duration of this growth failure has importance to the child's wellbeing (17).

Because of their sensitivity, measurements of velocity can show significant differences in quite a small sample. At present, there is no completely satisfactory reference for measurements of growth velocity in young children. Since the NCHS reference is cross-sectional, the difference between weights or heights at two ages in any percentile column provides an estimate of the expected gain in a child who starts in that percentile, but there is no estimate of the variability of gain, so that no statistical significance can be attached to any deviation from the expected rate (20).

Clinical Examination

Clinical examination can reveal specific signs of malnutrition, as well as providing an overall index of the nutritional status of the patient. Family and medical histories are also important, providing important information on health status as well as environmental and psychosocial factors that may indicate the need for additional nutritional evaluation. It is important to note, however, that many nutritional deficiencies, in their early stages, may be recognized only by laboratory evaluation (17).

Laboratory Evaluation

The laboratory can be a valuable adjunct to the nutritional evaluation of a patient. Appropriate selection of laboratory assessments is dependent on a knowledge of the purpose of each test, the normal values in the laboratory being used, and knowledge of other potential causes for abnormalities aside from nutritional status. Generally, only the body fluids, blood, and urine are used for determinations. Tissue samples in the form of biopsies or hair samples are rarely used and are not readily available.

The concentration of an essential nutrient in a body fluid can be low as a result of dietary deficiency, poor absorption, impaired transport, abnormal utilization, or a combination of any of these. Laboratory testing does not differentiate between these; further clinical investigation, including dietary and medical history, may be necessary.

Most laboratory techniques for assessing nutritional status measure (a) the nutrient level in blood; (b) the urinary excretion rate of the nutrient; (c) urinary metabolites of the nutrient; (d) abnormal metabolic products in blood; (e) changes in blood components or enzyme activities that can be related to intakes of the nutrient; and (f) response to a load, saturation, and isotopic test (17).

The tests for different nutrients are not equally valuable. Accuracy and precision, i.e., the ability to reproduce a value and the closeness of any reported value to the truth, vary. For example, direct tests of water-soluble vitamins in the blood are more sensitive than indirect tests of the excretion of a metabolite in the urine. The precision of a test can be measured by determining the coefficient of variation, that is, the standard deviation of a series of identical samples expressed as a percentage of the mean value of the sample. The smaller the coefficient of variation, the greater the precision of the test.

Dietary Evaluation

Epidemiological studies of diet and disease require extensive information from large numbers of subjects, a fact that makes the ability to draw statistically accurate epidemiological associations at best difficult and often unachievable.

Studies of dietary intake have been used, for example, to estimate nutrient requirements. For this purpose, nutrient intake was measured in a population free of nutritional deficiency. In general, when such quantitative data are required, prospective studies are preferred because they provide more precise information as to what is actually consumed during the period of study. Retrospective techniques are subject to errors of recall. On the other hand, retrospective studies may be appropriate for estimating usual intake during extended periods of time; prospective studies provide data only for the actual day or days of study.

Common methods of investigation include the following (22):

1. *The dietary history,* also called the "Burke method," was designed "to measure the average intake of an individual during a considerable period of time." The interviewer asks the subject or his caretaker about usual eating patterns, time, type, and composition of meals consumed, as well as snack consumption. Quantity of individual food consumption is calculated from the number of servings per interval times estimated size of servings. These data are cross-checked by extended interviewing.

   The dietary history intentionally does not ask about actual food consumption on the day or days prior to the survey, but attempts to reconstruct the subject's usual eating habits. This method requires a cooperative, intelligent informant, a skilled dietitian, and a relatively lengthy interview. Its advantage is that it provides data on the subject's usual intake while not requiring multiple visits to contend with day-to-day variations. Unfortunately, bias is created because of the exclusion of many people who do not have, or cannot describe, a consistent eating pattern. Furthermore, as explained below, attempts to validate this method have yielded disappointing results (23).

2. *The dietary recall* method requires that the subject report all of the foods consumed during an immediately preceding, fixed period of time. Although some investigators have conducted recall histories covering periods as long as 1 week, most believe that data are not reliable beyond 24 to 48 hr. Interview techniques vary. Some begin with the previous day's breakfast, usually a simple and easily remembered meal, and work forward through the activities of the day. Others begin with the last meal of the previous day and work backward. Some ask initially about main meals then probe additional intake.

   Photos or models of foods may be used to aid in the estimation of portion sizes, or subjects may be asked to weigh the actual foods. Although the latter appears most reliable, such quantification might simply be an illusion of accuracy in the face of unreliable memory (24).

   The advantage of the recall history is that it provides semiquantitative information on real intake during a fixed period of time. The interview is relatively simple and brief. Successful completion of recall histories by telephone will probably be limited in applicability in poorer communities. The major drawback of this technique, and of others that study a relatively short period of time, is normal day-to-day diversity in intake. In fact, multiple interviews are probably necessary to provide a valid estimate of an individual's "usual" intake (25).

3. *The dietary questionnaire* can be designed to elicit information similar either to the dietary history or to the recall history, or may only request information on the consumption of specific foods. The questionnaire is usually distributed by mail and is, therefore, very economical. There is, however, doubt about the validity of responses to any but the simplest types of questions, because of the problem of nonresponse, and because of the necessity that subjects be literate, a significant constraint in less-developed countries (26).

4. *The food-weighing technique* carried out by a trained observer is probably the most reliable method for determining the precise amounts of foods and nutrients consumed during the period of observation and is the standard against which other methods are generally evaluated. This method involves weighing all raw food ingredients that are either directly consumed or included in recipes. In the case of recipes ("menu items") composed of several food items, the final weight of the menu item minus plate waste is expressed as a proportion of the entire menu item so that the amounts of individual food items consumed can be calculated (27).

   Food-weighing studies of infants and young children pose special problems, however. Since children's feeding times often do not conform to a strict schedule, continuous observation must be maintained during the day and, ideally, throughout the night. Because 24-hr observation is usually not feasible, though, studies of children often employ a combination of food-weighing during the day and recall history of foods consumed at night. In addition, the consumption of breast milk and its components must be estimated for breast-fed infants (28).

   The advantage of food-weighing studies is the ability to precisely calculate intake. Disadvantages include the need for multiple days of observation, the unknown observer effect, and the cost of equipment and personnel (29).

The food diary is similar to the food-weighing technique, with the subject or a caretaker, rather than an "outside" observer, doing the weighing and record keeping. Even among highly educated, well-motivated subjects, no more than 80% successfully complete their diaries, and compliance tends to diminish rapidly after several days of study (30).

Other specialized techniques include the collection of duplicate diets and the preparation of preweighed diets for home delivery. This technique is tedious and costly but provides extremely accurate information without having to use food-composition tables. Furthermore, the analysis is completed on food "as eaten," thus correcting for any changes in nutrient concentrations during cooking (31).

Because of the tremendous range in the types and amounts of foods consumed by healthy individuals, attempts to quantify dietary intake must be concerned not only with measurement accuracy, but also with the issues of inter- and intrasubject variability. Apart from real differences in dietary intakes among individuals, other potential sources of variation include the day of the week (e.g., weekdays versus weekends), other day-to-day variability, the season of the year, the physiological status of the subject (age, sex, illness, etc.), and the study instrument. The study of a single day's intake—even if perfectly accurate—is not sufficient to define the habitual, or average, intake. Further, the degree of variability differs according to the nutrient studied (32).

NATIONAL MONITORING AND SURVEILLANCE SYSTEMS

The National Nutrition Monitoring System

The National Nutrition Monitoring System and other data sources provide information on (a) the national food supply, (b) food distribution, (c) food consumption, (d) nutrient utilization, and (e) health outcome.

A model that updates dietary and nutritional status in the United States describes 19 data sources in relationship to behavioral, environmental, and social factors (Fig. 2) (33).

The United States Department of Agriculture is responsible for providing (a) food composition measurements and the national nutrient data bank, (b) food supply determinants, (c) nationwide food consumption surveys, and (d) continuing survey of food intakes by individuals.

The Department of Health and Human Services (DHHS), through the National Center for Health Statistics (NCHS), is currently carrying out the third National Health and Nutrition Examination Survey (NHANES), scheduled to be completed in the mid-1990s. Completed and available now are (a) NHANES I, conducted in 1971–74, and (b) NHANES II, conducted in 1976–80. These surveys provide the basis for the currently utilized growth reference charts for children over 2 years of age. In addition, more detailed analyses of the data is reported as the NHANES I Epidemiologic Follow-Up Study. The center has carried out a similar study of Hispanics in the United States in 1982–84, the Hispanic HANES. The NCHS also provides important information through its vital statistics report as well as its periodically conducted maternal and infant health survey (14). In addition, the National Health Interview Survey (NHIS) provides other health-related information.

NHANES III is the most extensive survey to date. Subjects include a nationally representative sample of 40,000 individuals. Children, older persons, African-Americans, and Mexican-Americans are oversampled. Follow-up data will be collected on a regular basis including active tracking of the population. Dietary information will be collected directly from the subject by 24-hr recall, except from children under 6 years of age, for whom it will be given by a caretaker, and children between 6 and 12 years, for whom it will be given by the child and a caretaker. Anthropometric, biochemical, and hematological measures will provide the core of information. Other measurements will include an x-ray scan of the femur for bone age, ECG, spirometry, ophthalmological evaluation, selected skin testing, blood pressure, gallstone study, and data on reproductive history. The final survey will include information for research and evaluation of nutritional status in the United States including nutrient deficiencies and toxicities, normative reference data, prevalence of overweight and obesity, and nutrition risk factors (34).

CDC Nutrition Surveillance

The Division of Nutrition of the Centers for Disease Control (CDC) conducts (a) a pediatric nutrition surveillance system, (b) a pregnancy nutrition surveillance system, and (c) a behavioral risk factors surveillance system.

Surveillance data relating to nutritional status in low-income populations are collected from two high-risk groups: children and pregnant women. Demographic and birth weight data, as well as heights, weights, hematocrits, and hemoglobins, have been collected on children in public health clinics by the CDC Pediatric Nutrition Surveillance System since 1974. With 36 states participating, state-specific prevalences and current trends in short stature, overweight, obesity, low hematocrit, and low hemoglobin are reported by age and ethnic group. Monthly, quarterly, and annual reports are issued to participating states. The rapid availability of data specific to individual localities, and the capacity to identify individuals with abnormal values, make nutrition surveillance a useful resource for evaluation and planning. Aggregated data are reported annually (33).

The CDC Pregnancy Nutrition Surveillance System has, since 1979, collected similar information on pregnant women, in addition to birth outcome as it relates to smoking, vitamin and mineral intake, blood pressure and food stamp participation. Many of the 12 participating states, however, provide little data. State-specific

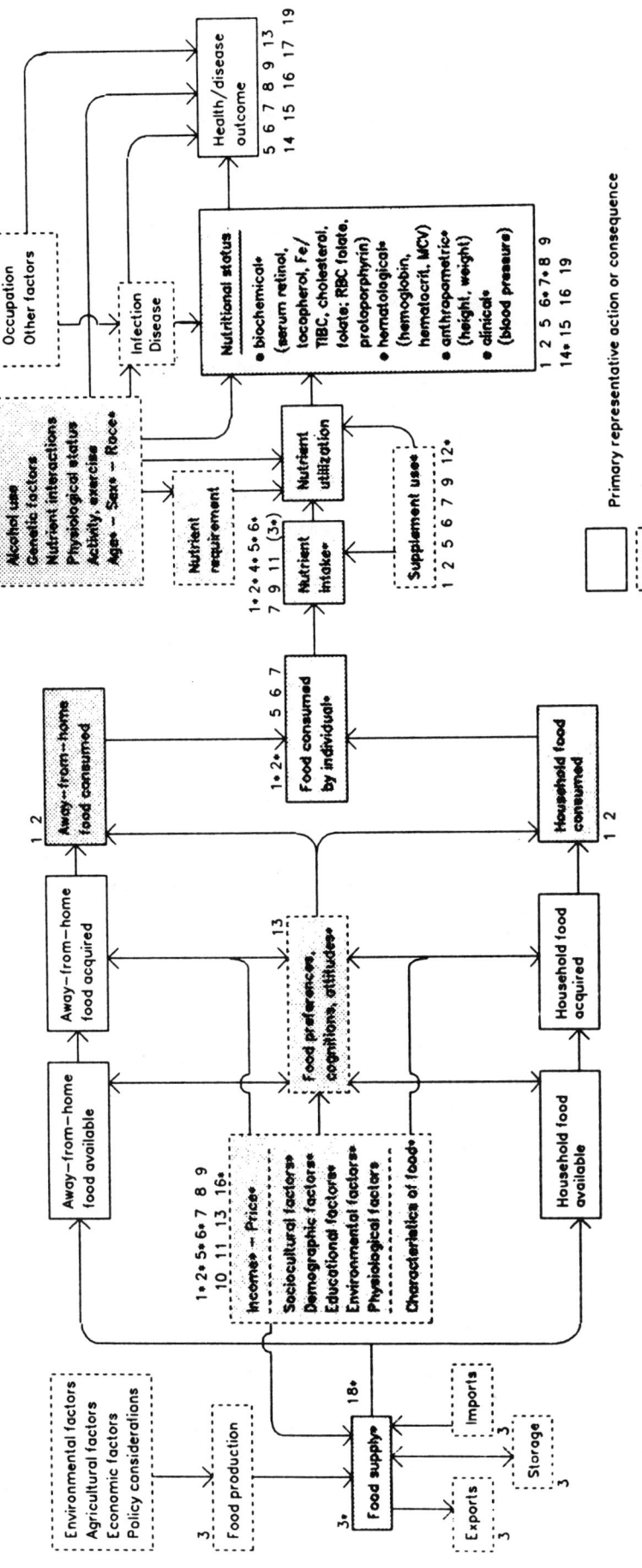

FIG. 2. A model of dietary and nutritional status in the United States in relationship to behavioral, environmental, and social factors and the information available from national nutrition monitoring systems and other data sources. (From ref. 33.) 1, continuing survey of food intakes by individuals; 2, nationwide food consumption survey; 3, U.S. food supply series; 4, national nutrient data bank; 5,6, national health and nutrition examination survey; 7, Hispanic health and nutrition examination survey; 8, NHANES I epidemiologic follow-up study; 9, national health interview survey; 10, food label and package survey; 11, total diet study; 12, vitamin mineral supplement intake survey; 13, health and diet study; 14, pediatric nutrition surveillance system; 15, pregnancy nutrition surveillance system; 16, behavioral risk factor surveillance system; 17, U.S. vital statistics; 18, alcohol epidemiologic data system; 19, national health examination survey.

prevalence and current trends in nutrition-related health problems during pregnancy and factors associated with low birth weight outcome are reported by age and ethnic group. Participating states receive a series of quarterly and cumulative quarterly reports.

Nationwide Food Consumption Survey

In addition to the dietary intake data from the NHANES surveys, from both a 24-hr recall and a food frequency, the United States Department of Agriculture (USDA) conducts a Nationwide Food Consumption Survey (NFCS). This is a survey of a cross-sectional sample of United States households and specific members of these households. Data include household food use, individual dietary intake, and demographic information related to food consumption. The two most recent NFCS surveys were completed in 1965–66 and 1977–78. Unlike the NHANES surveys, the NFCS does not collect nutritional status and health data, precluding analysis of nutritional status in relation to dietary intake.

No ongoing system for the surveillance of trends in dietary intake currently exists. However, the comparison of successive surveys of food consumption can provide some indication of trends in dietary practices.

Monitoring Behavioral Risk Factors

Behavioral risk factors that can affect nutrition and health are compiled via the NCHS National Health Interview Survey (NHIS), a nationwide sample survey that collects data through personal household interviews during an entire year. Information is collected on personal and demographic characteristics, behavioral health habits, illnesses, injuries, impairments, chronic conditions, and the utilization of health resources (6).

Another source for this data is the Behavioral Risk Factor Surveillance System (BRFSS), coordinated by CDC, and carried out in 35 states, plus the District of Columbia, during 1981–83. State-specific behavioral risk factor information related to the ten leading causes of death in the United States was collected using a standardized random-digit-dial telephone survey of adults (14,35). Behavioral risk factors surveyed included nutrition-related factors such as exercise and self-reported height and weight as well as alcohol consumption, smoking, stress, and seatbelt use.

These data sources have revealed a number of nutrition-related health problems of clinical, as well as, public health significance. Some of these health problems are related to undernutrition, especially in low-income populations and other high-risk groups. In recent years, however, the area of primary concern has been shifting from undernutrition to conditions related to nutritional excesses such as obesity, hypertension, and diabetes. These trends reflect the changing life-styles of the American population and have significant implications for directing the patient-education and intervention strategies of clinicians (6).

Nutrition Survey Results

The following subsections represent a brief review of the current knowledge of nutrition-related problems. They are problems which highlight the need for stronger interest in nutrition within the health care community.

Anemia

Iron deficiency anemia was prevalent in high-risk groups including young children, pregnant women, elderly men, and African-Americans in the 1971–74 NHANES I. It was associated with low income and low educational level of the head of the household (6,36).

The Pediatric and the Pregnancy Nutrition Surveillance Systems identified the same high-risk groups for anemia. Low-income children, ages 2 to 5 years, African-Americans, and pregnant women had higher prevalence of low hemoglobin and low hematocrit. Pregnant African-American women represented the most at-risk group. Data generally suggested a modest decline in the prevalence of low hematocrit and hemoglobin among white, African-American, and Hispanic children entering publicly supported health programs (37).

Growth Stunting

With the exception of children of Southeast Asian immigrants, African-American children under the age of 1 have the highest prevalence of decreased height-for-age in the Pediatric Nutrition Surveillance System. Linear growth of children of other ethnic groups in this age group were similar. Children with a history of low birth weight had a higher prevalence of growth stunting and of decreased weight-for-height, even at 2 to 4 years of age, in comparison to their normal birth weight counterparts (38,39).

In contrast to data for infants, African-American children in the CDC Pediatric Surveillance System have the *lowest prevalence* of short stature by 2 to 4 years of age, reflecting a more rapid rate of growth in early childhood. Growth stunting increases in prevalence with age among Hispanic and Native American children. Recent CDC data on stature of African-American children at school entrance in Washington, D.C., confirms the absence of growth stunting (40).

Low Birth Weight

Birth weight under 2,500 g is a standard indicator of poor pregnancy outcome. Low birth weight is associated with increased neonatal and infant mortality, poor growth, and increased rates of morbidity up to age 5 years. Data from the Pregnancy Nutrition Surveillance System have identified African-American women of all ages and women under the age of 20 years to be at a higher risk for delivering low birth weight infants. Pregnant women who smoked were at increased risk; they had nearly double the prevalence of low birth weight infants compared to nonsmoking pregnant women. The combination of smoking and being African-American placed a pregnant woman in one of the highest risk groups for poor pregnancy outcome.

Alcohol consumption, low prepregnancy weight, and low pregnancy weight gain have also been found to be contributing factors in low birth weight outcomes of pregnancy. For both alcohol and smoking during pregnancy, there is evidence of a dose-response effect.

Nutrient Deficiencies

Low intakes of nutrients including iron, calcium, vitamin B_6, and magnesium were documented in the 1977-78 NFCS survey. Females from adolescence through old age had deficient intakes of all four of these nutrients. Elderly men were at risk for low calcium intake and males of all ages were at risk for inadequate consumption of vitamin B_6.

Alcohol, Caffeine, Protein

High alcohol and caffeine consumption and low protein consumption may be additional risk factors.

Obesity

Obesity is related to significant morbidity and mortality in the United States population. In the NHANES I survey, adults had a high prevalence of being both obese (assessed by skin-fold thickness) and overweight (assessed by weight-for-height measurements). An increased prevalence with age was found beginning in the young adult years. Women, especially African-American women, were more likely to be obese than men at all ages. The CDC Pediatric Nutrition Surveillance System reported that Hispanic and Native American children had higher prevalences of obesity than other ethnic groups except in infancy. Trends show a modest decline in the prevalence of overweight for all ethnic groups under age 2 years. In contrast, no consistent pattern of change was observed in the 2 to 5 year age group.

Hypertension

Hypertension is a major health problem associated with heart disease and stroke. As in previous NCHS surveys, elevated blood pressure increased with age in the NHANES II survey population. Based on self-reports of blood pressure control, the BRFSS survey found a similar increase with age. A strong, consistent relationship existed between obesity and elevated blood pressure. Alcohol was also associated with elevated blood pressure. High-risk groups for hypertension include all adults, especially males, African-Americans, and obese or overweight women.

Sedentary Life-Styles

The lack of regular physical activity contributes to obesity and overweight and increases the risk for coronary heart disease. It also increases the risk for osteoporosis. The BRFSS found that men, more than women, increased sedentary living with age. About half of the respondents in the NHIS, in 1977, felt that their activity levels were about the same as others of the same age and sex. This self-perception correlated with income, i.e., as income increased, the percentage who reported being more active than their peers also increased.

Fat Intake

The NFCS and the NHANES I reported, respectively, an average 41% and 37% of total calories from fat. Current data indicate that the level of fat consumption has declined only slightly. Beef was the most popular meat consumed; other sources include poultry and fish.

Clinical Application

The practicing clinician can utilize survey and surveillance data in three major ways.

1. *Risk factors affecting specific populations:* Healthy individuals must know the potential risk factors associated with dietary intake related to age, sex, or other demographic characteristics. For example, parents must be aware of the necessity of including sources of dietary iron in their toddler's meals to prevent anemia as well as what those sources are. Females must be made aware of the ramifications of calcium deficiency combined with a lack of physical exercise including the eventual risk of osteoporosis. Prepregnancy education about the implications of maternal smoking and alcohol consumption on pregnancy outcome may be more effective in encouraging habit changes than last-minute advice during pregnancy.

Such information and guidance counseling should be provided as a routine component of health care.
2. *Changeable risk factors:* Individuals at risk should be made aware of those risk factors that are amenable to change and the appropriate methods of intervention. Such intervention in consistently overweight or obese individuals could significantly reduce their risk for hypertension, heart disease, and stroke.
3. *Changeable risk factors in nutrition-related health problems:* Identification of risk factors in individuals with a diagnosed nutrition-related health problem will enhance the clinician's ability to plan effective intervention to minimize the complications and consequences of the condition and to facilitate recovery.

In addition to the importance of the clinician's relationship to private patients is the essential role of community nutrition programs to assist low-income individuals to establish food consumption and behavioral health practices associated with optimal health.

COMMUNITY NUTRITION PROGRAMS

A number of federal food assistance programs assist high-risk, low-income populations, including pregnant and lactating women, infants, and preschool and school-age children.

Women, Infants, and Children (WIC)

The Special Supplemental Food Program for Women, Infants, and Children (WIC), which is federally funded, provides supplemental foods, nutrition education, and access to health services to low-income, high-risk pregnant and postpartum women as well as children from birth to 5 years of age. Households at or below 185% of the federally defined poverty level are eligible to receive benefits. About 40% of the eligible population is served. In 1990, national monthly participation averaged 3.4 million.

In 1972, the WIC program originated as a 2-year pilot project, an amendment to the Child Nutrition Act of 1966. The program's food assistance aspect was intended to complement existing prenatal and pediatric health care, in order to reduce nutrition-related health problems of pregnancy, infancy, and childhood. WIC's underlying premise continues to be that substantial numbers of pregnant, breast-feeding, and postpartum women, and infants and children from low-income families are at risk because of inadequate health care, poor nutrition, or both. In its attempt to ameliorate these problems, WIC has become an important step in integrating nutritional supplementation with health care delivery.

Program Implementation

At the federal level, WIC is administered by the Department of Agriculture's Food and Nutrition Service (FNS). FNS provides cash grants to authorized agencies in each of the 50 states, to Native-American populations, and to the United States territories.

Participants receive individually prescribed foods that are high in protein, iron, calcium, and vitamins A and C. Food packages contain items such as infant formula, milk or milk products, iron-fortified cereal, juice, eggs, and dried beans or peanut butter. WIC foods are intended to be a supplement to foods normally purchased by participants through other means such as family income or other feeding programs.

There are three principal food distribution systems—retail purchase, home delivery, and central distribution; some states use a combination of the three.

The results of two major national evaluations suggest that WIC has had a significantly positive, albeit modest, impact on mean birth weight, and has influenced a reduction in the proportion of low birth weight infants born to mothers who participate in the WIC program. A thorough analysis of WIC's impact has been hindered by methodological limitations of population-based studies, and the inability to successfully mount an experimental study design. Nevertheless, existing results, coupled with enthusiastic support from the health community, suggest it is a highly valued and effective program.

There are, however, a number of issues yet to be resolved within the WIC program. These include (a) supplemental food packages for children that exceed 100% of the RDA for many nutrients, (b) the limited types of foods provided, (c) foods that are high in fat and cholesterol, (d) ineffectual promotion of breast-feeding, and (e) the prevailing therapeutic approach to food supplementation as opposed to a preventive approach that encourages habit changing in order to reduce or eliminate risk.

In addition, although eligibility is predicated on an identified risk, supplemental food may not meet the specific need, e.g., iron deficiency anemia, the food package for a child 1 to 2 years of age is inadequate to remedy the problem. Moreover, many of the qualifying risk criteria, such as obesity or inadequate food group intake as determined from limited dietary recall data, are imprecise, inappropriate, or inconsistent.

Child Nutrition Programs

The United States Department of Agriculture supports child nutrition programs through state-level departments of education. These include school lunch and breakfast programs, as well as special milk programs, child care food programs, summer food programs, food distribution programs, and the nutrition education and training program. The types of services available include distribution of donated foods, and financial, supervisory, training, and technical assistance.

National School Lunch Program

The National School Lunch Program provides lunches that meet the nutritional standards established by the United States Department of Agriculture. The goal of this program, which may be sponsored by local educational agencies, private nonprofit schools or residential child care institutions, is to provide one-third of the recommended daily dietary allowances (RDA) for students.

School Breakfast Program

The School Breakfast Program encourages students to eat a nutritious breakfast and to understand the importance of this meal. Local educational agencies, private nonprofit schools, and residential child care institutions may sponsor this program.

Food Distribution Program

The Food Distribution Program has a twofold purpose: to improve the diets of schoolchildren, the poor, and the elderly as well as to distribute domestically produced foods acquired under surplus removal or price support operations.

Special Milk Program

The Special Milk Program encourages milk consumption by children in private nonprofit schools, including child care centers, settlement houses, and similar institutions that do not participate in a United States Department of Agriculture meal service program. Most programs are operated at sites that lack facilities to prepare meals. The Special Milk Program may also provide other food supplements.

Child Care Food Program

The purpose of this program is improved nutritional status in licensed nonresidential child care centers, family day care homes, and centers providing nonresidential care for functionally disabled adults. By initiating, maintaining, and/or expanding food service programs, it seeks to enable nonprofit day care institutions to integrate a nutritious food service with other existing services.

Summer Food Service Program for Children

This program provides nutritious meals to needy children during summer vacation. Local governmental agencies and boards of education operate and administer the program at specified sites. Other potential sponsors include public and private nonprofit organizations such as the Salvation Army, Boy Scouts, churches, and residential camps.

Nutrition Education and Training Program

This program attempts to improve well-being through nutrition education and training. Its ultimate goal is to teach children, teachers, and food service personnel about the relationship of dietary intake to good health not only for the present, but for long-term improved health prognosis.

Food Stamp Program

The Food Stamp Program is an entitlement program designed to assist low-income individuals to improve nutritional intake through improved purchasing ability. For eligibility, gross household income must be below 130% of poverty; net income must be below poverty. In 1986, monthly participation averaged 19.4 million. Amounts issued are dependent on family size and income; benefits average 50 cents a meal per person.

The Food Stamp Program was initiated in 1959 as a limited demonstration project. Originally, it had two purposes: (a) to provide food assistance to those in need, and (b) to dispense surplus food commodities accrued through the United States Department of Agriculture's price support operations. Eventually, however, the provision of food assistance to the poor has become its primary objective. It became a national program in 1975 and, gradually, the list of purchasable commodities has increased to the point that it has become the largest of the government's food assistance programs. From 1975 to 1987, federal food stamp expenditures have increased from approximately $4.6 billion to $12 billion.

The program has also grown more complex. Currently, to receive food stamps, households must pass a two-tiered income test. Exceptions include the elderly, disabled, or dependent children under 6 years of age. To qualify, the gross monthly income of a household must be less than an established amount adjusted for household size. When that qualification is met, specified deductions are calculated to determine whether the household's adjusted monthly income is below the net income ceiling.

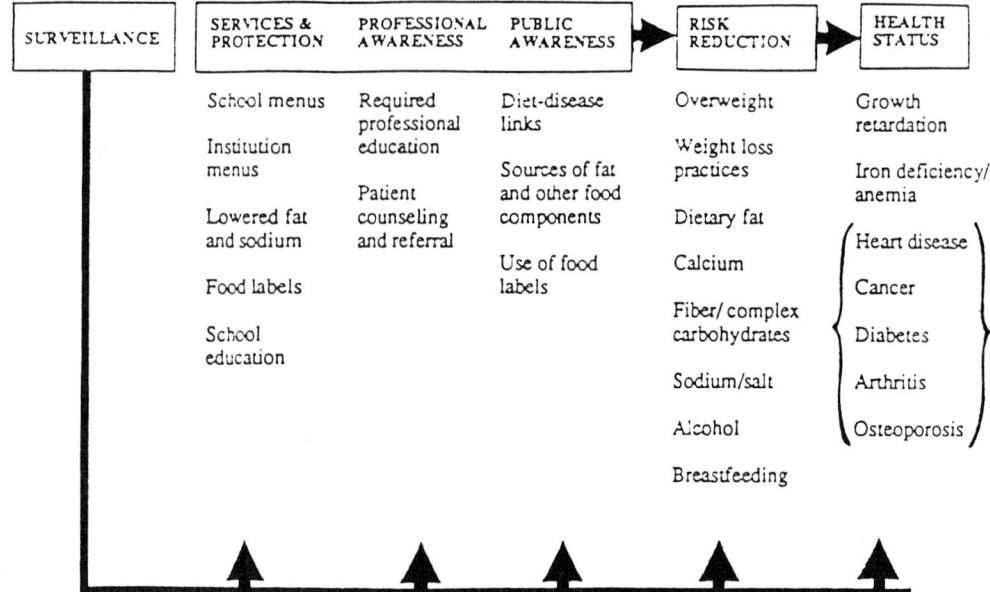

FIG. 3. Public and professional awareness of nutrition practices that reduce risks and improve health. (From ref. 41.)

FUTURE NATIONAL OBJECTIVES

The Public Health Service has designated this decade, leading to the year 2000, as a period in which improved health, and specifically nutritional health, is a priority goal for the United States. Recommendations include continued surveillance of national nutritional status, programs aimed at reducing growth retardation and iron deficiency anemia in young children, and programs to reduce the incidence of nutritionally related chronic diseases. Problems or population patterns that are being targeted include (a) overweight, (b) weight loss practices, (c) dietary fat intakes, (d) calcium intake, (e) fiber and complex carbohydrate intake, (f) sodium and salt intake, (g) alcohol consumption, and (h) breast-feeding frequency. Attention is directed at public and professional awareness as well as the provision of nutrition-related services (Fig. 3) (41).

REFERENCES

1. Habicht JP, Meyers LD, Brownie C. Indicators for identifying and counting the improperly nourished. *Am J Clin Nutr* 1982;35:1241–1254.
2. Methodology of nutritional surveillance (FAO-UNICEF report). WHO technical report series no. 593. 1976;53–54.
3. Wong F, Trowbridge F. Nutrition surveys and surveillance: their application to clinical practice. *Clin Nutr Suppl* 1984;1(3):94–99.
4. Nichaman MZ, Lane JM. Nutrition surveillance in developed countries: the United States experience. In: Alfin-Slater RB, Kritchevsky D, eds. *Human nutrition: a comprehensive treatise.* New York: Plenum Press, 1979;409–430.
5. Paige DM, Davis LR. Nutrition and health policy. In: Levine S, Lilienfeld A, eds. *Epidemiology and health policy.* New York: Tavistock, 1987;55–84.
6. Simopoulos AP. Assessment of nutritional status. *Am J Clin Nutr* 1982;35(suppl):1104–1110.
7. Jelliffe DB, Jelliffe EF. *Community nutritional assessment.* Oxford: Oxford University Press, 1989.
8. Owen AY, Frankle RT. *Nutrition in the community,* 2nd ed. St. Louis: Times Mirror/Mosby, 1986.
9. World Health Organization. *Weekly epidemiological record.* Geneva, Switzerland, 1987;7:37–52.
10. World Health Organization. *Weekly epidemiological record.* Geneva, Switzerland, 1987;9:53–60.
11. World Health Organization. *Use and interpretation of anthropometric indicators of nutritional status.* Geneva, Switzerland, 1986;64(6):929–941.
12. Scrimshaw SCM, Hurtado E. Field guide for the study of health-seeking behavior at the household level. *UNU Food Nutr Bull* 1984;6:27–37.
13. Jerome R, Kandel RF, Pelto GF. *Nutritional anthropology.* New York: Redgrave, 1980.
14. Paige DM, Egan M. Community nutrition. In: Walker A, Watkins J, eds. *Nutrition in pediatrics: basic science and clinical application.* Boston: Little, Brown, 1985;183–203.
15. Drummond JF. Clinical and laboratory diagnosis of nutritional problems. *Dent Clin North Am* 1976;20:585–594.
16. Willett W. *Nutritional epidemiology.* New York: Oxford University Press, 1990.
17. Trowbridge FL. Infants and children. In: Paige DM, ed. *Clinical nutrition,* 2nd ed. St. Louis: CV Mosby, 1988;119–136.
18. Griffiths M. *Growth monitoring,* 2nd ed. Washington, DC: American Public Health Association, 1985.
19. World Health Organization. *The growth chart. A tool for use in infant children care.* Geneva, Switzerland, 1986.
20. U.S. Department of Health and Human Services. *Health and nutrition examination survey (NHANES).* Washington, DC: Government Printing Office, 1975.
21. U.S. Department of Health and Human Services. *Health and nutrition examination survey (NHANES).* Washington, DC: Government Printing Office, 1980–84.
22. Burke BS. The dietary history as a tool in research. *J Am Diet Assoc* 1974;23:1041–1047.
23. Hubbard VS, Hubbard LR. Clinical assessment of nutritional status. In: Walker A, Watkins J, eds. *Nutrition in pediatrics: basic science and clinical application.* Boston: Little, Brown, 1985;121–150.

24. Beaton GH, Milner J, McGuire V, et al. Sources of variance in 24-hour recall data: implications for nutrition study and interpretation. *Am J Clin Nutr* 1983;37:986–995.
25. Karvetti R, Knuts L. Agreement between dietary interviews. *J Am Diet Assoc* 1981;79:654–658.
26. Sampson L. Food frequency questionnaires as a research instrument. *Clin Nutr* 1985;4:171–178.
27. Graham AM. Assessment of nutritional intake. *Proc Nutr Soc* 1982;41:343–351.
28. Jelliffe DB, Jelliffe EFP. *Human milk in the modern world,* 2nd ed. Oxford: Oxford University Press, 1989.
29. Kennedy ET. Dietary assessment. In: Paige DM. *Clinical nutrition,* 2nd ed. St. Louis: CV Mosby, 1988;148–164.
30. Burke MC, Pao EM. *Methodology for large scale surveys of household and individual diets.* Washington, DC: U.S. Department of Agriculture, 1976.
31. FAO. Household intakes. FAO, Rome, 1982.
32. Beaton GH, Milner J, Corey P, et al. Sources of variance in 24-hour dietary recall data: implications for nutrition study design and interpretation. *Am J Clin Nutr* 1979;32:2546–2549.
33. DHHS/USDA (Department of Health and Human Services/U.S. Department of Agriculture). *Nutrition monitoring in the United States.* DHHS No (PHS) 89-1255. Washington, DC: U.S. Government Printing Office, 1989.
34. DHHS/USDA (Department of Health and Human Services/U.S. Department of Agriculture). *Nutrition Monitoring in the United States: A Progress Report from the Joint Nutrition Monitoring Evaluation Committee* DHHS Pub. No (PHS) 86-1255. Washington, DC: U.S. Government Printing Office, 1986.
35. Institute of Medicine (U.S.) Subcommittee on nutritional status and weight gain during pregnancy. *Nutrition during pregnancy.* Washington, DC: National Academy of Sciences, 1990.
36. Life Sciences Research Office. *Assessment of the iron nutritional status of the U.S. population.* Bethesda, MD: Federation of American Societies for experimental biology, 1984;120.
37. Anda BF, Waller MN, Wotten KG et al. Behavioral risk factor surveillance. *MMWR* 1990, June 29;39:4371–4374.
38. Life Sciences Research Office. *Nutrition monitoring in the United States: An update report on nutrition monitoring.* Prepared for the U.S. Department of Agriculture and Human Services. DHHS Pub. No (PHS) 89-1225. Washington, DC: U.S. Government Printing Office, 1989.
39. Sandula MK, Herman D, Willamson DF, et al. Validity of clinic-based nutritional surveillance for prevalence estimation of undernutrition. *Bull WHO* 1987;65:529–533.
40. Trowbridge F, Wong F. Surveillance of severe pediatric undernutrition: conceptual and practical issues. *J Nutr* 1990;120(8):943–947.
41. U.S. Department of Health and Human Services. *The surgeon general's report on nutrition and health.* DHHS Pub. No (PHS) 88-50210. Washington, DC: U.S. Government Printing Office, 1988.

APPENDIX A

Pediatric Nutrition Guidelines

Rosanne Perlman Farris

This appendix includes general guidelines for implementing the specific recommendations discussed throughout this book. Information is provided in table form for purposes of easy reference and brevity, and is representative of current trends.

NORMAL DIETS

The recommended dietary allowances (RDA) specify levels of intake of essential nutrients adequate to meet the known nutritional needs of most healthy persons. Infant and child feeding recommendations are translated into guidelines to promote growth and development and to facilitate the adoption of healthy eating patterns early in life (1).

Recommended Daily Dietary Allowances

The recommended daily dietary allowances (RDA) were revised in 1989 to more accurately estimate an individual's daily nutrient requirements for energy, protein, vitamins, and minerals (Table 1) (2). These recommendations are for a healthy, moderately active, individual; adjustments must be made to accommodate any deviation in health status, size, or activity of the patient (Tables 2 and 3).

Feeding Guidelines

Oral, neuromuscular, and behavioral development are important components in early childhood feeding patterns (Table 4). A good nutrition plan for the first several years of life coordinates tastes, textures, and nutrient sources with the feeding skills associated with the various levels of development during the first 3 years of life. To create a positive feeding experience and ensure future success, mealtime expectations must be based on age-appropriate feeding behaviors. Specific feeding tools and methods are required for adequate nutritional support of the physically or mentally handicapped youngster. An appreciation of the enteral capacity of the infant is necessary to translate the RDA into household measurements.

Various opinions exist as to the optimal time at which solid foods should be introduced. With the current trend to breast-feeding, delaying introduction of solid foods appears to be more prevalent. Many mothers are skipping the transitional soft baby food stage and progressing from breast-feeding to toddler foods at 9 to 11 months. Current opinion delays the introduction of baby foods until 5 to 6 months of age (Table 5) (3,4).

Formulas

Table 6 is a list of currently available infant formulas, their nutrient compositions, and indications for their use. Table 7 is a list of commercially available, defined formula feedings and their nutrient compositions. Table 8 lists the components for enteral nutrition, including source, content, and calories.

Eating Patterns

The daily food plans and sample menus for normal healthy children ages 4 to 6 years and adolescent males ages 15 to 18 are shown in Tables 9 and 10. The aim of these diets is to maintain normal growth and development in healthy children and adolescents by providing adequate amounts of energy, protein, vitamins, minerals, and other nutrients.

R. P. Farris: Department of Pediatrics, Louisiana State University School of Medicine, New Orleans, Louisiana 70112.

TABLE 1. Food and Nutrition Board, National Academy of Sciences—National Research Council: Recommended Dietary Allowances,[a] Revised 1989, designed for the maintenance of good nutrition of practically all healthy people in the United States

Category	Age (years) or condition	Weight[b] (kg)	Weight[b] (lb)	Height[b] (cm)	Height[b] (in)	Protein (g)	Fat-soluble vitamins			
							Vitamin A (μg RE)[c]	Vitamin D (μg)[d]	Vitamin E (mg α-TE)[e]	Vitamin K (μg)
Infants	0.0–0.5	6	13	60	24	13	375	7.5	3	5
	0.5–1.0	9	20	71	28	14	375	10	4	10
Children	1–3	13	29	90	35	16	400	10	6	15
	4–6	20	44	112	44	24	500	10	7	20
	7–10	28	62	132	52	28	700	10	7	30
Males	11–14	45	99	157	62	45	1,000	10	10	45
	15–18	66	145	176	69	59	1,000	10	10	65
	19–24	72	160	177	70	58	1,000	10	10	70
	25–50	79	174	176	70	63	1,000	5	10	80
	51+	77	170	173	68	63	1,000	5	10	80
Females	11–14	46	101	157	62	46	800	10	8	45
	15–18	55	120	163	64	44	800	10	8	55
	19–24	58	128	164	65	46	800	10	8	60
	25–50	63	138	163	64	50	800	5	8	65
	51+	65	143	160	63	50	800	5	8	65
Pregnant						60	800	10	10	65
Lactating	1st 6 months					65	1,300	10	12	65
	2nd 6 months					62	1,200	10	11	65

From ref. 2.

[a] The allowances, expressed as average daily intakes over time, are intended to provide for individual variations among most normal persons as they live in the United States under usual environmental stresses. Diets should be based on a variety of common foods in order to provide other nutrients for which human requirements have been less well defined.

[b] Weights and heights of reference adults are actual medians for the United States population of the designated age, as reported by NHANES II. The median weights and heights of those under 19 years of age were taken from ref. 14. The use of these figures does not imply that the height-to-weight ratios are ideal.

[c] Retinol equivalents. 1 retinol equivalent = 1 μg retinol or 6 μg β-carotene.

[d] As cholecalciferol. 10 μg cholecalciferol = 400 IU of vitamin D.

[e] α-Tocopherol equivalents. 1 mg d-α-tocopherol = 1 α-TE.

[f] 1 NE (niacin equivalent) is equal to 1 mg of niacin or 60 mg of dietary tryptophan.

TABLE 2. Estimated safe and adequate daily dietary intakes of selected vitamins and minerals[a]

Category	Age (years)	Vitamins		Trace elements[b]				
		Biotin (μg)	Pantothenic acid (mg)	Copper (mg)	Manganese (mg)	Fluoride (mg)	Chromium (μg)	Molybdenum (μg)
Infants	0–0.5	10	2	0.4–0.6	0.3–0.6	0.1–0.5	10–40	15–30
	0.5–1	15	3	0.6–0.7	0.6–1.0	0.2–1.0	20–60	20–40
Children and adolescents	1–3	20	3	0.7–1.0	1.0–1.5	0.5–1.5	20–80	25–50
	4–6	25	3–4	1.0–1.5	1.5–2.0	1.0–2.5	30–120	30–75
	7–10	30	4–5	1.0–2.0	2.0–3.0	1.5–2.5	50–200	50–150
	11+	30–100	4–7	1.5–2.5	2.0–5.0	1.5–2.5	50–200	75–250
Adults		30–100	4–7	1.5–3.0	2.0–5.0	1.5–4.0	50–200	75–250

From ref. 2.

[a] Because there is less information on which to base allowances, these figures are not given in the main table of RDA and are provided here in the form of ranges of recommended intakes.

[b] Since the toxic levels for many trace elements may be only several times usual intakes, the upper levels for the trace elements given in this table should not be habitually exceeded.

Water-soluble vitamins							Minerals						
Vitamin C (mg)	Thiamin (mg)	Riboflavin (mg)	Niacin (mg NE)[f]	Vitamin B_6 (mg)	Folate (μg)	Vitamin B_{12} (μg)	Calcium (mg)	Phosphorus (mg)	Magnesium (mg)	Iron (mg)	Zinc (mg)	Iodine (μg)	Selenium (μg)
30	0.3	0.4	5	0.3	25	0.3	400	300	40	6	5	40	10
35	0.4	0.5	6	0.6	35	0.5	600	500	60	10	5	50	15
40	0.7	0.8	9	1.0	50	0.7	800	800	80	10	10	70	20
45	0.9	1.1	12	1.1	75	1.0	800	800	120	10	10	90	20
45	1.0	1.2	13	1.4	100	1.4	800	800	170	10	10	120	30
50	1.3	1.5	17	1.7	150	2.0	1,200	1,200	270	12	15	150	40
60	1.5	1.8	20	2.0	200	2.0	1,200	1,200	400	12	15	150	50
60	1.5	1.7	19	2.0	200	2.0	1,200	1,200	350	10	15	150	70
60	1.5	1.7	19	2.0	200	2.0	800	800	350	10	15	150	70
60	1.2	1.4	15	2.0	200	2.0	800	800	350	10	15	150	70
50	1.1	1.3	15	1.4	150	2.0	1,200	1,200	280	15	12	150	45
60	1.1	1.3	15	1.5	180	2.0	1,200	1,200	300	15	12	150	50
60	1.1	1.3	15	1.6	180	2.0	1,200	1,200	280	15	12	150	55
60	1.1	1.3	15	1.6	180	2.0	800	800	280	15	12	150	55
60	1.0	1.2	13	1.6	180	2.0	800	800	280	10	12	150	55
70	1.5	1.6	17	2.2	400	2.2	1,200	1,200	320	30	15	175	65
95	1.6	1.8	20	2.1	280	2.6	1,200	1,200	355	15	19	200	75
90	1.6	1.7	20	2.1	260	2.6	1,200	1,200	340	15	16	200	75

TABLE 3. *Median heights and weights and recommended energy intake*

Category	Age (years) or condition	Weight (kg)	Weight (lb)	Height (cm)	Height (in)	REE[a] (kcal/day)	Multiples of REE	Average energy allowance (Cal)[b] Per kg	Per day[c]
Infants	0.0–0.5	6	13	60	24	320		108	650
	0.5–1.0	9	20	71	28	500		98	850
Children	1–3	13	29	90	35	740		102	1,300
	4–6	20	44	112	44	950		90	1,800
	7–10	28	62	132	52	1,130		70	2,000
Males	11–14	45	99	157	62	1,440	1.70	55	2,500
	15–18	66	145	176	69	1,760	1.67	45	3,000
	19–24	72	160	177	70	1,780	1.67	40	2,900
	25–50	79	174	176	70	1,800	1.60	37	2,900
	51+	77	170	173	68	1,530	1.50	30	2,300
Females	11–14	46	101	157	62	1,310	1.67	47	2,200
	15–18	55	120	163	64	1,370	1.60	40	2,200
	19–24	58	128	164	65	1,350	1.60	38	2,200
	25–50	63	138	163	64	1,380	1.55	36	2,200
	51+	65	143	160	63	1,280	1.50	30	1,900
Pregnant	1st trimester								+0
	2nd trimester								+300
	3rd trimester								+300
Lactating	1st 6 months								+500
	2nd 6 months								+500

From ref. 2.
[a] Calculation based on FAO equations then rounded.
[b] In the range of light to moderate activity, the coefficient of variation is ±20%.
[c] Figure is rounded.

TABLE 4. Development of feeding skills

Age	Oral and neuromuscular development	Feeding behavior
Birth	Rooting reflex	Turns mouth toward nipple or any object brushing cheek
	Sucking reflex	Initial swallowing involves the posterior of the tongue; by 9–12 weeks, anterior portion is increasingly involved which facilitates ingestion of semisolid food
	Swallowing reflex	Pushes food out when placed on tongue; strong the first 9 weeks
	Extrusion reflex	By 6–10 weeks, recognizes the position in which he is fed and begins mouthing and sucking when placed in this position
3–6 months	Beginning coordination between eyes and body movements	Explores world with eyes, fingers, hands, and mouth; starts reaching for objects at 4 months but overshoots; hands get in the way during feeding
	Learning to reach mouth with hands at 4 months	Finger sucking—by 6 months, all objects go into the mouth
	Extrusion reflex present until 4 months	May continue to push out food placed on tongue
	Able to grasp objects voluntarily at 5 months	Grasps objects in mittenlike fashion
	Sucking reflex becomes voluntary and lateral motions of the jaw begin	Can approximate lips to the rim of cup by 5 months; chewing action begins; by 6 months, begins drinking from cup
6–12 months	Eyes and hands working together	Brings hand to mouth; at 7 months, able to feed self biscuit
	Sits erect with support at 6 months	Bangs cup and objects on table at 7 months
	Sits erect without support at 9 months	
	Development of grasp (finger to thumb opposition)	Holds own bottle at 9–12 months
		Pincer approach to food
		Pokes at food with index finger at 10 months
	Relates to objects at 10 months	Reaches for food and utensils including those beyond reach; pushes plate around with spoon; insists on holding spoon, not to put in mouth but to return to plate or cup
1–3 years	Development of manual dexterity	Increased desire to feed self
		15 months—begins to use spoon but turns it before reaching mouth; may hold cup, likely to tilt the cup rather than head, causing spilling
		18 months—eats with spoon, spills frequently, turns spoon in mouth; holds glass with both hands
		2 years—inserts spoon correctly, occasionally with one hand; holds glass; plays with food; distinguishes between food and inedible materials
		2–3 years—self-feeding complete with occasional spilling; uses fork; pours from pitcher; obtains drink of water from faucet

From ref. 13.

TABLE 5. Feeding guidelines

	0–2 weeks	2 weeks–2 months	2 months	3 months[a]	4–5 months	5–6 months
Formula						
Ounces per feeding	2–3 oz	3–5 oz	4–6 oz	4–6 oz	5–7 oz	5–7 oz
Average total ounces	22 oz	28 oz	29 oz	30 oz	32 oz	30 oz
Number of feedings	6–8	5–6	4–5	4–5	4–5	4–5
Food texture	Liquids	Liquids	Liquids	Baby soft	Baby soft	Baby soft
Food additions						
Orange juice		Give diluted juice, 1 oz juice and 1 oz water	2 oz, undiluted	3–4 oz	3–4 oz	3–4 oz

TABLE 5. Continued.

	0–2 weeks	2 weeks–2 months	2 months	3 months	4–5 months	5–6 months
Baby cereal, enriched				1 tsp, B & S	2 tbsp, B & S	2 tbsp, B & S
Strained fruits				1 tsp, B & S	1 tbsp, B & S	1½ tbsp, B & S
Strained vegetables					1–2 tbsp, L	2 tbsp, L
Strained meats						1 tbsp, L
Egg yolk or baby egg yolk						½ med or 1 tbsp
Teething biscuit						½–1
Total calories	440	475	610	659–674	751–772	777–843
Recommended calories 117 Cal/kg	410	410–608	608	667	725–784	784–878
Oral and neuromuscular development related to food intake	Rooting, sucking, swallowing →			Extrusion reflex diminishes; sucking becomes voluntary	Learning to reach hands to mouth; develops grasp	Chewing begins; can approximate lips to the rim of cup

	6–7 months	7–8 months	8–9 months	9–10 months	10–11 months	11–12 months
Whole milk						
Ounces per feeding	7–8 oz	8 oz	8 oz	8 oz	8 oz	8 oz
Average total ounces	28 oz	28 oz	24 oz	24 oz	24 oz	24 oz
Number of feedings	3–4	3–4	3	3	3	3
Food texture	Gradual increase →		Mashed →			Cut fine
Food items						
Orange juice	4 oz	4 oz	4 oz	4 oz	4 oz	4 oz
Fortified cereal	⅓ cup, B	⅓ cup, B	½ cup, B	½ cup, B	½ cup, B	½ cup, B
Fruit, canned or fresh	4 tsp, B, L, & S	4 tsp, B, L, & S	2 tbsp, L & S	2 tbsp, L & S	3 tbsp, L & S	3 tbsp, L & S
Vegetables	1½ tbsp, L & S	2 tbsp, L & S	2 tbsp, L & S	2 tbsp, L & S	3 tbsp, L & S	3 tbsp, L & S
Meat, fish, poultry	1 tbsp, L & S	2 tbsp, L & S	2 tbsp, L & S	2 tbsp, L & S	2½ tbsp, L & S	2½ tbsp, L & S
Egg yolk or baby egg yolk	1 medium yolk, or 2 tbsp	1 medium yolk, or 2 tbsp	1 medium yolk, or 2 tbsp	1 whole egg	1 whole egg	1 whole egg
Teething biscuit or bread	1 biscuit	1 biscuit	½ slice bread	½ slice bread	½ slice bread	½ slice bread
Starch—potato, rice, macaroni				2 tbsp, S	2 tbsp, S	2 tbsp, S
Dessert—custard, pudding			1 tsp	1 tsp	1 tsp	2 tbsp, S
Butter						1 tsp
Total calories	859	876	937	974	1037	1069
Recommended calories 108 Cal/kg	810–864	864–918	918–972	972–1,015	1,015–1,048	1,048–1,083
Oral and neuromuscular development related to food intake	Begins using cup →					
		Sits erect with support →		Without support →		
		Feeds self biscuit →				
				Holds bottle	Picks up small food items and releases	Will hold and lick spoon after dipped into food; self-feeding

From ref. 13.
[a] Current opinion is that the introduction of baby foods be delayed until 5 months of age.
B, breakfast, L, lunch; S, supper.

TABLE 6. Infant formulas[a]

Formula (manufacturer)	Cal per ml	Protein			Carbohydrate			Fat			Na mEq	K mEq	Ca mg	P mg	Fe mg	Osmolality mOsm/kg
		g	type	%cal	g	type	%cal	g	type	%cal						
Alimentum (Ross)	0.67	1.9	Hydrolized casein	11	6.9	Sucrose modified tapioca starch	41	3.8	MCT—50%, safflower oil—40%, soy oil—10%	48	1.3	2.0	71	51	1.20	370
Follow-Up Formula (Carnation)	0.67	2.0	82% casein; 18% whey	12	8.9	Lactose and corn syrup	53	2.6	Palm, corn, and high oleic safflower oil	35	1.2	2.3	118	61	1.30	345
Good Start (Carnation)	0.67	1.6	Enzymatically hydrolyzed reduced minerals whey and whey protein concentrate	9.6	7.4	Lactose and maltodextrin	44	3.4	Palm olein, soy, coconut and high oleic safflower oil	3.6	0.7	1.7	43	24	1.00	265
Cow's milk—whole	0.67	3.3	80% casein, 20% whey	21	4.7	Lactose	30	3.3	Butterfat	49	2.1	3.9	79	40	0	260
Enfamil 20 with Fe (MJ)	0.67	1.5	Nonfat cow's milk, reduced minerals whey	9	6.9	Lactose	41	3.8	Coconut and soy oil	50	0.8	1.86	46	32	1.28	300
Enfamil 24 with Fe (MJ)	0.8	1.8	Nonfat cow's milk, reduced minerals whey	9	8.3	Lactose	41	4.6	Coconut and soy oil	50	1.0	2.2	55	38	1.52	360
Enfamil premature formula (MJ)	0.67	2.0	Whey protein concentrate, nonfat milk solids	12	7.4	Corn syrup solids, lactose	44	3.4	MCT—40%, soy—40%, coconut oils—20%	44	1.1	1.7	112	56	1.28	260

Formula																
Enfamil Premature Formula 24 with Fe (MJ)	0.8	2.4	Whey protein concentrate, nonfat milk solids	12	9.0	Corn syrup solids, lactose	44	4.1	MCT—40%, soy and coconut oils	44	1.4	2.1	134	68	1.52	310
Human milk	0.67	1.0	20% casein, 80% whey	6	6.9	Lactose	39	4.4	Human milk fat	55	0.7	1.3	30	14	<0.10	273
Isomil (Ross)	0.67	1.8	Soy protein isolate	11	6.8	Corn syrup and sucrose	40	3.7	Soy and coconut oil	49	1.3	1.9	71	51	1.21	240
MJ 3232A (MJ)	0.42	1.9	Casein hydrolysate	17	2.8	Tapioca starch, mono- and disaccharide free	25	2.8	MCT—87%, corn oils—13%	57	1.3	1.9	63	42	1.26	250
Nursoy (Wyeth)	0.67	2.1	Soy protein	12	6.9	Sucrose	40	3.6	Coconut, safflower, soy oils	48	0.9	1.9	63	44	1.20	266
Nutramigen (MJ)	0.67	1.9	Casein hydrolysate, amino acid premix	11	9.1	Corn syrup solids and corn starch	54	2.6	Corn oil	48	1.4	1.9	63	43	1.28	320
Portagen (MJ)	0.67	2.3	Sodium	14	7.8	Corn syrup solids, sucrose, lactose	46	3.3	MCT—85%, corn oil—15%	40	1.6	2.2	64	48	1.28	230
Pregestimil (MJ)	0.67	1.9	Casein hydrolysate, cystine, tryosine, and tryptophan	11	6.9	Corn syrup solids, dextrose, corn starch	41	3.8	MCT—60%, corn oil—20%, high oleic safflower oil—20%	48	1.2	1.9	64	43	1.28	340
ProSobee (MJ)	0.67	2.0	Soy protein isolate methionine	12	6.8	Corn syrup solids	40	3.6	Soy and coconut oil	48	1.0	2.1	64	50	1.28	200

continued

TABLE 6. Continued.

Formula (manufacturer)	Cal per ml	Protein g	Protein type	%cal	Carbohydrate g	Carbohydrate type	%cal	Fat g	Fat type	%cal	Na mEq	K mEq	Ca mg	P mg	Fe mg	Osmolality mOsm/kg
Ross Carbohydrate Free (Ross)	0.4	2.0	Soy protein isolate	20				3.7	Soy and coconut oils	80	1.4	2.0	70	50	0.15	74
Similac 20 with Fe (Ross)	0.67	1.5	Nonfat cow's milk	9	7.2	Lactose	43	3.6	Coconut and soy oil	48	0.83	1.87	51	39	1.20	300
Similac 24 with Fe (Ross)	0.8	2.2	Nonfat cow's milk	11	8.5	Lactose	42	4.3	Coconut and soy oil	47	1.22	2.74	73	57	1.50	380
Similac Special Care (Ross)	0.67	1.8	Nonfat cow's milk and whey	11	7.1	Lactose and hydrolyzed corn starch	42	3.6	MCT–50%; coconut and soy oils	47	1.3	2.2	122	61	0.25	250
Similac Special Care 24 (Ross)	0.8	2.17	Nonfat cow's milk and whey	11	8.5	Lactose and hydrolyzed corn starch	42	4.3	MCT–50%; coconut and soy oils	47	1.5	2.7	146	73	1.5	300
Similac PM 60/40 (Ross)	0.67	1.6	Whey sodium caseinate	9	6.9	Lactose	41	3.8	Coconut and soy oil	50	0.7	1.5	38	19	0.15	280
SMA 20 with Fe (Ross)	0.67	1.5	Nonfat cow's milk demineralized whey	8.8	7.2	Lactose	42	3.6	Coconut, safflower, and soy bean oil	48	0.7	1.4	42	28	1.2	300
SMA Preemie (Wyeth)	0.8	2.0	Nonfat cow's milk: 60% whey, 40% casein	10	8.6	Lactose and glucose polymers	42	4.4	MCT, soy, and coconut oils	48	1.4	1.9	75	40	0.3	300
Soyalac (Loma Linda)	0.67	2.1	Soy protein solids	12	6.8	Corn syrup, sucrose soy bean CHO	39	3.7	Soy oil	49	1.3	2.0	64	37	1.3	215
I-Soyalac (Loma Linda)	0.67	2.0	Soy protein	12	6.8	Sucrose tapioca	40	3.6	Soy oil	48	1.4	2.0	70	50	1.2	206

Adapted from ref. 32.
[a] Analysis per 100 ml.
MJ, Mead Johnson.

TABLE 7. External feeding formulas[a]

Formula (Manufacturer)	Cal per ml	Protein g	Protein type	Protein %cal	Carbohydrate g	Carbohydrate type	Carbohydrate %cal	Fat g	Fat type	Fat %cal	Na mEq	K mEq	Ca mg	P mg	Fe mg	GI Solute load mOsm/kg
Compleat Modified (Sandoz)	1	43	Beef, vegetable	16	140	Maltodextrins, fruit	53	37	Corn oil	31	44	36	670	870	12.0	300
Enrich (Ross)	1	39	Na and Ca caseinates, soy protein isolate	15	160	Hydrolyzed corn starch, sucrose soy fiber	55	37	Corn oil	30	36	43	708	708	12.8	480
Ensure (Ross)	1.0	37	Na and Ca caseinates; soy protein isolate	14	143	Corn syrup, sucrose	55	47	Corn oil	31	36	37	521	521	9.4	470
Ensure Plus (Ross)	1.5	54	Na and Ca caseinates, soy protein isolate	15	197	Corn syrup, sucrose solids	53	53	Corn oil	32	49	53	696	696	12.5	690
Isocal (MJ)	1.1	34	Na and Ca caseinates; soy protein	13	133	Maltodextrins	50	44	Soy oil, MCT oil	37	23	24	630	530	0.5	300
Jevity (Ross)	1.0	44	Na and Ca caseinates	17	150	Hydrolyzed corn starch, soy fiber	53	36	MCT—50%, corn oil, soil oil	30	40	39	896	746	13.4	310
Osmolite (Ross)	1.0	37	Casein, soy protein isolate	14	143	Hydrolyzed corn starch	55	38	MCT—50%, corn oil, soil oil	31	27	26	521	521	9.4	300
Pediasure (Ross)	1.0	30	Na caseinate, whey, protein concentrate	12	110	Hydrolyzed corn starch, sucrose	44	50	High oleic safflower oil—50%, soy oil—30%, MCT—20%	44	17	33	970	800	14	325
Peptamen (Clintec)	1.0	40	Hydrolyzed whey	16	127	Maltodextrins	51	39	MCT, safflower	33	22	32	800	800	12.0	270
Pulmocare (Ross)	1.5	63	Na and Ca	17	106	Sucrose, hydrolyzed corn starch	28	92	Corn oil	55	57	49	1057	1057	19.0	520
Sustacal (MJ)	1.0	61	Na and Ca caseinates, soy protein isolate	24	140	Sucrose, corn syrup solids	55	23	Partially hydrolyzed soy oil	21	41	54	1010	930	16.9	620
Sustacal HC (MJ)	1.5	61	Na and Ca caseinates	16	190	Corn syrup solids, sucrose	50	58	Corn oil	34	36	38	850	850	15.0	650
Tolerex (Norwich-Eaton)	1.0	21	Free amino acids	8	226	Maltodextrins	91	1	Safflower	1	20	30	556	556	10.0	550
Travasorb MCT (Clintec)	1.0	49	Lactalbumin K caseinate	20	123	Corn syrup solids	50	33	Sunflower oil—20%, MCT—45%	30	15	26	500	500	9.0	250
Vital HN (Ross)	1.0	49	Partially hydrolyzed whey, meat soy, amino acids	17	185	Hydrolyzed corn starch, sucrose	74	11	Safflower oil, MCT—45%	9	20	34	667	667	12.0	500
Vivonex TEN (Norwich-Eaton)	1.0	38	Free amino acids	15	206	Maltodextrins	82	3	Safflower oil	3	20	20	500	500	9.0	630

Adapted from ref. 32.
[a] Analysis per liter.

TABLE 8. Single components for enteral nutrition

Component	Source	Content	Calories
Protein			
Casec	Calcium caseinate	88 g/100 g powder	370 cal/100 g
Promod	Whey protein	75 g/100 g powder	425 cal/100 g
Propac	Whey protein	75 g/100 g powder	395 cal/100 g
Carbohydrate			
Moducal	Corn starch hydrolysate	95 g/100 g powder	380 cal/100 g
Polycose	Corn starch hydrolysate		
Liquid		50 g/100 cc liquid	200 cal/100 cc
Powder		94 g/100 g powder	380 cal/100 g
Fat			
MCT	Fractionated coconut oil—90%, C8 and C10 triglycerides	93 g/100 cc	770 cal/100 cc
Microlipid	Safflower oil (50% emulsion)	50 g/100 cc	450 cal/100 cc
Vegetable oils	Corn, olive, peanut, etc.	100 g/100 cc	Approximately 830 cal/100 cc

Adapted from ref. 18.

TABLE 9. Menu pattern and sample meals for a child between 4 and 6 years of age (72 g protein, 1,800 Cal)

Daily Food Plan	Sample Menu Pattern	Sample Meals
Milk group[a]		A.M.
2–3 cups milk	1 citrus fruit or ½ cup juice	Orange juice
Meat group[b]	½ cup cereal with milk and sugar[d]	Enriched farina with milk and sugar[d]
3 equivalents[b]; 1 equivalent equals 1 oz meat (edible portion weighed after cooking)	1 slice toast with fortified margarine[d]	Toast with fortified margarine
	1 cup milk	Milk, low fat
Vegetable and fruit group		Noon
4 servings, including a dark green or deep yellow vegetable for vitamin A and a citrus fruit or other fruit rich in vitamin C daily	1 meat equivalent	Sliced turkey
	Vegetables, raw or cooked	Shredded lettuce
	Fruit	Baked apple
	1 slice enriched or whole grain bread with fortified margarine[d]	Bread with fortified margarine[d]
Bread-cereal-potato-legume group[c]	½ cup milk	Milk, low fat
5 servings		P.M.
Fats and sweets[d]	2 meat equivalents	Broiled ground beef
(Without this group the diet contains 1,355 Cal)	½ cup potato or substitute	Baked potato
	Dark green or deep yellow vegetable	Carrot rings
	Dessert[c]	Ice milk
	1 slice enriched or whole grain bread with fortified margarine[d]	Bread with fortified margarine[d]
	½ cup milk	Milk, low fat
		Between meals
	½ cup milk	Milk, low fat

Adapted from refs. 1 and 19.

[a] Vitamin D (400 IU) should be used as a concentrate if not contained in milk. Choose low fat (1%) or skim milk, non fat or low fat yogurt or cheese.

[b] If additional meat is desired, 1 serving of bread group (as 1 slice of bread) may be omitted for each 1 oz meat added, without changing the caloric value or reducing nutrient content substantially. Choose lean, well-trimmed meats and poultry without skin.

[c] Choose whole grain.

[d] One teaspoon sugar adds 20 Cal; 1 tsp fat or oil adds 45 Cal. Such desserts as ice cream, pudding, and gelatin may add 150–300 Cal. Choose margarine made from unsaturated oils, light or diet margarine.

TABLE 10. *Menu pattern and sample meals for an adolescent male between 15 and 18 years of age (100 g protein, 2,800 Cal)*

Daily Food Plan	Sample Menu Pattern	Sample Meals

Milk group[a]
   1 qt whole milk
 Meat group[b]
   5 equivalents[b]; 1 equivalent equals 1 oz meat (edible portion) weighed after cooking
 Vegetable and fruit group
   4 servings or more daily, including a dark green or deep yellow vegetable daily for vitamin A and a citrus or other fruit rich in vitamin C
 Bread-cereal-potato-legume group
   7 servings
 Fats and sweets[c]
   (Without this group the diet contains 1,645 Cal)
	1 citrus fruit or ½ cup juice
	 ½ cup cooked cereal or ¾ cup flake-type with milk and sugar[d]
	 1 slice enriched or whole grain toast with fortified margarine[d]
	 1 cup milk
	
	 2 meat equivalents
	 Vegetable
	 2 slices enriched or whole grain bread or substitute with fortified margarine[d]
	 1 cup milk
	
	 3 meat equivalents
	 ½ cup potato or substitute[b]
	 Dark green or deep yellow vegetable
	 Other vegetable
	 Fruit
	 2 slices enriched or whole grain bread with fortified margarine[d]
	 1 cup milk
	
	 1 cup milk
		A.M.
		   Grapefruit
		   Flakes with milk and sugar[d]
		   Toast with fortified margarine[d]
		   Milk, low fat
		
		 Noon
		   Sandwich—turkey on bread with fortified margarine[c]
		   Sliced tomatoes
		   Milk, low fat
		
		 P.M.
		   Meat loaf
		   Baked potato
		   Carrots
		   Cabbage slaw
		   Apple
		   Rolls with fortified margarine
		   Milk, low fat
		
		 Between meals
		   Milk, low fat

Adapted from refs. 1 and 19.

Notes: The recommended dietary allowances for adolescence may be met by this pattern, with the exception of iron; iron rich foods may be used to augment this level.

[a] Choose low fat (1%) or skim milk, non fat or low fat yogurt or cheese. The use of skim milk would result in a reduction of 320 Cal. Vitamin D (400 IU) should be used as a concentrate if not contained in milk.

[b] If additional meat is desired, 1 serving of the bread group (as 1 slice bread) may be omitted for each 1 oz meat added, without changing the caloric value or reducing nutrient content substantially. Choose lean, well-trimmed meats and poultry without skin.

[c] Choose whole grain.

[d] One teaspoon sugar adds 20 Cal; 1 tsp fat or oil adds 45 Cal. Desserts such as ice cream, pudding, and gelatin may add 150–300 Cal. Cake or pie may add 300–700 Cal. Adjustments in this group should be made to suit individual caloric needs. Choose margarine made from unsaturated oils, light or diet margarine.

THERAPEUTIC DIETS

It is important to understand that there is no specific doctrine dictating the nutritional management of the sick child. A thorough understanding of the altered metabolism as well as of age-appropriate requirements and socioeconomic status will help in formulating the best therapeutic nutrition plan for the well or sick child.

Celiac Disease

Gluten-sensitive enteropathy is a malabsorptive syndrome resulting from abnormal mucosal response to the protein fraction in grain gliadin. Elimination of foods containing gluten leads to a reversal of symptoms and permits normal gastrointestinal absorption. Vitamin and calcium supplementation are recommended in doses proportional to the severity of the malabsorption (Table 11).

TABLE 11. *Gluten-restricted diet*

Foods containing these grains contain gluten[a]	
Avoid:	alfalfa
	barley
	buckwheat
	oats
	rye
	wheat
Gluten-free grains and flour substitutes	
Use:	corn flour
	cornstarch
	cornmeal
	gluten-free wheat starch
	gluten-free bread mix
	lima bean flour
	potato flour
	rice
	rice flour
	soy flour

[a] Many prepared products contain one or more of these grains or their derivatives as a product ingredient. Therefore, it is advisable to counsel the gluten-restricted individual to carefully read all product labels in order to identify those items containing any of the restricted grains.

TABLE 12. *Nutrient guidelines for children with cystic fibrosis*

Age	Calories	Protein	Fat	
Infants (to 1 year old)	150–200 Cal/kg/day	4 g/kg/day	Infants	
Children (1–9 years)	130–180 Cal/kg/day	3 g/kg/day	Normal	30–60 g/day
Males (9–18 years)	100–130 Cal/kg/day		Moderate	30–50 g/day
Females (9–18 years)	80–110 Cal/kg/day	2.5–3 g/kg/day	Low-fat	30–40 g/day
			Older children	
			Normal	50–120 g/day
			Moderate	50–70 g/day
			Low-fat	30–50 g/day

Adapted from ref. 15.

Cystic Fibrosis

Nutrient guidelines for children with cystic fibrosis have been recommended by the National Cystic Fibrosis Foundation (Table 12). Energy requirements should be adjusted to accommodate the child's activity level and nutritional status.

Lactose Intolerance

Diet therapy for specific carbohydrate intolerance includes a lactose-free diet. The lactose content of dairy products listed in Table 13 may be used to design a dietary regimen for children with lactose deficiency. Such a diet is limited in calcium. Aged cheese, an excellent source of dietary calcium, may be included in a lactose-free diet because of its low lactose content. Calcium carbonate, a common ingredient in antacid preparations, is also a good source of dietary calcium.

Cardiac Disease

The National Cholesterol Education Program has published recommendations for preventive and therapeutic diets. The recommendations encourage the use of a "prudent" diet in an effort to decrease the incidence of coronary disease (5). The recommendations are as follows:

1. Caloric level should be adequate to promote normal growth and development and to achieve and maintain desirable weight.
2. Fat content should be less than or equal to 30% of total daily calories, with saturated fat and polyunsaturated fat each accounting for less than 10% of total calories. Remaining fat calories should be monounsaturated (Tables 14 and 15).
3. Dietary cholesterol should be less than 300 mg/day (Table 14).
4. Carbohydrate content should be 55% of total calories.

Renal Disease

Nutritional management must be individualized according to the severity of the renal disease and the individual patient's nutrient requirements (6–9). Predialysis patients are encouraged to consume adequate protein and calories for growth. Laboratory values dictate dietary sodium, potassium, phosphorus, and protein restrictions (Tables 16 and 17). All efforts are made to provide a liberal diet for the predialysis patient to ensure compliance and optimal growth while maintaining serum chemistries within normal limits.

The aim of dietary treatment for dialysis patients is to provide for optimal growth and to control fluid retention between dialyses. Daily dietary recommendations for the dialysis patient at the Boston Children's Hospital Medical Center (CHMC) dialysis unit are:

1.) calories   100–105/kg
2.) protein   2 g/kg (minimum)
3.) sodium   2 g/kg (adjust higher for Na^+ losses)
4.) potassium   2 g/kg
5.) phosphorus Low (400–600 mg)

TABLE 13. *Lactose content of selected dairy products*

Dairy product	Unit of measure	Lactose content (g)
Whole milk	1 cup	11.8
Low-fat milk (2%)	1 cup	9–13
Buttermilk	1 cup	9–11
Skim milk	1 cup	12–14
Low-fat yogurts	1 cup	11–15
Cottage cheese	1 cup	5–6
Aged cheddar cheese	1 oz	0.4–0.6
Butter	1 tbs	0.15
Margarine	1 tbs	0
Ice cream	1 cup	9
Sherbert	1 cup	4

From ref. 16.

TABLE 14. Saturated fat and cholesterol values of foods

Food product	Serving	Cholesterol (mg)	Saturated fat (g)	
Milk				
Whole	1 cup	34	5.1	
2% fat	1 cup	22	2.9	
Skim	1 cup	5	0.3	
Ice cream	½ cup	27	8.9	For 10% fat ice cream
Cheese				
Cottage, regular	¼ cup	12	1.6	
Hard	1 oz	28	5.3	Creamed, 4% cream fat as cheddar, Swiss
Vegetables	½ cup	0	0	Unless prepared with butter, cheese, milk, or other animal products
Fruits	½ cup	0	0	
Breads	1 slice	0	0.2	
Meats				
Beef pot roast				
Regular	1 oz	31	2.3	
Lean	1 oz	26	0.7	
Ground beef				
21% fat	1 oz	27	2.4	
10% fat	1 oz	26	1.3	
Sirloin steak				
Regular	1 oz	27	3.8	
Lean	1 oz	25	0.9	
Chicken				
Dark meat (skinless)	1 oz	25	0.6	
Light meat (skinless)	1 oz	18	0.3	
Fish	1 oz	20	0.1	
Shellfish				
Clams	3 oz	55	1.0	
Shrimp	3 oz	96	0.1	
Lobster	¼ cup	29	0.1	
Crab	¼ cup	85	0.2	
Eggs				
Whole	1	252	1.7	
Whites	1	0	0	
Fats				
Butter	1 tsp	12	2.5	All vegetable sources of fat are cholesterol free
Bacon	1 strip	16	1.3	
Cream, light	1 tbsp	10	2.9	

Seizure Disorder

Ketogenic diets have been used successfully in controlling myoclonic and akinetic seizures (10). Ketosis can be achieved by providing 50% to 70% of calories as protein. Medium-chain triglycerides have been used in ketogenic diets and can be incorporated into palatable frappes and desserts (11). A 24- to 74-hour period of fasting prior to initiation of the ketogenic diet is necessary to successfully achieve ketosis. All food must be accurately weighed and eaten to ensure a 3:1 ratio of ketogenic to nonketogenic calories. Daily urine testing for ketones is necessary to monitor the degree of ketosis.

Obesity

A balanced reduced-calorie deficit diet (Table 18) is optimally diagnosed through the use of food groupings.

TABLE 15. Fatty acid composition of fats and oils

Fat or oil	Saturated (%)	Polyunsaturated (%)	Monounsaturated (%)
Beef fat	51	4	44
Butter	54	4	30
Canola	6	31	62
Chicken fat	30	22	47
Coconut	77	2	6
Corn	13	62	25
Cottonseed	27	54	19
Lard	41	12	47
Olive	14	9	77
Palm	51	10	39
Palm kernel	81	1	11
Peanut	13	33	49
Safflower	9	78	12
Sesame	15	40	40
Soybean	15	61	24
Sunflower	11	69	20
Vegetable shortening	25	25	43

From ref. 17.

TABLE 16. *Foods high in sodium*

Breads, cereals, and sauces

Bread stuffing	Salted popcorn
Potato chips	Salted nuts
Pretzels	Snack items such as Bugles, corn chips, etc.
Salted crackers	

Fats

Bacon drippings	Salt pork
Commercial salad dressings except mayonnaise	

Meats, fish, poultry, cheese

All canned, cured, dried meats such as:	Frozen items such as:
Bacon	Frozen fish in brine
Cold cuts and luncheon meats	Fish sticks
Chipped and corned beef	Meat pies
Frankfurters	TV dinners
Ham	All cheese (processed and spreads) except cream cheese
Pastrami	
Sardines	
Sausage	
Tuna, canned in oil	

Soups

Bouillon	Canned soups
Canned broth	Dehydrated soups
Canned chowder	

Vegetables

Baked beans	Sauerkraut
Frozen prepared vegetables with butter, cream, or cheese sauces	Tomato juice
	Tomato puree

Miscellaneous items

Canned, dehydrated, or frozen potato, macaroni, spaghetti, or noodle products	Chinese food
	Italian food

Seasonings

Catsup	Onion salt
Celery flakes	Prepared gravies
Celery salt	Pickles
Chili powder	Poultry seasoning
Chili sauce	Relish
Garlic salt	Salt
Meat tenderizers	Soy sauce
Mustard, prepared	Seasoned coatings for meat
Monosodium glutamate	
Olives	Steak sauce
	Worcestershire sauce

TABLE 17. *Foods and beverages high in potassium*

Beverages

Brewed coffee	Milk, whole or skim
Postum	Low-sodium milk

Fruits and juices (200 mg or more K+/100 g)

Apricot	Orange
Avocado	Papaya
Banana	Peach, fresh
Cantaloupe	Rhubarb
Casaba melon	Orange juice
Dried fruits: apricot, date, fig, prune, raisin	Prune juice
	Tomato juice
Honeydew melon	

Meats, fish, poultry

All meats, fish, poultry

Vegetables (300 mg or more K+/100 g)

Artichokes	Mushrooms
Beans, lima	Parsnips, cooked
Carrots, raw	Parsley, raw
Celery, raw	Potato, baked, French fried, chips
Chicory, raw	
Chard, Swiss, cooked	Spinach, raw
Cress, cooked	Radish
Collards	Squash: winter—baked, acorn, butternut
Dandelion and beet greens	

Miscellaneous

Coconut	Peanut butter
Chocolate and cocoa	Salt substitute
Nuts	Bran
Molasses	

Foods are categorized into seven groups based on the American Diabetic Association exchange system (Appendix B) (12). Foods within each group have approximately the same protein, fat, carbohydrate, and caloric values. A food may be substituted for any other food in the same group in the serving size specified. For example, in the bread group, 1 slice of bread may be substituted for $\frac{1}{2}$ cup of cooked rice (Appendix B).

Caloric levels are adjusted during weight reduction to accommodate activity level, growth requirements, and expected rate of weight loss. Diets providing less than 1,200 kilocalories (Cal) per day are considered inadequate to supply the pediatric RDA for energy, iron, calcium, and several trace minerals. Weight reduction regimens of less than 1,200 Cal should be carefully monitored and supplemented with the limited nutrients (Table 18).

A multidisciplinary, physician-supervised approach to childhood obesity incorporating a protein sparing modified fast, physical activity and behavioral skills has been used extensively at the Children's Hospital in New Orleans (20). This program has been studied in adolescents

TABLE 18. Balanced calorie deficit diet

1,200 cal Proteins, 73 g Fat, 35 g Carbohydrate, 145 g	1,500 cal Protein, 79 g Fat, 50 g Carbohydrate, 186 g	1,800 cal Protein, 110 g Fat, 65 g Carbohydrate, 192 g
8 oz skim milk $\frac{1}{2}$ cup unsweetened cereal $\frac{1}{2}$ cup unsweetened orange juice	8 oz skim milk 1 cup unsweetened cereal $\frac{1}{2}$ cup unsweetened orange juice	8 oz skim milk 1 cup unsweetened cereal $\frac{1}{2}$ cup unsweetened juice
3 oz meat 2 slices bread 4 oz whole milk 1 piece fruit	3 oz meat 2 slices bread 8 oz whole milk 1 piece fruit	3 oz meat 2 slices bread $\frac{1}{2}$ tsp margarine 8 oz whole milk 1 piece fruit
1 piece fruit	Diet soda 1 oz cheese 5 saltines	4 oz skim milk 1 oz cheese 5 saltines
8 oz skim milk 3 oz meat $\frac{1}{2}$ cup vegetable salad/low-cal dressing	8 oz skim milk 3 oz meat $\frac{1}{2}$ cup potato $\frac{1}{2}$ cup vegetables Salad/low-cal dressing 1 piece fruit	8 oz skim milk 5 oz meat $\frac{1}{2}$ cup potato $\frac{1}{2}$ cup cooked vegetable $\frac{1}{2}$ tsp margarine Salad/low cal dressing 1 piece fruit
$\frac{1}{2}$ cup skim milk 2 graham crackers	Diet soda 1 oz meat or 1 tbsp peanut butter 1 slice bread or 5 crackers	Diet soda 1 oz meat or 1 tbsp peanut butter 1 slice bread or 5 crackers

TABLE 19A. Protein-sparing modified fast

600 to 800 kcal/day
1.5 to 2.0 g protein/kg ideal body weight/day
No carbohydrates   Low starch vegetables
Water or calorie-free fluids at least 2 liter/day
Daily supplements: Ca 800 mg/day (4 Tums/day), KC1 25 meq/
day multivitamins with minerals

TABLE 19B. *Foods allowed*

Protein

lean beef (fat trimmed and unmarbled) such as roast, stead, ground round (hamburger)
chicken, turkey (remove skin)
fish (if canned, water-packed)
seafood such as shrimp, lobster, oyster, clam

Vegetables

Serving size 4 ounces

okra	broccoli	artichokes	cabbage (cooked)
beets	radishes	sauerkraut	brussell sprouts
onion	eggplant	cauliflower	spinach (cooked)
squash	chickory	tomato juice	mushroom (cooked)
tomato	asparagus	bamboo shoots	beans, green or wax
rhubarb	water cress	vegetable juice	pepper, green or red
carrots			

Serving size 8 ounces

			greens:	
lettuce	endive			
cabbage	spinach	chard		mustard
cucumber	romaine	collard		turnip
zucchini	mushroom	dandelion		kohlrab
celery	chinese cabbage			
hot pepper	green onion			

Free Food

tea	rennet	clear broth
lime	spices	dill or sour pickle
salt	mustard	artificial sweetener
lemon	bouillon	gelatin (unsweetened)
coffee	vinegar	low calorie salad dressing
pepper	diet sodas	catsup (limit to 1 tbsp/day)
		BBQ sauce (limit to 1 tbsp/day)

TABLE 19C. *Foods to avoid*

oil	liver	cereals	hamburger	fried foods
nuts	sugar	sausage	cold cuts	peanut butter
eggs	cream	cheese	avocados	flour, cornmeal
pork	fruits	breads	mayonnaise	starchy vegetables
milk	butter	weiners	margarine	regular chewing gums
bacon	olives			

by several investigators to assess safety and efficacy (21,22). The goal is the selective loss of body fat without negative impact on lean body mass or linear growth. One advantage is that weight loss is more rapid and there is less hunger than with balanced calorie deficit diets. This is particularly useful for children who are morbidly obese, or who have experienced repeated failures with traditional diets. The diet consists of 800 calories per day, including 2 grams of high biological quality protein per kilogram of ideal body weight. Daily supplements include 800 milligrams per day of calcium, 25 meq per day of potassium and a multivitamin/mineral supplement (Tables 19A,B,C).

Diabetes Mellitus

See Appendix B: Exchange lists for planning pediatric diabetic diets.

REFERENCES

1. American Dietetic Association. *Handbook of clinical dietetics.* New Haven: Yale University Press, 1981.
2. Food and Nutrition Board. *Recommended dietary allowances, revised 1989.* Washington, DC: National Academy of Sciences National Research Council, 1989.
3. Fomon SJ. *Infant nutrition.* Philadelphia: WB Saunders, 1974.
4. Fomon SJ. *Pediatrics* 1975;56:350–354.

5. National Cholesterol Education Program. Highlights of the report of the expert panel on blood cholesterol, levels in children and adolescents. Washington, DC: National Institutes of Health, NHLBI, 1981.
6. Berger MA. *J Am Diet Assoc* 1977;70:498–505.
7. Burton BT. *J Am Diet Assoc* 1974;65:623.
8. Burton BT. *J Am Diet Assoc* 1977;70:479–482.
9. Spinozzi NS, Grupe WE. *J Am Diet Assoc* 1977;70:493–497.
10. Segnore JM. *J Am Diet Assoc* 1973;62:285–290.
11. Huttenlocker PR, Wilboum AJ, Segnore JM. *Neurology* 1971;21:1097–1103.
12. American Diabetic Association and the American Dietetic Association. *Exchange lists for weight management.* Chicago: 1989.
13. Getchell EL, Howard RB. In: Sciplen GM, et al., eds. *Comprehensive pediatric nursing.* New York: McGraw-Hill, 1975;220.
14. Cystic Fibrosis Foundation. *Guide to diagnosis and management of cystic fibrosis.* 1974.
15. *Am J Clin Nutr* 1978;31:595.
16. Department of Agriculture. *Composition of foods* (handbook no. 8-5). Washington, DC: United States Department of Agriculture, 1979.
17. Green MG (ed): *The Harriet Lane Handbook,* 12th edition. Mosby Year Book, Inc: St. Louis, 1991.
18. National Cholesterol Education Program. Report of the expert panel on blood cholesterol levels in children and adolescents. US Department of Health and Human Services, National Institutes of Health. NIH publication no. 91-2732, September, 1991.
19. Figueroa-Colon R, von Almen TK, Suskind RM. Clinical considerations in the treatment of childhood obesity IN: Giorgi PL, Suskind RM, Catassi C (eds); The obese child. *Pediatr Adolesc Med Basel,* Karger, 1992;(2):181–196.
20. Merritt RJ, Bistrian BR, Blackburn GL, Suskind RM. Consequences of modified fasting in obese pediatric and adolescent patients. Protein sparing modified fast. *J Pediatr* 1980;96:13–19.
21. Pencharz PB, Clarke R, Archibald EH, Vaisman N. The effect of a weight reducing diet on the nitrogen metabolism of obese adolescents. *Can J Physiol Pharmacol* 1988;66:1469–74.

APPENDIX B

Exchange Lists for Meal Planning from the American Diabetes Association, Inc. and the American Dietetic Association[1]

EXCHANGE LISTS

The reason for dividing food into six different groups is that foods vary in their carbohydrate, protein, fat, and calorie content. Each exchange list contains foods that are alike—each choice contains about the same amount of carbohydrate, protein, fat, and calories.

The following chart shows the amount of these nutrients in one serving from each exchange list.

Exchange List	Carbohydrate (grams)	Protein (grams)	Fat (grams)	Calories
Starch/Bread	15	3	trace	80
Meat				
Lean	—	7	3	55
Medium-Fat	—	7	5	75
High-Fat	—	7	8	100
Vegetable	5	2	—	25
Fruit	15	—	—	60
Milk				
Skim	12	8	trace	90
Lowfat	12	8	5	120
Whole	12	8	8	150
Fat	—	—	5	45

As you read the exchange lists, you will notice that one choice often is a larger amount of food than another choice from the same list. Because foods are so different, each food is measured or weighed so the amount of carbohydrate, protein, fat, and calories is the same in each choice.

You will notice symbols on some foods in the exchange groups. Foods that are high in fiber (3 grams or more per exchange) have a † symbol. High-fiber foods are good for you. It is important to eat more of these foods.

Foods that are high in sodium (400 milligrams or more of sodium per exchange) have an * symbol; foods that have 400 mg or more of sodium if two or more exchanges are eaten have a ★ symbol. It's a good idea to limit your intake of high-salt foods, especially if you have high blood pressure.

If you have a favorite food that is not included in any of these groups, ask your dietitian about it. That food can probably be worked into your meal plan, at least now and then.

STARCH/BREAD LIST

Each item in this list contains approximately 15 grams of carbohydrate, 3 grams of protein, a trace of fat, and 80 calories. Whole grain products average about 2 grams of fiber per exchange. Some foods are higher in fiber. Those foods that contain 3 or more grams of fiber per exchange are identified with the fiber symbol†.

You can choose your starch exchanges from any of the items on this list. If you want to eat a starch food that is not on this list, the general rule is that:

- $\frac{1}{2}$ cup of cereal, grain or pasta is one exchange
- 1 ounce of a bread product is one exchange

Your dietitian can help you be more exact.

CEREALS/GRAINS/PASTA

† Bran cereals, concentrated (such as Bran Buds®, All Bran®)	$\frac{1}{3}$ cup
† Bran cereals, flaked	$\frac{1}{2}$ cup
Bulgur (cooked)	$\frac{1}{2}$ cup
Cooked cereals	$\frac{1}{2}$ cup
Cornmeal (dry)	$2\frac{1}{2}$ Tbsp.
Grape-Nuts®	3 Tbsp.
Grits (cooked)	$\frac{1}{2}$ cup
Other ready-to-eat unsweetened cereals	$\frac{3}{4}$ cup

---

[1] The Exchange Lists are the basis of a meal planning system designed by a committee of the American Diabetes Association and The American Dietetic Association. While designed primarily for people with diabetes and others who must follow special diets, the Exchange Lists are based on principles of good nutrition that apply to everyone. Copyright (c) 1989 by American Diabetes Association Inc., and The American Dietetic Association.

Pasta (cooked)	½ cup
Puffed cereal	1½ cup
Rice, white or brown (cooked)	⅓ cup
Shredded wheat	½ cup
† Wheat germ	3 Tbsp.

DRIED BEANS/PEAS/LENTILS

† Beans and peas (cooked) (such as kidney, white, split, blackeye)	⅓ cup
† Lentils (cooked)	⅓ cup
† Baked beans	¼ cup

STARCHY VEGETABLES

† Corn	½ cup
† Corn on cob, 6 in. long	1
† Lima beans	½ cup
† Peas, green (canned or frozen)	½ cup
† Plantain	½ cup
Potato, baked	1 small (3 oz.)
Potato, mashed	½ cup
† Squash, winter (acorn, butternut)	1 cup
Yam, sweet potato, plain	⅓ cup

BREAD

Bagel	½ (1 oz.)
Bread sticks, crisp, 4 in. long × ½ in.	2 (⅔ oz.)
Croutons, lowfat	1 cup
English muffin	½
Frankfurter or hamburger bun	½ (1 oz.)
Pita, 6 in. across	½
Plain roll, small	1 (1 oz.)
Raisin, unfrosted	1 slice (1 oz.)
Rye, pumpernickel	1 slice (1 oz.)
Tortilla, 6 in. across	1
White (including French, Italian)	1 slice (1 oz.)
Whole wheat	1 slice (1 oz.)

* 3 grams or more of fiber per exchange

CRACKERS/SNACKS

Animal crackers	8
Graham crackers, 2½ in. square	3
Matzoh	¾ oz.
Melba toast	5 slices
Oyster crackers	24
Popcorn (popped, no fat added)	3 cups
Pretzels	¾ oz.
† Rye crisp, 2 in. × 3½ in.	4
Saltine-type crackers	6
† Whole-wheat crackers, no fat added (crisp breads, such as Finn®, Kavli®, Wasa®)	2–4 slices (¾ oz.)

STARCH FOODS PREPARED WITH FAT

(Count as 1 Starch/Bread Exchange, Plus 1 Fat Exchange.)

Biscuit, 2½ in. across	1
Chow mein noodles	½ cup
Corn bread, 2 in. cube	1 (2 oz.)
Cracker, round butter type	6
French fried potatoes, 2 in. to 3½ in. long	10 (1½ oz.)
Muffin, plain, small	1
Pancake, 4 in. across	2
Stuffing, bread (prepared)	¼ cup
Taco shell, 6 in. across	2
Waffle, 4½ in. square	1
† Whole-wheat crackers, fat added (such as Triscuit®)	4–6 (1 oz.)

MEAT LIST

Each serving of meat and substitutes on this list contains about 7 grams of protein. The amount of fat and number of calories vary, depending on what kind of meat or substitute you choose. The list is divided into three parts based on the amount of fat and calories: lean meat, medium-fat meat, and high-fat meat. One ounce (one meat exchange) of each of these includes:

	Carbohydrate (grams)	Protein (grams)	Fat (grams)	Calories
Lean	0	7	3	55
Medium-Fat	0	7	5	75
High-Fat	0	7	8	100

You are encouraged to use more lean and medium-fat meat, poultry, and fish in your meal plan. This will help decrease your fat intake, which may help decrease your risk for heart disease. The items from the high-fat group are high in saturated fat, cholesterol, and calories. You should limit your choices from the high-fat group to three (3) times per week. Meat and substitutes do not contribute any fiber to your meal plan.

* Meats and meat substitutes that have 400 milligrams or more of sodium per exchange are indicated with this symbol.

* Meats and meat substitutes that have 400 mg or more of sodium if two or more exchanges are eaten are indicated with this symbol.

TIPS

1. Bake, roast, broil, grill, or boil these foods rather than frying them with added fat.

2. Use a nonstick pan spray or a nonstick pan to brown or fry these foods.
3. Trim off visible fat before and after cooking.
4. Do not add flour, bread crumbs, coating mixes, or fat to these foods when preparing them.
5. Weigh meat after removing bones and fat, and after cooking. Three ounces of cooked meat is about equal to 4 ounces of raw meat. Some examples of meat portions are:
   2 ounces meat (2 meat exchanges) =
     1 small chicken leg or thigh
     $\frac{1}{2}$ cup cottage cheese or tuna
   3 ounces meat (3 meat exchanges) =
     1 medium pork chop
     1 small hamburger
     $\frac{1}{2}$ of a whole chicken breast
     1 unbreaded fish fillet
     cooked meat, about the size of a deck of cards
6. Restaurants usually serve prime cuts of meat, which are high in fat and calories.

LEAN MEAT AND SUBSTITUTES

(One Exchange is Equal to Any One of The Following Items.)

Beef:	USDA Select or Choice grades of lean beef, such as round, sirloin, and flank steak; tenderloin; and chipped beef*	1 oz.
Pork:	Lean pork, such as fresh ham; canned, cured or boiled ham*; Canadian bacon*, tenderloin.	1 oz.
Veal:	All cuts are lean except for veal cutlets (ground or cubed). Examples of lean veal are chops and roasts.	1 oz.
Poultry:	Chicken, turkey, Cornish hen (without skin)	1 oz.
Fish:	All fresh and frozen fish	1 oz.
	Crab, lobster, scallops, shrimp, clams (fresh or canned in water)	2 oz.
	Oysters	6 medium
	Tuna ★ (canned in water)	$\frac{1}{4}$ cup
	Herring ★ (uncreamed or smoked)	1 oz.
	Sardines (canned)	2 medium
Wild Game:	Venison, rabbit, squirrel	1 oz.
	Pheasant, duck, goose (without skin)	1 oz.
Cheese:	Any cottage cheese ★	$\frac{1}{4}$ cup
	Grated parmesan	2 Tbsp.
Other:	Diet cheeses* (with less than 55 calories per ounce)	1 oz.
	95% fat-free luncheon meat*	$1\frac{1}{2}$ oz.
	Egg whites	3 whites
	Egg substitutes with less than 55 calories per $\frac{1}{2}$ cup	$\frac{1}{2}$ cup

* 400 mg or more of sodium per exchange
★ 400 mg or more of sodium if two or more exchanges are eaten

MEDIUM-FAT MEAT AND SUBSTITUTES

(One Exchange is Equal to Any One of The Following Items.)

Beef:	Most beef products fall into this category. Examples are: all ground beef, roast (rib, chuck, rump), steak (cubed, Porterhouse, T-bone), and meatloaf.	1 oz.
Pork:	Most pork products fall into this category. Examples are: chops, loin roast, Boston butt, cutlets.	1 oz.
Lamb:	Most lamb products fall into this category. Examples are: chops, leg, and roast.	1 oz.
Veal:	Cutlet (ground or cubed, unbreaded)	1 oz.
Poultry:	Chicken (with skin), domestic duck or goose (well drained of fat), ground turkey	1 oz.
Fish:	Tuna ★ (canned in oil and drained)	$\frac{1}{4}$ cup
	Salmon ★ (canned)	$\frac{1}{4}$ cup
Cheese:	Skim or part-skim milk cheeses, such as:	
	Ricotta	$\frac{1}{4}$ cup
	Mozzarella	1 oz.
	Diet cheeses* (with 56–80 calories per ounce)	1 oz.
Other:	86% fat-free luncheon meat ★	1 oz.
	Egg (high in cholesterol, limit to 3 per week)	1
	Egg substitutes with 56–80 calories per $\frac{1}{4}$ cup	$\frac{1}{4}$ cup
	Tofu ($2\frac{1}{2}$ in. × $2\frac{3}{4}$ in. × 1 in.)	4 oz.

	Liver, heart, kidney, sweetbreads (high in cholesterol)	1 oz.

* 400 mg or more of sodium per exchange

★ 400 mg or more of sodium if two or more exchanges are eaten

HIGH-FAT MEAT AND SUBSTITUTES

Remember, These Items are High in Saturated Fat, Cholesterol, and Calories, and Should Be Used Only Three (3) Times Per Week.

(One Exchange is Equal to Any of The Following Items.)

Beef:	Most USDA Prime cuts of beef, such as ribs, corned beef ★	1 oz.
Pork:	Spareribs, ground pork, pork sausage* (patty or link)	1 oz.
Lamb:	Patties (ground lamb)	1 oz.
Fish:	Any fried fish product	1 oz.
Cheese:	All regular cheeses, such as American*, Blue*, Cheddar★, Monterey Jack★, Swiss	1 oz.
Other:	Luncheon meat*, such as bologna, salami, pimento loaf	1 oz.
	Sausage*, such as Polish, Italian smoked	1 oz.
	Knockwurst*	1 oz.
	Bratwurst★	1 oz.
	Frankfurter* (turkey or chicken)	1 frank (10/lb.)
	Peanut butter (contains unsaturated fat)	1 Tbsp.

Count as One High-Fat Meat Plus One Fat Exchange:

	Frankfurter* (beef, pork, or combination)	1 frank (10/lb.)

* 400 mg or more of sodium per exchange

★ 400 mg or more of sodium if two or more exchanges are eaten

VEGETABLE LIST†

Each vegetable serving on this list contains about 5 grams of carbohydrate, 2 grams of protein, and 25 calories. Vegetables contain 2-3 grams of dietary fiber. Vegetables which contain 400 mg or more of sodium per exchange are identified with a * symbol.

Vegetables are a good source of vitamins and minerals. Fresh and frozen vegetables have more vitamins and less added salt. Rinsing canned vegetables will remove much of the salt.

Unless otherwise noted, the serving size for vegetables (one vegetable exchange) is:

$\frac{1}{2}$ cup of cooked vegetables or vegetable juice
1 cup of raw vegetables

Artichoke ($\frac{1}{2}$ medium)	Mushrooms, cooked
	Okra
Asparagus	Onions
Beans (green, wax, Italian)	Pea pods
	Peppers (green)
Bean sprouts	Rutabaga
Beets	Sauerkraut*
Broccoli	Spinach, cooked
Brussels sprouts	Summer squash (crookneck)
Cabbage, cooked	
Carrots	Tomato (one large)
Cauliflower	Tomato/vegetable juice*
Eggplant	
Greens (collard, mustard, turnip)	Turnips
	Water chestnuts
Kohlrabi	Zucchini, cooked
Leeks	

Starchy vegetables such as corn, peas, and potatoes are found on the Starch/Bread List.

For free vegetables, see Free Food List on page 22.

* 400 mg or more of sodium per exchange

FRUIT LIST

Each item on this list contains about 15 grams of carbohydrate and 60 calories. Fresh, frozen, and dried fruits have about 2 grams of fiber per exchange. Fruits that have 3 or more grams of fiber per exchange have a † symbol. Fruit juices contain very little dietary fiber.

The carbohydrate and calorie content for a fruit exchange are based on the usual serving of the most commonly eaten fruits. Use fresh fruits or fruits frozen or canned without sugar added. Whole fruit is more filling than fruit juice and may be a better choice for those who are trying to lose weight. Unless otherwise noted, the serving size for one fruit exchange is:

$\frac{1}{2}$ cup of fresh fruit or fruit juice
$\frac{1}{4}$ cup of dried fruit

FRESH, FROZEN, AND UNSWEETENED CANNED FRUIT

Apple (raw, 2 in. across)	1 apple
Applesauce (unsweetened)	$\frac{1}{2}$ cup
Apricots (medium, raw)	4 apricots
Apricots (canned)	$\frac{1}{2}$ cup, or 4 halves
Banana (9 in. long)	$\frac{1}{2}$ banana
† Blackberries (raw)	$\frac{3}{4}$ cup
† Blueberries (raw)	$\frac{3}{4}$ cup
Cantaloupe (5 in. across)	$\frac{1}{3}$ melon
(cubes)	1 cup
Cherries (large, raw)	12 cherries
Cherries (canned)	$\frac{1}{2}$ cup
Figs (raw, 2 in. across)	2 figs
Fruit cocktail (canned)	$\frac{1}{2}$ cup
Grapefruit (medium)	$\frac{1}{2}$ grapefruit
Grapefruit (segments)	$\frac{3}{4}$ cup
Grapes (small)	15 grapes
Honeydew melon (medium)	$\frac{1}{8}$ melon
(cubes)	1 cup
Kiwi (large)	1 kiwi
Mandarin oranges	$\frac{3}{4}$ cup
Mango (small)	$\frac{1}{2}$ mango
† Nectarine ($2\frac{1}{2}$ in. across)	1 nectarine
Orange ($2\frac{1}{2}$ in. across)	1 orange
Papaya	1 cup
Peach ($2\frac{3}{4}$ in. across)	1 peach, or $\frac{3}{4}$ cup
Peaches (canned)	$\frac{1}{2}$ cup or 2 halves
Pear	$\frac{1}{2}$ large, or 1 small
Pears (canned)	$\frac{1}{2}$ cup, or 2 halves
Persimmon (medium, native)	2 persimmons
Pineapple (raw)	$\frac{3}{4}$ cup
Pineapple (canned)	$\frac{1}{3}$ cup
Plum (raw, 2 in. across)	2 plums
† Pomegranate	$\frac{1}{2}$ pomegranate
† Raspberries (raw)	1 cup
† Strawberries (raw, whole)	$1\frac{1}{4}$ cup
† Tangerine ($2\frac{1}{2}$ in. across)	2 tangerines
Watermelon (cubes)	$1\frac{1}{4}$ cup

DRIED FRUIT

† Apples	4 rings
† Apricots	7 halves
Dates	$2\frac{1}{2}$ medium
† Figs	$1\frac{1}{2}$
† Prunes	3 medium
Raisins	2 Tbsp.

FRUIT JUICE

Apple juice/cider	$\frac{1}{2}$ cup
Cranberry juice cocktail	$\frac{1}{3}$ cup
Grapefruit juice	$\frac{1}{2}$ cup
Grape juice	$\frac{1}{3}$ cup
Orange juice	$\frac{1}{2}$ cup
Pineapple juice	$\frac{1}{2}$ cup
Prune juice	$\frac{1}{3}$ cup

† 3 or more grams of fiber per exchange

MILK LIST

Each serving of milk or milk products on this list contains about 12 grams of carbohydrate and 8 grams of protein. The amount of fat in milk is measured in percent (%) of butterfat. The calories vary, depending on what kind of milk you choose. The list is divided into three parts based on the amount of fat and calories: skim/very lowfat milk, lowfat milk, and whole milk. One serving (one milk exchange) of each of these includes:

	Carbohydrate (grams)	Protein (grams)	Fat (grams)	Calories
Skim/Very Lowfat	12	8	trace	90
Lowfat	12	8	5	120
Whole	12	8	8	150

Milk is the body's main source of calcium, the mineral needed for growth and repair of bones. Yogurt is also a good source of calcium. Yogurt and many dry or powdered milk products have different amounts of fat. If you have questions about a particular item, read the label to find out the fat and calorie content.

Milk is good to drink, but it can also be added to cereal, and to other foods. Many tasty dishes such as sugar-free pudding are made with milk (see the Combination Foods list). Add life to plain yogurt by adding one of your fruit exchanges to it.

SKIM AND VERY LOWFAT MILK

skim milk	1 cup
$\frac{1}{2}$% milk	1 cup
1% milk	1 cup
lowfat buttermilk	1 cup
evaporated skim milk	$\frac{1}{2}$ cup
dry nonfat milk	$\frac{1}{3}$ cup
plain nonfat yogurt	8 oz.

LOWFAT MILK

2% milk	1 cup fluid
plain lowfat yogurt (with added nonfat milk solids)	8 oz.

WHOLE MILK

The whole milk group has much more fat per serving than the skim and lowfat groups. Whole milk has more than $3\frac{1}{4}$% butterfat. Limit your choices from the whole milk group as much as possible.

whole milk	1 cup
evaporated whole milk	$\frac{1}{2}$ cup
whole plain yogurt	8 oz.

FAT LIST

Each serving on the fat list contains about 5 grams of fat and 45 calories.

The foods on the fat list contain mostly fat, although some items may also contain a small amount of protein. All fats are high in calories and should be carefully measured. Everyone should modify fat intake by eating unsaturated fats instead of saturated fats. The sodium content of these foods varies widely. Check the label for sodium information.

UNSATURATED FATS

Avocado	$\frac{1}{8}$ medium
Margarine	1 tsp.
★ Margarine, diet	1 Tbsp.
Mayonnaise	1 tsp.
★ Mayonnaise, reduced-calorie	1 Tbsp.
Nuts and Seeds:	
Almonds, dry roasted	6 whole
Cashews, dry roasted	1 Tbsp.
Pecans	2 whole
Peanuts	20 small or 10 large
Walnuts	2 whole
Other nuts	1 Tbsp.
Seeds, pine nuts, sunflower (without shells)	1 Tbsp.
Pumpkin seeds	2 tsp.
Oil (corn, cottonseed, safflower, soybean, sunflower, olive, peanut)	1 tsp
★ Olives	10 small or 5 large
Salad dressing, mayonnaise-type	2 tsp.
Salad dressing, mayonnaise-type, reduced-calorie	1 Tbsp.
★ Salad dressing (oil varieties)	1 Tbsp.
* Salad dressing, reduced-calorie	2 Tbsp.

(Two tablespoons of low-calorie salad dressing is a free food.)

SATURATED FATS

Butter	1 tsp.
★ Bacon	1 slice
Chitterlings	$\frac{1}{2}$ ounce
Coconut, shredded	2 Tbsp.
Coffee whitener, liquid	2 Tbsp.
Coffee whitener, powder	4 tsp.
Cream (light, coffee, table)	2 Tbsp.
Cream, sour	2 Tbsp.
Cream (heavy, whipping)	1 Tbsp.
Cream cheese	1 Tbsp.
★ Salt pork	$\frac{1}{4}$ ounce

* 400 mg or more of sodium per exchange

★ 400 mg or more of sodium if two or more exchanges are eaten

FREE FOODS

A free food is any food or drink that contains less than 20 calories per serving. You can eat as much as you want of those items that have no serving size specified. You may eat two or three servings per day of those items that have a specific serving size. Be sure to spread them out through the day.

Drinks:

Bouillon * or broth without fat
Bouillon, low-sodium
Carbonated drinks, sugar-free
Carbonated water
Club soda
Cocoa powder, unsweetened (1 Tbsp.)
Coffee/Tea
Drink mixes, sugar-free
Tonic water, sugar-free

Nonstick pan spray

Fruit:

Cranberries, unsweetened ($\frac{1}{2}$ cup)
Rhubarb, unsweetened ($\frac{1}{2}$ cup)

Vegetables:
(raw, 1 cup)
Cabbage
Celery
Chinese cabbage†
Cucumber
Green onion
Hot peppers
Mushrooms
Radishes
Zucchini†

Salad greens:
Endive
Escarole
Lettuce
Romaine
Spinach

Sweet Substitutes:
Candy, hard, sugar-free
Gelatin, sugar-free
Gum, sugar-free
Jam/Jelly, sugar-free (less than 20 cal./2 tsp.)
Pancake syrup, sugar-free (1-2 Tbsp.)
Sugar substitutes (saccharin, aspartame)
Whipped topping (2 Tbsp.)

Condiments:
Catsup (1 Tbsp.)
Horseradish
Mustard
Pickles *, dill, unsweetened
Salad dressing, low-calorie (2 Tbsp.)
Taco sauce (3 Tbsp.)
Vinegar

Seasonings can be very helpful in making food taste better. Be careful of how much sodium you use. Read the label, and choose those seasonings that do not contain sodium or salt.

Basil (fresh)
Celery seeds
Chili powder
Chives
Cinnamon
Curry
Dill
Flavoring extracts (vanilla, almond, walnut, peppermint, butter, lemon, etc.)
Garlic
Garlic powder
Herbs
Hot pepper sauce
Lemon
Lemon juice
Lemon pepper
Lime
Lime juice
Mint
Onion powder
Oregano
Paprika
Pepper
Pimento
Spices
Soy sauce*
Soy sauce*, low-sodium ("lite")
Wine, used in cooking ($\frac{1}{4}$ cup)
Worcestershire sauce

† 3 grams or more of fiber per exchange
* 400 mg or more of sodium per exchange

COMBINATION FOODS

Much of the food we eat is mixed together in various combinations. These combination foods do not fit into only one exchange list. It can be quite hard to tell what is in a certain casserole dish or baked food item. This is a list of average values for some typical combination foods. This list will help you fit these foods into your meal plan. Ask your dietitian for information about any other foods you'd like to eat. The American Diabetes Association/American Dietetic Association Family Cookbooks and the American Diabetes Association Holiday Cookbook have many recipes and further information about many foods, including combination foods. Check your library or local bookstore.

Food	Amount	Exchanges
Casseroles, homemade	1 cup (8 oz.)	2 starch, 2 medium-fat meat, 1 fat
Cheese pizza*, thin crust	$\frac{1}{4}$ of 15 oz. or $\frac{1}{4}$ of 10″	2 starch, 1 medium-fat meat, 1 fat
Chili with beans †, * (commercial)	1 cup (8 oz.)	2 starch, 2 medium-fat meat, 2 fat
Chow mein* (without noodles or rice)	2 cups (16 oz.)	1 starch, 2 vegetable, 2 lean meat
Macaroni and cheese*	1 cup (8 oz.)	2 starch, 1 medium-fat meat, 2 fat
Soup:		
Bean†, *	1 cup (8 oz.)	1 starch, 1 vegetable, 1 lean meat
Chunky, all varieties*	10$\frac{3}{4}$ oz. can	1 starch, 1 vegetable, 1 medium-fat meat
Cream* (made with water)	1 cup (8 oz.)	1 starch, 1 fat
Vegetable* or broth-type*	1 cup (8 oz.)	1 starch

Spaghetti and meatballs* (canned)	1 cup (8 oz.)	2 starch, 1 medium-fat meat, 1 fat
Sugar-free pudding (made with skim milk)	½ cup	1 starch
If beans are used as a meat substitute:		
Dried beans†, peas†, lentils†	1 cup (cooked)	2 starch, 1 lean meat

† 3 grams or more of fiber per exchange
* 400 mg or more of sodium per exchange

FOODS FOR OCCASIONAL USE

Moderate amounts of some foods can be used in your meal plan, in spite of their sugar or fat content, as long as you can maintain blood-glucose control. The following list includes average exchange values for some of these foods. Because they are concentrated sources of carbohydrate, you will notice that the portion sizes are very small. Check with your dietitian for advice of how often and when you can eat them.

Food	Amount	Exchanges
Angel food cake	$\frac{1}{12}$ cake	2 starch
Cake, no icing	$\frac{1}{12}$ cake, or a 3″ square	2 starch, 2 fat
Cookies	2 small (1 $\frac{3}{4}$″ across)	1 starch, 1 fat
Frozen fruit yogurt	$\frac{1}{3}$ cup	1 starch
Gingersnaps	3	1 starch
Granola	$\frac{1}{4}$ cup	1 starch, 1 fat
Granola bars	1 small	1 starch, 1 fat
Ice cream, any flavor	$\frac{1}{2}$ cup	1 starch, 2 fat
Ice milk, any flavor	$\frac{1}{2}$ cup	1 starch, 1 fat
Sherbet, any flavor	$\frac{1}{4}$ cup	1 starch
Snack chips *, all varieties	1 oz.	1 starch, 2 fat
Vanilla wafers	6 small	1 starch

* 400 mg or more of sodium if two or more exchanges are eaten

Subject Index

Abetalipoproteinemia, 65
Absorbed energy, 376
Accelerator globulin, 68
N-acetyl-*L* tyrosine, 227, 235
Acrodermatitis enteropathica
   in AIDS, 152, 451
   cardinal features, 121
   and immune function, 150
   treatment, 123
   zinc deficiency, 120–121, 150
ACTH
   adaptation to malnutrition, 164–165
   psychosocial dwarfism, 276–277
Actinomycin, 419
Acute diarrhea, 325–329
Acute nonlymphocytic leukemia, 422
Acute pancreatitis, 367
Acute renal insufficiency, 396–397
Adaptation, and hormones, 162–163, 165, 169
Adherence
   childhood obesity intervention, 283–284
   exercise programs, 288
Adiposity, and lipoprotein levels, 297
Adolescent pregnancy, birth weight, 2
Adolescents, 257–264
   nutritional needs, 257–258
   risk conditions, 260–263
   year 2000 goals, 258–260
Adrenal gland, and malnutrition, 164–165
Adriamycin, 419
African-American, 524–525
   growth-stunting, 524
   lipoprotein levels, 296
Age factors, lipoprotein levels, 296
AIDS, 447–453. *See also* HIV infection
   clinical picture, 447–448
   costs, 447
   immunologic dysfunction, 448–450
   nutritional status, 152, 440, 450–452
   and protein-energy malnutrition, 449
Alanine
   burn patients, 219
   in oral rehydration solution, 328
Alberta Children's Hospital diet, 110
Albumin
   critically ill children, 212
   in nutritional status assessment, 199
Albumin supplementation, 222
Alcohol intake, and lipoproteins, 297
Alcoholism, thiamine deficiency, 78
Aldosterone, 164–165
Alkaptonuria, 87, 474

All-rac-α-tocopherol, 62–63
Allergic eosinophilic gastroenteritis, 462–463
Allergic reactions. *See* Food allergy
Amenorrhea
   and obesity, 282
   vegetarian diets, 187–188
American Diabetes Association diet, 286, 544–545, 549–556
American Dietetic Association exchange lists, 549–556
Amino acid mixture, complete, 402
Amino acid infusions, 202
Amino acid profiles
   anorexia nervosa, 267
   in nutritional status assessment, 201
Amino acids. *See also* Essential amino acids
   acute renal insufficiency, 397
   breast milk versus formulas, 14–15
   burn patients, 219
   inborn errors of metabolism, 471–484
   liver disease, 357
   in parenteral regimens, 226–227, 233–236
   term newborn requirements, 13–15
Ampicillin, 135, 444
Amylase
   pancreatic concentrations, 364
   secretion in obesity, 368
   in term newborn, 12–13
Amylase deficiency, 367
Anabolic steroids, 262–263
Anaphylaxis, 457–458, 462–467. *See also* Food allergy
Anasarca, 395–396
Anemia, 91–103. *See also* Iron deficiency anemia
   congenital heart disease, 389
   definition, 91–92
   juvenile arthritis, 411
Animal fat, 506
Animal models, 173–174
Anorexia
   and AIDS, 448, 451
   in juvenile arthritis, 412
   and malignancy, 417–419
Anorexia nervosa, 265–272
   definitions, 265–266
   and diabetes, 319
   epidemiology, 266
   home treatment, 269–270
   mortality rate, 268
   nutritional assessment, 267–268
   nutritional rehabilitation, 269–271
   premorbid nutritional status, 266–267

   tube feedings, 267–271
   tumor necrosis factor, 146
Anthropometric measures, 518–522
   evaluation of, 195–196
   interpretation, 519
Antibiotics
   and enteral feeding, 243–244
   immunocompromised children, 444
   malnourished children, 135, 444
Antibody-mediated immunity
   deficiencies, 438–439, 441
   in HIV infection, 151–152
   malnourished children, 147
   mechanisms, 141–142
Anticonvulsants
   in developmentally disabled, 488
   folate deficiency, 101
   lipoprotein levels, 297
   nutrient interactions, 251–253
   and rickets, 488
   vitamin K deficiency, 70
Antidepressants, bulimia nervosa, 272
Antigen-antibody complexes, 459–460
Antigenic food components, 458–460
Antihemophilic globulin, 68
Antihistamines, 467
Antioxidant hypothesis, 64
Apo B/Apo A-I levels, 296
Appetite, drug effects, 248–249
Arachidonic acid
   inflammatory mediator source, 144
   and parenteral nutrition, 236
Arginase deficiency, 472
Argininemia, 472–473
Argininosuccinate lyase deficiency, 472
Argininosuccinate synthetase deficiency, 472
Argininosuccinic aciduria, 472
Arthus reaction, 459
Ascorbic acid. *See* Vitamin C
Aspartame, diabetic diet, 318
Asplanchna, 64
Asthma, 462
Asymmetric tonic neck reflex, 489
Ataxia telangiectasia, 439
Atelectasis, 211
Atherosclerotic lesions, 295, 389
Athletes, risks, 262–263
Atopic dermatitis, 463–464
   breast-fed children, 41
   breast milk fatty acids, 35
   clinical syndrome, 463
   etiology, 463–464
Atopy, 460–461, 466

558 / Subject Index

Atrioventricular septal defect, 384–385
Attachment behavior, 108
Attention-deficit disorder, 175–177
Attentional processes
    food additive effects, 108–110
    iron deficiency, 108
    malnutrition long-term effects, 175–177
    sugar effects, 111–112
Auditory evoked potentials, 174–175
Autocanabalism, 208–209
Aversion to food, 418, 422
Azidothymidine (AZT), 451

B lymphocytes
    antibody production, 143
    critically ill children, 211
    in host defense, 141–142
    and malnutrition, 132
    maturation pathways, 142–143
Baby foods, 531, 534–535
Bactrim, 451
Balanced caloric deficit diet, 542–544
Barbados longitudinal study, 176–177
Bardet-Biedl syndrome, 281
Barnard's observational scale, 44–45
Basal metabolism
    critically ill children, 209–210, 213
    newborn, 10
    in pregnancy, 2
Basophil histamine release test, 465
BCG immunization
    immunodeficient children, 443
    and malnutrition, 153
Beef consumption, 513–514
Behavior, 173–177
    effects of breakfast, 110–111
    food additives, 108–110
    and iron deficiency, 95, 107–108
    malnutrition effects, 173–177
    and sugar, 111–112
Behavior modification, and obesity, 288–289
Behavioral Risk Factor Surveillance System, 524
Beriberi. *See* Thiamine deficiency
Bifidobacteria, 17
Biguanides, 248–250
Bile acid-binding resins, 304–305
Bile acid metabolism, 357
Binge eating, 266. *See also* Eating Disorders
Biochemical assessment techniques, 199–202
Bioelectrical impedance analysis, 197–198
Biotin, 85–86
    dependency syndromes, 86
    dietary sources, 85
    in human milk and formulas, 76
    parenteral intake, 76, 230
    pharmacologic use, 75
    recommended daily allowances, 74, 85–86, 532
    toxicity, 86
Biotin deficiency, 85
Birth defects, 4
Birth weight, 2. *See also* Low birth weight
Black Hebrews, 186–187
Blacks *See* African-American

Blalock-Taussig shunt, 390
Blenderized feedings, 244
Blood glucose, and diabetes, 320
Blount disease, 282
Body composition
    biochemical indices, 202
    indirect assessment methods, 196–199
    model of, 196–197
Body fat
    and body composition assessment, 196–197
    newborn infants, 26
    and tumors, 418
Body image, 265
Body mass index, 519
    and birth weight, 3
    childhood obesity, 279
    prenatal care, 4
Body surface area formula, 219–220
Body temperature, burn patients, 218
Body water
    in body composition, 196–197
    term newborn, 9, 11–12
Body weight, 9, 196
Bogalusa Heart Study, 511–514
Bonding, and breast-feeding, 46–47
Bone age, and obesity, 281
Bone density, anorexia nervosa, 267–268
Bone marrow transplantation, 423, 442
Bone metabolism, 58–60
Boric acid poisoning, 75, 80
Bottle-feeding. *See also* Infant formulas
    and bonding, 46–47
    and dental caries, 495–496
Bovine-based formulas. *See also* Cow's milk formulas
    energy intake and growth, 39–40
    trace minerals, 37
"Bowel rest," 328, 347, 350
Brain, energy requirements, newborn, 10
Brain
    development, 136
    energy requirements, newborn, 10
    mass, anorexia nervosa, 267–268
    weight, 174
Branched-chain amino acids
    burn patients, 219
    critically ill children, 208–209, 214
    liver disease, 357, 360
Branched-chain ketoaciduria, 476
Brazelton examination, 45
Bread exchanges, 549–550
Bread group, trace elements, 116
Breakfast
    and behavior, 110–111
    Bogalusa Heart Study, 512–513
    school programs, 527
Breast-feeding. *See also* Human milk; Lactation
    atopy development, 466
    and bonding, 46–47
    diabetes protection, 311
    energy requirements, 6
    fluoride supplements, 499
    HIV transmission, 440
    iron needs, 96
    mother-infant interaction, 43–47

    secondary immunodeficiency prevention, 155
Brittle diabetic, 320
Bronchopulmonary dysplasia, 29
Brown fat, newborn infant, 26
Bulimia nervosa, 265–272
    antidepressants in, 271
    definitions, 265–266
    dental complications, 268
    epidemiology, 266
    nutritional assessment, 268–269
    nutritional rehabilitation, 271–272
    premorbid nutritional status, 266–267
"Burke method." *See* Dietary history
Burn patient, 217–222
    "ebb" and "flow" phases, 217–219
    metabolism, 217–219
    nutritional requirements, 219–221
"Burning foot" syndrome, 84

C-reactive protein, 132
C3 levels, 147
Calbindin, 58–59
Calcium
    adolescent needs, 257–259
    bone content, gestational age, 28
    drug interactions, 252–253
    human milk and formulas, 34, 36–37
    parenteral nutrition, 229–230
    in pregnancy, 5, 183
    premature infant, 28
    recommended intake, 533
    term newborn, 18–19
    vegetarian diets, 183–185
    year 2000 goals, adolescents, 259
Calcium-binding protein, 58–59
Calcium homeostasis, 58–60
Calcium intake, 511, 533
Calcium phosphate, 229–230
Calcium supplements, vegetarians, 185
Caloric intake. *See* Energy intake
Caloric requirements
    AIDS patients, 452–453
    burn patients, 219–220
    critically ill children, 210, 213–214
    and malnutrition, 134
    parenteral nutrition, 227–228, 235
    pregnancy, 2
    premature infant, 24
Calorimetry
    human milk and formulas, 39
    methodology, 193
Cancer. *See* Malignancies
"Cancer enteropathy," 419
Candidiasis, 442
Candy consumption, 514
Carbamoyl phosphate synthase deficiency, 472
Carbohydrate intolerance, 356
Carbohydrate loading, athletes, 262
Carbohydrates
    adolescent athletes, 262
    Bogalusa Heart Study, 512–514
    cystic fibrosis, 377
    diabetic diet, 314–316, 319
    human milk and formulas, 34

Subject Index / 559

intake in critically ill, 213–214
and lipoprotein levels, 297
and liver disease, 356–357
premature infant requirements, 25
and renal failure, intake, 401–402
term newborn requirements, 12–13
α-Carboxyglutamic acid, 67–68
Cardiac arrhythmias
hypocaloric diets, 282
parenteral nutrition, 388
Cardiac cachexia, 383
Cardiac disease. *See* Cardiovascular disease;
Congenital heart disease
Cardiac habituation, 174
Cardiac output, burn patients, 218
Cardiac surgery, 388, 390
Cardiac transplants, 389
Cardiovascular disease
lipoprotein levels, 295–296
therapeutic diets, 542–543
Cardiovascular system, malnutrition, 211–214
Caretaker-infant interactions, 174
Carnitine
and diarrhea, 331–332
in parenteral nutrition, 229
requirements in term newborn, 15–16
vegetarian diets, 185, 187
Carnitine deficiency, 480
Carnosinemia, 473
Carotene
in premature infants, 29
recommended allowances, 55
retinol synthesis, 51–52
Carpel tunnel syndrome, 82
Caseins
breast milk versus formulas, 13–14, 36
premature infant, 27
Catch-up cognitive function, 176–177, 390
home environment, 177
Catch-up growth
congenital heart disease, 390
Crohn's disease, 344, 346
and malnutrition, 135–136, 177
home environment, 177
Catecholamines, 164–165
Catheter-related complications, 232–233
CD4 cells
in HIV infection, 151–152
and malnutrition, 147
T cell activation, 143
CD4/CD8 cell ratio
in HIV infection, 152, 448–449
and malnutrition, 147
CD8 cells, 143, 147, 152
CDC nutrition surveillance, 522
Celiac disease, 333–334, 463
description of, 463
and lymphoma, 419
nutritional considerations, 333–334
recommended diet, 541–542
Cellular hypoxia, 385
Cellular immunity
critically ill children, 211
deficiencies, 438
in HIV infection, 151–152, 448–450
interaction with nutrition, 130–131

iron deficiency role, 149
and malnutrition, 147
mechanisms, 141–142
nucleotide role, 17
Center for Disease Control programs, 522
Central vein parenteral nutrition, 225–226, 231, 422–423
Cephalosporin, 135, 444
Cereal
exchange lists, 549–550
iron absorption, infants, 96
iron fortification, 97
trace element content, 116
Cerebellar ataxia, 65
Cerebral atrophy, 136
Cerebral palsy, 486–487
Ceruloplasmin
biological functions, 117
cystic fibrosis, 378–379
Challenge tests, 465, 467
Cheeses, 497, 556
Cheilosis, 500
Chemotherapy
megaloblastic anemia cause, 103
nutritional considerations, 419–420, 422
Child abuse/neglect, 275–278
Child Care Food Program, 527
Childhood malignancies. *See* Malignancies
Childhood obesity. *See* Obesity
"Chinese restaurant syndrome," 466
Chlorine
human milk and formulas, 34, 37
in term newborn, 18
Cholecalciferol, 58
Cholecystitis, 281
Cholecystokinin, 364
Cholestasis, 358
Cholestasis, chronic childhood, 65, 75, 79, 380–381, 397–399, 438
Cholesterol. *See also* Total cholesterol
Bogalusa Heart Study, 512–514
in breast milk and formulas, 16, 35
dietary modification, 300–304
health risks, 263–264, 295–296
screening, 298–299
Cholestyramine, 248, 250–251, 304
Choline, 76
Chromium
body content, 117
intravenous intake, 123
recommended daily intake, 19, 29, 124, 532
toxicity, 124
Chromium deficiency, 119–120, 122–123
Chronic childhood cholestasis, 65
Chronic diarrhea, 329–334
Chronic lactic acidosis, 75, 79
Chronic mucocutaneous candidiasis, 438
Chronic obstructive lung disease, 380–381
Chronic renal insufficiency, 397–399
Chylomicrons, 49
Cigarette smoking
lipoprotein levels, 297, 304
premature birth determinant, 2
Cimetidine, 248
Cirrhosis. *See also* Liver disease
carbohydrate metabolism, 356
Citrullinemia, 472–473

"Clear liquid" solutions, 328
Clotting factors, 68–70
Cobalamin. *See* Vitamin B_{12}
Cocarboxylase, 77
Coffee, and iron absorption, 93
Cognition
effects of breakfast, 110–111
iron deficiency, 95, 107–108
and malnutrition, 136, 175–177
sugar effects, 111–112
Colchicine, 248
Colic, 461–462
infant, 461–462
Colonocytes, 332
Colostrum
fat composition, 16
trace mineral concentrations, 37
Common variable hypogammaglobulinemia, 438, 442
Community nutrition, 517–528
Complement system
deficiencies, 437
and malnutrition, 133, 147
mechanisms, 141–142
Complete amino acid mixture, 402
Computerized dietary analysis, 508–509
Computerized tomography, brain, 175
Congenital heart disease, 383–390
caloric needs, 386
drug-nutrient interaction, 388–389
growth failure etiology, 384–385
management, 386–388
nasogastric feedings, 387
nutritional assessment, 385–386
prognosis, 389–390
surgery, 388
Congenital methylmalonic acidemia, 476
Congenital pernicious anemia, 102
Congenital tryptophanuria, 75, 84
Congestive heart failure
anemia, 389
cardiac cachexia, 383
and parenteral nutrition, 388
prognosis, 389–390
Constipation, 245
Continuous enteral feedings, 243, 402
Continuous Performance Test, 111
Contraceptives
oral, and lipoproteins, 298
Convulsions, 543
pyridoxine treatment, 75, 82
Copper
absorption and metabolism, 117–118
biological functions, 117
body content, 117–118
cystic fibrosis, 378–379
dietary sources, 115–116
human milk concentrations, 37
intravenous intake, 123
and liver disease, 359–360
recommendations, 19, 29, 123–124, 523
toxicity, 123–124
Copper deficiency, 115–124
clinical features, 120–122
diagnosis, 122
etiology, 118–120

Copper deficiency (*contd.*)
   and immune function, 150–151
   treatment, 123
Corn diets, and niacin, 83
Corn oil, 301
Corneal clouding, 55
Coronary artery disease, 295–296, 389
Corticosteroids
   food hypersensitivity treatment, 467
   in juvenile arthritis, 412
Cortisol
   adaptation to malnutrition, 164–165
   psychosocial dwarfism, 276–277
Cortisol receptor, 53–54
Costochondral beading, 87
Coumadin, 389
Cow's milk formulas
   carbohydrates, 12, 34
   and diarrhea, 329, 331
   hypersensitivity, 462
   and iron depletion, 96–97
   nutritional composition, 34
   proteins, 13–14, 34
   vitamin C, 74
Creatinine height index, 202
Critical illness
   metabolic response, 208–209
   nutritional considerations, 207–214
   versus starvation, metabolism, 209
Crohn's disease
   assessment, 341–342
   and breast feeding, 41
   catch-up growth, 344, 346
   elemental diet therapy, 344–350
   growth failure, 341–350
   nutritional considerations, 332–333, 341–350
   surgery, 344, 350
   total parenteral nutrition, 344, 350
Cromolyn sodium, 467
Crying patterns, 174
Cryptosporidium, 326
Crystalline amino acids, 226–227
Cue elimination, weight reduction, 289
Cyanocobalamin. *See* Vitamin B_{12}
Cystathionine β-synthase deficiency, 473
Cystathioninuria, 75, 82, 473
Cysteine
   parenteral nutrition, 227, 235
   premature infant, 27
   term newborn, 13
Cystic fibrosis, 375–381
   clinical features, 365, 375–376, 379
   diagnosis, 365–366, 375
   energy needs, 376–377
   nutrient guidelines, 542
   pancreatic insufficiency, 365–366, 376
   pancreatic microspheres in, 369, 377–380
   prognosis, 375–376
   pulmonary function, 380–381
Cystic fibrosis transmembrane conductance regulation, 365
Cystinosis, 473
Cystinuria, 473

Dairy products
   consumption in United States, 505–506, 513
   diabetic diet, 314–315

Dark adaptation, vitamin A, 56
Dehydration, athletes, 262
7-Dehydrocholesterol, 58
Delayed type hypersensitivity, 147, 459–460
Dennison Inventory of Nutrition Evaluation, 508–509
Densitometry, 198
Dental caries, 494–497
   chewing gum, 496–497
   and fruit juices, 496
   "Gummi bears", 497
Dental fluorosis, 499–500
Dental-oral health, 493–502
   and bulimia nervosa, 268
   and fluoride, 497–500
   nutrients and diet role, 494–498
Depletion of iron stores, 92
Dermatitis herpetiformis, 463
Dessert consumption, 514
Developmental disabilities, 485–490
   anthropometric data, 487
   causes, 486–487
   effects on caretakers, 490
   feeding, 489–490
Developmental effects, malnutrition, 136
Dextran plaque, 494
Dextrose/water solution, 133–134
Diabetes mellitus, 309–321. *See also* Insulin-dependent; Thyroid function, and diabetes mellitus; Non-insulin dependent diabetes mellitus
   dietary needs, 263
   team treatment, 312
   therapy, 312–320
   viral infections, 311
Diabetic diet, 314, 549–556
Diabetic ketoacidosis, 310, 313
Dialysis, 397, 399–402
Diarrhea
   acute, 325–329
   chronic, 329–334
   invasive, 326–327
   osmotic, 326–327, 453
   rotavirus and secretory, 326–327, 453
   secretory, 326–327, 453
      Lactic acidosis, 75, 79
      Mucocutaneous candidiasis, 438
      Obstructive lung disease, 380–381
      Renal insufficiency, 397–399
   "toddler", 334
   toxigenic, 326
      in AIDS, 448, 450, 453
      enteral nutrition complication, 243–244
      immunocompromised children, 443–444
      and malnutrition, 130
      nutritional considerations, 325–334, 443–444
Diary records. *See* Food diary
Dibasic-aminoaciduria, 473
Dicarboxylic acidurias, 477
Diet diaries. *See* Food diary
Dietary analysis, computerized, 508–509
Dietary fat. *See also* Fat
   cystic fibrosis, 368, 380
   diabetes, 317
   and lipoprotein levels, 297
   United States trends, 505–506

Dietary history
   "Burke Method",
   childhood obesity, 280
   evaluation, 521
   intake observation method, 193
   malnutrition assessment, 191–193, 508, 521
   "Product Identification Notebook", 511
   questionnaire, 521
   recall method, 521
   recall method, electronic, 509
   "Recall phenomenon", 419
   tape-recorded, 509
   telephone recall, 509
   twenty-four hour, 192, 506–507, 521
   weighed food method, 506, 521
Dietary Intervention Study in Children, 304
Dietary questionnaire, 521
Dietary recall method, 521
Dietary sweeteners, 317–318
Dieting behavior, adolescents, 260–261
Diets *See also* Menu patterns; *See* Alberta Children's Hospital; American Diabetes Association; American Dietetic Association Exchange Lists; Balanced calorie deficit diet; Corn, and niacin; Elemental; High-carbohydrate, high-fiber; High-fiber, diabetes; High-protein; High-protein, low-carbohydrate; Hypocaloric; Lacto-ovovegetarians; Lactovegetarians; Low protein; Mediterranean; Protein-sparing modified fast; Shriners' burn; Soybean. *See* Lipoprotein patterns; "Traffic light"; Vegan; Vegetable protein; Vegetarian
"Difficult" temperament, 174–175
DiGeorge syndrome, 389
Dihomo-gamma-linolenic acid, 35
Dihydroliopoyl dehydrogenase deficiency, 477
Dihydropteridine reductase deficiency, 474
Dihydrotachysterol, 58
1,25-Dihydroxycholecalciferol, 57–59
5,8 Dimethyl tocol, 63
7,8 Dimethyl tocol, 63
5,8 Dimethyl tocotrienol, 63
Diphenylhydantoin, 70
Diphyllobothrium latum, 102
Direct calorimetry, 193
Disaccharides, 25
Docosahexanoic acid, 16–17
"Doping," 262
Double-blind food challenge, 465
Doubly labeled water method, 193, 195
Drug metabolism, and food, 253–254
Drug-nutrient interactions, 247–255
Dumping syndrome, 242
Duodenal resection, 420
Duration of malnutrition, 173
Dyslipidemia, 295–305
   health risks, 295–296
   screening, 298–299
   therapy, 300–305

"Easy" temperament, 174–175
Eating behavior, 505–515

Eating disorders. *See* Anorexia nervosa; Bulimia nervosa; Purgers; Binge eating
Edema, in pregnancy, 1
EEG, and malnutrition, 174–175
Electrolyte therapy, 133–134, 443
Electronic dietary recall methods, 509
Elemental diet
  Crohn's disease, 344–350
  enteral feedings, 242
Elimination diet, 465
Emotions, and iron deficiency, 108
Enamel hypoplasia/hypocalcification, 493–494
Encopresis, childhood obesity, 281
Endocrine changes, malnutrition, 161–170
Energy
  absorbed, 39–40
Energy expenditure
  assessment, 193–195
  critically ill children, 209–210
Energy intake
  in adolescence, recommendations, 258
  Bogalusa Heart Study, 512–514
  human milk and formulas, 39–40
  juvenile arthritis, 409–410
  parenteral nutrition, 227–228
  recommendations, 533
  and renal disease, 397, 399–402
Energy requirements
  and malnutrition, 134
  parenteral nutrition, 235
  pregnancy, 1–2
  premature infants, 24
  term newborn, 10–11
Enfamil
  carbohydrate source, 12
  fat composition, 16, 35
  protein composition, 14
Enteral feedings
  continuous, 243, 402
  full strength, 242–243
  graded, 242–243
  intermittent, 243
Enteral nutrition, 239–245. *See also* Nasoenteral feedings
  acute renal insufficiency, 396–397
  administration, 242–243
  algorithm, 240
  anorexia nervosa, 269–272
  assessment, 243
  burn patients, 222
  complications, 243–245
  components, 540
  congenital heart disease, 387–388
  continuous, 243, 402
  Crohn's disease, 344–350
  formulas, 242, 540
  full-strength, 242–243
  graded, 242–243
  indications, 239–240
  malignancies, 422
  psychological effects, 270, 422
  route of administration, 240–242
Enteric-coated encapsulated microspheres, 369
Enterocytes
  burn patients, 219
  and glutamine, 332
Enterokinase deficiency, 366

Enterostomy feedings
  complications, 245
  indications, 240–242
Eosinophilic gastroenteritis, 462–463
Epithelial tissues, and vitamin A, 53–54
Ergocalciferol, 57–58
Ergosterol, 57–58
Erythrocyte protoporphyrin, 98–99
Escherichia coli, 325–327
Esophagitis, in AIDS, 451
Essential amino acids *See also* Amino acids
  premature infant, 27
  renal failure diet, 402
  requirements in term newborn, 13–15
Essential fatty acids *See also* Fatty acids
  cystic fibrosis, 377
  in premature infant, 26
  in term newborn, 16–17
Estradiol, and lipoprotein levels, 296
Ethanol, thiamine deficiency, 78
Evaporated milk, folate deficiency, 101
Exchange diets, 544–545, 549–556
Exercise
  adherence problem, 288
  diabetes management, 313, 318–319
  lipoprotein levels, 304
  and obesity, 282–283, 288, 304
  year 2000 goals, adolescents, 259–260
Exercise-induced anaphylaxis, 462, 464
Exercise tolerance, 95
Extended Table of Nutrient Values, 508–509, 511
Extracellular fluid, 197

Failure to thrive
  and AIDS, 448, 451–453
  inborn errors of metabolism, 472, 478
  and mother-infant relationship, 47
Familial hypercholesterolemia
  dietary modification, 300
  drug therapy, 304–305
Familial hypophosphatemia, 60
The Family Environment Scale-Form R, 290
Family intervention
  dyslipidemia, 300
  and obesity, 282–284, 291
The Farm, 182–183
Fasting
  adolescent athletes, 262
  fuel supply mechanism, 161–162
Fat. *See also* Animal fat; Body fat; Brown, in newborn; Dietary fat; Fat intake; Polyunsaturated fatty acids; Saturated fatty acids; Unsaturated fats
  in body composition assessment, 196–197
  in breast milk, 16, 34–35
  exchange lists, 554
  infant formulas, 34–35
  and liver disease, 357–358
  premature infant, 25–26
  term newborn, 15–17
Fat digestion
  human milk function, 38
  and liver disease, 357–358
Fat free body mass
  body composition model, 196–197
  childhood obesity, 281

Fat intake
  Bogalusa Heart Study, 512–514
  exchange lists, 554
  and heart disease, 542–543
  nutrition surveys, 525
  United States trends, 505–506, 514–515, 525
  year 2000 goals, adolescents, 259
Fat malabsorption
  chronic diarrhea, 330–331
  cystic fibrosis, 377
  vitamin E deficiency, 65
Fat-soluble vitamins, 49–71
  absorption and distribution, 49–50
  Crohn's disease, 247–248
  cystic fibrosis, 377–378, 380
  drug interactions, 250–251
Fatty acids. *See also* Polyunsaturated fatty acids; Saturated fatty acids
  in breast milk and formulas, 16–17, 34–35
  digestion, and human milk, 38
  in fats and oils, 543
  lactating vegetarians, 185
  parenteral nutrition, 228–229, 236
  positional distribution, human milk, 38
  premature infant requirements, 26
  term newborn requirements, 15–17
  in United States food supply, 506–507
Fatty streaks, and dyslipidemia, 295
Feeding. *See also* Infant feeding
  developmentally disabled, 489–490
Feingold hypothesis, 108–110
Ferritin
  depletion of, 92
  iron deficiency test, 98–99
Ferrous sulfate, 97, 99
Fetal growth, 6
Fiber, diabetic diet, 316
Fibric acid derivatives, 304
Fibronectin, 201
Fibrous plaques, 295
Fish group, trace elements, 116
Fish oil, 155
"Flat-slope" syndrome, 192
Flavin absorption, 250
Fluid therapy, 133–134, 443
Fluoride, dental health, 497–500
Fluorine
  metabolism, 118
  recommended intake, 19–20, 29
Fluorine deficiency, 119, 123
Fluorosis, 499–500
Focal biliary cirrhosis, 376
Folic acid
  drug interactions, 249–250
  in human milk and formulas, 76
  parenteral intake, 76, 230
  pregnant/lactating adolescents, 258–259
  recommended intake, 74, 100
Folic acid deficiency
  birth defects, 4
  Crohn's disease, 347
  diagnosis and treatment, 101–102
  dietary causes, 100–101
  drug interactions, 101
  gingival disease, 501
  immune system effects, 149
Folic acid supplementation, 5
Follicle-stimulating hormone, 168

Follicular hyperkeratosis, 56
Food additives
    and attentional processes, 108–110
    challenge studies, 109
    double-blind studies, 109
    hypersensitivity, 465–466
Food allergy, 457–467
    and arthritis, 408–409
    clinical manifestations, 461–462
    definition, 457
    diagnosis, 464–466
    family history, 466
    milk, 408–409
    prevention, 466
    treatment, 466–467
Food antigens, hypersensitivity, 458–460
Food aversion, 418, 422
Food challenge, 465, 467
    weight-reduction programs, 289
Food Distribution Program, 527
Food frequency method, 192, 507–508
Food hypersensitivity, 457–467. See also Food allergy
Food Stamp Program, 527
Foods. See Beef consumption; Candy consumption, Cheeses; Dairy products; Desserts; Fruit; Meat group; Pork consumption; Poultry intake; Snack consumption; Vegetables
Food-weighing technique, 506, 521
Formiminoglutamic aciduria, 473
Formula milk. See Infant formulas
Free fatty acids, 229
Fructose, diabetic diet, 317
Fruit
    Bogalusa Heart Study, 513
    diabetic diet, 315, 552–553
    exchange list, 552–553
Full-strength enteral feedings, 242–243

Gag reflex, 489–490
Galactosemia, 489
Gastrectomy, 420
Gastric aspirate volumes, 243
Gastroenteritis, 130
Gastroenteritis, allergic eosinophilic, 462–463
Gastrointestinal antisepsis, 444
Gastrointestinal tract
    and parenteral nutrition, 232
    term newborn, 9
Gastrostomy
    acute renal insufficiency, 397
    cystic fibrosis, 380
    developmentally disabled, 488
    indications, 240–241
Gentamicin, 135, 444
Giardia lamblia, 326
Giardiasis, 442
Gingival diseases, 500–501
Globulin
    accelerator, 68
Glomerular filtration rate, 393–396
Glucagon, 165–166
Glucocorticoid receptor, 53–54
Glucocorticoids
    effects on nutrients, 162
    influence on pancreas, 364

Gluconeogenesis
    burn patients, 217, 219
    critical illness response, 209
    term newborn, 13
    and tumors, 418
Glucose
    adaptation to malnutrition, 165–166
    burn patients, 219
    parenteral nutrition, 226, 228, 234
    in term newborn, 12–13
    tumor consumption, 418
Glucose intolerance, 3, 356
Glutamine
    burn patients, 219
    intestinal lumen nutrient, 332
Glutaric acidemia, 477
Gluten-restricted diet, 541
Gluten-sensitive enteropathy. See Celiac disease
Glycemic index, 315–316
-Glyceric acidemia, 477
Glycosylated hemoglobin, 320
Goat milk, 34
Gonadal hormones, 168
Good Start, 12, 14, 16
Graded enteral feedings, 242–243
Grains, exchange lists, 549–550
Growth. See also Growth retardation
    and anorexia nervosa, 268
    assessment, 518–520
    catch-up studies, 135–136, 177
    and human milk properties, 38
    hypocaloric diets, 287–288
    obesity effects, 281
    parenteral nutrition, 231–232
    term newborn, 10–11
    zinc deficiency effects, 121
Growth charts, 519
Growth failure. See also Growth retardation
Growth hormone
    effects on nutrients, 162
    in juvenile arthritis, 411
    and malnutrition, 166–167
    in psychosocial dwarfism, 276–278
Growth retardation
    cardiac surgery, 390
    catch-up, 135–136
    congenital heart disease, 384–386, 388, 390
    cystic fibrosis, 368, 379
    developmentally disabled 487–488
    inflammatory bowel disease, 341–350
    intrauterine, 2–3
    juvenile arthritis, 410–411
    low-fat, low-cholesterol diets, 303
    malnutrition consequences, 135–136, 161
    psychosocial dwarfism, 277
    renal failure, 400
Growth spurt
    anorexia nervosa, 268
    sex differences, adolescence, 258
Growth stunting
    African-American children, 524
    anthropometric measurements, 195–196
    catch-up studies, 135–136
    definition, 128, 195
    malnutrition consequences, 135–136
    surveys, 524

Growth velocity
    assessment, 520
    hypocaloric diets, 287–288
    inflammatory bowel disease, 342–343

Halitosis, food additives, 110
Hanes. See Health and Nutrition Examination Survey; Health and Nutrition Examination Survey, Hispanic; National Health and Examination Survey
Hartnup disease, 475
    niacin treatment, 75, 84
Head circumference
    congenital heart disease, 386
    developmentally disabled, 487
    and malnutrition, 136, 175
Headache
    food additives, 110
    and obesity, 281–282
Health and Nutrition Examination Survey, 513. See also Health and Nutrition Examination Survey, Hispanic; National Health and Nutrition Examination Survey
Health and Nutrition Examination Survey, Hispanic, 522
Health education, 290
Health food diets, 74
Heart disease. See Congenital heart disease; Cardiovascular disease
Heart surgery, 388, 390
Heart transplants, 389
Heat-treated milk formulas, 101
Height-for-age, 195–196
    as anthropometric measure, 195–196
    childhood obesity, 281
    congenital heart disease, 386
    liver disease assessment, 355
    malnutrition consequences, 135–136, 161
    nutritional measure, 127–128
    renal failure, 400
Heiner's syndrome, 463
Helper T cells
    activation, 143
    in HIV infection, 151–152
    in host defense, 141–142
    and malnutrition, 147
Hematocrit, 92, 98
Heme iron, 93
Hemodialysis, 397
    nutritional aspects, 397, 399–402
    taste perception, 400
Hemoglobin
    and anemia, 91–92, 98
    changes during development, 94–95
Hemolytic anemia, 65
Hemophilia, HIV infection, 452
Hemorrhagic disease, 70
Hepatic disease. See Liver disease
HHH syndrome, 474
High birth weight, 3
High-carbohydrate, high-fiber diets, 316
High-density lipoprotein cholesterol
    and atherosclerosis, 295
    levels of, 296–298
High-fiber diets, diabetes, 316

High-protein diets, 220
High protein-low carbohydrate diet, 254
Hip replacement, 213
Hirsutism, and obesity, 282
Hispanic HANES, 522
Histidinemia, 473
HIV infection, 447–453
   diagnosis, 441–442
   immunologic abnormalities, 151–152, 441, 448–450
   nutritional status, 152, 439–440, 450–452
   nutritional support, 452–453
   pathogenic process, 440
   psychological deficits, 452
HMG CoA reductase inhibitors, 304
Homeorrhesis, 162
Homeostasis, 162
Homocystinuria, 473
   pyridoxine treatment, 75, 82
Homogentisic aciduria, 87
Hormonal changes, malnutrition, 161–170
Hormones
   adaptation, 162–163, 165, 169
   human growth, 411
Hospitalized child, enteral support, 239–245
Human growth hormone, 411
Human milk, 33–41
   carbohydrates, 12, 34
   choice of, consequences, 40–41
   composition, 33–41
   diabetes protection, 311
   and diarrhea, advantage, 328–329
   energy intake and growth, 39–40
   fat composition, 16, 34–35
   versus formulas, protein, 14
   functional role, 33, 37–38
   iron absorption, 93, 96–97
   mineral composition, 18–20, 34, 36–37
   nucleotides, 17–18
   protective function, 37
   proteins, 13–15, 34
   secondary immunodeficiency prevention, 155, 442–443
   and vegetarian diets, 184–185
   vitamin concentrations, 36, 73–74, 76
   and weight gain, 11, 39–40
Human rotavirus, and diarrhea, 325–327
Humoral immune response, 132
Hydralazine, 81
Hydrolysate formulas, 466
1α-Hydroxycholecalciferol, 58
3-Hydroxy-3-methylglutaric acidemia, 475
25-Hydroxyvitamin D, 57–58
Hyperactivity, 108–112
Hyperammonemia
   inborn errors of metabolism, 480
   parenteral nutrition complication, 233
Hypercholesterolemia
   dietary modification, 300–304
   and nicotinic acid, 84
Hyperglycemia, burn patients, 219
Hyperglycerolemia, 477
Hyperhydroxyprolinemia, 475
Hyperkalemia, 28
Hyperkeratosis, 56
Hyperlipidemias. See also Dyslipidemia
   cardiac transplants, 389
   year 2000 goal, 259–260

Hypermethioninemia, 474
Hypernatremia, 27
Hyperoxaluria, 75
Hyperphenylalaninemia, 474
Hyperprolinemia, 475
Hypersegmented neutrophils, 100
Hypersensitivity reactions, 457–460
Hypertension
   childhood obesity, 281
   control of, adolescents, 263–264
   in diabetes, 318
   nutrition surveys, 525
Hypervitaminosis A, 56–57
Hypervitaminosis D, 62
Hypervitaminosis E, 66
Hypervitaminosis K, 70
Hyperzincuria, 119–120
Hypoalbuminemia
   burn patients, 222
   and edema, 199
Hypocaloric diets, 286–288
Hypogammaglobulinemia, common variable, 438, 442
Hypokalemia, 389
Hypolactasia, 334
Hypomagnesemia, 378
Hyponatremia
   cystic fibrosis, 378
   premature infants, 27
Hypophosphatemia
   burn patients, 220
   total parenteral nutrition, 271
Hypoplastic left heart syndrome, 388
Hypoxemia, 384, 389–390
Hypoxic ventilatory response, 211

"Idiopathic hypercalcemia," 62
Idiopathic intestinal pseudoobstruction syndrome, 327
IgA deficiency, 438–439, 442. See also Secretory IgA
IgE levels, 148
IgE-mediated food reactions, 459–461, 464–466
IgG levels, 442, 466
IgG replacement therapy, 442–443
Iminoglycinuria, familial, 475
Immune abnormalities, 141–155, 437–447
   and cancer, 421–422
   critically ill children, 211
   differential diagnosis, 154–155, 440–442
   and forms of malnutrition, 146–151
   HIV infection, 151–152, 448–450
   in iron deficiency, 95
   prevention, 155, 442
   treatment, 442–444
Immune complexes, 459–460
Immune globulin, 442
Immunization, 443
Immunodeficiency, severe combined, 349
Immunodeficiency syndromes, 437–445
Immunoprotective factors, human milk, 38
Inborn errors of metabolism, 471–484
   clinical presentation, 471
   diagnostic workup, 471–472, 478
   trace metal metabolism, 120
   treatment/management, 478–480

Infant feeding
   as behavioral indicator, 45
   developmentally disabled, 489–490
   guidelines, 531, 534–535
   maternal interactions, 43–47
Infant formulas, 33–41. See also soy-based
   versus breast milk, proteins, 14
   carbohydrates, 12, 34
   choice of, consequences, 40–41
   congenital heart disease, 387
   efficiency of energy utilization, 11
   energy expenditure patterns, 40
   fats, 16, 34–35
   heat-treated milk, 101
   iron fortification, 96–97
   list of, 531, 536–539
   and malnutrition, 134–135
   milk-based, 34
   mineral composition, 18–20, 34, 36–37
   nucleotides, 17–18
   proteins, 13–15, 34–36
   vitamin content, 76
   and weight gain, 39–40
Infantile convulsions, 75, 82
Infection, 133, 153–154
Infection resistance, 95
Inferior vena cava catheters, 226
Inflammatory bowel disease. See also Crohn's disease; Ulcerative colitis
   growth failure treatment, 341–350
   and nutrition, 332–333, 341–350
Inflammatory response, downregulation, 155
Inositol, 76
Insulin
   adaptation to malnutrition, 165–166
   effects on nutrients, 162
Insulin-dependent diabetes mellitus
   breastfeeding, effects of, 41
   classification and diagnosis, 309–310
   dietary strategies, 313–319
   emotional-behavioral components, 319–320
   epidemiology, 310
   etiology, 310–311
   hypertension management, 318
   pathophysiology, 311–312
   therapy, 312–320
Insulin-like growth factor-1
   growth hormone relationship, 166–167
   juvenile arthritis, 411
   in psychosocial dwarfism, 276
"Insulin pump," 313
Insulin resistance, 356
Insulin therapy, 312–313, 319
   openloop infusion, 313
Intake observation method, 193
Intellectual performance
   iron deficiency, 95, 108
   and malnutrition, 136, 175
Intensive care unit, 207–214
Interleukin 1
   critical illness response, 209
   malnutrition effect, 131
   and tumor necrosis factor, 145–146
   and tumors, 418
Interleukin 2
   differential diagnostic use, 154–155, 441

Interleukin 2 (*contd.*)
  and malnutrition, 131–132
  in T lymphocyte activation, 143
Intermittent enteral feedings, 243
Intestinal antisepsis, 444
Intestinal lymphangiectasia, 439
Intestinal malabsorption syndromes
  AIDS, 451–452
  trace element deficiencies, 119
  and tumors, 418–419
Intestinal mucosa
  antigen penetration, 461
  iron homeostatic regulation, 93
  and nutrition, diarrhea, 332–334
  radiation-induced injury, 420
Intracellular fluid, 197
Intradermal allergen testing, 464
Intrauterine growth retardation, 2–3
Invasive diarrhea, 326–327
Iodine
  metabolism, 118
  recommended allowances, 19, 29, 123, 533
  toxicity, 124
Iodine deficiency
  birth defects, 4
  diagnosis and treatment, 122–123
  etiology, 119
  and thyroid, 167
"Iowa Breakfast Studies," 110–111
IQ tests. *See* Intellectual performance
Iron
  absorption, 93–95, 117, 444
  adolescent needs, 257–259
  depletion, 92
  developmental changes in needs, 94–95
  dietary sources, 93, 115
  and emotions, 108
  human milk content, 37
  low birth weight infants, requirements, 97
  metabolism, 118, 360
  nonheme, 93
  normal homeostasis, 92–94
  poisoning, 99–100
  recommended intake, 533
  requirements, 18–19, 28–29, 123
  in vegan diets, 183
Iron deficiency, 92–100. *See also* Iron deficiency anemia
  in AIDS, 152, 450
  behavioral effects, 95, 107–108
  breast- and formula-fed infants, 96–97
  causes, 94, 119
  definition, 92
  and emotions, 108
  in developing countries, 97–98
  developmentally disabled, 488
  diagnosis, 98–99, 122
  and immune function, 149–150, 450
  manifestations, 95, 120
  in mother, consequences, 94
  prevalence, 98
  prevention, 95–96
  treatment, 99
  and work performance, 95
Iron deficiency anemia, 92–100
  Crohn's disease, 348
  cystic fibrosis, 378

definition, 92
diagnosis, 98–99
and immune function, 149
juvenile arthritis, 411
low birth weight infants, 29
manifestations, 95
nutrition surveys, 524
in pregnancy, 5
prevalence, 98, 524
treatment, 99
vegan diets, 183, 187
year 2000 goals, 259
Iron-fortified formula, 96–97
Iron supplementation
  versus fortification, 97
  immunodeficient children, 444
  low birth weight infants, 97
  in malnourished children, 134–135, 444
  pregnancy, 5
Isoleucine metabolism, 476, 478
Isonicotine hydrazine, 81–82
Isovaleric acidemia, 475

Jamaican study, 177
Jejunostomy feeding
  complications, 245
  cystic fibrosis, 380
  indications, 240–242
Johanson-Blizzard syndrome, 366
Juvenile arthritis, 407–413
  anemia, 411
  anorexia, 412
  food allergies, 408–409
  growth disturbance, 410–411
  nocturnal nasogastric feeding, 412
  nutritional assessment, 409–410
  nutritionist's role, 413
  symptoms, 407
Juvenile pernicious anemia, 102

Kangaroo care, 47
Kaposi's sarcoma, 451
Keshan disease, 118, 122
2-Ketoadipic acidemia, 477
Ketogenic diets, 543
Ketonuria, 4
Ketosis, 478
β-Ketothiolase deficiency, 476
"Ketotic hyperglycinemia," 86
Ketotifen, 467
Kidney function. *See* Renal function
Kwashiorkor. *See also* Protein-energy malnutrition
  clinical classification, 128–130
  cognitive function, 136, 176
  hormone changes, 163–165, 168–170
  immunologic abnormalities, 146
  long-term consequences, 135–136, 176
  pathogenesis, 129–130
  and tuberculosis, 153
Kynurenic acid excretion, 82

Laboratory assessment, 191–203, 521
α-Lactalbumin, 35

Lactase, and gestational age, 25
Lactase deficiency, 334, 465
Lactation. *See also* Breast feeding; Human milk
  adolescent nutritional needs, 259
  energy requirements, 6
  vegetarian diet effects, 184–185
Lactic acidosis, 75, 477
Lactoferrin, human milk, 35–36
Lacto-ovovegetarians, 182, 183, 185–187
Lactose
  in dairy products, 542
  human milk, 34
  in term newborn, 12
Lactose intolerance, 34, 542
Lactovegetarians, 182, 185–187
Lactulose/mannitol recovery ratio, 330
Language development, 174–175
Lead poisoning
  birth defects, 4
  and iron deficiency, 95
Learned food aversion, 418, 422
Left-to-right cardiac shunts, 384, 386–387
Leigh's encephalopathy, 75, 79
Leucine, inborn errors of metabolism, 475
Leukemia
  acute nonlymphocytic, 422
Leukemia-lymphoma, 422
Leukopenia, 55
Leukotrienes, 144
Linoleic acids
  cystic fibrosis, 368, 377
  in human milk, 35
  intake in critically ill, 213
  parenteral nutrition requirements, 236
  premature infant, 26
  soybean oil emulsions, 229
  term newborns, 16–17
  United States' food supply, 506
Lipases
  human milk, 38
  pancreatic concentrations, 364, 366
  premature infant, 26
  supplements, 369
Lipid emulsions, 228–229, 236
Lipid peroxidation, 64
Lipids. *See* Fat
Lipoprotein patterns
  adiposity, 297
  age factors, 296
  alcohol intake, 297
  contraceptives, oral, 298
  dietary modification, 300–304
  influencing factors, 296–298
  medication effects, 304–305
  screening, 298–299
  Soybean diet, 300–302
  tracking, 295
Liquid diets, 286
Liquid supplements, 270
Liver disease, 353–361. *See also* Cirrhosis
  anthropometry, 355
  assessment, 353–355
  nutritional considerations, 355–361
  and parenteral nutrition, 234
  vitamin deficiencies, 77

Long-chain polyunsaturated fatty acids
  and dietary nucleotides, 17
  human milk, 34–35
  inflammation downregulation, 155
  premature infant, 26
  term newborn, 16–17
Long-chain triglyceride, 331
Low birth weight
  determinants, 2–3
  iron needs, 97
  mothers-infant interaction, 46
  nutritional requirements, 23–29
  surveillance systems, 524–525
  vitamin intake, 74
Low-density lipoprotein cholesterol
  cardiovascular health risks, 295–296
  dietary modification, 300–304
  drug therapy, 304–305
  screening, 298–299
Low protein diets, 254
Lung parenchyma, 211
Luteinizing hormone, 168
Lymphocyte proliferation, 147
Lymphocyte stimulation test, 465
Lymphocyte transformation, 131
Lymphokines, 143
Lymphoma, and breast feeding, 41
Lysinuric protein intolerance, 474
Lysozyme, 36, 38

Macrophage function
  HIV infection, 151–152
  in host defense, 141–142
  and malnutrition, 131–132
Macrosomia, 3
Magnesium. *See also* Hypomagnesemia
  adolescent needs, 257–259
  drug interactions, 252
  human milk and formulas, 34, 36–37
  premature infant, 28
  recommended intake, 533
  supplements, 133–134, 443
  term newborn, 18
Malabsorption syndrome. *See* Intestinal malabsorption syndromes
Malignancies, 417–423
  nutritional assessment, 421
  nutritional support, 422
  side effects of treatment, 419–421
Malnutrition. *See* Protein-energy malnutrition
Maltase, 25
Manganese
  intravenous intake, 123
  metabolism, 118
  premature infant, 29
  recommended daily intake, 124, 532
  term newborn, 19
  toxicity, 124
Maple syrup urine disease, 75, 476, 482
Marasmic-kwashiorkor. *See also* Protein-energy malnutrition
  clinical classification, 128–130
  immunologic abnormalities, 146

Marasmus. *See also* Protein-energy malnutrition
  clinical classification, 128–130
  cognitive function, 176
  hormone changes, 163–165, 168–169
  immunologic abnormalities, 146
  pathogenesis, 129–130
Mastication, 489
Maternal malnutrition, 44–45
Maternal weight, 2–3, 5–6
Mayan Indians, 174
Measles, 146
Meat group
  Bogalusa Heart Study, 513–514
  exchange lists, 550–552
  trace element content, 116
Mediterranean diet, 317
Medium-chain triglycerides, 331
Megaloblastic anemia
  diagnosis, 100
  and folate deficiency, 100–102
  pyridoxine treatment, 82
  thiamine treatment, 75, 79
  and vitamin B_{12} deficiency, 102–103
Menadione, 66
Menaquinones, 66–67
Menarche
  childhood obesity effect, 281
  and malnutrition, 136
  vegetarian diets, 187
Menkes's steely-hair syndrome, 120, 122
Menstrual cycle, 187–188
Mental development, 173–177
Mental retardation, 487
Menu patterns, 531, 540
Mercury contamination, 4
Metabolic acidosis, 479–480
Metabolic carts, 213
Metarhodopsin II, 53–54
Metformin, 248
Methionine, 227, 235
Methotrexate
  folate deficiency, 101
  gastrointestinal toxicity, 418–419
  megaloblastic anemia, 103
8-Methyl tocol, 63
3-Methylcrotonylglycinemia, 475
β-Methylcrotonylglycinuria, 75, 86
Methylenetitrahydrofolate reductase deficiency, 473
2-Methyl-3-hydroxybutyric acidemia, 476
Methylmalonic acidemia, congenital, 476
N^1-Methylnicotinamide, 83
Methyltransferase deficiency, 473
Microcytic-hypochromic anemia, 82, 121
Microspheres, 369, 379–380
Midarm circumference, 195
Milk allergy, 408–409
Milk-based formulas, 34
Milk/egg group
  Bogalusa Heart Study, 512–514
  exchange lists, 553–554
  trace element content, 116
Milk-induced immune reactions, 460, 463
Mineral oil, 247–248, 250–253
Mineral requirements
  burn patients, 220

  premature infants, 27–29
  term infants, 17–20
Minerals
  and birth defects, 4
  body composition, 197–198
  drug interactions, 251–253
  in human milk and formulas, 34, 36–37
  parenteral intakes, 229–230
Molybdenum
  intravenous intake, 123
  recommended intake, 19, 29, 124, 532
  toxicity, 124
Molybdenum deficiency, 119, 123
Monocytes, 141–142
Monosodium glutamate, 466
Monounsaturated fatty acid
  in fats and oils, 543
  and lipoprotein levels, 300–302, 317
Mother-child interaction, 43–47
  bonding controversy, 46–47
  malnutrition effects, 44–45, 174–175
  premature infants, 46
  synchrony in, 45–46
Motor disabilities, 486–487
Motor skills
  iron deficiency, 107–108
  recovery from malnutrition, 175
Multiple acyl-CoA dehydrogenase deficiency, 477
Multiple carboxylase deficiency, 476
Mumps infection, 311
Muscle catabolism
  burn patients, 219
  critically ill children, 210
Mustard operation, 390
Mycobacterial infections, 152–153
Mycobacterium tuberculosis, 152–153
Myelination, 486

Nasoenteral feedings
  complications, 244–245
  congenital heart disease, 387
  Crohn's disease, 344–346
  indications, 240–241
  juvenile arthritis, 412
  malignancies, 422
  uremia, 402
National Health and Nutrition Examination Survey (NHANES), 522. *See also* Health and Nutrition Examination Survey; Health and Nutrition Examination Survey, Hispanic, 522
National Health Interview Survey, 522
National Nutrition Monitoring System, 522
National School Lunch Program, 527
Nationwide Food Consumption Survey, 524
Natural killer cells, 131
"Near-SIDS" patients, 478
Neomycin, 248–250
Neoplasms. *See* Malignancies
Neopterin, 152
Nephron damage, 398
Nephrotic syndrome, 395–396
Neuroblastoma, 421–422
Neutron activation method, 198–199

Neutropenia, 437–438
NHANES, 522
Niacin, 82–84
   dietary sources, 83
   in human milk and formulas, 76
   parenteral intake, 76
   pharmacologic use, 75
   recommended allowances, 74, 82, 533
   requirements, 84
   toxicity, 84
Niacin deficiency, 83–84
Nicotinamide. *See* Niacin
Nicotinic acid. *See also* Niacin
   high-density lipoprotein effect, 304
   in niacin dependency syndromes, 84
   toxicity, 84
Night blindness, 56
Nitrogen
   critically ill children, 208, 210, 214
   in parenteral regimens, 226–227, 235
   premature infant, 27
   term newborn, 13–14
Nitrogen balance
   critically ill children, 214
   in nutrition assessment, 202
   renal disease, 397, 401–402
Nocturia, childhood obesity, 281
Nonheme iron, 93
Non-insulin-dependent diabetes mellitus, 309–321. *See also* Diabetes mellitus
Nonketotic hyperglycinemia, 473
Norwalk virus, 325
Norwood operation, 390
Nosocomial cachexia, 383
Nucleotides
   and intestinal function, 331
   in term newborn, 17–18
Nutrition Coordinating Center, 508–509
Nutrition education, obesity, 290
Nutrition guidelines, 531–547
Nutrition surveys, 518
Nutritional surveillance, 517–526
Nuts/legumes, trace elements, 116

Obesity. *See also* Overweight
   adherence problems, diet, 283
   in adolescents, United States, 261, 263
   balanced caloric diet, 543–545
   and birth weight, 3
   behavior modification, 288–290
   dietary history, 280
   dietary modification, 282, 286–288
   exercise, 288
   family history, 280
   family prototypes, 283
   and female puberty onset, 258
   genetics, 285
   intervention, 282–291
   lipoprotein levels, 297
   and mother-infant relationship, 47
   nutrition education, 290
   nutrition surveys, 525
   pancreatic function, 368
   and parental obesity, 283
   peritoneal dialysis effect, 401–402
   physical examination, 281–282
   and pregnancy, 5
   prevalence, 285
   psychosocial consequences, 280–281
   school-based programs, 289–290
   team treatment, 289–290
Ocular manifestations, 121
25-OH vitamin D, 359
Oleic acid, 506
Olive oil, 301
Omega-3 fatty acid
   and dietary nucleotides, 17
   parenteral nutrition, 236
   requirements in newborn, 16–17
Omega-6 fatty acid
   in burn patients, 219
   and dietary nucleotides, 17
   parenteral nutrition requirements, 236
   requirements in newborn, 16–17
Oral allergy syndrome, 464
Oral contraceptives, lipoproteins, 298
Oral cromolyn sodium, 467
Oral mucosa, 500
Oral reflexes, 489–490
Oral rehydration solution, 327–328
Orange juice, iron absorption, 93, 96
Ornithine, inborn metabolic errors, 474
Ornithine carbamoyl transferase deficiency, 472
Osmotic diarrhea, 326–327, 453
Osteoblasts, and vitamin D, 60
Osteomalacia, 60
Osteopenia, and steroids, 412
Overeaters Anonymous, 272
Overweight, 259, 261. *See also* Obesity
5-Oxoprolinemia, 477
Oxygen consumption
   congenital heart disease, 384–385
   critically ill children, 210, 214
   term newborn, 10

Palmitic acid, 38
Pancreas
   adaptation to malnutrition, 165–166, 367–368
   influences on function, 363–365
Pancrease MT-4, 369, 379
Pancreatic disease, 363–370
Pancreatic insufficiency
   cystic fibrosis, 365–366, 376–377
   nutritional management, 368–369
Pancreatic microspheres, 369, 379–380
Pancreatitis
   acute, 367
Pantothenate deficiency, 84–85
Pantothenic acid
   dietary sources, 84
   in human milk and formulas, 76
   parenteral intake, 76, 230
   recommended daily allowances, 74, 84, 532
   toxicity, 85
Parathyroid hormone, 57–59
Parenteral nutrition, 225–236. *See also* Enteral nutrition; Total parenteral nutrition
   acute renal insufficiency, 396–397
   amino acid requirements, 235–236
   central versus peripheral vein, 226, 231
   complications, 232–233
   composition, 226–230
   congenital heart disease, 387–388
   critically ill children, 213–214
   delivery, 230–232
   indications, 231
   lipid requirements, 236
   malignancies, 422–423
   monitoring, 233–234
   techniques, 225–226
   weight gain, 232
Parents, and childhood obesity, 291
Partial combined immunodeficiencies, 439
Patent ductus arteriosus, 384–385
Pauciarticular juvenile arthritis, 407–411
Peanut oil, 301
Pediatric AIDS. *See* AIDS
Pediatric Nutrition Surveillance System, 522, 524
Pellagra, 83–84
Penicillamine, 411–412
Penicillin, 135, 444
Pentamidine, 451
Percentiles, 519–520
Percutaneous endoscopic gastrostomy, 241
Periodontitis, 500–501
Peripheral hyperalimentation solution, 387–388
Peripheral vein parenteral nutrition, 226, 231
Peritoneal dialysis, 397, 401–402
Pernicious anemia, congenital, 102
Persistent hyperlysinemia, 474
Persistent hyperphenylalaninemia, 474
Phenolphthalein, 248
Phenylalanine
   inborn errors of metabolism, 474, 482
   parenteral nutrition, 227, 235
Phenylketonuria, 474, 482
   nutritional plan, 263
Phospholipids, 15–16
Phosphorus
   in human milk and formulas, 34, 36–37
   parenteral nutrition, 229–230
   recommended intake, 18, 28, 533
   and renal insufficiency, 398–399
Photoexcited rhodopsin, 53–54
Phototherapy, and riboflavin, 80
Phylloquinone. *See* Vitamin K
Physical activity. *See also* Exercise
   childhood obesity, 282–283, 288
   diabetes, 313, 318–319
   lipoprotein levels, 297, 304
   in pregnancy, 2
   year 2000 goals, 259–260
Physical education programs, 290
Physical examination, 195
Physical fitness, 261
Plaque, 494
Plasma amino acid profile, 14
Plasma osmolality, 234
cis-Platinum, 419
Pneumocystis carinii
   and AIDS, 448, 450
   malnutrition association, 422

Pneumonia, antibiotics, 444
Polio vaccine, 443
Polyarticular juvenile arthritis, 407–408
  growth retardation, 410–411
  malnutrition, 409
Polycystic ovary disease, 282
Polymeric formulas, 242
Polymorphonuclear leukocytes
  activation, 143–144, 146–147
  in host defense, 141–142
  and malnutrition, 132–133
Polyunsaturated fatty acids. See also Long-chain polyunsaturated fatty acids
  adverse effects, 317
  dietary modification effect, 300–302
  in fats and oils, 543
Polyurethane feeding tubes, 242–243
Polyvinyl catheters, 226
Polyvinylchloride feeding tubes, 243
Pork consumption, 513–514
Postpartum care, 6
Potassium
  body composition, 197–198
  burn patients, 220
  drug interactions, 251–252
  food values, 544
  human milk and formulas, 34, 36–37
  parenteral nutrition, 229
  premature infants, 28
  in renal insufficiency, 398
  supplements in malnutrition, 133–134, 443
  term newborn, 18
Potassium chloride, 248
Poultry intake, 514
Prealbumin, 200–201
Preconception care, 4
"Predigested" formula, 242
Pregestamil, liver disease, 360
Pregnancy
  adolescent, 2
  edema in, 1
  energy requirements, 1–2
  preconception care, 4
  prenatal care, 4–5
  vegetarian diets in, 182–183
  vitamin requirements, 77
  weight gain, 2–6
Pregnancy Nutrition Surveillance System, 522, 524
Premature infants
  developmental aspects, 23–24
  energy requirements, 24
  and maternal weight gain, 2–3
  mineral requirements, 27–29
  mother-infant interactions, 46
  nutritional requirements, 23–29
  protein requirements, 26–27
  trace element deficiencies, 119
  vitamin recommendations, 29, 76
  weight gain, 24
Prenatal care, 4–5
"Product Identification Notebook," 511
Proglutamic acidemia, 477
Prolactin, and malnutrition, 168
Proline, inborn errors of metabolism, 475
Propionic acidemia, 476
  biotin treatment, 75, 86

Protein
  adolescent needs, 257–259
  body composition, 197–198
  diabetic diet, 316–317
  in human milk and formulas, 34–36
  intake in critically ill, 214
  and lactation, 35–36
  liver disease, 357
  recommended dietary allowances, 532
  vegetarian diets, 185–187
Protein C, 68
Protein-energy malnutrition, 127–136. See also Thyroid gland in malnutrition
  age factors, 173
  anthropometric classification, 127–128
  clinical classification, 128–130
  critically ill children, 209–210
  duration, effect of, 173
  hospitalized children, 239
  immune system interaction, 130–133, 146–151
  infection interaction, 151–153
  long-term consequences, 135–136
  neurological signs, soft, 175
  pancreatic effects, 367–368
  pathogenesis, 129–130
  prognosis and mortality, 128–129
  renal function effects, 393–394
  renal insufficiency similarity, 399
  timing, effect of, 173
  timing importance, 173
  treatment, 133–136
  tuberculosis, 152–153
Protein-induced gastroenteropathy, 462
Protein malabsorption, 377
Protein requirements
  AIDS patients, 453
  burn patients, 220
  and premature infant, 26–27
  term newborn, 9, 13–15
Protein intake
  Bogalusa Heart Study, 512
  chronic renal insufficiency, 397–398
  nephrotic syndrome, 396
  renal failure, 401
Protein S, 68
Protein-sparing modified fast, 286–288
Proteinuria, nephrotic syndrome, 396
Proteolysis, 208–209
Prothrombin, 67–69
Prothrombin time, 70–71
Psychomotor development, 95, 107–108
Psychosocial-deprivation dwarfism, 275–278
  diagnosis, 276–277
  etiology, 275–276
  versus protein-energy malnutrition, 278
  treatment, 277–278
Psychostimulation, 135–136
Puberty
  early malnutrition effect, 136
  nutritional needs, 257–258
  sex differences, 258
  vegetarian diets, 188
Pulmonary artery hypertension
  growth retardation, 384
  infections, 387

Pulmonary function
  critically ill children, 211
  cystic fibrosis, 380–381
Purgers
  eating disorder characteristics, 265–267
  metabolic needs, 268
4-Pyridoxic acid, 81–82
Pyridoxine (vitamin B_6), 81–82
  drug interactions, 249–250
  in human milk, 36, 76
  parenteral intake, 76, 230
  pharmacologic use, 75, 82
  recommended daily allowances, 74, 81, 533
  requirements, 81
  toxicity, 82
Pyridoxine deficiency, 81–82
  clinical features, 81
  diagnosis, 81–82
  immune function effects, 148–149
  treatment, 82
Pyridoxine-responsive anemia, 82
Pyruvate decarboxylase, 79

Questionnaires, 521
Quetelet index, 4, 519

Racial factors, lipoproteins, 296
Radiation therapy, 420
Radioallergosorbent test, 464–465
RAST, 464–465
Rastafarians, 186–187
"Recall phenomenon," 419
Recombinant growth hormone, 411
Recommended dietary allowances
  current guidelines, 531–532
  as dietary standard, 510–511
Recumbent length, 487
Red cell distribution width, 98
Reference growth charts, 519
Reference population, 519
Rehydrating fluid, 443
Renal concentrating ability, 394–395
Renal dialysis, 397
  nutritional aspects, 399–402
  taste perception, 400
Renal disease, 393–402, 542, 544
Renal failure, 396–402
Renal function
  diabetes mellitus, 320
  in malnutrition, 393–394
  term newborn, 9
Renal growth/maturation, 394–395
Renal insufficiency, acute, 396–397
Renal plasma flow, 393–394
Respiratory conditions
  critically ill children, 211
  food allergy, 462
Respiratory quotient, 209–210
Resting metabolic rate, 10–11
  nutritional assessment, 267–268
Retinoic acid, 53–54
Retinol, 51–57. See also Vitamin A
  isomers, 51
  metabolism, 51–53
  structure, 51
11-cis Retinol, 51, 53–54

Retinol-binding protein
  in nutritional status assessment, 201
  in retinol metabolism, 52–53
Retinopathy, 65
Reverse-T_3, 167–168
Rhinitis, 110
Rhodopsin, 53–54
Riboflavin, 79–80
  dependency syndromes, 80
  dietary sources, 79
  drug interactions, 250
  in human milk and formulas, 76
  parenteral intake, 76, 230
  pharmacologic use, 75
  phototherapy, 80
  recommended daily allowances, 74, 79, 533
  requirements, 80
  toxicity, 80
Riboflavin deficiency, 79–80
Rice glucose polymers, 330
Rice water, 328
Rickets
  clinical manifestations, 60–61
  vegetarian diets, 184, 187
  vitamin D deficiency, 60
Risk factor surveillance, 524
"Roid rage," 262
Rotavirus infection, 442
RRR-α-tocopherol, 62–64
"Rule out sepsis" patients, 471–472, 481

Saccharin, diabetic diet, 317–318
Safflower oil emulsions, 228–229
Salt intake, 398
Sarcosinemia, 475
Saturated fatty acids
  Bogalusa Heart Study, 512, 514
  computerized analysis, 508
  dietary modification effect, 300–304
  in fats and oils, 543
  food values of, 543
  and lipoprotein levels, 297
  United States' food supply, 506
Schilling test, 103
School-based programs, obesity, 289–290
School Breakfast Program, 527
School lunches, 511–513, 527
School performance, malnutrition, 175–176
Scurvy
  clinical features, 86–87
  developmentally disabled 488
  diagnosis, 87
Scurvy line, 87
Secretin, 364
Secretory diarrhea, 326–327, 453
Secretory IgA
  and food hypersensitivity, 460
  human milk, 35–36
  and malnutrition, 132, 148
Sedentary life-style, 525
Seizure disorder, 543
Selenium
  intravenous intake, 123
  premature infant, 29
  recommended intake, 533

in term newborn, 19
  toxicity, 124
Selenium deficiency
  in AIDS, 152, 450–451
  clinical features, 120, 122
  cystic fibrosis, 379
  diagnosis, 122
  etiology, 118–119
  immune function, 151
  treatment, 123
Self-monitoring, weight reduction, 289
Sepsis
  antibiotics, 444
  diagnosis, 133
Serum ferritin, 98–99
Serum protein measures, 199–201
Severe combined immunodeficiency, 439
  differential diagnosis, 154–155, 440–442
  and interleukin-2 administration, 155
  nutritional evaluation, 439
  treatment, 442
Sex differences
  adolescent nutritional needs, 258
  eating disorders, 266
Short-chain fatty acid, 332
Short-chain polymers of glucose, 330
Shriners' burn diet, 220
Shwachman-Diamond syndrome, 366
Sialorrhea, 500
Sideroblastic anemia, 366
  pyridoxine treatment, 75, 82
Siderophores, 150
Silastic catheters, 226
Silicone feeding tubes, 243
Similac
  carbohydrate source, 12
  fat composition, 16
  protein composition, 14
Skimmed milk, 34
Skin-fold measurements, 195–196. See also
      Triceps skin-fold.
Skin manifestations, food allergy, 462
Skin-prick testing, 464
Skin puncture, 98
Skin test response, malnutrition, 147
Sleep apnea, obesity, 281
Sleeping metabolic rates, 39–40
Small bowel resection, 421
Small for gestational age
  interactive behavior effect, 44
  nutritional requirements, 23–29
Snack consumption, 511–513
Social environment, and catch-up, 176–177
Social support, and obesity, 291
Sodium. See also Hypernatremia,
      Hyponatremia
  burn patient requirements, 220
  diabetic diet, 318
  drug interactions, 251
  foods values, 544
  human milk and formulas, 34, 36–37
  intake trends, United States, 514
  parenteral nutrition, 229
  in pregnancy, 5
  recommended intake, 510
  in rehydration solution, 327–328

renal disease restrictions, 396, 398
  renal handling, malnutrition, 394
  and renal insufficiency, 398
  term newborn requirements, 18
Sodium bicarbonate, 248
Sodium chloride
  and renal growth, 395
  requirements in preterm infant, 27
Somatomedin-C. See Insulin-like growth
      factor-1
Sorbitol, 317
Soy-based formulas
  carbohydrates, 12, 34
  and diarrhea, 329
  hypersensitivity, 466
  nutritional composition, 34
Soybean diet, lipoprotein levels, 300–302
Soybean oil emulsions, 228–229
Special Milk Program, 527
Spinocerebellar ataxia, 65
Stable isotope techniques, 197, 202
"Stagnant anoxia," 385
Starch exchanges, 549–550
Starvation
  versus critical illness, metabolism, 209
  tumor necrosis factor, 146
Steatohepatitis, 281
Steatorrhea, 331, 377
Steroid-resistance, 349–350
Steroids, athletes, 262–263
Stimulus control, weight reduction, 289
"Stoplights," 303
Storage iron, 92
Stress
  hormonal adaptation, 162–163, 165
  metabolic response, 208–209
Stunting. See Growth stunting
Subacute necrotizing encephalopathy, 75, 79
Suck-pause phenomenon, 45
Sucrase, and gestational age, 25
Sucrose
  behavioral effects, 111–112
  dental caries, 495
  term newborn, 12
Sudden infant death syndrome, 462, 478
Sugar
  behavioral effects, 111–112
  dental caries, 495
Sugar alcohols, 496–497
Sulfasalazine, 248, 250
Summer Food Service Program, 527
Sunflower oil, 301
"Super-ORS," 328
Superior vena cava catheters, 225–226
Suppressor T cells
  activation, 143
  in host defense, 142
  and malnutrition, 147
Surveillance programs, 517–526
Survey methods, 518
Swallowing, 489–490
Sweeteners, diabetic diet, 317–318
Synthetic diets
  and renal failure, 402
  trace element deficiencies, 119
Systemic juvenile arthritis, 407–411

T-cell receptor, 143
T lymphocytes
  activation pathways, 143
  food allergy role, 459–460
  HIV infection, 151–152, 448–450
  in host defense, 141–42
  and iron deficiency, 149
  malnutrition interaction, 131
  maturation pathways, 142–143
Tachypnea, tube feeding, 387
Tape recorded food records, 509
Taste perception
  and malignancies, 418
  in uremia, 400
  zinc deficiency, 121
Taurine
  importance in premature infant, 27
  parenteral nutrition, 227, 235
  in term newborn, 13, 15
Team treatment
  childhood obesity, 289–290
  diabetes mellitus, 312
Telephone diet recall, 509
Television, and childhood obesity, 281
Temperament, malnutrition effects, 174–175
  "difficult", 174–175
  "easy", 174–175
Temporomandibular joint, 412
Testosterone
  and lipoprotein levels, 296
  and malnutrition, 168
Tetralogy of Fallot, 384–385
Thermic effects of feeding
  breast- and formula-fed infants, 39–40
  term newborn, 10
Thiamine (vitamin B_1), 77–79
  dependency syndromes, 79
  dietary sources, 77
  in human milk and formulas, 76
  parenteral intake, 76, 230
  pharmacological use, 75
  recommended daily allowances, 74, 77, 533
  requirements, 78
  toxicity, 79
Thiamine deficiency (beriberi), 77–78
Thiamine pyrophosphate, 77, 79
Thiamine triphosphate, 79
Thrombophlebitis, 233
Thymic atrophy
  and malnutrition, 130–131
  zinc deficiency, 150
Thyroid function, and diabetes, 320
Thyroid gland, in malnutrition, 167–168
Thyroid hormone receptor, 53–54
Thyroid hormones, nutrient effects, 162
Thyroid-stimulating hormone, 167
Thyroxine (T_4), 167
Tocols, structure, 62–63
α-Tocopherol, 62–66. See also Vitamin E
Tocopherol hydroquinone, 62–63
Tocopherol quinone, 62–63
D-α-Tocopherol polyethylene glycol-1000 succinate, 358
Tocopheroxide, 62–63
"Toddler diarrhea," 334
Tomography, brain, computerized, 175

Total body water, 197
Total cholesterol
  dietary modification, 300–304
  drug therapy, 304–305
  factors influencing levels of, 296–298
  and health risks, 295–296
  screening, 298–299
Total enteral nutrition. See Enteral nutrition
Total parenteral nutrition
  anorexia nervosa, 269–271
  Crohn's disease, 344, 350
  cystic fibrosis, 380
  malignancies, 423
  medical risks, 271
  water soluble vitamins, 76–77
Toxigenic diarrhea, 326
Trace mineral deficiencies, 115–124
  cystic fibrosis, 378–379
  etiology, 118–120
  liver disease, 359–360
Trace minerals
  biological functions, 115–116
  bread group, 116
  in diabetes, 318
  human milk, 37
  parenteral intake, 230
  premature infants, 29
  term newborn, 19–20
"Traffic-light" diet, 286, 303
Transferrin saturation test, 98–99, 199, 201
Transient hypogammaglobulinemia of infancy, 438–439
Transposition of the great arteries, 384–385, 390
Transpyloric feedings, 240–242
Triceps skin-fold. See also Skin-fold measurements
  childhood obesity, 279
  liver disease assessment, 355
  nutritional status measure, 128
Trienols, 62–63
Triglycerides
  breast milk and formulas, 16, 38
  parenteral nutrition, 228–229
  positional distribution, human milk, 38
  requirements in term newborn, 15
Triiodothyronine (T_3), 167–168
Trimethoprim, 101
5,7,8 Trimethyl tocol, 63
5,7,8 Trimethyl tocotrienol, 63
Trypsin, 364, 369
Trypsinogen deficiency, 366
Tryptophanuria, 475
  congenital, 75, 84
Tube enterostomy. See Enterostomy feedings
Tube feedings. See Enteral nutrition
Tuberculin reactivity, 153
Tuberculosis
  immunocompromised children, 443
  susceptibility, 152–153
Tumor necrosis factor
  acute phase response to infection, 146
  critical illness response, 209
  in HIV infection, 151–152, 449, 452
  immunity role, 144–146
  and malnutrition, 131–132

  recombinant form, 145
  and tumors, 418
Twenty-hour recall method, 192, 506–507, 521
Twins, maternal weight gain, 3–4
Type I diabetes, 41. See Insulin-dependent diabetes
Tyrosine, 227, 235
Tyrosinemias, 477–478

Ulcerative colitis
  assessment, 341–342
  growth failure, 341–350
  nutritional considerations, 332–334, 341–350
Unsaturated fats, 554
Urea clearance, 394
Urea cycle defects, 471–484
Uremia
  growth failure, 400
  malnutrition similarity, 399
  nutritional aspects, 399–402
  taste perception, 400
Urinary creatinine excretion, 202
Urinary pH, and diet, 254
Urine-diluting capacity, 9
Urine volume, term newborn, 11–12

Vegan diets, 181–188
Vegetable protein diet, 300–302
Vegetables
  Bogalusa Heart Study, 513
  trace element content, 116
Vegetarian diets, 181–188
  B vitamins, 74
  classification, 182
  exchange list, 552
  in infants, 186–187
  and lactation, 184–185
  nutritional implications, 181–188
  in pregnancy, 182–183
Velocity of growth. See Growth velocity
Venipuncture, 98
Ventricular function, 212
Ventricular septal defect, 384–385, 389–390
Vinblastine, 419
Visual cycle, and vitamin A, 53–54
Vitamers, 49
Vitamin A, 51–57
  absorption and transport, 50–51
  adolescent needs, 257–259
  chemistry, 51
  drug interactions, 250–251
  epithelial function, 53–54
  in human milk and formulas, 76
  metabolism, 51–53
  overdosage, 4, 56–57
  parenteral intake, 76, 230
  premature infant recommendations, 29
  receptor structure domain, 53–54
  recommended daily allowances, 55, 74, 532
  structure, 51
  visual function, 53–54

Vitamin A deficiency
  clinical findings, 55–56
  Crohn's disease, 347
  cystic fibrosis, 368, 377–378
  and immune function, 148, 450
  interleukin levels, 132
  liver disease, 358–359, 361
Vitamin A supplementation
  cystic fibrosis, 368
  liver disease, 361
Vitamin B_1. See Thiamine
Vitamin B_2. See Riboflavin
Vitamin B_5. See Pantothenic acid
Vitamin B_6. See Pyridoxine
Vitamin B_{12}
  drug interactions, 249–250
  in human milk, 36, 76
  parenteral intake, 76, 230
  recommended daily allowances, 74, 533
  vegetarian diets, 184–185
Vitamin B_{12} deficiency
  in AIDS, 451
  Crohn's disease, 347
  cystic fibrosis, 378
  diagnosis, 103
  dietary causes, 102
  inherited defects, 103
  pathogenesis, 102–103
  supplementation recommendations, 36
  treatment, 103
  in vegetarians, 184–185, 187
Vitamin C, 86–88
  adolescent needs, 257–259
  dietary sources, 86
  in human milk and formulas, 76
  and iron absorption, 93, 96
  parenteral intake, 76, 230
  pharmacologic use, 75, 87
  recommended daily allowances, 74, 86, 533
  requirements, 87
  toxicity, 4, 87–88
Vitamin C deficiency, 86–87
  clinical features, 86–87
  Crohn's disease, 347
  developmentally disabled, 488
  diagnosis, 87
  gingival diseases, 501
  immune system effects, 149
  treatment, 87
Vitamin D, 57–62
  absorption and transport, 50, 57
  bone metabolism, 58–60
  calcium homeostasis role, 58–60
  chemistry, 57
  drug interactions, 250, 252
  history, 57
  in human milk and formulas, 76
  immunoregulatory role, 144
  metabolism, 57–58
  overdose effects, 4, 62
  parenteral intake, 76, 230
  in premature infant, 29
  recommended daily allowances, 20, 55, 60, 74, 532
  in term newborn, 20, 60
  vegetarian diets, 183–184

Vitamin D deficiency
  clinical manifestations, 60–61
  Crohn's disease, 347–348
  cystic fibrosis, 368, 378
  liver disease, 359, 361
  tuberculosis predisposition, 152–153
  vegetarian diets, 183–184
Vitamin D receptor
  DNA binding domain, 53–54, 58
  and rickets, 60
Vitamin D-resistant rickets, 6
Vitamin D supplementation
  cystic fibrosis, 368
  liver disease, 361
  premature infants, 29
  prenatal care, 5
  recommendations, infants, 36, 60
  vegetarians, 184
Vitamin E, 62–66
  absorption and transport, 50, 62–63
  antioxidant hypothesis, 64
  chemistry, 62
  genetic regulatory function, 64
  human milk and formulas, 76
  immunity effects, 148
  and iron-fortified formula, 97
  metabolism, 63–64
  parenteral intake, 76, 230
  physiological function, 64
  premature infant requirements, 29, 64
  recommended allowances, 55, 64–65, 74, 532
  toxicity, 66
Vitamin E deficiency
  in AIDS, 152, 440, 451
  and antioxidant hypothesis, 64
  clinical features, 65–66
  cystic fibrosis, 368–369, 378
  and immune function, 148
  liver disease, 358, 361
  premature infants, 65
Vitamin E supplementation, 361, 369
Vitamin K, 66–71
  absorption and transport, 50, 67
  anticoagulation function, 67–68
  chemistry, 66–67
  drug interactions, 250–251
  history, 66
  human milk concentrations, 36, 70, 76
  in infant formulas, 76
  metabolism, 67
  parenteral intake, 76, 230
  premature infants, 29, 70
  metabolism, 67
  recommended allowances, 55, 69, 74, 532
  requirements, 69
Vitamin K cycle, 69
Vitamin K deficiency
  cystic fibrosis, 369, 378
  general characteristics, 69–70
  liver disease, 361
Vitamin K-dependent carboxylation, 68
Vitamin K supplements
  liver disease, 361
  preterm infant, 29, 70
  recommendations, infants, 36, 69

Vitamins
  and birth defects, 4
  and chronic diarrhea, 332
  drug interactions, 248–251
  human milk concentrations, 36
  parenteral intakes, 229–230
Vivonex, Crohn's disease, 345–350
Vomiting, and enteral feeding, 244–245

Wasting
  and AIDS, 448, 450
  anthropometric measurements, 195–196
  definition, 128, 195
  hospitalized patients, 196, 210
  immune function impairment, 450
Water. See also Body water
  premature infants, 24–25
  term newborn, 11–12
Water soluble vitamins
  Crohn's disease, 347
  cystic fibrosis, 378, 380
  disorders of, 73–88
  drug interactions, 249–250
Waterlow's classification, 195
Weaning, and vegetarian diets, 186
Weighed-food record method, 506, 521
Weight-for-age
  as anthropometric indices, 194–195
  and malnutrition, 161
Weight-for-height, 195–196
  as anthropometric measure, 195–196
  congenital heart disease, 386
  hospitalized patients, 196
  nutritional status measure, 127–128, 161
  renal failure, 400
Weight gain
  human milk and formulas, 39–40
  maternal, 2–6
  in mothers, 2–3, 5–6
  parenteral nutrition, 232
  premature infants, 24
  term newborns, 11
  with twins, 3–4
Weight loss, AIDS, 450
Weight reduction, self-monitoring, 289
Whey protein
  breast milk versus formulas, 13–14, 35
  premature infant, 27
WIC program, 3, 526
Wilson's disease, 360
Wiskott-Aldrich syndrome, 442
Women, Infants, and Children program (WIC), 3, 526
Work performance, iron deficiency, 95
Wound healing
  vitamin C, 87
  zinc therapy, 121

X-linked agammaglobulinemia, 438, 442
Xanthurenic acid excretion, 82
Xanthurenic aciduria, 75, 82

Xerophthalmic, 55
Xerostomia, 500
Xylitol, 496

Yellow nail syndrome, 152, 451

Z scores, 519–520
Zen macrobiotic diet, 74
Zinc
    absorption and metabolism, 117–118
    adolescent needs, 257–259
    biological functions, 116–117
    body content, 117–118
    and chronic diarrhea, 332
    dietary sources, 115–116
    DNA metabolism importance, 53–59, 116
    drug interactions, 253
    excessive secretion, 120
    human milk concentrations, 37
    intravenous intake, 123
    liver disease, 360
    parenteral intake, 230
    premature infants, 29, 123
    recommended intake, 533
    requirements, 123–124
    term newborn, 19
    toxicity, 124
Zinc deficiency, 115–124
    in AIDS, 152, 440, 450–451
    and birth defects, 4
    chronic diarrhea, 332
    clinical features, 120–121
    Crohn's disease, 348
    cystic fibrosis, 378
    diagnosis, 122
    etiology, 119–120
    and immune function, 150, 450
    liver disease, 359–360
    ocular manifestations, 121
    treatment, 122–123
Zinc supplementation
    immunodeficient children, 444
    and malnutrition, 135